Clinical Nuclear Medicine

Clinical Nuclear Medicine

SECOND EDITION

Edited by

M. N. Maisey
Guy's Hospital
London

K. E. Britton
St Bartholomew's Hospital
London

D. L. Gilday
The Hospital for Sick Children
Toronto

CHAPMAN & HALL MEDICAL
London · New York · Tokyo · Melbourne · Madras

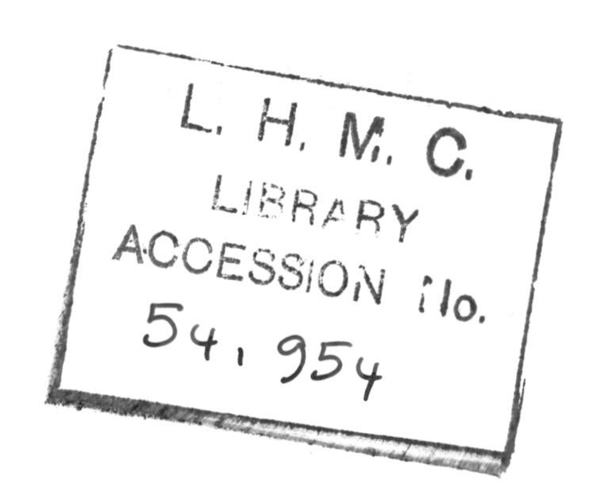

UK Chapman & Hall, 2–6 Boundary Row, London SE1 8HN

JAPAN Chapman & Hall Japan, Thomson Publishing Japan, Hirakawacho Nemoto Building, 7F, 1-7-11 Hirakawa-cho, Chiyoda-Ku, Tokyo 102

AUSTRALIA Chapman & Hall Australia, Thomas Nelson Australia, 102 Dodds Street, South Melbourne, Victoria 3205

INDIA Chapman & Hall India, R. Seshadri, 32 Second Main Road, CIT East, Madras 600 035

First edition 1983
Second edition 1991

Typeset in 9½/11½ Palatino by
Rowland Phototypesetting Ltd
Bury St Edmunds, Suffolk
Printed in Great Britain at the
University Press, Cambridge

ISBN 0 412 27900 2

British Library Cataloguing in Publication Data
Clinical nuclear medicine.
1. Nuclear medicine
I. Maisey, M. N. (Michael Norman) II. Britton, K. E. (Keith Eric) III. Gilday, D. L. (David L.)
616.07575

ISBN 0 412 27900 2

Contents

Contributors

D. Ackery, MB, MSc
Department of Nuclear Medicine
Southampton General Hospital
Southampton, UK

J. Ash, MD
Department of Nuclear Medicine
The Hospital for Sick Children
Toronto
Ontario, Canada

D. A. Brennand-Roper, MA, MRCP
Department of Cardiology
West Hill Hospital
Dartford
Kent, UK

A. B. Brill, MD, PhD
Department of Nuclear Medicine
University of Massachusetts Medical Center
Worcester
Massachusetts, USA

K. E. Britton, MD, MSc, FRCP
Department of Nuclear Medicine
St Bartholomew's Hospital
London, UK

S. E. M. Clarke, MBBS, MRCP, MSc
Department of Nuclear Medicine
Guy's Hospital
London, UK

A. J. Coakley, MSc, FRCP
Consultant in Nuclear Medicine
Department of Nuclear Medicine
Kent and Canterbury Hospital
Canterbury
Kent, UK

D. N. Croft, MA, DM, FRCP, FRCR
Department of Nuclear Medicine
St Thomas' Hospital
London, UK

P. J. Ell, MD, MSc, PD, MRCP, FRCR
Institute of Nuclear Medicine
University College and Middlesex Hospital
Medical School
London, UK

A. T. Elliott, BA, PhD
Department of Clinical Physics and
Bioengineering
Western Infirmary
Glasgow, UK

A. J. Fischman, MD, PhD
Division of Nuclear Medicine
Massachusetts General Hospital
Boston
Maryland, USA

I. Fogelman, MD, FRCP
Department of Nuclear Medicine
Guy's Hospital
London, UK

D. L. Gilday, BEng, MD, FRCP (C)
The Hospital for Sick Children
Toronto
Ontario, Canada

M. Granowska, MD, MSc
Department of Nuclear Medicine
St Bartholomew's Hospital
London, UK

N. D. Greyson, MD, FRCP (C)
Department of Nuclear Medicine
St Michael's Hospital
Toronto
Ontario, Canada

M. D. Gross, MD
Department of Internal Medicine
University of Michigan and Veteran's Administration Medical Center
Ann Arbor
Michigan, USA

A. J. W. Hilson, MB, MSc, MRCP
Department of Nuclear Medicine
Royal Free Hospital
London, UK

S. Howle, MD
The Hospital for Sick Children
Toronto
Ontario, Canada

J. Hutton, BSc, BPhil
Centre for Health Economics
University of York
York, UK

R. F. Jewkes, MB, FRCP
Department of Nuclear Medicine
Charing Cross Hospital
London, UK

F. A. Khafagi, MB BS, FRACP
Division of Nuclear Medicine
Department of Internal Medicine
University of Michigan
Ann Arbor
Michigan, USA

C. Lazarus, B Pharm, PhD, MPS
Department of Nuclear Medicine
Guy's Hospital
London, UK

S. M. Lewis, FRCPath
Department of Haematology
Royal Postgraduate Medical School
Hammersmith
London, UK

M. N. Maisey, MD, FRCP, FRCR
Department of Nuclear Medicine
Division of Radiological Sciences
Guy's Hospital
London, UK

N. J. Marshall, PhD
Department of Chemical Pathology
University College Hospital
London, UK

B. J. McNeil, MD
Department of Radiology
Harvard Medical School
Cambridge
Massachusetts, USA

R. Mistry
Department of Nuclear Medicine
Guy's Hospital
London, UK

A. M. Noyek, MD, FRCPC
Radiology Department
University of Toronto
Faculty of Medicine
Ontario, Canada

A. M. Peters, MD, MRCPath, MSc
Department of Diagnostic Radiology
Royal Postgraduate Medical School
Hammersmith
London, UK

M. Prentice, MD, MRCP
Department of Chemical Pathology
University College Hospital
London, UK

H. D. Royal, MD
Harvard Medical School
Cambridge
Massachusetts, USA

R. H. Secker-Walker, MD, MRCP
Division of Health Sciences
University of Vermont
Vermont, USA

B. Shapiro, MB ChB, PhD
Division of Nuclear Medicine
University of Michigan Medical Center
Ann Arbor
Michigan, USA

A. Sheldrake
Department of Chemical Pathology
University College Hospital
London, UK

P. Shepherd, MB, BS, MRCP
Department of Immunology
Guy's Hospital
London, UK

H. W. Strauss, MD
Division of Nuclear Medicine
Massachusetts General Hospital
Boston
Massachusetts, USA

N. Tamaki, MD
Division of Nuclear Medicine
Massachusetts General Hospital
Boston
Massachusetts, USA

H. N. Wagner, Jr, MD
Division of Nuclear Medicine
The Johns Hopkins Medical Institutions
Baltimore
Maryland, USA

P. Wells, BSC, MSc
Department of Medical Physics
Kent and Canterbury Hospital
Canterbury
Kent, UK

J. C. Williams, MA, MSc, FRCP
School of Postgraduate Studies in Medical and Healthcare
University College of Swansea
Swansea, UK

Preface to the first edition

Nuclear medicine is the bridge between a particular clinical problem and a relevant test using radionuclides. It began as a minor technical tool used in a few branches of medicine, notably endocrinology and nephrology. However, throughout the world it has now become established as a clinical discipline in its own right, with specific training programmes, special skills and a particular approach to patient management. Although the practising nuclear medicine physician must necessarily learn a great deal of basic science and technology, a sound medical training and a clinical approach to the subject remains of fundamental importance. It is for this reason that we have attempted in this book to approach the subject from a clinical standpoint, including where necessary relevant physiological material.

There exist many excellent texts which cover the basic science and technology of nuclear medicine. We have, therefore, severely limited our coverage of these aspects of the subject to matters which we felt to be essential, particularly those which have been less well covered in other texts – for example, the contents of Chapter 20 on Measurement by Royal and McNeill. Similarly, we have limited details of methodology to skeletal summaries of protocol (Appendix 1) and have included at the end of some chapters descriptions of particular techniques where we and the authors felt that it would be helpful. In order to emphasize the clinical approach of this book we have inverted the traditional sequence of material in chapters, presenting the clinical problems first in each instance. For similar reasons we have placed the chapters on Radiopharmaceuticals and Practical Instrumentation towards the end of the book.

Since medicine concerns the investigation, care and management of sick people who have specific problems, the virtues of a problem-orientated approach to the subject are becoming more widely recognized, particularly in the education of undergraduates. This approach has therefore been adopted in each chapter, making the overall structure of the book closer to that of a conventional textbook of medicine rather than a scientific treatise.

The contributors to this book come from both the United Kingdom and North America. As editors, in addition to requiring that authors should be expert in their field, we also wanted them to be particularly concerned about the day to day care of patients. We have endeavoured to emphasize the problem-orientated approach to clinical situations, whilst providing textual uniformity, without at the same time reducing the essentially individual contributions of each author.

We hope this textbook will be of value to a wide variety of medical professionals, including nuclear medicine clinicians in training, radiologists and clinicians from other specialities who use nuclear medicine in some form or other and require to know how it can help in solving their clinical problems. Finally, believing that medical students prefer the style of a textbook of medicine rather than that of a textbook of physics, we hope that the clinical priorities which have dictated the production of this book will encourage them to consult it.

M.N.M., K.E.B., London
D.L.G., Toronto

Preface to the second edition

Although adaptability and evolution are the key to growth, in medicine growth of a specialty is not an end in itself unless it contributes positively to patient care. Nuclear medicine is adapting to the changes in medicine and evolving to meet new challenges in a way which will ensure the discipline an important role in clinical medicine during this decade. Since the first edition of this textbook was published in 1984, significant changes have taken place in the way we practice our specialty. These changes have resulted from the development of new radiopharmaceuticals (^{99m}Tc-Sesta MIBI, ^{99m}Tc-HMPAO, ^{99m}Tc-MAG3 etc.), the development of improved instrumentation, new clinical applications for established radionuclide imaging methods and a wider appreciation and understanding of its benefits.

We believe that nuclear medicine is concerned with the way that the application of its investigative techniques to clinical problems can assist patient management and ultimately benefit patient outcome. We hope this is again reflected in this new edition. First the clinical problem is identified and this initiates the nuclear medicine investigation or treatment, whose pathophysiological role is explained and evaluated.

There are new areas of development in the speciality which we expect to have a clinical impact and which are likely to be incorporated into clinical practice during the lifetime of this edition. These have been included; in particular single photon and positron emission topography, immunoscintigraphy, single photon receptor imaging and new approaches to unsealed radioactive source therapy.

The practice of nuclear medicine is well established, but continuously changing. We hope that this edition will go some way towards consolidating the developments of the second half of the 1980s, provide some guidance to those of the early 1990s and even some pointers to the 21st century.

M.N.M., K.E.B., London
D.L.G., Toronto

CHAPTER ONE

Radionuclide imaging of the heart

N. Tamaki, A. J. Fischman and H. William Strauss

1.1 INTRODUCTION

Approximately 43 million Americans have one or more forms of acquired heart or blood vessel disease: high blood pressure occurs in 38 million adults; coronary artery disease occurs in 4.5 million adults; rheumatic heart disease occurs in 2 million; and stroke in 1.9 million. Myocardial infarction caused approximately 555 000 deaths (25% of all mortality) in 1982. Some aspect of the pathophysiology of each of these diseases can be evaluated with radionuclide techniques. The disorders involving the heart produce the following abnormalities which can be evaluated with radionuclide techniques: (a) myocardial ischaemia (a reversible condition, caused by a temporary deficiency in the supply of oxygen to the myocardium due to atherosclerotic narrowing of the vessel); (b) myocardial infarction (an irreversible condition leading to death of a portion of the myocardium, most commonly caused by acute thrombotic coronary occlusion superimposed on pre-existing severe coronary atherosclerotic narrowing); and (c) cardiomyopathy (a category of diseases of unknown cause associated with either thickening of the myocardium (hypertrophic or infiltrative myopathy) or thinning of the muscle resulting in altered function).

Radionuclide studies of the heart and circulation are amongst the oldest uses of radioactive tracers in human subjects. In the mid-1920s, Herrmann Blumgart and his associate Soma Weiss embarked on a number of experiments to measure the velocity of blood in man (Blumgart and Weiss, 1927). To make these measurements 'non-invasively', they injected **radium C** into the vein of one arm and identified the arrival of the tracer by observing a cloud chamber (described a few years earlier by Wilson *et al.*) placed over an artery of the other arm.

Following the Second World War, the increased availability of radioisotopes for medical use and the introduction of sophisticated radiation detection instruments gave cardiovascular nuclear medicine the impetus for rapid growth. Prinzmetal *et al.* used the Geiger counter and radioiodinated albumin in 1948 to record the radiocardiogram, a technique for measuring right and left heart transit times and cardiopulmonary blood volume. Ten years later Rejali *et al.* (1958) described the first *in vivo* imaging procedure in cardiovascular nuclear medicine: the blood pool scan for the detection of pericardial effusion. In the early 1960s, rapid advances were made. In a three-year period from 1962 to 1965 the concepts of myocardial perfusion imaging, acute myocardial infarct imaging, fatty acid imaging and radionuclide angiocardiography were described. Over the next two decades these procedures were refined, improved, and found to be of significant value in the management of patients with heart diseases. Now, both single-photon and positron approaches are available for the evaluation of cardiac function, perfusion and metabolism as described in the following sections:

1. Anatomy and physiology
2. Blood pool imaging
   - (a) Equilibrium studies
     - (i) Radiopharmaceutical
     - (ii) Planar image recording
     - (iii) Analysis
   - (b) First-pass imaging
     - (i) Injection technique
     - (ii) Analysis
   - (c) Clinical applications
     - (i) Diagnosis and evaluation of coronary artery disease
     - (ii) Acute infarction
     - (iii) Aneurysm
     - (iv) Right ventricular abnormalities in infarction

(v) Prognosis
(vi) Cor pulmonale
(vii) Valvular disease
(viii) Cardiomyopathy
(ix) Pericardial effusion
(d) Tomography
(e) Non-imaging probe
3. Perfusion imaging
(i) Coronary injection
(ii) Intravenous injection
(iii) Characteristics of thallium
(iv) Data recording
(v) Interpretation
(vi) Dipyridamole
(vii) Sensitivity and specificity
(a) Clinical applications
4. Infarct avid imaging
(i) Non-specific agents for imaging myocardial necrosis
(ii) ^{99m}Tc-labelled pyrophosphate
(iii) Antimyosin
5. New radiopharmaceuticals
6. Positron emission tomography

1.2 ANATOMY

The adult heart weighs about 300 g and holds approximately 500 ml of blood. The heart is located in the lower portion of the thoracic cavity between the lungs. It is covered by a clear fibrous sac, the pericardium. The pericardium contains a minimal amount of fluid to act as a lubricant between the moving surface of myocardium and the other structures in the chest.

The atria serve as temporary reservoirs of blood returned to the heart. The atria are separated by a thin muscular wall, the atrial septum, while the ventricles are separated by the thicker, muscular, interventricular septum.

The right side of the heart receives venous blood (pO_2 about 40 mmHg) returning via the superior and inferior venae cavae to the right atrium. The blood traverses the tricuspid valve and enters the pyramid-shaped right ventricle. The right ventricle expels blood through the pulmonic valve into the pulmonary artery and lungs. Blood returns from the lungs (pO_2 about 100 mmHg) via the four pulmonary veins to the left atrium. The blood traverses the mitral valve, and enters the left ventricle. The left ventricle expels blood through the aortic valve into the aorta.

The myocardium receives its oxygen supply from the right and left coronary arteries. The left coronary artery divides into two main branches: the left anterior descending artery and left circumflex artery. The left anterior descending artery branches to supply the interventricular septum and anterolateral wall of the left ventricle. The left circumflex artery supplies the left atrium and posterior and lateral ventricular walls of the left ventricle. The right coronary artery supplies the right atrium, right ventricle and the inferior wall of the left ventricle. The true posterior wall of the left ventricle is supplied by the posterior descending coronary artery which is most commonly a branch of the right coronary artery, but may arise from the left circumflex (10%). Blood drains from the myocardium to the coronary veins which terminate in the coronary sinus of the right atrium.

1.3 PHYSIOLOGY

1.3.1 CIRCULATION

Deoxygenated venous blood, transporting carbon dioxide and metabolic waste products, flows from the tissues towards the heart via the veins. Although venous pressure is low, resistance to blood flow is also low, and blood flows through the large veins at 40 cm s^{-1} on its way to emptying into the right atrium at a pressure of <5 mmHg. Blood is expelled from the right ventricle at a pressure of 25 mmHg into the lungs. In the enormous capillary bed of the lungs, the velocity of blood slows to 1 mm s^{-1}, carbon dioxide is eliminated and oxygen is taken up. The oxygenated blood returns to the heart at a pressure of <5 mmHg. The left ventricle provides sufficient kinetic energy in the form of a systolic pressure of 120 mmHg, and flow rate of 50 cm s^{-1}, to permit the blood to travel to the furthest capillary bed and return to the heart. As in the pulmonary capillaries, the velocity of blood slows at the tissue capillaries, to permit the exchange of nutrients for waste products.

The valves in the heart prevent backflow. The blood is forced forward with such force that the tricuspid and mitral valves are anchored by muscle strands – chordae tendinae – into the ventricular walls to prevent the valve leaflets from prolapsing into the atria.

Starting in early diastole, the atria and ventricles are relaxed. Atrial pressure is slightly higher than ventricular pressure, the tricuspid and mitral valves are open and blood passes from the atria to the ventricles. The aortic and pulmonary valves are closed, preventing backflow of blood. The majority (80–90%) of ventricular filling takes place in this passive fashion. Atrial contraction serves to 'top off' the ventricles with the last 10–20% of blood volume. The quantity of blood in the ventricle at the end of diastole (following atrial contraction) is called the end-diastolic volume (about 150 ml).

Ventricular systole starts as the myofibrils shorten and ventricular pressure rises. The initial rise in pressure causes the tricuspid and mitral valves to close. As the myofibrils continue to shorten, pressure in the ventricles rises at a rapid rate. The interval following atrioventricular (AV) valve closure, but prior to the generation of sufficient pressure to open the pulmonary and aortic valves, is the interval of isovolumetric contraction. Continued shortening of the myofibrils causes the ventricular pressure to exceed pulmonary and aortic pressure; the pulmonary and aortic valves open and ventricular ejection begins. During the 250–300 ms interval when the myofibrils shorten to their minimal length (ventricular systole), approximately one-half to two-thirds of the end-diastolic volume is ejected. The fraction of the end-diastolic blood volume ejected during the systolic interval is called the **ejection fraction** (normal values by blood pool imaging range from 50% to 65%). Blood returning to the left heart during the interval of ventricular ejection, when the tricuspid and mitral valves are closed, is stored in the atria. As a result, both the atrial volumes and pressures rise slightly during the interval of ventricular ejection. At the conclusion of ventricular ejection ventricular pressure falls rapidly, the pulmonary and aortic valves close, the ventricle continues to relax with no change in volume (isovolumetric diastole) until the interventricular pressure drops below the pressure in the atria and the tricuspid and mitral valves open, to commence the filling phase. At resting heart rates, filling occurs rapidly for the first half of diastole, as atrial pressure and volume decrease. The slow filling phase follows, with atrial systole contributing 15–20% of the stroke volume. At high heart rates, the slow filling phase disappears, and the atrial contribution is reduced.

A normal 70 kg adult has a stroke volume of 80–100 ml beat^{-1}; at a heart rate of 60–70 beats min^{-1} this provides a cardiac output of 5–7 l min^{-1}. The cardiac output is distributed to the organs in proportion to their oxygen requirements, which change from rest to exertion. The usual distribution of cardiac output at rest and during exercise is listed in Table 1.1.

1.3.2 HEART BEAT

The myocardium has an intrinsic rhythm of contraction. The sinoatrial (SA) node, a small mass of specialized cells embedded in the right atrium near the entrance of the superior vena cava (SVC), has the fastest inherent rhythm and supersedes other similar sites in the heart. As a result, the SA node usually serves as the impulse generator for the remainder of the heart. To coordinate contraction the myocardium has a conducting system, consisting of specific muscle fibres which carry an electrical message from the SA node through the AV node to the ventricles. The wave of depolarization begins in the SA node and spreads to the surrounding atrial myocardial fibres. There are no specialized conduction fibres in the atria, but the wave of excitation spreads from cell to cell and covers the atria within 0.08 s. Atrial systole requires approximately 0.1 s. To permit the completion of mechanical atrial systole and effect maximal ventricular filling, the electrical signal enters the AV node, where it is held, prior to spreading over the surface of the ventricles via the specialized conducting system. The rapid conduction along the His–Purkinje system and the left and right bundle branches and their ramifications causes depolarization of all the right and left ventricular cells to occur almost simultaneously.

Abnormalities of conduction are quite common and may have substantial effects on radionuclide studies of ventricular function (see below).

Table 1.1

Organ	*Fraction of cardiac output* Rest (5 l min^{-1})	Exercise (17.5 l min^{-1})
Brain	15%	4%
Heart	4%	5%
Kidneys	20%	3%
Liver	10%	<2%
GI tract	15%	<1%
Skeletal muscle	20%	70%
Skin	6%	10%
Other	10%	5%

After McArdle *et al.* (1981).

1.4 BLOOD POOL IMAGING

Blood pool imaging comprises a series of radionuclide techniques to determine global and regional ventricular function. Four measurements can be made from these scans: (1) the ejection fraction (EF) – i.e. the amount of blood ejected each beat (stroke volume) divided by the amount of blood in the ventricle at the end of diastole (end-diastolic volume) – is the single most important indicator of global ventricular performance; (2) the motion of the walls of the left and right ventricles; (3) the relative size of the chambers (end-diastolic volumes); and (4) rates of filling and emptying of the ventricles.

Ventricular function can be measured either during the initial passage of radiopharmaceutical through the heart (first pass), or following equilibration of the tracer in the blood pool (equilibrium-gated blood pool imaging). The two approaches differ in the radiopharmaceuticals, techniques of data recording and data analysis. The values obtained for ejection fraction, however, are comparable. The equilibrium method averages information from several hundred cardiac cycles to produce a high count density image, which permits detection of subtle wall motion abnormalities. The first-pass approach is better suited to recording cardiac function under circumstances of rapid change. Overall, both methods provide an accurate assessment of cardiac chamber size and global function.

1.4.1 EQUILIBRIUM-GATED BLOOD POOL IMAGING

(a) Radiopharmaceutical

Equilibrium imaging requires a radiopharmaceutical that is retained within the blood pool such as ^{99m}Tc-labelled human serum albumin or autologous red blood cells. The former is available as a multi-dose kit radiopharmaceutical, while the latter is prepared for each patient. Red cells may be labelled either *in vitro* (Smith and Richards, 1976) *in vivo* (Pavel *et al.*, 1977), or by a modified *in vivo* approach (Callahan *et al.*, 1982).

The *in vivo* method involves the injection of approximately 1 mg of stannous ion (usually in the form of stannous pyrophosphate) intravenously to prime the red cells, followed at 20–30 min by 550–750 MBq (15–20 mCi) of ^{99m}Tc-pertechnetate to label the erythrocytes.

The modified *in vivo* approach provides a higher labelling efficiency than the *in vivo* method, without the usual requirement for centrifugation of the cells in the *in vitro* methods. The modified *in vivo* method involves the injection of approximately 1 mg of stannous ion (usually in the form of stannous pyrophosphate) intravenously to prime the red cells, followed at 20–30 min by withdrawal of 3–5 ml of whole blood into a heparinized, shielded syringe containing 550–750 MBq (15–20 mCi) of ^{99m}Tc-pertechnetate to label the erythrocytes. The cells are allowed to incubate at room temperature in the syringe for 10–15 min prior to reinjection.

The labelling efficiencies of the *in vitro* and *in vivo* methods are both over 90% (Hamilton and Alderson, 1977).

(b) Data collection

Frame mode The R wave of the patient's electrocardiograph (ECG) is usually employed as the physiological trigger. Following an R wave, images are recorded for a preset time/frame, usually 10–50 ms, until the next R wave occurs. The time/frame should be selected to permit the average cardiac cycle to fill all frames (e.g. to record a 16-frame gated scan in a patient with a heart rate of 60, a time/frame of $1000/16 = 62.5$ ms should be employed). Relatively few counts (<5000) are recorded in each frame during a single cycle. At the time of the next R wave, the information from the first portion of this cardiac cycle is added to that from the previous cycle, the second portion is added in phase, etc. The process is repeated each time the triggering signal is received and information input into the appropriate set of computer frames or files over a period of about 10 min until a series of composite pictures is accumulated, each comprising the data from a sufficient number of cardiac cycles to record 200 000–400 000 counts per frame (usually 500–1000 beats). This method of data accumulation is referred to as 'frame mode' acquisition (Figure 1.1).

To ensure that the gated blood pool data will be an accurate representation of cardiac function the patient's condition must be stable during acquisition. To optimize the likelihood of detecting small wall motion abnormalities, pixel size in the computer should be <5 mm. The computer should be able to acquire the data with sufficient temporal resolution (<50 ms per frame at a heart rate of 80, <25 ms per frame at a heart rate of 160) that permits accurate calculation of the ejection frac-

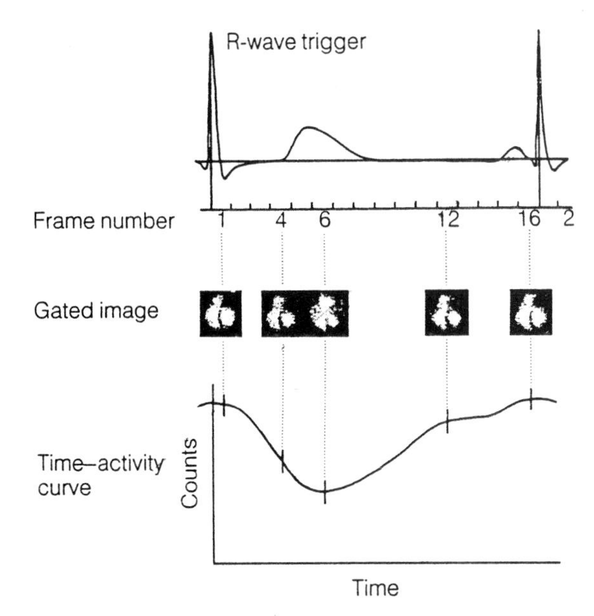

Figure 1.1 Diagram of 'frame mode' collection of a multigated scan. Selected images from a scan in a normal patient, recorded in the left anterior oblique position, are shown in the middle panel. The electrocardiogram (ECG) is shown in the top panel, and the time–activity curve derived from analysis of the blood pool images is shown in the bottom panel. The end-diastolic (ED) and end-systolic (ES) frames are marked.

tion (to compute filling rates the time/frame must be halved).

List mode When atrial fibrillation, marked sinus arrhythmia or multiple ectopic beats occur the R–R interval will vary. The data collected from short beats is terminated by the arrival of another R wave before the last few frames receive data. This results in terminal frames that contain fewer counts than the early frames with consequent degradation of the image quality. This may be partly overcome by computer rejection of short cycles or by setting the R–R interval for the computer at a time equal to the shortest beats. These approaches improve the visual quality of the images but do not permit accurate calculation of filling phase parameters because beats of different rates are averaged. Another method of dealing with the problem of an irregular heart rate is to acquire the study in 'list mode'. In list mode acquisition, the computer records the position of each photon recorded by the camera in sequence. When the acquisition is complete, this sequential list of data can be sorted by beat length, or the relationship of one beat to another. In addition, the data can be formatted either forward (from end-diastole through systole to the next diastole) or backwards (from end-diastole back through the previous systole). Backward-formatted data on beats of selected lengths provide a better assessment of the filling phase of the cardiac cycle than forward formatted data (Bonow *et al.*, 1981).

(c) Image recording

Rest A general all-purpose collimator with a regular or large field of view gamma camera provides an acceptable trade-off between sensitivity and resolution. After injection of the radiopharmaceutical, the patient is placed supine on the imaging table. Gated images are usually acquired in three views: (1) anterior; (2) left anterior oblique (LAO; optimized to best define the septum and maximize separation of the right and left ventricles); and (3) either the left lateral or left posterior oblique view (Figure 1.2). The left posterior oblique view is particularly useful for visualizing the inferobasal region of the left ventricle and the left atrium. Three views are necessary to visualize wall motion at the base, apex, septal and posterior walls of the left ventricle.

Exercise Left ventricular functional reserve can be measured by recording the blood pool scan during exercise. Since the duration of exercise is limited, data are usually recorded only in the LAO view during stress, to permit calculation of the changes in ejection fraction from rest to stress.

The patient should arrive in the laboratory in the fasted state, wearing light clothing, prepared for physical exertion. To minimize patient motion during physical exertion, the patient pedals a bicycle ergometer equipped with shoulder restraints and hand grips in either the supine or semi-supine position. Data are recorded for the last 2 min of each 3 min stage of exercise. The limited time for data collection usually requires a change from the all-purpose to a high-sensitivity collimator (a sensitivity improvement of a factor of two). The ECG and blood pressure are monitored throughout the procedure. Prior to exercise, images are obtained in both the anterior and LAO projections as described above. Exercise is started at 25 or 50 W and increased by regular increments of 25 W at 3 min intervals. The usual end points for the exercise test are:

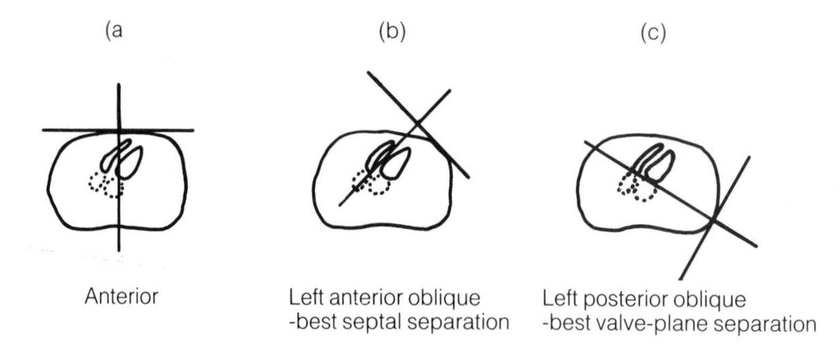

Figure 1.2 Diagram of positions employed for data collection in typical blood pool images. (a) The anterior view is recorded with the collimator of the scintillation camera just touching the anterior chest, with the patient in the supine position. (b) The left anterior oblique view is recorded with the patient in the supine position by rotating the detector to a position perpendicular to the axis of the septum (indicated by the dotted line). (c) The left posterior oblique view is recorded with the collimator parallel to the long axis of the left ventricle (indicated by the dotted line), with the patient rotated into the right lateral decubitus position.

1. severe angina pectoris;
2. hypotension;
3. significant arrhythmias;
4. severe fatigue;
5. achievement of 85% of predicted maximal heart rate.

Alternative approaches to large muscle dynamic exercise, such as isometric exercise (hand-grip) or immersion of the hand in ice-cold water ('cold pressor' test) are not as useful as large muscle dynamic exercise: isometric exercise may alter preload (via the Valsalva manoeuvre), and the cold pressor response may invoke reflexes which can depress cardiac function independent of ischaemia. As a result, large muscle dynamic leg exercise remains the method of choice for evaluating the functional reserve of the heart.

(d) Analysis

Gated blood pool scans are analysed in two parts: inspection of the data while they are displayed as an endless cinematic loop of the cardiac cycle, and quantification of volumes and function.

From inspection of the cinematic display the size of the chambers and great vessels is determined, regional wall motion is assessed, thickness of the muscular wall is estimated, and evidence is sought for pericardial effusion, spaces or masses. Normal subjects empty at least half the end-diastolic volume of their right and left ventricles each beat (normal left ventricular ejection fraction (LVEF) ranges from 50% to 65%); shorten the long axis of their left ventricle by >25% and the short axis by >45%; and have left ventricular end-diastolic volumes of <200 ml (114 ml m^{-2}). Inspection permits the subjective grading of regional wall motion into normal (regional shortening of a radius of at least 25%), hypokinetic (regional shortening of a radius of 10–25%), akinetic (regional shortening of 0–5%) and dyskinetic (systolic expansion), based on a comparison of end-diastolic to end-systolic outlines (Figure 1.3). When multiple images are recorded, or previous studies are compared to a new examination, the images should be examined side by side in simultaneous display to assess changes in cardiac size or regional wall motion.

Ejection fraction The ejection fraction (EF) is usually calculated by measuring the stroke counts and the background-corrected end-diastolic counts from regions of interest placed over the left ventricular blood pool data recorded in the LAO view (Parker *et al.*, 1972; Burow *et al.*, 1977) (Figure 1.1).

When the data are collected using the R wave for synchronization, the first frame of the collection corresponds to end-diastole. End-systole, the nadir of the curve, usually occurs between one-third and half-way through the series of images.

Prior to calculation of the EF, the counts in each frame of the data collection should be normalized, and a spatial and temporal smoothing of the data should be performed. A background region, located at about 3–6 o'clock from the left ventricle, free of branches of the pulmonary artery, left atrium and spleen, is selected, and the counts/

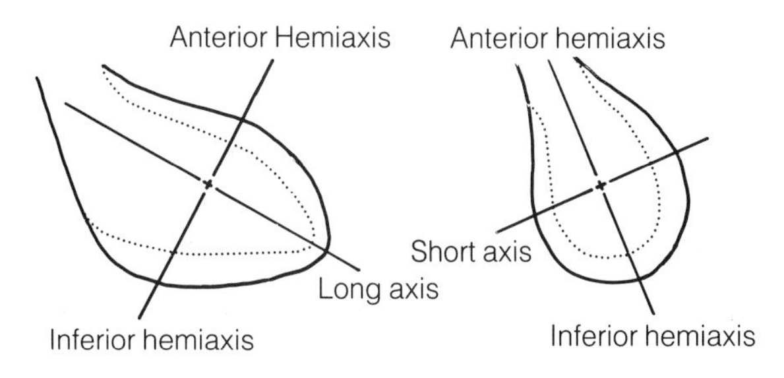

Figure 1.3 Diagram of end-diastolic outline (solid line) and end-systolic outline (dashed line) in (a) anterior view and (b) left anterior oblique view. The long and short axes are indicated by the heavy lines. Normal shortening is 50% of a radius in the short axes of the anterolateral, inferior and posterior walls. The septum should move posteriorly and thicken, but radial shortening may be limited to <15%.

picture element in the lung determined. A typical value for lung background is between 30% and 60% of left ventricular end-diastolic counts (depending on the radiopharmaceutical, window setting and collimator). This value is then subtracted from each picture element in the image. The background subtraction step is crucial to the subsequent calculation of the correct EF. Subtraction of too much background will result in a falsely elevated EF, while subtraction of too little background will result in a falsely depressed EF. The region of the left ventricle is then identified to the computer, and using either a manual, threshold or second derivative algorithm the edges of the left ventricle are identified on each frame. The total background-corrected counts in the left ventricle on each frame are used to generate the time–activity curve. The EF is calculated from the time–activity curve. In addition to the EF the time of filling, emptying, and ejection and filling rates can be readily computed from these curves. Filling and emptying rates of the left ventricle, important indexes of diastolic and systolic performance (Bonow *et al.*, 1981), are calculated from the time–activity curve by measuring either the average or peak slope of the desired phase.

An alternative approach to the calculation of EF uses a single region of interest, based on the end-diastolic frame, to calculate the background-corrected time–activity curve. The LVEF calculated by this approach is usually about 5% lower than that obtained with the variable region of interest method. The method has the advantage of producing a smoother curve, which is more useful for calculating the filling and emptying rates.

The EF derived from background-corrected gated blood pool scan correlates well with that derived from contrast ventriculography (Bacharach *et al.*, 1979). The intra-observer variation in calculation of EF is about 3%, while the inter-observer variation is <5%. Similarly, calculation of right ventricular EF using a count-based method has been described (Maddahi *et al.*, 1979). However, the right atrial contribution to the right ventricular time–activity curve in the LAO view makes these data less reliable.

Ventricular volumes Left ventricular volumes can be calculated by either a geometric (area/length) method (Strauss *et al.*, 1979) or by a count-based method. The geometric method requires calibration of the gamma camera to determine the relative size of the left ventricle in each of two views in the image. The volume of the chamber is then calculated using either an area/length formula or the Simpson rule approach (to calculate the volume of irregularly shaped objects). A minimum error of about 20% can be expected with the geometric approach, due to operator variation in defining the borders of the chamber. The count-based method requires a blood sample as a counting standard and correction for attenuation of blood pool activity by overlying chest wall. The count-based method has better precision than the geometric approach (minimum error of about 10%) (Massie *et al.*, 1982), but may have substantial inaccuracy due to the difficulty of computing attenuation.

Quantification of regional wall motion can be achieved either by measuring regional radial shortening (Yasuda *et al.*, 1981; Tamaki *et al.*, 1986a) as in contrast angiography, or by calculation of regional EF (Maddox *et al.*, 1979). The digital nature of the data lends itself to the generation of functional images, such as EF images (Maddox *et al.*, 1978), paradox image (Holman *et al.*, 1979), and amplitude and phase images (Adam *et al.*, 1979; Links *et al.*, 1980) that can be used to characterize regional asynergy and asynchrony.

Phase analysis Functional images can reduce complex information to a single image representing both anatomy and physiology. The stroke

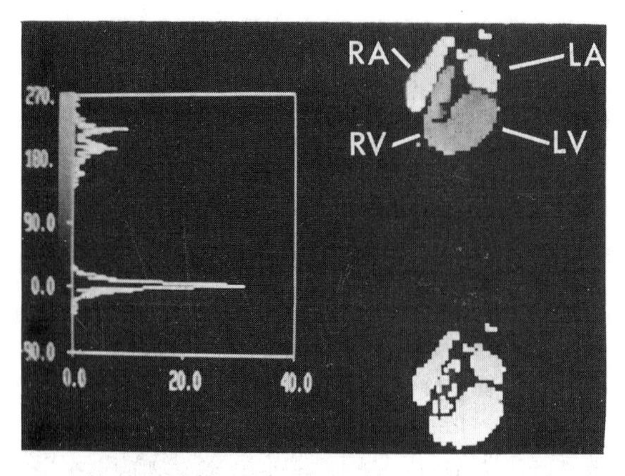

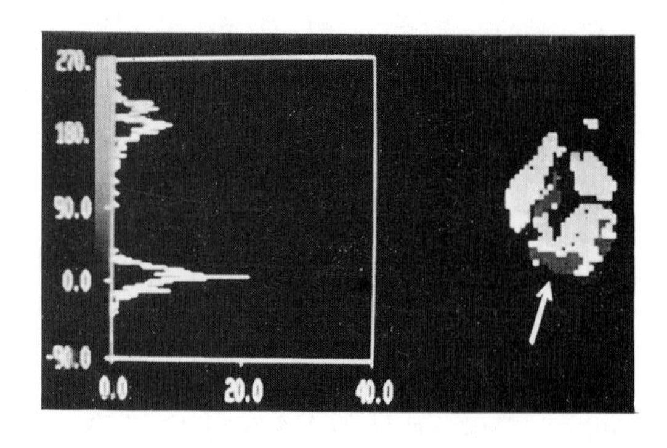

Figure 1.4 Phase-analysis images and histograms in the left anterior oblique position of two patients: (a) normal subject; (b) patient with coronary artery disease with left ventricular aneurysm. The time of onset of change in activity is indicated by the shading of the image. The regional differences in onset of contraction are apparent in the patient in (b).

volume image and the paradox image provide useful data, but do not take full advantage of the cyclic nature of the gated blood pool scan. A more general method of data evaluation is provided by the technique of Fourier analysis. Briefly, any periodic function can be represented mathematically by a sum of sinusoidal and cosinusoidal curves of various amplitude and frequency. This concept has been applied to many fields ranging from music to magnetic resonance imaging. In music, a complex tone can be exactly duplicated by striking a series of tuning forks in just the right order with just the right force. In the language of Fourier analysis, the force with which the tuning forks are struck determines the amplitude of the pure tone, and the onset of a pure tone relative to other tones determines the phase of the tone. Each pure tone with its associated amplitude and phase is referred to as a Fourier component. Mathematically, this process can be represented by the following equation:

$$f(t) = \sum_{n=1}^{\infty} A_n \cos(n\pi/T)t + \sum_{n=1}^{\infty} B_n \sin(n\pi/T)t$$

where t = time, T = period, amplitude = + $(A_n^2 + B_n^2)^{1/2}$ and phase = arctan (A/B).

For an arbitrary waveform, many different Fourier components need to be combined to faithfully reproduce the pattern. To generate functional images of the heart, Fourier analysis is employed to approximate the volume curve with the first Fourier harmonic, a pure sine or cosine function with a period equal to the period of the cardiac cycle. The amplitude and phase of this function is adjusted to best match the left ventricular time–activity curve. This matching process can be best appreciated by an example. In order to fit an arbitrary left ventricular time–activity curve with a pure cosine function (the first harmonic), two adjustments to the cosine curve have to be made. First the amplitude of the cosine curve has to be scaled to equal the maximal excursion of the time–activity curve. Second, the cosine function must be moved to the left or right along the time axis so that the temporal evolution of activity is also matched by the cosine function. The degree of translation that optimizes the fit to the time–activity curve is the phase. For example, if a cosine curve had to be shifted to the right by 25% of the cardiac cycle length to achieve the best fit, the phase associated with this curve would be $0.25 \times 360° = 90°$. Similarly, a cosine curve requiring no shift would have zero phase. By convention 180° are added to all phase values to avoid negative values when the curve has to be translated to the left.

Analysis of a time–activity curve by Fourier transformation yields the best-fit values for amplitude and phase. When this analysis is performed for each pixel in an image, amplitude and phase images are obtained. The amplitude image is qualitatively similar to the stroke volume image, but has two important differences: (1) the stroke volume image is calculated from only two points in the cardiac cycle, while the amplitude image is computed from the entire time–activity curve of each pixel; (2) the atria are detectable in the amplitude image (unlike the stroke volume image where negative changes in activity are ignored, amplitude image values are always positive since, by convention, the positive square root is always taken).

The phase image reflects the timing of regional ejection and is not determined solely by any particular cardiac event, but depends on function in general. Since the amplitude and phase images are computed from entire local time–activity curves, they possess smaller uncertainties than simpler images such as the stroke volume image. In addition to the pictorial representation, phase data can also be represented in histogram format. In this representation, the number of pixels in an image with a particular phase is plotted against phase (Figure 1.4).

Fourier analysis of gated blood pool data will never replace the subjective evaluation of the cinematically displayed data by an experienced observer, but the additional quantification provided by this technique has important clinical applications. The analysis of wall motion is dependent on changes in edges, while phase and amplitude data primarily reflect changes in regional volume. These two phenomena are often similar, but are not necessarily identical. As a result it is not useful to consider phase and amplitude analysis as a quantitative means of assessing regional wall motion. Phase analysis may be useful for following subtle changes in ventricular function following medical and/or surgical intervention and has been particularly useful for evaluating premature ventricular contraction (Botvinick *et al.*, 1982) and accessory conduction pathways (Nakajima *et al.*, 1984).

1.4.2 FIRST-PASS BLOOD POOL IMAGING

First-pass radionuclide angiography measures indices of cardiac function from the initial transit of the radiotracer through the heart. This technique provides a means of assessing (1) transit time (2) cardiac output, (3) intracardiac shunt, (4) right ventricular function and (5) global and regional left ventricular function.

(a) Instrumentation and radiopharmaceuticals

During the passage of a bolus of activity through the heart extremely high count rates are generated (Figure 1.5). Although Anger cameras produced after 1985 have the ability to handle these high count rates, multicrystal cameras were designed for this purpose (Bender and Blau, 1963; Jengo *et al.*, 1978).

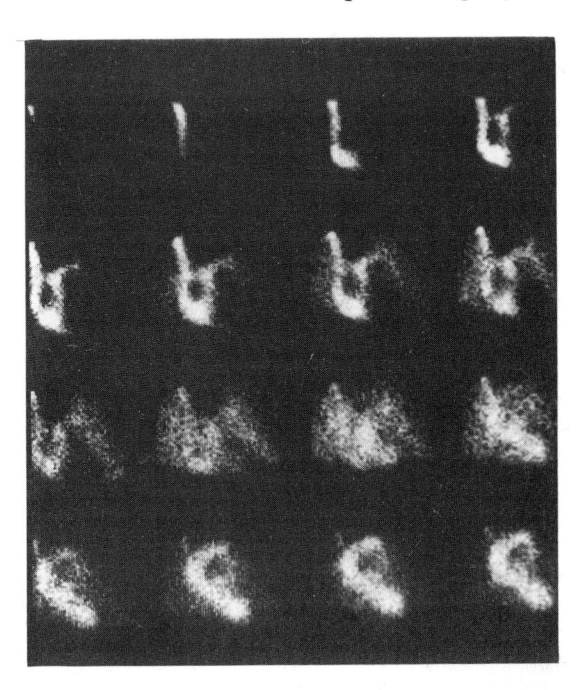

Figure 1.5 Sequential images recorded in the anterior position at 2 s per frame, delineating the superior vena cava, right atrium and ventricle, lungs, left atrium and ventricle, and aorta.

Almost any non-particulate tracer may be used, but radiopharmaceuticals that are rapidly cleared from the blood pool, such as ^{99m}Tc-labelled diethylenetriaminepentaacetic acid (DTPA) or ^{99m}Tc-labelled sulphur colloid, are advantageous if multiple studies are to be performed as the background activity will be lower.

(b) Injection technique

For optimum separation of the left and right sides of the heart, a compact bolus is required. This is usually achieved by administering the dose at a time of maximal limb hyperaemia induced by ischaemic vasoconstriction.

Typically, a butterfly needle (20 gauge or larger) is placed in the basilic vein, attached to a three-way stopcock filled with saline, connected to two syringes – the first containing the activity in a volume <1 ml, the second containing a saline flush (usually 5–10 ml). A blood pressure cuff is placed on the arm, inflated to below diastolic pressure for about 1 min to suffuse the veins, inflated above systolic pressure for 1–2 min to render the limb ischaemic and provoke maximal reactive vasodilatation, the radionuclide is injected, followed by cuff release and saline flush (Oldendorf *et al.*, 1965).

(c) Analysis

The ejection fraction is calculated by placing a computer-derived region of interest over the left ventricle and generating a time–activity curve with a temporal resolution of at least a 25 frames s^{-1}. The peaks of the curve correspond to end-diastole while the troughs correspond to end-systole. The six to seven cardiac cycles that contain the maximum activity are then summed in phase and a composite curve made from the data. The time–activity curve is analysed as described above. Left ventricular end-diastolic and end-systolic volumes can be calculated using the area/length method (assuming a prolate ellipsoidal shape) as described by Dodge.

The advantages of the first-pass study are the rapidity of imaging, high target-to-background ratio, temporal separation of the right and left ventricles, and assessment of transit time. A disadvantage of the first-pass method is that each injection only permits recording in one view – at a specific point in time – requiring multiple injections for multiple measurements.

Exercise testing can be performed as described above for equilibrium blood pool images, but with the first-pass technique the images are obtained over a shorter period of time and do not represent the average of 2–3 min of exercise. The disadvantage of this technique is that it is more difficult to obtain sequential studies during each stage of exercise as further amounts of radionuclide have to be given and background correction becomes more of a problem.

(d) First-pass gated scans

At times, it is helpful to combine the rapid data acquisition and high count rate abilities of the first-pass technique with the equilibrium gated approach. This approach is particularly useful to measure right ventricular function. During the first pass of activity through the cardiac chambers, gated images are recorded with termination of one acquisition when activity reaches the lungs so that the right-sided structures alone are imaged (McKusick *et al.*, 1978) followed immediately by a second acquisition as the activity passes through the left side. By this means, the two ventricles are separated temporally; though the count statistics are inferior to conventional equilibrium images, the quality is similar to that recorded with first-pass studies.

1.4.3 CLINICAL APPLICATIONS OF BLOOD POOL IMAGING

(a) Diagnosis and evaluation of coronary artery disease

Ventricular function is usually measured either for the detection/characterization of coronary disease, or to verify the effect of therapy on ventricular function. Since myocardial ischaemia causes a reduction in local contractile function, a decrease in either regional wall motion, global EF or both from rest to exercise identifies patients with myocardial ischaemia. Borer *et al.* (1977) investigated the effects of maximal supine exercise on ventricular function in normal subjects and patients with coronary artery disease: the normal group increased their EF by at least 5%, whereas patients with coronary artery disease either showed a fall in EF or failed to show a 5% rise.

Jones *et al.* (1981) noted that the magnitude of a fall in EF with exercise appears to increase with the severity of disease. The development of regional wall motion abnormalities, an infrequent finding, is relatively more specific for coronary artery disease than a fall in EF. The sensitivity and specificity of a decrease in EF is lower in women than in men. In addition, normal subjects with EF at rest over 65%, or who are over 60 years of age, may not increase their EF during exercise (Port *et al.*, 1980). Rozansky *et al.* (1982) also reported declining specificity of the exercise blood pool scan for diagnosing coronary artery disease, probably due to different patient populations.

Diastolic performance is altered by ischaemia (Hammermeister and Warbasse, 1974). Bonow *et al.* (1981) reported that peak diastolic filling rate at rest can be used to distinguish patients with coronary disease and normal systolic function from control subjects. Hayes *et al.* (1983) demonstrated that exercise/rest peak filling rates are a sensitive and specific index of coronary artery disease. Furthermore, asynchronous left ventricular function in addition to global diastolic dysfunction is observed in these patients (Bonow *et al.*, 1985). However, the presence of an age-dependent decrease in peak filling rate in subjects without coronary artery disease may decrease the specificity of filling rate measurements for detecting coronary artery disease in the elderly.

Regional wall motion abnormalities at rest may be due to scar or ischaemia. The term 'hibernating myocardium' is often applied to severely ischaemic areas which are akinetic on wall motion studies. The exercise blood pool scan is often useful for making this differentiation. Rozansky *et al.* (1982) reported that in most patients with surgically reversible regional myocardial dysfunction regional wall motion abnormalities improve on images recorded immediately after exercise compared to rest.

Right ventricular function may also show abnormalities in response to exercise in patients with coronary artery disease. A decrease in right ventricular function with exercise may occur either from ischaemia of the right ventricular myocardium (usually secondary to a severe stenosis of the right coronary artery with poor collateral flow) or secondary to left ventricular failure with an elevation of the wedge pressure. Johnson *et al.* (1979) reported that the extent of decrease in right ventricular function appears to be more dependent on the severity of left ventricular dysfunction than on the presence of significant right coronary artery stenosis. Another effect of left ventricular dysfunction which may be observed in blood pool scans is a rise in pulmonary blood volume. Okada *et al.* (1979) demonstrated increased diagnostic accuracy for coronary artery disease when an exercise-induced fall in EF is accompanied by a rise in pulmonary blood volume, as compared to fall in EF alone.

(b) Acute infarction

The spectrum of abnormalities in ventricular function following myocardial infarction range from nothing (very small non-transmural infarcts), to local wall motion abnormalities (small transmural infarcts), to extensive wall motion abnormalities with global ventricular dysfunction (massive infarction) (Rigo *et al.*, 1974b; Sandford *et al.*, 1982) (Figure 1.6). Blood pool imaging has been used to differentiate diffuse hypokinesis of the left ventricle from a focal abnormality such as an evolving left ventricular aneurysm as the cause of left ventricular failure.

The effect of acute interventions on both left and right ventricular global function and regional wall motion may be assessed at the bedside as has been shown for the intra-aortic balloon pump (Nichols *et al.*, 1978). Patients with unstable angina pectoris or extensive myocardial infarction were imaged on and off the pump and LVEF and wall motion abnormalities determined. Those with unstable angina showed a significant reduction of ventricular akinesis when on balloon support, whereas those with established infarction showed no significant change. Similarly, the potential of drug therapy, such as propranolol for the reduction of acute and long-term effects on left ventricular function, can be investigated by blood pool imaging.

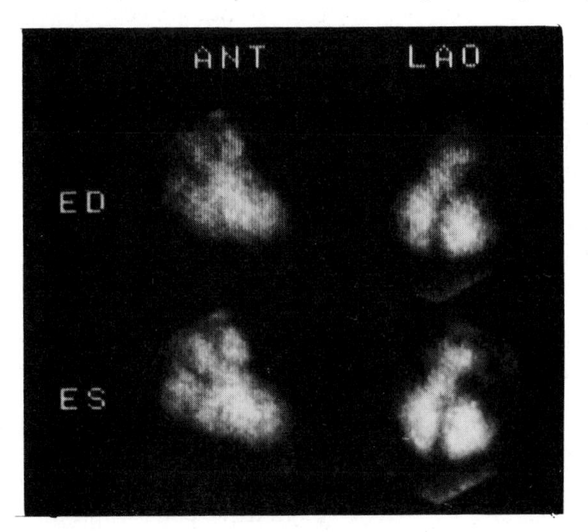

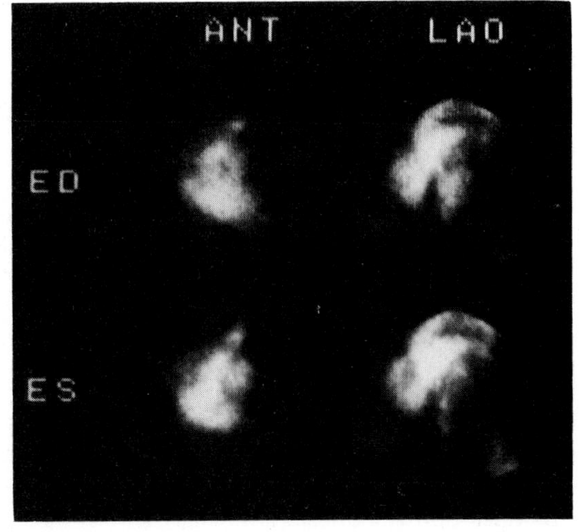

Figure 1.6 Gated scans (end-diastole and end-systole) in the anterior position and left anterior oblique position in two patients with infarction: (a) diffuse hypokinesis due to extensive left anterior descending coronary artery occlusion; (b) focal left ventricular aneurysm.

The location of the infarct has a direct bearing on the extent of left ventricular dysfunction. Those patients with anterior infarction have lower EF than those with inferior infarction (34% against 50%) (Reduto *et al.*, 1978). In the absence of residual ischaemia, the reduction of EF and wall motion abnormalities remain virtually unchanged over the first two weeks after infarction. Thereafter, with progressive return to normal activity there may be an increase in end-diastolic volume, compensatory hypertrophy of uninvolved walls of the left ventricle and increased vigour of contraction. Most of the improvement in left ventricular function will occur within three months of the acute event.

Successful thrombolytic therapy frequently converts episodes of infarction into episodes of severe ischaemia. As a result, early determination of ventricular function in patients treated with thrombolysis frequently demonstrate marked wall motion abnormalities and depression of ventricular function, 'stunned myocardium', which exhibit striking resolution on studies performed at ten days.

Aneurysm

An aneurysm is defined as a break in the contour of the diastolic outline of the ventricle. Left ventricular aneurysms, though usually discovered weeks to months following infarction, can be detected within the first week. Left ventricular aneurysms should be suspected in patients with persistent left ventricular failure, recurrent arrhythmias, embolic phenomena, or persistent ST elevation on ECG.

Both first-pass and equilibrium blood pool imaging are very effective for the recognition of left ventricular aneurysms (Rigo *et al.*, 1974b; Dymond *et al.*, 1979; Borer *et al.*, 1980) and may be used as a screening test to select patients for contrast angiography. The presence of dyskinesis alone does not constitute an aneurysm. There is often a well-defined junction between the aneurysmal zone and the more normally contracting ventricle (Figure 1.6). Multiple views of the heart are essential (especially the left posterior oblique view) to measure residual ventricular function, as preserved motion at the ventricular base may be entirely obscured by the overlying aneurysm (in the LAO view) and right ventricle (in the anterior view). Apical aneurysms can cause the calculated EF to be artefactually low, since the large blood pool in the aneurysm obscures the retained wall motion at the base of the ventricle.

Occasionally, a small rupture of the infarcted wall will appear but be contained by the pericardium and give rise to the formation of a false aneursym. This abnormality may be identified by its saccular appearance, almost as a second ventricular chamber with a very thin narrow neck (Botvinick *et al.*, 1976; Sweet *et al.*, 1979; Katz *et al.*, 1979). Contrast examination may demonstrate the cavity only poorly because of the slow exchange of blood through the narrow neck and the equilibrium blood pool images may be extremely valuable for exact delineation.

(d) Right ventricular abnormalities in infarction

Right ventricular infarction occurs in about 30% of patients with inferior wall necrosis (Figure 1.7). While it is uncommon for the right ventricle to be the only site of necrosis, right ventricular involvement may be the major cause of decreased cardiac output in patients with inferior wall infarction. Involvement of the right ventricle is identified by disproportionate right ventricular enlargement, a reduced EF of the right ventricle and focal zones of akinesis (Reduto *et al.*, 1978).

The gated blood pool scan is also valuable for determination of response to therapy, such as thrombolysis (Anderson *et al.*, 1983; Khaja *et al.*, 1983) and angioplasty (Bonow *et al.*, 1985; Liu *et al.*, 1986). The lack of an increase in LVEF after intervention suggests ultimate failure of therapy.

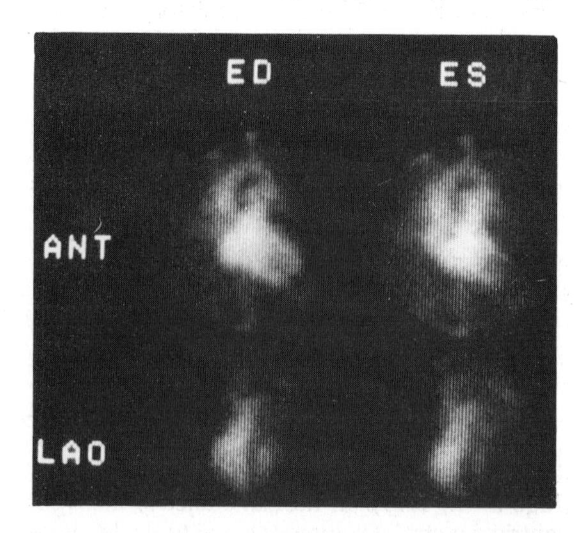

Figure 1.7 Selected end-diastolic and end-systolic views of a gated scan of a patient with right ventricular dysfunction. The large right ventricle is apparent on both the anterior and left anterior oblique views.

(e) Prognosis

Several studies have demonstrated the prognostic importance of the resting LVEF as a predictor of subsequent development of congestive heart failure and early death (Schulze *et al.*, 1977; Shah *et al.*, 1980; Mukharji *et al.*, 1984). On the other hand, Schelbert *et al.* (1976) reported spontaneous changes in left ventricular function after acute myocardial infarction. These changes in global and regional function may also add prognostic information (Meizlish *et al.*, 1984; Tamaki *et al.*, 1985c). Additional prognostic information may be obtained from submaximal exercise study prior to discharge from hospital to select patients at high risk for subsequent complications (Corbett *et al.*, 1981) (based on a decrease in their EF from rest to exercise).

(f) Cor pulmonale

When right ventricular afterload increases in an adult, the right ventricle dilates and has a reduced EF. When the overload becomes chronic, the right ventricle hypertrophies, but rarely returns to normal function. Patients with cor pulmonale (Berger *et al.*, 1978) had a significant reduction in right ventricular EF (35 $\pm$ 2%) compared with 17 controls (57 $\pm$ 2%). Blood pool imaging allowed differentiation of patients with severe ventilatory impairment into those with concomitant right ventricular dysfunction (cor pulmonale), who are at higher risk of developing secondary problems from any additional loss of ventilatory function, from those with well-maintained right ventricular function, who are more stable. Matthay *et al.* (1980) demonstrated that abnormal right ventricular exercise reserve is present in 80% of patients with chronic obstructive pulmonary disease. In contrast, left ventricular response to exercise is generally normal.

(g) Valvular disease

Blood pool imaging rarely provides a specific diagnosis in valvular heart disease, but deductions about aetiology may be made from the secondary effects on chamber size and function. The severity of regurgitation may be estimated from a region-of-interest analysis of the relative stroke volume of the right and left ventricles in the LAO position (Rigo *et al.*, 1979). In normal subjects, the right ventricular stroke volume is equal to the left ventricular stroke volume, whereas in aortic and mitral regurgitation the left ventricular stroke volume increases and the left-to-right stroke index becomes greater than one. Due to differences in the relationship of the right atrium to the right ventricle compared to that of the left atrium to the left ventricle, the calculated value of left to right stroke counts in normal subjects may be up to 1.6. A refined method for making this measurement, which utilizes both first-pass and equilibrium techniques, was described by Klipzig *et al.* (1986). Clearly, when there is a regurgitant lesion on the right side as well as on the left, such as tricuspid plus mitral regurgitation, this approach is no longer valid. Fortunately, this is a relatively rare occurrence. Rigo's data suggest that regurgitation cannot be diagnosed until it amounts to >30% of the stroke volume.

(h) Aortic stenosis

Compensated aortic stenosis may be recognized by left ventricular hypertrophy, manifest by an increase in the photon-deficient area around the left ventricular cavity. There may also be widening of the aortic root due to post-stenotic dilatation. The cavity frequently takes on an elongated shape in pure aortic stenosis, often likened to a spearhead. The base of the left ventricle appears to contract earlier than the apex so that there may be a small region of retained activity at the apex. Occasionally a supranormal EF is seen with excessive hypertrophy suggesting the appearance of associated hypertrophic cardiomyopathy (Nanda *et al.*, 1974). The right side remains normal until the late stages of the disease when left ventricular decompensation supervenes. Late in the course of aortic stenosis, when EF has decreased below 40%, the ventricle dilates and wall motion becomes diffusely abnormal. Gated images are particularly helpful pre-operatively when the patient is too ill to have a contrast ventriculogram, or the aortic valve cannot be traversed by the catheter. Following aortic valve replacement, the left ventricular hypertrophy regresses and left ventricular function returns towards normal (Schuler *et al.*, 1979).

(i) Aortic regurgitation

Compensated aortic regurgitation is manifest by left ventricular dilatation, an increased stroke volume and slight hypertrophy. The aorta is dilated and may pulsate. As the severity of regurgitation increases, the left ventricular cavity becomes globular. Patients with aortic regurgitation have decreased left ventricular reserve during exercise even in the absence of symptoms and normal resting function (Borer *et al.*, 1978). Schuler *et al.* (1982) reported that the asymptomatic patients with aortic regurgitation may be uncovered by determination of the end-systolic pressure–volume relation or left ventricular exercise reserve. Shen *et al.* (1985) demonstrated that the slope of the pressure–volume curve during stress is a reliable indicator of left ventricular dysfunction. Since these patients occasionally have a normal rest EF and may respond abnormally to exercise, these parameters may be useful as a sensitive index of myocardial contractile state and may help in the difficult clinical decision on the timing of aortic valve replacement in asymptomatic patients.

(j) Mitral stenosis

The most striking feature of mitral stenosis is left atrial enlargement, which is best observed in the left posterior oblique projection. Since the left ventricle is relatively unaffected by an inflow problem, left ventricular function is usually preserved, though in some patients there is a reduction of EF, possibly due to rheumatic cardiomyopathy, underfilling of the left ventricle, or rigidity of the mitral valve apparatus which restricts the mobility of the adjacent left ventricle (Heller and Carleton, 1970). The right ventricle is frequently dilated because of associated pulmonary hypertension. If pulmonary hypertension is severe, the right ventricle will dilate and may cause tricuspid regurgitation.

(k) Mitral regurgitation

In mitral regurgitation left ventricular dilatation is the dominant response, with some myocardial hypertrophy. The stroke volume and end-diastolic volumes are increased in direct proportion to the degree of regurgitation. The left atrium may show very marked dilatation, and associated mitral stenosis may give rise to the signs of pulmonary hypertension. Patients with compensated mitral regurgitation have a normal or increased EF. During exercise, however, the EF may fall, due to changes in loading conditions and/or contractile reserve, even in the absence of coronary disease. As a result, a reduction in left ventricular function during exercise in a patient with mitral regurgitation should not be interpreted as an indication of concomitant coronary artery disease. As the disease progresses the end-diastolic volume will continue to increase, but the end-systolic volume will remain constant until decompensation occurs (Phillip *et al.*, 1981).

(l) Tricuspid valve disease

Tricuspid valve disease is usually manifest by massive enlargement of the right atrium. During first-pass studies, reflux of activity into the jugular vein and hepatic veins may be seen. The reflux will occur during atrial diastole with tricuspid regurgitation and atrial systole with stenosis. Regurgitation is associated with right ventricular volume overload and tricuspid stenosis with a small right ventricle.

(m) Dilated cardiomyopathy

The term encompasses a number of pathological causes of heart failure associated with an enlarged left ventricular chamber and profoundly depressed LVEF. The right ventricle is frequently involved and there is often myocardial hypertrophy. The cause of the disease is commonly undetermined (idiopathic cardiomyopathy) but may be due to alcohol-induced damage to the heart, viral infection, drug induced or a number of less frequent causes. The distinction between congestive cardiomyopathy of undetermined cause and the cardiomyopathy due to coronary artery disease is important as the latter may benefit from surgery if there is significant rest ischaemia. Unfortunately, it is difficult to distinguish between these two entities by blood pool imaging alone, though congestive cardiomyopathy frequently shows greater dilatation of the right ventricular cavity (Bulkley *et al.*, 1977a) and the observation of dyskinesis of the left ventricular wall is more often associated with an ischaemic aetiology.

One other important cause of cardiomyopathy is that due to therapy with the cardiotoxic antineoplastic agent doxorubicin. Alexander *et al.* (1979) have used sequential cardiac blood pool imaging and measurement of the EF to determine the amount of doxorubicin that can be administered to an individual patient to achieve the maximal potential antineoplastic effect but avoiding induction of severe cardiotoxicity. Doxorubicin cardiotoxicity is dose related, usually manifest when cumulative doses exceed 400 $mg\,kg^{-1}$. As a result, patients receiving doses in this range should be tested prior to additional therapy to determine their EF. Cardiotoxicity should be suspected if the EF falls more than 5% on sequential determinations, or if the EF falls below 45%.

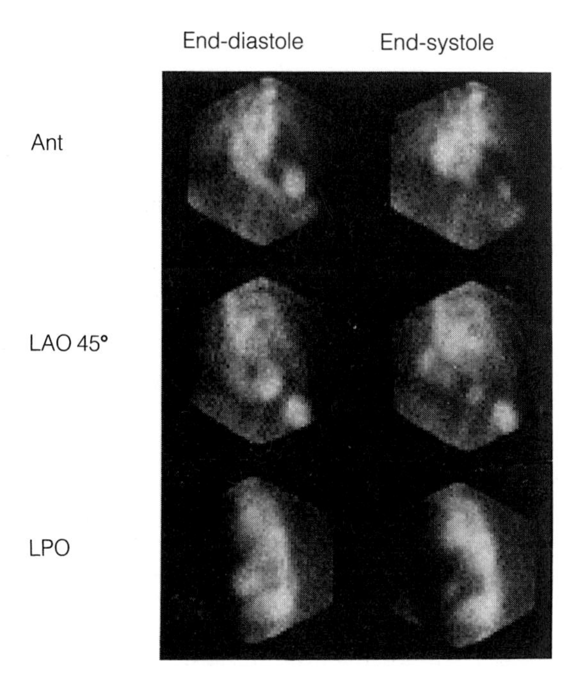

Figure 1.8 Selected end-diastolic and end-systolic views of a gated scan of a patient with IHSS. The thick muscle is apparent as a zone of decreased blood pool activity seen surrounding the left ventricle on all three images.

(n) Hypertrophic cardiomyopathy

Idiopathic hypertrophic subaortic stenosis (IHSS) (hypertrophic obstructive cardiomyopathy or asymmetric septal hypertrophy) is a familial disease of unknown aetiology characterized by asymmetric hypertrophy of the left ventricular myocardium, systolic anterior motion of the mitral valve and sudden death due to dynamic outflow obstruction (Figure 1.8).

The choice of the correct LAO projection is critical to the assessment of septal thickness as the septum has a spiral geometry, with the higher septum being more prominent in the higher oblique views. Multiple views are essential for correct evaluation as the septal thickening may be obscured by incorrect positioning. In the normal blood pool image, the septum is seen as a curvilinear region of relative photon deficiency with its concavity directed towards the left ventricular cavity. In 22 patients studied by Pohost *et al.* (1977) straightening of the septum was seen in 73%, disproportionate upper septal thickening (DUST) in 50%, a defect in the left ventricular outflow tract due to the thickened upper septum in 73% and cavity obliteration in 77%.

The availability of ultrasound and the ease with which the thickness of the septum and posterior wall can be measured makes it the imaging modality of choice for the diagnosis of IHSS.

(o) Cardiac tumours

Intracavitary tumours, such as atrial myxoma, may cause heart failure by obstructing the entry of blood into a cardiac chamber or give rise to emboli (in the pulmonary bed – right atrial lesions; or the systemic circulation – left atrial lesions). It is possible for a left ventriculogram alone to miss these tumours and there is always the chance of a piece of the tumour being dislodged during catheterization. Usually, left atrial myxomata are seen in the laevo phase of a pulmonary angiogram, but if identified with confidence on both echocardiogram and blood pool images surgery can probably be performed without recourse to catheterization unless knowledge of the coronary anatomy is required (Bonte and Curry, 1967; Pohost *et al.*, 1977).

Rarely, malignant tumours involving the pericardium or myocardium can compress the cardiac chambers and cause heart failure because of restriction to inflow of blood, reduction of ventricular function or obstruction to outflow. Pericardial or myocardial involvement should be suspected when patients with lymphoma, oat cell or breast carcinoma develop unexplained heart failure. The blood pool scan can identify the site and extent of chamber compression and/or wall motion abnormality, and permits a simple means of following therapy (Pitcher *et al.*, 1980).

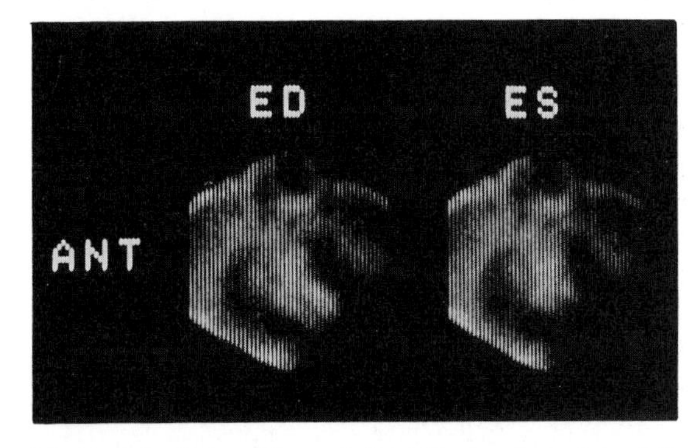

Figure 1.9 Selected end-diastolic and end-systolic views of a gated scan in the anterior projection of a patient with pericardial effusion. The 'halo' surrounding the entire heart is seen on both images.

(p) Pericardial effusions

Large pericardial effusions may cause congestive heart failure because of restriction of blood entry into the cardiac chambers. Effusions can be recognized as a 'halo' of decreased activity surrounding the cardiac blood pool (Figure 1.9). The 'halo' should separate the cardiac blood pool from that in the surrounding lungs and liver. It may, on occasion, be difficult to distinguish pericardial fat pads and ventricular hypertrophy from loculated effusions. When the effusion is very large the cardiac chambers may seem to rock sideways with each contraction within the pericardial cavity. The ventricular cavities may be reduced in volume and the filling phase of the ventricle brief with a long diastolic plateau. The gated scan can detect effusions of >100 ml.

1.4.4 BLOOD POOL TOMOGRAPHY

Recording data from gated blood pool scans with SPECT offers an opportunity to reconstruct the data in orientations that cannot be recorded with conventional planar images (Fischman *et al.*, 1989) (Figure 1.10): (1) an apical four-chamber view can be obtained to provide simultaneous information about atrial and ventricular wall motion; (2) a true left ventricular long axis view can be reconstructed to provide information about left ventricular wall motion without overlying right ventricular activity; (3) the short axis of the ventricle can be sampled at multiple points, to permit independent assessment of motion at the base and apex of the left ventricle. This approach can be particularly useful in patients with apical aneurysms and left ventricular failure, to determine if retained function at the base is sufficient to warrant surgery (Corbett *et al.*, 1985; Gill *et al.*, 1986b; Maublant *et al.*, 1983; Tamaki *et al.*, 1983).

1.4.5 NON-IMAGING NUCLEAR PROBE

A non-imaging nuclear probe can be used to monitor cardiac function (Wagner *et al.*, 1976). The probe has the major advantage of portability, decreased cost and high sensitivity. Thus, a beat-to-beat volume curve of high temporal resolution can be recorded. Excellent correlation between probe measurement of LVEF and those recorded with the gamma camera have been reported (Berger, *et al.*, 1981).

The probe concept was extended from a bedside method to one that could be used continuously while the patient performed activities of daily living (Strauss *et al.*, 1979). An instrument was constructed that consisted of two small radionuclide detectors, an ECG recorder and associated electronics placed in a garment which is worn like

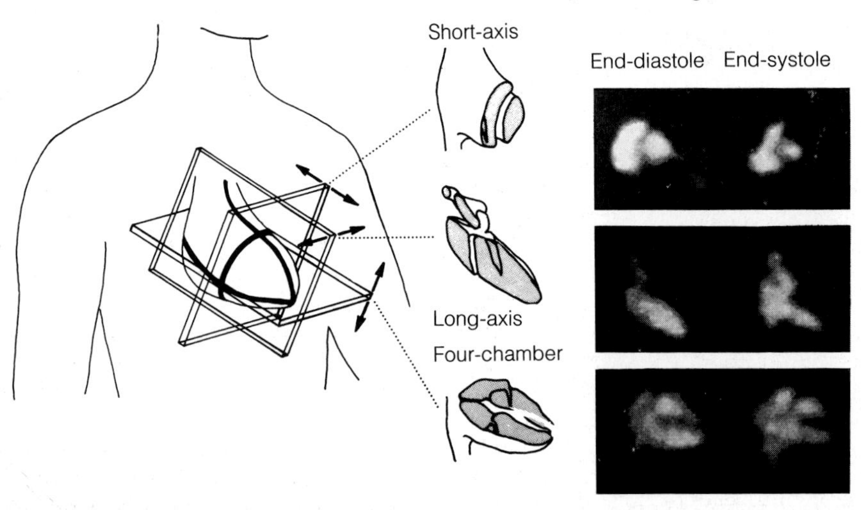

Figure 1.10 Schematic representation of oblique planes through the heart. Also shown are corresponding short-axis, long-axis, and apical four-chamber slices through mid-ventricle at end-diastole and end-systole in a normal subject. In the short-axis oblique slice, the right ventricle and the infundibulum are on the viewer's left. The long-axis slice is through the mid-portion of the left ventricle. The apical four-chamber view has been rotated 90° clockwise to correspond to the diagram. Right atrium and ventricle are superior and left atrium and ventricle are inferior. The AV valve plane, atria and aorta are well appreciated at end-systole. Septal thickening is also seen at end-systole.

a vest (Figure 1.11) (hence the name of the device – VEST). The VEST records beat-to-beat left ventricular time–activity curves over several hours (Figure 1.12). Preliminary studies have demonstrated changes in LVEF during non-stressful daily activities (Wilson *et al.*, 1983) and rapid sequential changes in EF during treadmill exercise in normal subjects (Tamaki *et al.*, 1987a). When ventricular function was monitored in patients with coronary artery disease, transient decreases in EF with or without ECG changes were frequently observed normal during daily activity (Tamaki *et al.*, 1986b).

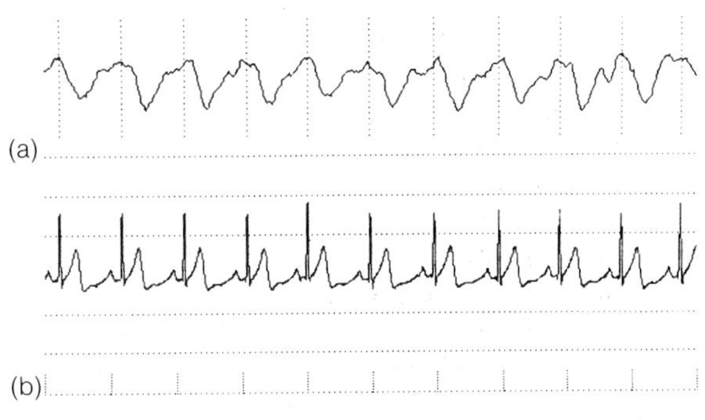

Figure 1.12 (a) Time–activity curve and (b) ECG recorded with the VEST.

1.5 PERFUSION IMAGING

Perfusion imaging comprises a series of radionuclide techniques to measure the distribution of regional blood flow at the capillary level in the heart. The techniques are usually applied to the detection and localization of myocardial ischaemia or scar.

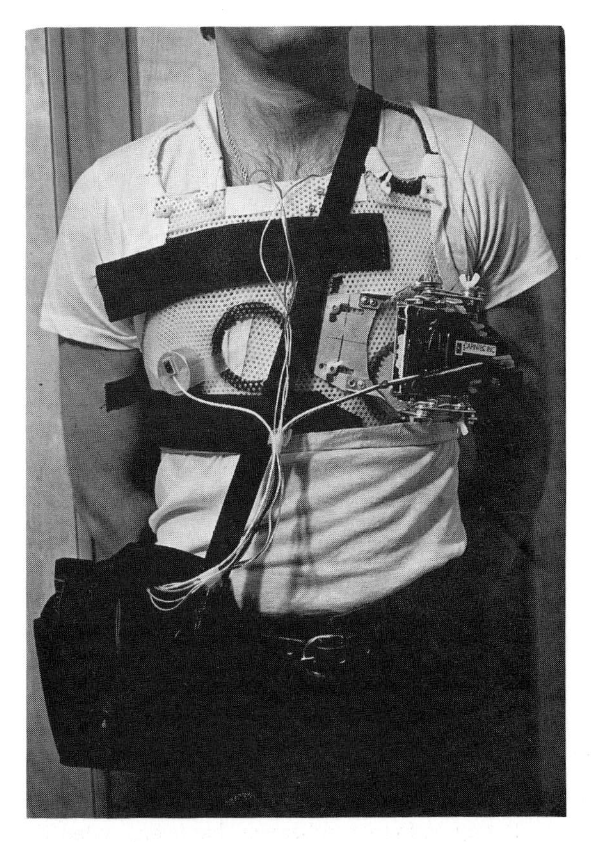

Figure 1.11 Photograph of a subject wearing the VEST. The detector is the circular object located over the patient's left ventricle.

1.5.1 INTRACORONARY INJECTION

Imaging of the myocardium can be performed invasively with labelled microspheres (Endo *et al.*, 1970) introduced into the coronary circulation via a catheter. While the coronary arteries have limited collaterals, obstruction of a small fraction of the precapillary arteriolar bed is safe, as indicated by the work of Grames *et al.* (1975) where up to 800 000 particles of ^{131}I-labelled macro-aggregated albumin (35 μm diameter) and up to 30 000 particles of ^{99m}Tc-labelled macro-aggregated albumin (30 μm diameter) were injected without untoward occurrence. The particles impact in myocardial precapillary arterioles and reflect perfusion at the time of injection. Once the particles have impacted, their distribution can be recorded several hours later. Consequently, imaging at a site remote from the catheterization laboratory is possible. This method allows the demonstration of relative perfusion within an arterial distribution and, when two different labels are used, the relative contribution of right and left coronary arteries to myocardial blood supply (hence the presence of collaterals may be determined).

An alternative approach to the measurement of regional myocardial perfusion is the use of an inert gas such as ^{133}Xe dissolved in saline. When injected into the coronary arteries, ^{133}Xe rapidly equilibrates with the perfused myocardium supplied by that vessel. Since clearance is dependent on perfusion, measurement of the rate of washout gives a measure of the rate of blood flow to the myocardium (Kolibash *et al.*, 1979; Cannon *et al.*, 1972). Studies in patients with normal coronary arteries revealed myocardial perfusion rates between 50 and 100 ml min^{-1} per 100 g of tissue. Using the same technique, Korbuly *et al.* (1975)

demonstrated increased myocardial perfusion following left anterior descending coronary artery bypass grafting, not only to the bypassed territory but also to the unbypassed circumflex territory.

1.5.2 INTRAVENOUS INJECTION

Non-invasive imaging of myocardial perfusion has been accomplished with the monovalent cations ^{131}Cs (Carr, 1964), ^{43}K (Hurley *et al.*, 1971), ^{81}Rb (Zaret *et al.*, 1974) and ^{201}Tl (Lebowitz *et al.*, 1975). Following intravenous injection, these ions are distributed in proportion to cardiac output (Sapirstein, 1956), where well-perfused zones of myocardium receive a larger amount of tracer than areas of ischaemia or scar. Administration of these tracers under basal (resting) conditions is an insensitive approach to the detection of ischaemia, however, because coronary narrowings have to reduce the lumen by more than 90% to diminish perfusion at rest. To detect ischaemia, it is necessary to increase the myocardial oxygen demands and coronary blood flow, either by exercise or by pharmacological means.

The pioneering studies of Zaret *et al.* (1973) used a two-part approach to make this measurement. At the peak of treadmill exercise, ^{43}K was injected intravenously and images were recorded immediately. Regions of ischaemia and zones of scar had decreased tracer concentration. In a separate rest-injected study (usually performed several days later), zones of myocardium supplied by moderately stenosed vessels were well perfused, while zones of scar remained abnormal.

The relatively high energy of ^{43}K was well suited for the rectilinear scanner, but could not be effectively imaged with the gamma camera. Two radiopharmaceuticals, ^{81}Rb and ^{201}Tl, were suggested as alternatives. It was not until Lebowitz *et al.* developed a practical means of producing ^{201}Tl in 1972 (Lebowitz *et al.*, 1975), however, that routine imaging of the myocardium with a gamma camera would occur.

1.5.3 PRINCIPLES OF THALLIUM IMAGING

^{201}Tl is produced by cyclotron bombardment of stable ^{203}Tl with protons to produce radioactive ^{201}Pb ($t_{1/2}$ physical = 9.4 h), which decays by electron capture to form ^{201}Tl:

$$^{203}\mathrm{Tl}\,(p, 3n)\,^{201}\mathrm{Pb} \rightarrow {}^{201}\mathrm{Tl}\ (t_{1/2}\ \text{physical} = 74\ \text{h})$$

^{201}Tl decays via electron capture to stable ^{201}Hg with the production of the 69–80 keV mercury X-rays (100% abundant), and gamma photons of 135 and 167 keV (2% and 8% abundance, respectively). The 74 h physical half-life of ^{201}Tl, coupled with the long biological half-life of this agent, limits the amount that can be administered to <3 mCi (111 MBq). This administered dose results in a radiation burden of about 5 rad to the kidneys.

Thallium is actively transported into tissue by the sodium–potassium adenosine triphosphate system (Na^+–K^+ ATPase) (Britton and Blank, 1968; Sessler *et al.*, 1986), with 88% extraction in one pass through the coronary circulation (Weich *et al.*, 1977). Thallium has a higher affinity for this transport system than other monovalent cations, resulting in a higher extraction of thallium by the myocardium than that of potassium or rubidium. After intravenous injection with the patient at rest approximately 3.5% of the injected dose localizes in the myocardium (Svensson *et al.*, 1982); after injection during exercise this increases to approximately 4.4% (Svensson *et al.*, 1982), while administration of dipyridamole causes 8–10% of the dose to concentrate in the myocardium.

Myocardial ischaemia can be identified in thallium scans by comparing the results of rest- and exercise-injected studies (Strauss *et al.*, 1975), or more commonly by comparing initial and 'redistribution' images after exercise injection (Pohost *et al.*, 1980). Thallium redistribution is defined as the relative increase in regional thallium concentration in an area of ischaemia in the images acquired several hours after injection compared to the immediate post-exercise images. This apparent 'redistribution' is usually due to a difference in clearance of thallium, with the normally perfused zones clearing more rapidly than the ischaemic areas (Figure 1.13). After intravenous injection, thallium is rapidly cleared from the blood (half-life <30 s). During the first 10 min after injection, more than 99% of the activity in blood is cleared into the tissues, leaving a small reservoir of about 0.5% of the injected dose in the total blood volume (Pohost *et al.*, 1980). The thallium in the myocardium is in dynamic equilibrium with that in the blood. In zones of normal perfusion, the intracellular thallium concentration is high compared with the residual amount in the blood, and a net loss of thallium occurs. In zones of ischaemia, where the initial concentration of thallium is relatively low, the gradient between intra- and extracellular environments is lower and the rate of loss is much slower (Pohost *et al.*, 1980).

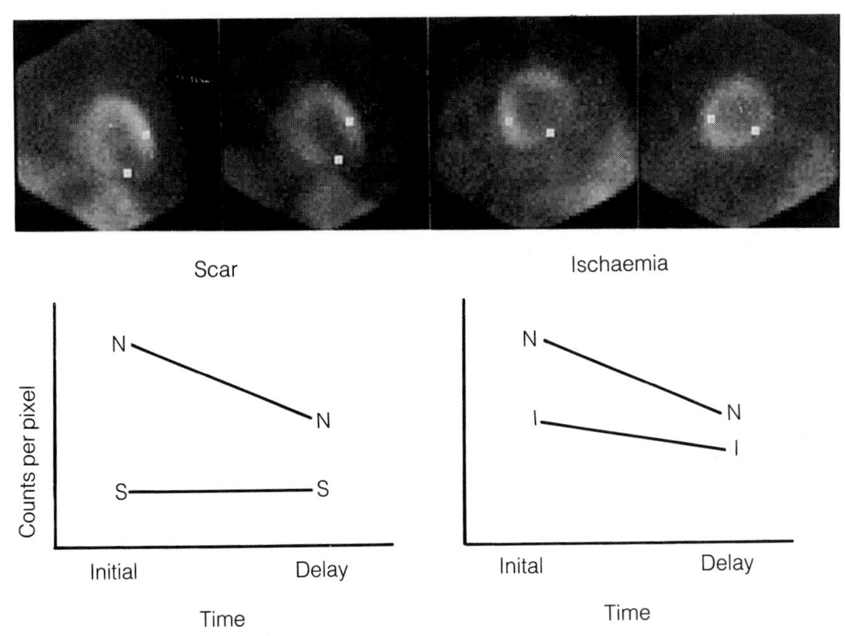

Figure 1.13 Thallium scans in the anterior position recorded immediately after injection (left), and 3 h later (right) in patients with ischaemia and a patient with scar. Regions of interest placed over the normal zone of myocardium (N) and the areas of ischaemia (I) and scar (S) are graphed as counts per pixel. Note the relatively rapid clearance of activity from the normal myocardium, compared to the much slower rate of clearance from the ischaemic area.

Ischaemia produced after thallium injection does not cause any demonstrable difference in clearance (Gewirtz *et al.*, 1979). Similarly, hyperaemia produced after thallium administration is associated with a minimal (10–15%) change in clearance rate (Leppo *et al.*, 1985). Areas of fibrosis have minimal perfusion and hence low initial concentration of thallium. The loss of thallium from these areas occurs at about the same rate as the loss from normal myocardium. As a result no differential clearance (redistribution) is observed.

Although most ischaemic lesions exhibit redistribution, about 25% of patients with ischaemia fail to redistribute (Liu *et al.*, 1985). After restoration of blood flow by means of bypass surgery or angioplasty, many of these lesions return to normal. The reasons for this phenomenon remain unclear, but may be due to differences in metabolism between acutely and chronically ischaemic tissue. These observations have led to a new approach to thallium imaging methodology: when an apparently fixed perfusion defect is seen on the 4 hour redistribution image either a second ^{201}Tl injection is given with immediate reimaging or the patient is reimaged at 24 hours. This approach reduces the incidence of fixed defects when there is viable myocardial ischaemia from about 25% to 10–15% and is now widely practised (Pieri *et al.*, 1990). Rarely, an abnormal scan can be seen in the absence of large-vessel coronary artery disease. This has been reported in hypertrophic cardiomyopathy (Bulkley *et al.*, 1975), congestive cardiomyopathy (Bulkley *et al.*, 1977a), sarcoidosis (Bulkley *et al.*, 1977b; Makler *et al.*, 1981), aortic stenosis (Bailey *et al.*, 1977a), Chagas' disease (E. Kushnir, personal communication), and left bundle branch block (McGowan *et al.*, 1976). The cause of these abnormalities is not clear but may involve many factors, such as changes in the size and shape of the ventricular cavity (Gewirtz *et al.*, 1979), or it may represent disease at either the level of the myocyte or the capillary/sarcolemma interface.

In addition to ischaemia, at least two other factors can alter the rate of thallium clearance from the heart.

First, glucose and insulin cause an accelerated loss of thallium from both normal and ischaemic myocardium (Wilson *et al.*, 1983a; Wilson *et al.*, 1986). The mechanism may be related to insulin driving potassium into tissues, causing enhanced turnover of intracellular potassium and thallium. Evidence for this comes from the observation of increased blood thallium levels during insulin infusion in experimental animals. The rapid clearance can cause areas of ischaemia to appear as 'fixed' lesions (Wilson *et al.*, 1986). This phenomenon can occur if patients eat food that cause an insulin response between initial and delayed imaging. To avoid this problem, patients should not eat any carbohydrate-containing foods between their initial post-exercise scans and the redistribution images.

Second, the heart rate achieved during exercise is inversely proportional to the rate of thallium myocardial clearance (Brown *et al.*, 1984; Kaul *et al.*, 1986). This may be due to altered cellular thallium kinetics secondary to elevated catecholamines or the redistribution of cardiac output from the splanchnic bed to skeletal muscle during intense exercise, with a concomitant reduction in blood levels. Since thallium in skeletal muscle is cleared slower than thallium in the splanchnic bed, blood activity is reduced following injection at high levels of exercise compared with activity following injection at rest. This creates a higher gradient between the intra- and extracellular environments, leading to more rapid clearance. In review of the global thallium clearance, the level of exercise should be considered. When thallium is injected at a heart rate of 100 beats min^{-1}, the clearance half-life from the myocardium is approximately 8 h, while at heart rates greater than 160 beats min^{-1} the half-life is less than 4 h.

(a) Imaging characteristics of thallium

The limited photon flux and the relatively poor spatial resolution of the gamma camera for the 69–83 keV mercury X-rays of thallium, as well as problems with scatter and attenuation, contribute to a procedure that requires 8–10 min to record an image. Thallium images should be recorded with an all-purpose collimator using a 20% window centred on the mercury X-rays using a 0.25-inch crystal gamma camera. The gamma photons should also be used, if a camera with multiple windows is available, since they increase the overall count rate by 12%, and improve image resolution. The images should be recorded for a preset time to permit measurement of myocardial thallium clearance from initial to delayed images.

(b) Data recording

Prior to exercise, an intravenous line is placed in a vein of the forearm and a blood pressure cuff is secured on the contralateral arm. Baseline 12-lead ECGs are recorded while supine, standing, and during hyperventilation. A multistage exercise is performed according to a standardized protocol with continuous monitoring of ECG, blood pressure and the subject's overall condition. Approximately 1 min prior to the end of exercise (see indications to terminate exercise testing above) a bolus of 2–3 mCi ^{201}Tl is administered intravenously and exercise continued for at least one additional minute. The subject is then placed on a stretcher, sequential recovery ECGs and blood pressures are recorded and imaging commences.

1.5.4 PLANAR IMAGING

Myocardial perfusion data are recorded in at least three projections: anterior, 45° LAO, and a steep LAO view (either 70° or lateral) with the patient in the supine position. Rotating the camera, instead of the patient, minimizes the problem of repositioning for the delayed images. In patients with an elevated left hemidiaphragm, however, the inferior wall of the heart may be obscured by the diaphragm when the images are recorded with the patient in the supine position. Under this circumstance, a left lateral view should be recorded with the patient in the right lateral decubitus position. Data are recorded for preset time on a computer at a spatial resolution of at least 64 × 64 matrix.

The patient is then discharged from the laboratory, told to refrain from eating any carbohydrate-containing foods (see above) and asked to return three hours later for redistribution images. On the patient's return, the imaging sequence is repeated.

1.5.5 SINGLE PHOTON EMISSION COMPUTED TOMOGRAPHY (SPECT)

The patient is placed supine on the SPECT table, with the left arm raised over the head (to avoid attenuation artefacts). SPECT images are recorded with a 180° acquisition (30° right anterior oblique to 30° left posterior oblique at 6° increments for 30 s per angle in either a circular or non-circular orbit (non-circular preferred). Transverse tomograms are reconstructed by filtered back-projection at 1 cm intervals. Sagittal, coronal and optimal short- and long-axis images are reconstructed for interpretation.

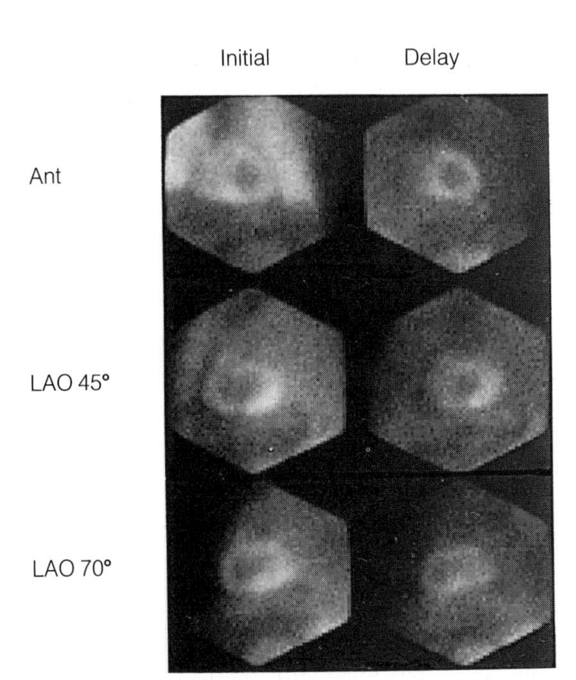

Figure 1.14 Thallium scan recorded after injection at stress in a patient with left ventricular dysfunction at the time of injection. Top: anterior views; centre: left anterior oblique views; bottom: left posterior oblique views recorded immediately (left) and 3 h later (right). The dilatation of the left ventricular cavity and increased lung uptake are seen on the initial images.

1.5.6 INTERPRETATION

(a) Planar imaging

Thallium images are reviewed for:

1. homogeneity of regional myocardial activity;
2. change in left ventricular cavity size from initial to delayed scan;
3. lung uptake;
4. changes in the regional distribution of thallium from initial to delayed scan.

The sequence in which thallium images are recorded is important, since left ventricular dysfunction can be identified by two evanescent scan findings; (1) increase in lung uptake; or (2) increase in the apparent size of the left ventricular cavity (Figure 1.14). To increase the likelihood of detecting these changes, it is best to record the anterior image first. The relative concentration of thallium in the myocardium compared with that in the lungs on the anterior view has been correlated with the pulmonary capillary wedge pressure at the time of injection. When the thallium concentration in the lungs is equal to that in the myocardium, the wedge pressure is markedly elevated. Studies in dogs (Bingham *et al.*, 1980) have revealed that the lung uptake also correlates with prolonged pulmonary transit time, another indicator of left ventricular dysfunction. The clearance of thallium from the lung is very rapid compared with its clearance from the myocardium. Within 20 min of injection, increased lung uptake is no longer seen in about one-third of patients who manifested this finding on their initial images. Similarly, the finding of transient cavity dilatation is best seen in the anterior view. Typically the left ventricle returns to its basal size within 10–20 min after cessation of exercise. The combination of the transient nature of these findings and the ease of positioning patients for the anterior view makes a strong case in favour of obtaining this view first.

The images are reviewed on the computer, where the contrast, brightness, size and sequence of the images can be adjusted by the observer. The computer also permits quantification of the images (Berger *et al.*, 1981; Maddahi *et al*, 1981; Lim *et al.*, 1984). The quantitative methods require background subtraction to define the 'true' appearance of activity in the myocardium. Although the methods of background subtraction vary in the specific weighting factors applied to the structures adjacent to the myocardium, the outcomes are similar. The 'background-corrected'

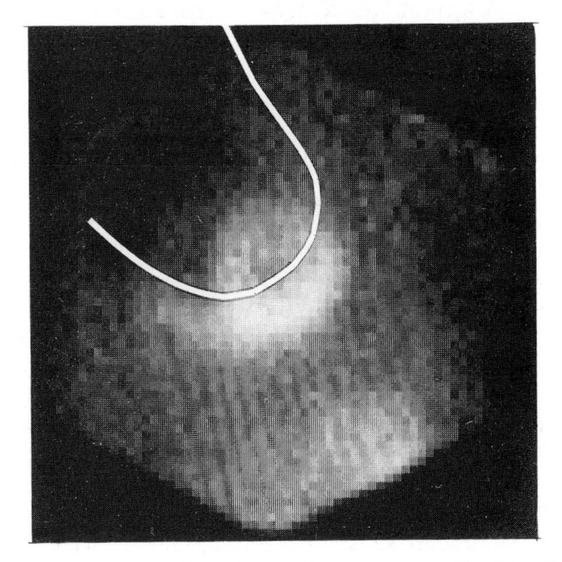

Figure 1.15 Thallium scan demonstrating the breast attenuation artefact. The breast outline is indicated by the white line.

image is then evaluated for its peak counts per pixel in either a radius, segment or slice profile. The activity in the maximal myocardial element is set to 100%, and the activity in the other zones is compared with this. Typically at least two criteria are applied to the quantitative data: (1) activity in a zone is compared with activity in neighbouring zones; and (2) the change in activity in a zone from initial to the delayed scan is determined. The quantitative approaches improve the reliability of interpretation, especially for physicians who do not perform a great many studies (Wackers *et al.*, 1985). However, they offer little improvement in the reliability of experienced observers. Present computer programs cannot differentiate artefacts, such as decreased activity due to breast or stomach attenuation (Figure 1.15), from true decreases in myocardial activity. In addition, only two major criteria are used by the quantitative programs (relative activity and change of activity from initial to delayed imaging) to detect ischaemia, while the experienced observer can utilize lung uptake, changes in cavity size, and alterations in regional wall thickness in addition to relative activity and regional clearance rates as criteria for detection of disease. As a result, the programs should be used as an adjunct to qualitative interpretation of the images, after careful subjective review by an experienced observer.

A ratio of lung/heart of >0.5 is abnormal when thallium is administered at heart rates exceeding 140 beats min^{-1}, while a value greater than 0.65 is abnormal when thallium is injected at heart rates between 80 and 100 beats min^{-1}. The clearance of thallium from the myocardium should exceed 25% over the 3 h interval between initial and delayed images.

(b) SPECT

The diagnostic quality of thallium images may be improved by SPECT imaging (Gill *et al.*, 1986a; Tamaki *et al.*, 1982) by enhancing the contrast between lesions and normal tissue. While the enhanced contrast is important, a potentially more valuable attribute of SPECT is the capability of reconstructing the data in both the true long-axis and short-axis projections. Unfortunately, the limited photon flux and substantial attenuation of the mercury X-rays do not allow SPECT to reach its full potential. Most investigators now think that SPECT will not enhance the sensitivity for detection of disease but can provide additional data about the location of lesions, and hence help differentiate multi-vessel from single-vessel disease. As with planar images, quantitative programs can be applied to the reconstructed projection data. One unique approach to the presentation of quantitative data creates a 'bull's eye' by portraying the data from each successive section as a concentric ring (Garcia *et al.*, 1985). The advantage of this approach is the ease of appreciating the relationship of lesions in multiple sections to each other. Since this presentation is several steps removed from the raw data, however, the quantitative presentations should not be used for interpretation without a complete evaluation of the data from which it is derived.

1.5.7 CLINICAL APPLICATIONS

Thallium imaging has gained clinical acceptance in three areas: (1) detection of coronary artery disease; (2) prognostication of the likelihood of a major ischaemic event (sudden death, infarction, or the onset of unstable angina); and (3) post-therapy follow-up study.

Because thallium imaging is a physiological test identifying differences in regional perfusion, discordance between the results of the anatomical and physiological evaluation may occur. Not every case of luminal diameter narrowing greater than 50% is detected, and, conversely (Gould, 1978; Bailey *et al.*, 1977b), thallium perfusion defects can occur in cases of less than 50% stenosis (Brown *et al.*, 1985). A regional difference in perfusion of >25% is required for detection by thallium imaging (Gould, 1978).

Since myocardial oxygen consumption/contraction is related to the tension developed by the myofibrils, and oxygen consumption per minute is related to the heart rate, the heart rate–systolic blood pressure product provides insight into the ability of the heart to increase its oxygen supply (myocardial perfusion) in response to exercise. Hence a normal thallium scan obtained with injection at a heart rate of 170 beats min^{-1} and a blood pressure of 200/100 mmHg has greater prognostic value than the same normal scan obtained with injection at a heart rate of 100 beats min^{-1} and a blood pressure of 130/85 mmHg.

In patients with unstable forms of coronary artery disease, information on the extent of disease is extremely important but exercise testing may be dangerous. If possible, thallium imaging should be delayed until the patient is able to exercise. However, thallium imaging, even with injection at rest, is sensitive for detection of acute myocardial infarction (Wackers, 1980) and can identify areas of severe ischaemia in situations in which the ECG is of no value (Brown *et al.*, 1983a). Thallium imaging following injection at rest is typically performed in patients hospitalized for unstable coronary artery disease who have already undergone arteriography to separate ischaemic dysfunction from myocardial scar.

(a) Dipyridamole

An alternative means of detecting coronary artery disease in patients who cannot exercise does not involve the production of ischaemia but instead detects regional differences in perfusion induced by a potent coronary vasodilator, such as dipyridamole (Gibson *et al.*, 1983; Leppo *et al.*, 1989). Normal vessels respond with a marked (three- to fivefold) increase in flow, while vessels with haemodynamically significant stenoses cannot respond with the same increase in perfusion. Thallium administration at the time of peak vasodilatation is distributed to the myocardium in proportion to the distribution of perfusion. As with exercise thallium imaging, zones of relatively decreased thallium concentration indicate areas supplied by stenosed vessels or scar.

The most common indications for using dipyridamole–thallium scanning are in patients with peripheral vascular disease and claudication, arthritis, neurological deficit, amputation, myopathy or poor conditioning who cannot exercise. Dipyridamole is contraindicated in patients with bronchospasm and chronic long disease who are receiving theophylline preparations. Administration of dipyridamole should be carefully considered in these patients, since it may cause a sudden increase in bronchospasm (Ranhosky and Kempthorne-Rawson, 1990).

Although the dipyridamole–thallium scan is a sensitive procedure, the information about rate–pressure product, exercise capacity, etc., is important for patient management. Therefore, exercise thallium imaging is preferred in those patients that can exercise.

(b) Sensitivity and specificity

The sensitivity and specificity of myocardial perfusion imaging have been compared to electrocardiography for the detection of coronary artery disease, using the coronary arteriogram as the final arbiter. The average sensitivity of the electrocardiogram is about 58%, and the average sensitivity of either qualitative or quantitative thallium imaging is about 85%. The sensitivity of thallium changes with the number of vessels diseased: 80% for single-vessel disease, 83% for two-vessel disease, and 96% for three-vessel disease (Gibson and Beller, 1982). Inadequate levels of stress decrease the sensitivity for the detection of coronary artery disease (Wharton *et al.*, 1980).

The specificity of exercise thallium imaging for the detection of coronary artery disease is about 85%, compared with 82% for electrocardiography (Kaul *et al.*, 1985; Ritchie *et al.*, 1978). Thallium imaging is particularly useful under two circumstances: (1) when the rest electrocardiogram is either difficult or impossible to interpret due to left ventricular hypertrophy, digitalis therapy or left bundle branch block; and (2) when disease is suspected in areas where the ECG is insensitive – the posterior and inferior regions of the myocardium. When the rest ECG is interpretable, and disease is suspected in the territory of the left anterior descending coronary artery, the advantage of thallium imaging over electrocardiography is less definitive (Kaul *et al.*, 1985; Ritchie *et al.*, 1978; Bailey *et al.*, 1977c).

1.5.8 CLINICAL PROBLEMS

(a) Extent of ischaemia in patients with known coronary disease

These studies are performed because of the increased awareness of the role of silent ischaemia as a predictor of cardiac events. Patients identified using the stress thallium scan as having ischaemic potential and being at increased risk for future cardiac events are seriously considered as candidates for interventional procedures to restore coronary blood flow. In these patients restoration of perfusion provides both relief of symptoms and increased survival (Loop *et al.*, 1986).

When patients experience angina or hypotension within the first 3 min of exercise at a low heart rate they are known to have a high risk of acute cardiac event. Such patients get little or no diagnostic benefit from the addition of the thallium procedure.

(b) Establishing the diagnosis of coronary artery disease

Stress-injected thallium imaging is most beneficial in the following groups of patients:

1. atypical chest pain or non-specific rest ST segment abnormalities (in whom the electro-

cardiographic response to stress alone is of little value);
2. multiple and severe coronary risk factors (family history of coronary disease, elevated cholesterol/lipoprotein levels, etc. – where the sensitivity of electrocardiographic stress testing may not be sufficient to detect disease);
3. ST segment depression during the stress test without pain, and those with chest pain and a negative or non-diagnostic electrocardiographic stress test.

(c) Post-therapy testing

Both the mechanical interventions of angioplasty and bypass surgery and the consequences of medical therapy can be studied to determine whether the therapy has masked or suppressed the ischaemia. Since bypassed vessels may occlude, and angioplastied vessels may restenose, serial testing with exercise thallium imaging (usually biannually) is helpful to document the continued success of these interventions.

(d) Prognostication

In stable patients free of severe congestive heart failure, severe depression of left ventricular function, or ventricular tachyarrhythmias, two findings have been reported as powerful indicators of future cardiac events: (1) perfusion defects that redistribute (unmasked by stress) (Brown *et al.*, 1983a; Gibson *et al.*, 1983; Miller *et al.*, 1985b; Ladenheim *et al.*, 1986; Boucher *et al.*, 1985); and (2) increased lung uptake of thallium (Kaul *et al.*, 1984).

1.6 INFARCT AVID IMAGING

Infarct avid imaging comprises radionuclide imaging techniques to detect the site and extent of acute myocardial necrosis (Botvinick, 1990).

Acute myocardial infarction will be clinically 'silent' in about 25% of patients. In many of these subjects the infarct will be detected only in retrospect, by the discovery of a 'scar' on myocardial perfusion scan; a zone of abnormal wall motion on radionuclide ventriculogram, echocardiogram, or contrast ventriculogram; or an abnormality on resting ECG. In some patients admitted to hospital for suspected infarction, diagnosis can only be made by laboratory studies. In the current era of acute reperfusion therapy, however, it is becoming far more difficult in the acute situation to determine whether substantial myocardial necrosis has occurred: enzyme levels may be elevated even when myocardial preservation has been achieved, segmental wall motion may remain abnormal for several days despite successful reperfusion, and arrythmias may occur either as a result of reperfusion or because of ongoing ischaemia. As recent studies suggest that thrombolytic therapy for acute myocardial infarction improves survival it becomes important to be able to assess the extent of acute myocardial salvage (or, conversely, to be able to demonstrate the extent of irreversible myocardial necrosis) to determine whether thrombolysis is successful or whether further procedures must be performed to revascularize the myocardium.

1.6.1 NON-SPECIFIC AGENTS FOR IMAGING MYOCARDIAL NECROSIS

Radiopharmaceuticals which show non-specific uptake in infarcted myocardium include ^{201}Hg-labelled chlormerodrin (Carr *et al.*, 1962), ^{201}Hg-labelled fluorescein (Malek *et al.*, 1967), ^{99m}Tc-labelled tetracycline (Holman *et al.*, 1973) and ^{99m}Tc-labelled glucoheptonate (Rossman *et al.*, 1975). The mechanism of localization of these agents is not completely understood, and none is widely used for the detection of infarction in human subjects. The most commonly used agent, ^{99m}Tc-labelled pyrophosphate (^{99m}Tc-PYP) has been evaluated in more detail.

(a) ^{99m}Tc-PYP

Mechanism The observation that intracellular calcium accumulation occurred in irreversible myocardial cell injury (Shen and Jennings, 1972) prompted Bonte *et al.* (1974) to investigate ^{99m}Tc-labelled stannous PYP for the detection of myocardial infarction in humans. PYP uptake in damaged tissue appears to be related to influx of calcium into the infarcted zone. The proposed mechanism of localization is the formation of a complex of PYP with calcium in crystalline and subcrystalline form within the damaged myocardial tissue (Buja *et al.*, 1977); an alternative explanation is that this bone-seeking chelate combines with macromolecules within the necrotic cells. Unlike ^{99m}Tc-labelled tetracycline, the uptake of PYP bears a non-linear relationship to the reduction of blood flow, the peak occurring when flow is reduced by 60–70% (Zaret *et al.*, 1976), and the uptake then decreases as the blood flow is further reduced. Consequently, in large infarcts, there is maximal uptake in ischaemic areas in the peri-infarct zone with less than maximal uptake occurring in the central infarcted area, and the concentration of PYP correlates poorly with the extent of infarction. This accounts for the so-called 'doughnut' pattern of the massive anteroseptal infarct where there is a rim of uptake around the border of the lesion, corresponding to predominantly ischaemic myocardium and a relatively photon-deficient centre where there is necrotic tissue with grossly impaired perfusion. Serial injection and imaging reveals a tendency for the uptake to gradually increase in the centre as uptake in the periphery decreases. The zone of necrosis may remain persistently positive for months following infarction.

Time course and extent of uptake In animals, increased activity is present in infarcted myocardial tissue within 6 h after coronary occlusion but is not detectable by imaging until about 12 h (Parkey *et al.*, 1977). In man maximum infarct uptake is seen at 48–72 h post-infarction and gradually fades so that most infarcts show no uptake by ten days after infarction. Serial imaging at 24 and 72 h after the onset of the infarct increases diagnostic accuracy as sequential changes can be observed (Parkey *et al.*, 1977). Rarely, uptake will only be observed at four days after the infarct so that repeat injection and imaging is occasionally necessary when the initial study is negative.

There is a correlation between the size of infarction and the area of PYP uptake and it has been possible both in dogs (Stokely *et al.*, 1976) and in man (Willerson *et al.*, 1977) to measure infarct size by computer reconstruction from planimetered outlines of the infarcted area. Anteriorly located infarcts lend themselves more readily to this than inferior lesions (Lewis *et al.*, 1977).

Sensitivity and specificity The sensitivity for detection of transmural myocardial infarction is 95–100% (Lyons *et al.*, 1980) if patients are studied between three and ten days following the infarction. The sensitivity falls slightly when only a localized pattern is accepted as evidence of infarction rather than a diffuse pattern. The sensitivity for detection of non-transmural myocardial infarction is much lower, between 40% and 88% depending on whether a localized or diffuse pattern is accepted as evidence of positivity.

There are numerous causes of uptake of PYP in a region of the myocardium in the absence of acute infarction, including: residual blood pool activity; left ventricular aneurysm; recent cardioversion; contusion of the myocardium; infarction in the previous nine months; calcification in the pericardium and valve rings; ongoing myocardial necrosis; stable and unstable angina; cardiomyopathy; cardiac tumour; renal failure; and tumour metastatic to overlying ribs.

The incidence of false-positive studies ranges from 8% (Parkey *et al.*, 1977) to 26% (Lyons *et al.*, 1980), though the figure quoted by the later authors includes a preponderance of patients with unstable angina and patients who had been resuscitated with electrical countershock. If these patients are excluded, the false-positive rate is reduced to 14%. This incidence of false positivity can be reduced by eliminating the diffuse pattern from the positive group, but at an inevitable expense of sensitivity.

Prognosis PYP imaging may identify those patients with a poor prognosis. Patients with a persistently positive scan, those with extensive, intense uptake (Holman *et al.*, 1977), and those with a doughnut pattern (Ahmad *et al.*, 1979), have a higher incidence of cardiac death and congestive heart failure than those whose PYP scans return to negative.

SPECT Further improvement in accuracy may come from SPECT imaging. Planar imaging cannot visualize infarcts less than 3 g in size, infarcts located subendocardially or those that are imaged too late (five or more days after the acute event). In contrast, with SPECT imaging, infarcts as small as 1 g can be detected (Corbett *et al.*, 1984). Comparisons of the sensitivity and specificity of planar versus SPECT imaging have demonstrated improved sensitivity and specificity of SPECT (Corbett *et al.*, 1984).

Indications Most transmural infarcts are apparent from electrocardiographic and enzyme changes alone and do not require further confirmation. Small transmural infarcts, recent transmural infarcts, infarcts adjacent to old scars, subendocardial infarcts, true posterior infarcts and infarction in the presence of left bundle block may be diagnostic problems, as well as when cardiac enzyme analysis is useless. In these patients, ^{99m}Tc-PYP imaging is likely to be of diagnostic value.

(b) Antimyosin

Severe ischaemia, trauma, severe electrical shock, immunological rejection and inflammatory disease can all cause sarcolemmal damage, which proceeds in stages. Early in the injury process, the cellular changes can be reversed. Clinically, it is important to have markers of cell injury that can differentiate reversibly injured tissue from that which is irreparably damaged. In a test of ^{99m}Tc-PYP uptake in injured myocytes, Fischman *et al.* (1986) demonstrated accumulation of ^{99m}Tc-PYP in the face of both reversible injury and irreversibly damaged cells. As a result, ^{99m}Tc-PYP uptake is not a specific marker of irreversible necrosis, but a marker of both severe injury and irreversible damage. A marker of irreversible damage must utilize a different mechanism of localization than ^{99m}Tc-PYP. One of the hallmarks of irreversible injury is the appearance of frank holes in the myocyte membrane. The large holes in the membrane permit macromolecules to escape from the cell, and permit the entry of large molecules into the intracellular environment.

Cardiac myosin, the major protein component of cardiac muscle, is exposed to the extracellular environment under circumstances of irreversible injury. The exposed cardiac myosin can be detected by administration of radiolabelled antibodies directed against this protein. The Fab fragment of antimyosin monoclonal antibodies labelled with ^{99m}Tc (Khaw *et al.*, 1986) and ^{111}In (Khaw *et al.*, 1987) (Figure 1.16) have been used to image myocardial necrosis in human subjects. In a series of 54 patients with acute myocardial infarction, gamma-scintigraphic images with ^{111}In-labelled antimyosin Fab predicted the location of the infarct as defined by electrocardiogram, contrast ventriculography and coronary angiography in 50 patients. Although the lesions were in many cases visualized as early as 6–7 h after intravenous administration of the radiolabelled antibody, the best time for imaging was 18–24 h after injection, which allows for optimal contrast after clearance of blood pool activity.

In addition to acute myocardial infarction, myocyte necrosis associated with sarcolemmal disruption may also be caused by acute myocarditis (Figure 1.17) and cardiac transplant rejection. In a series of 28 patients with suspected myocarditis (Yasuda *et al.*, 1987) every patient who had an endomyocardial biopsy positive for myocarditis also had a positive ^{111}In-labelled monoclonal antimyosin Fab scan, and every patient with a negative scan had a negative biopsy. However, there was a puzzling group of patients who had positive scans associated with negative biopsies. In one of these patients, a second biopsy (performed after a positive scan) was positive for myocarditis. It is possible that the sampling error inherent in endomyocardial biopsy may account for this discrepancy. ^{111}In-labelled antimyosin Fab was

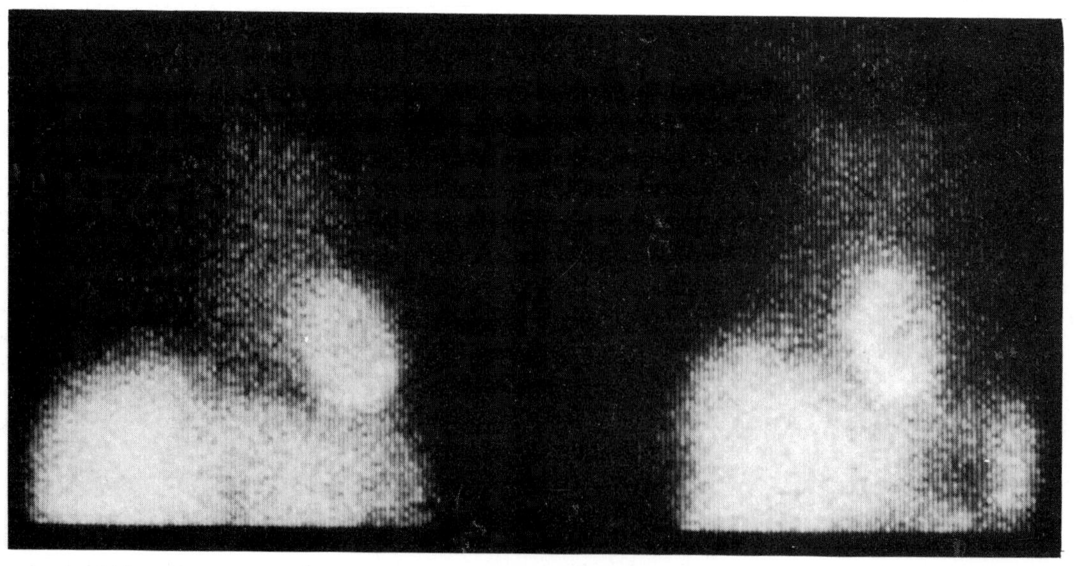

Figure 1.16 ^{111}In-labelled antimyosin scan for myocardial necrosis recorded in the anterior (left), and left anterior oblique (right) positions in a patient with anterior infarction.

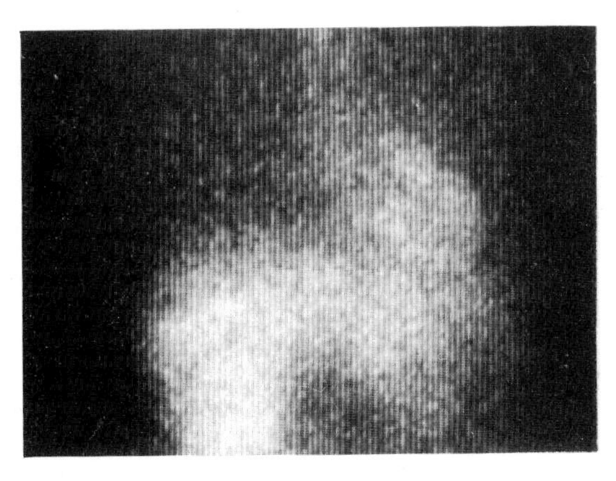
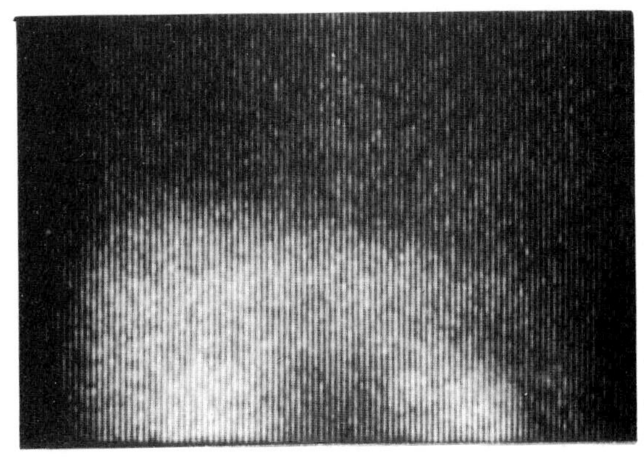

Figure 1.17 Serial ^{111}In-labelled antimyosin scans in a patient with myocarditis. The extensive myocardial uptake seen on the initial scan (left) is not visible on the image recorded six months later (right).

administered to patients who had received transplants from ten days to four years earlier (First *et al.*, 1986). Gamma camera images obtained 48 h after intravenous administration showed increased ^{111}In-labelled antimyosin activity in the hearts of all transplanted patients. Concurrent with acute episodes of rejection, the intensity of ^{111}In uptake increased significantly over basal levels. Thus it appears that non-invasive imaging with radiolabelled antimyosin may be an alternative to endomyocardial biopsy as an initial means of screening for acute heart transplant rejection. It is also being evaluated for infarct sizing and risk stratification.

1.7 NEW SINGLE-PHOTON RADIOPHARMACEUTICALS

1.7.1 BLOOD POOL RADIOPHARMACEUTICALS

Four new radiopharmaceutical generator systems have been developed and tested in human subjects for blood pool imaging: (1) ^{191}Os/^{191m}Ir; (2) ^{195}Hg/^{195m}Au; (3) ^{178}W/^{178}Ta; and (4) ^{81}Rb/^{81m}Kr. The combination of short daughter half-life and relatively high photon abundance make these systems attractive for repeated measurements of ventricular function at a very low radiation burden.

(a) Iridium-191m

Iridium-191m (^{191m}Ir) has a half-life of 4.7 s, and emits a 129 keV gamma-photon and 65 keV X-rays. The parent ^{191}Os is reactor produced and has a half-life of 15 days. The radiation burden of 3–5 mrad mCi^{-1} permits injection of large quantities of iridium (typically 50–150 mCi per injection) with a low radiation burden. The major contribution to the radiation burden comes from column breakthrough of the parent ^{191}Os into the eluate. Improvement in column design in the future may reduce the radiation burden by 10- to 100-fold (Brihaye *et al.*, 1985).

This tracer was originally described by Yano and Anger (1968) for the determination of pulmonary perfusion. Treves *et al.* (1980a, 1980b) described its clinical use for paediatric angiocardiography. The combination of high photon flux and low radiation burden is well suited for the evaluation of cardiac shunts and ventricular function in the paediatric patient population.

Although ^{191m}Ir can be used in adults, the relatively long pulmonary transit time (6–8 s) as compared to the physical half-life (4.7 s) results in a photon flux from the right heart that is two- to fourfold higher than that from the left heart. The extremely high photon flux from the right heart presents a problem for imaging with Anger-type scintillation cameras due to the dead time of the camera and the non-linear relationship between the actual activity in the field of view and the recorded counts. In this regard, multicrystal cameras or multiwire proportional chambers (Lacy *et al.*, 1985) can take advantage of the high count rate offered by ^{191m}Ir.

(b) Gold-195m

Gold-195m (^{195m}Au) is a 30.5 s half-life radionuclide that is eluted from a column containing the 40.5 h half-life cyclotron-produced ^{195}Hg. ^{195m}Au emits a 262 keV gamma-photon that is 68% abundant. The relatively long half-life of ^{195m}Au with reference to the central circulation time permits high-quality studies of right and left ventricular function. Mena *et al.* (1983) first described the clinical application of ^{195m}Au for sequential first-pass angiography. Co-injection of ^{195m}Au and ^{201}Tl at peak exercise and imaging with a special dual-energy collimator permits the simultaneous evaluation of ventricular function and myocardial perfusion (Kipper *et al.*, 1985). An exercise first-pass study was performed during bolus injection of the tracers using the ^{195m}Au window. After waiting 5 min for the ^{195m}Au to decay, ^{201}Tl perfusion images were recorded in the thallium window. ^{195m}Au has also been shown to be useful for the sequential evaluation of left ventricular function during exercise (Caplin *et al.*, 1986).

Unfortunately, the decay product, ^{195}Au, builds up on the column between elutions. The radiation burden from this agent creates a slight potential risk of renal and hepatic radiotoxicity.

(c) Tantalum-178

Tantalum-178 (^{178}Ta) is a 9.3 min half-life radionuclide eluted from a tungsten-178 (^{178}W) generator. It decays from the parent ^{178}W (half-life 28 days), emitting 55–65 keV X-rays. The critical organ is the kidney which receives 2.9 mrad mCi^{-1}, which is approximately 1/20 of the dose from ^{99m}Tc. Thus, ^{178}Ta can be used for low-dose paediatric imaging, high count density first-pass imaging, and because ^{178}Ta binds to plasma proteins it can also be used for equilibrium imaging.

Lacy *et al.* (1986) employed ^{178}Ta with a multiwire gamma camera for first-pass angiography. This procedure yielded high-quality left and right ventricular images and time–activity curves and the whole-body radiation dose was one-tenth of that delivered with ^{99m}Tc imaged with a multicrystal camera.

(d) Krypton-81m

Yano and Anger (1968) first proposed the use of a rubidium-81 (^{81}Rb)/krypton (^{81m}Kr) generator for blood-pool imaging. The 4.7 h half-life ^{81}Rb is absorbed to a column and the 13 s half-life daughter ^{81m}Kr is eluted in a saline solution.

The 190 keV of ^{81m}Kr is well suited for imaging with low- or medium-energy collimation. After intravenous injection of a ^{81m}Kr-labelled saline solution of the tracer, it passes through the right heart and evolves from the blood into the alveolar gas during its passage through the lung. This property makes ^{81m}Kr particularly useful for the repetitive evaluation of right ventricular function (Neinaber *et al.*, 1985).

1.7.2 MYOCARDIAL PERFUSION AGENTS

(a) ^{99m}Tc-labelled isonitriles

Because of the relatively long physical half-life and poor imaging characteristics of ^{201}Tl, ^{99m}Tc-labelled perfusion agents have been investigated as alternatives. Deutsch *et al.* (1981) pioneered the development of a new class of radiopharmaceuticals, the lipid-soluble ^{99m}Tc complexes, as a potential replacement for ^{201}Tl. The initial agents tested, ^{99m}Tc-labelled dimethylphosphoethane complex (DMPE) and a diarsenical complex (DiARS) worked well in animals but had very disappointing results in human subjects. Jones *et al.* (1982, 1984) developed several compounds in the hexakis (alkylisonitrile) technetium(I) cation family that concentrated in the human myocardium (Holman *et al.*, 1984). Approximately 2% of the injected dose localizes in the myocardium. Following intravenous administration, a significant amount of the tertiary butylisonitrile (TBI) localizes in the lungs. However, clearance from the lung is more rapid than from the heart, permitting myocardial imaging at about 1 h post-injection.

To minimize the uptake of TBI in liver and lung relative to myocardium a number of other isonitriles were investigated. Two compounds, ^{99m}Tc-labelled carbomethoxy isonitrile (CPI) and ^{99m}Tc-labelled 2-methoxy 2-methylpropyl isonitrile (MIBI), were tested in human subjects. CPI, which has both high myocardial uptake and rapid clearance from liver and lung, can be used to acquire high-quality myocardial images as early as 10 min after injection (Holman *et al.*, 1987). With this agent myocardial activity falls to about 76% of the initial level by one hour after injection. MIBI also has high myocardial uptake combined with rapid clearance from blood pool, liver and lung. With this agent high-quality myocardial images can be obtained at 5–10 min after injection, and retention of the tracer in the myocardium is longer than CPI (Mousa *et al.*, 1986; McKusick *et al.*, 1986).

The isonitrile compounds combine the properties of high lipid solubility and technetium chelation. The mechanism of accumulation of these agents in myocardium is not fully under-

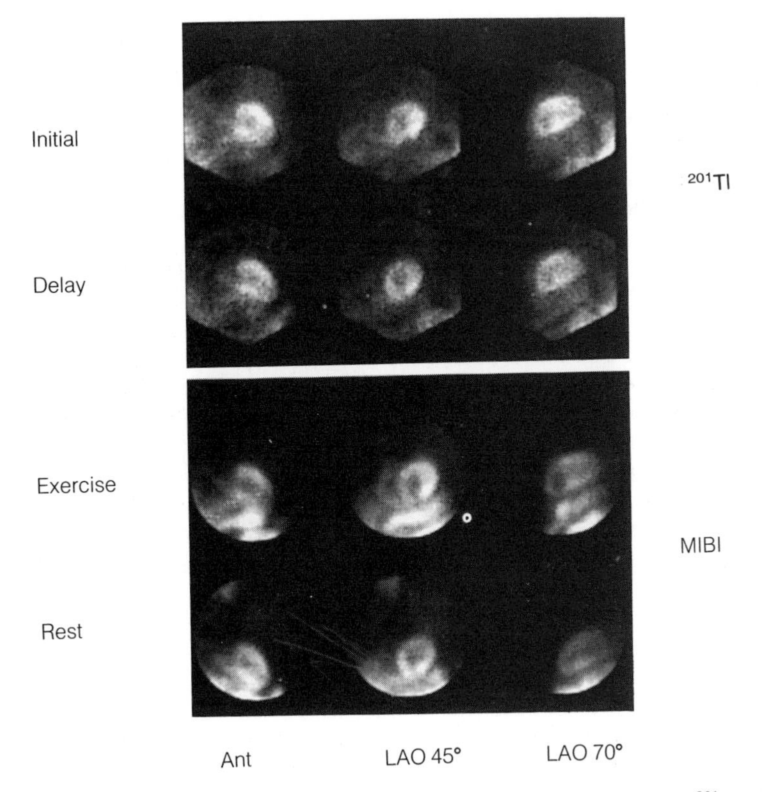

Figure 1.18 Myocardial perfusion scans in the same patient recorded after injection of ^{201}Tl at peak exercise and 3 h later (upper two panels) and after injection of ^{99m}Tc-labelled SestaMIBI during exercise and at rest (bottom two panels), in the anterior, 45° left anterior oblique and 70° left anterior oblique positions.

stood, but appears to be passive diffusion with binding in the cytosol. There are considerable potential advantages of a ^{99m}Tc-labelled perfusion agent which is fixed in the myocardium as an alternative to ^{201}Tl in clinical practice.

The photon energy and half life of ^{99m}Tc give better imaging characterization with a higher photon yield and lower radiation doses, decreased soft tissue attenuation and scatter advantages which have proved particularly important in SPECT imaging. The slow myocardial clearance in addition to being an advantage with SPECT allows patients to be imaged geographically distant from the site of exercise testing and is proving to be particularly valuable in acute myocardial infarction when the injection of ^{99m}Tc-Sesta MIBI can be given before thrombolytic therapy with subsequent imaging providing information on the jeopardized myocardium without any delay in instituting treatment (Pellikk *et al.*, 1990). The improved imaging characteristics have permitted good quality gated acquisition which can provide global and wall motion data as well as the myocardial perfusion study from the first pass as well as the delayed images.

Clinical studies performed to date have shown excellent correlation with ^{201}Tl with SPECT studies using ^{99m}Tc-Sesta MIBI being generally superior (Kiat *et al.*, 1989; Maisey *et al.*, 1990). Other applications are under extensive trial at the present time. As the ^{99m}Tc isonitriles do not significantly redistribute it was initially thought that a second day injection at rest would be necessary. However, recent trials have shown that 2 injections (rest and exercise) can be given on the same day without significant loss of diagnostic accuracy (Taillefer *et al.*, 1989).

(b) Metabolic agents

The rationale for measuring myocardial metabolism stems from the heart's requirement for a constant source of high-energy phosphate to provide fuel for contraction. In an aerobic environment, the catabolism of long-chain fatty acids provides the most efficient means of generating energy for contraction (one molecule of palmitate provides 129 ATPs, while one molecule of glucose provides 38) (Opie, 1984). When oxygen availability decreases (i.e. during ischaemia), catabolism of fatty acids is reduced. Decreased beta-oxidation of fatty acids, therefore, can serve as a sensitive marker of oxygen availability. When ischaemia occurs oxidation of fatty acids decreases and glycolytic flux increases (Opie, 1968). Glucose metabolism may remain largely aerobic, but becomes anaerobic when oxygen availability becomes severely limited. Persistence of some residual blood flow is critical for removal of lactate and maintenance of glycolysis. When flow is markedly impaired, increases in lactate and hydrogen ion in the cytosol inhibit residual glycolysis. This downward course of biochemical events may progress to complete cessation of energy production, and thus to irreversible cell injury.

Both single-photon and PET approaches have been described for the evaluation of regional metabolic activity. Precise catabolic measurements require PET (see below), but clinically useful (though less quantitative) data can be derived from single-photon measurements.

(c) Fatty acids and analogues

Long-chain fatty acids supply 80–90% of myocardial contractile energy requirements under aerobic conditions. In contrast, under anerobic conditions, glucose consumption is increased with suppression of fatty acid utilization. Thus comparing regional perfusion and regional fatty acid accumulation may be useful for identifying sites of relative oxygen deprivation.

Several radiolabelled free fatty acids have been proposed for the non-invasive assessment of myocardial fatty acid metabolism with single-photon agents including ^{123}I-labelled hexadecenoic acid, *p*-iodophenyl pentadecanoic acid (IPPA), and recently the branched-chain fatty acid beta-methyl *p*-iodophenyl pentadecanoic acid (BMIPP) (van der Wall *et al.*, 1981; Knapp *et al.*, 1981, Livni *et al.*, 1982).

Once in the myocardium, IPPA has a clearance half-time of 20 min and is catabolized by beta-oxidation. Recently Kennedy *et al.* (1986) reported on the clinical application of stress ^{123}I-IPPA imaging in patients with coronary artery disease, showing non-homogeneous distribution and delayed clearance in ischaemic areas.

In contrast, branched-chain fatty acids have a mean residence time of more than 60 min because they cannot undergo beta-oxidation (Figure 1.19). When ischaemia is present in viable myocardium, restoration of perfusion is associated with an increase in local fatty acid uptake, probably due to an increase in triglyceride content of the previously ischaemic zone. Combined imaging of BMIPP and ^{201}Tl demonstrate discordant distribution of these two radiopharmaceuticals in ischaemic but viable myocardium and matched decrease of uptake in infarcted myocardium (Strauss *et al.*, 1987).

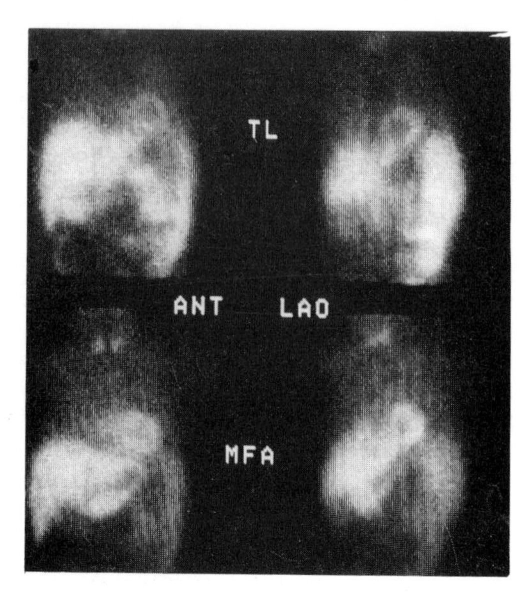

Figure 1.19 Comparison of regional perfusion to regional modified fatty acid distribution in a patient with myocardial ischaemia. Note the reduction of thallium uptake in the anterior wall, while fatty acid concentration is relatively increased in this zone.

1.7.3 ATHEROMA DETECTION

Lipoproteins interact with plaques to transport cholesterol in and out of the lesions. Some studies (Lees *et al.*, 1985) indicate that radiolabelled low-density lipoprotein localizes in atheromatous plaques in human subjects. This technique offers a means of identifying plaques based on their metabolic activity instead of their haemodynamic significance.

1.7.4 RECEPTORS

The adrenergic receptor compound ^{123}I/^{131}I-MIBG has been used to image and quantify the myocardial adrenergic receptors (Kulkarni and Corbett, 1990). Clear clinical indications have not as yet emerged but it has been shown that the distribution reflects myocardial ischaemia and is significantly altered in cardiomyopathies and after cardiac transplantation.

1.8 POSITRON EMISSION TOMOGRAPHY

Positron emission tomography (PET) is a technique of radionuclide imaging which utilizes annihilation radiation from positron-emitting nuclides to record tomographic images. PET can make all measurements that can be recorded with single-photon agents and offers precise quantification that is not available with single-photon techniques.

1.8.1 ADVANTAGES OF PET

The 'electronic collimation' utilized in PET imaging devices to localize the origin of radiation gives three major advantages to this method:

1. The sensitivity for the detection of events is approximately 1000-fold greater than that of a collimated single-photon imaging device.
2. Resolution at the centre of a tomographic slice through the heart is <7 mm, about twice as good as SPECT.
3. A true attenuation correction can be applied to the data, which allows the activity–concentration within an image to be determined accurately.

In addition to the advantages of instrumentation, organic substrates can be labelled with ^{11}C, ^{13}N or ^{15}O without altering their physiological properties. Thus, metabolic information, such as the changes in regional distribution of glucose, fatty acids or amino acids, can be determined. This information can be applied to kinetic models to translate the regional concentrations in the image to assess physiological and metabolic process.

1.8.2 DATA ACQUISITION AND ANALYSIS

Most PET devices record multiple images (3–18 slices) simultaneously. The patient is prepared for radiopharmaceutical administration with venous and arterial lines and positioned in the imaging device. The high resolution of PET instruments requires gating of the data collection to optimize image quality. If precise quantification is required, a transmission image is recorded with a positron emitting source (usually ^{68}Ga or ^{18}F), prior to administration of the positron-emitting radiopharmaceutical.

Most PET procedures do not require arterial sampling or precise attenuation correction, since the regional distribution of radiopharmaceutical is sufficient for clinical purposes. The use of relative radiopharmaceutical distribution makes the PET imaging procedure similar to single-photon data acquisition.

The serial transverse slices are used to generate true long-axis and short-axis images. This technique is particularly useful for evaluating regional abnormalities of the inferior wall (Senda *et al.*, 1986).

Tracer kinetic models can be applied to PET data to calculate regional blood flow and rates of metabolism. These calculations usually require precise information about the arterial input function to the myocardium (both from regions of interest placed over the appropriate areas of the image (Tamaki *et al.*, 1985a) and from direct measurement of the concentration of tracer in arterial blood (Henze *et al.*, 1983)).

1.8.3 SPECIFIC PET MEASUREMENTS

(a) Perfusion

Three approaches have been employed to measure regional perfusion in human subjects with PET: (1) $^{13}NH_3$ ($T_{1/2}$ physical = 10 min); (2) $H_2{}^{15}O$ ($T_{1/2}$ physical = 2 min); and (3) ^{82}Rb ($T_{1/2}$physical = 1.2 min). The short half-life of these agents makes it necessary to use two separate injections – one at rest and the other during stress or pharmacological intervention – to detect ischaemia. The first two agents require an on-site cyclotron to produce the radionuclide, while ^{82}Rb is available from an ^{82}Sr ($T_{1/2}$physical = 25 days) generator.

$^{13}NH_3$ PET studies at rest and after stress have demonstrated segmental reduction in tracer uptake during stress-induced ischaemia. This technique is accurate for detecting coronary artery disease and identifying stenosed vessels (Tamaki *et al.*, 1985b; Yonekura *et al.*, 1987). The accuracy for detecting fixed coronary lesions is similar to ^{201}Tl SPECT; however, the accuracy for identifying ischaemia is higher (Tamaki *et al.*, 1987b). Dipyridamole-induced vasodilatation has also been used in conjunction with $^{13}NH_3$ for detecting coronary stenosis (Gould *et al.*, 1979). This combination has allowed the detection of 47% diameter stenosis in animal studies.

$H_2^{15}O$ (Knabb *et al.* 1985) and ^{82}Rb (Selwyn *et al.*, 1982; Gould, 1990), have been used in similar fashion for the detection of coronary artery stenosis. Measured regional blood flow with ^{82}Rb during physical stress in patients with coronary artery disease remained depressed during stress and even after the acute ECG changes and chest pain resolved, reflecting delayed recovery of blood flow and cation uptake after the acute ischaemic episode (Wilson *et al.*, 1987). The sensitivity of PET myocardial imaging was tested by Deanfield *et al.* (1984), who demonstrated a segmental decrease in ^{82}Rb uptake in 97% of patients with ischaemic ST segments. Similarly, Goldstein *et al.* (1986) and Gould *et al.* (1986) demonstrated that ^{82}Rb can predict myocardial viability after reperfusion and can detect coronary narrowings of 47% of luminal diameter. In addition, this technique can be applied to assess the collateral circulation (Demer *et al.*, 1986).

(b) Assessment of myocardial metabolism

PET measurements of both fatty acid utilization and glycolysis have been performed using a variety of radiolabelled fatty acids and glucose analogues (including ^{11}C-palmitate and ^{18}F-labelled deoxyglucose).

Mild ischaemia which impairs beta-oxidation can be demonstrated by abnormal ^{11}C-palmitate kinetics. In ischaemic segments, the early rapid clearance of ^{11}C decreases (Schon *et al.*, 1982b; Grover *et al.*, 1984). Schwaiger *et al.* (1985) observed a decrease in regional myocardial free fatty acid (FFA) metabolism lasting several days following 3 h of balloon occlusion of the left anterior descending vessel (LAD), despite prompt return of perfusion. This impaired FFA oxidation is associated with increased utilization of exogenous glucose.

The loss of metabolic integrity assessed *in vivo* by ^{11}C-palmitate imaging is well correlated with infarct size determined morphologically and by creatine phosphokinase (CPK) depletion (Weiss *et al.*, 1977). In animal studies, Bergmann *et al.* (1982) evaluated the relationship between the time of ischaemia and the beneficial effects of reperfusion. Thrombolysis after 1–2 h of occlusion produced a 50% reduction in metabolic infarct size assessed by ^{11}C-palmitate, while reperfusion after 4–6 h of occlusion had no effect on infarct size.

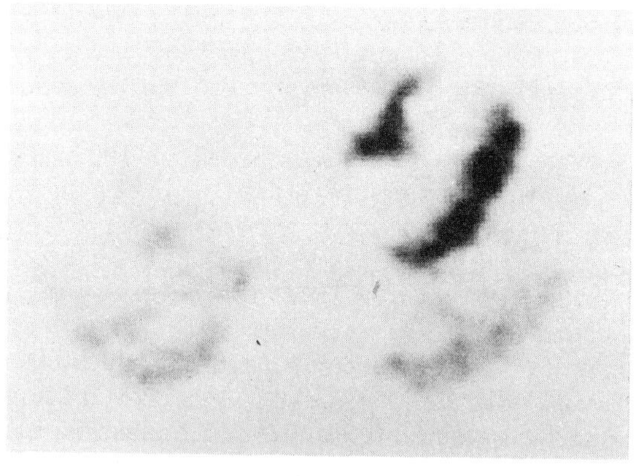

$^{13}NH_3$

^{18}FDG

Figure 1.20 PET transverse section images comparing regional perfusion measured with $^{13}NH_3$, to glucose metabolism measured with ^{18}F-labelled deoxyglucose (^{18}FDG). The zone of decreased perfusion has increased glucose concentration, suggesting ischaemia.

Myocardial ischaemia does not cause a uniform change in glycolytic flux. A modest perfusion decrease is usually associated with an augmented glycolytic flux, as demonstrated by a focal increase in ^{18}F-labelled deoxyglucose relative to perfusion (Figure 1.20). In severe ischaemia, segmental perfusion and exogenous glucose utilization both decrease. Such 'mismatch' may reflect ischaemic but viable myocardium (Marshall *et al.*, 1981). The pattern of increased exogenous glucose utilization relative to blood flow has been observed in acute ischaemia and post-ischaemic stunned myocardium in animal studies (Schwaiger *et al.*, 1985). This mismatch is often seen in myocardial segments with stress-induced hypoperfusion (Yonekura *et al.*, 1986). The mismatch often persists into the post-exercise state, indicating persistent impairment of metabolic processes after exercise (Camini *et al.*, 1986).

Tillisch *et al.* (1986) demonstrated the value of this mismatch pattern for predicting tissue viability prior to coronary artery bypass surgery. Improvement of regional function after revascularization was observed in 85% of segments with mismatches, while function failed to improve in 92% of matched segmental defects. The mismatch pattern is observed in one-third of segments with chronic Q wave infarction (Brunken *et al.*, 1986), and in about one-half of segments with acute Q wave infarction (Schwaiger *et al.*, 1986). Over a two-month follow-up period, function failed to improve in matched abnormal segments, while function improved spontaneously in about half of the mismatched segments and remained unchanged or worsened in the other half.

Other substrates have also used for the PET assessment of myocardial metabolism during ischaemia. Delayed clearance of ^{11}C-acetate in patients with coronary artery disease (Selwyn *et al.*, 1981) suggests impairment of tricarboxylic acid cycle activity. Recent animal studies demonstrated a close correlation between ^{11}C-acetate clearance measured by PET and myocardial oxygen utilization (Brown *et al.*, 1987). Thus, ^{11}C-acetate PET has potential for accurate estimation of regional myocardial oxygen consumption *in vivo*. PET applications in myocardial ischaemia have been reviewed (Schelbert, 1989).

1.8.4 CARDIOMYOPATHY

Deficiency of specific enzymes or other metabolic defects have been identified as the cause of some cardiomyopathies, i.e. carnitine transferase deficiencies. However, these diseases are rare and the more common cardiomyopathies may be unrelated to a primary metabolic derangement. Characterization of the metabolic state of the abnormal myocardium may, however, provide insights into the disease mechanism.

Dilated cardiomyopathy has been evaluated with ^{11}C-palmitate PET (Geltman *et al.*, 1983). In this study, the distribution of ^{11}C-palmitate in the myocardium was heterogeneous, while ^{201}Tl uptake was homogeneous, suggesting patchy impairment of FFA metabolism. Recently, Schelbert *et al.* (1986) evaluated the effect of substrate manipulation on the regional uptake and clearance of ^{11}C-palmitate in patients with cardiomyopathy. With glucose loading, about half of the patients with cardiomyopathy shifted from FFA to glucose utilization (a normal response), while the other half responded paradoxically, with accelerated utilization of FFA. These results may support the hypothesis of an impairment in substrate utilization in diseased myocardium and metabolic imaging with PET offers an opportunity to clarify the underlying pathology.

Duchenne's muscular dystrophy, as a model of cardiomyopathy, is a unique disease involving specific regions of the myocardium. In this disorder, post-mortem examination often reveals fibrotic degeneration of the posterobasal and lateral myocardial segments. In a PET study of patients with this disorder, Perloff *et al.* (1984) demonstrated reduced $^{13}NH_3$ uptake and increased ^{18}F-labelled deoxyglucose uptake in posterolateral segments.

In hypertrophic cardiomyopathy Grover *et al.* (1986) demonstrated a decrease in exogenous glucose utilization with relatively normal blood flow and FFA utilization in asymmetrically hypertrophied septa.

The constellation of enhanced resolution, wide range of radiopharmaceuticals, and opportunity to identify early metabolic indicators of disease, make it likely that PET imaging will have increasing clinical applications in the future.

REFERENCES

Adam, W. E., Tarkowska, A., Bitter, F. *et al.* (1979) Equilibrium (gated) radionuclide ventriculography. *Cardiovasc. Radiol.*, **2**, 161–73.

Ahmad, M., Dubiel, J. P., Logan, K. W., Verdon, T. A. and Martin, R. H. (1977) Limited clinical diagnostic specificity of Tc-99m stannous pyrophosphate myocardial imaging in acute myocardial infarction. *Am. J. Cardiol.*, **39**, 50–4.

Alexander, J., Dainiak, N., Berger, H. J. *et al.* (1979) Serial assessment of doxorubicin cardiotoxicity with quantitative radionuclide angiocardiography. *N. Engl. J. Med.*, **300**, 278–83.

Anderson, J. L., Marshal, H. W., Bray, B. E. *et al.* (1983) A randomized trial of intracoronary streptokinase in the treatment of acute myocardial infarction. *N. Engl. J. Med.*, **308**, 1312–18.

Bacharach, S. L., Green, M. V., Borer, J. S. *et al.* (1979) Left ventricular peak ejection rate, filling rate and ejection fraction: frame rate requirements at rest and exercise. *J. Nucl. Med.*, **20**, 189–93.

Bailey, I. K., Come, P. G., Kelly, D. T. *et al.* (1977a) Thallium-201 myocardial perfusion imaging in aortic valve stenosis. *Am. J. Cardiol.*, **40**, 889–99.

Bailey, I. K., Griffith, L. S. C., Rouleau, J. *et al.* (1977b) Thallium-201 myocardial perfusion imaging at rest and exercise: comparative sensitivity to electrocardiography in coronary artery disease. *Circulation*, **55**, 79–87.

Bailey, I. K., Rouleau, J. R., Griffith, L. S. C. *et al.* (1977c) Myocardial perfusion imaging to detect patients with single and multivessel disease. *Herz*, **62**, 192–9.

Bender, M. A. and Blau, M. (1963) The autofluoroscope. *Nucleonics*, **21**, 52–3.

Berger, H. C., Watson, D. D., Taylor, G. J. *et al.* (1981) Quantitative thallium-201 exercise scintigraphy for detection of coronary artery disease. *J. Nucl. Med.*, **22**, 585.

Berger, H. J., Matthay, R. A., Lohe, J. *et al.* (1978) Assessment of cardiac performance with quantitative radionuclide angiocardiography: right ventricular ejection fraction with reference to findings in chronic obstructive pulmonary disease. *Am. J. Cardiol.*, **41**, 897–905.

Berger, H. J., Davies, R. A., Batsford, W. P. *et al.* (1981) Beat-to-beat left ventricular performance assessed from the equilibrium cardiac blood pool using a computerized nuclear probe. *Circulation*, **63**, 133–42.

Bergmann, S. R., Lerch, R. A., Fox, K. A. A. *et al.* (1982) Temporal dependence of beneficial effects of coronary thrombolysis characterized by positron tomography. *Am. J. Med.*, **73**, 753–81.

Bingham, J. B., McKusick, K. A., Strauss, H. W. *et al.* (1980) Influence of coronary disease on pulmonary uptake of thallium-201. *Am. J. Cardiol.*, **46**, 821–6.

Blumgart, H. L. and Weiss, S. (1927) Studies on the velocity of blood flow. VII. The pulmonary circulation time in normal resting individuals. *J. Clin. Invest.*, **4**, 399–425.

Bonow, R. O., Bacharach, S. L., Green, M. V. *et al.* (1981) Impaired left ventricular diastolic filling in patients with coronary artery disease: assessment with radionuclide angiography. *Circulation*, **65**, 315–20.

Bonow, R. O. Vitale, D. R., Bacharach, S. L. *et al.* (1985) Asynchronous left ventricular regional function and impaired global diastolic filling in patients with coronary artery disease: reversal after coronary angioplasty. *Circulation*, **71**, 297–307.

Bonte, F. J. and Curry, T. S. (1967) Tc-99m HSA blood pool scan in diagnosis of a intracardiac myxoma. *J. Nucl. Med.*, **8**, 35–9.

Bonte, F. J., Parkey, R. W., Graham, K. D., Moore, J. and Stokely, E. M. (1974) A new method for radionuclide imaging of myocardial infarcts. *Radiology*, **111**, 473–4.

Borer, J. S., Bacharach, S. L., Green, M. V. *et al.* (1977) Real-time radionuclide cineangiography in the noninvasive evaluation of global and regional left ventricular function at rest and during exercise in patients with coronary-artery disease. *N. Engl. J. Med.*, **296**, 839–44.

Borer, J. S., Bacharach, S. L., Green, M. V. *et al.* (1978) Exercise-induced left ventricular dysfunction in symptomatic and asymptomatic patients with aortic regurgitation: assessment with radionuclide cineangiography. *Am. J. Cardiol.*, **42**, 351–7.

Borer, J. S., Jacobstein, J. G., Bacharach, S. L. and Green, M. V. (1980) Detection of left ventricular aneurysm and evaluation of effects of surgical repair: the role of radionuclide cineangiography. *Am. J. Cardiol.*, **45**, 1103–6.

Botvinick, E. H., Shames, D., Hutchinson, J. C. *et al.* (1976) Noninvasive diagnosis of a false left ventricular aneurysm with radioisotope gated cardiac blood pool imaging. *Am. J. Cardiol.*, **37**, 1089–93.

Botvinick, E. H., Sceinman, M., Hattner, R. S. *et al.* (1982) An accurate means of detecting and characterizing abnormal patterns of ventricular activation by phase image analysis. *Am. J. Cardiol.*, **50**, 289–98.

Botvinick, E. H. (1990) 'Hot spot' imaging agents for acute myocardial infarction. *J. Nucl. Med.*, **31**, 143–6.

Boucher, C. A., Brewster, D. C., Darling, R. C. *et al.* (1985) Determination of cardiac risk by dipyridamole–thallium imaging before peripheral vascular surgery. *N. Engl. J. Med.*, **312**, 389–94.

Brihaye, C., Knapp, F. F., Butler, T. A. *et al.* (1985) A new osmium-191/iridium-191m generator system (abstract). *J. Nucl. Med.*, **26**, P27.

Britton, J. S. and Blank, M. (1968) Thallium activation of the (Na^+-K^+) activated ATPase of rabbit kidney. *Biochim. Biophys. Acta*, **159**, 160.

Brown, K. A., Boucher, C. A., Okada, R. D. *et al.* (1983a) Prognostic value of exercise thallium-201 imaging in patients presenting for evaluation of chest pain. *J. Am. Coll. Cardiol.*, **1**, 994–1001.

Brown, K. A., Boucher, C. A., Okada, R. D. *et al.* (1984) Quantification of pulmonary thallium-201 activity following upright exercise in normal subjects: importance of peak heart rate and propranolol usage in defining normal values. *Am. J. Cardiol.*, **53**, 1678–82.

Brown, K. A., Osbakken, M., Boucher, C. A. *et al.* (1985) Positive exercise thallium-201 test responses in patients with less than 50% maximal coronary stenosis: angiographic and clinical predictors. *Am. J. Cardiol.*, **55**, 54–7.

Brown, M. A., Myears, D. W., Marshall, D. R. *et al.* (1987) Assessment of regional myocardial oxygen utilization by positron tomography with ^{11}C-acetate (abstract). *J. Am. Coll. Cardiol.*, **9**, 73A.

Brunken, R., Tillisch, J., Schwaiger, M. *et al.* (1986) Regional perfusion, glucose metabolism and wall motion in patients with chronic electrocardiographic Q wave infarctions: evidence of persistence of viable tissue in some infarct regions by positron emission tomography. *Circulation*, **73**, 951–963.

Buja, L. M., Tofe, A. J., Kulkarni, P. V., Mukherjee, A., Parkey, R. W., Francis, M. D., Bonte, F. J. and Willerson, J. T. (1977) Sites and mechanisms of localization of Technetium-99m phosphorus radiopharmaceuticals in acute myocardial infarcts and other tissues. *J. Clin. Invest.*, **60**, 724–40.

Bulkley, B. H., Rouleau, J., Strauss, H. W. and Pitt, B. (1975) Idiopathic hypertrophic subaortic stenosis: detection by thallium-201 myocardial perfusion imaging. *N. Engl. J. Med.*, **293**, 1113–16.

Bulkley, B. H., Hutchins, G. M., Bailey, I. K. *et al.* (1977a) Thallium-201 imaging and gated blood pool scans in patients with ischemic and idiopathic congestive cardiomyopathy. *Circulation*, **55**, 753–60.

Bulkley, B. H., Rouleau, J. R., Whitaker, J. Q. *et al.* (1977b) The use of Tl-201 for myocardial perfusion imaging in sarcoid heart disease. *Chest*, **72**, 27–32.

Burow, R. D., Strauss, H. W., Singleton, R. *et al.* (1977)

Analysis of left ventricular function from multiple gated acquisition cardiac blood pool imaging: comparison to contrast angiography. *Circulation*, **56**, 1024–8.

Callahan, R. J., Froelich, J. W., McKusick, K. A. *et al.* (1982) A modified method for the *in-vivo* labeling of red blood cells with Tc-99m. *J. Nucl. Med.*, **23**, 315–18.

Camini, P., Araujo, L. I., Spinks, T. *et al.* (1986) Increased uptake of ^{18}F-fluorodeoxyglucose in postischemic myocardium of patients with exercise-induced angina. *Circulation*, **74**, 81–8.

Cannon, P. H., Dell, R. B. and Dwyer, E. M. (1972) Measurement of regional myocardial perfusion in man with Xe-133 and a scintillation camera. *J. Clin. Invest.*, **51**, 964–77.

Caplin, J. L., Dymond, D. S., O'Keefe, J. C. *et al.* (1986) Relation between coronary anatomy and serial changes in left ventricular function on exercise: a study using first pass radionuclide angiography with gold-195m. *Br. Heart J.*, **55**, 120–8.

Carr, E. A. (1964) The direct diagnosis of myocardial infarction by photoscanning after administration of cesium-131. *Am. Heart J.*, **68**, 627–36.

Carr, E. A., Jr, Beierwaltes, W. H., Patno, M. E. *et al.* (1962) The detection of experimental myocardial infarcts by photoscanning. *Am. Heart J.*, **64**, 650–60.

Corbett, J. R., Dehmer, G. J., Lewis, S. E. *et al.* (1981) The prognostic value of submaximal exercise testing with radionuclide ventriculography before hospital discharge in patients with myocardial infarction. *Circulation*, **64**, 535–44.

Corbett, J. R., Jansen, D. E., Lewis, S. E. *et al.* (1985) Tomographic gated blood pool radionuclide ventriculography: analysis of wall motion and left ventricular volumes in patients with coronary artery disease. *J. Am. Coll. Cardiol.*, **6**, 349–58.

Deanfield, J. E., Shea, M., Ribiero, P. *et al.* (1984) Transient ST-segment depression as a marker of myocardial ischemia during daily life. *Am. J. Cardiol.*, **54**, 1195–200.

Demer, L. L., Goldstein, R., Mullani, N. *et al.* (1986) Coronary steal by non-invasive PET identifies collateralized myocardium (abstract). *J. Nucl. Med.*, **27**, 977.

Deutsch, E. W., Glavan, R. A., Nishiyama, H. *et al.* (1981) Tc-99m complexes a potential myocardial imaging agents. *J. Nucl. Med.*, **22**, 897–907.

Dymond, D. S., Jarritt, P. H., Britton, K. E. and Spurrell, R. A. J. (1979) Detection of postinfarction left ventricular aneurysms by first pass radionuclide ventriculography using a multicrystal camera. *Br. Heart J.*, **41**, 68–78.

Endo, M., Yamazaki, T., Konno, S. *et al.* (1970) The direct diagnosis of human myocardial ischemia using I-131-MAA via the selective coronary catheter. *Am. Heart J.*, **80**, 498–506.

Fischman, A. J., Scott, J. A., Rabito, C. A. *et al.* (1986) Demonstration of Tc-99m pyrophosphate uptake in reversibly injured neonatal myocytes. *J. Nucl. Med.*, **27**, P993.

Fischman, A. J., Moore, R. H., Gill, J. B. and Strauss, H. W. (1989) Gated blood pool tomography: a technology whose time has come. *Sem. Nucl. Med.*, **19**, 13–21.

Garcia, E. V., Van Train, K., Maddahi, J. *et al.* (1985) Quantification of rotational thallium-201 myocardial tomography. *J. Nucl. Med.*, **26**, 17–26.

Geltman, E. M., Smith, J. L., Beecher, D. *et al.* (1983) Altered regional myocardial metabolism in congestive cardiomyopathy detected by positron emission tomography. *Am. J. Med.*, **74**, 773–85.

Gewirtz, H., Grotte, G. J., Strauss, H. W. *et al.* (1979) The influence of left ventricular volume and wall motion on myocardial images. *Circulation*, **59**, 1172–7.

Gibson, R. S. and Beller, G. A. (1982) in *Controversies in Coronary Artery Disease* (eds S. H. Rahimtolla and A. M. Brest), Davis, Philadelphia, pp. 1–31.

Gibson, R. S., Watson, D. D., Craddock, G. B. *et al.* (1983) Prediction of cardiac events after uncomplicated myocardial infarction: a prospective study comparing pre-discharge exercise thallium-201 scintigraphy and coronary angiography. *Circulation*, **68**, 321–36.

Gill, J. B., Miller, D. D., Boucher, C. A. and Strauss, H. W. (1986a) Clinical decision making: dipyridamole thallium imaging. *J. Nucl. Med.*, **27**, 132–7.

Gill, J. B., Moore, R. H., Tamaki, N. *et al.* (1986b) Multigated blood-pool tomography: new method for the assessment of left ventricular function. *J. Nucl. Med.*, **27**, 1916–24.

Goldstein, R. A., Kirkeeide, R., Demer, L. *et al.* (1986) Assessment of coronary flow reserve with positron tomography: a comparison with quantitative coronary arteriography (abstract). *J. Nucl. Med.*, **27**, 943.

Gould, K. L. (1978) Noninvasive assessment of coronary artery stenosis with myocardial perfusion imaging during pharmacological coronary vasodilatation. I. Physiologic basis and experimental validation. *Am. J. Cardiol.*, **41**, 267.

Gould, K. L., Schelbert, H. R., Phelps, M. E. and Hoffman, E. J. (1979) Noninvasive assessment of coronary stenosis with myocardial perfusion imaging during pharmacological vasodilatation. V. Detection of 47 percent diameter coronary stenosis with intravenous nitrogen-13 ammonia and emission-computed transaxial tomography in intact dogs. *Am. J. Cardiol.*, **43** 200–8.

Gould, K. L., Goldstein, R. A., Mullani, N. A. *et al.* (1986) Noninvasive assessment of coronary stenosis by myocardial perfusion imaging during pharmacological coronary vasodilation. VIII. Clinical feasibility of positron cardiac imaging without a cyclotron using generator produced rubidium-82. *J. Am. Coll. Cardiol.*, **7**, 775–89.

Gould, K. L. (1989) Clinical cardiac PET using generator-produced Rb-82: a review. *Cardiovasc. Intervent. Radiol.*, **12**, 245–51.

Grames, G. M., Jansen, C., Gander, M. P. *et al.* (1975) Safety of the direct coronary injection of radiolabelled particles. *J. Nucl. Med..*, **15**, 2–6.

Grover, M., Schwaiger, M., Sochor, H. *et al.* (1984) C-11 palmitic acid kinetics and positron emission tomography detect pacing-induced ischemia in patients with coronary artery disease (abstract). *Circulation*, **70**, II–340.

Grover, M., Schwaiger, M., Krivokapich, J. *et al.* (1986) Regional myocardial blood flow and metabolism determined by positron emission tomography in patients with hypertrophic cardiomyopathy (abstract). *J. Nucl. Med.*, **27**, 933.

Hamilton, R. G. and Alderson, P. O. (1977) A comparative evaluation of techniques of rapid and efficient *in vivo* labeling of red cells with Tc-99m-pertechnetate. *J. Nucl. Med.*, **18**, 1010–13.

Hammermeister, K. E. and Warbasse, J. R. (1974) The rate of change of left ventricular volume in man. II. Diastolic events in health and disease. *Circulation*, **49**, 739–47.

Hayes, D., Borer, J. S., Mosee, J. W. and Carter, J. (1983) Exercise induced systolic abnormalities predicted by diastolic measurements using a nonimaging radionuclide probe (abstract). *J. Am. Coll. Cardiol.*, **1**, 643.

Heller, S. J. and Carleton, R. A. (1970) Abnormal left ventricular contraction in patients with mitral stenosis. *Circulation*, **42**, 1099–110.

Henze, E., Huang, S. C., Ratib, O. *et al.* (1983) Measurements of regional tissue and blood flow radiotracer concentrations from serial tomographic images of the heart. *J. Nucl. Med.*, **24**, 987–996.

Holman, B. L., Dewanjee, M. K., Idoine, J., Fliegel, C. P., Davis, M. A., Treves, S. and Eldh, P. (1973) Detection and localization of experimental myocardial infarction with 99m-Tc-Tetracycline. *J. Nucl. Med.*, **14**, 595–9.

Holman, B. L., Wynne, J., Idoine, J. *et al.* (1979) The paradox image: a noninvasive index of regional ventricular dyskinesis. *J. Nucl. Med.*, **20**, 1237–42.

Holman, B. L., Jones, A. G., Lister-James, J. *et al.* (1984) A new Tc-99m-labeled myocardial imaging agent, hexakis (t-butylisonitrile)-technetium(I): initial experience in the human. *J. Nucl. Med.*, **25**, 1350–5.

Holman, B. L., Sporn, V., Jones, A. G. *et al.* (1987) Myocardial imaging with technetium-99m CPI: initial experience in the human. *J. Nucl. Med.*, **28**, 13–18.

Hurley, P. H., Cooper, M., Reba, R. C. *et al.* (1971) ^{43}KCl: a new radiopharmaceutical for imaging the heart. *J. Nucl. Med.*, **12**, 515–19.

Jengo, J. A., Mena, I., Blaufuss, A. and Criley, J. M. (1978) Evaluation of left ventricular function (ejection fraction and segmental wall motion) by single pass radioisotope angiography. *Circulation*, **57**, 327–32.

Johnson, L. L., McKarthy, D. M., Sciacca, R. R. and Cannon, P. J. (1979) Right ventricular ejection fraction during exercise in patients with coronary artery disease. *Circulation*, **60**, 1284–91.

Jones, A. G., Davison, A., Abrams, M. J. *et al.* (1982) Investigations on a new class of technetium cations (abstract). *J. Nucl. Med.*, **23**, P16.

Jones, A. G., Abrams, M. J., Davison, A., *et al.* (1984) Biological studies of a new class of technetium complexes: the hexakis (alkylisonitrile technetium (I) cations. *Int. J. Nucl. Med. Biol.*, **11**, 225–34.

Jones, R. H., McEwan, P., Newman, G. *et al.* (1981) The accuracy of diagnosis of coronary artery disease by radionuclide measurements of left ventricular function during rest and exercise. *Circulation*, **64**, 586–601.

Katz, R. J., Simpson, A., DiBianco, R. *et al.* (1979) Noninvasive diagnosis of a left ventricular pseudoaneurysm. *Am. J. Cardiol.*, **44**, 372–7.

Kaul, S., Boucher, C. A., Newell, J. B. *et al.* (1984) Computer analysis of thallium images: correlates of coronary artery disease. *Circulation*, **70**, 286.

Kaul, S., Chesler, D. A., Pohost, G. M. *et al.* (1986) Influence of peak exercise heart rate on normal thallium-201 clearance. *J. Nucl. Med.*, **27**, 26–30.

Kaul, S., Kiess, M., Liu, P. *et al.* (1985) Comparison of exercise electrocardiography and quantitative thallium imaging for one-vessel coronary artery disease. *Am. J. Cardiol*, **56**, 257–61.

Kayden, D. S., Wackers, F. J. and Zaret, B. L. (1988) The role of nuclear cardiology in assessment of acute myocardial infarction. *Cardiol. Clin.*, **6**, 81–95.

Kennedy, P. L., Corbett, J. R., Kularni, P. V. *et al.* (1986) Iodine 123-phenylpentadecanoic acid myocardial scintigraphy: usefulness in the identification of myocardial ischemia. *Circulation*, **74**, 1007–15.

Khaja, F., Walton, J. A., Brymer, J. F. *et al.* (1983) Intracoronary fibrinolytic therapy in acute myocardial infarction: report of a prospective randomized trial. *N. Engl. J. Med.*, **308**, 1305–11.

Khaw, B. A., Gold, H. K., Yasuda, T. *et al.* (1986) Scintigraphic quantification of myocardial necrosis in patients after intravenous injection of myosin-specific antibody. *Circulation*, **74**, 501–8.

Kiat, H., Maddahi, J., Roy, L. T., van Train, K., Friedman, J., Resser, K. and Berman, D. S. (1989) Comparison of technetium 99m methoxy isobutyl isonitrile and thallium 201 for evaluation of coronary artery disease by planar and tomographic methods. *Am Heart J.*, **117**, 1–11.

Kipper, S. L., Ashburn, W. L., Nooris, S. L. *et al.* (1985) Gold-195m first-pass radionuclide ventriculography, thallium-201 single-photon emission CT, and 12 lead ECG testing as a combined procedure. *Radiology*, **156**, 817–21.

Klipzig, H., Standke, R., Maul, F. D. *et al.* (1986) Combined first pass and equilibrium radionuclide ventriculography for non-invasive quantitation of aortic and or mitral regurgitation: comparison of left and right ventricular stroke count ratio. *Z. Cardiol.*, **75** (suppl. 2), 24–7.

Knabb, R. M., Fox, K. A. A., Sobel, B. E. and Bergmann, S. R. (1985) Characterization of the functional significance of subcritical coronary artery stenosis with $H_2{}^{15}O$ and positron-emission tomography. *Circulation*, **71**, 1271–8.

Knapp, F. F., Ambrose, K. R., Callahan, A. P. *et al.* (1981) Effect of chain length and tellurium position on the myocardial uptake of Te-123m fatty acids. *J. Nucl. Med.*, **22**, 988–93.

Kolibash, A. J., Goodenow, J. S., Bush, C. A. *et al.* (1979) Improvement of myocardial perfusion and left ventricular function after coronary bypass grafting in patients with unstable angina. *Circulation*, **59**, 66–74.

Korbuly, D. E., Formanek, A., Gypser, G. *et al.* (1975) Regional myocardial blood flow measurements before and after coronary artery bypass surgery. *Circulation*, **52**, 38–45.

Kulkarni, P. V. and Corbett, J. R. (1990) Radioiodinated tracers for myocardial imaging. *Semin. Nucl. Med.*, **20**, 119–29.

Lacy, L. J., Verani, M. S., Packard, A. *et al.* (1985) Minute to minute assessment of left ventricular function with a new multiwire gamma camera and an ultra-short lived isotope Ir-191m (abstract). *J. Am. Coll. Cardiol.*, **5**, 405–9.

Lacy, L. J., Verani, M. S., Ball, M. E. *et al.* (1986) First-pass radionuclide angiocardiography with the multiwire gamma camera and Ta-178 compared with the multicrystal camera and Tc-99m in patients (abstract), *J. Nucl. Med.*, **27**, 911.

Ladenheim, M. L., Pollock, B. H., Rozanski, A. *et al.* (1986) Extent and severity of myocardial hypoperfusion as predictors of prognosis in patients with suspected coronary artery disease. *J. Am. Coll. Cardiol.*, **7**, 464.

Lebowitz, E., Greene, M. W., Fairchild, R. *et al.* (1975) Thallium-201 for medical use I. *J. Nucl. Med.*, **16**, 151–60.

Lees, R. S., Lees, A. M., Strauss, H. W. *et al.* (1985) The distribution and metabolism of Tc-99m low density lipoprotein in human subjects (abstract). *J. Nucl. Med.*, **26**, P35.

Leppo, J. A., Boucher, C. A., Okada, R. D. *et al.* (1982) Serial thallium-201 imaging following dipyridamole infusion: diagnostic utility in detecting coronary stenosis and relationship to regional wall motion. *Circulation*, **66**, 649–57.

Leppo, J. A., Okada, R. D., Strauss, H. W. and Pohost, G. M. (1985) Effect of hyperemia on thallium-201 redistribution in normal canine myocardium. *Cardiovasc. Res.*, **19**, 679–85.

Leppo, J. A. (1989) Dipyridamole-Thallium imaging: the lazy man's stress test. *J. Nucl. Med.*, **30**, 281–7.

Lewis, M., Buja, L. M., Saffer, S., Mishelevich, D., Stokely, E., Lewis, S., Parkey, R., Bonte, F. and Willerson, J. (1977) Experimental infarct sizing using computer processing and a three dimensional model. *Science*, **197**, 167–9.

Lim, Y. L., Okada, R. D., Chesler, D. A. *et al.* (1984) A new approach to quantitation of exercise thallium-201 scintigraphy before and after an intervention: application to define the impact of coronary angioplasty on regional myocardial perfusion. *Am. Heart J.*, **108**, 917–25.

Links, M. J., Douglass, H. K. and Wagner, N. H., Jr (1980) Pattern of ventricular emptying by Fourier analysis of gated blood-pool studies. *J. Nucl. Med.*, **21**, 978–82.

Liu, P., Kiess, M. C., Okada, R. D. *et al.* (1985) The persistent defect on exercise thallium imaging and its fate after myocardial revascularization: does it represent scar or ischemia? *Am. Heart J.*, **110**, 996–1001.

Liu, P., Kiess, M.C., Strauss, H. W. *et al.* (1986) Comparison of ejection fraction and pulmonary blood volume ratio as markers of left ventricular function change after coronary angioplasty. *J. Am. Coll. Cardiol.*, **8**, 511–16.

Livni, E., Elmaleh, D. R., Levy, S. *et al.* (1982) Beta-methyl ($1-{}^{11}C$) heptadecanoic acid: a new metabolic tracer for positron emission tomography. *J. Nucl. Med.*, **23**, 169–75.

Loop, F. D., Lytle, B. W., Cosgrove, D. M. *et al.* (1986) Influence of internal-mammary-artery graft on 10-year survival and other cardiac events. *N. Engl. J. Med.*, **314**, 1–6.

Lyons, K. P., Olson, H. G. and Aronow, W. S. (1980) Pyrophosphate myocardial imaging. *Semin. Nucl. Med.*, **10**, 168–77.

Maddahi, J., Berman, D. S., Matsuoka, D. T. *et al.* (1979) A new technique for assessing right ventricular ejection fraction using rapid multiple-gated equilibrium cardiac blood pool scintigraphy: description, validation and findings in chronic coronary disease. *Circulation*, **60**, 581–9.

Maddahi, J., Garcia, E. V., Berman, D. C. *et al.* (1981) Improved noninvasive assessment of coronary artery disease by quantitative analysis of regional stress myocardial distribution and washout of thallium-201. *Circulation*, **64**, 925.

Maddox, D. E., Holman, B. L., Wynne, J. *et al.* (1978) A noninvasive index of regional left ventricular wall motion. *Am. J. Cardiol.*, **41**, 1230–8.

Maddox, D. E., Wynne, J., Uren, R. *et al.* (1979) Regional ejection fraction: a quantitative radionuclide index of regional left ventricular performance. *Circulation*, **59**, 1001–9.

Maisey, M. N., Mistry, R. and Sowton, E. (1990) Planer Imaging Techniques used with Technetium 99m Sesta MIBI to evaluate chronic myocardial ischaemia. *Amer. J. Card.*, **66** (13).

Makler, P. T., Lavine, S. J., Denenberg, B. S. *et al.* (1981) Redistribution on the thallium scan in myocardial sarcoidosis: concise communication. *J. Nucl. Med.*, **22**, 428–32.

Malek, P., Ratusky, J., Vavrejn, B., Kronrad, L. and Kolc, J. (1967) Ischaemia detecting radioactive substances for scanning cardiac and skeletal muscle. *Nature*, **214**, 1130–1.

Marshall, R. C., Tillisch, J. H., Phelps, M. E. *et al.* (1981) Identification and differentiation of resting myocardial ischemia and infarction in man with positron computed tomography ${}^{18}F$-labeled fluorodeoxyglucose and N-13 ammonia. *Circulation*, **65**, 766–78.

Massie, B. M., Kramer, B. L., Gertz, E. W. and Henderson, S. G. (1982) Radionuclide measurements of left ventricular volume: comparison of geometric and count based methods. *Circulation*, **65**, 725–30.

Matthay, R. A., Berger, H. J., Davies, R. A. *et al.* (1980) Right and left ventricular exercise performance in chronic obstructive pulmonary disease: radionuclide assessment. *Ann. Intern. Med.*, **93**, 234–9.

McArdle, W. D., Katch, F. I. and Katch, V. L. (1981) in *Exercise Physiology* (eds W. D. McArdle, F. I. Katch and V. L. Katch), Lea and Febiger, Philadelphia, ch. 17, pp. 219–33.

McGowan, R. L., Welch, T. G. Zaret, B. L. *et al.* (1976) Noninvasive myocardial imaging with potassium-43 and rubidium-81 in patients with left bundle branch block. *Am. J. Cardiol.*, **38**, 422–8.

McKusick, K. A., Bingham, J. B., Pohost, G. M. and Strauss, H. W. (1978) The gated first pass radionuclide angiogram: a method for measurement of right ventricular ejection fraction (abstract). *Circulation*, **57**, 58-II 130.

McKusick, K. A., Holman, B. L., Jones, A. G. *et al.* (1986) Comparison of 3-Tc-99m isonitriles for detecting ischemic heart disease in humans (abstract). *J. Nucl. Med.*, **27**, 878.

Meizlish, J. L., Berger, H. J., Plankey, M. *et al.* (1984) Functional left ventricular aneurysm formation after acute anterior transmural myocardial infarction. *N. Engl. J. Med.*, **311**, 1001–6.

Mena, I., Narahara, A., deJong, R. and Maublat, J. (1983) Gold-195m, an ultrashort-lived generator produced radionuclide: clinical application in sequential first pass ventriculography. *J. Nucl. Med.*, **24**, 139–44.

Miller, D. D., Gill, J. B., Barlai-Kovach, M. *et al.* (1985a)

Identification of the ischemic border zone in reperfused canine myocardium using iodinated fatty acid analogues. *Clin. Res.*, **33**, 211A.
Miller, D. D., Liu, P., Block, P. C. *et al.* (1985b) Prognostic value of exercise thallium imaging early after percutaneous transluminal angioplasty (PTCA): quantitative and qualitative analysis. *J. Am. Coll. Cardiol.*, **5**, 532.
Mousa, S. A., Morgan, R. A., Carroll, T. R. and Meheu, L. J. (1986) Pharmacology of Tc-99m isonitriles: agents with favorable characteristics for heart imaging (abstract). *J. Nucl. Med.*, **27**, 877.
Mukharji, J., Rude, R. E., Pool, W. K. *et al.* (1984) Risk factors for sudden death after acute myocardial infarction: two-year follow-up. *Am. J. Cardiol.*, **54**, 31–6.
Nakajima, K., Bunko, H., Tada, A. *et al.* (1984) Phase analysis in the Wolff–Parkinson–White syndrome with surgically proven accessory conduction pathways. *J. Nucl. Med.*, **25**, 7–13.
Nanda, N. C., Gramiak, R., Shah, P. M. *et al.* (1974) Echocardiography in the diagnosis of idiopathic hypertrophic subaortic stenosis co-existing with aortic valve disease. *Circulation*, **50**, 752–7.
Neinaber, C. A. Spielman, R. P., Wasmus, G. *et al.* (1985) Clinical use of ultrashort lived radionuclide Kr-81m for noninvasive analysis of right ventricular performance in normal subjects and patients with right ventricular dysfunction. *J. Am. Coll. Cardiol.*, **5**, 678–98.
Nichols, A. B., Pohost, G. M., Gold, H. K. *et al.* (1978) Left ventricular function during balloon pumping assessed by multigated cardiac blood pool imaging. *Circulation*, **88** (suppl. I, Cardiovasc. Surg.), 176–83.
Okada, R. D., Pohost, G. M., Kirshenbaum, H. D. *et al.* (1979) Radionuclide-determined change in pulmonary blood volume with exercise. *N. Engl. J. Med.*, **301**, 569–76.
Oldendorf, W. H., Kitano, M. and Shimizy, S. (1965) Evaluation of a simple technique for abrupt intravenous injection of radionuclide. *J. Nucl. Med.*, **6**, 205–9.
Opie, L. H. (1968) Metabolism of the heart in health and disease. *Am. Heart J.*, **76**, 685–98.
Opie, L. H. (1984) in *The heart* (ed. L. H. Opie), Grune and Stratton, New York, ch. 9.
Parker, A. J., Secker-Walker, R., Hill, R. *et al.* (1972) A new technique for the calculation of left ventricular ejection fraction. *J. Nucl. Med.*, **13**, 649–651.
Parkey, R. W., Bonte, F. J., Buja, L. M., Stokely, E. M. and Willerson, J. T. (1977) Myocardial infarct imaging with Technetium-99m phosphate. *Semin. Nucl. Med.*, **7**, 15–28.
Pavel, D., Zimmer, A. M. and Patterson, V. N. (1977) *In vivo* labeling of red blood cells with Tc-99m: a new approach to blood pool visualization. *J. Nucl. Med.*, **18**, 305–8.
Pellikka, P. A., Behrenbeck, T., Veranc, M. S., Mahmarian, J. J., Wackers, F. J. and Gibbons, R. J. (1990) Serial changes in myocardial perfusion using tomographic Technetium 99m-Hexakis-2-Methoxy-2-Methylpropyl-Isonitrile imaging following Reperfusion therapy of myocardial infarction. *J. Nucl. Med.*, **31**, 1269–75.
Perloff, J. K., Henze, E. and Schelbert, H. R. (1984) Alteration in regional myocardial metabolism, perfusion and wall motion in Duchenne's muscular dystrophy studied by radionuclide imaging. *Circulation*, **69**, 33–42.
Phillip, H. R., Levine, F. H., Carter, J. E. *et al.* (1981) Mitral valve replacement for isolated mitral regurgitation: analysis of clinical course and late postoperative left ventricular ejection fraction. *Am. J. Cardiol.*, **48**, 647–54.
Pieri, P., Abraham, S. A., Katayma, H. and Yasuda, A. (1990) Thallium-201 myocardial scintigraphy: Single infection reinjection or 24 hour delayed imaging. *J. Nucl. Med*, **31**, 1390–6.
Pohost, G. M., Vignola, P. A., McKusick, K. A. *et al.* (1977) Hypertrophic cardiomyopathy: evaluation by gated blood pool scanning. *Circulation*, **55**, 92–9.
Pohost, G. M., Alpert, N. M., Ingwall, J. S. and Strauss, H. W. (1980) Thallium redistribution mechanism and clinical utility. *Semin. Nucl. Med.*, **10**, 70–93.
Port, S., Cobb, F. R., Coleman, R. W. and Jones, R. H. (1980) Effect of age on the response of the late ventricular ejection fraction to exercise. *N. Engl. J. Med.*, **303**, 1133–7.
Prinzmetal, M., Corday, E., Bergman, H. C. *et al.* (1948) Radiocardiography: a new method for studying the blood flow through the chambers of the heart in human beings. *Science*, **108**, 340–1.
Ranhosky, A. and Kempthorne-Rawson, J. (1990) The safety of intravenous dipyridamole thallium myocardial perfusion imaging. Intravenous Dipyridamole Thallium Imaging Study Group. *Circulation*, **81**, 1205–9.
Reduto, L. A., Berger, H. J., Cohen, L. S. Gottschalk, A. and Zaret, B. L. (1978) Sequential radionuclide assessment of left and right ventricular performance after acute transmural myocardial infarction. *Ann. Intern. Med.*, **89**, 441–7.
Rejali, A. M., MacIntyre, W. J. and Friedell, H. L. (1958) Radioisotope method of visualization of blood pools. *Am. J. Roentgenol.*, **79**, 129–37.
Rigo, P., Murray, M., Strauss, H. W. and Pitt, B. (1974a) Scintiphotographic evaluation of patients with suspected left ventricular aneurysm. *Circulation*, **50**, 985–91.
Rigo, P., Murray, M., Strauss, H. W. *et al.* (1974b) Left ventricular function in acute myocardial infarction evaluated by gated scintiphotography. *Circulation*, **50**, 678–84.
Rigo, P., Alderson, P. O., Robertson, R. M. *et al.* (1979) Measurement of aortic and mitral regurgitation by gated blood pool scans. *Circulation*, **60**, 306–12.
Rossman, D. J., Strauss, H. W., Siegel, M. E. and Pitt, B. (1975) Accumulation of 99m-Tc-Glucoheptonate in acutely infarcted myocardium. *J. Nucl. Med.*, **16**, 875–8.
Rozansky, A., Berman, D., Gray, R. *et al.* (1982) Preoperative prediction of reversible myocardial asynergy by postexercise radionuclide ventriculography. *N. Engl. J. Med.*, **307**, 212–16.
Sandford, C. F., Corbett, J., Nicod, P. *et al.* (1982) Value of radionuclide ventriculography in the immediate characterization of patients with acute myocardial infarction. *Am. J. Cardiol.*, **49**, 637–44.
Sapirstein, L. A. (1956) Fractionation of the cardiac output of rats with isotopic potassium. *Circ. Res.*, **4**, 689–92.

Schelbert, H. R., Henning, N., Ashburn, W. L. *et al.* (1976) Serial measurements of left ventricular ejection fraction by radionuclide angiography early and late after myocardial infarction. *Am. J. Cardiol.*, **38**, 407–15.

Schelbert, H. R., Henze, E., Sochor, H. *et al.* (1986) Effects of substrate availability on myocardial C-11 palmitate kinetics by positron emission tomography in normal subjects and patients with ventricular dysfunction. *Am. Heart J.*, **111**, 1055–64.

Schelbert, H. R. (1989) Myocardial ischemia and clinical applications of positron emission tomography. *Am. J. Cardiol.*, **64**, 46E–53E.

Schon, H. R., Senekowitsch, R., Berg, D. *et al.* (1986) Measurement of myocardial fatty acid metabolism: kinetics of iodine-123 heptadecanoic acid in normal dog heart. *J. Nucl. Med.*, **27**, 1449–55.

Schuler, G., Peterson, K. L., Johnson, A. D. *et al.* (1979) Serial non-invasive assessment of left ventricular hypertrophy and function after surgical correction of aortic regurgitation. *Am. J. Cardiol.*, **44**, 585–94.

Schuler, G., von Olshausen, K., Schwarz, F. *et al.* (1982) Noninvasive assessment of myocardial contractility in asymptomatic patients with severe aortic regurgitation and normal left ventricular ejection fraction at rest. *Am. J. Cardiol.*, **50**, 45–53.

Schulze, R. A., Strauss, H. W. and Pitt, B. (1977) Sudden death in the year following myocardial infarction: relation to ventricular premature contractions in the late hospital phase and left ventricular ejection fraction. *Am. J. Med.*, **62**, 192–9.

Schwaiger, M., Schelbert, H. R., Keen, R. *et al.* (1985) Retention and clearance of C-11 palmitic acid in reperfused myocardium. *J. Am. Coll. Cardiol.*, **6**, 311–20.

Schwaiger, M., Brunken, R., Grover, M. *et al.* (1986) Regional myocardial metabolism in patients with acute myocardial infarction assessed by positron emission tomography. *J. Am. Coll. Cardiol.*, **8**, 800–8.

Shen, A. C. and Jennings, R. B. (1972) Myocardial calcium and magnesium in acute ischaemic injury. *Am. J. Path*, **67**, 417–33.

Selwyn, A. P., Allan, R. M., Pike, V. *et al.* (1981) Positive labeling of ischemic myocardium: a new approach to patients with coronary artery disease (abstract). *Am. J. Cardiol.*, **47**, 81.

Selwyn, A. P., Allan, R. M., L'Abbate, A. *et al.* (1982) Relation between regional myocardial uptake of rubidium-82 and perfusion: absolute reduction of cation uptake in ischemia. *Am. J. Cardiol.*, **50**, 112–21.

Senda, M., Yonekura, Y., Tamaki, N. *et al.* (1986) Interpolating scan and oblique-angle tomograms in myocardial PET using nitrogen-13 ammonia. *J. Nucl. Med.*, **17**, 1830–6.

Sessler, M. J., Geck, P., Maul, F. D. *et al.* (1986) New aspects of cellular thallium uptake: Tl+ – Na+ – 2Cl – cotransport is the central mechanism of ion uptake. *Nuklearmedizin*, **25**, 24–7.

Shah, P. K., Pichler, M., Berman, D. S. *et al.* (1980) Left ventricular ejection fraction and first third ejection fraction determined by radionuclide ventriculography in early stages of first transmural myocardial infarction: relation to short-term prognosis. *Am. J. Cardiol.*, **45**, 542–6.

Shen, W. F., Roubin, G. S., Choong, C. Y. *et al.* (1985) Evaluation of the relationship between myocardial contractile state and left ventricular function in patients with aortic regurgitation. *Circulation*, **71**, 31–8.

Smith, T. D. and Richards, P. (1976) A simple kit for the preparation of Tc^{99m} labelled red blood cells. *J. Nucl. Med.*, **17**, 126–32.

Stokely, E. M., Buja, L. M., Lewis, S. E., Parkey, R. W., Bonte, F. J., Harris, R. A. and Willerson, J. T. (1976) Measurement of acute myocardial infarcts in dogs with 99m-Tc-stannous pyrophosphate scintigrams. *J. Nucl. Med.*, **17**, 1–5.

Strauss, H. W., Lazewatsky, J., Moore, R. H. *et al.* (1979a) The VEST: a device for the continuous monitoring of cardiac function in ambulatory patients (abstract). *Circulation*, **59**, II-246.

Strauss, H. W., McKusick, K. A., Boucher, C. A. *et al.* (1979b) Of linens and laces: the eighth anniversary of the gated blood pool scan. *Semin. Nucl. Med.*, **9**, 296–309.

Strauss, H. W., Yasuda, T., Gold, H. K. *et al.* (1987) Potential role of combined fatty acid and thallium imaging in patients with myocardial ischemia and infarction (abstract). *J. Nucl. Med.*, **28**, P632.

Svensson, S. E., Lomsky, M., Olsson, L. *et al.* (1982) Non-invasive determination of the distribution of cardiac output in man at rest and during exercise. *Clin. Physiol.*, **2**, 467–77.

Sweet, S. E., Sterling, R., McCormick, J. R. *et al.* (1979) Left ventricular false aneurysm after coronary bypass surgery: radionuclide diagnosis and surgical resection. *Am. J. Cardiol.*, **43**, 154–7.

Taillefer, R., Gagnon, A., Laflamme, L., Grégoire, J., Léveille, J. and Phaneuf, D.-C. (1989) Same day injections of Tc-99m methoxy isobutyl isonitrile (hexamibi) for myocardial tomographic imaging: Comparison between rest-stress and stress-rest injection sequences. *Eur. J. Nucl. Med.*, **15**, 113–17.

Tamaki, N., Mukai, T., Ishii, Y. *et al.* (1982) Comparative study of thallium emission myocardial tomography with 180° and 360° data collection. *J. Nucl. Med.*, **23**, 661–6.

Tamaki, N., Mukai, T., Ishii, Y. *et al.* (1983) Multiaxial tomography of heart chambers by gated blood-pool emission computed tomography using a rotating gamma camera. *Radiology*, **147**, 547–54.

Tamaki, N., Senda, M., Yonekura, Y. *et al.* (1985a) Dynamic positron computed tomography of the heart with a high sensitivity positron camera and nitrogen-13 ammonia. *J. Nucl. Med.*, **26**, 567–75.

Tamaki, N., Yonekura, Y., Senda, M. *et al.* (1985b) Myocardial positron computed tomography with ^{13}N-ammonia at rest and during exercise. *Eur. J. Nucl. Med.*, **11**, 246–51.

Tamaki, N., Leinbach, R. C., McKusick, K. A. *et al.* (1985c) Prognostic importance of changes in regional wall motion in patients with acute myocardial infarction (abstract). *Circulation*, **72**, III-481.

Tamaki, N., Yasuda, T., Leinbach, R. C. *et al.* (1986a) Spontaneous changes in regional wall motion abnormalities in acute myocardial infarction. *Am. J. Cardiol.*, **58**, 406–10.

Tamaki, N., Yasuda, T., Moore, R. H. *et al.* (1986b) Ambulatory monitoring of left ventricular function in patients with severe coronary artery disease (abstract). *Circulation*, **74**, II-479.

Tamaki, N., Gill, J. B., Moore, R. H. *et al.* (1987a) Cardiac response to daily activities and exercise in normal subjects assessed by an ambulatory ventricular function monitor. *Am. J. Cardiol.*, **59**, 1164–9.

Tamaki, N., Yonekura, Y., Senda, M. *et al.* (1987b) Is stress N-13 ammonia PET imaging superior to Tl-201 SPECT (abstract). *J. Nucl. Med.*, **28**, 567.

Tillisch, J., Brunken, R., Marshall, R. *et al.* (1986) Reversibility of cardiac wall-motion abnormalities predicted by positron tomography. *N. Engl. J. Med.*, **314**, 884–8.

Trevers, S., Cheng, C., Samuel, A. *et al.* (1980a) Iridium-191m angiocardiography for the detection and quantitation of left to right shunting. *J. Nucl. Med.*, **21**, 1151–7.

Trevers, S., Fogle, R. and Lang, P. (1980b) Radionuclide angiography in congenital heart disease. *Am. J. Cardiol.*, **46**, 1247–55.

van der Wall, E. E., Heidendal, G. A. K., den Hollander, W. *et al.* (1981) Metabolic myocardial imaging with ^{123}I-labeled heptadecanoic acid in patients with unstable angina pectoris. *Eur. J. Nucl. Med.*, **6**, 391–94.

Wackers, F. J. T. (1980) Thallium-201 myocardial scintigraphy in acute myocardial infarction and ischemia. *Semin. Nucl. Med.*, **10**, 127–45.

Wackers, F. J. T., Fetterman, R. C., Mattera, J. A. and Clements, J. P. Quantitative planar thallium-201 stress scintigraphy: a critical evaluation of the method. *Semin. Nucl. Med.*, **15**, 46–6.

Wagner, H. N., Jr, Wake, R., Nickoloff, E. and Natarajan, T. K. (1976) The nuclear stethoscope: a simple device for generation of left ventricular volume curves. *Am. J. Cardiol.*, **38**, 747–50.

Weiss, E. S., Ahmed, S. A., Welch, M. J. *et al.* (1977) Quantification of infarction in cross sections of canine myocardium *in vivo* with positron emission transaxial tomography and ^{11}C-palmitate. *Circulation*, **55**, 66–73.

Weich, H., Strauss, H. W. and Pitt, B. (1977) The extraction of thallium-201 by the myocardium. *Circulation*, **56**, 188–91.

Wharton, T. P., Neill, W. A. Oxenidine, J. M. and Painter, L. N. (1980) Effect of duration of regional myocardial ischemia and degree of reactive hyperemia on the magnitude of the initial thallium-201 defect. *Circulation*, **62**, 516–21.

Willerson, J. T., Parkey, R. W., Stokely, E. M., Bonte, F. J., Lewis, S., Harris, R. A., Blomqvist, G., Poliner, L. R. and Buja, L. M. (1977) Infarct sizing with technetium-99m stannous pyrophosphate scintigraphy in dogs and man; relationship between scintigraphic and precordial mapping estimates of infarct size in patients. *Cardiovasc. Res.*, **11**, 191–8.

Wilson, R. A., Okada, R. D., Strauss, H. W. and Pohost, G. M. (1983a) Effect of glucose–insulin–potassium infusion on thallium clearance. *Circulation*, **68**, 203–9.

Wilson, R. A., Sullivan, P. J., Moore, R. H. *et al.* (1983b) An ambulatory ventricular function monitor: validation and preliminary results. *Am. J. Cardiol.*, **52**, 601–6.

Wilson, R. A., Sullivan, P. J., Okada, R. D. *et al.* (1986) The effect of eating on thallium myocardial imaging. *Chest*, **89**, 195–8.

Wilson, R. A., Shea, M., deLandsheere, C. *et al.* (1987) Rubidium-82 myocardial uptake and extraction after transient ischemia: PET characterization. *J. Comp. Assis. Tomogr.*, **11**, 60–6.

Yano, T. and Anger, H. O. (1968) Ultrashort lived radioisotopes for visualizing blood vessels and organs. *J. Nucl. Med.*, **9**, 2–6.

Yasuda, T., Alpert, N., Gold, H. K. *et al.* (1981) Quantitative regional wall motion analysis of multigated blood pool scans: validation (abstract). *Circulation*, **64**, IV-250.

Yasuda, T., Palacios, I. F., Dec, G. W. *et al.* (1987) Indium 111-monoclonal antimyosin antibody imaging in the diagnosis of acute myocarditis. *Circulation*, **76**, 306–11.

Yonekura, Y., Senda, M., Saji, H. *et al.* (1986) Increased accumulation of fluorodeoxyglucose in stress induced myocardial ischemia (abstract). *J. Nucl. Med.*, **27**, 933.

Yonekura, Y., Tamaki, N., Senda, M. *et al.* (1987) Detection of coronary artery disease with ^{13}N-ammonia and high-resolution positron emission computed tomography. *Am. Heart J.*, **113**, 645–54.

Zaret, B. L., Dicola, V. C., Donabedian, R. K., Puri, S., Wolfson, S., Freedman, G. S. and Cohan, L. S. (1976) Dual radionuclide study of myocardial infarction. *Circulation*, **53**, 422–8.

Zaret, B. L., Strauss, H. W., Martin, N. D., Wells, H. P. and Flamm, M. D. (1973) Non-invasive regional myocardial perfusion with radioactive potassium. *New Engl. J. Med.*, **288**, 809–12.

FURTHER READING

Brunken, R. C. and Schelbert, H. R. (1989) Positron emission tomography in clinical cardiology. *Cardiol. Clin.*, **7**, 607–29.

Dilsizian, V., Rocco, T. P., Bonow, R. O., Fischman, A. J., Boucher, C. A. and Strauss, H. W. (1990) Cardiac blood-pool imaging II: Applications in noncoronary heart disease.. *J. Nucl. Med.*, **31**, 10–22.

Nunn, A. D. (1990) Radiopharmaceuticals for imaging myocardial perfusion. *Semin. Nucl. Med.*, **20**, 111–18.

Pohost, G. M. and Henzlova, M. J. (1990) The value of thallium-201 imaging. *New Engl. J. Med.*, **323**, 190–2.

Rocco, T. P., Dilsizian, V., Fischman, A. J. and Strauss, H. W. (1989) Evaluation of ventricular function in patients with coronary artery disease. *J. Nucl. Med.*, **30**, 1149–65.

Schelbert, H. R. and Czernin, J. (1990) Noninvasive quantification of regional myocardial blood flow: assessment of myocardial perfusion reserve and collateral circulation. *J. Nucl. Med.*, **31**, 271–3.

CHAPTER TWO

Exercise electrocardiogram testing and thallium scintigraphy

D. A. Brennand-Roper

2.1 INTRODUCTION

Since 1918 when electrocardiogram (ECG) changes were first described during an attack of angina (Bousfield) the exercise ECG has become the most commonly used non-invasive test to identify those patients with coronary artery disease. The purpose of the test is to determine whether the coronary circulation will allow an increased oxygen supply to the myocardium in response to increased demand during exercise as well as assessing the overall exercise capacity of the patient. Initial results from exercise ECG studies suggested an extremely accurate test which could clearly distinguish between those patients with normal arteries and those patients with coronary disease (Mason *et al.*, 1967). These studies were, however, derived in a patient population where the prevalence of disease was high and since then different authors have reported different predictive values for the exercise ECG depending on the patient population studied and the criteria of abnormality adopted (Redwood *et al.*, 1976; Baron *et al.* 1980; Epstein, 1978).

Bruce and his colleagues from Seattle (Bruce, 1974; Bruce *et al.*, 1980) emphasize that analysis of the tests should look not only at the ECG changes but also haemodynamic data and other important variables as an aid to correct diagnosis, and it is only by adopting a Bayesian approach (Hamilton, 1979; Diamond and Forrester, 1979; Epstein 1980) to the analysis of these non-invasive tests that their accuracy can be maintained, particularly in groups of patients where the prevalence of disease is relatively low. This is particularly important when considering thallium scintigraphy where the results of exercise testing in a particular individual provide the pre-test probability of disease when analysing the thallium images, thereby increasing the accuracy of the study.

2.2 PROTOCOL FOR EXERCISE TESTING

All studies should be carried out in the presence of a qualified doctor and the following should be available:

Equipment
Exercise machine (treadmill/bicycle ergometer)
ECG machine
Sphygmomanometer
Cardiac monitor
Defibrillator
Couch and chair
Syringes and needles
Ambu-bag/endotracheal tube
Intravenous-giving set and dextrose saline

Drugs
Intravenous β-blockers
Intravenous nitroglycerine or isosorbide dinitrate
Verapamil
Frusemide
Amiodarone
Digoxin
Heparin
Glucose
Sodium bicarbonate
Calcium chloride
Isoprenaline
Adrenaline 1 : 10 000
Atropine 0.6 mg
Potassium chloride
Lignocaine
Glyceryl trinitrate

Data from the study may be recorded from a single V5 chest lead or from the three CM leads on a multiple lead system. The predicted accuracy of the test may be improved by using multiple leads but this is only seen clearly when the group of patients studied has a high pre-test probability of coronary disease. Continuous blood pressure recordings must be assessed as an index of left ventricular response to stress. An inability to increase systolic blood pressure indicates severely compromised left ventricular function and this observation by itself was the best predictor of prognosis in the early Seattle Heart Watch study.

All patients should be advised to take a light diet four hours prior to the study and testing should not be carried out on those patients with intercurrent infections. The following precautions should be taken to minimize any morbidity and mortality associated with the study.

(a) The clinical history, examination and resting ECG findings should always be reviewed before starting the test. This should identify those high-risk groups with valvar heart disease, recent myocardial infarction, systemic hypertension, a history of ventricular arrhythmias or conduction abnormalities and any patient with severely impaired left ventricular function. Any necessary precautions can then be taken and a limited study performed if clinically appropriate (Bruce, 1974; Bruce *et al.*, 1980).

(b) The ECG, pulse rate and blood pressure response must be carefully monitored throughout the study.

The following are absolute and relative end points for terminating the study:

Absolute end points

Progressive angina at least as severe as that which would normally cause the patient to stop exercise activity
Fall in systolic blood pressure or heart rate
Severe dyspnoea or faintness especially if the patient looks pale and clammy
Ventricular tachycardia (or fibrillation)

Relative end points

Chest pain in the absence of ST segment change
Fatigue
Unsteadiness (reassurance or repeat test often necessary in the elderly)
Marked ST segment depression > 3 mm
Atrial arrhythmias, ventricular extrasystoles
Marked elevation of blood pressure (unless the patient is an athlete)
Attainment of predicted maximal heart rate
Development of high-grade atrioventricular (AV) block

The nature and purpose of the study should be fully explained to the patient beforehand and in many centres informed consent is mandatory. Each patient is instructed to exercise until forced to stop because of general fatigue, dyspnoea, chest pain, muscle fatigue or other symptoms, and in the vast majority of tests these subjective end points prevent further exercise (Bruce *et al.*, 1980).

(c) All patients should be examined after completing the exercise test to detect any transient abnormality of left ventricular function, such as an added third or fourth heart sound.

(d) No changes should be made in drug therapy before the test. If β-blockade is withdrawn, not only is the risk of possible myocardial infarction increased but predictive accuracy of the study may be lessened (Marcomichelakis *et al.*, 1980).

2.3 MAXIMAL EXERCISE PROTOCOLS

The following may be used.

1. Bicycle ergometer:
   (a) initial stage of 25 W (150 kpm) min^{-1} for 3 min;
   (b) increasing workload every 3 min by 25 W min^{-1} until a standard end point has been achieved.
2. Calibrated motor-driven treadmill. Of the different protocols available, the following are most commonly used:
   (a) Bruce protocol (Seattle Heart Watch treadmill test) varying speed and gradient:

Test phase	*Duration (min)*	*Speed (mile h^{-1})*	*Grade (%)*
1	3	1.7	10
2	3	2.5	12
3	3	3.4	14
4	3	4.2	16
5	3	5.0	18
6	3	5.5	20
7	3	6.0	22

(*cont'd*)

Table 2.3 cont'd

(b) Modified Bruce protocol – varying speed and/or gradient:

1	3	1.7	0
2	3	1.7	5
3	3	1.7	10
4	3	2.5	12
5	3	3.4	14
6	3	4.2	16
7	3	5.0	18
8	3	5.5	20
9	3	6.0	22

(c) Unit MET protocol – varying speed and/or gradient:

1	3	1	0
2	3	2	0
3	3	2	3.5
4	3	2	7.0
5	3	2	10.5
6	3	2	14.0
7	3	2	17.5
8	3	3	12.5
9	3	3	15.0
10	3	3	17.5
11	3	3	20.0
12	3	3	22.5

Any of these protocols may be used for submaximal exercise testing if appropriate. The only additional end points to those already described are a suitable workload limitation (e.g. 100 W min^{-1}: test phase 5) or the achievement of 70% of the age-predicted maximal heart rate for that individual as shown in the table below.

Age	*Predicted maximal heart rate*	
	Male	*Female*
20	200	195
30	190	186
40	180	178
50	170	166
60	160	157
70	150	148
80	140	138

1.4 ANALYSIS OF RESULTS

The following ECG changes should be evaluated.

1. Changes in the ST segment. These should be recorded from the preceding PQ segment. Significant ST depression includes:
   (a) horizontal or downsloping shift of 1 mm or more persisting 1 min or longer into the recovery phase of the test;
   (b) ST shift which although upsloping remains depressed by 1 mm or more 0.08 s from the end of the QRS complex and which persists for 3 min or more into the recovery period (Bruce *et al.*, 1980). ST segment elevation should be measured 0.06 s from the preceding QRS complex and is significant when greater than or equal to 1 mm.

The following criteria may be considered for further information.

2. Changes in R wave amplitude. In normal patients, the R wave amplitude decreases with exercise. Recent studies (Berman *et al.*, 1980; Bonoris *et al.* 1978a, 1978b; Yiannikas *et al.*, 1981) suggest that when the sum of R wave amplitudes remains the same or increases during exercise this identifies those patients with coronary artery disease (CAD) as accurately as measuring ST segment changes, although these results were obtained in patient populations where the prevalence of disease was high. R wave analysis may be particularly helpful in assessing patients with bundle branch block (Uhl and Hopkirk, 1979) or those taking digitalis (Berman *et al.*, 1980), where the interpretation of ST segment changes is unreliable.
3. Duration of exercise and total work performed.
4. Development of anginal chest pain or discomfort at maximal exercise.
5. Appropriate haemodynamic response to exercise.
6. ST segment/heart rate relationship. Linden and Mary from the University of Leeds suggested in the late 1970s that careful analysis of the maximal ST/heart rate slope would not only accurately identify those patients with coronary disease but also subdivide them into those with single, double and triple vessel disease. Their approach is clearly summarized in a recent review article (Bishop *et al.*, 1987) although there are conflicting results from other groups who have not been able to report these findings in different patient populations (Thwaites *et al.*, 1986; Kligfield *et al.*, 1986). More data from different centres are needed before this approach can be recommended for general

use, particularly since the analysis is time consuming. It will be interesting to see if the overall specificity declines in new published series as the tested population changes, as described in the declining specificity for exercise radionuclide ventriculography during the last ten years (Rozanski *et al.*, 1984). The results from the Seattle Heart Watch study (Bruce, 1971) suggest that the only variables of value in predicting possible myocardial infarction within five years were significant ST changes, a failure to achieve 70% of the age-predicted heart rate, the development of chest pain or limited duration of exercise. Indeed, any patient unable to complete more than 6 min of the modified Bruce protocol on the treadmill had significant impairment of left ventricular function if limited by dyspnoea of cardiac origin.

2.4 INTERPRETATION OF RESULTS

The predictive accuracy of any non-invasive test in correctly identifying those patients with coronary artery disease depends not only upon the sensitivity and specificity of the test but also upon the prevalence of disease in the population studied.

Results of exercise testing in a varied population (Chaitman *et al.*, 1979; Chaitman and Hanson, 1981; Epstein *et al.*, 1979) emphasize the importance of a Bayesian approach to the analysis of any non-invasive test. When using this concept of conditional probability to improve diagnostic information a positive or negative test result is of little value unless related to the pre-test probability of disease in that individual. For example, given a positive test result, the post-test probability of CAD in a 16-year-old girl with atypical chest pain is minimal, yet the same findings in a 55-year-old man who smokes heavily and has typical anginal pain make it virtually certain that he has obstructive CAD.

All post-test probability statements of disease are based upon the detection sensitivity and specificity figures for that particular test. The assumption that these figures remain constant over a wider range of clinical subgroups with different disease prevalences has been queried (Ransohoff and Feinstein, 1978; Weiner *et al.*, 1979) particularly by a recent study from Duke University (Hlatky *et al.*, 1984). The importance of a correct approach to the analysis of the data has been clearly summarized by Diamond (1986a,b), and reference criteria for disease should be established for different subgroups studied by the individual

Table 2.1 Sensitivity and specificity of diagnostic tests for angiographically significant coronary artery disease (data from Diamond and Forrester, 1979)

Procedure	*No. of patients*	*Criterion*	*Sensitivity (% ± 1 SEP)**	*Specificity (% ± 1 SEP)*
Electrocardiographic stress	4838	Flat or downsloping ST depression 0.08 min after R wave		
		0.5 mm	14.3 ± 3.3	37.5 ± 5.7
		1.0 mm	20.8 ± 3.4	77.3 ± 5.8
		1.5 mm	23.3 ± 2.5	89.0 ± 1.4
		2.0 mm	8.8 ± 2.9	97.9 ± 1.3
		2.5 mm	13.3 ± 2.3	98.8 ± 0.8
		2.5 mm	19.5 ± 1.6	99.5 ± 0.5
Cardiac fluoroscopy	507	Coronary calcification (vessels)		
		0	42.0 ± 2.5	3.9 ± 1.7
		1	23.5 ± 2.2	97.7 ± 1.3
		2	20.1 ± 2.1	98.4 ± 1.1
		3	14.5 ± 1.8	100.0 ± 0.0
Stressed thallium scintigraphy	1132	Perfusion defect		
		None	14.7 ± 1.7	16.4 ± 3.1
		Fixed	14.6 ± 2.6	89.7 ± 3.4
		Reversible	70.7 ± 1.9	93.9 ± 1.3

*SEP, standard error of percentage.

Table 2.2 Asymptomatic 50-year-old man: pre-test likelihood of coronary artery disease = 9.7 ± 0.4%

Test performed	*Result*	*Post-test likelihood*	
Exercise ECG stress	ST depression 2 mm		
Chest X-ray	Calcification in right coronary artery	99.3	0.8%
Thallium scintigraphy	Normal study	96.1	4.3%
Thallium scintigraphy	Abnormal study	99.9	0.1%

laboratory if the predictive accuracy of the test is to be maintained.

Before analysing the results of any test, the pre-test likelihood of disease should therefore be assessed from a careful clinical history and physical examination (Diamond and Forrester, 1979). The appropriate detection sensitivity and specificity figures for exercise testing in that particular population are then used to define the post-test probability of disease given a positive or negative test result, using the criteria already discussed (Table 2.1). This probability estimate may then be used as the pre-test probability figure when interpreting the results of further non-invasive studies in the same patient such as ^{201}Tl scintigraphy. This scheme is best illustrated by the example in Table 2.2 from Diamond and Forrester's original paper.

In this way the minimum number of these less-than-perfect tests can be used to derive the maximum diagnostic information, offering savings both in time and cost of the studies for an individual patient. Those patients with typical symptoms in whom the pre-test probability of disease is extremely high should be offered coronary arteriography to delineate the anatomical extent of their disease if clinically appropriate, since this will to a large extent determine their subsequent medical or surgical management. This will also identify the small number of patients with entirely normal coronary arteries in this group who cannot be categorically reassured following non-invasive testing. When patients present with atypical symptoms, however, and the pre-test probability of disease is much lower, coronary arteriography may be premature since many of this group have normal coronary arteries and can be spared an invasive investigation by appropriate use of non-invasive tests. This approach to the investigation of patients presenting with chest pain precludes a simple 'yes' or 'no' diagnostic statement to the referring physician but does provide a reliable assessment of the probability that an individual patient has normal coronary arteries or significant CAD.

REFERENCES

Baron, D. W. *et al.* (1980) Maximal 12 lead exercise testing for prediction of severity of coronary artery disease. *Eur. J. Cardiol.*, **11**, 259–67.

Berman, J. L. *et al.* (1980) Multiple lead QRS changes with exercise testing: diagnostic value and haemodynamic implications. *Circulation*, **61**, 53–61.

Bishop, N., Adlakha, M. L., Boyle, R. M. *et al.* (1987) The segment/heart rate relationship as an index of myocardial ischaemia. *Int. J. Cardiol.* **14**, 281–93.

Bonoris, P. E., Greenbergh, P. S., Castallanet, M. J. and Ellestad, M. M. (1978a) Significance of changes in R wave amplitude during treadmill stress testing: angiographic correlation. *Am. J. Cardiol.*, **41**, 846–51.

Bonoris, P. E., Greenbergh, P. S., Christison, G. W. *et al.* (1978b) Evaluation of R wave amplitude changes versus ST segment depression in stress testing. *Circulation*, **57**, 904–10.

Bousfield, G. (1918) Angina pectoris: variations in electrocardiograms during paroxysm. *Lancet*, 195: 457.

Bruce, R. A. (1971) Exercise testing of patients with coronary heart disease: principles and normal standards for evaluation. *Ann. Clin. Res.*, **3**, 323–32.

Bruce, R. A. (1974) Values and limitations of exercise electrocardiography. *Circulation*, **50**, 1–3.

Bruce, R. A. *et al.* (1980) Value of maximal exercise tests in risk assessment of primary coronary heart disease events in healthy men: 5 years experience of the Seattle Heart Watch study. *Am. J. Cardiol.*, **46**, 371–8.

Chaitman, B. R. and Hanson, J. S. (1981) Comparative sensitivity and specificity of exercise electrocardiographic lead systems. *Am. J. Cardiol.*, **47**, 1335–49.

Chaitman, B. R. *et al.* (1979) The importance of clinical subsets in interpreting maximal treadmill exercise test results: the role of multiple lead systems. *Circulation*, **59**, 560–70.

Diamond, G. A. (1986a) Monkey business. *Am. J. Cardiol.*, **57**, 471–5.

Diamond, G. A. (1986b) Reverend Bayes' silent majority: an alternative factor affecting sensitivity and specificity of exercise electrocardiography. *Am. J. Cardiol.*, **57**, 1175–80.

Diamond, G. A. and Forrester, J. S. (1979) Analysis of probability as an aid in clinical diagnosis of coronary artery disease. *N. Engl. J. Med.*, **300**, 1350–8.

Epstein, S. E. (1978) Value and limitations of the electrocardiographic response to exercise in the assessment of patients with coronary artery disease. *Am. J. Cardiol.*, **42**, 667–74.

Epstein, S. E. (1980) Implications of probability analysis on the strategy used for non-invasive detection of coronary artery disease. *Am. J. Cardiol.*, **46**, 491–9.

Epstein, S. E. *et al.* (1979) Strategy for evaluation and surgical treatment of the asymptomatic or mildly symptomatic patient with coronary artery disease. *Am. J. Cardiol.*, **43** 1015–25.

Hamilton, G. W. (1979) Myocardial imaging with thallium-201: the controversy over its clinical usefulness in ischaemic heart disease. *J. Nucl. Med.*, **20**, 1201–5.

Hlatky, M. A., Pryor, D. B., Marrell, F. E. *et al.* (1984) Factors affecting sensitivity and specificity of exercise electrocardiography: multivariable analysis. *Am. J. Med.*, **77**, 64–71.

Kligfield, P., Okin, P. M., Ameisen, O. and Borer, J. S. (1986) Evaluation of coronary artery disease by an improved method of exercise electrocardiography: the ST segment/heart rate slope. *Am. Heart J.*, **112**, 589–98.

Marcomichelakis, J. *et al.* (1980) Exercise testing after beta blockade: improved specificity and predictive value in detecting coronary heart disease. *Br. Heart J.*, **43**, 252–61.

Mason, R. E. *et al.* (1967) Multiple lead exercise electrocardiography: experiences in 107 normal subjects and 67 patients with angina pectoris and comparison with coronary cinearteriography in 84 patients. *Circulation*, **36**, 517–25.

Redwood, D. R. *et al.* (1976) Whither the ST segment during exercise. *Circulation*, **54**, 703–6.

Rojanski, A., Diamond, G. A., Forrester, J. S. *et al.* (1984) Alternative referent standards for cardiac normality. *Ann. Intern Med.*, **101**, 164–71.

Thwaites, B. C. (1986) Comparison of the ST/heart rate slope with the modified Bruce exercise test in the detection of coronary artery disease. *Am. J. Cardiol.*, **57**, 554–6.

Uhl, G. S. and Hopkirk, A. C. (1979) Analysis of exercise induced R wave amplitude changes in detection of coronary artery disease in asymptomatic men with left bundle branch block. *Am. J. Cardiol.*, **44**, 1247–50.

Weiner, D. A. *et al.* (1979) Correlations among history of angina, ST segment respone and prevalence of coronary artery disease in the coronary artery surgery study *N. Engl. J. Med.*, **301**, 230–5.

Yiannikas, J. *et al.* (1981) Analysis of exercise induced changes in R wave amplitude in asymptomatic men with electrocardiographic SR-T changes at rest. *Am. J. Cardiol.*, **47**, 238–43.

CHAPTER THREE

Lung scanning

S. E. M. Clarke and R. H. Secker-Walker

3.1 INTRODUCTION

For many years, the main use of radionuclide lung imaging has been the detection of pulmonary emboli. Recently, the development of new ventilation tracers has broadened the clinical use of lung scanning to include the investigation of regional ventilation, the assessment of alveolar clearance and the evaluation of patients prior to surgery.

3.1.1 ANATOMY AND PHYSIOLOGY

Respiration, the primary function of the lung, involves the gaseous exchange of oxygen and carbon dioxide by diffusion between the alveoli and the pulmonary capillary blood. During breathing, air enters by the nose and mouth and passes through the glottis to the trachea and thence by the main bronchi and their branches, the bronchioles, to the terminal or respiratory bronchioles. The respiratory bronchioles in turn give rise to alveolar ducts which lead to alveoli. The 300 million pulmonary alveoli consist of thin epithelial cells which lie in immediate proximity to the numerous pulmonary capillaries.

The gaseous exchanges across the alveolar–capillary membrane occur solely by diffusion which in turn depends on the difference in partial pressure of the gas across the membrane and on the area and thickness of the membrane.

The lungs are divided into self-contained fundamentally independent units of lung tissue called bronchopulmonary segments – each segment is supplied by a bronchus and a branch of one of the pulmonary arteries. The pulmonary veins, however, lie between bronchopulmonary segments and each segment is drained by more than one vein. The bronchopulmonary segment therefore constitutes a respiratory unit within the lung but is not a bronchovascular unit.

During quiet breathing a healthy man inspires and expires about 500 ml of air. The inspiratory reserve volume is the maximal volume of air that can be inspired from the end-inspiratory position (2000–3200 ml) and the expiratory reserve volume is the maximal volume of air that can be expired after normal tidal inspiration (750–1000 ml). The remaining volume of gas remaining in the lungs after a maximal expiration is the residual volume (1200 ml).

Efficient gaseous exchange between alveoli and pulmonary capillary blood necessitates perfusion of the alveoli by the pulmonary capillary bloodstream. Since approximately 4 litres of air ventilate the alveoli each minute and 5 litres of blood pass through the pulmonary capillaries in the same time, the mean ventilation perfusion ratio is 4/5 or 0.8.

3.1.2 REGIONAL VENTILATION

The regional distribution of ventilation depends on regional compliance and regional airways resistance. In healthy human lungs, in the upright position, ventilation per unit lung volume increase 1.5- to 2-fold from the upper zones to the bases. The compliance of an alveolus determines, in part, its volume and airways characteristics. The volume of an alveolus is determined by the balance between its inflation pressure and the elastic recoil of its wall. The alveolar compliance is measured by its volume change in response to a given pressure change (V/P). Low compliance due to interstitial fibrosis or fluid results in the exchange of a large fraction of alveolar volume with each respiration whereas alveoli with increased compliance, as found in chronic obstructive airways disease, have reduced wall integrity and exchange a smaller fraction of their internal volume during respiration.

Regional airways resistance is another factor influencing the distribution of lung ventilation. For a given change in inflation pressure, gas flow is usually related to airways resistance. Increased airways resistance may be caused by bronchospasm, foreign bodies, extrinsic airways compression, parenchymal strictures, increased secretions and loss of supporting lung tissue.

Other factors that influence the distribution of ventilation include minute ventilation rate, inhalation rate, lung volume and patient position. Patient position in particular has a significant effect on the distribution of pulmonary ventilation because of the gravitational influences on alveolar size. In the upright position, the lung bases are compressed by the weight of the lung itself and the alveoli are less distended than those at the lung apices where the more negative intrapleural pressure makes the alveoli larger and less compliant. The effect of these changes in intrapleural pressure is that the alveoli at the apices ventilate less well than those at the bases. In the supine position regional ventilation changes so that lower-most alveoli ventilate more efficiently than the upper.

3.1.3 REGIONAL PERFUSION

Regional distribution of the blood flow depends on the relationship between alveolar pressure, pulmonary artery pressure and interstitial pressure. It is influenced by gravity and by the structural support of the lungs within the chest. Local pulmonary blood flow is affected by intravascular and perivascular pressures and vascular resistance. Conditions that cause local changes in vascular resistance such as hypoxia, perivascular oedema or pulmonary emboli will reduce local blood flow.

3.1.4 PULMONARY EPITHELIAL PERMEABILITY

The alveolar capillary membrane is composed of the capillary endothelium and the alveolar epithelium. Gas exchange occurs across segments of the membrane where epithelium and endothelium are fused to form a common basement membrane. Fluid exchange in the lung is determined by the diffences in intravascular and interstitial hydrostatic and oncotic pressure and by the permeability of the capillary endothelium and alveolar membrane. Changes in the integrity of either membrane will cause an increase in movement of fluid and protein and may result in high-permeability pulmonary oedema. Hyaline membrane disease in the infant and adult respiratory distress syndrome (ARDS) are both clinical examples of high-permeability pulmonary oedema. More recently increased permeability has been demonstrated in patients with interstitial lung disease, asbestosis and sarcoidosis and also in cigarette smokers.

3.2 RADIOTRACERS

3.2.1 PERFUSION

Perfusion lung imaging depends on the embolization of radiolabelled particles, 20–40 μm in diameter, in the pulmonary arterial circulation. The pulmonary arterioles act as a sieve so that the amount of particulate matter impacted is proportional to the pulmonary artery flow to that region. An area of reduced perfusion will be visualized as an area of decreased activity on the image. Although embolization by labelled particles causes a transient reduction in blood flow, this is physiologically insignificant as only 200 000–500 000 particles are distributed into approximately 280 million pulmonary arterioles. Since the particles are biodegradable, the occlusion is temporary and the breakdown products are phagocytosed by the cells of the reticuloendothelial system.

The most commonly used radiotracer is ^{99m}Tc-labelled macroaggregates; 90% have a diameter within 10–40 μm. ^{99m}Tc-labelled microspheres, diameter 20–40 μm, may also be used although allergic reactions have occasionally been reported.

3.2.2 VENTILATION

In 1955 Knipping *et al.* pioneered the use of ^{133}Xe to study lung ventilation. Since then, a number of radiotracers have been used, each with different characteristics and each having specific advantages and disadvantages.

^{133}Xe remains the most commonly used means of ventilation imaging, as it is inexpensive, readily available and has a convenient half-life. By imaging during the wash-in phase, at equilibrium and during xenon wash-out, functional information may be obtained about global and regional ventilation with the distribution of activity in the equilibrium image corresponding to aerated lung volume and areas with impaired ventilation showing as areas of reduced activity on wash-in views and as areas of retention on the wash-out images. ^{133}Xe has several disadvantages, however, including a low principal γ-energy (80 keV) which makes soft tissue absorption a greater problem than with a higher energy of ^{99m}Tc (140 keV), and β-particle emission which increases the radiation dose to the patient and makes the safe discharge of the exhaled gas essential to minimize radiation doses to staff. Furthermore, images in one projection only can be obtained and it is generally accepted that this should be performed before the perfusion studies are undertaken.

^{127}Xe is now widely available. It has the advantages of a higher photon energy (172 keV) and can therefore be used after perfusion images have been acquired. Its long half-life (36.3 days) gives it an advantage of availability but the combination of some high γ-emissions with the long half-life increase the radiation burden to patients and staff and necessitate the use of a higher-energy collimator.

^{81m}Kr has become the ventilation imaging agent of choice in many centres. The 190 keV γ-photon is ideal for imaging and yield images that are similar in quality to the ^{99m}Tc perfusion images. Its short half-life of 13 s requires its administration by constant inhalation and the distribution of activity therefore represents regional ventilation per unit lung volume. No wash-in or wash-out information can be obtained from an ^{81m}Kr study, but imaging in multiple projections can be obtained. A serious disadvantage of ^{81m}Kr is that it is obtained from an ^{85m}Rb generator which is cyclotron produced and its availability is limited to centres which are reasonably close to a supplying cyclotron. It is also usually only available once or twice per week.

A ^{99m}Tc-labelled ventilation agent is obviously highly desirable and attempts to produce such an agent have resulted in the development of ^{99m}Tc-labelled aerosols first used by Pircher *et al.* (1965) and Taplin and Poe (1965). The technology of aerosol production has now advanced enough to ensure the consistent production of submicrometre monodispersed particles that will penetrate the lung peripheries with minimal central deposition. Whilst aerosols provide adequate information in the majority of patients, the images do not represent the pattern of ventilation within the lungs and pathology such as airways narrowing will result in aerosol deposition centrally which may seriously affect image quality.

A further new development is that of ^{99m}Tc-labelled fine carbon particles, which are smaller in size than aerosols and therefore penetrate more efficiently to the lung peripheries. Clinical trials on this new agent are now in progress.

3.3 PULMONARY EMBOLISM

The clinical suspicion of pulmonary emboli remains in the early 1990s the chief indication for the performance of ventilation perfusion scanning in most nuclear medicine departments. The clinical significance of pulmonary emboli has been assessed by Benotti *et al.* in the large USA survey in 1983. They demonstrated that the annual incidence in the USA is 630 000 cases with 11% of these patients dying within the first hour of the acute event. In one-third of the remaining cases, a diagnosis will be confirmed and treatment instigated, with a death rate in the treated group of 8%. In the two-thirds of cases where no diagnosis is made, and therefore no treatment instigated, 120 000 will die subsequently, of which it is estimated that 100 000 deaths could be avoided with diagnosis and treatment.

The method of detection of pulmonary emboli has surprisingly changed little in the past twenty years, with radionuclide methods offering the only non-invasive technique with an acceptable sensitivity. The invasive alternative of pulmonary angiography remains the diagnostic gold standard, with its attendant morbidity.

3.3.1 PATHOLOGY OF PULMONARY EMBOLI

Pulmonary emboli originate from thrombi developing in the deep veins of the legs or pelvis. Patients are particularly at risk of developing deep-vein thrombosis during periods of prolonged bed rest and at the time of surgery, particularly gynaecological or orthopaedic involving the hips. Because of the high incidence of deep-vein thromboses and subsequent pulmonary emboli in these at-risk groups, prophylaxis in the form of antithrombotic stockings, early post-operative mobilization, physiotherapy and low-dose heparin have reduced the morbidity and mortality from pulmonary emboli over the last twenty years.

3.3.2 CLINICAL FEATURES

The classical symptoms of pulmonary embolus include sudden onset of pleuritic chest pain, acute shortness of breath, haemoptysis and, in the case of large pulmonary emboli occluding more than 50–60% of the pulmonary circulation, syncope. Death occurs suddenly if more than 80% of the circulation is blocked. Signs are those of tachypnoea and right heart strain with elevation of the jugular venous pressure, right third or fourth heart sound and on auscultation of the chest a pleural rub. An electrocardiogram (ECG) will confirm right heart strain and the chest X-ray may demonstrate an oligaemic segment of the lung if the embolus is large, or a small basal effusion with a linear atelectasis with smaller emboli. In many cases of proven pulmonary emboli, however, the presentation is far from classical, with gradual onset of breathlessness and minimal chest pain. Since there is a significant mortality in untreated patients, the diagnosis of pulmonary embolus is clinically important and it is for this reason that radionuclide imaging techniques for the detection of pulmonary emboli have gained widespread acceptance.

3.3.3 MANAGEMENT

Following the diagnosis of a pulmonary embolus, resuscitation techniques may be used in the case of large emboli to maintain right ventricular filling pressure and cardiac output. The patient is anticoagulated using an intravenous infusion of heparin and anticoagulation maintained using oral warfarin. The duration of anticoagulation will vary with the circumstances of the patient but a minimum of six weeks is generally accepted and the usual duration of treatment is three to six months. Throughout this period, the prothrombin time is regularly monitored to ensure that the patient remains anticoagulated without running the risks of haemorrhage from overtreatment.

3.3.4 DIAGNOSIS OF PULMONARY EMBOLISM USING VENTILATION–PERFUSION IMAGING

The diagnosis of pulmonary embolic disease using radionuclide techniques is achieved by straining images of both perfusion and ventilation of the lungs. In pulmonary emboli occlusion of segmental arterioles occurs but ventilation to these areas of lungs with reduced perfusion is virtually unchanged. The images will therefore demonstrate areas of mismatch, i.e. areas of lung that are ventilated but not perfused. Although these lesions may be solitary, the classical appearance is of bilateral segmental perfusion defects, tending to affect the basal segments more than the apical. Views in multiple projections should be obtained to adequately visualize all lung segments; the six usual projections are anterior, posterior, right and left lateral, and right and left posterior oblique (Figure 3.1). Wellman *et al.* (1968) have shown that 12% of pulmonary emboli will be missed if oblique views are not performed. Although the presence of multiple perfusion defects in both lungs is highly suggestive of pulmonary emboli in the presence of a normal X-ray with a true positive rate of 75–80%, the true negative rate is only 64% (Alderson *et al.* 1976, 1980). If a ventilation scan is performed at the same time as the perfusion scan, however, the true positive and true negative rates are increased to 90% (Figures 3.2 and 3.3).

The need to perform ventilation–perfusion imaging as soon as possible after the onset of symptoms must be stressed. Large pulmonary emboli commonly break down and disperse to the lung peripheries within several days of the acute event and a delay in imaging will reduce the sensitivity of the technique. If a perfusion scan is performed initially without ventilation, the perfusion scan should be repeated when the ventilation scan is performed to ensure a true comparison of ventilation and perfusion.

It is a common misconception that the sensitivity for the detection of pulmonary emboli in patients with chronic obstructive airways disease is low. Whilst the classical changes of parenchymal lung disease are matched ventilation–perfusion defects, the finding of normal perfusion in a patient with chronic obstructive airways disease will make the probability of that patient having pulmonary emboli extremely low. It is also possible to distinguish segmental areas of

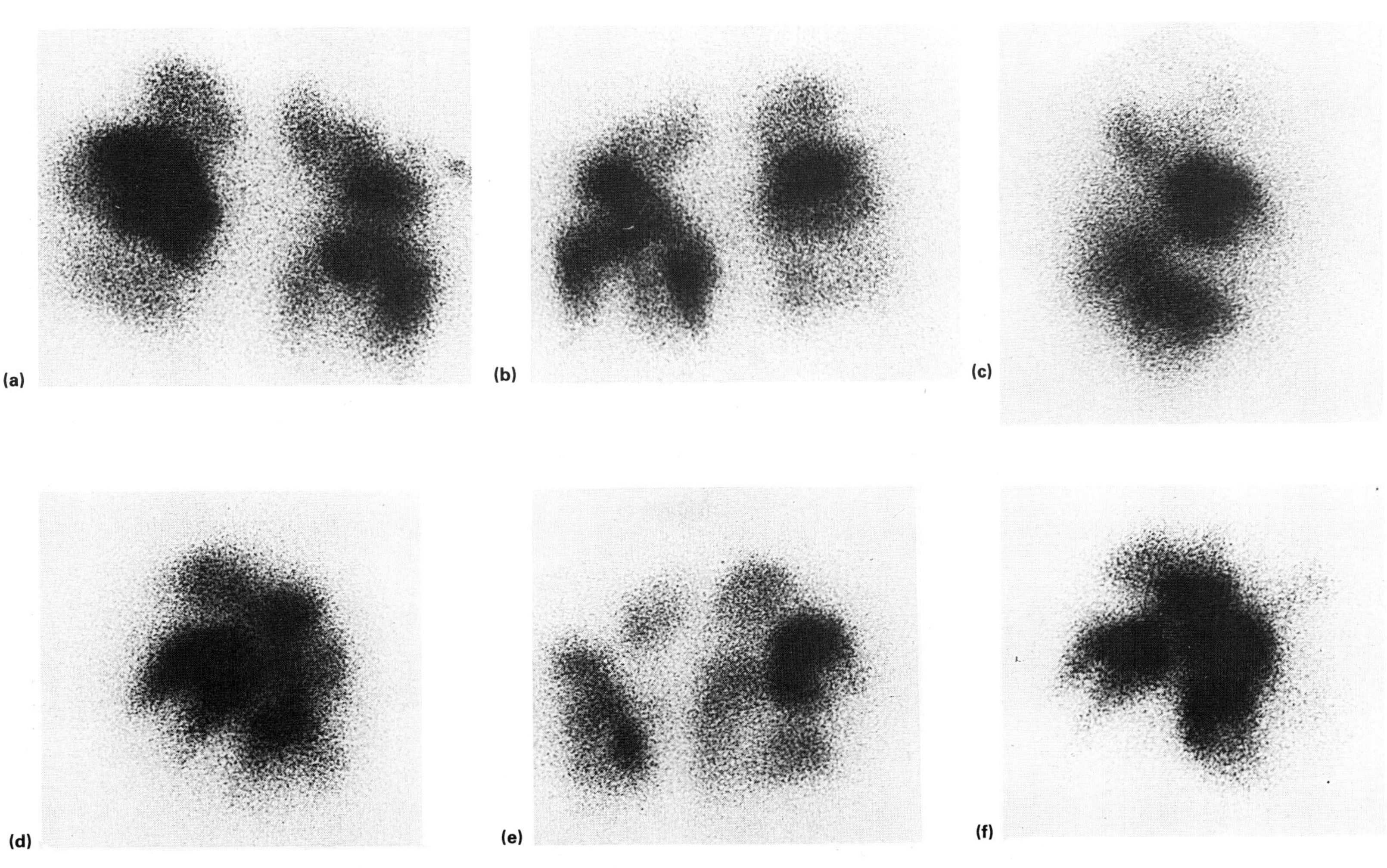

Figure 3.1 Female, 43 years old, with sudden onset of severe pleuritic chest pain and a normal chest X-ray. Perfusion lung scans show multiple bilateral segmental defects. Diagnosis of multiple pulmonary emboli made. (a) Anterior; (b) posterior; (c) right lateral; (d) left lateral; (e) right posterior oblique; and (f) left posterior oblique projections.

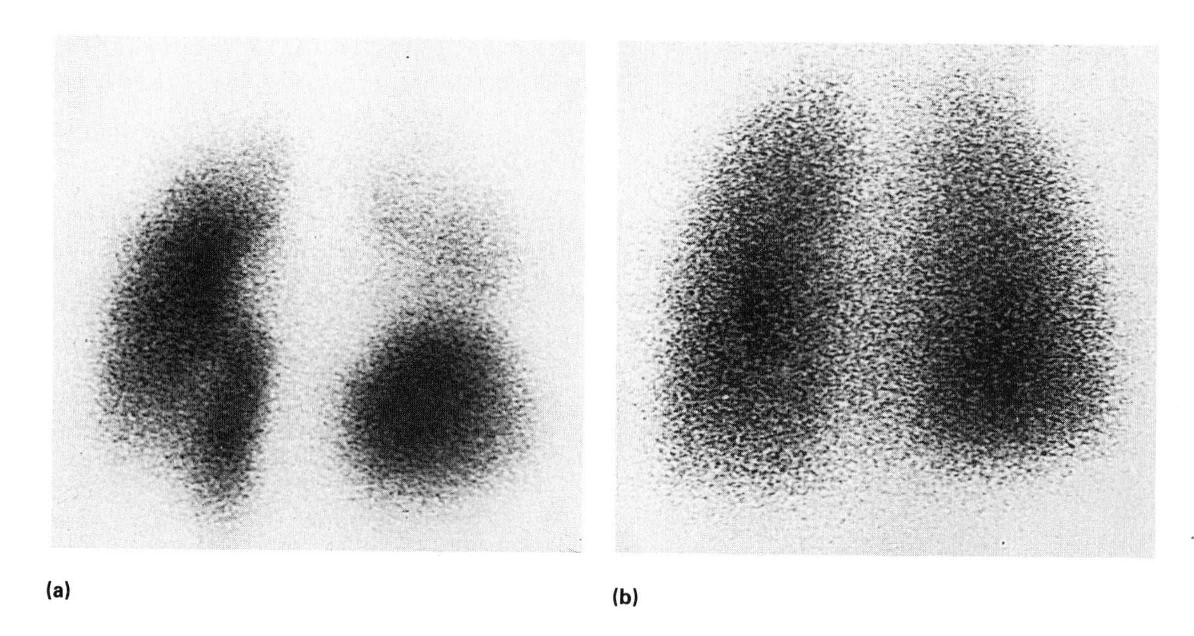

(a) (b)

Figure 3.2 Female, 72 years old, with known carcinoma of the rectum, with bone and groin lymph node metastases and lymphoedema of the left leg. Two-day history of pleuritic chest pain, dyspnoea and ECG changes. Posterior perfusion imaging (a) demonstrates multiple segmental perfusion abnormalities in both lung fields, with normal ^{81m}Kr ventilation (b) confirming multiple pulmonary emboli.

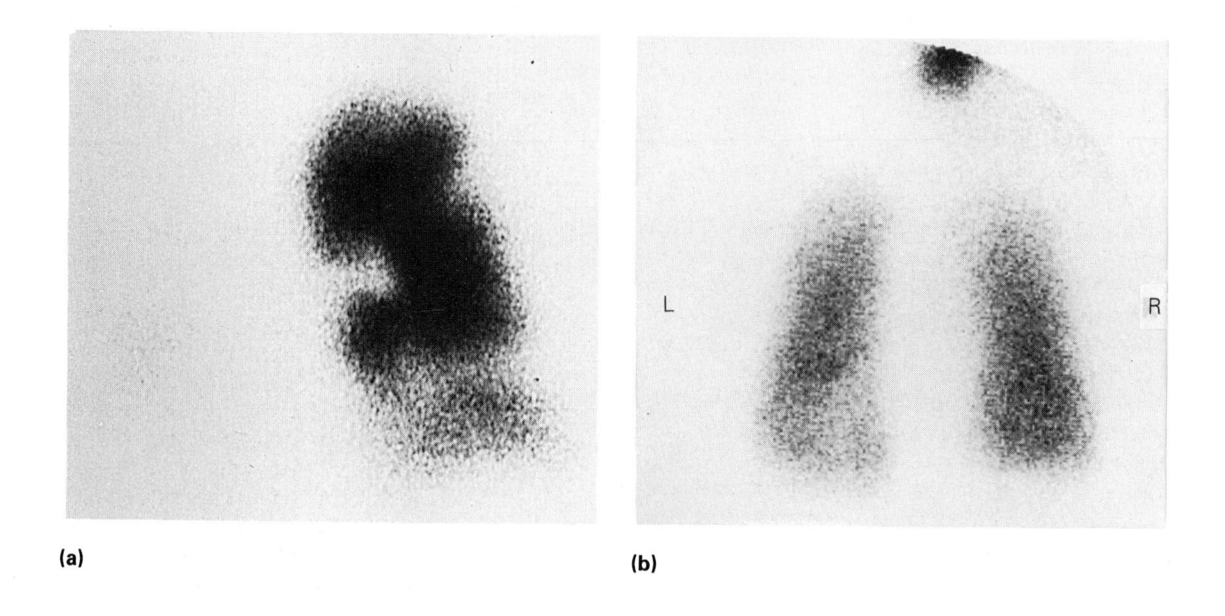

(a) (b)

Figure 3.3 Female, 93 years old, with clinical evidence of deep vein thrombosis (DVT) in the right leg and a sudden onset of chest pain and collapse. Posterior perfusion image (a) shows virtually absent perfusion of the left lung with further segmental defects in the right lung. The posterior ventilation image (b) was normal, confirming multiple pulmonary emboli including a major embolus obstructing the left main pulmonary artery.

mismatch, coexistent with matched defects in patients with pulmonary emboli and chronic obstructive airways disease. A diagnosis of chronic obstructive airways disease therefore is not a contraindication to performing a ventilation–perfusion scan for the detection of pulmonary emboli (Figure 3.4).

3.3.5 DIAGNOSTIC CRITERIA

A number of studies have been reported that attempt to define the interpretative criteria that should be used to ascribe a probability rating for diagnosing pulmonary emboli. Bogren *et al.* (1978) compared the relative size of the defect on ventilation and perfusion imaging and defined low- and high-probability studies and an equivocal group. Biello *et al.* (1979) included a current chest X-ray in the assessment of probability and defined three categories: low, intermediate and high probability. In a retrospective study of 146 patients, Biello established that patients with two moderate areas of mismatch (25–75% of a segment) or a large area of mismatch (greater than one segment) have a high probability of pulmonary emboli that is greater than 90%. A low probability for pulmonary emboli exists when the perfusion defects are small and constitute less than 25% of a pulmonary segment, when there are matched focal ventilation–perfusion defects or when there are perfusion defects that are significantly smaller than the X-ray abnormality (Figure 3.5). The probability for the presence of pulmonary emboli is deemed to be intermediate in the presence of severe diffuse airways disease regardless of the nature of the perfusion defect, when the perfusion defects matched the X-ray changes or with a single moderate-sized perfusion defect despite normal ventilation and X-ray. The significance of a single unmatched moderate-sized perfusion defect has been assessed by several groups. Neumann *et al.* (1980) found that these single defects have an intermediate probability of pulmonary emboli. Rosen *et al.* (1985) commented on the problem of the single defect and again found an intermediate probability of pulmonary emboli in patients in this group.

3.3.6 THE RELATIONSHIP OF RADIONUCLIDE IMAGING AND PULMONARY ANGIOGRAPHY

Although pulmonary angiography is the generally accepted gold standard in the diagnosis of pulmonary emboli, a false-negative rate of 5–10% has been demonstrated. False negatives are kept to a minimum by the use of oblique projections with selective injections and magnifications. The complementary nature of the ventilation–perfusion lung scan may thus be appreciated as it provides the information required for the selective placement of the catheter (Bookstein, 1986). The morbidity associated with contrast pulmonary angiography arises from the volume of contrast used and its use in patients with high right atrial pressures (greater than 25 mmHg). The use of selective injection will obviously reduce the volume of contrast required and the use of the new non-ionic contrast media will also reduce the morbidity, although increasing the cost of the procedure. The new technique of digital subtraction angiography has yet to establish its place in the diagnosis of pulmonary emboli.

3.3.7 MANAGEMENT OF PATIENTS FOLLOWING VENTILATION PERFUSION SCAN

Patients in whom the ventilation–perfusion scan demonstrates a high probability of pulmonary emboli should be anticoagulated with intravenous heparin, ideally by slow infusion, followed by oral warfarin, assuming there are no contraindications to anticoagulation. Patients in whom the scan indicates a low probability of pulmonary emboli should be followed by conventional X-rays if their symptoms persist. In the majority of cases, an abnormality will appear with time on X-ray, confirming the parenchymal nature of the pathology. Patients with a scan that yields a result of intermediate probability should be managed according to the *a priori* clinical probability of pulmonary emboli. If a pulmonary embolus remains a high clinical probability, then the patient should either commence anticoagulation therapy immediately or undergo pulmonary angiography to confirm or refute the clinical diagnosis. Hull *et al.* (1986) showed that patients with prior estimates of high probability had an incidence of pulmonary emboli of 79% on pulmonary angiography, those with low probability had an incidence of 15%, and those with intermediate probability an incidence of 38%. In the patient in whom the diagnosis of pulmonary emboli has been made and anticoagulation commenced, a follow-up ventilation–perfusion scan should be

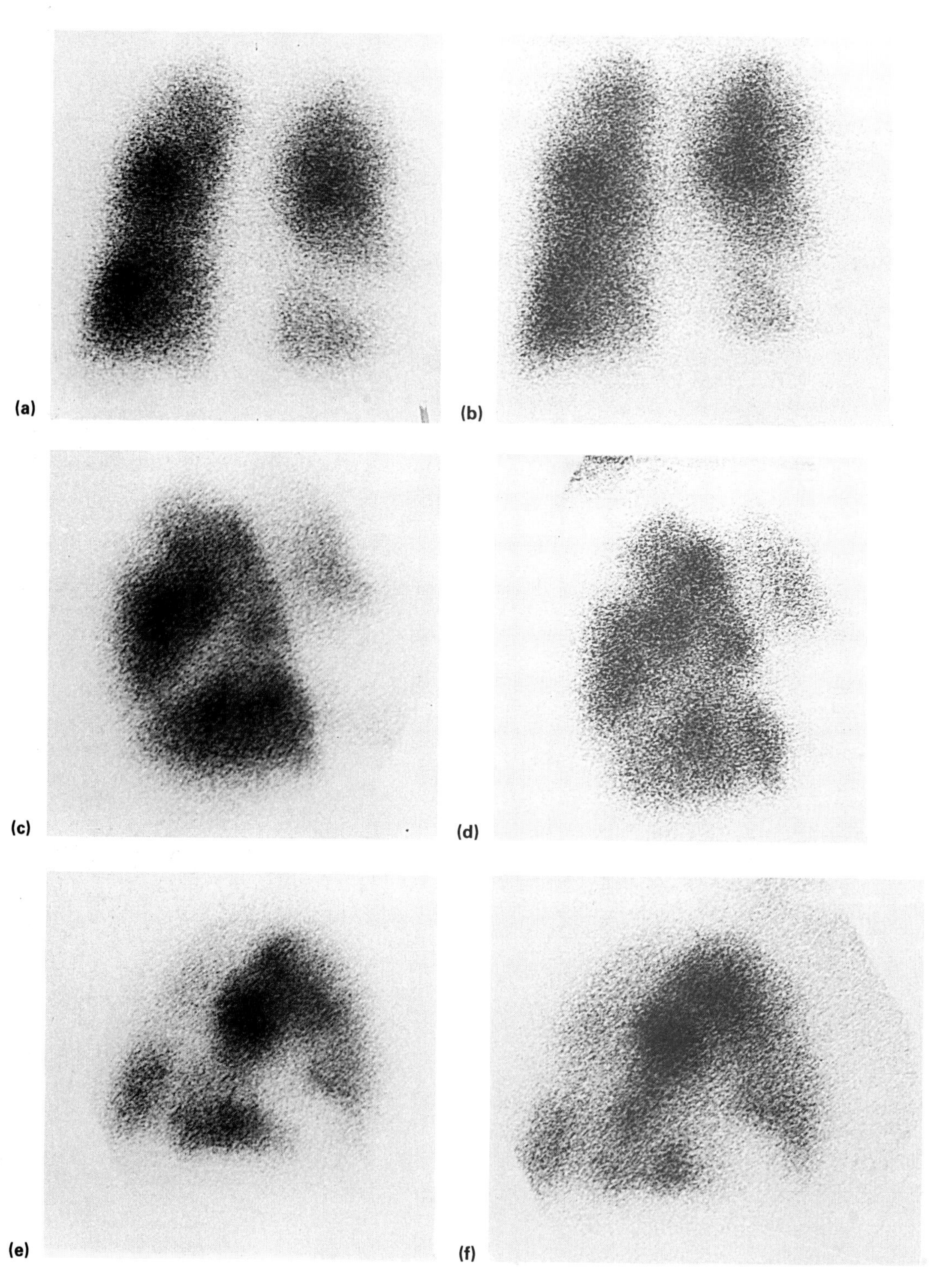

Figure 3.4 Male, 63 years old. Known chronic bronchitic with recent increase in dyspnoea. Perfusion imaging (a, c, e) and ventilation imaging with ^{81m}Kr (b, d, e) in posterior, left posterior oblique and right posterior oblique projections demonstrated matched defects in both lungs. No mismatch seen. Low probability of pulmonary emboli.

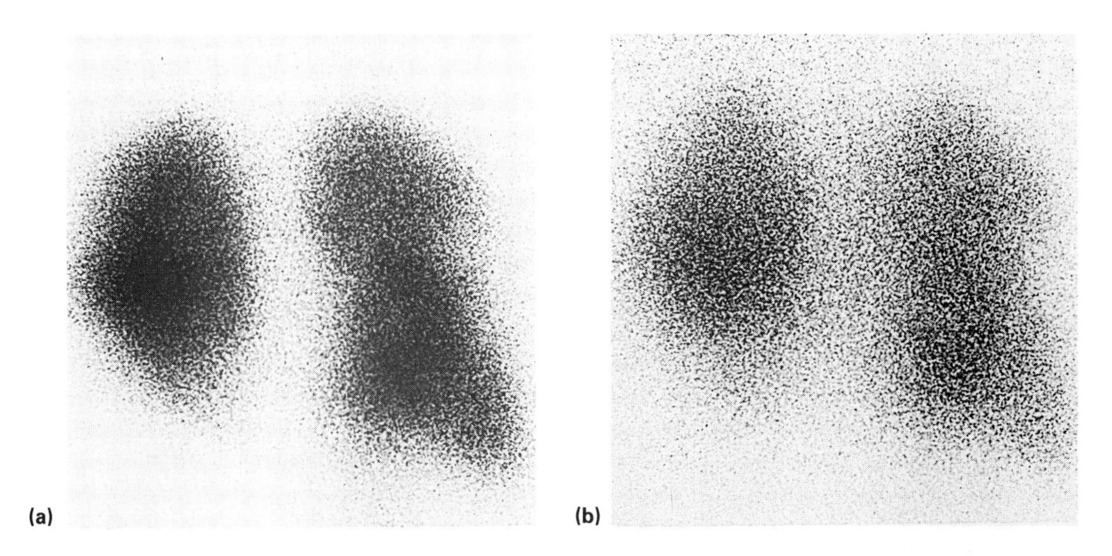

Figure 3.5 a, b. Male, 77 years old, with past history of pulmonary emboli and IVC filter *in situ*. Presented with breathlessness query recurrent pulmonary emboli. Perfusion–ventilation imaging in posterior and right posterior oblique projections shows matched defects in both lung fields. Low probability of pulmonary emboli.

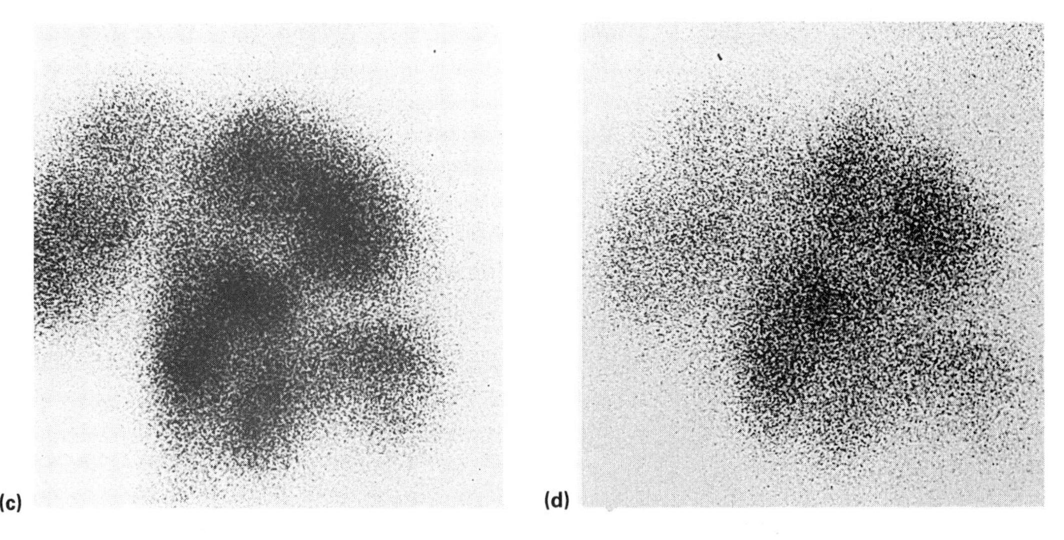

Figure 3.5 c, d. Male, 16 years old. Renal transplant on ventilator, collapsed lower lobe on X-ray. Ventilation–perfusion imaging in left posterior oblique projection shows reduced ventilation to the left lung with normal perfusion.

performed at the end of the anticoagulation period to assess the degree of resolution (Figures 3.6 and 3.7). Unless this follow-up study is performed it may prove extremely difficult to assess future scans should the patient develop further symptoms. Repeat scanning is also indicated, whilst the patient is anticoagulated if further symptoms develop (Figure 3.8). Evidence of new perfusion defects in an adequately anticoagulated patient may indicate a need to consider more drastic treatment methods such as tying off pelvic veins, plication of the inferior vena cava (IVC) or the use of an IVC umbrella.

Saenger *et al.* (1985) have performed the interesting exercise of assessing the effects of ventilation–perfusion lung scan results on further management. They demonstrated that 23% of patients had their management changed after scanning, 15% of whom had anticoagulation discontinued (Figure 3.9). Mercandetti *et al.* (1985), in a similar study, confirmed that ventilation–perfusion imaging resulted in a net reduction in the use of anticoagulation and also demonstrated that on long-term follow-up the morbidity from the pulmonary emboli in the low-probability group was very low.

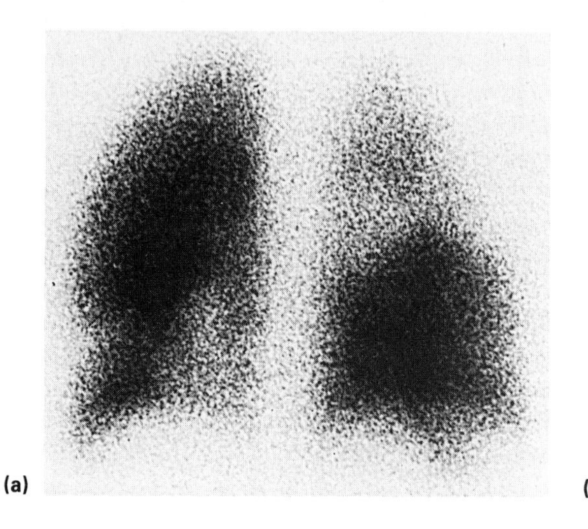

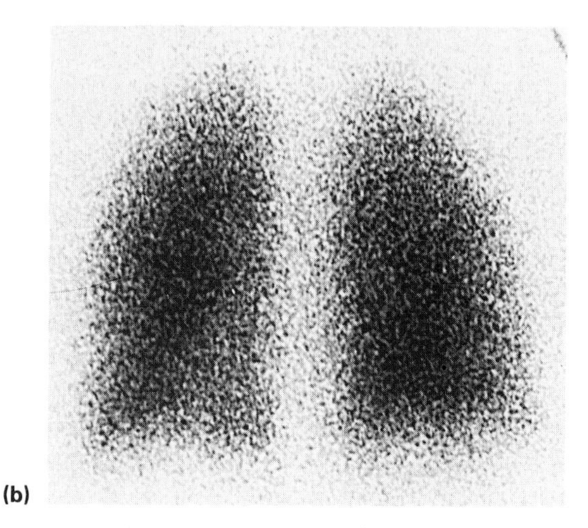

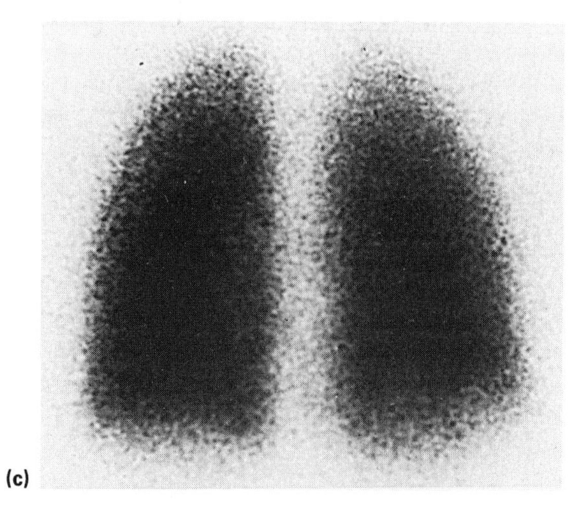

Figure 3.6 Female, 32 years old, with sudden onset of central chest pain and tachycardia two days after hysterectomy. Images show bilateral segmental defects on the posterior perfusion image (a) with normal ^{81m}Kr ventilation imaging (b), high probability of pulmonary emboli. Posterior perfusion image six months later had returned to normal (c).

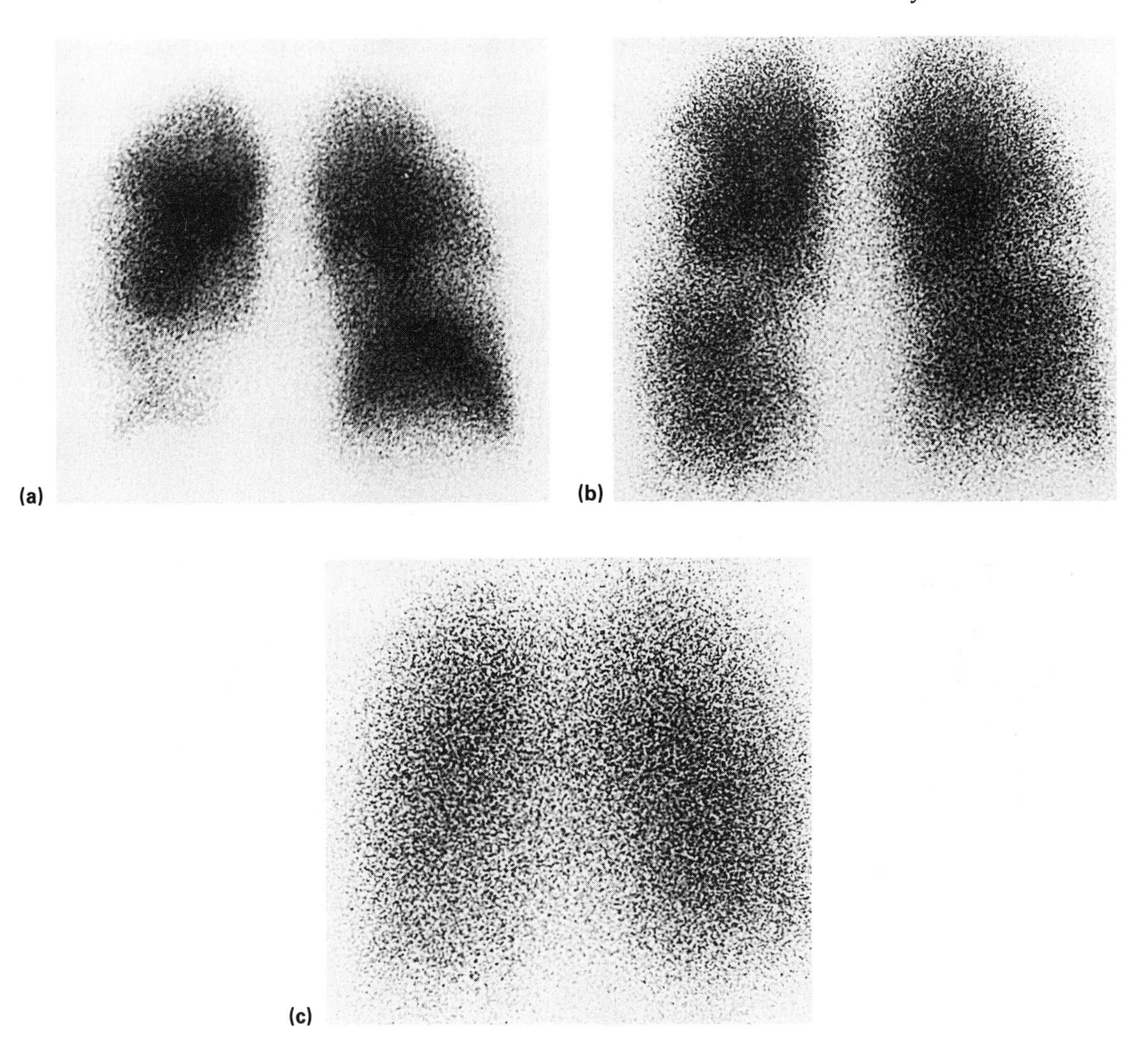

Figure 3.7 Female, 63 years old, with a history of DVT and chest pain. Perfusion image (a) showed abnormal perfusion at the left base and right mid-zone. Ventilation was normal. Diagnosis pulmonary emboli. Repeat imaging two months later demonstrated partial resolution with improved perfusion at the left base but persistent mid-zone abnormalities (b). Ventilation imaging remained normal (c).

3.3.8 THE CHOICE OF RADIOTRACERS IN THE DIAGNOSIS OF PULMONARY EMBOLI

There is little debate about the choice of the radiopharmaceutical for the assessment of lung perfusion since the majority of scans are performed with macroaggregates of albumin. Macroaggregates have the advantage over microspheres of improved biodegradability and fewer reported adverse reactions.

In the choice of radiotracers for ventilation, however, there is still significant debate. The characteristics of an ideal radiopharmaceutical for ventilation imaging will be an agent whose pattern of distribution is that of ventilation with good imaging characteristics, low radiation dose to patients and staff, easily disposable, cheap, and with the ability to perform multiple views. Unfortunately, no agent currently available is able to fulfil all these criteria. ^{133}Xe remains the most widely used ventilation imaging agent, does not possess good imaging characteristics and can only be imaged in a single projection. Disposal is also a problem with potential high radiation doses to staff and patient unless disposal is efficient.

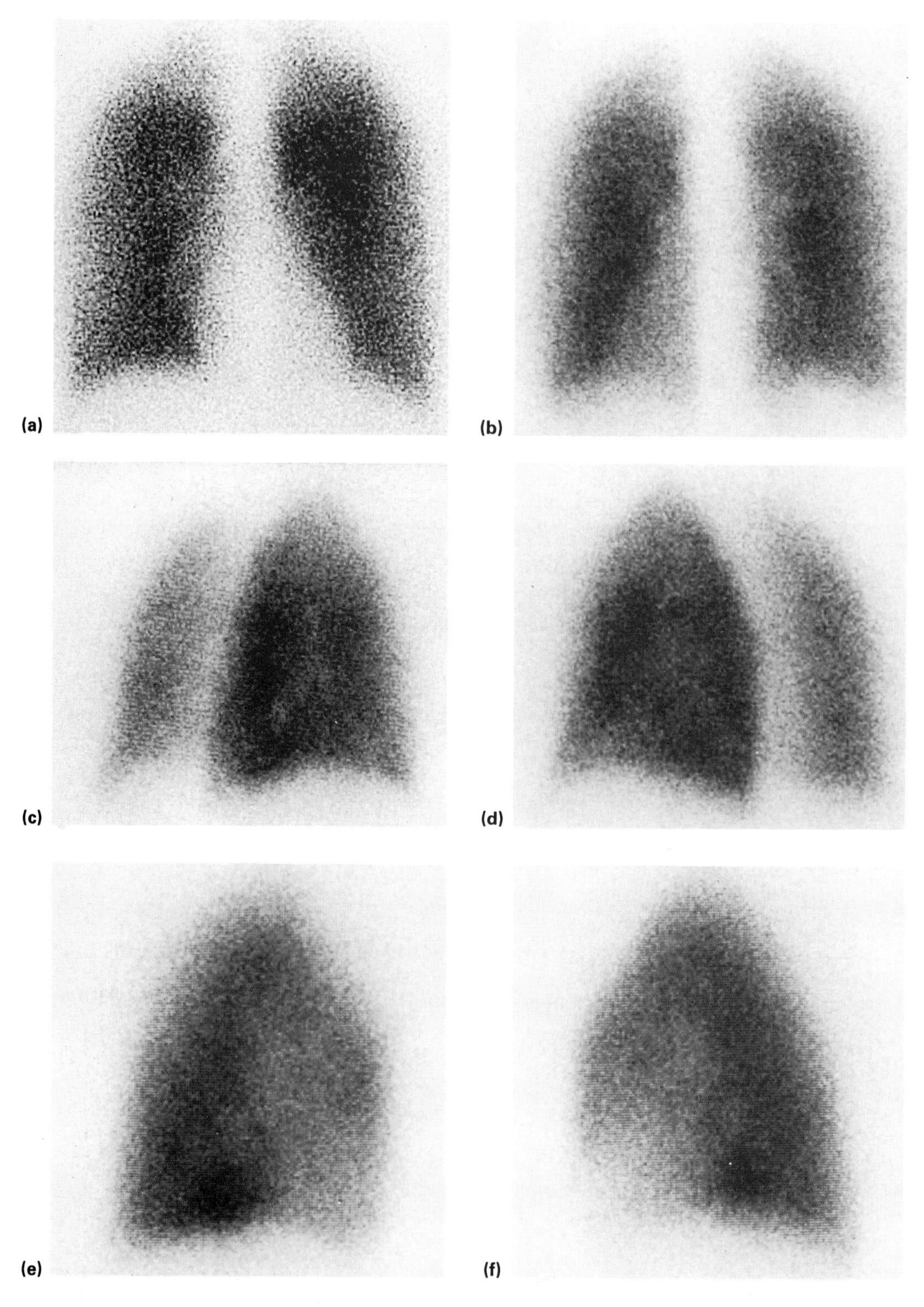

Figure 3.8 Male, 43 years old on warfarin, with a three-day history of pleuritic chest pain and a past history of pulmonary emboli. Perfusion imaging showed no defects, therefore low probability of new pulmonary emboli.

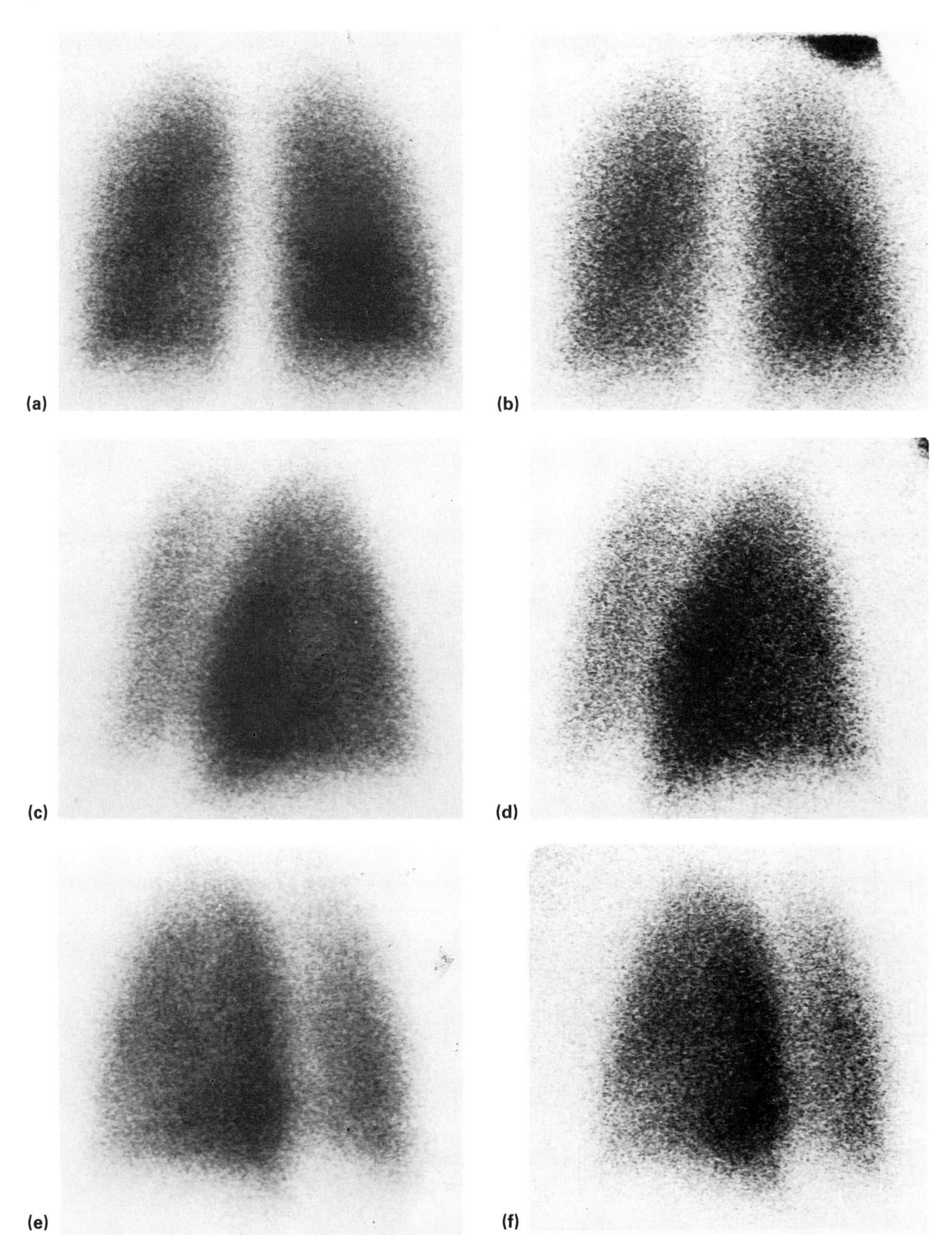

Figure 3.9 Female, 33 years old, with acute dyspnoea one month post-partum. Patient was heparinized and ventilation–perfusion imaging performed. Paired ^{81m}Kr ventilation and perfusion images. In posterior, right posterior oblique and left posterior oblique views displayed with normal results. Anticoagulation was discontinued and symptoms resolved spontaneously.

^{81m}Kr is an excellent ventilation but is restricted by availability. Probably the best current agent for widespread application is the new ^{99m}Tc-labelled carbon preparation – Technegas.

3.3.9 CONDITIONS THAT MAY MIMIC PULMONARY EMBOLI ON THE VENTILATION – PERFUSION SCAN

Whilst mismatch between perfusion and ventilation is the classical finding in patients with pulmonary emboli, other clinical conditions may produce ventilation–perfusion scan defects that mimic those of pulmonary emboli, i.e. a defect in which perfusion is impaired but ventilation is normal. As might be expected, the majority of these disease processes producing ventilation–perfusion mismatch involve the pulmonary arteries and include arteritic processes such as collagen vascular diseases, tuberculosis, sarcoidosis, pneumonia and radiation-induced arthritis (Alderson *et al.*, 1980). Congenital abnormalities of the vasculature (Figure 3.10), pulmonary artery stenosis or agenesis and anomalous origins of the pulmonary artery may result in similar areas of segmental or lobar mismatch. Vascular damage due to intravenous drug abuse, vascular occlusion due to bronchial carcinoma or infestation with dog heart worm and other rare conditions such as pulmonary artery sarcoma and haemangioendotheliomatosis may also mimic pulmonary emboli.

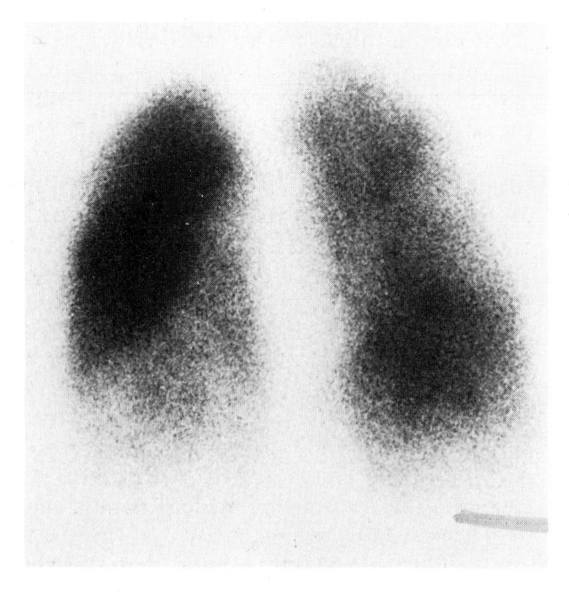

Figure 3.10 Male, 17 years old, with known multiple peripheral pulmonary stenosis. Posterior perfusion scan with patchily reduced perfusion in both lung fields consistent with known diagnosis.

3.3.10 NON-THROMBOTIC EMBOLI

Air embolism produces defects in blood flow in the lungs which are related to posture and to the rate and amount of air which enters the venous system. Segmental defects are seen with rapid entry of moderate amount of air whereas a pattern of peripheral loss is seen when air enters the system more slowly. The defects are seen in the region of the lung that are uppermost at the time the air enters the system and, providing the patient survives the event, the defects resolve without anticoagulant therapy (Carrol *et al.*, (1977).

Fat embolism has been shown by Park *et al.* (1986) to produce multiple small areas of mismatch throughout the lungs in the early stages of the disease with a normal chest X-ray. In more longstanding emboli, Skarzynaki *et al.* (1986) have shown diffuse areas of mismatch with accompanying X-ray changes.

3.4 RADIONUCLIDE IMAGING IN CARCINOMA OF THE BRONCHUS

Carcinoma of the bronchus remains the commonest form of cancer in men and with the increased incidence of smoking in women since the Second World War it has become the second commonest cancer in women, secondary only to breast cancer. Carcinomas of the lung are divided histologically into squamous carcinoma which are commonly central tumours, small cell carcinomas frequently found in the lung periphery, adenoma carcinomas and large cell tumours which occur throughout the lungs.

3.4.1 PRIMARY DIAGNOSIS

A diagnosis of carcinoma of the lung may be suspected on clinical grounds with a history of cough, haemoptysis and weight loss. Clinical examination may reveal signs of consolidation with bronchial breathing or, if airways are narrowed, a localized ronchus. Finger clubbing and palpable supraclavicular lymph nodes are also significant findings, as is the presence of Horner's syndrome in patients with apical tumours. Carcinoma of the lung may, however, be suspected following the chance finding on X-ray of a circumscribed lesion in the lung field. The diagnosis will be confirmed with sputum cytology or brushings taken at bronchoscopy. With peripheral lesions, biopsy under X-ray control may be required to obtain a histological diagnosis and rarely mediastinoscopy or thoracoscopy will be used. Following histological diagnosis, management will depend on the operability of the lesion, the patient's symptoms and the presence or absence of metastases.

3.4.2 THE ROLE OF PERFUSION SCANNING IN CARCINOMA OF THE BRONCHUS

Although perfusion imaging has little to contribute in the establishment of a primary diagnosis, it may provide valuable information about unsuspected areas of decreased perfusion implying central disease that has not been demonstrated by other techniques (Wagner 1965). The low specificity of the technique precludes its use for diagnosing or staging disease. In patients in whom surgery is contemplated, however, perfusion imaging will define the extent of an abnormality and confirm that the uninvolved lung tissue is normal.

Because cigarette smoking is also the major cause of chronic bronchitis and emphysema, many patients with lung cancer have chronic airflow obstruction and impaired pulmonary function. The assessment of individual lung function used to require differential bronchospirometry; this may now be accomplished by ventilation–perfusion imaging. When a patient is to have a pneumonectomy, post-operative lung function can be predicted with considerable accuracy from a pre-operative perfusion scan. The best correlation for the prediction is obtained from a perfusion scan done in the upright position during exertion, although a perfusion scan done in the upright position at rest is almost as good. Ventilation studies in the upright position are less satisfactory (Kristersson, 1974). After pneumonectomy, the post-operative forced expiratory volume in one second (FEV_1) can be predicted from the product of the pre-operative FEV_1 and the relative perfusion of the lung which will remain post-operatively (Boysen *et al.*, 1977).

Carcinomas of the bronchus receive their blood supply from the bronchial arterial system. Small tumours, less than 2 cm in diameter, are not usually detected by ventilation–perfusion imaging unless they impinge on the pulmonary vasculature or cause bronchial obstruction. Larger tumours may produce defects in blood flow and ventilation in proportion to their size, but the defects in ventilation, which are produced by bronchial obstruction, tend to be smaller than those of blood flow because there is often greater extrabronchial spread of the tumour than intrabronchial protrusion or tracheal compression.

Disturbances of ventilation and blood flow are common in the contralateral lung, delayed clearance of ^{133}Xe being recognized in up to 65% of patients and abnormalities of blood flow in about 50%. These are usually due to the associated chronic airflow obstruction, but pulmonary embolism or malignant invasion of the contralateral vessels may occur.

3.4.3 OTHER RADIONUCLIDE TECHNIQUES IN CARCINOMA OF THE LUNG

(a) Gallium-67 imaging

^{67}Ga has been evaluated in the primary diagnosis of bronchogenic carcinoma and has been shown by many workers to be taken up by malignant tissue. Although the sensitivity of detection is high, with 80–90% of bronchial tumours concentrating ^{67}Ga, the specificity is unfortunately low. Inflammatory tissue and granulomatous tissue have also been shown to concentrate ^{67}Ga. Alazraki *et al.* (1978) have shown, in a study comparing the results of ^{67}Ga imaging with the results of mediastinoscopy, that the ratio of true-positive ^{67}Ga scan to true-positive mediastinoscopies was 100%, whereas the value of true-negative ^{67}Ga scan to true-negative mediastinoscopies was only 71%. Waxman *et al.* (1984) evaluated patients undergoing thoracotomy for primary lung cancer. Two separate sets of criteria were used to determine the specificity and sensitivity of the gallium scan. The first set of criteria was that described by Alazraki *et al.* which considered a gallium scan positive if activity in the hilar and/or mediastinal region was increased. The second set of criteria was defined by Demeester *et al.* (1979), who only considered increased activity in the mediastinum as positive. Waxman *et al.* concluded that when the mediastinum is evaluated selectively the sensitivity for detection is low, while the specificity is high. High specificity is also associated with unilateral hilar uptake. If the hilum and/or mediastinum are considered together the sensitivity for the ^{67}Ga study is high, but the specificity falls considerably.

(b) Other agents

^{99m}Tc Methylene diphosphonate (MDP) bone scanning is frequently used as a staging procedure in patients with proven carcinoma of the bronchus, as is ^{99m}Tc liver colloid imaging and ^{99m}Tc brain imaging. The demonstration of metastases using any of these techniques would obviously alter management if a patient appeared otherwise suitable for surgery. If there is clinical or biochemical evidence of spread to any of these roles, approximately two-thirds to three-quarters of the relevant scans will be positive (Ramsdel *et al.*, 1977; Hooper *et al.*, 1978); if a patient has no clinical or biochemical evidence of disease, then the pick-up rate of about 5% suggests there is no clear role for bone, liver or brain scanning in this group. Thallium-201 chloride has been evaluated in several studies in patients with a variety of pulmonary diseases, including primary lung cancer. Salvatore *et al.* (1976) reported on 43 patients with lung cancer, of whom 23 had hilar metastases. Of these patients 20 showed thallium uptake in the hilar disease and 18 of 20 patients had uptake in peripheral lesions. Tonami and Hisada (1977) imaged six patients with lung cancer, with thallium uptake in five of the six patients. Hisada *et al.* (1978) reported positive scans in 40 of 57 patients studied. A further nine studies were reported as equivocal.

3.4.4 POSITRON IMAGING TOMOGRAPHY IN LUNG CARCINOMA

Positron emission tomography (PET) imaging using radiolabelled amino acids has been used by Kubota *et al.* (1985) in patients with lung cancers and benign tumours. Using L-methionine ^{11}C they successfully imaged eight patients with lung cancer. Activity in the malignant tumours was significantly higher than in benign tumours. With the development of new positron imaging radiopharmaceuticals it will prove possible to study a variety of tumour characteristics including protein synthesis, glucose metabolism and blood flow. Recently anti-CEA antibodies have been used with the same success. Johnson *et al.* (1988) have used ^{111}In-labelled diethylenetriaminepentaacetic acid (DTPA) anti-carcinoembryonic antigen (CEA) monoclonal antibody in patients with lung carcinoma and shown that using cold antibody does not increase the sensitivity of the technique. Liewendahl *et al.* (1988) have used ^{111}In-labelled DTPA anti-CEA F(ab)2 fragments in 17 patients with recurrent or metastatic lung cancer; using pulmonary and liver spleen subtraction 46 out of 48 lesions were identified.

3.5 CHRONIC OBSTRUCTIVE AIRWAYS DISEASE

Irreversible airways obstruction is the significant pathological feature in chronic bronchitis and emphysema. In healthy lungs, most of the resistance to airflow is in the larger bronchi, where air flow is transitional or turbulent. Only about 10–20% of resistance can be attributed to the smaller airways – those less than 2 mm in diameter. Considerable damage or dysfunction can take place in the smaller bronchi and bronchioles, with little effect on overall resistance to air flow. The forced vital capacity, forced expiratory volume in 1 s and airway resistance may be normal, while more sensitive tests of airways function such as closing volume or measurements of the change of flow–volume relationship can detect even early changes in the small airways. Chronic bronchitis and emphysema are common complications of cigarette smoking. Other causative factors may be industrial exposure to cotton or hemp dust, and air pollutants have also been implicated.

The airway obstruction in chronic bronchitis is due to the reduced bronchiole lumen associated with increased bronchial mucous glands and bronchial secretions. Associated inflammation and oedema serve to narrow the conducting airways and increase the resistance to flow.

In emphysema, dilatation and destruction of the alveoli beyond the terminal bronchioles occurs, which leads not only to loss of the available alveolar surface area and its contained pulmonary capillary bed but also to loss of the support of airways by their surrounding alveoli, so that they collapse more readily on expiration. Narrowing of the conducting airways with dilatation of the alveoli results in air trapping in the emphysematous regions.

Patients with chronic bronchitis present with a history of chronic productive cough and increasing dyspnoea. Examination of the chest reveals coarse crepitations and the patient may be clinically cyanosed. In emphysematous patients, symptoms of dyspnoea predominate and auscultation may reveal poor air entry. In both, signs of right ventricular failure may be present, particularly in patients with longstanding disease. Chest X-rays may appear normal, particularly in the early stages of the disease. In later stages the hyperinflated lungs will cause flattening of the diaphragm and bullous change may be observed. Lung function tests will reveal increased total lung capacity, increased residual volume and a reduced transfer factor.

3.5.1 RADIONUCLIDE IMAGING IN CHRONIC OBSTRUCTIVE AIRWAYS DISEASE

The use of radioactive gases for the study of lung function is well established. ^{81m}Kr distribution throughout the lung fields is proportional to regional ventilation. However, when minute ventilation is greater than normal, ^{81m}Kr regional count rates become more dependent on regional lung volume than ventilation. ^{81m}Kr images will therefore underestimate ventilation in regions with high ventilatory flow. With its γ-energy well suited to the gamma camera, good-quality images in multiple projections may be obtained, enabling small areas of abnormal ventilation to be visualized. In general ventilation abnormalities in chronic obstructive airways disease affect both lungs and can affect the upper or lower zones. ^{81m}Kr images show decreased activity in regions of obstructive airways disease (Figures 3.11 and 3.12). Fazio *et al.* (1978) compared ^{81m}Kr images with findings on chest X-ray in 75 patients with pulmonary disease and found that the chest X-ray underestimated full functional impairment in emphysema, chronic bronchitis and asthma. Patients with radiographic evidence of emphysema showed patchy areas of reduced ^{81m}Kr ventilation. Some deficiencies were associated with bullae and others were in areas that appeared normal radiographically. Matching ventilation and perfusion defects were characteristic. In bronchial diseases such as chronic bronchitis and asthma, both patchy and segmental ventilation defects may be seen, often associated with a normal chest X-ray. Mismatched ventilation–perfusion defects are occasionally seen in asthma (Feinmann *et al.* 1978). ^{133}Xe and ^{127}Xe ventilation studies provide a sensitive means of detecting regional airways disease. Alderson *et al.* (1974a) compared the findings of chest X-ray, ^{133}Xe ventilation imaging and lung spirometry. Of patients with abnormal ^{133}Xe studies 40% had normal chest X-rays, and spirometry in these patients confirm the presence of mild abnormalities. Data suggest that ^{133}Xe imaging provides a means of detecting mild airways disease in patients with normal X-rays.

Since a xenon study gives wash-in, equilibrium and wash-out information, Alderson *et al.* (1979) compared the sensitivity of single-breath ^{133}Xe inhalation with the wash-out phase. The wash-out phase study was demonstrated to be clearly superior to the single-breath study, detecting 94%

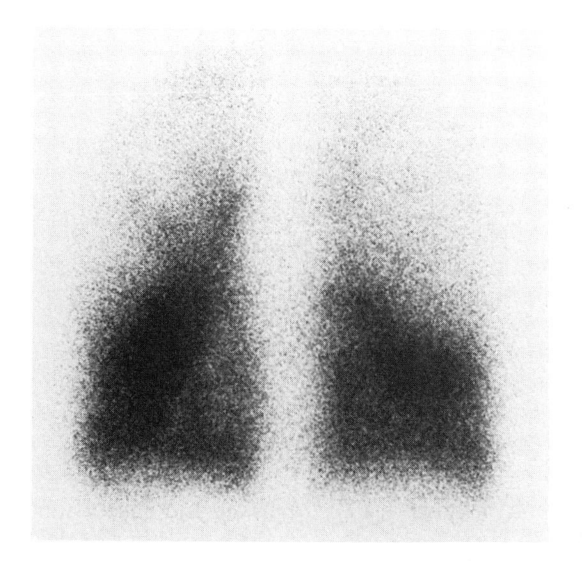

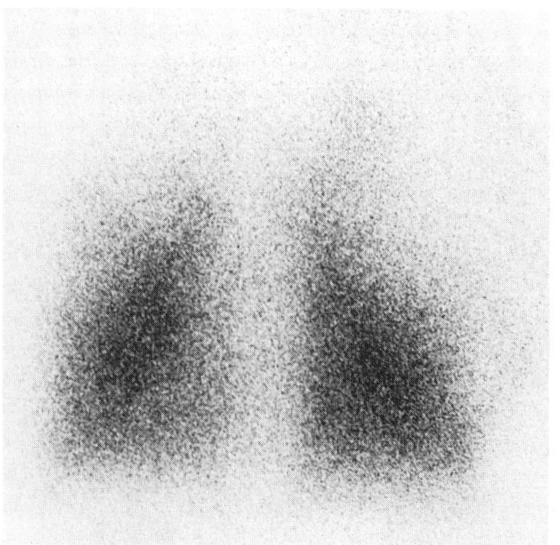

Figure 3.11 Female, 61 years old, with history of shortness in breath and known apical bullous emphysema. Ventilation–perfusion imaging demonstrates matched defects at both apices at sites of emphysema but no mismatched tissue to suggest emboli.

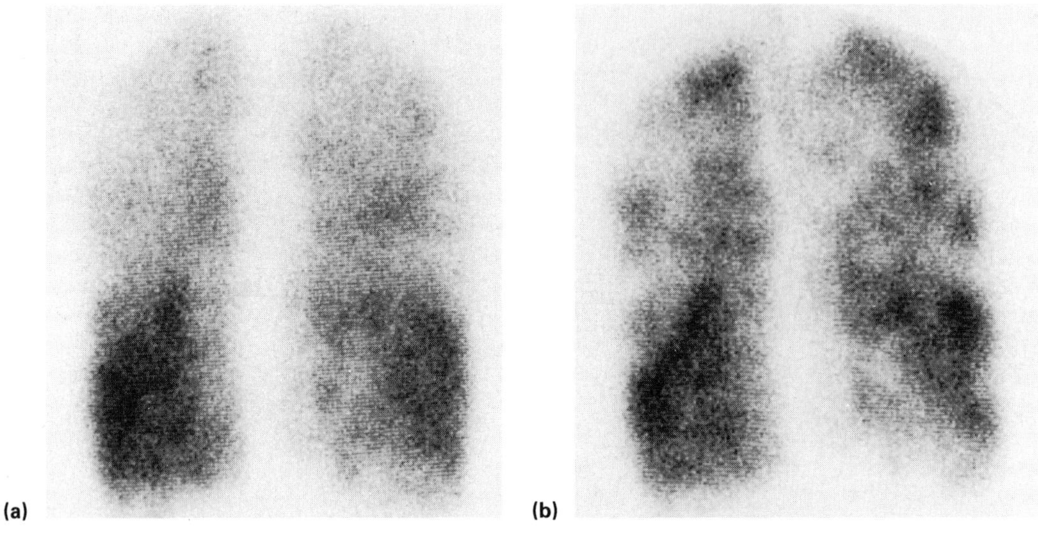

Figure 3.12 Female, 63 years old, with α_1-antritrypsin deficiency and recurrent chest pain. Ventilation–perfusion imaging shows matched ventilation–perfusion defects at both lung bases consistent with known basal emphysema. No mismatch identified. Low probability of pulmonary emboli.

of abnormal zones, compared with 64% detected by a single breath. Another disadvantage of the single-breath technique is its effort dependence; 10–15% of patients are unable to perform the manoeuvre.

Few comparative studies of ^{133}Xe and ^{127}Xe have been performed. Atkins *et al.* (1977) concluded, following a study, that ^{127}Xe was preferable because of increased count rates, lower patient radiation dose and long shelf life. Coates and Nahmias (1977) found that ^{127}Xe was able to resolve smaller lesions than ^{133}Xe.

The use of ^{99m}Tc-labelled aerosols to investigate patients with obstructive airways disease has been studied by Taplin and Chopras (1978). They demonstrated that areas of poor aerosol penetration correspond to areas of reduced activity or poor ventilation in the gas inhalation images. Unlike xenon images, aerosol images show not only the regional ventilatory abnormality but also indicate the site of obstruction. In mild airways disease such as early bronchitis or mild asthma, aerosol patterns show increased central deposition and near-normal peripheral ventilation. In more severe obstructive pulmonary disease, the pattern is different, with gross central deposition plus areas of poor or nearly absent aerosol penetration to the lung periphery. α_1-Antitrypsin deficiency patients characteristically show reduced aerosol penetration to both lower lung fields associated with matched perfusion impairment. Bullae in bullous emphysema are demonstrated as areas of reduced activity on inhalation lung scans. It is not possible to demonstrate airways trapping by this technique as it is with xenon imaging.

3.6 PARENCHYMAL LUNG INFECTION

The diagnosis of interstitial lung infection or pneumonia is usually made on the basis of the patient's history, clincial signs and chest X-ray. The differentiation between bacterial, fungal and viral pneumonias depends on optimum culture and the measurement of viral antibody titres. Transbronchial biopsy or open lung biopsy may be required in some atypical pneumonias. In the areas of consolidated lung, the consequent local hypoxia leads to vasoconstriction and results in shunting with consequent hypoxaemia. Ventilation–perfusion imaging identifies the area or areas of lung with absent ventilation and reduced perfusion (Figure 3.13). In tuberculosis, the pulmonary arterial blood flow is markedly reduced in the affected areas and the extent of the perfusion defect frequently exceeds that of the X-ray abnormality. ^{67}Ga imaging has been used to distinguish between pulmonary infection and infarction but is of no use in differentiating infection from malignancy. In patients with known tuberculosis, the

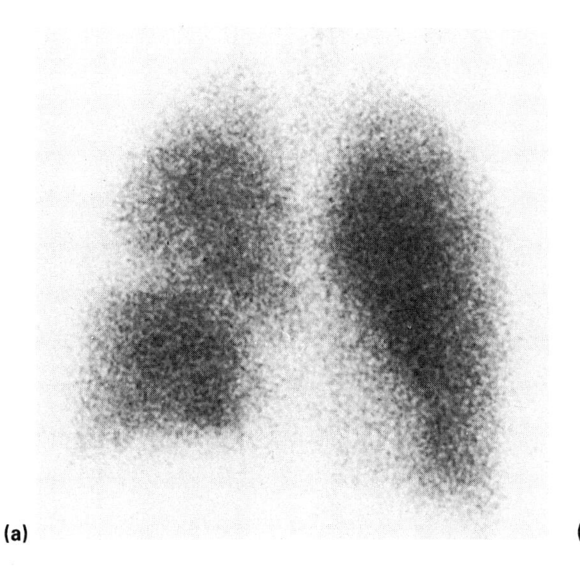

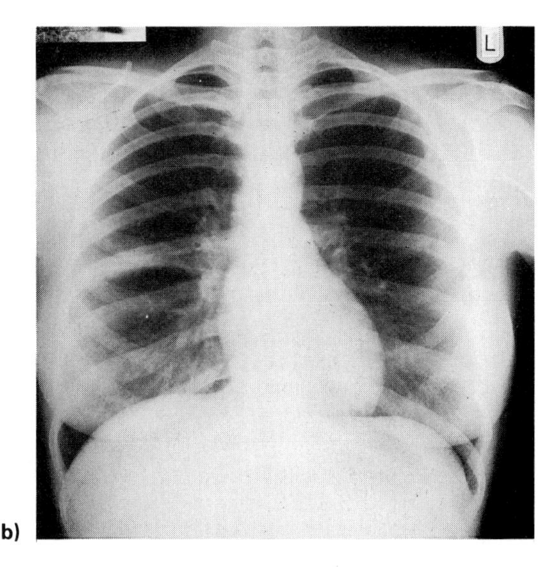

Figure 3.13 Female, 27 years old, with a history of sudden onset of dyspnoea and cough. Ventilation imaging with ^{81m}krypton (a) demonstrates a segmental abnormality in the right mid-zone which corresponds to an area of consolidation on the chest X-ray (b).

degree of activity of the infection may be assessed using ^{67}Ga, since only sites of active infection are gallium avid.

3.6.1 PULMONARY INFECTION IN AIDS

Since 1981, when Gottlieb first described acquired immunodeficiency syndrome (AIDS) in five young homosexual men, more than 70 000 cases had been reported by 1988 in 130 countries. During 1990 one million total cases of AIDS are expected.

The causative agent in this disease is a human T-cell lymphotropic retrovirus (human immunodeficiency virus, HIV). AIDS patients are predisposed to a wide variety of opportunistic infections which may be protozoan (*Pneumocystis carinii* pneumonia), bacterial (*Myobacterium avium intracellulare*), fungal, viral or helminthic. They are also likely to develop unusual cancers, Kaposi's sarcoma, lymphoreticular neoplasms, Burkitt's lymphoma and oral or rectal squamous cell carcinoma associated with herpesvirus infection.

3.6.2 ASSESSMENT OF ALVEOLAR CLEARANCE IN AIDS

The alveolar clearance of ^{99m}Tc-labelled DTPA aerosol has been shown to be increased in several conditions such as interstitial lung disease (Maini *et al.*, 1987), cigarette smoke (Jones *et al.*, 1980), asbestosis (Gellert *et al.*, 1985) and sarcoidosis (Jacobs *et al.*, 1985).

O'Doherty *et al.* (1987) have used ^{99m}Tc-labelled DTPA aerosols in patients with HIV antibody positivity and shown that alveolar clearance was increased in patients with *Pneumocystis carinii* infections proved on transbronchial biopsy and that the lung transfer curves were biphasic, unlike the monophasic curves in non-affected patients. They suggested that ^{99m}Tc-labelled DTPA clearance data could be used to diagnose *Pneumocystis carinii* in early stages of the disease.

3.6.3 GALLIUM IMAGING OF LUNGS IN AIDS

Since ^{67}Ga scanning is widely used in the detection of lung inflammation, several studies have now been reported assessing its use in the diagnostic evaluation of pulmonary manifestation in AIDS patients. Tuazon *et al.* (1985) demonstrated lung uptake of ^{67}Ga in 100% of AIDS patients with *Pneumocystis carinii* including those with subclinical infection. Barron *et al.* (1985) investigated the validity and reliability of ^{67}Ga scanning for the diagnosis of *Pneumocystis carinii*. They demonstrated that the overall sensitivity of the technique is high at 94% but the specificity is only 74%. They concluded that if a patient has AIDS and is suspected of having *Pneumocystis carinii* and the ^{67}Ga scan is negative there is only a 7% chance that *Pneumocystis carinii* pneumonia is present.

Kramer *et al.* (1987) have correlated the patterns of ^{67}Ga distribution in the lungs of patients with AIDS with their respective aetiologies. *Pneumocystis carinii* is associated with diffuse lung uptake as are cytomegalovirus and *Cryptococcus* infections. In 10–15% of patients with AIDS who have pulmonary complications, the uptake of ^{67}Ga by the lung is localized to a pulmonary segment or lobe. Segmental or lobar uptake usually indicates a bacterial infection, such as *Klebsiella* or *Staphylococcus aureus* (Kramer *et al.*, 1987). It has also been shown by Kramer *et al.* (1987) that the association of a positive chest X-ray with a negative ^{67}Ga scan often indicates Kaposi's sarcoma.

3.7 PAEDIATRIC LUNG DISEASE

Lung disease in children ranges from hyaline membrane disease in premature neonates to aspiration of foreign bodies in toddlers. Radionuclide lung scanning provides a sensitive method of assessing regional ventilation and perfusion and alveolar permeability.

3.7.1 HYALINE MEMBRANE DISEASE

Although membrane disease is frequently an obvious diagnosis in the premature neonate, other causes of respiratory failure such as pneumonia or patent ductus arteriosus exist. Jefferies *et al.* (1984) have used ^{99m}Tc-labelled DTPA aerosol clearance rates to distinguish hyaline membrane disease from other causes of neonatal respiratory failure. They have shown that the clearance curve in hyaline membrane disease is biphasic whereas the curves in respiratory failure from other causes are monoexponential.

3.7.2 CYSTIC FIBROSIS

Cystic fibrosis usually presents in early childhood with failure to thrive and recurrent pulmonary infections, pneumonias and episodes of bronchitis. An increasing number of children are living into late teenage or early adult life, and some mildly afflicted individuals are being diagnosed in adult life. The secretions from most of the exocrine glands of the body are abnormal, including the sweat glands, with their high sodium content of sweat, the pancreas with its failure to produce the proper pancreatic enzymes, and the bronchial tubes in which a more viscid mucus is secreted which leads to widespread airflow obstruction with frequent episodes of bronchial infection, bronchopneumonia, local scarring, fibrosis and bronchiectasis.

Diffuse patchy infiltrates are usually seen radiographically and regional ventilation and perfusion become more and more disorganized the more advanced the condition. The upper lobes tend to be more severely afflicted than the lower lobes, but the disturbance of function is rarely symmetrical. Perfusion scans show a prominent fissure sign in about half of the affected children. The overall clearance of ^{133}Xe from both lungs has been shown to correlate reasonably well with peak flow and the forced expiratory volume at 1 s (Alderson *et al.*, 1974b).

There is nothing that distinguishes these findings from those seen during an attack of bronchial asthma. Ventilation–perfusion studies play no part in the diagnosis of this condition.

Nebulized aerosol therapy is still given to some children with cystic fibrosis even though less than 10% of the material reaches the bronchial tubes. The material deposited within the lungs is distributed in proportion to regional ventilation so that the poorly ventilated areas get very little. The clearance rate of the aerosol through mucociliary action is normal (Sanchis *et al.*, 1972).

3.7.3 INHALED FOREIGN BODY

Inhalation of foreign bodies may provide a diagnostic dilemma in the toddler with respiratory distress or unexplained pneumonia. Inhalation of a solid object causing obstruction of a bronchus may be demonstrated as a defect in ventilation imaging using ^{81}Kr or ^{133}Xe. Perfusion in this area will be normal. Inhalation of a peanut results in a localized chemical pneumonitis and both ventilation and perfusion will be impaired (ventilation more than perfusion).

3.7.4 CONGENITAL LUNG ABNORMALITIES

Hypoplasia or agenesis of a pulmonary artery may be suspected from the oligaemic appearance of the lung fields on X-ray. Hypoperfusion of one lung or lung segment may be confirmed on perfusion lung imaging. Similarly, agenesis of the lung can be confirmed on ventilation imaging when both ventilation and perfusion will be absent on the affected side. Pulmonary sequestration, a segment of the lung with aberrant arterial supply, on X-ray may appear as a focal lesion at the base of the lung. Perfusion imaging will demonstrate a defect corresponding to the X-ray abnormality, and Kawakami *et al.* (1978) showed that the delayed perfusion in the sequestrated segment could be demonstrated following injection of ^{99m}Tc albumin and dynamic imaging.

3.8 RESTRICTIVE LUNG DISEASE

In restrictive lung disease stiffness of the lungs is due to interstitial lung abnormalities. Studies of regional ventilation and blood flow are of no diagnostic value in interstitial lung diseases, nor do they help in the management of patients suffering from this diverse group of conditions. ^{127}Xe imaging, however, has been used experimentally by Bradley *et al.* (1979), who showed that using a single-breath inhalation technique ventilation abnormalities could be detected in the irradiated lungs of dogs. Patients with a diffuse interstitial pulmonary fibrosis have been studied in an attempt to understand the mechanisms of hypoxaemia in these conditions. Blood flow is reduced to the bases of the lungs and the regions of infiltrate seen radiographically. Patchy or subsegmental defects may be seen, and there is redistribution of blood flow towards the upper parts of the lungs. Regional lung volume is reduced in the area of infiltrates but regional ventilation is usually preserved. Occasionally there may be some delay in the clearance of ^{133}Xe from the bases. Ventilation–perfusion ratios tend to be low in the more normal parts of the lung because of the redistribution of blood flow. The reduction in blood flow to the bases has been shown to correlate well with oxygen tension and also with the alveolar–arterial oxygen tension differences. The low ventilation–perfusion ratios in the upper zones are positively correlated with oxygen tension, while the high ones at the bases are negatively correlated with oxygen tension, lending credence to the idea that it is this redistribution of blood flow in relation to ventilation that accounts for much of the hypoxaemia (McCarthy and Chemiak, 1973; Crystal *et al.*, 1976).

3.8.1 SARCOIDOSIS

Studies using ^{133}Xe have shown that regional ventilation tends to be increased in sarcoidosis. When fibrotic changes appear, regional ventilation returns to normal. Regional blood flow is reduced towards the mid-zone and bases in patients with fibrotic sarcoidosis (Wietzenblum *et al.*, 1977).

Perfusion scans using macroaggregated albumin show a variety of defects in blood flow which bear little relationship to the accompanying radiographic findings (Shibel *et al.*, 1969). In diffuse interstitial pulmonary fibrosis and sarcoidosis ^{67}Ga may be used to assess the activity of the disease process. Semi-quantitative methods of grading the uptake of ^{67}Ga in the lungs which take into account the percentage of lung involved, the intensity of the uptake and the distribution of abnormalities have been shown to correlate with semi-quantitative methods of grading the alveolar and interstitial cellularity of material obtained by lung biopsy. As the biopsy material shows less inflammatory or granulomatous response and more fibrosis so the uptake of ^{67}Ga decreases.

3.8.2 PNEUMOCONIOSIS

In coal workers' pneumoconiosis, there is little disturbance in blood flow as might be expected because non-smoking coal workers with uncomplicated coal workers' pneumoconiosis have only minimal changes on pulmonary function testing. Abnormalities of ventilation and blood flow are seen in relation to the associated chronic bronchitis and emphysema that is found in smoking coal workers. When progressive, massive fibrosis develops the defects in perfusion correspond to the radiographic abnormalities (Seaton *et al.*, 1971). Similar findings are found in silicosis.

With the development of interstitial fibrosis, perfusion of the bases of the lungs is reduced and small subsegmental or ragged defects appear. There is diminished filling of the bases during a ^{133}Xe ventilation study associated with the loss of lung volume in this fibrotic area and clearance may be normal or only slightly delayed from this region.

In smoking asbestos workers, additional defects in ventilation and blood flow may be seen in other parts of the lung, as well as those involved radiographically by fibrosis. These are due to the associated chronic bronchitis and emphysema (Secker-Walker and Ho, 1979).

Table 3.1 Radioactive gases used for ventilation studies

Agent	*Dosage*	*Physical half-life*	*Principal γ-energy (keV)*	*Radiation absorbed dose per 37 MBq* (mSv)*
^{81m}Kr†	10 mCi	13 s	190	90
^{13}N	5 mCi	10 min	511	110
^{15}O	5 mCi	2 min	511	140
^{127}Xe	0.5–1 mCi litre^{-1} (up to 10 mCi for a single-breath study)	36.4 d	172 203 375	1000
^{133}Xe	1 mCi litre^{-1} for rebreathing technique (up to 30 mCi for a single-breath study)	5.3 d	80	3000
^{135}Xe	0.2 mCi litre^{-1}	9.1 h	250	2500

*The radiation absorbed dose has been estimated by assuming a rebreathing time of 5 min. For single-breath studies it would be much smaller.
†^{81m}Kr is eluted from a 10 mCi ^{81}Rb generator (Fazio and Jones, 1975).

3.9 TECHNIQUES

3.9.1 REGIONAL VENTILATION

Radionuclide gases are the best tracers for studies of regional ventilation. Some of the gases available are shown in Table 3.1. ^{133}Xe is one of the most widely used ventilation imaging agents despite its low γ-ray energy, β-emission and fat solubility. ^{127}Xe, which has more desirable energy peaks, delivers less radiation to the patient and also provides images of comparable if not better quality (Atkins *et al.*, 1977; Coates and Nahmias, 1977), however, remains an expensive imaging agent and has therefore failed to achieve the popularity of ^{133}Xe. ^{81m}Kr, which is obtained from a ^{81}Rb generator, has a 13 s half-life. This half-life is less than that for lung clearance, which means that continuous administration of ^{81}Kr during tidal breathing results in an equilibrium being reached when the count rate is almost directly proportional to regional ventilation. Images can be made in the same projection as the perfusion images, and these allow much better comparison than is possible with ^{133}Xe studies (Fazio and Jones, 1975). The difficulties of obtaining ^{81m}Kr however, have restricted its use to centres within reasonable proximity of a cyclotron centre. Alternative agents for ventilation imaging are the recently developed ^{99m}Tc aerosols. The use of these agents to examine pulmonary ventilation was reported as early as 1965 (Pircher, 1965), but it is only in recent years that the problems of uneven distribution of radiolabelled aerosols have been overcome by the ability now to produce a submicrometre monodispersed particle which will deposit evenly in the distal airways and hopefully penetrate the alveoli. Modern systems use technetium-labelled DTPA, labelled with 30–50 mCi of ^{99m}Tc and produced the aerosol through the Bernoulli effect on the solution using standard hospital compressed oxygen systems. The system is self-contained for closed-circuit breathing by the patient, producing submicrometre particles said to be down to 0.25 μm in size, which theoretically should have monodispersion through the airways. Only the smaller particles will reach the patient's airways system, and due to the inefficiency of most systems only 1 mCi of activity is ultimately delivered for imaging after breathing on the apparatus for several minutes. The DTPA aerosols have relatively short half-lives in the lung, approximately 20 min, with the DTPA being absorbed readily by the normal alveolar–capillary membrane and even more rapidly by abnormal areas of the lung. A major problem with aerosol ventilation studies is that of central airways narrowing due to chronic obstructive airways disease, which leads to central airways deposition of aerosols, poor peripheral distribution of the aerosol and therefore technically inadequate studies.

A recent development in ventilation imaging has been the production of a new ultrafine agent with a particle size of 50–200 Å produced from ^{99m}Tc-pertechnetate and graphite in an argon environment. Although particulate in nature this agent is transported and perfused like a gaseous agent. There is therefore no central deposition and good peripheral visualization of the lung. Sullivan *et al.* (1988) have recently reported a comparison of this agent, 'Technegas', with ^{133}Xe in 50 patients and high-quality images were obtained with the new agent, with better patient compliance. It has been widely accepted as the optimal ventilation agent especially in Australia where over 22 000 patients have been studied (Murray, 1990, personal communication).

3.9.2 EQUIPMENT

For ventilation imaging a large field of view, a gamma camera should be used with a general all-purpose collimator. Commercially available rebreathing systems are available for ^{133}Xe and ^{127}Xe imaging and good exhaust ventilation should be provided. With ^{81}Kr imaging fans should be used to disperse the gas and care should be taken to disperse the activity away from the camera to avoid excessive background. Commercial delivery equipment is available for the administration of ^{99m}Tc-labelled DTPA aerosols. In all delivery equipment, dead space should be kept to a minimum. An integrated data processor is only necessary if divided pulmonary function or data on regional ventilation are required.

3.9.3 TECHNIQUES

(a) Xenon imaging

^{133}Xe and ^{127}Xe are administered via a face mask to the patient sitting with his or her back against the camera face. With the single-breath technique, a single breath of xenon is inhaled to total lung capacity and an image of the gas distribution in the lungs made during a breath of 10–20 s. Serial images of wash-out are made while the patient breathes air. The rate at which the xenon is inhaled must be controlled, as the distribution at slow inhalation depends on local compliance whereas fast inhalation will be more influenced by regional airway resistance (Milic-Emili, 1971). Regional ventilation can be assessed during tidal breathing by having patients breath xenon from a rebreathing circuit with a carbon dioxide absorber and oxygen inlet. A wash-in period of 3–5 min is satisfactory, followed by a wash-out period of up to 10 min.

(b) Krypton

^{81m}Kr is administered via a face mask during tidal breathing and images of regional ventilation may be acquired in multiple projections.

3.9.4 REGIONAL PERFUSION

The vast majority of regional perfusion studies are performed by using either macroaggregated human serum albumin (Taplin, 1964; Wagner *et al.*, 1964) or human albumin microspheres labelled with ^{99m}Tc (Rhodes *et al.*, 1971) (Table 3.2).

(a) Equipment

As with ventilation imaging, a large-field gamma camera with a general all-purpose collimator is the equipment of choice.

Table 3.2 Radiopharmaceuticals used for perfusion lung scanning*

Agent	*Dosage*	*Physical half-life*	*Biological half-life*	*Principal γ-energy (keV)*	*Particle size*	*Radiation absorbed dose per 37 MBq (MSv)*
^{113m}In-labelled ferric hydroxide	1–3 mCi	1.7 h	27 h	393	5–60 μm	5500–7500
^{131}I-labelled macroaggregated albumin	250–300 μCi	8 d	2–9 h	364	5–100 μm	1–6.3 × 104
^{99m}Tc-labelled macroaggregated albumin	1–3 mCi	6 h	2–9 h	140	5–100 μm	1500
^{99m}Tc-labelled albumin microspheres	1–3 mCi	6 h	7 h	140	20–40 μm	4000–6000
^{99m}Tc-labelled ferric hydroxide	1–3 mCi	6 h	27 h	140	5–60 μm	1500–6200
^{133}Xe	5–10 mCi	5.3 d	30 s	80	Gaseous	1000
^{81m}Kr†	10 mCi	13 s	30 s	190	Gaseous	90

*Adapted from Taplin and MacDonald (1971).
†The ^{81m}Kr is eluted from a 10 mCi ^{81}Rb generator (Fazio and Jones, 1975).

(b) Technique

A standard adult dose of ^{99m}Tc macroaggregates should contain approximately 400 000 particles and have an activity of 70–200 MBq. The dose is reduced in children in accordance with their body surface area. In patients who are suspected of having a right to left cardiac shunt or known pulmonary hypertension, the dose should be reduced by 50%.

Imaging technique is important. The syringe should be shaken prior to injection to disperse the particles. The dose should be drawn up immediately before injection to avoid particles adhering to the walls of the syringe and should then be injected slowly with the patient supine. Injection through plastic tubing should be avoided. Blood must not be drawn back into the syringe during the procedure as labelling of small clots may occur, with resultant hot spots appearing on the scan. Imaging should take place as soon as possible after the injection. A current chest X-ray must always be available at the time of reporting.

3.9.5 ALTERNATIVE PERFUSION TECHNIQUES

In patients with severe pulmonary hypertension in whom perfusion imaging with labelled particles is relatively contraindicated, intravenous ^{133}Xe in saline or infusion of ^{81m}Kr may be safely used. When ^{133}Xe is given intravenously it passes through the right heart, into the pulmonary arteries and comes out of solution in the air-containing alveoli. Its distribution during a breath hold shortly after injection is proportional to capillary blood flow to these alveoli. Areas of atelectasis or pneumonia will appear to have no blood flow.

When ^{81m}Kr is given by continuous intravenous infusion, the count rate at equilibrium is proportional to regional blood flow. Because the gas has been removed partly by ventilation and partly by decay, defects in the pattern of blood flow in poorly ventilated areas are less well defined than those obtained by particle perfusion images (Ciofetta *et al.*, 1978).

3.9.6 MEASUREMENTS OF REGIONAL VENTILATION

(a) Quasi-static methods

Measurements of regional ventilation can be made in several ways, none of which is entirely satisfactory. The simpler methods, or quasi-static methods, compare the distribution of a single breath of ^{133}Xe at total lung capacity with its distribution after rebreathing to equilibrium and the breath held a second time at total lung capacity. The counts in each image are then normalized and regional ventilation is expressed as the distribution of activity in the single-breath image divided by that at equilibrium; the figures in any region of the lung then represent relative ventilation per unit lung volume. Ball *et al.* (1962) also took into account the concentration of ^{133}Xe in the spirometer and the volume of air in the lungs to derive indices of ventilation that allowed more accurate comparisons between the same individual on different occasions and also between different individuals.

Figures for the relative distribution of ventilation per unit lung volume may also be derived from a wash-in procedure by using the integrated counts of the distribution of activity during the first 30–40 s, which represents the distribution of a tidal breath, and dividing this by the equilibrium distribution obtained at functional residual capacity (Secker-Walker *et al.*, 1974).

In a similar fashion the distribution of blood flow may be obtained following the intravenous administration of ^{133}Xe in saline. The measurements can be made at total lung capacity or during tidal breathing at functional residual capacity. If ^{99m}Tc-labelled particles are used it must be remembered that their distribution will reflect blood flow at the time of injection, and that the geometry of the system will be different from that using ^{133}Xe because of the differences in energy. ^{127}Xe is more satisfactory in this respect. Regional blood flow per unit lung volume can be obtained by dividing by the normalized ^{133}Xe equilibrium lung volume image, and the differences in geometry ignored if ^{99m}Tc-labelled particles were used for blood flow.

These measurements of regional lung volume tend to be slightly underestimated at the bases because the greater blood flow in normal subjects removes more of the ^{133}Xe compared to the upper parts of the lung. Of greater significance is the failure to reach equilibrium during the relatively short wash-in periods used in clinical practice (3–5 min) in patients with moderate to severe obstructive airflow diseases. Such regions can be recognized as defects on the wash-in image, and figures for regional ventilation per unit lung volume or

Table 3.3 Ventilation and perfusion indices using ^{133}Xe

Ventilation index $= V/E \times B/A \times 100$
Perfusion index $= I/E \times B/J \times 100$

where V = measured count rate during single breath after inhalation of ^{133}Xe
E = measured count rate during equilibrium
B = concentration of ^{133}Xe in spirometer × lung volume at time of measurement
A = concentration of ^{133}Xe in spirometer × volume of air inspired for single breath less anatomical and instrument dead space
I = measured count rate during single breath after intravenous injection of ^{133}Xe
J = quantity of ^{133}Xe injected

Regional ventilation and blood flow quasi-static method:

$$\mathrm{SBr} = \frac{\mathrm{Ctrsb}}{\mathrm{CtTsb}} \times 100$$

$$\mathrm{Vr} = \frac{\mathrm{CtrEq}}{\mathrm{CtTEq}} \times 100$$

$$\mathrm{Qr} = \frac{\mathrm{Ctrq}}{\mathrm{CtTq}} \times 100$$

Regional ventilation = SBr/Vr
Regional blood flow = Qr/Vr
Regional ventilation/perfusion = SBr/Qr

where Ct = count rate
r = regional
T = total
sb = single breath
Eq = equilibrium
q = blood flow
SB = normalized value for single breath
V = normalized value for lung volume
Q = normalized value for blood flow

regional blood flow per unit lung volume will be overestimated in these areas. The calculations for ventilation and perfusion indices are shown in Table 3.3.

Ventilation–perfusion images may also be obtained by dividing the normalized distribution of ventilation by that of blood flow. Because normalized count rates are used for these calculations, i.e. regional counts are expressed as a proportion of total counts in the image, the ventilation–perfusion ratios are relative and the overall ratio obtained for both lungs is unity. These calculations are shown in Table 3.3. Measurements of alveolar ventilation and cardiac output would have to be incorporated into the calculations to obtain more appropriate physiological ventilation–perfusion ratios.

(b) Dynamic methods

Several methods have been used to measure regional ventilation during tidal breathing using wash-in–equilibrium–wash-out procedures. Some make use of the time to reach 50% or 90% of the equilibrium count rate during the wash-out since the longer the time the more impaired the ventilation. Ventilation is the exchange of air and has the dimensions of flow (litres min^{-1}) whereas ventilation per unit lung volume has the dimensions of flow/volume or the reciprocal of time. Thus the dimensions of regional ventilation are the same as those of a rate constant.

Three methods have been applied to analyse wash-in and wash-out curves:

1. fitting a straight line to a semi-logarithmic plot of the initial part of the wash-out data, the first 50% or 60% of the curve (MacIntyre *et al.*, 1970; Jones *et al.*, 1971);
2. performing a least-squares fit of a model to the wash-in or wash-out data (Bunrow *et al.*, 1979);
3. using the Stewart–Hamilton equation for the wash-out data (Secker-Walker and Siegle, 1973; Alpert *et al.*, 1976).

The first of these has been used for wash-out data

following inhalation to equilibrium and also from the wash-out of injected ^{133}Xe. In both, the later parts of the wash-out curve are ignored and the more poorly ventilated regions will be underestimated. The least-squares fitting technique for both wash-in and wash-out data has the same accuracy as a modified Stewart–Hamilton technique which uses the wash-out data alone. Both procedures have been shown to have relative errors of less than 5% and coefficients of variation between 10% and 20%, when regions with equilibrium count rates of 3 counts s^{-1} and clearance times between 10 and 90 s were examined. The modified Stewart–Hamilton approach is somewhat simpler and the calculations can be carried out considerably faster than the least-squares curve-fitting method. Its main sources of error are terminating the wash-in or wash-out too soon and, more importantly, the tissue background activity (Matthews and Dollery, 1965). The larger this is as a proportion of the equilibrium count rate, and the shorter the clearance time, the greater the error. Wash-in and wash-out periods should be at least three times the largest clearance time and the equilibrium counts should be collected for between 25 s and 50 s (Bunrow *et al.*, 1979).

Approximately one-quarter of the background activity comes from the xenon dissolved in the tissues of the chest wall and the remainder from that dissolved in the blood (Ronchetti *et al.*, 1975).

The quasi-static methods and the dynamic methods give similar results for regional ventilation in normal subjects but tend to differ significantly in patients with airflow obstruction, because each is measuring a different aspect of ventilation. The quasi-static methods show how much air enters a region of the lung in comparison to the local lung volume, which may not be the same as how much air is actually exchanged. The dynamic methods estimate how much air is exchanged in relation to local lung volume and are more sensitive to abnormalities in ventilation.

(c) ^{81m}Kr images

As Fazio and Jones (1975) showed, the images obtained while breathing ^{81m}Kr are, for practical purposes, images of relative regional ventilation per unit lung volume (see Table 3.3). Although possible, it is not practical to obtain an image of lung volume with this gas, so that attempts to quantify these images in terms of the actual exchange are difficult. Rebreathing ^{85}Kr to equilibrium has been proposed as one solution (Jones *et al.*, 1978).

It should also be pointed out that, although ^{81m}Kr images and ^{99m}Tc particle perfusion scans may look similar, the latter show relative blood flow and not relative blood flow per unit lung volume.

Once a data collection and analysis system is set up, it is possible to generate figures for relative blood flow or ventilation, to calculate regional ventilation or perfusion indices and to determine regional ventilation–perfusion ratios. The output may be prepared in tables or presented more conveniently as parametric images in grey scan, colour, contours, three dimensions or as cinematic images. A critical comparison of the impact of these computer-assisted techniques on the decision-making process in patient care versus careful scrutiny of the original images has yet to be undertaken.

REFERENCES

Alazraki, N. P., Ramsdell, J. W., Taylor, A., Friedman, P. J., Peters, R. M. and Tisi, G. M. (1978) Reliability of gallium scan chest radiography compared to mediostinoscopy for evaluating mediastinal spread in lung cancer. *Am. Rev. Resp. Dis.*, **117**, 415–20.

Alderson, P. O., Secker-Walker, R. H. and Forrest, J. V. (1974a) Detection of obstructive pulmonary disease: relative sensitivity of ventilation–perfusion studies and chest radiography. *Radiology*, **112**, 643–8.

Alderson, P. O., Secker-Walker, R. H. and Strominger, D. B. (1974b) Pulmonary deposition of aerosols in children with cystic fibrosis. *J. Pediatr.*, **84**, 479–84.

Alderson, P. O., Rujanavech, N., Secker-Walker, R. H. and McKnight, R. C. (1976) The role of ^{133}xenon ventilation studies in the scintigraphic detection of pulmonary embolism. *Radiology*, **120**, 633–40.

Alderson, P. O., Lee, H. and Summer, W. L. (1979) Comparison of xenon 133 washout and single breath imaging for the detection of ventilation abnormalities. *J. Nucl. Med.*, **20**, 917–22.

Alderson, P. O., Biello, D. R., Khan, A. R., Barth, K. H., McKnight, R. C. and Siegel, B. A. (1980) A comparison of ^{133}Xenon single-breath and washout imaging with scintigraphic diagnosis of pulmonary embolism. *Radiology*, **137**, 481–6.

Alpert, N. M., McKusick, K. A., Correia, J. A. *et al.* (1976) Initial assessment of simple functional image of ventilation. *J. Nucl. Med.*, **17**, 88–92

Atkins, H. L., Susskind, H. and Klopper, J. F. (1977) A clinical comparison of xenon 127 and xenon 133 for ventilation studies. *J. Nucl. Med.*, **18**, 653–9.

Ball, W. C., Steward, P. B., Newsham, L. G. and Bayes, D. V. (1962) Regional pulmonary function studies with xenon-133. *J. Clin. Invest.*, **41**, 519–31.

Barron, T. F., Brinbaum, N. S. A. and Shane, L. B. (1985) *Pneumocystis carinii* pneumonia studied by gallium 67 scanning. *Radiology*, **154**, 791–3.

Benotti, R., Ockene, I. S., Alpert, S. and Daklen, J. E. (1983) The clinical profile of unresolved pulmonary embolism. *Chest*, **84**, 669–78.

Biello, D. R., Mattar, A. G., McKnight, R. C. and Siegel, B. A. (1979) Ventilation–perfusion studies in suspected pulmonary embolism. *Am. J. Radiol*, **133**, 1033–7.

Bogren, H. G., Berman, D. S., Viemara, L. A. and Mason, D. T. (1978) Lung ventilation perfusion scintigraphy in pulmonary embolism. *Acta. Radiol. Diagnosis*, **19**, 933–44.

Bookstein, S. J. (1986) Segmental arteriography in pulmonary embolism. *Radiology*, **93**, 619–34.

Boysen, P. G., Block, G. A., Olsen, G. N., Moulder, P. V., Harris, J. O. and Rawitscher, R. E. (1977) Prospective evaluation of pneumonectomy using the ^{99m}technetium quantitative perfusion lung scan. *Chest*, **72**, 422–5.

Bradley, E. W., Alderson, P. O. and Deye, J. A. (1979) Effects of fractionated doses of fast neutrons and photons on the normal canine lung-RBE values obtained by radionuclides. *Int. J. Radiat. Oncol.*, **5**, 197–207.

Bunrow, B., Line, B. R., Horton, M. R. and Weiss, G. H. (1979) Regional ventilatory clearance by xenon scintigraphy: a critical evaluation of two estimation procedures. *J. Nucl. Med.*, **20**, 703–10.

Carrol, R. G., Albin, M., Waterman, P. and Gummerman, L. W. (1977) Lung scan patterns in fifty cases of proven pulmonary air embolism. *J. Nucl. Med.*, **18**, 606.

Ciofetta, G., Pratt, T. A. and Hughes, S. J. M. B. (1978) Regional pulmonary perfusion assessed with continuous intravenous infusion of ^{81m}krypton: a comparison with technetium^{99m} macroaggregates. *J. Nucl. Med.*, **18**, 221–5.

Coates, G. and Nahmias, L. (1977) Xenon-127, a comparison with xenon-133 for ventilation studies. *J. Nucl. Med.*, **18**, 21–6.

Crystal, R. G., Fulmer, J. D., Roberts, W. C. *et al.* (1976) Idiopathic pulmonary fibrosis: clinical histologic radiographic physiologic scintigraphic, cytologic and biochemical aspects. *Ann. Intern. Med.*, **85**, 769–88.

Demeester, T. R., Goloms, M. M., Kircher, P. *et al.* (1979) The role of Ga-67 scanning in the clinical staging and preoperative evaluation of patients with carcinoma of the lung. *Ann. Thorac. Surg.*, **28**, 451–64.

Fazio, F. and Jones, T. (1975) Assessment of regional ventilation by continuous inhalation of radioactive krypton-81m. *Br. Med. J.*, **3**, 673–676.

Fazio, F., Lavender, P. J. and Steiner, R. E. (1978) ^{81m}Krypton ventilation and ^{99m}Tc perfusion scans in chest disease: comparison with standard radiographs. *Am. J. Roentgenol.*, **130**, 421–8.

Feinmann, R., Testa, H. J. and Prescott, M. (1978) Krypton 81m: its use in the clinical assessment of lung disease. *Br. J. Radiol.*, **15**, 112–17.

Gellert, A. R., Langford, J. A., Winter, R. J. D. *et al.* (1985) Asbestosis assessment by bronchial lavage and measurement of epithelial permeability. *Thorax*, **40**, 508–14.

Hisada, K., Tonami, N., Miyamae, E. Hiraki, Y., Yamazak, T., Maeda, T. and Nakajo, M. (1978) Clinical evaluation of tumour imaging with ^{201}thallium chloride. *Radiology*, **129**, 492–500.

Hooper, R. G., Beechler, C. R. and Johnson, M. C. (1978) Radioisotope scanning in the initial staging of bronchogenic carcinoma. *Am. Rev. Resp. Dis.*, **118**, 279–86.

Hull, R. D., Karkob, G. E. and Hirsh, J. (1986) The diagnosis of clinical suspected pulmonary embolism. *Chest*, **89** (suppl.), 4175–255.

Jacobs, M. P., Baughan, R. P., Huges, J. and Fernandez-Ulloa, M. (1985) Residual lung clearance in patients with active pulmonary sarcoidosis. *Am. Rev. Resp. Dis.*, **131**, 687–9.

Jefferies, A. L., Coates, G. and O'Brodovich, H. (1984) Pulmonary epithelial permeability in hyaline-membrane disease. *N. Engl. J. Med.*, **311**, 1075–1080.

Johnson, L., Krishnamurthy, S., Gilbert, S. *et al.* (1988) Effect of two levels of unlabelled antibody on lung tumour uptake of 111-In-anti CEA MOAb. *J. Nucl. Med.*, **29**, 825.

Jones, T., Clark, J. C., Rhodes, C. G., Heather, J. and Tofts, P. (1978) Combined use of krypton 81m and 85m in ventila-studies, in *Clinical and Experimental Application of Krypton 81m* (ed. J. Peter Lavender), British Institute of Radiology, London, pp. 46–50.

Jones, J. G., Lawler, P., Crawley, J. N. C. *et al.* (1980) Increased alveolar epithelial permeability in cigarette smokers. *Lancet*, **i**, 66–8.

Jones, R. H., Coulson, C. M. and Goodrich, J. K. (1971) Radionuclide quantitation of lung function in patients with pulmonary disorders. *Surgery*, **70**, 891–903.

Kawakami, K., Tada, S., Kalsuyama, N. and Machizuki, S. (1978) Radionuclide study in pulmonary sequestration. *J. Nucl. Med.*, **19**, 287–9.

Kramer, E. L., Sanger, J. J. and Garay, S. M. (1987). Gallium 67 scans of the chest in patients with AIDS. *J. Nucl. Med.*, **28**, 1107–14.

Kristersson, S. (1974) Prediction of lung function after lung surgery: a ^{133}Xenon radiospirometric study of regional lung function in bronchial cancer. *Scand. J. Thorac. Cardiovasc. Surg. (Suppl.)*, **18**, 5–44.

Kubota, K., Matsuzawa, T., Ito, M. *et al.* (1985) Lung tumour imaging by positron emission tomography using C-11 L methionine. *J. Nucl. Med.*, **26**, 37–42.

Liewendahl, K., Kairemo, K., Brownell, A. L. and Manty L. A. M. (1988) in *Nuclear Medicine: Trends and possibilities in Nuclear Medicine* (eds H. A. E. Schmidt and G. L. Buraggi), Schatlaker, Stuttgart, New York, 353–6.

MacIntyre, W. J., Inkley, J. R. and Roth, E. (1970) Spatial recording of disappearance constants of xenon-133 washout from the lung. *J. Lab. Clin. Med.*, **76**, 701–12.

Maini, C. L., Pistelli, R., Bonetti, M. G. *et al.* (1987) ^{99m}Technetium DTPA radio aerosol scintigraphy in progressive systemic sclerosis. *Nucl. Comp.*, **18**, 119–25.

Matthews, C. M. E. and Dollery, C. T. (1965) Interpretation of 133Xe lung washin and washout curves using an analogue computer. *Clin. Sci.*, **28**, 573–90.

McCarthy, D. and Chemiak, R. M. (1973) Regional ventilation–perfusion and hypoxia in cryptogenic fibrosing alveolitis. *Am. Rev. Resp. Dis.*, **107**, 200–8.

Mercandetti, A. J., Kipper, M. S. and Moser, K. M. (1985) Influence of perfusion and ventilation scans on therapeutic decision making and outcome in cases of possible embolism. *West. J. Med.*, **142**, 108–213.

Milic-Emili, J. (1971) Radioactive xenon in the evaluation of regional lung function. *Semin. Nucl. Med.*, 1246–62.
Neumann, R. D., Sostman, R. D. and Gottshalk, A. (1980) A current status of ventilation perfusion imaging. *Semin. Nucl. Med.*, **10**, 198–217.
O'Doherty, M. J., Page, C. G., Barlow, D. *et al.* (1987) Lung ^{99m}Technetium DTPA transfer in HIV antibody positive patients with *Pneumocystis carinii* pneumonia. *Nucl. Med. Comm.*, **8**, 308.
Park. H. M., DuCret, R. P. and Brindley, D. C. (1986) Pulmonary scintigraphy in fat embolism syndrome. *Clin. Nucl. Med.*, **11**, 521–2.
Pircher, F. J., Temple, J. R. and Kirsch, W. J. (1965) Distribution of pulmonary ventilation determined by radioisotope scanning. *Am. J. Roentgenol.*, **94**, 807–14.
Ramsdell, J. W., Peters, R. M. and Taylor, A. T. (1977) Multi organ scanning for staging lung cancer correlation with clinical evaluation. *J. Thorac. Cardiovasc. Surg.*, **73**, 653–9.
Rhodes, B. A., Stem, H. S. and Buchanan, J. W. (1971) Lung scanning with ^{99m}Technetium microspheres. *Radiology*, **99**, 613–21.
Ronchetti, R., Ewan, P. W., Jones, T. and Hughes, J. M. B. (1975) Use of ^{13}N for regional clearance curves compared with ^{133}Xe. *Bull. Européen Physiopath. Resp.*, **11**, 124–5.
Rosen, J. M., Biello, D. R., Siegel, B. A., Seldin, D. W. and Alderson, P. O. (1985) ^{81m}Kr ventilation imaging: clinical utility in suspected pulmonary embolism. *Radiology*, **154**, 787–90.
Saenger, E. L., Buncher, C. R., Specker, B. C. and McDevitt, R. A. (1985) Determination of clinical efficiency: nuclear medicine as applied to lung scanning. *J. Nucl. Med.*, **26**, 793–806.
Salvatore, M., Carratu, L. and Porta, E. (1976) Thallium-201 as a positive indicator for lung neoplasm: preliminary experiments. *Radiology*, **121**, 487–8.
Sanchis, J., Dolovich, M. and Chalmers, R. (1972) Quantitation of regional aerosol clearance in the normal human lung. *J. Appl. Physiol.*, **33**, 757–62.
Seaton, A., Lapp, N. L. and Change, C. H. J. (1971) Lung perfusion scanning in coal workers pneumoconiosis. *Am. Rev. Resp. Dis.*, **103**, 338–49.
Secker Walker, R. H. and Ho, J. E. (1979) Regional lung function in asbestosis workers. *J. Nucl. Med.*, **29**, 621.
Secker Walker, R. H. and Siegle, B. A. (1973) The use of nuclear medicine in the diagnosis of chest disease. *Radiol. Clin. N. Am.*, **11**, 215–241.
Secker Walker, R. H., Alderson, P. O. and Forrest, J. V. (1974) Detection of obstructive pulmonary disease. *Radiology*, **112**, 643–8.
Shibel, E. M., Tisi, G. M. and Moser, K. M. (1969) Pulmonary photoscan–roentgenographic comparisons in sarcoidosis. *Am. J. Roentgenol.*, **106**, 770–7.
Skarzynaki, J. J., Slavin, J. D., Spencer, R. P. and Karimeddini, M. K. (1986) Matching ventilation/perfusion imaging in fat embolism. *Clin. Nucl. Med.*, **11**, 40–41.
Sullivan, P. J., Burke, W. M., Burch, W. M. and Lomas, F. E. (1988) A clinical comparison of Technegas and xenon-133 in 50 patients with suspected pulmonary emboli. *Chest*, **94**, 300–4.
Taplin, G. V. (1964) Lung photoscan with macroaggregates of human serum albumen: experimental basis and initial clinical trials. US AEC University of California at Los Angeles Medical School. *Lab. Nucl. Med.*, **5**, 1–46.
Taplin, G. V. and Chopras, K. (1978) in *Progress in Nuclear Medicine*, Vol. 5 (ed. M. Guter), Karger, Basel, pp. 119–43.
Taplin, G. V. and MacDonald, N. S. (1971) Radiochemistry of macroaggregated albumin and newer lung scanning agents. *Semin. Nucl. Med.*, **1**, 132–52.
Taplin, G. V. and Poe, N. D. (1965) A dual lung scanning technique for evaluation of pulmonary function. *Radiology*, **85**, 363–8.
Tonami, N. and Hisada, K. (1977) Clinical experience of tumour imaging with 201-thallium chloride. *Clin. Nucl. Med.*, **2**, 75–81.
Tuazon, C. V., Delaney, M. D. and Simon, G. L. (1985) Utility of gallium 67 scintigraphy and bronchial washings in the diagnosis and treatment of *Pneumocystis carinii* pneumonia in patients with AIDS. *Am. Rev. Resp. Dis.*, **132**, 1087–92.
Wagner, H. N., Jr (1965) Radioisotope scanning of lungs in early diagnosis of bronchogenic carcinoma. *Lancet*, **i**, 344.
Wagner, H. N., Sabiston, D. C. and McAfee, J. A. (1964) Diagnosis of massive pulmonary embolism in man by radioisotope scanning. *N. Engl. J. Med.*, **271**, 377–384.
Waxman, A. D., Julien, P. S., Brachman, M. B. *et al.* (1984) Gallium scintigraphy in bronchogenic carcinoma: the effect of tumour location on sensitivity and specificity. *Chest*, **86**, 178–83.
Wellman, H. N., Mack, J. F. and Saenger, E. L. (1968) Clinical experience with oblique views in pulmonary perfusion scintigraphy in normal and pathological anatomy. *J. Nucl. Med.*, **9**, 374.
Wietzenblum, E., Moysis, B., Hirth, C. *et al.* (1977) Regional pulmonary function in sarcoidosis. *Scand. Resp. Dis.*, **58**, 17–26.
Zimmer, A. M., Rosen, S. T. and Spies, S. M. (1985) Radioimmuno imaging of human cell lung carcinoma with I-131 tumour specific monoclonal antibody. *Hybridoma*, **4**, 1–14.

CHAPTER FOUR

Peripheral vascular disorders

N. D. Greyson

4.1 INTRODUCTION

The widely prevalent problem of phlebitis, with its potentially fatal complication of pulmonary embolism, remains an important clinical problem both for the hospitalized and ambulatory patient. Peripheral vascular disease, resulting from atherosclerosis or other forms of vasculitis, with the complications of chronic cutaneous ulceration, pain, atrophy and gangrene, results in significant morbidity and incapacitation of the geriatric population.

After history and clinical assessment, the most widely used technique for assessing the peripheral circulation is opacification of the arterial or venous systems by angiography. The resultant radiographs are high-resolution images providing anatomical detail often necessary for specific diagnosis and treatment planning, especially when surgical reconstruction of diseased vessels is contemplated.

However, these invasive procedures are generally time consuming and expensive, and require the use of a special radiographic procedure suite, with its quasi-operating room ambiance, which may be intimidating to the patient. With the recent introduction of non-ionic contrast agents and digital subtraction angiography, the incidence of systemic effects of iodinated contrast agents has been reduced, and intravenous injections may frequently replace direct arterial catheterizations. These procedures are still not easily applicable for diagnostic screening procedures.

The use of radionuclide angiography provides an accurate, fast and simple method of detecting major vascular channel patency. Local tissue perfusion patterns and the presence of arteriovenous shunting may be detected using intra-arterial injections of labelled macroaggregates, analogous to performing a perfusion lung scan. ^{201}Tl and the newer technetium-labelled agents localize in tissues according to local blood flow and demonstrate perfusion and viability at the cellular level, without the need for intra-arterial injections.

Venous occlusion, or thrombophlebitis, may be detected by techniques which demonstrate the patency of venous channels using radionuclide venography, or by the use of various labelled agents which localize in thrombi, according to metabolic processes associated with thrombosis.

Radionuclide studies permit rapid, non-invasive diagnosis which might obviate or confirm the need for the more complex, but generally more definitive angiographic procedures.

Initial assessment by nuclear medicine techniques is performed with negligible discomfort or risk to the patient, and follow-up serial studies are possible with greater convenience and patient acceptability. In many situations, the combined use of multiple non-invasive procedures, such as radionuclide scanning and Doppler ultrasound or plethysmography, will increase the accuracy of detection of exclusion of disease to such a high confidence level that contrast angiography is now less frequently performed, except in cases of discordant results, or for pre-operative evaluation.

Table 4.1 lists a variety of procedures and applications of radionuclide studies.

4.2 RADIONUCLIDE ANGIOGRAPHY

Following a rapid intravenous injection of 10–20 mCi (370–740 MBq) of a ^{99m}Tc-labelled radiopharmaceutical, the bolus of activity passes through the route of least resistance toward the heart, outlining in turn the peripheral veins, superior or inferior vena cava, right atrium, right ventricle and lung fields. It returns to the arterial side of the

Table 4.1 Applications of nuclear medicine to peripheral vascular disorders

Clinical problem	*Nuclear technique*	*Route of administration**	*Radiopharmaceutical*
SVC obstruction Lung tumour staging Patency of aorta and branches Graft patency Vascular trauma	Radionuclide angiogram ('flow study')	i.v.	^{99m}Tc-pertechnetate ^{99m}Tc-albumin ^{99m}Tc-colloid ^{99m}Tc-phosphates
Haemangioma Vascularity of mass	Blood pool image (equilibration)	i.v.	^{99m}Tc-RBC
Tissue perfusion Ulcer healing Amputation level Pre- and post-op. evaluation	Capillary blockade or tissue perfusion scanning	i.a. i.m.	^{99m}Tc-albumin MAA ^{201}Tl-chloride ^{99m}Tc-isonitriles
Quantify blood flow	Xenon clearance	i.m., s.c.	^{133}Xe
A-V shunts	Lung uptake	i.a.	^{99m}Tc-albumin MAA
DVT IVC obstruction	Radionuclide venogram Venous blood pool imaging	i.v. i.v.	^{99m}Tc-MAA ^{99m}Tc-RBC
DVT Old vs. new thrombi	Thrombus seekers	i.v.	^{131}I-, ^{125}I-, ^{125}I-fibrinogen ^{99m}Tc-urokinase ^{99m}Tc-streptokinase ^{99m}Tc-plasmin ^{111}In-platelets

*i.v., intravenous; i.m., intramuscular; i.a., intra-arterial; s.c., subcutaneous.

circulation through the pulmonary veins, and after exiting the left ventricle it outlines the aorta and peripheral arterial branches.

Depending on the position of the gamma camera and sequence of imaging, the venous or arterial pathways are visualized, producing a quick, low-resolution vascular image.

The patency of mediastinal great vessels may be determined in patients with lung or hilar neoplasms, to assist in staging operability. Obstruction, stasis and collateral vessels are easily recognized (Figure 4.1). Serial assessment is possible to determine the progress of the disease or efficacy of treatment, without the need for repeated exposure to angiographic contrast material (Hartshorne *et al.*, 1984; Krishnamurthy *et al.*, 1973; Miyamae, 1973).

The thoracic aorta is best seen in a marked left anterior oblique position which unfolds the aorta. The abdominal aorta and iliac vessels are well seen in the anterior view positioned over the abdomen or pelvis. The presence of aneurysmal dilatation or obstruction of major vessels can be recognized in a few seconds after the intravenous injection (Figures 4.2 and 4.3). Aortic aneurysms are usually detected as a serendipitous finding in an abdominal flow study. Best evaluation for a suspected aneurysm is using ultrasound, which shows not only the patent channel but also the presence of mural thrombi and atherosclerotic plaques which would not be seen on the radionuclide flow study.

In the detection of major arterial obstruction, arteriovenous malformations, graft patency (Meindock, 1972) and vascular trauma (Diamond *et al.*, 1973; Rosenthall, 1974) the screening procedure is rapid and efficacious.

Immediate blood pool images taken after equilibration demonstrate the vascular compartment, including venous, arterial and capillary blood volumes, and the distribution of blood spaces within the organ. Some vascular malformations, such as cavernous haemangiomas, have rather slow circulation, despite the relatively large blood pool capacity. These lesions may not be demonstrated on the usual first-pass flow study, but may be delineated on delayed images when ^{99m}Tc-labelled red blood cells are used (Front *et al.*, 1983).

Visual inspection of the arterial phase of the

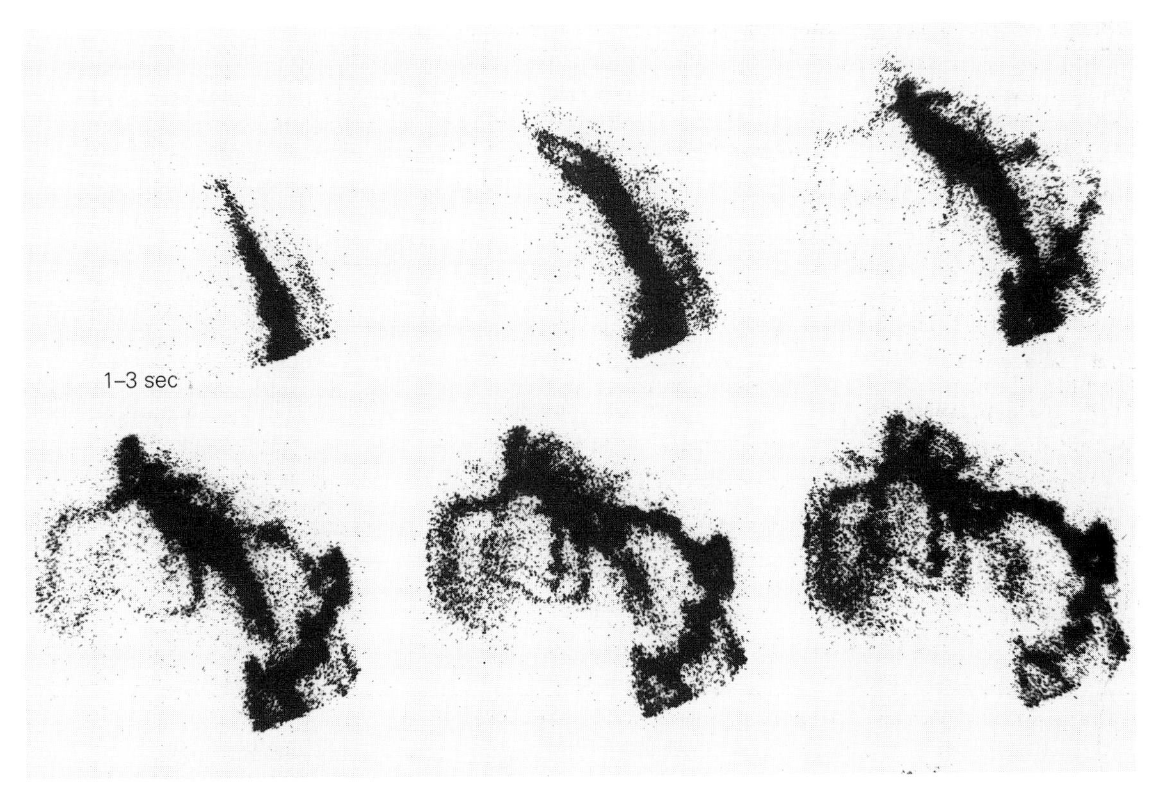

Figure 4.1 Mediastinal venogram. Left antecubital vein injection of ^{99m}Tc-pertechnetate in a 42-year-old renal dialysis patient with sudden onset of swelling of the left arm. The bolus of activity follows a slow tortuous course in the upper arm and over the chest wall. The innominate vein is not visualized. This patient had angiographically proven innominate and subclavian thrombosis, possibly a complication of the dialysis fistula.

images or computer quantification will demonstrate the relative but not absolute flow rates through the vessels, and permits comparison of flow through paired structures.

The radionuclide angiogram does not compare with conventional angiography in resolution or specificity. The procedure is, however, very rapid, without discomfort or side effects and requires no hospitalization. It may be used in conjunction with other organ imaging such as liver, bone or lung scans, to outline perfusion to these organs, to assess the vascularity of lesions within the organ, or to demonstrate venous or arterial pathways en route to these organs.

4.3 DETECTION OF THROMBOPHLEBITIS

Thrombophlebitis and pulmonary embolism are common causes of hospitalization and major complications of prolonged bed rest, orthopaedic surgery and cardiac disease. Pulmonary emboli and deep venous thrombosis are found in more than 50% of post-mortem examinations, usually clinically unsuspected. As most pulmonary emboli arise from a source in the lower extremities or abdomen, and about half the patients with clinical thrombophlebitis in the extremities have pulmonary emboli, suspicion of either problem justifies performing both lung scanning as well as an assessment of the venous system (Dorfman *et al.*, 1987; Kistner *et al.*, 1972).

The clinical diagnosis of thrombophlebitis may be in error, particularly when the obstruction is partial, and involves the proximal veins. Nonphlebitic lesions simulating deep venous thrombosis include musculoskeletal diseases, muscle infarcts, haematomas, lymphoedema, congestive heart failure, cellulitis and ruptured Baker's cyst.

Thrombophlebitis can be demonstrated indirectly by the demonstration of occlusion of the deep system and collateral pathways, indicating intraluminal thrombosis, or by the direct visualization of actively forming thrombi using thrombus-seeking agents such as ^{125}I-, ^{131}I- or ^{123}I-labelled fibrinogen, ^{111}In-labelled platelets, (Fenech *et al.*, 1981; Moser *et al.*, 1984; O'Connor *et al.*, 1986) and other technetium-labelled thrombus precursors or antagonists.

Non-nuclear adjunctive diagnostic methods include contrast venography, plethysmography and Döppler ultrasound.

4.3.1 FLOW VENOGRAM

Using ^{99m}Tc-labelled macroaggregates of albumin injected into a superficial vein of the foot, a radionuclide venogram may be added to the lung scan (Vlahos *et al.*, 1976). Tourniquets are applied above the knee and at the ankle to occlude the superficial system. Technetium-labelled macroaggregates of albumin (3–4 mCi (110–150 MBq) in less than 1 ml volume) are injected into a vein on the dorsum of the foot using a small-gauge needle. Using a gamma camera, the bolus of activity is followed through the deep system of the lower extremity to the inferior vena cava. Variations in the technique utilize larger volumes with slow infusion to fill the venous system more completely; repeat injections with the camera positioned at different levels; and single, multiple, or no tourniquets (Gomes *et al.*, 1982; Hayt *et al.*, 1977; Henkin *et al.*, 1974; Ryo *et al.*, 1977; Sy *et al.*, 1978a). Either technique demonstrates the bolus following a single, slightly curvaceous deep channel in the central portion of the extremity, sweeping medially above the inguinal ligament to join the contralateral iliac vein at the midline, forming the inferior vena cava. This appearance is that of an inverted 'Y' or wishbone, with an

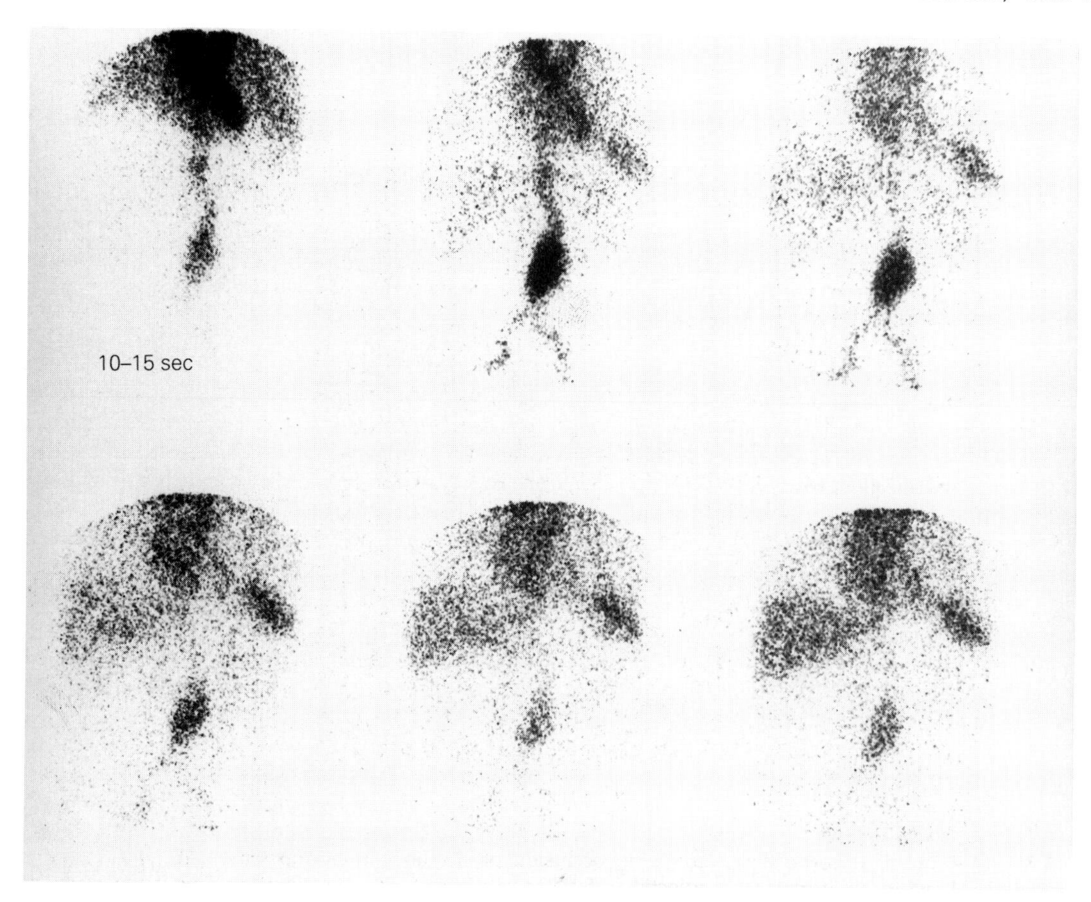

Figure 4.2 Abdominal aortic flow. A fusiform aortic aneurysm above the iliac bifurcation is demonstrated in conjunction with a ^{99m}Tc colloid liver and spleen scan.

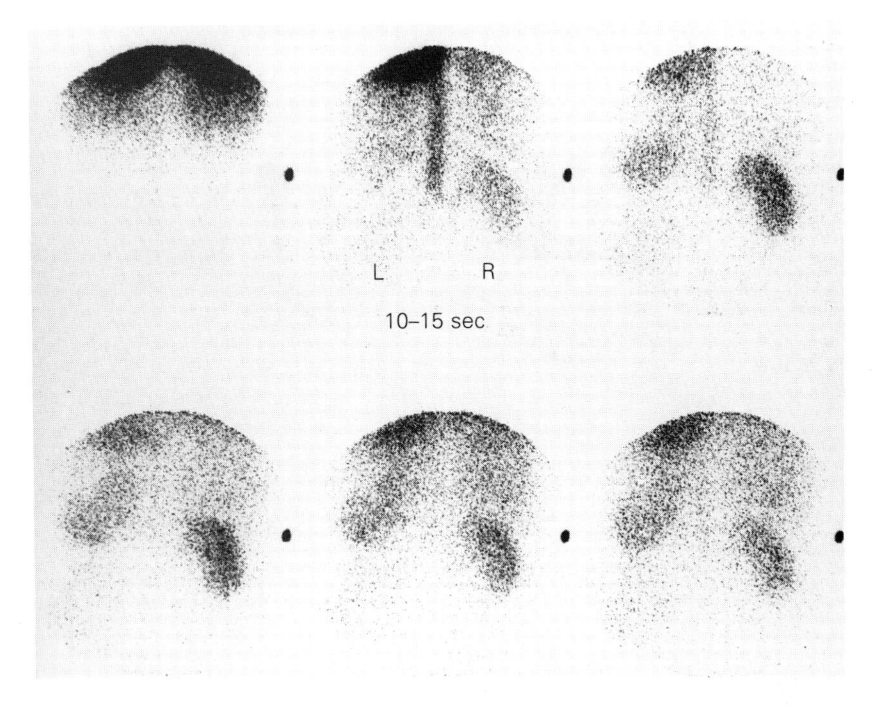

(a)

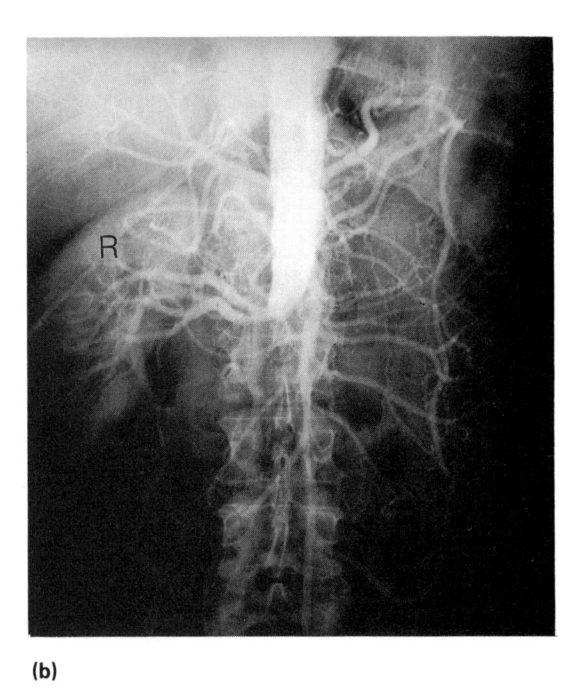

(b)

Figure 4.3 (a) Abdominal aortic flow. Complete occlusion of the abdominal aorta and left renal artery is demonstrated following an intravenous injection of ^{99m}Tc-labelled DTPA. (b) Abdominal aortic angiogram. Contrast opacification of the abdominal aorta via an intra-arterial catheter defines the aortic obstruction initially detected by radionuclide flow study.

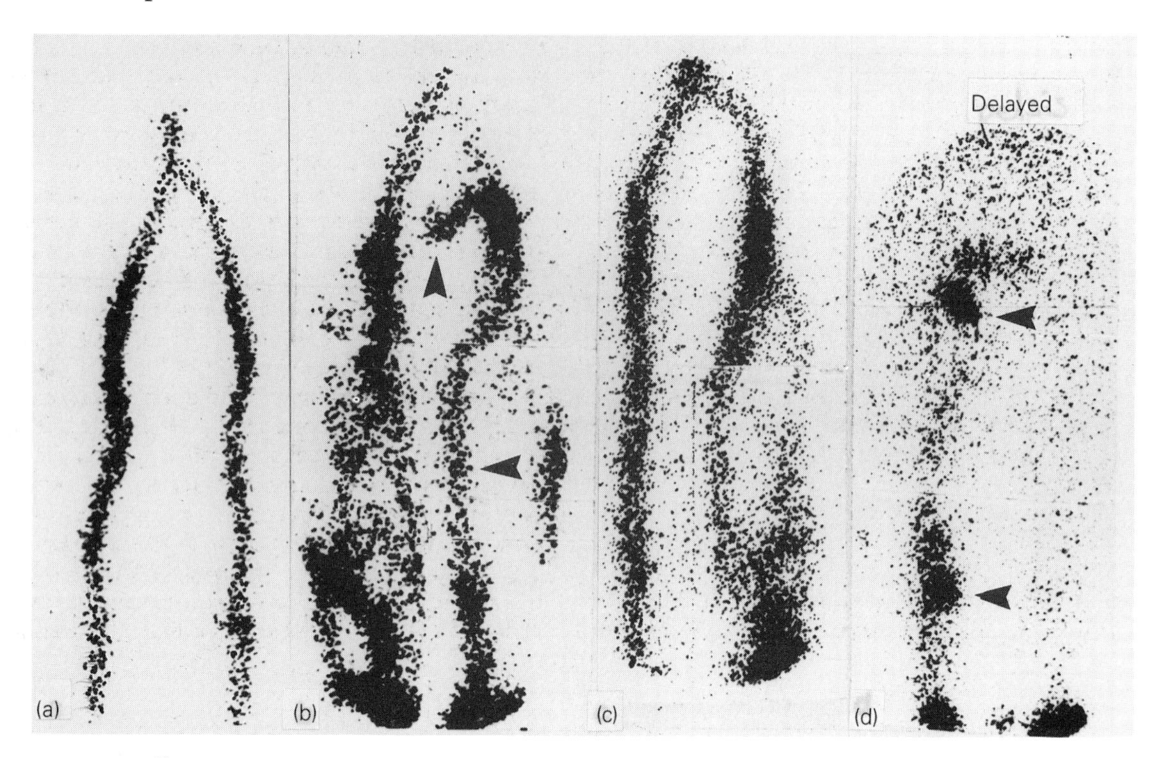

Figure 4.4 ^{99m}Tc-labelled macroaggregate lower extremity venogram patterns. (a) Normal. Note uncomplicated 'wishbone' appearance of the single-channel deep systems joining to form the inferior vena cava. (b) Bilateral multifocal deep vein thrombosis. Cross pelvic collateral (vertical arrow) indicates obstruction of left common iliac. Left femoral–popliteal occlusion results in absent flow through the deep system, with collateral flow through the long saphenous (horizontal arrow). Right DVT with numerous superficial collaterals. (c) Left popliteal occlusion with superficial collateral flow through long and short saphenous veins while tourniquet is on. Right deep system is normal. (d) Delayed scan in patient with multiple intraluminal thrombi of the right leg (arrows). Focal stasis did not clear with exercise or leg raising.

hourglass-shaped lower portion (Figure 4.4(a)). Images are repeated with the tourniquets off, producing an almost identical pattern although superficial veins may be observed, usually medial to the deep system at the skin surface. Images of the extremity following the time interval necessary to perform the lung scan, and after elevated leg exercise, if necessary, show no significant focal retained activity.

When deep venous thrombosis exists, it may be detected by the slowed passage of the bolus due to resistance to flow, and incompletely filled deep channels due to partial occluding intraluminal defect. With complete obstruction, there is no visualization of the deep system, but flow is seen in the superficial system, while the tourniquet is on. Collateral flow through the superficial system may be recognized by the medial location of the pathway, along the skin surface, close to the midline. Other collaterals may take any bizarre course (Figure 4.4(b) and (c)). Varicose veins and incompetent perforators may be misinterpreted as representing deep venous thrombosis, but the deep system should be observable.

Occlusion of the common iliac vein results in cross-pelvic collateral pathways, and the appearance suggesting a broken wishbone, or incomplete 'A' appearance. Obstruction of the inferior vena cava may produce numerous superficial abdominal collaterals or a wide double channel following the paravertebral plexus (Dhekne *et al.*, 1982; Sy *et al.*, 1978b).

The presence of focal stasis following exercise suggests intraluminal thrombi with the particles of labelled albumin entrapped on the fibrin network on the surface of the clot (Webber *et al.*, 1969, 1974) (Figure 4.4(d)). Delayed labelling is not always present in deep vein thrombosis (DVT), as a totally occluded vessel may prevent the particles from coming in contact with and adhering onto the thrombus (Rosenthall and Greyson, 1970).

Because the test demonstrates only the haemodynamic alterations and flow through pathways of least resistance, false-positive studies may be found in extrinsic compression, varicosities, and in the presence of incompetent perforating vessels. The technique does not differentiate old from new thrombi, but does separate high-risk patients with venous disease from the non-risk group. Although some false positives do occur (5–8%) the incidence of false negatives is even less, which is an acceptable situation in a screening procedure (Uphold *et al.*, 1980).

4.3.2 BLOOD POOL VENOGRAM

Radionuclide venograms using macroaggregates of albumin demonstrate the antegrade flow of the bolus through the interconnecting venous channels downstream from the injection site. As there are multiple deep channels below the knee (anterior and posterior tibial, and peroneal veins) and muscular branches (sural, soleal, gastrocnemius, etc.), many of these veins will not be opacified by injection into a superficial foot vein. The presence of oedema, cellulitis or dermatitis, or interference from a plaster cast or other dressing, may preclude an injection site in the affected limb.

Lisbona has demonstrated a method of detection of venous pathology by means of high-resolution imaging of the venous blood pools of the lower limbs, iliac veins and inferior vena cava (Lisbona, 1986; Lisbona *et al.*, 1982, 1985). The patient's red blood cells are labelled with ^{99m}Tc using a stannous reduction technique (Strivastava and Chervu, 1984). After pre-tinning the patient, 10–20 mCi (370–740 MBq) of pertechnetate may be injected into the foot to produce a 'flow' radionuclide venogram, or into another available vein, or the blood may be labelled *in vitro*. Circulating

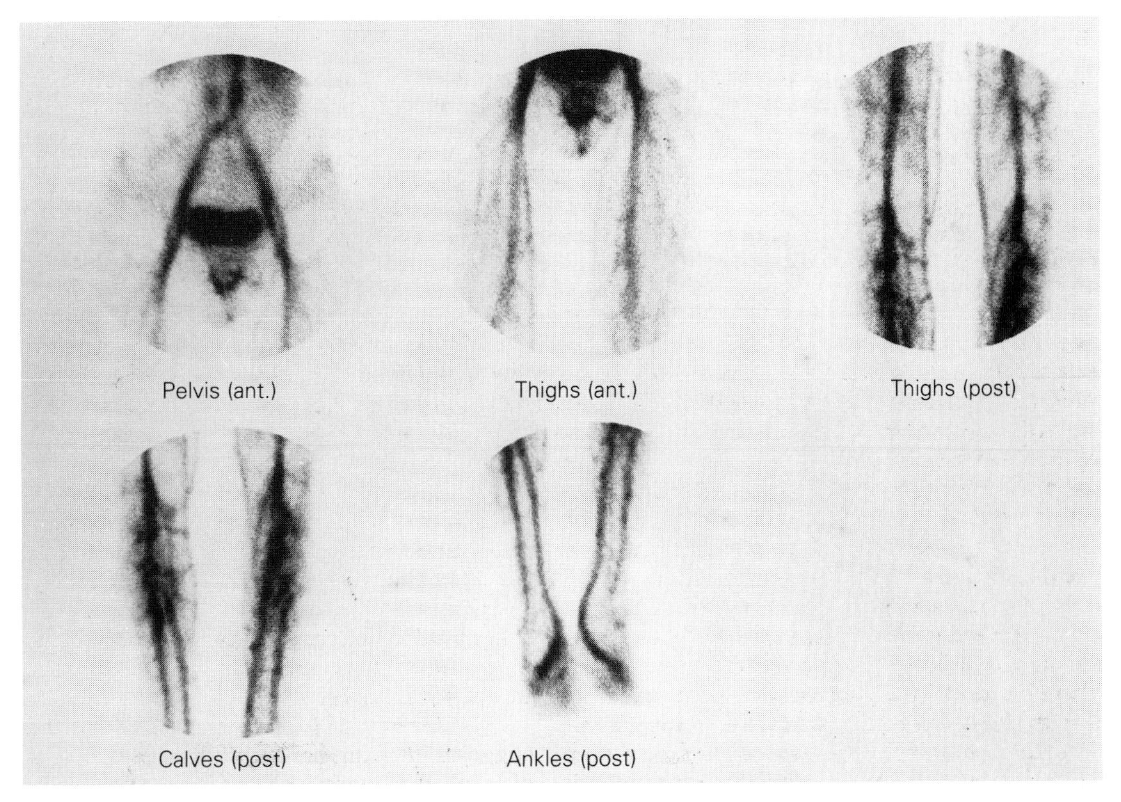

Figure 4.5 ^{99m}Tc-labelled red blood cell (RBC) venogram. Normal visualization of the deep and superficial venous system by this technique shows symmetrical, sharply defined appearance of major veins throughout the lower extremities. Multiple deep calf veins are imaged with the patient prone, to prevent compression by calf muscles.

labelled red blood cells are imaged in the inferior vena cava, iliac and upper femora on the anterior view, while the lower femora, popliteal and calf areas are imaged posteriorly with the patient prone to minimize extrinsic pressure caused by the weight of the legs on the calf vessels.

Normal images demonstrate at least two parallel deep veins in the calf (the posterior tibial on the medial side, and peroneal vein laterally). The sural vein extends downward and medially just below the knee. These join to form the popliteal vein. The femoral, common iliac and inferior vena cava are well visualized. The smaller muscular, superficial and cutaneous veins are seen variably. Internal iliac, pelvic and anterior tibial veins are not normally seen. The appearance should be symmetrical, with venous outlines being intense and sharply defined (Figure 4.5).

In DVT, the venous channel is filled with thrombus, thus labelled red blood cells are displaced, accounting for focal defects, thinning or non-visualization of the abnormal vessel. Collateral or superficial channels are more prominent in affected limbs. The leg may be swollen, and inflammation results in focal hyperaemia with soft tissue blood pool obscuring the normally clear definition of the vein wall (Figures 4.6–4.8).

False positives may occur with extrinsic compression (haematoma, pelvic mass, Baker's cyst and muscle contractions). An abnormal scan does not differentiate old from new DVT, and small, non-obstructing thrombi may not be resolved. However, with meticulous labelling, and the use of a high-resolution collimator, a sensitivity of 95% and specificity of 85% may be achieved. Even below the knee, 80% of calf DVT may be detected (Lisbona *et al.*, 1985).

While dynamic venography is superior in defining collateral pathways, particularly in the iliac area where abnormalities may be subtle (McCalley and Braunstein, 1987), this technique has the advantage of excellent anatomical visualization of venous channels remote from the injection site. Superior sagittal sinus thrombosis has been detected (Front *et al.*, 1986), and diagnostic manipulation (i.e. expressing a Baker's cyst) is possible with equilibration images (Littlejohn *et al.*, 1985). Sequential studies during therapy will demonstrate resolution or progression of disease.

4.3.3 THROMBUS LOCALIZATION

A fundamental principle of nuclear medicine is the use of metabolic processes to actively localize the radiotracer within the system under investigation. A number of different thrombus-seeking agents are in clinical use or under investigation.

Fibrinogen, labelled with one of several available radio-iodines, retains the biological property of being incorporated into fresh thrombi (Palko *et al.*, 1964; DeNardo *et al.*, 1977; DeNardo and DeNardo, 1981). This technique has been widely used as a method of detecting active thrombophlebitis (DeNardo and DeNardo, 1977; Kakkar, 1977).

^{99m}Tc-labelled agents such as streptokinase (Kempi *et al.*, 1974), urokinase (Millar and Smith, 1974; Asavavekinikul *et al.*, 1977) and plasmin

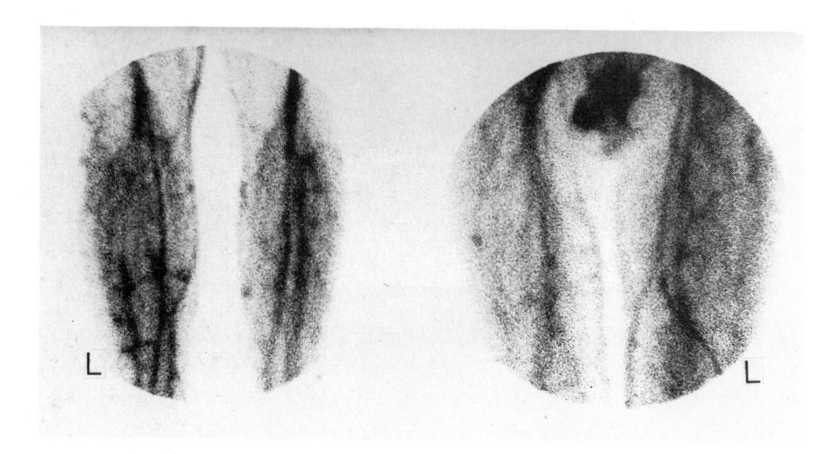

Figure 4.6 Left leg DVT. Poor definition of the left femoral vein, and deep veins below the knee. Hyperaemia associated with inflammation is apparent. Preferential flow through superficial veins.

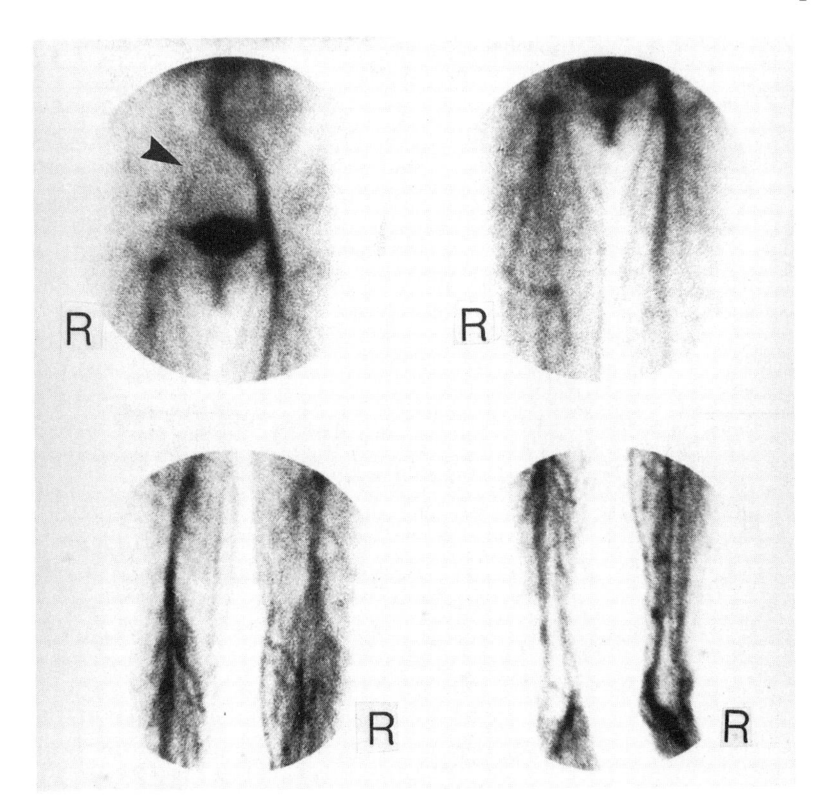

Figure 4.7 ^{99m}Tc-labelled RBC venogram. Right iliac occlusion. Cross-pelvic collateral channels not apparent on this study.

(Deacon *et al.*, 1980; Olsson *et al.*, 1982) have had mixed results.

^{111}In-labelled monoclonal antibodies have been used experimentally (Som *et al.*, 1986). Imaging the thrombus with ^{111}In-labelled platelets is the most physiological approach, but this technique is time consuming, with a complex extraction and labelling process, and the cost of indium is extremely high (Loken *et al.*, 1985). These drawbacks are shared with ^{123}I-labelled fibrinogen.

The use of ^{99m}Tc-, ^{111}In- or ^{123}I-labelled products permits visualization of the thrombus by a gamma camera (Figure 4.9). However, ^{131}I, because of the low doses necessary to minimize radiation exposure, or ^{125}I, because of its low energy, does not permit efficient gamma camera imaging. Thus, the use of iodofibrinogen is generally performed with external counting techniques.

Following an intravenous injection of 100 μCi (370 mBq) of ^{125}I-labelled fibrinogen into a peripheral vein, external counting over previously marked 5 cm intervals in the thigh and calf are made. Count rates are recorded and compared to the contralateral side, and cardiac blood pool, each of which acts as a control. The leg is slightly elevated to reduce venous pooling. Sequential counting is made daily, or more often, to observe local increases in count rate, indicating sequestration of the fibrinogen in an active thrombus. An increased count rate of about 20% compared with control is considered positive.

The technique is very effective in the calf and lower thigh, but loses sensitivity in the upper thigh and abdomen due to attenuation of the low keV ^{125}I, and overlapping splanchnic blood pool and bladder activity. Regrettably, it is of little use in the iliac vessels or inferior vena cava where thrombi are of greatest clinical threat (Moser and LeMoine, 1981).

Active thrombi may be detected as early as 1 h post-injection, or within several hours of the onset of thrombosis in a prospective screening. Below the upper thigh there is about 20% false-negative and 10% false-positive rates compared with venography (Morris, 1977).

Older thrombi with minimal fibrinogen turn-

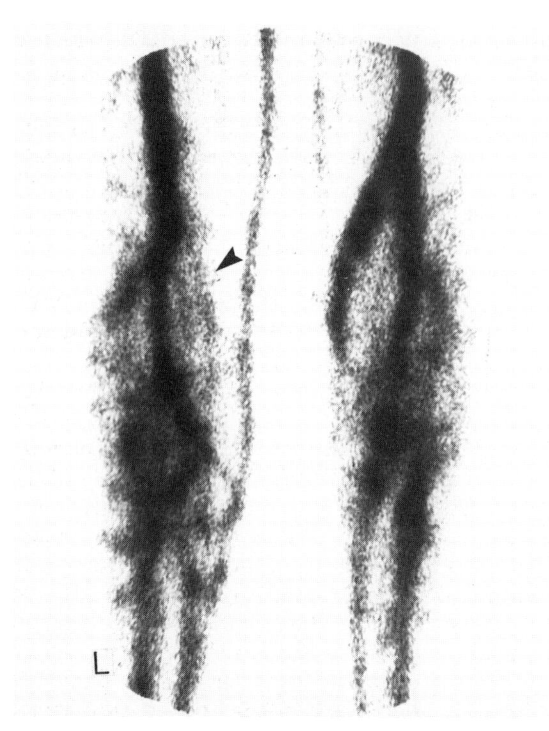

Figure 4.8 ^{99m}Tc-labelled RBC venogram. Left calf thrombophlebitis. The left sural vein is occluded (arrow). The long saphenous vein is dilated. Below the knee, the normal peroneal veins (lateral) and posterior tibial veins (medial) are well demonstrated.

over may be missed. However, in fresh thrombi, using high specific activity ^{131}I-labelled fibrinogen, the thrombus : serum ratio may be as high as 50 : 1, permitting imaging of the thrombus (Harwig *et al.*, 1975). False-positive misinterpretations occur in areas of cellulitis, haematoma or recent surgery. This is of particular significance considering the high percentage of thrombi developing near the site of femoral neck fractures, or in pelvic veins following abdominal surgery. In a general hospital, the test may be performed prospectively on the high-risk population such as following stroke or myocardial infarction, or orthopaedic surgery. This, however, is relatively time consuming and expensive if performed on large numbers of patients. Because of its high sensitivity for small thrombi in the calf, it may result in a therapeutic dilemma when the test becomes positive (Morris, 1977). As better agents are developed, positive imaging of thrombi using radiotracers and the gamma camera should enhance diagnosis. At present the method for non-invasive detection of thrombophlebitis varies with the local availability of expertise in the various modalities such as Doppler ultrasound (Comerota, 1985; Vogel *et al.*, 1987) and plethysmography (Hull *et al.*, 1981; Ramchandani *et al.*, 1985; Strandness, 1977). Frequently, more than one non-invasive test is used, combined with one or other nuclear medicine procedure.

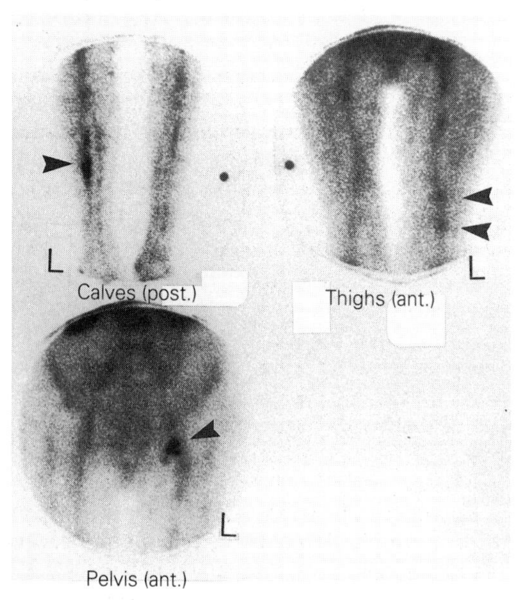

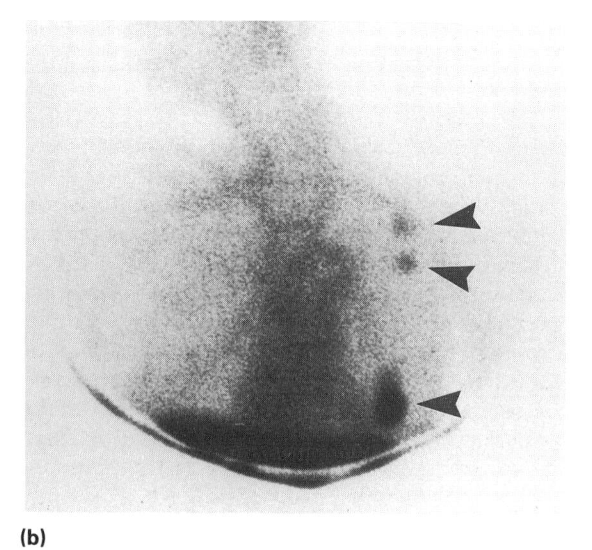

Figure 4.9 Thrombus seeking by ^{99m}Tc-labelled plasmin. (a) Leg images showing focal activity in left peroneal, femoral and inguinal regions (arrows). (b) Chest image shows focal activity indicating pulmonary emboli (arrows). (Courtesy of Dr S. Houle, Toronto General Hospital.)

Our approach, following clinical assessment, is to combine radionuclide venography with either Döppler or plethysmography. When these modalities agree, appropriate treatment is instituted. When there is disagreement, and there is a clinical requirement for more exact diagnosis, such as contraindication to anti-coagulants or when inferior vena cava plication is considered, then conventional radiographic venography is the final arbiter. If there is a question of the age of detected thrombi, the iodofibrinogen uptake test is used to separate old from active thrombi (Coleman *et al.*, 1975; Pollak *et al.*, 1975).

4.4 ASSESSMENT OF PERIPHERAL PERFUSION

The radionuclide angiogram discussed above is non-quantitative, although the rate of accumulation of activity within a limb or organ may be recorded using a computer and area of interest program. The resultant time–activity curve shows relative blood flow to each limb, but does not accurately measure absolue blood flow in terms of volume of flow per gram of tissue per unit time.

Blood pool images with labelled blood cells, albumin or transferrin show the activity within the vascular compartment, and the intensity of activity is a reflection of the local volume of blood, but this is not synonymous with blood flow and does not show perfusion at the capillary level.

4.4.1 CAPILLARY BLOCKADE AND TISSUE PERFUSION SCANNING

Images of the distribution of perfusion may be obtained following the intra-arterial injection of ^{99m}Tc-labelled albumin macroaggregate. This is analogous to performing a perfusion lung scan (Seigel and Wagner, 1976; Wagner *et al.*, 1969). Following intra-arterial injection, the particles are distributed distally in proportion to the arterial blood flow through each vascular segment. The particles are larger than capillaries (15–50 μm compared with 15 μm capillary diameter) and are thus trapped on the first pass through the capillary bed, permitting imaging with a gamma camera. This distribution reflects tissue perfusion at the physiologically significant capillary level.

The particles do not significantly affect blood flow to the limb as the total number of particles injected is normally less than 500 000, which is small compared with the number of capillaries in the extremity.

Radiographic angiography shows arterial anatomy to a diameter of 1–2 mm, and the presence of intraluminal disease, obstruction and collateral circulation may be recognized. The two modalities are thus complementary. Radiography shows gross vascular anatomy necessary before any surgical intervention, while the perfusion scan shows the resultant peripheral distribution of blood flow and the microcirculation.

Tissue perfusion may also be demonstrated using the intravenous injection of ^{201}Tl, which localizes in myocardial and skeletal muscle, according to local blood flow and viability of tissue. A similar distribution of perfusion within the muscles is seen by either thallium or capillary blockade techniques, but the thallium images do not require intra-arterial injection and may be performed at rest and following stress (Seigel and Stewart, 1984). This enhances the usefulness of the technique, as stressing permits the detection of mildly abnormal areas which are sufficiently perfused at rest, but unable to compensate for the increased oxygen demands of exercise.

In the normal individual, the pattern of activity is similar to the muscle bulk, with most activity localized in the thigh and calf, with less activity at the knee and ankle (Figure 4.10(a)). With diffuse small vessel disease, this 'muscular' distribution is lost and the appearance is more uniform or inhomogeneous (Figure 4.10(b)). When major arterial occlusions are present, the segmental perfusion defect may be recognized because of reduced flow through the high resistance of stenotic vessels (Figure 4.10(c)). The patency of specific 'run-off' vessel territories below the knee may be recognized. In the presence of iliac stenosis, the ratio of activity between the two limbs permits quantification of the degree of stenosis, or the patency of bypass grafts used to correct this condition (Rhodes *et al.*, 1973; Seigel *et al.*, 1975a).

Comparison of the perfusion patterns and the arteriographic anatomy is valuable in assessing patients with peripheral vascular disease. Despite the presence of large-vessel disease, the scan may appear normal if the microcirculation is intact and adequate collateral circulation is present. When abnormalities of the microcirculation coexist with large arterial abnormalities, reparative surgery is less successful in restoring normal tissue perfusion. The demonstration of normal capillary

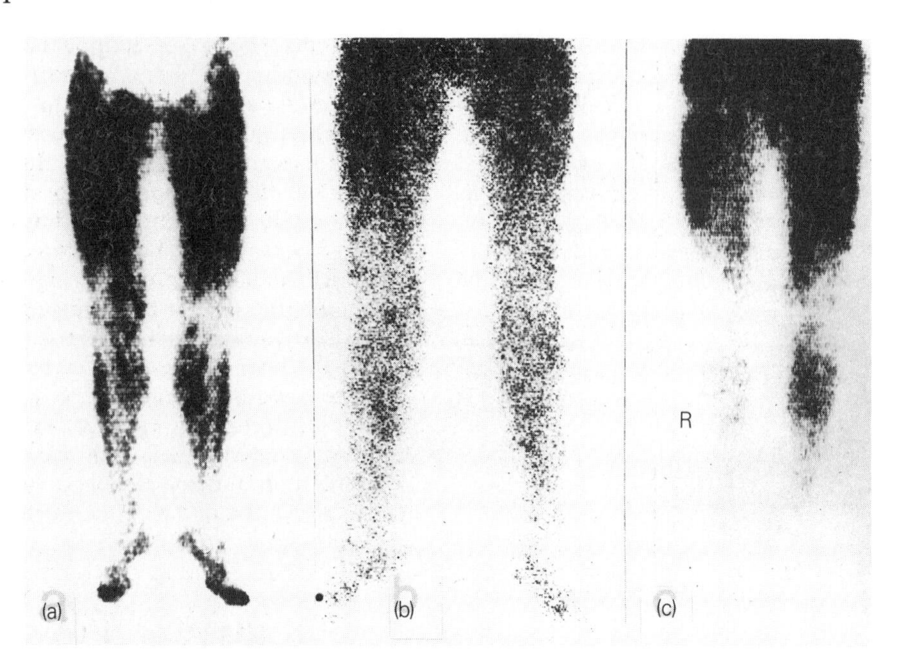

Figure 4.10 ^{99m}Tc-labelled macroaggregates. (a) Normal bilateral femoral artery injections show symmetrical distribution with 'muscular distribution'. (b) Diffuse peripheral vascular disease with disordered microcirculation resulting in a more uniform 'cutaneous' distribution. The patient did not respond well to reconstruction of large vessel abnormalities found on angiogram. (c) Iliac occlusion with marked asymmetric flow. Normal 'muscle' pattern despite severe large vessel disease indicates intact microcirculation. Good results followed aorto-iliac graft. Percentage flow to each limb may be measured.

perfusion distal to an obstruction suggests that the re-establishment of good flow to the extremity may be beneficial, while diseased microcirculation is of poor prognostic significance.

Pre- and post-treatment studies show the effect of vasodilating medication, sympathectomy and vascular reconstruction.

Peripheral perfusion scans are useful in the assessment of chronic cutaneous ulcers. Arterial insufficiency may coexist with chronic venous stasis, and diabetics may have a combination of peripheral vascular disease, infection, and peripheral neuropathy complicating the presence of an ulcer. It may be clinically difficult to separate out these aetiological factors requiring different forms of treatment.

Tissue perfusion scans demonstrate the presence or absence of hyperaemia around the ulcer bed (Figure 4.11). When the count rate in the area of an ulcer is approximately three times or greater than the activity of the adjacent portion of the limb, or contralateral similar site, this indicates that there is still sufficient capillary reserve to mobilize hyperaemia for repair (Seigel *et al.*, 1975b, 1981; Seigel and Stewart, 1984; Ohta, 1985). If this vascular reserve is inadequate, the high oxygen level required to promote healing cannot be obtained (Hunt *et al.*, 1968) and there is little likelihood that the ulcer will be healed by conservative means.

The presence of hyperaemia demonstrated by perfusion scanning correlates better with the potential to heal than the clinical assessment of the pulses. Some patients with hyperaemia fail to heal by conservative treatment and require surgery due to infection or pain, or to prevent prolonged immobilization. The majority of those patients without hyperaemia require amputation. Prolonged hospitalization and further complications can be prevented in this group by an earlier decision for surgical intervention, as determined by the perfusion scan.

The level of amputation site may be evaluated by establishing the level at which the microcirculation is abnormal. Following amputation, if there is delayed closure of the incision, perfusion scans may demonstrate a lack of hyperaemia indicating a poor prognosis for healing. The presence of

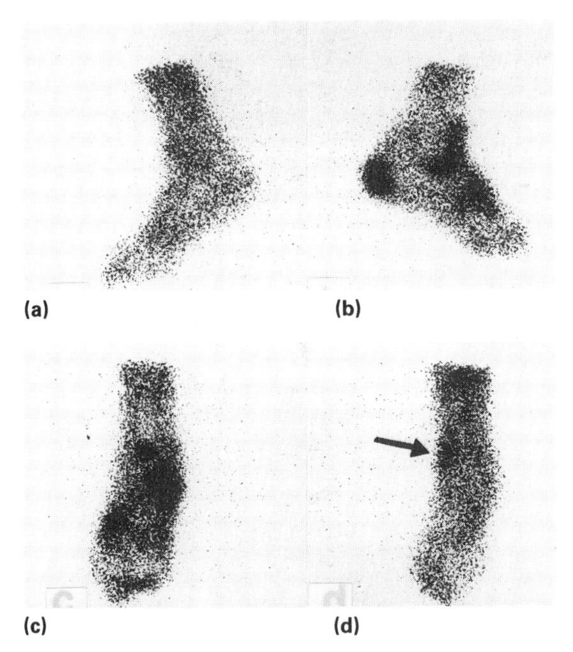

Figure 4.11 Assessment of chronic foot ulcers by ^{99m}Tc-labelled macroaggregate perfusion scanning. (a) Normal foot. (b, c) Multiple chronic ulcers in diabetic. Note marked increased activity around ulcer bed indicating hyperaemia of repair, suggesting healing is in progress. (d) Chronic ulcer of ankle (arrow) showing negligible hyperaemia. This suggests poor prognosis for healing. Amputation required 3 months later.

sufficient hyperaemia suggests that healing could progress, but that other local factors such as secondary infection may be inhibiting healing.

Newly developed ^{99m}Tc-labelled isonitriles have an intramuscular distribution which parallels blood flow, and images are similar to ^{201}Tl, but no redistribution occurs with time (Holman *et al.*, 1984; Schwartzkopff *et al.*, 1986). Images of the ^{99m}Tc label are slightly superior to the ^{201}Tl with its lower energy (Figure 4.12). These radiopharmaceuticals may have a future role in imaging peripheral vascular disease.

4.4.2 BLOOD FLOW MEASUREMENTS BY XENON CLEARANCE

^{133}Xe is a lipophilic inert gas whose clearance from local tissues permits direct measurement of blood flow rate (Lassen *et al.*, 1965; Silberstein *et al.*, 1983). Following direct subcutaneous or intramuscular injection, the soluble xenon diffuses out of the injection site into the bloodstream, and is carried to the lungs where it is exhaled preventing recirculation. The rate of disappearance of xenon is dependent on the rate of blood flow washing the xenon from the area, and the solubility of xenon in the injected tissue (partition coefficient).

The skin clearance rate of xenon has been used to diagnose vascular insufficiency, predict ulcer healing, and localize amputation levels (Moore *et al.*, 1981; Harris, 1986). A mean skin blood flow of less than 1 ml 100 g^{-1} min^{-1} suggested that an amputation flap will not heal, while patients with a mean flow of 2.4 ml 100 g^{-1} min^{-1} or greater healed. This ratio between positive and negative response is similar to that found in microsphere and thallium techniques for prediction of healing.

Although measurements are accurate, the determinations indicate blood flow only for the local area of injection and not for the entire limb as a

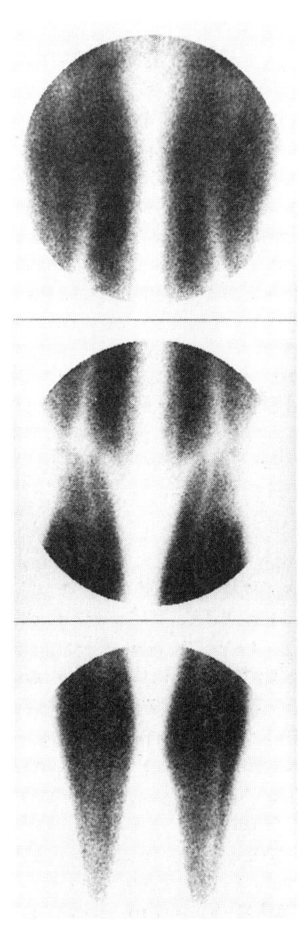

Figure 4.12 ^{99m}Tc-labelled isonitrile perfusion images. Analogous to ^{201}Tl, distribution of activity is dependent on muscle blood flow following intravenous injection. This patient had normal blood flow to both limbs in this post-exercise image.

whole. More complete assessment of the entire limb perfusion distribution requires multiple injections. A combination of a tissue perfusion scan with thallium or intra-arterial macroaggregates to outline the distribution of perfusion, coupled with xenon clearance flow rate determinations of selected areas, is a useful approach to the total assessment of the extremity.

4.4.3 ARTERIOVENOUS SHUNT MEASUREMENTS

Actual or potential arteriovenous (A-V) shunts exist in the skin and muscles of humans, and in some species are important in local tissue perfusion and temperature regulation. The presence of A-V shunts has been suspected or implicated in a number of peripheral vascular problems such as chronic ulcers, varicose veins, peripheral vascular disease, traumatic or congenital arteriovenous malformations and Paget's disease (Giargiana *et al.*, 1974; Lopez-Majano *et al.*, 1969; Rhodes *et al.*, 1972; Rosenthall *et al.*, 1970).

A-V shunts may be easily detected by arterial and venous oxygen measurements, but are more difficult to quantify by these methods. In the presence of A-V shunts, venous oxygen levels are abnormally high because arterial oxygen is diverted through shunts and not utilized. However, A-V shunting may be easily measured by determining the proportion of particles which become localized in the lungs following an intra-arterial injection of 5 mCi (185 MBq) of technetium-labelled particles 15–50 μm in diameter. Virtually 100% of the particles should become lodged in the distal capillary bed, but if A-V communications larger than capillaries are present then a proportion of the particles will bypass the capillary bed and enter the venous circulation and return to the lungs. The deposition of radioactivity in the lungs can be monitored with a simple scintillation detector. A second intravenous injection of particles simulates a 100% shunt. Thus, the percentage shunted from the extremities can be simply calculated.

Another approach utilizes a whole-body camera system. The count rate within the area supplied by the intra-arterial injection is evaluated. This is compared with the whole-body count rate and the percentage shunted outside of the area of investigation may be determined.

This has research applications in determining the response of peripheral circulation to various vasoactive medications, determining the presence of A-V shunts in a variety of diseases and conditions, and in the pre- and post-operative assessment of surgically corrected peripheral A-V shunts.

REFERENCES

Asavavekinikul, S., Forbes, C. D. and McDougall, I. R. (1977) Is ^{99m}Tc-urokinase a useful agent for detection of deep venous thrombosis? *Clin. Nucl. Med.*, **2**, 235–8.

Coleman, R. E., Harwig, S. S. L., Harwig, J. F. *et al.* (1975) Fibrinogen uptake by thrombi: effect of thrombus age. *J. Nucl. Med.*, **16**, 370–3.

Comerota, A. J. (1985) Diagnostic methods for deep vein thrombosis: venous doppler examination, phleborheography, iodine-125 fibrinogen uptake and phlebography. *Am. J. Surg.*, **150**, 14–25.

Deacon, J. M., Ell, P. J., Anderson, P. *et al.* (1980) Technetium-99m-plasmin: a new test for the detection of deep vein thrombosis. *Br. J. Radiol.*, **53**, 673–7.

DeNardo, G. L. and DeNardo, S. J. (1981) Thrombosis detection: fibrinogen counting and radionuclide venography. *Clin. Nucl. Med.*, **6**, 37–45.

DeNardo, S. J. and DeNardo, G. L. (1977), Iodine-123-fibrinogen scintigraphy. *Semin. Nucl. Med.*, **3**, 245–51.

DeNardo, G. L., DeNardo, S. J., Barnett, C. A. *et al.* (1977) Assessment of conventional criteria for the early diagnosis of thrombophlebitis with the 125-I fibrinogen uptake test. *Radiology*, **125**, 765–8.

Dhekne, R. D., Moore, W. H. and Long, S. E. (1982) Radionuclide venography in iliac and inferior vena caval obstruction. *Radiology*, **144**, 597–602.

Diamond, A. B., Meng, C. H., Wolenske, A. C. *et al.* (1973) Radionuclide demonstration of traumatic arterial injury. *Radiology*, **109**, 623–6.

Dorfman, G. S., Cronen, J. J., Tupper, T. B. *et al.* (1987) Occult pulmonary embolism: a common occurrence in deep venous thrombosis. *Am. J. Roentgenol.*, **148**, 263–6.

Fenech, A., Hussey, J. K., Smith, F. W. *et al.* (1981) Diagnosis of deep vein thrombosis using autologous indium-111-labelled platelets. *Br. Med. J.*, **282**, 1020–2.

Front, D., Israel, O., Joachims, H. *et al.* (1983) Evaluation of hemangiomas with technetium-99m-labelled RBC's: perfusion–blood pool mismatch. *JAMA*, **249**, 1488–90.

Front, D., Israel, O., Even-Sapir, E. *et al.* (1986) Superior sagittal sinus thrombosis: assessment with Tc-99m labelled red blood cells. *Radiology*, **158**, 453–6.

Giargiana, F. A., Greyson, N. D., Rhodes, B. A. *et al.* (1974) Absence of arteriovenous shunting in peripheral arterial disease. *Invest. Radiol.*, **9**, 222–6.

Gomes, A. S., Webber, M. M. and Bufkin, D. (1982) Contrast venography vs. radionuclide venography: a study of discrepancies and their possible significance. *Radiology*, **142**, 719–28.

Harris, J. P. (1986) Skin blood flow measurement with xenon-133 to predict healing of lower extremity amputations. *NZ J. Surg.*, **56**, 413–15.

Hartshorne, M. F., Bauman, J. M., Telepak, R. J. *et al.*

(1984) Chest radionuclide angiography in the evaluation of pulmonary masses. *Clin. Nucl. Med.*, **9**, 502–5.
Harwig, J. F., Coleman, E., Harwig, S. *et al.* (1975) A new look at thrombus localizing agents. *J. Nucl. Med.*, **16**, 756–63.
Hayt, D. B., Blatt, C. J. and Freeman, L. M. (1977) Radionuclide venography: its place as a modality for the investigation of thromboembolic phenomenon. *Semin. Nucl. Med.*, **7**, 263.
Henkin, R. E., Yao, J. S. T., Quinn, J. L. III *et al.* (1974) Radionuclide venography (RNV) in lower extremity venous disease. *J. Nucl. Med.*, **15**, 171–5.
Holman, B. L., Jones, A. G., Lister, J. J. *et al.* (1984) A new Tc-99m labelled myocardial imaging agent, hexakis (*t*-butylisonitrile) technetium (1) [Tc-99m TBI]: initial experience in the human. *J. Nucl. Med.*, **25**, 1350–55.
Hull, R., Hirsh, J., Sackett, D. L. *et al.* (1981) Replacement of venography in suspected venous thrombosis by impedance plethysmography and ^{125}I fibrinogen leg scanning: less invasive approach. *Ann. Intern. Med.*, **94**, 12–15.
Hunt, T. K., Zederfeldt, B. and Dunphy, J. E. (1968) Role of oxygen tension in healing. *Q. J. Surg. Sci.*, **4**, 279–83.
Kakkar, V. V. (1977) Fibrinogen uptake test for detection of deep vein thrombosis: a review of clinical practice. *Semin. Nucl. Med.*, **7**, 229–44.
Kempi, V., Van Der Linden, W. and Von Scheale, C. (1974) Diagnosis of deep vein thrombosis with ^{99m}Tc-streptokinase: clinical comparison with phlebography. *Br. Med. J.*, **4**, 748–9.
Kistner, R. L., Ball, J. S., Nordyke, R. A. *et al.* (1972) Incidence of pulmonary embolism in the course of thrombophlebitis of the lower extremities. *Am. J. Surg.*, **124**, 169–76.
Krishnamurthy, G. T., Blahd, W. T. and Winston, M. A. (1973) Superior vena caval syndrome: scintigraphic evaluation of response to radiotherapy. *Am. J. Roentgenol.*, **117**, 609–14.
Lassen, N. A., Lindbjerg, I. F. and Dahn, I. (1965) Validity of the Xe 133 method for measurement of muscle blood flow evaluated by simultaneous venous occlusion plethysmography. *Circ. Res.*, **16**, 287–93.
Lisbona, R. (1986) Radionuclide blood-pool imaging in the diagnosis of deep-vein thrombosis of the leg. *Nucl. Med. Annual*, **1986**, 161–93.
Lisbona, R., Stern, J. and Derbekyan, V. (1982) Technetium-99m red blood cell venography in deep vein thrombosis of the leg: correlation with contrast venography. *Radiology*, **143**, 771–3.
Lisbona, R., Derbekyan, V., Novales-Diaz, J. A. *et al.* (1985) Tc-99m red blood cell venography in deep venous thrombosis of the lower limb: an overview. *Clin. Nucl. Med.*, **10**, 208–24.
Littlejohn, G. O., Brand, C. A., Ada, A. *et al.* (1985) Popliteal cysts and deep venous thrombosis: Tc-99m red blood cell venography. *Radiology*, **155**, 237–40.
Loken, M. K., Clay, M. E., Carpenter, B. A. *et al.* (1985) Clinical use of indium-111 labelled blood products. *Clin. Nucl. Med.*, **12**, 902–11.
Lopez-Majano, V., Rhodes, B. A. and Wagner, H. N. Jr (1969) Arteriovenous shunting in extremities. *J. Appl. Physiol.*, **27**, 782–6.
McCalley, M. G. and Braunstein, P. (1987) Diagnosing iliofemoral vein occlusion from radionuclide blood pool venography. *Clin. Nucl. Med.*, **12**, 180–4.
Meindock, H. (1972) Visualization of arterial graft patency by intravenous radionuclide angiography. *J. Can. Med. Assoc.*, **106**, 1180–2.
Millar, W. T. and Smith, J. F. B. (1974) Localization of deep venous thrombosis using technetium-99m labelled urokinase. *Lancet*, **ii**, 695–6.
Miyamae, T. (1973) Interpretation of ^{99m}Tc superior vena cavograms and results in 92 patients. *Radiology*, **108**, 339–52.
Moore, W. S., Henry, R. E., Malone, J. M. *et al.* (1981) Prospective use of xenon-133 clearance for amputation level selection. *Arch. Surg.*, **116**, 86–88.
Morris, G. K. (1977), Does the ^{125}I-fibrinogen uptake test help us to understand and manage venous thromboembolism? *Clin. Nucl. Med.*, **2**, 334–5.
Moser, K. M. and Fedullo, P. F. (1984) Imaging of venous thromboemboli with labelled platelets. *Semin. Nucl. Med.*, **14**, 188–97.
Moser, K. M. and LeMoine, J. R. (1981) Is embolic risk conditioned by location of deep venous thrombosis? *Ann. Intern. Med.*, **94**, 439–44.
O'Connor, M. K., Brennan, S. S. and Shanik, D. G. (1986) Indium-111 labelled platelet deposition following transfemoral angiography. *Radiology*, **158**, 191–4.
Ohta, T. (1985) Noninvasive technique using thallium-201 for predicting ischaemic ulcer healing of the foot. *Br. J. Surg.*, **72**, 892–5.
Olsson, C. G., Albrechtsson, U., Darte, L. *et al.* (1982) Technetium-99m plasmin for rapid detection of deep venous thrombosis. *Nucl. Med. Comm.*, **3**, 41–52.
Palko, P. D., Nanson, E. M. and Federuk, S. O. (1964) The early detection of deep vein thrombosis using I-131 tagged human fibrinogen. *Am. J. Surg.*, **110**, 613–16.
Pollak, E., Webber, E. and Victery, W. (1975) Radioisotope detection of venous thrombosis: venous scan vs. fibrinogen uptake test. *Arch. Surg.*, **110**, 613–16.
Ramchandani, P., Soulen, R. L., Fedullo, L. M. *et al.* (1985) Deep vein thrombosis: significant limitations of non-invasive tests. *Radiology*, **156**, 47–9.
Rhodes, B. A., Greyson, N. D., Hamilton, C. R. *et al.* (1972) Absence of anatomic arteriovenous shunts in Paget's disease of bone. *N. Engl. J. Med.*, **287**, 686–9.
Rhodes, B. A., Greyson, N. D., Seigel, M. E. *et al.* (1973) The distribution of radioactive microspheres after intra-arterial injection in the legs of patients with peripheral vascular disease. *Am. J. Roentgenol.*, **118**, 820–5.
Rosenthall, L. (1974) Intravenous angiography in the diagnosis of trauma. *Semin. Nucl. Med.*, **4**, 395–409.
Rosenthall, L. and Greyson, N. D. (1970) Observations on the use of ^{99m}Tc albumin macroaggregates for detection of thrombophlebitis. *Radiology*, **94**, 413–16.
Rosenthall, L., Greyson, N. D., Herba, M. J. *et al.* (1970) Measurement of lower extremity arteriovenous shunting with ^{131}I macroaggregates of albumin. *J. Can. Assoc. Radiol.*, **21**, 153–5.
Ryo, U. Y., Qzai, M., Srikantaswany, S. *et al.* (1977) Radionuclide venography: correlation with contrast venography. *J. Nucl. Med.*, **18**, 11–17.
Schwartzkopff, B., Szabo, Z., Losse, B. *et al.* (1986)

Effect of stress on the myocardial kinetics of T-butylisonitrile-technetium (Tc-99m-TIBI). *Eur. J. Nucl. Med.*, **12**, 534–5.

Siegel, M. E. and Stewart, C. A. (1984) The role of nuclear medicine in evaluating peripheral vascular disease. *Nucl. Med. Annual*, **1984**, 227–71.

Siegel, M. E. and Wagner, H. N., Jr (1976) Radioactive tracers in peripheral vascular disease. *Semin. Nucl. Med.*, **6**, 253–78.

Seigel, M. E., Giargiana, F. A., White, R. I. *et al.* (1975a) Peripheral vascular perfusion scanning: correlation with the arteriogram and clinical assessment in the patient with peripheral vascular disease. *Am. J. Roentgenol.*, **125**, 628–37.

Siegel, M. E., Williams, G. M., Giargiana, F. A. *et al.* (1975b) A useful, objective criterion for determining the healing potential of an ischemic ulcer. *J. Nucl. Med.*, **16**, 993–5.

Siegel, M. E., Steward, C. A., Wagner, W. *et al.* (1981) New objective criterion for determining, non-invasively, the healing potential of an ischemic ulcer. *J. Nucl. Med.*, **22**, 187–9.

Silberstein, E. B., Thomas, S., Cline, J. *et al.* (1983) Predictive value of intracutaneous xenon clearance for healing of amputation and cutaneous ulcer sites. *Radiology*, **147**, 227–9.

Som, P., Oster, Z. H., Zamora, P. O. *et al.* (1986) Radioimmunoimaging of experimental thrombi in dogs using technetium-99m-labelled monoclonal antibody fragments reactive with human platelets. *J. Nucl. Med.*, **27**, 1315–20.

Strandness, D. E. (1977) Thrombosis detection by ultrasound, plethysmography, and phlebography. *Semin. Nucl. Med.*, **7**, 213–18.

Strivastava, S. C. and Chervu, R. L. (1984) Radionuclide-labelled red blood cells: current status and future prospects. *Semin. Nucl. Med.*, **14**, 68–82.

Sy, W. M., Lao, R. S., Bay, R. *et al.* (1978a) (^{99m}Tc) pertechnetate radionuclide venography: large volume injection without tourniquet. *J. Nucl. Med.*, **19**, 1001–6.

Sy, W. M., Lao, R. S., Nissen, A. *et al.* (1978b) Occlusion of inferior vena cava: features by radionuclide venography. *J. Nucl. Med.*, **19**, 1007–12.

Uphold, R. E., Knopp, R. and Paulo, A. L. (1980) Radionuclide venography as an outpatient screening test for deep venous thrombosis. *Ann. Emerg. Med.*, **9**, 613–16.

Vlahos, L., MacDonald, A. F. and Causer, D. A. (1976) Combination of isotope venography and lung scanning. *Br. J. Radiol.*, **49**, 840–51.

Vogel, P., Laing, F. C., Jefferey, R. B., Jr *et al.* (1987) Deep venous thrombosis of the lower extremity: US evaluation. *Radiology*, **163**, 747–51.

Wagner, H. N., Jr, Rhodes, B. A., Sasaki, Y. *et al.* (1969) Studies of the circulation with radioactive microspheres. *Invest. Radiol.*, **4**, 374–86.

Webber, M. M., Bennett, L. R., Cragin, M. *et al.* (1969) Thrombophlebitis demonstrated by scintillation scanning. *Radiology*, **92**, 620–3.

Webber, M. M., Pollak, E. W., Victery, W. *et al.* (1974) Thrombosis detection by radionuclide particle (MAA) entrapment: correlation with fibrinogen uptake and venography. *Radiology*, **111**, 645–50.

CHAPTER FIVE

Renal radionuclide studies

K. E. Britton, M. N. Maisey and A. J. W. Hilson

5.1 ANATOMY AND PHYSIOLOGY

The easiest way to locate the kidneys is to feel for the lumbar spine and the costal margins following the line of the ribs medially and cranially. A disc 10 cm in diameter may then be set with its medial edge towards the lumbar spine and the lowest rib overlying a quarter of its surface. The kidneys move with respiration and with change of posture, falling forward in the prone and sitting forward positions, so investigations are best performed with the patient reclining. In this position the two kidneys are at approximately equal depths, less than 1 cm difference in 75% of cases. The actual depth of the kidney in any individual varies from 4 cm–11 cm, therefore it is usual to calculate individual renal function as a fraction or percentage of the total, and measure the total function separately to avoid the need to measure the absolute radiotracer content of each kidney. To correct for tissue attenuation, renal depth may be estimated directly or indirectly. In each kidney there are about a million nephrons, composed of a glomerulus, proximal tubule, loope of Henle and distal tubule connected to the collecting duct. It is not known exactly how the kidneys work, but it is clear that the physical arrangement of the filters, tube and loops made up of living cells is important; that the interaction of physical phenomena – forces, resistances, filtration, diffusion, osmosis, pressure gradients and flows with active transport mechanisms – enable the system to work; and that a hierarchy of control systems – the cell and intercellular channels, tubuloglomerular balance, nephron autoregulation, the juxtaglomerular apparatus, intrarenal flow distribution and hormonal interactions – maintain not only the functioning kidney but also conserve and support the internal environment of the body. The maintenance of salt and water balance and the control of osmolality and acidity of the body and the levels of plasma potassium, calcium and phosphate ions are essential functions. Important substrates such as glucose and amino acids are retained while unnecessary metabolites such as uric acid, urea, sulphate, creatinine and guanidine derivatives are excreted.

Classical renal physiology emphasizes the differences between glomerular filtration and tubular function. Inulin, ^{51}Cr-labelled ethylenediaminetetraacetate (EDTA) or pure ^{99m}Tc-labelled diethylenetriaminepentaacetate (DTPA) are excreted from the kidney only through glomerular filtration and, being neither reabsorbed nor metabolized by the kidney, may be used to measure glomerular filtration rate (GFR). Para-aminohippurate (PAH), radio-iodinated orthoiodohippurate (OIH) and ^{99m}Tc-labelled mercaptoacetyl triglycine (MAG3) are primarily secreted by the tubules and may be used to provide an index of renal plasma flow since the major part of such compounds entering the peritubular capillary blood finish up in the tubules. However, an overall look at blood–kidney exchange of compounds shows that the amount per unit time taken up by the kidneys of all the compounds mentioned above depends on their supply rate to the kidneys, and the kidneys' extraction efficiency for each (E). The amount in the plasma supplied per unit time, t (the supply rate) is given by the renal plasma flow (RPF) multiplied by the plasma concentration (P_t) at unit time. Thus the amount taken up by the kidneys, Q, per unit time is given by

$$Q_t = \text{RPF} \times P_t \times E \qquad (5.1)$$

For OIH and PAH, RPF × E is usually called the effective renal plasma flow (ERPF) to take account of the fact that these compounds are not 100% extracted – about 80% extraction is usually accepted. For the glomerular filtered agents, the fraction filtered (the filtration fraction, FF) is given by the fraction of RPF of GFR. Thus the extraction efficiency, *E*, for these compounds equals FF equals GFR/RPF. Thus

$$Q_t = \text{RPF} \times P_t \times \text{GFR/RPF} \quad (5.2)$$
$$= \text{GFR} \times P_t$$

for glomerular filtered compounds.

In the kidney, tubule function and GFR are maintained in balance through the control of the juxtaglomerular apparatus, so that not too little filtrate is reabsorbed and not too much filtration is allowed to occur. This is called tubuloglomerular balance and depends on a feedback control loop. If either tubular disease alone or glomerular disease alone affects a nephron, tubuloglomerular balance is disrupted and the nephron in effect shuts down. This phenomenon is the basis of the 'intact nephron hypothesis' of Bricker (1969) which proposed that 'surviving nephrons of the diseased kidney largely retain their essential functional integrity'. If this hypothesis is correct then the GFR/RPF ratio (FF) for a diseased kidney of 100 000 nephrons should be the same as the ratio of its normal partner with a million nephrons. Thus, although the overall FF may vary from 0.15 to 0.4 it is the same for each kidney.

These findings have the following important consequences for work with renal radiopharmaceuticals. First, if one writes $GFR_L = 25$, $RPF_L = 125$, $RPF_R = 250$, it is easy to see that $GFR_R = 50$ ml min^{-1}, where L and R refer to left and right. Second, if one measures the individual contribution of one kidney to total function under steady-state conditions, it does not matter whether a GFR agent or an ERPF agent is used, the percentage contribution of each kidney to total function will be the same. Third, the intact nephron hypothesis, by implying that nephrons are either working or not working, also implies that the working nephrons are working similarly whichever kidney they are in. This in turn implies that each is responding to a common stimulus in such a way that it either self-regulates or is self-regulated so as to preserve its individual balance of GFR and RPF independent of their absolute values. It would also account for why a renogram from a normal kidney with hundreds of thousands of nephrons or from half a normal kidney has a sharp peak and why both kidneys when normal have the peaks of their renograms at the same time. For if nephrons all worked differently, their tracer transit times would differ and no sharp peak could occur.

Nephrons are of two distinct types, although there is overlap between them. Cortical nephrons make up about 85% and their glomeruli lie in the outer two-thirds of the cortex. Each cortical nephron has a juxtaglomerular apparatus (JGA), which is formed as a syncytium between the muscular afferent arteriole and the early part of the distal tubule, the macula densa, of the same glomerulus, together with some interstitial mesangial cells and the almost amuscular efferent arteriole. The muscle fibres of the afferent arterioles bear granules containing the enzyme, renin, probably as a precursor.

The substrate for renin is a globulin called angiotensinogen, present in plasma. Enzymic breakage by renin produces a decapeptide, angiotensin I, which in turn forms the substrate for a plasma and tissue converting enzyme which converts it into angiotensin II, an octapeptide. This is both a potent constrictor of arterioles and a stimulus to aldosterone release by the adrenals. All the enzymes necessary to produce angiotensin II are apparently bound to larger molecules in the isolated JGA. The angiotensin-converting enzyme (ACE) inhibitor captopril inhibits the production of angiotensin II both locally in the kidney and systemically.

The resistance to the flow of blood to cortical nephrons depends on the tone of the muscular wall of the afferent arteriole. Paradoxically this tone depends on the renal perfusion pressure itself in the following way. A fall in perfusion pressure reduces the peritubular capillary pressure around the proximal tubule and this enhances salt and water reabsorption. Less salt and water is delivered to the JGA, which senses this and in turn reduces the local release of renin and thence angiotensin, so that the afferent arteriole tends to relax. This reduces the afferent resistance, thereby maintaining flow at a lower renal perfusion. This ability to maintain flow in spite of variation in perfusion pressure between physiological limits is called autoregulation.

The autoregulatory response sets off a further control loop. The lack of requirement for renin locally leads to its release into renal venous blood in response to a fall in blood pressure. The production of angiotensin II in the circulation stimulates the release of aldosterone from the adrenal cortex. Aldosterone enhances sodium reabsorption in the distal tubule, which with the systemic vasoconstrictor effects of angiotensin II tends to reverse the drop in perfusion pressure.

Afferent arteriolar vasoconstriction occurs in response to a rise in perfusion pressure through increased delivery of salt to the JGA. Increased tone can be initiated additionally by a rise in sympathetic activity, which can override the autoregulatory response. Certain systemic disorders, such as renovascular hypertension, occur when pathology affects these renal self-regulatory mechanisms, and certain renal disorders such as acute renal failure in shock result from an overriding of their local autoregulatory system by changes in the systemic control systems.

In the normal resting state afferent arterioles are relaxed and the resistance to flow through cortical nephrons is less than the resistance to flow through juxtamedullary nephrons. This, as well as their greater numbers, accounts for the higher blood flow through cortical nephrons. Reduction in flow by 20% can occur in normal daily life, for example from sudden noise, change in posture or mild stress, therefore a relaxed atmosphere is essential for reliable renal studies.

The afferent arterioles to juxtamedullary (JM) nephrons are poorly muscular and the main control site is at the efferent arterioles. They respond to antidiuretic hormone (ADH), which also increases the permeability of the collecting duct to water, to circulating angiotensin II and to sympathetic activity by vasoconstriction. They relax in response to prostaglandin activity. Radioiodinated OIH uptake by JM nephrons is determined by efferent, not afferent, arteriolar flow. Relaxation of efferent arteriolar tone, for example due to the ACE inhibitor captopril, will cause a fall in JM glomerular filtration but an increase in delivery of OIH to the JM proximal tubules. This may explain the increased sensitivity with the use of a filtered agent, DTPA, over OIH in the 'captopril test' for renovascular disorder. The fall in GFR due to loss of JM efferent arteriolar tone through captopril coupled with the fall in blood pressure and renal perfusion pressure causes impaired renal function which is usually but not always reversible. The long venous vasa recta descend, associated with the long loops of Henle, towards the tip of the medulla. The interactions of the flows of salt, water and urea between, up and down these tubes and the collecting ducts whose permeabilities vary for these different solutes lead to the conservation of water in dehydration. The traditional counter-current hypothesis of urinary concentration is insufficient because it requires the single effect of active transport to be present both in the thick and thin parts of the ascending limbs of the loop of Henle, yet there is no substantive evidence for active transport of salt out of the thin ascending limb.

There is no way that the cortical and JM nephrons can be separated by external imaging as their convolutions and loops overlap, although only glomeruli of cortical nephrons are likely to reside in the outer third of the cortex and only long loops of Henle of the JM nephrons reside in the inner medulla. Investigative separation of these two populations therefore depends on their functional differences.

The mechanism of salt and water reabsorption in the proximal tubule depends on both active and passive transport. Whereas active transport accounts for the greater part of salt reabsorption and a natriuretic hormone is invoked for its control, alteration in the passive component of sodium reabsorption is affected by blood flow, and a solute such as OIH or DTPA is concentrated in the tubules and the transit times of these compounds along the nephrons is increased and can be estimated to assess this renovascular disorder.

In the situation of increased resistance to the outflow of urine, as with pelviureteric junction obstruction, the pressure gradient from the glomerulus to the site of resistance changes to maintain the rate of urine flow. The force comes from the cardiac output through glomerular filtration, and the intraluminal pressure rises as one component of the change in pressure in response to the resistance to outflow. The intraluminal pressure thereby exceeds the peritubular capillary pressure, salt and water reabsorption is increased and the transit times of OIH and DTPA are prolonged through the parenchyma. An index of the prolongation of parenchymal tracer transit time may be used to distinguish the presence or absence of obstructive nephropathy in a kidney with a dilated renal pelvis.

Just as conservation of salt is the major function of the cortical nephrons, so the conservation of water is the main purpose of the JM nephrons. Their function determines the urine flow, which has a large influence on renal parenchymal transit time. The relationship between transit time and urine flow is hyperbolic. No mean transit time shorter than 120 s occurs however fast the urine flow, whereas at slow flows, less than 0.4 ml

min^{-1}, the mean transit time becomes disproportionately prolonged.

A somewhat inverse linear relationship occurs between mean transit time and urine flows of 1–3 ml min^{-1}. Since the collecting ducts are common to both cortical and JM nephrons and the transit time through the collecting ducts depends on the urine flow rate, a correction to the mean parenchymal transit time is made to account for variations in urine flow between patients by subtracting from it a minimum transit time common to all nephrons to leave the parenchymal transit time index (PTTI), which will more accurately represent the effect of changes in salt and water reabsorption. The minimum transit time represents the obligatory minimum time of transit through the tubules and loop of Henle and the component due to variation in water reabsorption in the collecting ducts.

The renal transit times can be summarized as follows. The very short time for ^{99m}Tc-labelled DTPA to pass the glomerular filter and the slight difference in timing between this and the secretion of ^{99m}Tc-labelled MAG3 or ^{123}I-labelled OIH into the proximal tubular lumen are quite lost in consideration of the nephron transit times when the usual data sampling interval is 10 s. The whole kidney transit time (WKTT) is given by the total transit time through renal parenchyma and pelvis. The mean parenchymal transit time (MPTT) is that through the whole of the parenchyma and together with the pelvic transit time (PVTT) equals WKTT. The mean parenchymal transit time is made up of a minimum transit time (MinTT) common to all nephrons, and parenchymal transit time index (PTTI). The whole kidney transit time corrected for the minimum transit time is called the whole kidney transit time index (WKTTI). Thus

$$\begin{aligned} \text{WKTT} &= \text{MPTT} + \text{PVTT} \\ \text{MPTT} &= \text{MinTT} + \text{PTTI} \\ \text{WKTT} &= \text{MinTT} + \text{WKTTI} \end{aligned}$$

Normal ranges are for: PTTI = 10–156 s; MPTT = 100–240 s; WKTTI = 20–170 s.

The normal pelvis has effectively laminar flow with a mean residence time of 5–10 s. However, if the pelvis is dilated, whether floppy walled and unobstructed or with its outlet obstructed, then eddying and mixing of tracer results and the mean residence time may be over 3 min. Any method increasing the flow rate of urine will reduce the pelvic transit time in the absence of obstruction to outflow and this forms the basis for the use of diuretics such as frusemide or mannitol in making this distinction.

The normal ureter contracts at three to six times per minute, helping to massage the urine to the bladder, but ureteric contraction is not essential to urine flow since, with an aperistaltic ureter as in retroperitoneal fibrosis, urine will flow normally under the influence of gravity. Because of the arrangement of the smooth muscle bundles and the angled path of the ureter through the bladder wall, the opening and closing of the vesicoureteric valve comes about as a natural consequence of ureteric peristalsis. This may be disrupted by inflammation or overdistension of the bladder wall, and lead to reflux of urine from the bladder towards the kidney.

5.1.1 RENAL MODELS

There are two types of measurement, 'descriptive' and 'physiological', that can be made from renal radionuclide studies. First, there are at least twenty different points or times that have been taken from the renogram, such as the time for the curve to fall from peak to half its height, the height of the curve at the end of the first phase and so on. Such measurements are descriptive, and enable one to classify the shape of the curve and to compare one curve with another. It should not be expected that such values have inherent physiological significance. This has to be demonstrated empirically by clinical observation and correlation with other tests applied to the kidney. This is also true of the classification technique called principal component analysis (Oppenheim and Appledorn, 1981). Secondly, there are those measurements that relate directly to the physiology and pathophysiology of the kidney through a 'physiological model'.

It is crucial to understand that the application of mathematics or a mathematical model to the analysis of data depends on the physiological model that represents as simply and truly as possible the reality of the clinical situation. A crude example is the statement that blood is in a space (compartmental) and that the kidney is made up of tubes (linear). The more anatomically and physiologically acceptable (isomorphic) the physiological model is, the more is one able to understand deviations from normal of data obtained in pathological situations. Conversely, data analysis based on an incorrect physiological model, while appearing correct in the original test system, may well give uninterpretable or wrongly interpreted results in pathophysiological situations. Just as there are rules for mathematics so there are for physiology and each model has its own rules and assumptions. Thus a conceptually isomorphic model gives both the physiological basis for interpreting a particular measurement and allows one to appreciate the biological assumptions and sources of error that are inherent in such an interpretation in the context of renal disorders. These are in addition to the more readily documented random and systematic measurement errors due to the physical basis of the external counting technique.

Two different models are typically used in assessing dynamic studies: the compartmental model and the linear system model. The compartmental model is most often isomorphic to fluid collections, for example, the interchange of tracer between blood and extracellular fluid. If a tracer that is only taken up by the organ under study is chosen, the rate of loss from, for example, blood plasma will equal the rate of uptake by the chosen organ which may be termed the **uptake function** of the organ.

The uptake function may also be determined relatively in paired organs, in parts of organs and in sites of suspected pathology. The popularity of compartmental models led to their attempted use in the kidney (De Grazia *et al.*, 1974), a situation in which they were hardly isomorphic. As well as all the assumptions required by indicator dilution theory, an important feature of a compartmental model is that the rate of mixing in one compartment is rapid compared to the rate of exchange between compartments. This situation is clearly reasonable for a tracer introduced into the blood, but hardly likely to occur in a kidney made up of tubes of nephrons which cross back and forth between the cortex, outer and inner medulla.

Provided that a compartmental model is justified, then the results of compartmental analysis of the data may be applied to the compartments. Compartmental (exponential) analysis may be applied to curves obtained from many different sites. It is only when they are obtained from a site with which a compartmental model is isomorphic that the results of the compartmental analysis may be meaningfully related to the model. As a result of these difficulties, the linear model is being increasingly used.

The linear system approach tends to consider an organ as a 'black box' containing a series of alternative pathways that the tracer may take between input and exit. Different path lengths take different times to traverse, causing different delays between input and output. The linear model thus concerns the transit times of tracer through an organ and the distribution of these transit times.

An organ containing a mixture of tubes like the kidney may be modelled if an appropriate tracer is used. The assumptions of a linear model of the kidney include stationarity: that the response of the system to an input given at one time will be the same if the same input is given at another time. This implies a steady-state situation and anxiety on the part of the patient is the most common source of disturbance. Another assumption is that the response of the system to a series of inputs will equal the sum of the responses that would have occurred if each input had been given individually. This latter statement is the key to the success of the linear model because it allows the blood clearance curve of OIH, MAG3 or DTPA to be considered as the sum of a series of ever-decreasing single inputs to the kidney. In this way the total response of the kidney to that complex input may be considered as the summation of the individual responses to the series of individual inputs entering the kidney over a chosen period of time.

Deconvolution analysis is the name of the

Table 5.1 Renal functions with radionuclide imaging

1. Uptake functions
   - Total renal function
     - Effective renal plasma flow
     - Glomerular filtration rate
     - Functioning mass
   - Individual kidney functions as a percentage of total
   - Relative cortical and juxtamedullary function in one kidney
2. Transit functions
   - Whole kidney transit time
   - Mean parenchymal transit time
   - Parenchymal transit time index
     - – measures of salt and water reabsorption
   - Pelvic transit time – an index of pelvic dilatation and status
3. Removal functions
   - Response to frusemide
   - Ureteric peristalsis
   - Reflux
4. Distribution of these functions

mathematical technique whereby the response of the kidney to an individual input from blood is derived. This means that, from the blood clearance curve recorded over the heart, the equivalent of a spike injection into a renal artery can be derived and the individual response of the kidney to this spike injection can be obtained. This response is called the renal (impulse) retention function. From it may be derived, by differentiation, the mean and distribution of tracer transit times through the kidney, from which the total response curve was originally obtained. It may thus be appreciated that measurement of renal uptake function, the quantity of tracer taken up in unit time by a kidney and the transit time through different parts of the kidney and the pelvis are physiologically relevant measurements (Table 5.1), none of which can be obtained directly from the 'descriptive' measurements of a renogram.

5.1.2 UPTAKE AND OUTPUT COMPONENTS

The activity–time curve recorded over a kidney using an externally placed detector or gamma camera represents the variation with time in the quantity of radiation arriving at the detector from radioactive material within its field of view. When the organ of interest is the kidney and a probe detector is used then the activity–time curve has been called the 'renogram' and the technique 'renography'. When the gamma camera is used, the term renal radionuclide study is preferred for the technique and 'renogram' is used loosely for the activity–time curve recorded from a region of interest taken to include the kidney. This 'renal' activity–time curve is a complex and composite curve, $R(t)$.

One component is the curve representing the variation with time of the quantity of activity in non-renal tissue in the chosen region of interest, mainly in front of and behind the kidney; another is the component representing activity in the renal vasculature not taken up by the kidney; and the important component of interest is how the amount of radiotracer activity taken up by the kidney varies with time, which is called the kidney activity–time curve, $K(t)$. This may be considered to have been derived or obtained theoretically as in an idealized situation free of blood and tissue background activity. In practice the kidney curve is obtained as the resultant activity–time curve after appropriate assumptions or corrections have been applied to the composite activity–time curve $R(t)$ obtained from the gamma camera for tissue and blood background activity, depth, attenuation and size of region of interest. The supply curve, i.e. the blood clearance curve $B(t)$ which is usually obtained from a region of interest posteriorly over the left ventricle in the field of view of the camera, decreases with time as DTPA is taken up by the kidneys.

Since the non-renal blood and tissue component of the composite externally recorded activity–time curve, $R(t)$, is proportional to the blood clearance curve, the relationship between $R(t)$ and $K(t)$ is given by

$$R(t) = K(t) + FB(t) \qquad (5.3)$$

F is a constant called the blood background subtraction factor. For probe renography the factor F was calculated using a prior injection of radiolabelled human serum albumin.

The kidney activity–time curve $K(t)$, also called the kidney content curve, is itself complex and it can be separated into uptake and removal components (Britton and Brown, 1971). Such a separation not only aids an understanding of the underlying physiology but also leads to new ways of analysis for determining renal blood flow (Rutland 1985; Rutland and Stuart, 1986; Peters *et al.*, 1987) and for determining the radiotracer output curve and response to frusemide (Nimmon *et al.*, 1988).

Taking ^{99m}Tc-labelled DTPA as an example, it is evident that before any DTPA leaves the kidney parenchyma to enter the pelvis in urine, the amount of DTPA in the kidney depends on the amount which has been supplied to it in the blood and the renal extraction efficiency. (For a filtered agent the extraction efficiency is equal to the filtration fraction, GFR/RPF.) The early part of the kidney activity–time curve during the minimum time of transit of DTPA from its glomerular uptake site along the nephron, before any urinary loss of DTPA activity occurs, represents the accumulation with time of DTPA in the kidney. The kidney is in effect integrating the uptake of the supplied and extracted DTPA. The DTPA supplied to the kidney in renal arterial blood can take one of two paths: either it remains in the intrarenal blood circulation returning via the renal vein, or it is filtered at the glomerulus. The renal artery to renal vein transit time is of the order of 4 s, with a range of about 3–20 s. As the rate of loss of DTPA from the intrarenal blood by glomerular filtration is clearly equivalent to the GFR, then the fraction of blood activity taken up per second, designated U (the uptake constant), will be proportional to the blood activity, and the total uptake (during the period of the minimum parenchymal transit time, t) will be proportional to the integral of the blood curve. This is the uptake component $Q(t)$ of $K(t)$:

$$Q(t) = UB(t) \qquad (5.4)$$

Then, combining Equations 5.1 and 5.2, during minimum transit time, t, when $K(t) = Q(t)$:

$$R(t) = UB(t)\mathrm{d}t + FB(t) \qquad (5.5)$$

Alternatively, dividing both sides of the equation by $B(t)$:

$$\frac{R(t)}{B(t)} = \frac{UB(t)\mathrm{d}t}{B(t)} + F$$

This is in the form $y = mx + c$, the equation of a straight line. The intercept F and the slope U can be obtained by plotting the actual externally detected renal $R(t)$ divided by the actual background $B(t)$ data against the integral of $B(t)$. This approach to the measurement of the background component and the individual kidney (1K) uptake constant (i.e. IKGFR for DTPA and IKERPF for radio-iodinated OIH) has been developed by Rutland (1985), and applied not only to renal events but also to the renal arterial inflow and outflow. The same logic has been applied to the separate determination of the extravascular and intravascular components of the non-renal activity in the renal region of interest by Peters *et al.* (1987), in selecting the most appropriate region for the background correction of $R(t)$ to give $K(t)$.

Since during the minimum transit time period $K(t)$ is proportional to $B(t)\mathrm{d}t$, consider a situation where no activity appears in the urine for a long time, as with complete outflow obstruction; then the kidney continues to integrate the supply for as long as this period and $K(t)$ becomes a 'zero output' curve. Therefore one considers the curve of the integral of the blood clearance curve $B(t)$ as a representation of the kidney curve that would have been obtained if no activity had left the kidney. Then by fitting (using a least-squares technique) the integral of the blood clearance curve to the uptake phase of a particular normal or abnormal kidney curve that decreases with time after a delay period, the difference between the two curves (fitted $B(t)\mathrm{d}t$ and $K(t)$) gives the cumulative output – the removal or output component $O(t)$. Differentiation of the renal component gives the tracer output curve, which is the variation with time of the quantity of tracer leaving the kidney. This should act as a reminder that the falling phase (third phase) of a kidney curve is not an excretory phase but an 'amount of tracer left behind in the kidney' phase. Only by deriving the tracer output curve in this way can the true 'excretory' activity time curve be obtained. By comparing the removal component with the uptake component an estimate of the efficiency of the process of excretion can be made. An isotope removal factor can be calculated for a series of renal transit times in order to make this comparison, for example a kidney recovering after operation for pelviuretic junction obstruction would show progressive improvement of the isotope removal factor with time.

This approach has been developed by Nimmon *et al.* (1988) to determine the appropriateness of the renal response to frusemide, particularly when renal function is impaired. The output component $O(t)$ is expressed as a percentage of the uptake component to give the output efficiency $OE(t)$%. The output efficiency may be calculated both before and after frusemide, $OE(t)$%. The normal range of $OE(t)$% post-frusemide in patients with a dilated pelvis is better than 75% and similar to the normal range in patients with no outflow disorder, $OE(t)$% of greater than 70%. An inappropriately impaired response to frusemide gives a value below 60% with a borderline range 60–75%.

5.2 RENAL RADIOPHARMACEUTICALS

5.2.1 ^{99m}Tc-labelled DTPA

^{99m}Tc-labelled DTPA has been the routine renal radiopharmaceutical for gamma camera studies for twenty years. It is a chelating agent able to bind reduced technetium firmly. Thus it may be formulated in a kit so that it is easy to prepare using a mix-and-shake procedure according to the kit manufacturers' instructions. Pure ^{99m}Tc-labelled DTPA is a glomerular filtered agent (Hauser *et al.*, 1970); however, Carlsen *et al.* (1980) warn that certain preparations may have contaminants and variable protein binding which may invalidate their use for the measurement of the true GFR.

The disadvantage of ^{99m}Tc-labelled DTPA is its low extraction efficiency. Being only glomerular filtered, it has a fourfold lower extraction efficiency than radio-iodinated OIH. This means that the tissue and blood background is always higher for ^{99m}Tc-labelled DTPA than for radio-iodinated OIH. Thus, when renal function is poor, inferior-quality images are obtained and data analysis is limited by the effects of background and the poor statistical quality of the data. The advantages of ^{99m}Tc-labelled DTPA are the ready availability of the ^{99m}Tc generator and a robust kit that is simple to prepare. The quality control is good since the renal-bound component of some previous DTPA kits has been largely eliminated and the preparation is easy to use.

5.2.2 ^{131}I-OIH

^{131}I-OIH has been an ideal tubularly secreted compound for probe renography for thirty years (Nordyke *et al.*, 1960). It is bought ready prepared and may be diluted from stock with sterile 0.9% physiological saline or preferably sterile sodium bisulphate solution. It can be resterilized by autoclaving for 30 min at two atmospheres pressure (120 °C). It should be kept cool and in dark glass bottles, since it has a tendency to dissociate in the light. It should be free of ^{131}I-labelled benzoic acid, and contain less than 2% free iodine, which is glomerular filtered. Special high-purity [^{131}I]OIH should be purchased and used when accurate ERPF measurements are required and should not be diluted. For probe renography and for ERPF 1.5 MBq (55 μCi) is usually sufficient but for gamma camera studies up to 20 MBq (500 μCi) are used.

^{131}I-OIH has the advantage of high extraction efficiency and cheapness, but ^{131}I is a poor radiolabel for the modern gamma camera and the β-emission and long half-life limit the administered activity so that image quality and the statistical quality of the data obtained are poor, particularly when renal function is reduced. The radiation dose is also high to the kidneys when there is retention of tracer in the kidney in the presence of outflow disorder and ^{131}IOIH should no longer be used for routine renal gamma camera studies.

Tubular secreted compounds have physiological problems, since many drugs can interfere with their excretion, including the penicillins, probenecid and some X-ray contrast media. Red cell uptake of OIH is about 45% at equilibrium. Weak protein binding around 70% in blood reduces the glomerular filtration OIH from 20% to 6% and the tubular extraction is between 80% and 87%. Hippurates are secreted from post-glomerular capillary blood into the proximal tubules of both cortical and JM nephrons (Nissen, 1968).

5.2.3 ^{123}I-OIH

^{123}I-OIH is a better renal imaging agent as it is tubular secreted and has a γ-ray energy (159 keV) suitable for the gamma camera and a 13 h half-life. ^{123}I-OIH may be prepared in-house by the technique of Hawkins *et al.* (1982). Briefly, 1 ml acetate buffer (pH 4, 0.2 M), 0.2 ml OIH in 50% ethanol (25 mg ml^{-1}), 0.2 ml cupric sulphate in water (5 mg ml^{-1}) and 1–5 ml ^{123}I in 0.02 M NaOH (activity 1.5–2 mCi) are transferred, in that order, to a 10 ml vial. This is autoclaved for 15 min at 121 °C (17 p.s.i.) and allowed to cool. Chromatography shows less than 2% free ^{123}I and less than 0.2% iodobenzoate. ^{123}I-OIH may now be purchased commercially. The main problems of ^{123}I-OIH are related to the availability of the compound and its expense. Excellent quality images may be obtained even when renal function is poor, provided the administered activity is related to that usually used for ^{99m}Tc-labelled DTPA. If 10 mCi (400 MBq) ^{99m}Tc-labelled DTPA are used then 2.5 mCi (100 MBq) ^{123}I-OIH will give similar count rate images, but because of its more rapid excretion the background of the ^{123}I-OIH image is much less than that from four times the quantity of ^{99m}Tc-labelled DTPA, so that it gives a better kidney signal-to-noise ratio.

5.2.4 ^{99m}Tc-labelled MAG3

The disadvantages of the current renal imaging agents ^{99m}Tc-labelled DTPA and radio-iodinated OIH have led many workers to search for a better agent. The properties of an ideal substitute for radio-iodinated OIH are as follows. It should be labelled with ^{99m}Tc. It should have an extraction efficiency three times greater than ^{99m}Tc-labelled DTPA (20%) and preferably better than radio-iodinated OIH. It should be a stable compound easily prepared from a robust kit, cheap to purchase and easy to use. It should show weak or no protein binding to improve glomerular filtration and tubular secretion. The development of a ^{99m}Tc tubular agent started with the work of Davidson *et al.* (1981) based on N_2S_2 compounds known as DADS. Initial disappointments occurred because good animal data did not lead to good human data, although the latest compound, CO_2 DADS, appeared promising (Klingensmith *et al.*, 1984). Then compounds based on N_3S were developed by Fritzberg *et al.* (1986), leading to MAG3, which was shown to be tubular secreted by probenecid inhibition studies and equivalent to radio-iodinated OIH.

The three nitrogens and the sulphur of MAG3 are in a ring structure and it is able to bind reduced technetium in a stable way. It also contains the appropriate combination of polar and non-polar groups that make it suitable for proximal tubular uptake and secretion as a potential technetium-labelled replacement for OIH. The MAG3 kit preparation contains a benzoyl group to protect the ring structure and this must be displaced by a boiling step to enable the binding of technetium in the ring.

MAG3 is supplied in the form of white powder in sealed glass vials. A lead-shielded water bath is prepared and brought to the boil. About 5 mCi (185 MBq) of $^{99m}TcO_4$ is eluted in the standard way from a technetium generator. Volume dilution of the pertechnetate stock to give the required activity should be only with physiological 0.9% saline. An amount should be calculated so that the volume to be added to the vial of MAG3 is not less than 4 ml and not more than 10 ml. The vial is then placed in the boiling water and left there for 10 min. It is then removed and cooled under running tap water or by immersion in cold water. Investigations of this method of preparation have shown that a number of modifications may be made to improve its convenience in routine use.

First, the addition of ^{99m}Tc to the MAG3 powder may take place at a time convenient to the radiopharmacist at the time of elution of the generator for routine dispensing. Up to 4 h may be allowed to elapse before the boiling step. It is, however, important to avoid the entrance of air into the system and to keep the product cold. After boiling for 10 minutes the kit can be divided into four portions using 4 sterile syringes. Each is capped and frozen at 4°C. When the patient arrives, the syringe is thawed under a table lamp and used. By spreading this arrangement through the day, eight renal studies can be prepared using two MAG3 vials.

Radiochromatography shows that the impurities increase with time after the boiling step but up to one hour less than 5% of non-tubular secreted MAG3 is present and this is made up of three or more components, two of which are slowly taken up by the liver and excreted in the bile and intestine. The amount of this hepatic excreted contaminant depends on the preparation conditions and the length of time between boiling and injection, and not on the level of renal function. The liver uptake does not interfere with the renal study, which is typically completed within 30 min. Accidental omission of the boiling step leaves benzoyl MAG3, which is a ^{99m}Tc-labelled DTPA-like renal agent. By 5 h without boiling much of the benzoyl group has dissociated and 90% is in the form of ^{99m}Tc-labelled MAG3. No adverse effects, either clinical or biochemical, have been demonstrated using ^{99m}Tc-labelled MAG3. ^{99m}Tc-labelled MAG3 shows between 78% and 93% of weak protein binding, which reduces its glomerular filtration in the same way as radio-iodinated OIH.

The clearance studies showed that MAG3 had a 65% smaller volume of distribution than ^{131}I-labelled hippuran and a similar blood clearance half-life (slow component ratio ^{99m}Tc-labelled MAG3 : ^{123}I-labelled hippuran is 1.09 : 1). The clearance relationship is

$$\text{ERPF hippuran} = 1.5 \times \text{ERPF } ^{99m}\text{Tc-labelled MAG3} + 40 \text{ ml min}^{-1}$$

Although clearance had a linear relationship with effective renal plasma flow, ^{99m}Tc-labelled MAG3 is not yet proposed as a substitute for the absolute measurement of GFR or ERPF by the appropriate agents.

Clinical studies performed have showed it to be a successful radiopharmaceutical for routine renal work, combining the physiological advantages of OIH with the benefits of using ^{99m}Tc label. It is, to date, free of side effects and has been used in the whole range of clinical studies (Jafri *et al.*, 1988, Al-Nahhas *et al.*, 1988). At an administered activity of 100 MBq (2.5 mCi) it is better than 400 MBq (10 mCi) DTPA and equivalent to 80 MBq (2 mCi) of ^{123}I-OIH for routine renal imaging, for relative function measurements, for renal transit time analysis and for frusemide diuresis studies. It is suitable for use for the measurement of the intrarenal plasma flow distribution (page 104).

5.2.5 ^{99m}Tc-LABELLED DIMERCAPTO-SUCCINATE (DMSA)

DMSA labelled with ^{99m}Tc is a representative of a class of compounds that are taken up by the kidneys and retained in the proximal tubules with less than 5% being excreted. In order to avoid urinary excretion and liver uptake attention to detail is required in the preparation. It is necessary to keep air (oxygen) out of the vials and to use the compound within 30 min of preparation. Poor preparations show high urinary loss which may interfere with the measurement of renal function. A typical kit, for example, contains DMSA, stannous chloride dihydrate, inositol and ascorbic acid. Without using an air bleed needle, 1–6 ml ^{99m}Tc-sodium pertechnetate solution is introduced and the vial is shaken vigorously for 8 min. It may be stored at 4 °C but should be used as soon as possible. The compound binds to plasma proteins and then is glomerular filtered and taken up by the kidney tubules. If renal function is poor, uptake by the liver may be seen. Acidosis also affects renal uptake (Yee *et al.*, 1981). A dose of 100 MBq (2.7 mCi) is administered intravenously and static images are taken at 1 h if renal function is good, or 6 or 3 h if renal function is poor. Recently single-photon emission computed tomography (SPECT) studies have indicated that they may have advantages over planar studies with DMSA (Williams *et al.*, 1986).

Many other radiopharmaceuticals have been used to evaluate renal function, but those described above will meet all routine clinical requirements.

5.3 MEASUREMENT OF INDIVIDUAL RENAL FUNCTION

When a restorative operation on a kidney or nephrectomy is about to be performed electively it is essential to know the contribution that the kidney makes to total renal function. In an adult with a total GFR of over 50 ml min^{-1} in the presence of obstructive nephropathy or renovascular disorder a kidney contributing less than 7% of total function is usually not worth preserving, but a kidney contribution over 16% is worth preserving by a restorative operation; between 7% and 16% the decision will be affected by other factors: pain, tuberculosis, surgical difficulty, etc. A kidney with better than 20% function may need nephrectomy in special circumstances for tumour or bleeding, for example. Generally kidneys work better than their radiological assessments would suggest and too many kidneys contributing substantial renal function have been removed unnecessarily, particularly in the context of obstructive nephropathy. This is because intravenous urography (IVU) is designed to give resolution of the anatomical and pathological detail of the cortical outline, calyces and outflow system. If urography had a 'grey scale' representing function levels, it would by its very nature obscure such detail by loss of contrast. The advances in urography have been to improve the demonstration of detail by high-contrast infusion and/or tomography when glomerular filtration is impaired, rather than to improve the measurement of the degree of impairment of GFR. Cortical thickness is also an unreliable guide to function since it varies so much from pole to pole. The other approach to measuring the contribution of each kidney to total function is by bilateral ureteric catherization combined with clearance studies. The invasive nature, the discomfort induced and the morbidity of this technique do not commend it.

It must be made clear, however, that there is no non-invasive method, based on the use of radionuclides, for obtaining a precise estimate of the absolute measure of any function from each kidney in man. This is because the organ of interest is not the sole organ in the field of view of the radiation detector, the uptake of radionuclide is time dependent and the distance of the organ from the detector varies from patient to patient.

The relative contribution of each kidney to total function can be reliably determined as follows. From the regions of interest over the two kidneys, activity–time curves are generated. These are each corrected for the effects of tissue background using the data from the superior and lateral background regions of interest (ROIs). From these it can be seen that a normal peak occurs at about 150–180 s, at which time the tracer is starting to be lost from the kidney. Therefore no analysis of percentage function can be taken after this time. During the first 90 s or so there are unstable conditions with mixing effects and therefore it is best to limit the consideration of relative renal function to that period when uptake is unaffected by these factors, usually between 90 s and 150 s in kidneys without outflow disorder. The time period may be later, e.g. 3–4 min, in kidneys that have outflow disorder. As described on page 92 the quantity in a kidney at such a time $Q(t)$ is given by the supply rate, which is RPF × plasma concentration, $P(t)$. This product is multiplied by the extraction efficiency, E, of the tracer. For radioiodinated OIH, RPF × E is called the effective renal plasma flow (ERPF). Thus $Q(t)$ = ERPF × $P(t)$. For ^{99m}Tc-labelled DTPA $Q(t)$ is RPF × the filtration fraction × the plasma concentration. The filtration is given by GFR divided by RPF and so this cancels down to the quantity in the kidney being equal to GFR × the plasma concentration.

Then for the left and right kidneys, the following apply:

For OIH	For DTPA
$Q_L = ERPF_L \times P$	$Q_L = GFR_L \times P$
$Q_R = ERPF_R \times P$	$Q_R = GFR_R \times P$

Since over a small time interval P is the same for each kidney and $FF_L = FF_R$ then by division

$$Q_L/Q_R = ERPF_L/ERPF_R = GFR_L/GRF_R$$

By rearrangement

$$\frac{Q_L}{Q_L + Q_R} = \frac{ERPF_L}{ERPF_L + ERPF_R} = \frac{ERPF_L}{\text{Total ERPF}}$$

or

$$\frac{GFR_L}{\text{Total GFR}}$$

Thus, if Q_L and Q_R are measured, the percentage contributions of each kidney to total renal uptake function may be obtained. The problem then is to estimate $Q(t)$, the quantity of OIH or DTPA in each kidney at a given time, in order to obtain $Q_L/Q_L + Q_R$. It is obtained using the regions of interest selected from the gamma camera as above. $Q(t)$ can be obtained by measuring the relative uptake components of each kidney using the techniques previously described (Rutland, 1985; Delcourt *et al.*, 1985; Peters *et al.*, 1987). The potential errors in measuring $Q(t)$ are not negligible. The most important assumption is that the kidneys are at equal depth so that the attenuation of ^{99m}Tc or radio-iodine may be considered to be equal. The most important requirement for this is that the kidneys are not falling forward during the study, thus the patient should be reclining back or even supine, although in that position placing the camera is more difficult. In such a situation 75% of kidneys have less than 1 cm difference in depth and the count rate loss is about 10% cm^{-1} for ^{99m}Tc or ^{123}I. Such a loss leads to an error of about ±3.5% for the measured percentage relative function. Corrections for depth may be undertaken using true lateral views of the kidney (Duffy *et al.*,1982; Lee *et al.*, 1982; Rutland, 1983), ultrasound (Shone *et al.*, 1984) or from a height–weight formula (Tonnesen *et al.*, 1975).

Errors due to variation of distribution of the radiopharmaceutical in the kidney are probably small: counting errors due to Poisson statistics require the use of ^{123}I-OIH rather than ^{131}I-OIH, with the gamma camera giving on average a twentyfold increase in count rate and a fivefold reduction in absorbed dose for the same administered activity. Reduction of non-renal-background activity by ROI selection does not eliminate the contribution from anterior and posterior to the kidney, but for ^{99m}Tc and ^{123}I, unlike ^{131}I, the mean effective equivalent source of background is from posterior to the kidneys, from the largely symmetrical muscle bulk. Background ROIs for conventional correction should be taken from two separate areas above and below each kidney (Peters, 1987). These ROIs should not include aorta or renal hilum. Testing the chosen background ROI using patients with unilateral nephrectomy is wise since differences in equipment, particularly collimation and data processing, give slightly differing results. The alternative approach is by interpolative background subtraction (Goris *et al.*, 1976; Brown, 1982). This gives reliable results in moderately well-functioning kidneys but may lead to gross errors when one kidney's contribution is less than 15% of total function – the very circumstances when such a correction is required.

The normal range for relative uptake function determined in practice and thus incorporating both biological variation and physical sources of error is 42.5–57.5% for one kidney's contribution. The accuracy of a particular figure depends on the overall renal function and the number of nephrons in a kidney but ranges from +4.5% at 40% of total uptake with a creatinine clearance of 90 ml min^{1-} to +7.5% at 20% of total uptake at a creatinine clearance of 20 ml min^{-1}. Nevertheless this accuracy is sufficient for most clinical applications since the usual decision is whether to perform nephrectomy or a restorative operation.

In order to obtain the flow to each kidney in millilitres per minute, the percentage relative function is applied to the total GFR or ERPF as appropriate. Because of the arguments set out above and the intact nephron hypothesis, the same equations apply to the relative function determined by ^{99m}Tc-labelled MAG3 (Jafri *et al.*, 1988; Russell *et al.*, 1988), or by the use of ^{99m}Tc-labelled DMSA (Nimmo *et al.*, 1987). The preferred method for determining relative function (RF) with ^{99m}Tc-labelled DMSA is to use the geometric mean of background corrected anterior (A) and posterior (P), left (L) and right (R) renal counts (C), taken between two and three hours after injection (Wujanto *et al.*, 1987):

$$RF_L\% = \frac{\sqrt{CLP \times CLA}}{\sqrt{CLP \times CLA + CRP \times CRA}} \times 100\%$$

Recently the use of SPECT has been advocated by Groshar *et al.* (1989).

5.4 ABSOLUTE MEASUREMENT OF EACH KIDNEY'S INDIVIDUAL FUNCTION

The difficulties in measuring absolute individual renal function include the rates of change of the renal input, the blood and tissue background and the renal uptake, the effects of different renal depths on the attenuation of the renal count rate, the problem of relating the detected activity to the injected activity, the sensitivity of the gamma camera and the dead time losses in count rate if a highly active syringe is counted on its face.

Many attempts have been made to overcome these problems so that an absolute measurement of the uptake by each kidney of an intravenously injected radiopharmaceutical may be made. Most published methods correct for some but not all of the above problems. Kidney depth may be measured directly as above or use a height–weight formula and assume them to be equal (Gates, 1982). Some avoid blood sampling (Piepsz *et al.*, 1987; Schlegel and Hamway, 1979; Lee *et al.*, 1982; Gates, 1984; Vivian and Gordon, 1983; Rutland, 1985). Others require one or more blood samples to calibrate the activity–time curves (Duffy *et al.*, 1982; Ginjaume *et al.*, 1985) but measurements with or without blood sampling tend to be made when the rate of change of activity in the blood is high. An estimate of blood volume from height and weight may also be used (Gates, 1984). This has an interesting effect when the clearance of ^{99m}Tc-labelled MAG3 is compared with [^{131}I]OIH. Since the volume of distribution of MAG3 is 65% of that of OIH, and the difference in clearance half-time is only a few per cent, the calculation of ERPF by the Gates (1982, 1984) method gives the same result for MAG3 or as OIH, whereas methods using blood sampling show that the clearance of MAG3 is about two-thirds that of OIH (Jafri *et al.*, 1988). Thus errors due to estimates of kidney depth or blood volume and errors due to failure to fulfil the assumptions of the indicator dilution theory may be added to those inherent in the relative function measurement. While these apparently direct methods give a pleasing computer print-out in terms of the GFR or ERPF of each kidney in millilitres per minute, it is more accurate and reliable in principle and probably in practice to measure the blood clearance properly in millilitres per minute and apply the relative uptake function percentage measurements to it to give the individual renal clearance (Duffy *et al.*, 1982; Ginjaume *et al.*, 1985).

The use of ^{99m}Tc-labelled DMSA is an alternative and more reliable approach to a direct measure of the absolute individual renal function since the conditions are much closer to a steady state at two or three hours than during the first 30 min. The geometrical mean method overcomes some of the problems of count attenuation due to different renal depths (Taylor, 1982; Wujanto *et al.*, 1987). In order to determine the absolute uptake the amount injected must be known either by preparing a proper standard or by counting the active syringe before and after injection on the camera face. Renal depth may be obtained by taking true lateral images of the kidneys or by ultrasound. Kidney phantom studies using different thicknesses of tissue-equivalent material give the relationship between depth, count rate and activity in the kidney, or else a linear attenuation coefficient taking scatter into account may be incorporated into the calculation.

It should be noted that ^{99m}Tc-labelled DMSA must be freshly prepared and used within 30 min, for oxidation increases the urinary loss, which may alter the estimation of function especially in the presence of obstructive nephropathy (Verboven *et al.*, 1987), although Pauwels *et al.* (1987) and Zananin *et al.* (1987) did not find this. The acid–base balance is also relevant for acidosis may reduce uptake (Yee *et al.*, 1981). The normal value for absolute uptake at 2 h is 27.0 ± 6.0% (Kawamura *et al.*, 1983), at 3 h 25.4 ± 8.9%, and at 6 h 30.0 ± 9.2% (mean ± SD patient injected activity in each kidney (Zananin *et al.*, 1987)).

The percentage uptake should rise gradually after successful treatment to one kidney to relieve inflow or outflow disorder assuming unchanging function in the other. The rate of improvement will depend on many factors, such as the length of time that an obstruction has been there before its successful relief. The uptake function is made up of two components: an irreversible component which depends on the number of nephrons present and which can only change for the worse when there is destruction of nephrons as, for example, by infection or tumour; and a reversible component in which nephron function such as ERPF or GFR falls as a physiological control response to some pathological process, to rise again when such a process is corrected. To take an example, a stone obstructing the renal outflow tract will lead to a reduction in GFR through its normal autoregulatory response to a rise in resistance to outflow, but when the stone is removed this resistance falls and GFR returns towards normal. However, if the obstructing stone is associated with infection in the kidney then the infection may cause nephron damage and thereby loss of functioning nephrons. Such a loss of nephrons will not be made up when the infection is treated by removal of the stone and by antibiotics, so that that component of uptake function will not improve.

In the context of bilateral outflow obstruction, for example due to bilateral stone disease, Sreenevasan (1974) showed that in deciding which kidney should have its obstruction relieved measurement of relative uptake function was crucial. The kidney with the better uptake function as demonstrated by renography was the kidney on which to operate first. Its better initial function would lead to a quicker recovery from obstruction and thus the clinical situation would be stabilized sooner.

5.5 INTRARENAL BLOOD FLOW DISTRIBUTION

The ratio of cortical nephrons to JM nephrons in anatomical terms is about 6:1. In physiological terms, the ratio of cortical nephron function to JM function is much more variable. The intralobular artery supplies an afferent arteriole to the JM nephrons before those to cortical nephrons, so flow through the glomeruli of JM nephrons precedes that through glomeruli of cortical nephrons.

Intrarenal distribution of blood flow has some importance in renal physiology. The conservation of water depends on medullary blood flow, which is controlled by the JM efferent arterioles. It is a general assumption that various drugs, particularly diuretics, act similarly on all nephrons, yet consideration of their differing effects on renal physiology, for example free-water clearance, may be explicable in terms of separate actions on cortical or JM nephrons. Certain diseases appear to affect the two populations differently. Examples mainly affecting JM nephrons are analgesic nephropathy, the atrophy of outflow obstruction and essential hypertension. Techniques requiring kidney slicing, for example using microspheres or ^{86}Rb, or direct kidney puncture for local gas wash-out studies are only applicable to experimental studies. The use of ^{133}Xe washout in man requires renal arterial catheterization and is subject to the following criticisms. A compartmental model is not appropriate for analysis of intrarenal distribution of ^{133}Xe since such a model is not isomorphic. The derivation of three of four components from the Xe wash-out curve does not have sufficient data points to do this reliably. The distribution of such components does not relate to the distribution of microspheres. An alternative non-invasive approach in man using probe renography and ^{131}I OIH was put forward by Britton and Brown (1971), who demonstrated changes of flow distribution with alteration of salt intake. Plasma renin activity was shown to increase as the 'cortical nephron' component of flow decreased (Wilkinson *et al.*, 1977) and the technique has been validated against microsphere distribution in animals (Wilkinson *et al.*, 1978; Britton *et al.*, 1980).

The measurement of intrarenal blood flow distribution between the cortical nephrons and the JM nephrons is based on the fact that the long loops of Henle of the JM nephrons have a longer mean transit time for non-reabsorbable solutes such as ^{123}I OIH than the short loops of Henle of the cortical nephrons. Therefore the OIH transit time distribution obtained from a kidney should be bimodal, the earlier larger mode representing the fraction of cortical nephron flow and the later smaller mode representing the fraction of JM nephron flow. Since the quantity of ^{123}I OIH administered is well below the tubular maximum, the uptake of ^{123}I OIH by each population of nephrons is proportional to flow, each population being identified by its nephron transit time. The technique has now been adapted to the use of ^{123}I OIH with the gamma camera (Gruenewald *et al.*, 1981; Britton *et al.*, 1986).

To make these measurements the renal parenchyma is first identified separate from the pelvis. To outline the pelvicalyceal area the computer is programmed to construct a mean time picture which is a functional image displaying the mean tracer time for each pixel of the 64 × 64 matrix, so the pixels with long mean times in the calyces and pelvis have high intensities. Further regions of interest are then constructed to exclude the high-intensity, easily identified renal pelvis and calyces from the parenchyma.

To emphasize the dominant components in each zone of the cortex to aid subsequent mathematical analysis, the parenchymal region is further divided into an outer zone which will contain a sample of glomeruli mainly of cortical nephrons but few glomeruli of JM nephrons, and a middle zone containing both cortical and JM nephron glomeruli. Using the activity–time curve from the heart region of interest or the probe over the chest as the renal input and curves from the outer and middle zones, separate deconvolution analysis by the inverse matrix algorithm method are performed to give the retention of activity in each zone. These impulse retention functions of each zone would result from a theoretical spike injection to the renal artery with recirculation. The earlier vascular component is excluded and differentiations of these corrected retention functions give the distribution of transit times through the outer and middle zones, respectively. After the data have undergone a noise reduction process using a cross-correlation technique the leading edge of outer zone transit time–distribution curve is fitted to the leading edge of the middle zone transit time–distribution curve. Subtraction of the two curves results in a new transit time –distribution curve which represents the transit of tracer through the JM nephrons. By comparing the heights of these cortical and JM nephron transit time–distribution curves, the flow to the cortical nephrons is obtained as a percentage of the total flow to the nephrons.

In summary, the fraction of flow that takes the shorter mean transit time is the fraction of flow to the cortical nephrons, and the fraction of flow that takes the longer mean transit time is the fraction of flow to the JM nephrons. These fractions are applied to the flows to each kidney to give the flows to each nephron population in each kidney in millilitres per minute. Simulation studies have shown that the standard deviation for these results is 6.8% when ^{123}I OIH is given in the dose used for this study. The technique requires high count rate data to reduce the statistical noise in the analysis and therefore is only applicable to kidneys with good function using tubularly secreted radiopharmaceuticals. When the mean transit times of the two populations are similar the differentiation of cortical from JM nephrons cannot be made. A 60 s difference is required for a 95% probability of separating the two components (Nimmon *et al.*, 1982).

5.6 CLINICAL PROBLEMS AND THE APPLICATIONS OF RENAL RADIONUCLIDE INVESTIGATIONS

The most important clinical areas where renal radionuclide studies may be of particular importance in patient management can be conveniently classified under the following headings:

1. Hypertension
2. Obstruction to outflow
3. Distribution of function
4. Acute renal failure
5. Mass lesions in the kidney
6. Transplantation

5.6.1 HYPERTENSION

For the patient, the taking of treatment for hypertension is essentially the paying of the premium of an insurance policy, in that long-term reduction of blood pressure reduces the incidence of the complications of heart failure, stroke and renal impairment. The incidence of myocardial infarction also falls if other risk factors are controlled at the same time. Depending on the selection of patients attending the general practitioner or the special clinic, and their age, so the incidence of causes for hypertension varies between one in 20 and one in eight. The commonest cause is bilateral renal disease. Depending on further selection, between 1% and 5% of hypertensives can be shown to have a renal or adrenal disorder whose correction by surgery will lead to amelioration of hypertension. Since virtually all hypertension responds to the right combination of drugs, the question is whether the pursuit of these few is worthwhile. This depends on whether the clinical tests demonstrating those likely to benefit from surgery are sufficiently simple, non-invasive, reliable and cost effective; and whether the patient should be denied the right to choose a possibility of cure, whether by surgery or angioplasty as an alternative to a life-time of drug taking. For those that answer these questions affirmatively the search for these few may be considered as a five-stage process: (1) identification of the hypertensives in the population; (2) selection of hypertensives that possibly have surgically correctable lesions; (3) demonstration of those with the functional pattern of renovascular disorder; (4) definition of the surgical anatomy; and (5) making the choice between angioplasty, a restorative operation and nephrectomy.

In renovascular hypertension the crucial clinical problem is whether successful correction of an arterial stenosis to one kidney is likely to relieve the hypertension. Renovascular hypertension suitable for surgical treatment may be defined as being present in those patients in whom an occlusive lesion (or lesions) of the large or small arteries is associated with a particular pattern of renal function and in whom angioplasty, surgical repair of the lesion, or nephrectomy is likely to relieve the hypertension. This functional pattern has three features relevant to radionuclide studies. First, there is an increased proximal tubular water and salt reabsorption related to the reduction in peritubular capillary pressure due to the occlusive arterial lesion or lesions. A non-reabsorbable solute such as ^{131}I-labelled hippuran will therefore become relatively concentrated within a pool of fluid that travels more slowly along the nephron. The time to peak of the renogram which represents a crude measure of the mean transit time of hippuran entering and leaving the kidney will be prolonged as compared with a normal kidney. In the absence of outflow system disorder and in a normally hydrated person a difference of over a minute between peak times in the two renograms is significant of prolonged hippuran transit. Second, the blood supply and therefore delivery of the radiopharmaceutical to the kidney with renovascular disorder is reduced below normal due to the occlusive arterial lesion or lesions. An uptake function less than 42% of total function is abnormal. It should, however, be noted that renal artery stenosis is not an all-or-none phenomenon and in the early 'unstable' stage only a difference in peak time may be seen, without reduction in function. The third requirement is that the 'non-affected' kidney has not itself undergone small vessel renovascular disorder as a consequence of hypertension. This may be demonstrated by the normality of the unaffected kidney. A non-affected kidney should have an ERPF of at least 300 ml min^{-1}.

The selection of hypertensives for those that might have a renovascular disorder used to be most simply undertaken by probe renography (Mogensen *et al.*, 1975; Giese *et al.*, 1975). These authors showed that 99.4% of 980 essential hypertensives with normal renograms were correctly assumed to be free of significant unilateral renal parenchymal or renovascular disease. They found no benefit in pursuing further investigations for renovascular disorder in hypertensives with normal results of renography. Taking angiography demonstration of renal artery stenosis as the gold standard, Britton and Brown (1971) showed that 90% of patients with a so-called false-positive renogram had elevated peripheral renins indicating the likelihood of small-vessel disorder causing 'high renin' essential hypertension. Renal radionuclide studies do not and cannot in principle distinguish small-vessel from large-vessel causes of renovascular disorder. Nordyke *et al.* (1969) found that 15% of their hypertensive patients had abnormal findings from standard renography, and in one-third of these after further tests surgery for renovascular disorder was undertaken and ameliorated hypertension. These findings may be contrasted with the use of rapid sequence IVU. One in four patients with successfully corrected renovascular disorder have an undiagnostic rapid-sequence IVU; hypertension *per se* is no longer an indication for an IVU. Ultrasound is used by some as a screen for unequal renal size and will also demonstrate pelvic dilatation, but it gives no functional information.

Using a conventional gamma camera technique different authors place different emphases on the features that are extractable from the study. A conventional region of interest around each kidney and a C-shaped background for each kidney

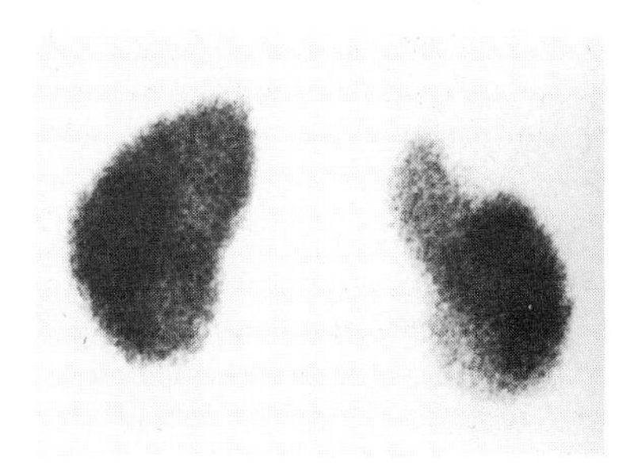

Figure 5.1 Loss of function at the upper pole of the right kidney due to a segmental stenosis confirmed at arteriography.

are used to obtain whole kidney background-corrected activity–time curves. Rapid recording of the initial arrival of activity at the kidney using 1 s frames and with a region of interest over the left ventricle or aorta demonstrates the aortic to renal 'appearance time', which may be prolonged if renal plasma flow is reduced. However, the technique is not reliable in diagnosis of renovascular disease. An 'appearance time' is a marker of the velocity of flow, which is typically more rapid through a stenosis and which relates to volume flow through the square of the radius, which itself varies along a vessel.

The distribution of uptake in the kidneys at 2 min is important and will be decreased in significant renovascular disorders. Reduction of size is typical of but not specific for renovascular disorder and normal-sized kidney does not exclude it. Parenchymal defects such as infarct, small or large cystic disease and pyelonephritic scars (Davies *et al.*, 1971) may be noted.

Functionally significant branch artery stenosis

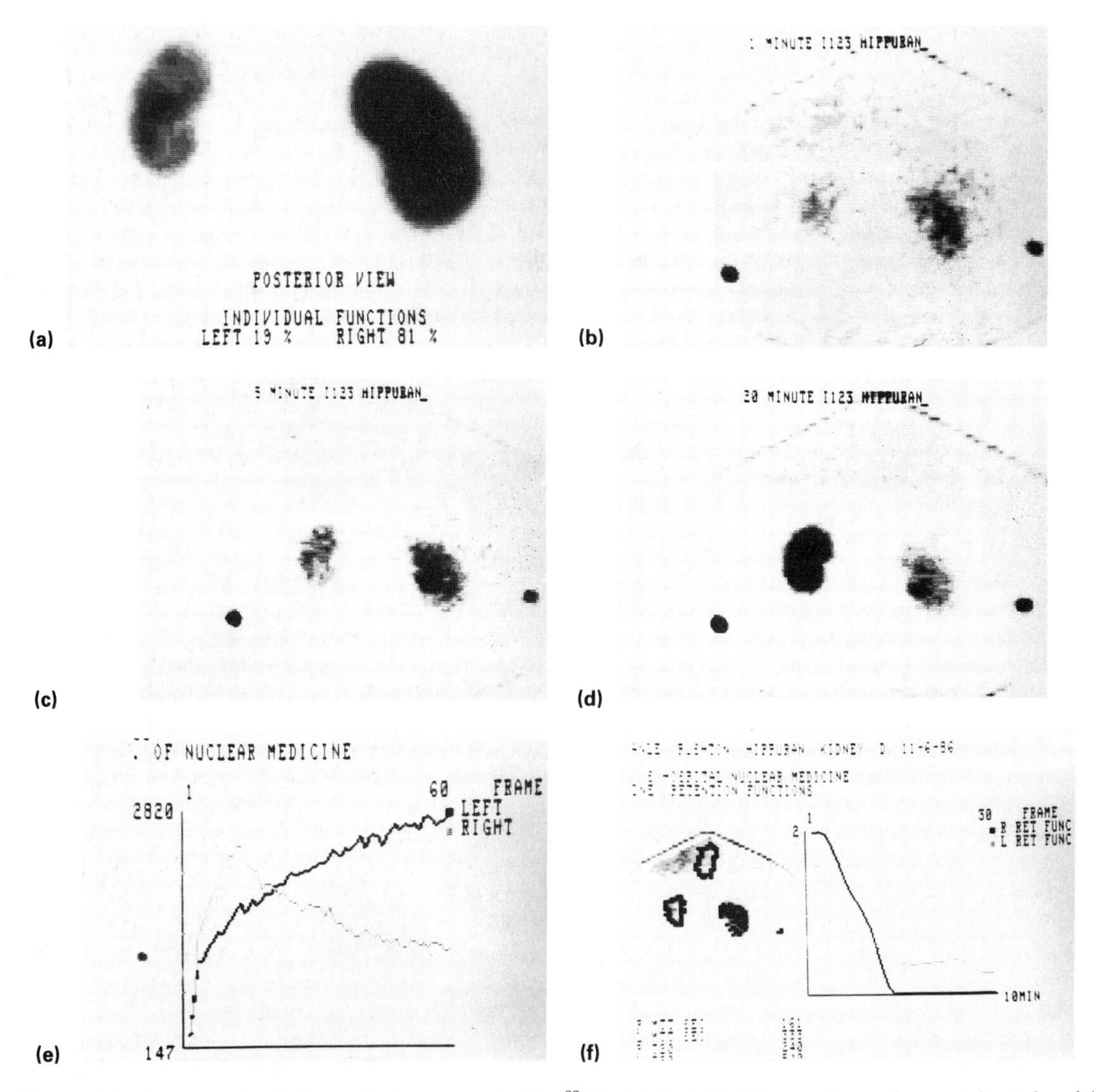

Figure 5.2 An example of left renal artery stenosis. The ^{99m}Tc-labelled DMSA scan shows decreased uptake of the left kidney (a). The ^{123}I-labelled hippuran study (b–d) shows decreased uptake on the left with prolonged parenchymal transit. Activity–time curves from the hippuran study (e) show delayed renogram peak on the left and the deconvolution study (f) a prolonged transit time (333 s versus 161 s).

may be identified as delayed parenchymal uptake at one pole of a kidney and this may also be noted with the patchy microangiopathy sometimes associated with use of the contraceptive pill (Figure 5.1). Such appearances are due to local prolongation of the tracer's parenchymal transit time. Duplex kidneys may be shown, one moiety of which is ischaemic.

The measurement of the relative uptake function of each kidney as a percentage of total uptake function is the first main reason for the study (Figure 5.2). Normal kidneys have equal 50/50 uptake with a range of 42–58%. Asymmetry of renal uptake function is the first step towards the demonstration of stable, unilateral, functionally significant renovascular disorder.

The second requirement is the demonstration of an abnormally prolonged parenchymal transit time which reflects the second renal function disorder in the ischaemic kidney: that of increased salt and water reabsorption due to a drop in peritubular capillary pressure relative to the intratubular luminal pressure in the proximal tubules. There is also an increase in medullary concentrating ability in the collecting ducts due to the reduction in JM nephron flow which cannot autoregulate in response to the fall in perfusion pressure and whose efferent arteriolar tone is heightened by the increased circulating angiotensin II. The flow of fluid in the collecting ducts is thus reduced. In consequence the **mean parenchymal transit time** (MPTT) is prolonged in renovascular disorder because of both the prolonged minimum transit time and a prolonged parenchymal transit time index (page 95). The separation of the MPTT from the WKTT (page 113) is important since it obviates the effect of changes in pelvic transit time by which the specificity of the whole kidney transit time or activity–time curve is reduced.

In a normal hydrated hypertensive patient, a mean **parenchymal** transit time over 240 s or, in a small kidney, over 1 min longer than that of a normal contralateral kidney taken together with an uptake function of less than 42% is strongly suggestive of functionally significant renovascular disorder.

Such finding does not distinguish between large-vessel and small-vessel disease. Normals (kidney donors) showed equal RF% (50 ± 8%) and MPTT of 171 ± 43 s. Hypertensive patients with radiologically significant unilateral renal artery stenosis showed RF% less than 30% and a prolonged MPTT of 344 ± 76 s. The contralateral unaffected kidney showed a normal MPTT of 186 ± 32 s, similar to hypertensive patients without renal artery stenosis, MPTT 222 ± 87 s. The prolonged MPTT in unilateral renal artery stenosis was significantly different from the other groups (Al-Nahhas *et al.*, 1989). Bilaterally prolonged MPTT was seen in patients with impaired renal function due to small-vessel disease. Bilateral functionally significant renal artery stenosis is rare and causes bilateral prolongation of MPTT. Renal activity–time curves and MPTT findings more usually demonstrate that one stenosis is significant at the time of the study when arteriography shows bilateral stenoses.

Congenitally small kidney and the small kidney due to pyelonephritis unilaterally will have normal parenchymal transit time if they are an incidental occurrence in a hypertensive patient. The unilaterally small pyelonephritic kidney with a prolonged parenchymal transit time may be considered usually to have renovascular disorder contributing to hypertension; Smith (1956) and Luke *et al.* (1968a) showed that between a quarter and half of nephrectomies for unilaterally small kidneys in hypertensives would relieve hypertension. It should also be noted that the demonstration of a renal artery stenosis incidentally in a hypertensive patient, for example undergoing aortography for peripheral vascular disease, does not mean it is necessarily contributing to hypertension, particularly in the elderly. Essential hypertension and atheroma are both common, and less than 1% of hypertension is due to renal artery stenosis. Another factor seen in both adults and the young is the demonstration of unilateral stenosis to a smaller kidney (usually through fibromuscular hyperplasia in the young) yet symmetrically impaired renal function and normal although often asymmetrical transit times. This implies subsequent bilaterally hypertensive damage causing partial loss of nephrons by the time of the study even though the stenosis may have been an initiating stimulus in the past. This is borne out by failure of the subsequent correction of the stenosis to relieve hypertension or change the function of the 'stenosed' kidney.

The captopril test (Figure 5.3) has been introduced as an alternative approach to improving the specificity of the changes in renal activity–time curves associated with renovascular disorder (Oei *et al.*, 1984; Wenting *et al.*, 1984; Dondi *et al.*, 1989). This short-acting ACE inhibitor acts on the

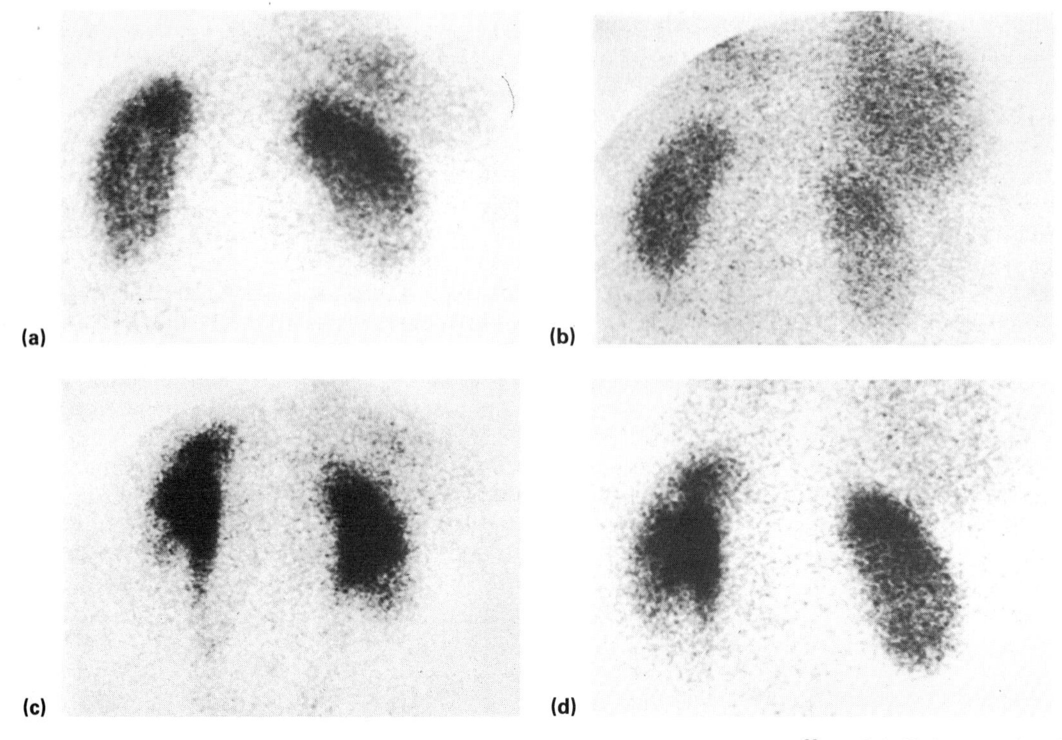

Figure 5.3 An example of a positive captopril test in a hypertensive patient. The ^{99m}Tc-labelled DTPA baseline study is (a, c) normal with a right individual GFR of 51%. After 25 mg of captopril the right GFR drops to 42% with a delayed transit time (b, d).

afferent arteriolar tone of cortical nephrons, which in renovascular disorder may well be already maximally dilated as an autoregulatory response to the reduction in perfusion pressure. Through inhibition of the local effect of circulating angiotensin II, it relaxes the efferent arterioles of JM nephrons, causing a fall in glomerular filtrate there. This is further to the already compromised flow due to the reduction in perfusion pressure. This effect of captopril, however, is not specific to renovascular disorder, only to a high circulating angiotensin II. Oei *et al.* (1987) using ^{99m}Tc-labelled DPTA and 25 mg captopril found three of 16 patients with normal activity–time curves from small kidneys which showed renovascular patterns after captopril. They showed an improvement in sensitivity from 75% to 94% and specificity from 84% to 100% using response to percutaneous angioplasty as the control. Six patients with renal artery stenosis but not responding to captopril showed no improvement after angioplasty. Sfankianakis *et al.* (1987) using 50 mg captopril found radio-iodinated OIH superior to DTPA in their series, although on theoretical grounds reduction of GFR should be more sensitive for renovascular disorder than reduction of plasma flow by captopril. A single dose of captopril can cause potentially dangerous hypotension in two circumstances: when renin levels are high and in the salt-depleted patient. The latter is typically related to diuretic therapy, which must be stopped for at least two days before the use of captopril intervention. Good hydration is important and the blood pressure must be monitored during the test. Because of the extra intervention it is recommended that a conventional gamma camera study is performed first and that the captopril intervention is then made subsequently before a repeat study so that the two may be compared. If the first study is normal the subsequent study is only undertaken if there is a high clinical likelihood of renovascular disorder. If one kidney appears smaller than the other but activity–time curve or MPTT are normal or borderline the captopril intervention may be recommended.

Once the triad of unilaterally reduced uptake, prolonged MPTT and a contralateral normal kidney is found in a patient with importunate or difficult to control hypertension, the next step is renal arteriography when the patient's blood pressure has been controlled as well as possible. This procedure should include a free aortic injection as well as selective catheterization to check the renal ostium and the number of renal arteries. Most authorities would follow angiography with selective renal vein sampling for plasma renin activity. As well as the renal vein samples, low and high inferior vena cava (IVC) samples are obtained. It should be noted that over three-quarters of the renin that leaves by the renal vein entered by the renal artery, so the correct estimation of renin output is given by individual kidney plasma flow × the renin arteriovenous difference. However, a renal vein renin activity twice that from the non-affected kidney is a strong indicator of renovascular disorder (Maxwell *et al.*, 1975).

The decision as to nephrectomy or not depends partly on the contribution that the affected kidney makes to total uptake function. A nephrectomy is indicated if this is less than 7% and a restorative operation if this is more than 16% of total function. Between these limits, the decision depends on other factors such as the complexity of the surgical anatomy, the overall renal function and the clinical state of the patient. In bilateral renal artery stenosis it is usual that only one is functionally significant and it is an unwise surgeon who attempts to revascularize both renal arteries at the same time, as the morbidity and mortality even in the best hands outweigh any likely benefits. The success of the MPTT measurement in predicting the outcome of angioplasty of the renal artery stenosis has been recently demonstrated when radiologically important renal artery stenoses are evaluated.

The importance of using MPTT in the follow-up to detect restenosis has also been demonstrated. Thus reliable screening for functionally significant, correctable renovascular disorder may be undertaken without pharmacological intervention through the use of the MPTT.

5.6.2 OBSTRUCTION TO OUTFLOW

Definitions are important and a distinction has to be made between the real state of the nephrourological system and what investigations of the state imply. An obstructing process may be considered to have three consequences: on structure as demonstrated by intravenous urography; on renal function as demonstrated by radionuclide studies; and on pressure–flow relationships as demonstrated by antegrade perfusion pressure measurements in the upper urinary tract and by urodynamic studies of the lower urinary tract. **Obstructive uropathy** is the effect of an obstructing process on the anatomy of the renal and urinary tract. **Obstructive nephropathy** is the effect of an obstructing process on nephron function. An obstructing process is considered to be present when there is a resistance to outflow that is greater than normal. This is usually accompanied initially by some changes in the renal parenchyma and outflow system so as to try to maintain a normal urine flow.

The force applied to the kidney results from the pumping action of the heart driving blood through the glomeruli, where part of the plasma is filtered, and through the peritubular capillaries from which certain substances are taken up and secreted by active transport. The resistance to this force is seen at several sites: in the afferent arterioles of cortical nephrons acting as a control point; at the efferent arterioles of JM nephrons acting as a control point; at the glomerular basement membrane; in the reduction in tubular luminal cross-section from the million nephrons to the 20–30 ducts of Bellini passing through the tips of the medullary pyramids; at the pelviureteric and vesicoureteric junctions; and at the bladder neck. When a force acts with a resistance in a contained space such as a nephron with its blood supply, a pressure is generated. As the resistance is dispersed variably along a nephron then a series of pressure gradients occur along the system. The pressures in the proximal tubular lumina and in the peritubular capillaries are slightly different but in balance so that the passive movement of salts and water from the lumen to peritubular capillaries occurs normally and accounts for about 30% of proximal tubular reabsorption. Pressure gradients with reducing pressure distally cause flow: the flow of blood from renal artery to vein and the flow of fluid along a nephron. The concept of 'obstruction' or better 'an obstructing process' can then be defined as an increase in resistance above normal in the system made up of the kidney and its outflow tract. Such an increase of resistance will consequentially affect pressures and thence flow. However, the renal system is not so simple because renal control systems tend to respond to changes from the steady state and because the system is not rigid. Thus a small increase in pelviureteric junction resistance causes a small increase in the pressure gradient from glomerulus to the site of resistance. This in turn leads to an increase in the passive reabsorption of salt and water from the proximal tubule, and depending on the capacity and compliance of the pelvis, to its dilatation. Thus increased resistance to outflow tends to reduce flow. The renal control systems then cause a reduction in arteriolar resistance, giving an increase in renal blood flow and glomerular filtration, so that there is an increase in force to overcome the resistance. This effect weakens with time and eventually there is a steady state, with reduction in renal blood flow and GFR and increased salt reabsorption.

In the context of renal radionuclide studies, these events affect the movement of radiotracer from the renal input to the renal output in the following ways. DTPA, MAG3 and radio-iodinated OIH are non-reabsorbable solutes; although DTPA is filtered and the others are tubularly secreted, their times of transfer from renal blood to the early proximal tubular lumen are similar and very short as compared to a typical data sampling rate of 10 s intervals. The time of transit of these non-reabsorbable solutes along the nephron from the early proximal tubule to the papillary ducts is of the order of 180 s under normal conditions of hydration. When there is an increased resistance to flow in obstruction the intratubular pressure gradient changes so that there is greater pressure difference between the lumen of the nephron and the peritubular capillary and as a consequence the passive component of salt and water reabsorption is increased. In this situation the increased fluid reabsorption concentrates the non-reabsorbable tracer in the tubular luminal fluid, reducing its flow rate so that its transit time along the nephron is prolonged. Thus DTPA, MAG3 or radio-iodinated OIH is concentrated in a smaller volume of fluid in the lumen of the nephron, the intranephron fluid flow rate is reduced and consequently the parenchymal transit time of these tracers is increased. It has been recognized for ten years that the PTTI may be used to indicate the presence or absence of obstructive nephropathy.

The prime symptom of an obstucting process is pain due to a rise in distending pressure in pelvis or ureter. The sensation of renal colic is not related to ureteric contractions, and recordings of ureteric pressure in the presence of a ureteric obstruction show that ureteric contractions become of lesser amplitude and greater frequency as the distending pressure rises. In this the ureter is unlike the colon and ureteric spasm does not occur.

It is a matter of debate as to whether there are also intrarenal pain receptors sited in the JGA and responsive to changes in stretch. Such would account for the temporary relief of pain obtained by anaesthetizing or section of the renal nerves. The combination of dilated pelvis and loin pain has led to an operation on the pelviureteric junction on the assumption that a dilated pelvis *per se* means obstruction to outflow and that the loin pain was due to this obstruction; now it is recognized that loin pain has many causes, pelvic dilatation is relatively common, and that such operations frequently failed to cure the presenting symptoms. It is now required to demonstrate the presence of increased resistance to outflow before such an operation is undertaken.

The nature of the resistance to outflow depends on the pathology. Stone and tumour are common examples. In hydronephrosis due to pelviureteric junction obstruction, most of the evidence points to a disorganization of the architecture of the muscular bundles and their innervation at this site. From any of these conditions the resulting resistance to flow may be severe or trivial when it may be overcome by increasing the force of flow by the use of a fluid load or osmotic diuretic. Clinical tests are based on the use of diuretic frusemide (diuretic renography), or by direct antegrade infusion of saline into the renal pelvis after percutaneous or peri-operative puncture while recording the pressure response (Whitaker's test). Antegrade perfusion pressure measurement (APPM) helps to categorize the strength of the resistance to outflow. These are different from and complementary to the assessment of the response of the nephrons to the outflow disorder by indices of renal function, the uptake function and the PTTI. The methods for evaluating the nephrourological disorder from an

Table 5.2 The evaluation of renal outflow disorder

1. Evaluation of resistance to outflow
   (a) Direct antegrade perfusion of the pelvis with pressure measurements
   (b) Indirect diuresis using frusemide
      – during intravenous urography
      – during radionuclide study
2. Evaluation of obstructive nephropathy
   Relative uptake function
   Parenchymal transit time index

obstructing process are summarized in Table 5.2.

Direct APPM requires the percutaneous insertion of a needle and tube through the renal cortex into the pelvis. Saline is perfused at 10 ml min^{-1} and the pressure rise recorded using a transducer on the inflow tube. A rise of over 15 cm water pressure represents a significant resistance to outflow. If no such rise is seen, saline is perfused at 20 ml min^{-1}, and the pressure measurement is repeated. Absence of a pressure rise indicates absence of an obstructing uropathy in a dilated renal pelvis. Problems include leakage around the tube so that a positive pressure rise is not recorded in the presence of important outflow resistance. This can be tested for by injecting contrast media after the measurement. The capacity and distensibility of the pelvis also affect the response. Nevertheless it is considered to be a standard against which other techniques should be tested.

Frusemide acts directly on the thick ascending limb of the loop of Henle, where it inhibits the active non-ATPase-dependent sodium pump. This active transport system, previously called the 'chloride pump', moves salt out of the lumen of the thick ascending limb into the interstitium without taking either water (leading to the hypotonicity of early distal tubular fluid) or urea. This active transport system aids the formation of the concentration gradients necessary for the concentration of urine through sodium-dependent and urea-dependent gradients set up in the medulla. The prevention of salt reabsorption by frusemide at this site creates a hypertonic distal tubule and forces an osmotic diuresis against the resistances to outflow. In order for frusemide to work, there must be a sufficient number of nephrons to produce a diuresis and the patient should not be chloride or sodium depleted. Thus frusemide diuresis is an unreliable test of outflow resistance when renal function is poor and when the patient has major electrolyte distances. Conversely, if renal function is good, there may be such a diuretic response that a nephrologically important but relatively slight outflow resistance may be overcome, leading to a false diagnosis of lack of obstruction when in fact obstructive nephropathy is present. The capacity and compliance of the pelvis also affect the response. The response may be lost in a grossly dilated pelvis and an inappropriately good response obtained if the pelvis is rigid, as has been shown by modelling the system (Zechmann, 1988), whereas variable correlations have been shown between the frusemide diuresis technique and APPM, from poor (Hay *et al.*, 1984) to good (O'Reilly *et al.*, 1987).

The use of frusemide during standard intravenous urography has become routine in many departments since the recognition that the IVU is an unreliable method of diagnosing upper urinary tract obstruction when pelvic dilatation is the main feature. The most reliable feature of obstructing uropathy using the diuretic IVU, frusemide being given intravenously 15 min after the start, is an increase in pelvic size by more than 22%. Patients with an increase in pelvic size between 10% and 22% are in the equivocally obstructed range and those in whom there was an increase of less than 10% did not have obstruction. Whitfield *et al.* (1979) showed that only 15% of cases remain in the equivocal range after the frusemide IVU. The major drawback inherent in all tests using frusemide is the effect of poor renal function since in these circumstances the diuretic response may be insufficient for the test to be definitive. It is now reasonable to undertake frusemide IVU in those patients in whom the request form indicates the possibility of outflow obstruction in the absence of uraemia.

Frusemide diuresis is applied before or during (18–20 min) conventional gamma camera renal radionuclide studies (Koff *et al.*, 1978) using ^{99m}Tc-labelled DTPA, ^{99m}Tc-labelled MAG3 or ^{123}I OIH. The test is applied in patients thought to have obstructive uropathy in order to determine the presence or absence of a non-trivial resistance to outflow. Visually the collection of activity in the renal pelvis is washed out by frusemide in the normal. An activity–time curve from the whole kidney may be normal, in which case frusemide diuresis makes little difference to a normal third (falling) phase. A good response to frusemide is a steepening of the rate of fall of an abnormal third phase or an interruption of a horizontal or rising curve with a concave rapidly falling third phase. No response to frusemide, with the curve continuing horizontally or continuing to rise, is taken as an indication of obstructing uropathy. A slight fall in the activity–time curve after frusemide is less easy to interpret. It is no good reporting the result as indicating 'partial obstruction' since that fails to inform the surgeon as to whether operation is or is not indicated for obstructing uropathy.

Since the measured change in activity with time is the basis of determining the response to frusemide, this response is also crucially dependent on the amount of activity taken up by the kidney and the rate of uptake. Thus the rate of fall of the activity–time curve by the kidney in response to frusemide is dependent on its previous rate of rise and one has to judge whether the rate of fall is appropriate for a given rate of rise. A moderately poorly functioning kidney would have a moderately impaired rate of rise and a moderately impaired but appropriate rate of fall in response to frusemide in the absence of obstructing uropathy. An inappropriately slow rate of fall in response to frusemide would then support the diagnosis of obstructing uropathy.

It is therefore necessary to evaluate the frusemide response not only as to whether it is good or poor but whether it is appropriate or not appropriate. A poor response is appropriate to a poorly functioning kidney and a nil response is appropriate to a non-functioning kidney and in neither case does the poor or nil frusemide response mean obstructing nephropathy. Poorly functioning kidneys are often those that provide a real problem to the surgeon evaluating possible outflow obstruction, and it is difficult to rely on the frusemide diuresis either visually, graphically or on numerical indices applied to the third phase (slopes, differentials, half-times, emptying times) and studies claiming their value have disproportionately few cases with poor renal function. The solution to the problem is to compare the frusemide response with the second (uptake) phase of the activity–time curve. The technique relates to the output component $O(t)$ (the cumulative output of activity) before and after frusemide with the uptake component $U(t)$ (the integral of the blood clearance curve fitted to the second phase representing the curve that would have been obtained with zero output). The efficiency of output before frusemide $OE(t)$% is given by $(O(t)/U(t)) \times 100$ (normally 70%) and the efficiency of output after frusemide $OE(t)$% is given by $(O(t))/U(t)) \times 100$ for each 10 s data point during the time period after the injection of frusemide. The normal value for $OE(t)$% is over 75%, indicating an appropriate response. With an inappropriate response $OF(t)$% is below 65%. The advantage of this relationship is that it is independent of the level of kidney function. In a series of patients (88 kidneys) under evaluation for possible obstructive nephropathy, visual assessment of the frusemide response for the images and activity–time curve was uncertain in ten as compared to this objective approach (Nimmon *et al.*, 1988). A further problem arises with severe renal tract dilatation when false positives occur frequently (Hunter *et al.*, 1987).

5.6.3 RELATIVE RENAL FUNCTION

In chronic obstructive nephropathy, a fall in renal function is a typical response to the outflow obstruction and is partly due to normal control loop response causing a reduction in GFR and RPF and partly due to a reduction in nephron population which occurs typically in the presence of infection. The extent that the response to obstruction is reversible depends on the degree to which that response is a physiological consequence of the nephron control loop. Through this mechanism, recovery of renal function is often much greater than expected previously, particularly when the appearance of the kidney or an estimate of cortical thickness was determined from the IVU. It has been shown that prolongation of the parenchymal transit time occurs before reduction in uptake function and shortening of the parenchymal transit time towards normal precedes an increase in uptake function after relief of the obstruction (Britton *et al.*, 1979).

(a) Parenchymal transit time index (PTTI)

The pathophysiological basis and linear model for the prolongation of the parenchymal transit time along the nephron of a non-reabsorbable solute in the presence of a resistance to outflow has already been described. Here three aspects of the measurement of PTTI are considered: the separation of a parenchymal region of interest from the pelvis; the method of deconvolution analysis; and the relationships between the renal transit times. The first requirement is to separate the parenchyma from all pelvic and calyceal elements so that the longer transit times that occur in these will not falsely increase the parenchymal transit time. It is not sufficient to draw a region of interest around a pelvis on a typical count rate image since when the pelvis is dilated the separation may not be clear. Furthermore regions of overlap of pelvis on parenchyma due to cortical scarring need to be avoided. The great advantage of 'time' as a variable is that it does not require that all the parenchyma is used for the analysis. Only a representative portion of parenchyma is needed to give the activity–time curve for subsequent deconvolution analysis, as one part of a kidney is representative of another due to the phenomenon of nephron autoregulation, tubuloglomerular balance and the intact nephron hypothesis.

The problem of obtaining parenchyma free of pelvic and calyceal contributions may be reliably solved by representing the data in the form of a 'mean time' image. This is determined by taking the mean time of the activity–time display matrix: a series of mini renograms. The mean time, $\bar{t}$, of each mini renogram is obtained from $\bar{t} = \Sigma_i tiNi/\Sigma_i Ni$, where Ni is the count recorded between the t_i and $t(i + 1)$. Each value of E is substituted for the mini renogram in the matrix using a grey or colour scale.

No activity appears in the pelvis until about 2.5 min after arrival of tracer at the kidney. When the distribution of mean times is displayed with a grey scale, the pelvis is clearly defined separate from the parenchyma and an ROI can be drawn generously round the pelvis. This is superimposed on the ROI drawn round the 2 min renal count distribution picture and the parenchymal ROI is demonstrated. The parenchymal activity–time curve is obtained directly from this ROI without background subtraction. It may be filtered using a 1–2–1 weighted smoothing. The activity–time curve from an ROI over the left ventricle is obtained and any irregular leading edge removed so that the first data point of the curve is the highest one. Then the parenchymal activity–time curve is used with this left ventricle activity–time curve for deconvolution analysis. The result of this is composite renal impulse retention function (Figure 5.4). The renal impulse retention function is composed of an initial peak representing the short transit times from renal artery to vein of tracer not taken up by the kidney. The peak appears narrower for OIH and MAG3 than for DTPA. A plateau follows, which may be short and may need computer assistance to define using gradient method, and the point at which the plateau becomes a falling curve is also determined. The minimum transit time runs up to this point, B, and the PTTI is the time beyond. The mean transit time (MPTT) is calculated for the parenchymal impulse retention function and is given by its area divided by the height of the plateau. The same process is applied to the activity–time curve obtained from the region of interest over the whole kidney including the pelvis to give the whole kidney transit time and, after subtracting the minimum transit time, the whole kidney transit time index (WKTTI). Comparison of the impulse retention functions from which the minimum transit times have been subtracted for the parenchyma and the whole kidney (Figure 5.5) shows diagrammatically the differentiation of a dilated non-obstructive pelvis from one that has an increased resistance to flow causing an obstructive nephropathy (Table 5.2). It is the parenchymal findings, not the whole kidney or pelvic changes, that make the distinction. This is more easily made numerically where a PTTI over 156 s indicates obstructive nephropathy with a sensitivity of 94% (52/55 correctly diagnosed as obstructive nephropathy) and a specificity of 98% (260/265 correctly diagnosed as not obstructed) in a study of 163 patients of whom six had a single

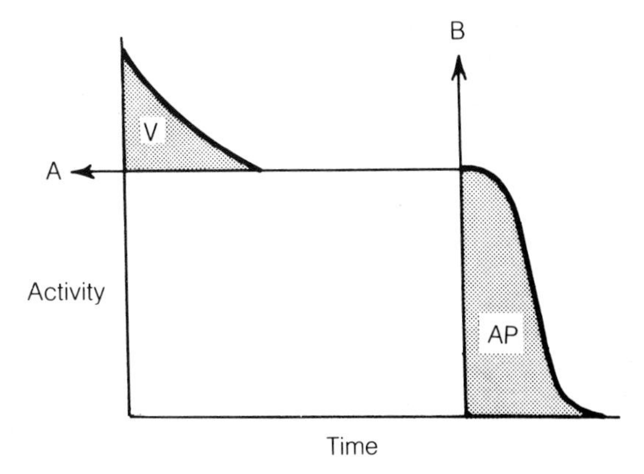

Figure 5.4 Parenchymal impulse retention function. A, extrapolation of the plateau of the impulse retention to exclude vascular component, V. B, time of the change from plateau to a falling activity which delineates the minimum transit time. The parenchymal transit time index is given by the area divided by the height of the impulse retention function for transit times longer than the minimum and is measured in seconds.

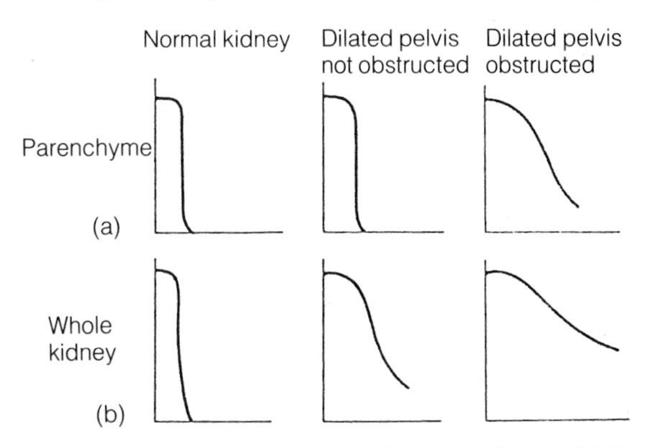

Figure 5.5 Impulse retention functions from which the min transit times have been subtracted for the parenchyma and whole kidney, a dilated non-obstructed pelvis and a dilated obstructed pelvis.

kidney. Against the 'gold' standard of APPM in 13 patients with hydronephrosis nine patients had a rise of over 15 cm water, confirming outflow obstruction, and four patients showed no such rise (less than 10 cm water); PTTI was correct in all (Britton *et al.*, 1979).

In a comparison of conventional frusemide diuresis and PTTI undertaken during the same study, it was shown that PTTI was more sensitive and specific than frusemide diuresis in patients with suspected obstructive nephropathy (Britton *et al.*, 1987). Sensitivity of PTTI over 156 s for obstructive nephropathy was 97% (35/36 correct), frusemide diuresis 90% (32/34 correct positive) and specificity of PTTI was 96% (24/25 correct negative), frusemide diuresis 92% (23/27 correct negative). When PTTI and frusemide diuresis are combined, care has to be taken if frusemide is given 18–20 min into the test because the estimation of WKTTI to give the pelvic transit time may be inappropriately shortened. Another empirical observation is that in vesicoureteric or distal ureteric potential obstruction a value of PTTI of over 130 s should be taken to indicate obstructive nephropathy probably because of some damping of the pressure changes by the capacity of the system and the distance from the site of resistance.

(b) Distribution of intrarenal function

The theoretical basis for the measurement of regional distribution of function within the kidney is the same as that for the distribution of function between the two kidneys as previously described. Measurement of the uptake function of the radiopharmaceutical at the appropriate time, i.e. ^{99m}Tc-labelled DMSA at 1–3 h, or ^{99m}Tc-labelled DTPA, ^{99m}Tc-labelled MAG3 and ^{123}I-labelled hippuran at 90–150 s, have been shown in a large number of studies to correlate well with GFR and RPF using conventional invasive methods. Thus the distribution of uptake function of these renal localizing radiopharmaceuticals in different areas of the kidney presents a functional image of the distribution of renal parenchyma. It must be emphasized that we are not considering the regional distribution of function in terms of parts of the nephron but simply the distribution of 'functioning renal parenchyma' as measured by GFR and RPF. It is essential that all assessments of distribution of function either within or between kidneys must be made in the light of a measurement of total renal function, usually ^{51}Cr-labelled EDTA measurement of GFR, without which serious errors may be made. No other method of renal investigation gives this functional information so the radionuclide studies are always complementary and never competitive with the structural studies of ultrasound or IVU. The clinical situation in which knowledge of distribution of renal function is helpful in the management of the patient will be considered.

(i) Reflux nephrolpathy The measurement of divided renal function is now an essential part of the investigation and follow-up of the patient with ureteric reflux as decisions about surgical management may depend on serial measurements of renal function. Urinary reflux may differentially affect parts of a single kidney, for example where there is a duplex system with reflux up one ureter only with consequent damage to that renal moiety (usually the lower moiety) of a duplex system. In this situation it is essential to know what proportion of function there is in each of the two moieties in order to make rational decisions about the need for partial nephrectomy, total nephrectomy or reconstructive surgery. A ^{99m}Tc-labelled DMSA scan performed at 3 h after injection will clearly display the regional variations in functional damage brought about by reflux and associated infection (Figure 5.6), and is currently the most sensitive method to show renal scarring (Monsour *et al.*, 1987).

(ii) Calculous disease The measurement of the contribution of each kidney to total function should always be performed in the assessment and follow-up of patients with intrarenal stone

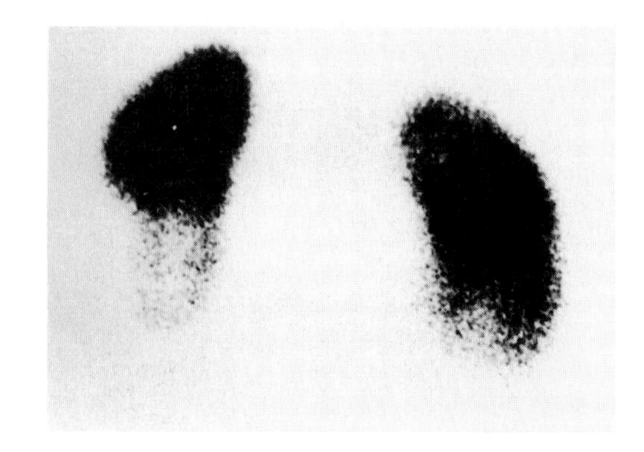

Figure 5.6 ^{99m}Tc-labelled DMSA scan showing the effect of reflux into a lower moiety of a duplex kidney on the left and a lower pole scar in the right kidney.

formation. Knowledge of the distribution of function within the kidney will be additionally helpful prior to surgical treatment to enable the surgical approach to be planned in such a way as to minimize surgical damage to the residual renal tissue and also to decide between total and partial nephrectomy or simple stone removal. Postoperative repeat assessment will be used to determine how successful the operation has been in preserving renal function and subsequent progress of the disease. Large masses of calcium lying between the kidney and the gamma camera may result in misinterpretation of the distribution of function so it is advisable to make anterior in addition to routine posterior images.

(iii) Hypertension due to local ischaemia Renal scanning with DMSA, DTPA, OIH or MAG3 may be helpful in defining an abnormal renal segment with poor function which is responsible for hypertension and which can be treated by partial nephrectomy or segmental angioplasty. The delayed DMSA scan (Figure 5.2) will show a focal area of decreased function and the DTPA or MAG3 scan may show an early uptake defect at 2 min with an increase later due to local delayed transit times secondary to local ischaemia and water reabsorption. This assessment will usually be performed together with regional venography for the measurement of segmental renin secretion and arteriography. The theoretical basis for these abnormalities are as described under renovascular hypertension.

(iv) Renal localization Although renal localization prior to biopsy is routinely performed under X-ray fluoroscopy control, occasionally localization using ^{99m}Tc-labelled DMSA may be preferable, for example when renal function is impaired so that contrast media localization is poor or when there is a particular region of the kidney which is functionally abnormal. It may also be valuable to localize the renal outline on the skin surface when planning radiotherapy of the abdomen in order to avoid unnecessary renal radiation.

(v) Pyelonephritic scarring Pyelonephritis is one of the commonest causes of end-stage renal failure and in children is often associated with reflux and/or asymptomatic bacteriuria. To follow up and treat these children and young adults appropriately with long-term antibiotics or ureteric reimplantation it is necessary to identify the presence or absence and progress of renal parenchymal scarring.

The identification of scar using urography is good when there is impeccable technique and good preparation, especially with nephrotomography. However, frequently bowel gas complicates the picture, too low a dose of contrast is used and nephrotomography is not employed. Merrick *et al.* (1980) has shown that excretion urography has a sensitivity of 86% and a specificity of 92%, whereas radionuclide imaging with ^{99m}Tc-labelled DMSA has a sensitivity of 96% and a specificity of 98%. Renal scanning, therefore, is an important adjunct in the identification of scars as well as in the measurement of divided function in children and young adults with reflux or urinary infections (Smellie *et al.*, 1988). Care must be taken in the presence of current infection as focal 'scars' may be due to focal nephritis and resolve with time, whereas true scars cannot resolve (Figure 5.7).

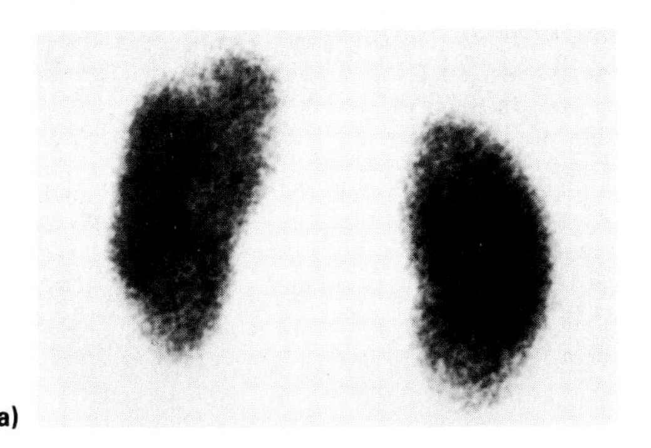

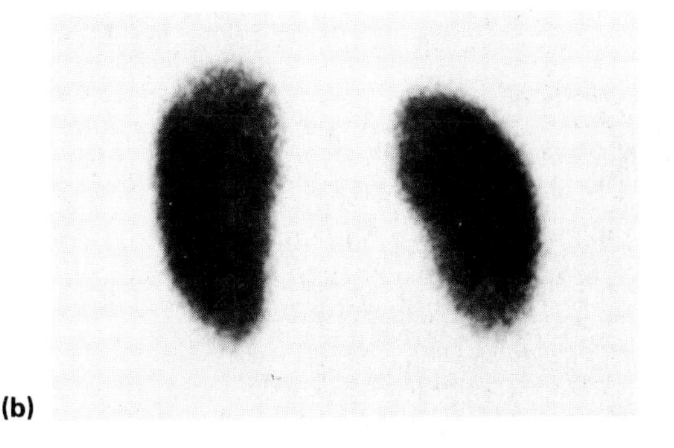

Figure 5.7 (a) Showing focal loss of function at the upper pole of the left kidney on a DMSA scan during an infection and (b) resolving a few months later with no scar formation.

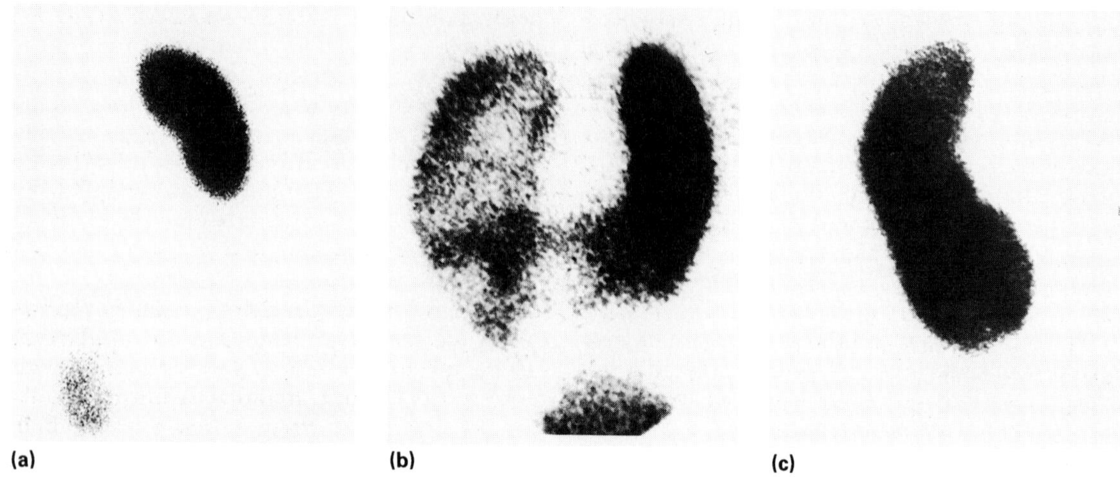

Figure 5.8 ^{99m}Tc-labelled DMSA scans showing (a) posterior view of a pelvic kidney, (b) anterior view of a horseshoe kidney with obstruction and (c) posterior view of crossed renal ectopia.

(vi) Congenital abnormalities Renal imaging with ^{99m}Tc-labelled DMSA is valuable for the proper assessment of many congenital abnormalities affecting the renal tract (Figure 5.8). Reflux and duplex kidneys with 'seesaw' reflux have already been mentioned; other examples include the assessment of horseshoe kidneys where the function of the 'bridge' can often be assessed very much more easily than with urography; ectopic kidneys, for example pelvic kidney, can usually be more easily identified and investigated because once the radiopharmaceutical has been given a whole-body search can be undertaken if necessary, whereas a small pelvic kidney, especially if it is poorly functioning, cannot always be seen against the background of the pelvic bone. Renal abnormalities and the assessment of divided function associated with neurological abnormalities such as meningomyelocele can easily be documented.

5.7 Renal failure

Renal failure is present when the urine output of metabolites and waste products is insufficient to maintain the normal body composition without alteration in body fluids. This may be a chronic process resulting in progressive renal insufficiency or it may be an acute clinical presentation. It is important to appreciate the role radionuclide studies may have in these conditions.

5.7.1 ACUTE RENAL FAILURE

Acute renal failure is usually a dramatic clinical event frequently complicating another medical or surgical condition. There is usually a rapid rise in blood urea and creatinine, the rate of rise depending on the degree of failure and associated catabolism or muscle damage, but is normally in the order of 10 mg per 100 ml per day of urea and 0.5 mg per 100 ml per day of creatinine. Oliguria is usually present although non-oliguric acute renal failure occurs in up to one-third of cases of acute renal failure and may frequently cause considerable diagnostic confusion. There is no clear definition of oliguria but less than 400 ml d^{-1} of urine is generally accepted as indicating oliguria and less than 50 ml d^{-1} represents anuria. The causes of acute renal failure are multiple and occur in all branches of medical subspecialities but broadly may be classified as shown in Table 5.3.

The mechanism of acute tubular necrosis is controversial and indeed probably should not be called acute tubular necrosis because it is now well established that necrosis is by no means always present or always necessary for the clinical picture of 'acute tubular necrosis' (ATN). The initial insult in all cases is probably decreased renal perfusion which results in a decrease in renal blood flow and renal ischaemia. As GFR is acutely dependent on renal blood flow so the GFR falls, resulting in a decrease in urine flow (oliguria). The renal ischaemia is then in some way self-perpetuating, possibly by arteriolar vasoconstriction due to angiotensin, obstruction to microcirculation due to swelling of the vascular endothelium or possibly a decrease in secretion of intrarenal vasodilators such as prostaglandins. Certainly if the ischaemia is severe or nephrotoxins are present actual tubular cell necrosis will occur, with consequent back-leakage of filtrate and also tubule obstruction by debris. Whatever the mechanism may be, recognition of the clinical picture is important. With ATN as with other causes of acute renal failure, correct recognition with appropriate vigorous treatment usually results in a return to normal renal function, even though this may take up to one year. On the other hand, a wrong diagnosis or inappropriate treatment may result in chronic renal failure, the need for long-term supportive treatment or death.

5.7.2 CLINICAL AND DIAGNOSTIC EVALUATION

In most instances a careful history and physical evaluation will elicit the cause, for example exposure to toxin or drug, recent surgery with hypotension, heart failure, sore throat. However, in a significant number of patients no cause of acute renal failure is ever established. Basic urine and serum biochemistry is also helpful in a number of cases but there are no formulae for classifying every case. Urine analysis may be helpful; anuria is not usual in ATN; intermittent changes in urine output suggest obstruction; tubular casts may be present in ATN and red cells and red cell casts are frequently found in acute glomerular nephritis. Urine composition may help to differentiate pre-renal oliguria from ATN and thereby allow the possibility of preventing progression of one to the other (Table 5.4).

Table 5.3 Classification of acute renal failure

1. Post-renal – obstruction, e.g. from calculi, prostate, urethral valves
2. Pre-renal
   (a) Hypovolaemia, e.g. haemorrhage, diarrhoea and vomiting, burns
   (b) Cardiac, e.g. heart failure, infarction
   (c) Vascular, e.g. sepsis, anaphylaxis, hypotension
3. 'Acute tubular necrosis' (ATN)
   (a) Post-ischaemia secondary to 2
   (b) Pigment precipitation, e.g. intravascular haemolysis, trauma, acute myositis
   (c) Nephrotoxins, e.g. heavy metals, ethylene glycol, drugs, radiographic contrast media
4. Parenchymal renal disease
   (a) Glomerulonephritis
   (b) Interstitial nephritis
   (c) Acute pyelonephritis and papillary necrosis
   (d) Intratubular precipitates, e.g. myeloma, sulphonamides
   (e) Vasculitis
   (f) Hepatorenal syndrome
5. Vascular
   (a) Arterial, e.g. thrombosis, embolus, aneurysm
   (b) Venous, e.g. IVC thrombosis, renal vein thrombosis

Table 5.4 Biochemical measurements in acute renal failure

	Pre-renal	*ATN*
Urine Na	Low	High
SG osmolarity	Higher than plasma	Lower than plasma
U/P creatinine ratio	High (>20)	Low (<10)

Unfortunately, however, history, examination and these simple measures fail to allow a firm diagnosis and therefore further imaging measures are required, including high-dose urography with tomography, ultrasound, retrograde pyelography, renal biopsy as well as radionuclide investigations.

The first problem is to decide what investigation to use first and, depending on the result of this initial investigation, what additional studies are necessary. The straight abdominal radiography is always necessary but frequently unhelpful. Stones, renal size, calcification or other unsuspected pointers may be identified.

Ultrasound examinations should always be performed early and will provide essential information about renal size, and should exclude obstruction as a cause of renal failure.

Intravenous urography with high dosage and early nephrotomography may be used although the disadvantages of a high osmolar load, possible sensitivity to contrast, high sodium content and nephrotoxicity must be weighed against the diagnostic information needed. The urogram will usually correctly estimate the renal size, correctly identify obstruction and often provide helpful diagnostic features of ATN. In ATN there is usually an early dense nephrogram which becomes progressively denser with time and is unassociated with a negative pyelogram and dilated calyces, whereas the obstructed kidney builds up contrast slowly and progressively with a negative pyelogram showing dilated calyces; if there is enough contrast excreted the site of obstruction may be demonstrated. In cases which might have a vascular basis angiography may be required to demonstrate the anatomical lesion but like the IVU carries the risk of further renal damage, even though the modern contrast media are superior in this respect to the older ones. A combination of ultrasound examination and radionuclide functional study will usually provide all the necessary information for clinical management, with no fear of associated toxicity and consequent further deterioration of renal function which might be associated with contrast agents. A dynamic ^{99m}Tc-labelled DTPA or ^{99m}Tc-labelled MAG3 scan is the method of choice, possibly with the addition of a ^{99m}Tc-labelled complex radiopharmaceutical such as DMSA.

The radionuclide study provides information about renal perfusion (first pass), the handling of the glomerular filtered agent and if there is sufficient urine flow the collecting systems. The frequency of renal visualization on the radionuclide study when there is no visualization on the IVU is variable, but we have found this to be quite common – more so if ^{99m}Tc-labelled DMSA is also used. Radionuclide imaging also provides prognostic information concerning eventual recovery. The single most useful role of the dynamic radionuclide scan is to make a firm diagnosis of ATN, which has a good prognosis given adequate dialysis from other causes of acute renal failure. Well-perfused kidneys which have a typical ATN pattern are likely to return to adequate function given adequate supportive treatment including dialysis.

It may also be available to differentiate the early onset phase of ATN which may be reversible by fluid and electrolye correction from the established phase of ATN. The typical images seen in ATN (Figure 5.9) using ^{99m}Tc-labelled DTPA are: a practically normal perfusion phase during the first transit followed by a moderately good visualization of the kidneys at 90–180 s which represents a blood pool image of the kidneys; as the tracer diffuses into the larger extracellular space from the vascular space the renal image diminishes without the appearance of tracer into the collecting system. Early signs of recovery are:

1. Increasing retention of tracer in the kidney, as the GFR returns to normal and is superimposed on the blood pool image.
2. Progressive concentration as glomerular filtration continues to improve but intrarenal transit remains grossly prolonged.
3. Excretion as at the onset of the diuretic phase of ATN.

These progressive appearances are shown diagrammatically in Figure 5.10.

The findings associated with acute obstruction are a decreased perfusion image during first transit and poor early uptake image with progressive parenchymal accumulation due to the grossly delayed intrarenal transit. Dilated calyces are frequently seen on the early images as negative photon-deficient areas which then progressively accumulate tracer over several hours. These findings, although characteristic, should be confirmed with ultrasound prior to surgical treatment and the absence of evidence of obstruction on a ^{99m}Tc-labelled DTPA scan should never be used to exclude it without ultrasound confirmation.

(a)

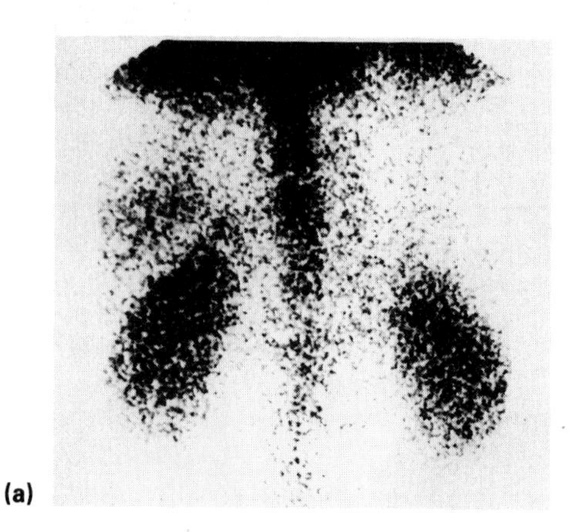

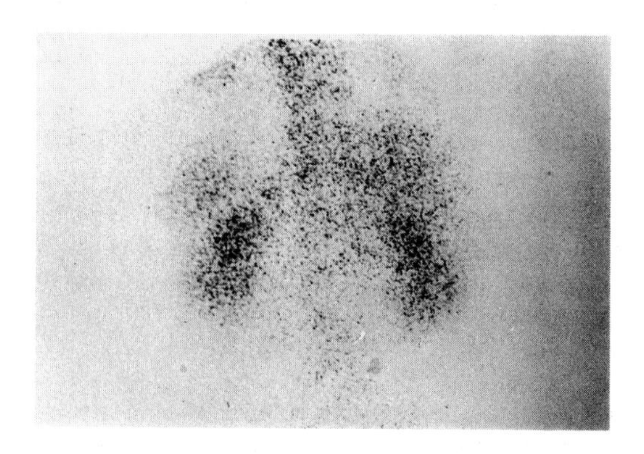

Figure 5.9 A ^{99m}Tc-labelled DTPA scan in a patient with ATN: (a) shows a good perfusion to both kidneys but does not concentrate DTPA (b) and the image fades as the tracer distributes into the larger extracellular space.

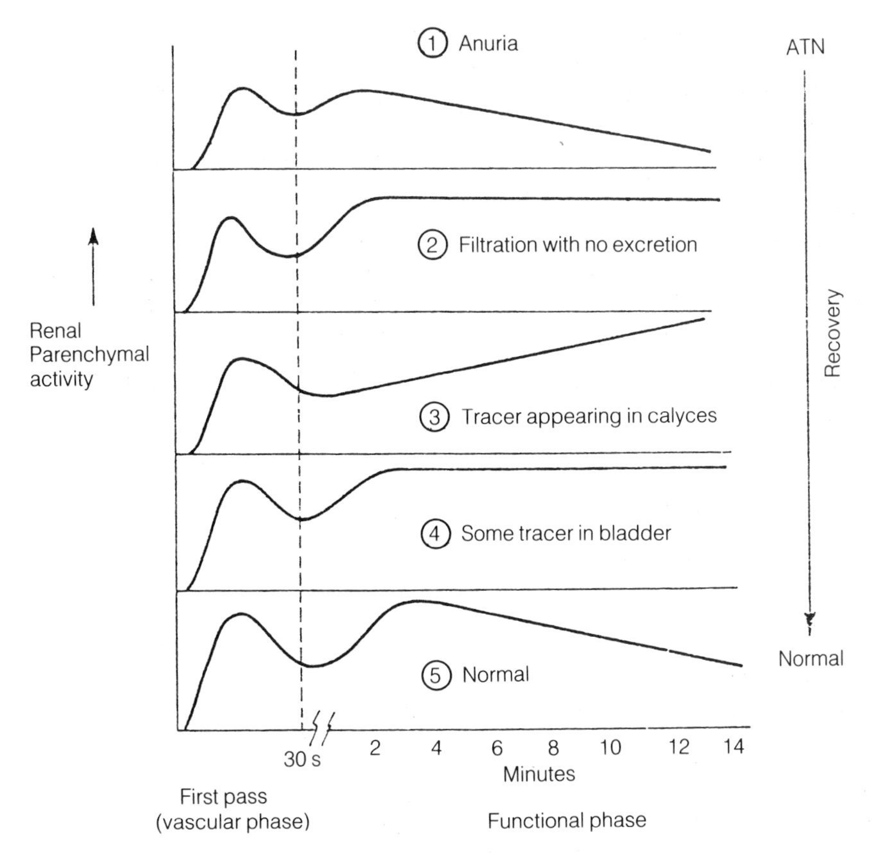

Figure 5.10 ^{99m}Tc-labelled DTPA renal parenchymal time–activity curves during phases of recovery from ATN.

Pre-renal failure associated with acute oliguria due to, for example, dehydration or hypovolaemia but before the established phase of ATN, is identical to phase 2 or 4 of the ATN recovery pattern, i.e. well-perfused kidneys with a significant secretory peak representing glomerular filtration, markedly delayed parenchymal transit but with some excretion of tracer which may only appear in the calyces towards at the end of the normal 20–30 min period of imaging.

Acute nephritis and most other renal parenchymal diseases usually show significantly worse perfusion as compared to ATN, with markedly decreased uptake at 2 min with either no accumulation or slow progressive accumulation in the renal parenchyma but without significant excretion.

In addition to these patterns representing the majority of cases of acute renal failure, other causes may be diagnosed, such as acute loss of perfusion unilaterally associated with renal artery embolus. In aortic obstruction (Figure 5.11) there

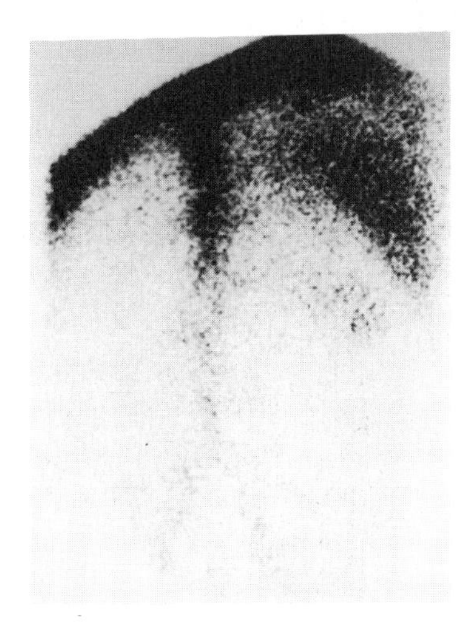

Figure 5.11 An example of severe loss of perfusion which is complete on the left and almost complete on the right due to vascular complications during aortic surgery for aneurysm.

will be lack of visualization of the aorta as well as grossly diminished renal perfusion; aneurysm if associated with a large lumen will be identified as a large abdominal blood pool; venous thrombosis decreases perfusion but to a lesser extent than arterial occlusion.

When the visualization is very poor or absent with ^{99m}Tc-labelled DTPA or MAG3 a repeat image following ^{99m}Tc-labelled DMSA usually demonstrates better visualization and may possibly be a better guide to eventual prognosis. However, no systematic studies are available at the present time to answer this important question.

5.7.3 CHRONIC RENAL FAILURE

Chronic renal insufficiency is usually the result of progressive renal disease, the commonest being chronic pyelonephritis, malignant hypertension, chronic glomerulonephritis, diabetic nephropathy and polycystic disease. In many cases an exact diagnosis beyond end-stage contracted kidneys is not possible and frequently the exact diagnosis is not of great importance in management, which consists essentially of delaying the effects of renal failure to excrete waste products and metabolites prior to supportive treatment with chronic dialysis or renal transplantation. Chronic obstruction is an obvious exception where relief and drainage may restore a very useful amount of renal function.

Ultrasound examination remains the best initial investigation in chronic renal failure and may indicate the aetiology, for example irregularly scarred kidneys of pyeonephritis or reflux, the enlarged kidneys of polycystic disease, the small uniformly contracted kidneys of chronic glomerulonephritis, and the dilated ureters, collecting system and enlarged kidneys of chronic obstruction. Radionuclide investigations certainly visualize chronically damaged kidneys in this situation and to a very limited extent predict the degree of recoverable function. Only occasionally would radionuclide imaging be of any clinical value and then is best performed with ^{123}I-labelled hippuran, ^{99m}Tc-labelled MAG3 or ^{99m}Tc-labelled DMSA.

5.8 RENAL MASS LESIONS

When renal parenchyma is replaced by a space-occupying lesion, whether it is a tumour, cyst, infarct or scar, it can be identified by a loss of functioning renal tissue compared to the surrounding normal renal parenchyma together with the presence or absence of changes in local perfusion during the angiographic phase. This is the basis for the use of radionuclide methods. Early studies with ^{99m}Tc-labelled DTPA and ^{99m}Tc-labelled DMSA concentrated on the detection of tumours and cysts of the kidney but with the development of improved structural imaging techniques (high-dose nephrotomography, ultrasonography and computed tomography (CT) scanning) together with a more widespread use of diagnostic cyst puncture with cytological examination, the role of nuclear medicine techniques has changed markedly.

In the vast majority of cases there is no real problem therefore and most patients receive the appropriate investigative sequence and treatment. Radionuclide scans, which for the purpose of this particular problem are always ^{99m}Tc-labelled DMSA scans usually with first-pass radionuclide angiography, are used in three clinical situations.

1. The ultrasound examination does not confirm a mass lesion or is equivocal. This is not often a problem with quality ultrasound examination, but when it does arise the renal scan is the next best investigation to confirm or exclude a tumour. The renal scan may also help to answer the related question 'is it a single or multiple lesion?' Lateral and oblique views of the kidney are often helpful and should always be performed. These images should be reviewed in conjunction with the IVU in order to correlate the abnormality on the IVU with the scan and to identify the site and size of the calyces on the renal scan, because with current high-resolution images of the renal parenchyma normal calyces may be confused with a space-occupying lesion.
2. The second situation when renal scanning may be helpful is in the further evaluation of a definite lesion on IVU which is solid on ultrasound but could possibly be a pseudo-tumour. In this situation, if it is possible to demonstrate that the 'tumour' is functionally normal renal tissue without resorting to arteriography, that is an advantage. Examples of pseudo-tumours are the lump from splenic pressure, fetal lobulation, compensatory hypertrophy, and prominent columns of Bertin.
3. Occasionally when arteriography and surgery

are contraindicated for other reasons the renal scan with particular emphasis on the first-pass arteriographic phase may help to establish the diagnosis. Increased blood flow in the lesion indicates a high probability of tumour; no flow in a large lesion increases the likelihood of a cyst but there are a significant number of cases in which the tumour has a relatively poor supply and the differentiation of benign and malignant is not possible. Finally it must be emphasized that this is a small part of the investigation of such patients and the radionuclide scan must not be used as just one more test to document the lesion when it is not going to influence the management of the patient.

5.9 VESICOURETERIC REFLUX

The micturating cystogram remains the preferred method and is the 'gold standard' for the diagnosis of vesicoureteric reflux. This investigation is usually necessary to establish the diagnosis and to achieve the anatomical information necessary for patient management. The micturating cysto-urogram (MCU) does, however, have the disadvantages of being an unpleasant investigation to perform, increasing the risk of infection due to bladder catheterization and carrying a relatively high radiation dose to the child. Radionuclide methods therefore are used and have a place, particularly in the follow-up of children with established reflux in whom the anatomical information has been obtained from the MCU.

There are two methods in routine use.

5.9.1 INDIRECT METHOD (Figure 5.12)

A standard dynamic ^{99m}Tc-labelled DTPA renal scan is performed with the generation of appropriate images, renogram curves and measurements of total and individual renal function. At the end of the study, instead of emptying the bladder the child is encouraged to drink fluids until the bladder is full and there is a desire to micturate. At this point the child stands (boys) or sits (girls) with the back against the gamma camera, with the field of view including both kidneys and the bladder. After a baseline period of data acquisition the bladder is emptied with continuous data acquisition and continued for several minutes after the bladder has been emptied. ROIs are placed over each kidney and over the bladder; the ureters can also be separated, which will show peaks occurring in the renal area if radiolabelled urine refluxes up as far as the kidney. The detection of lesser degrees of reflux by using the ureters is possible but generally more prone to error. The bladder curve will show the rapid emptying phase if it is a good study and a partial refilling phase if the refluxed

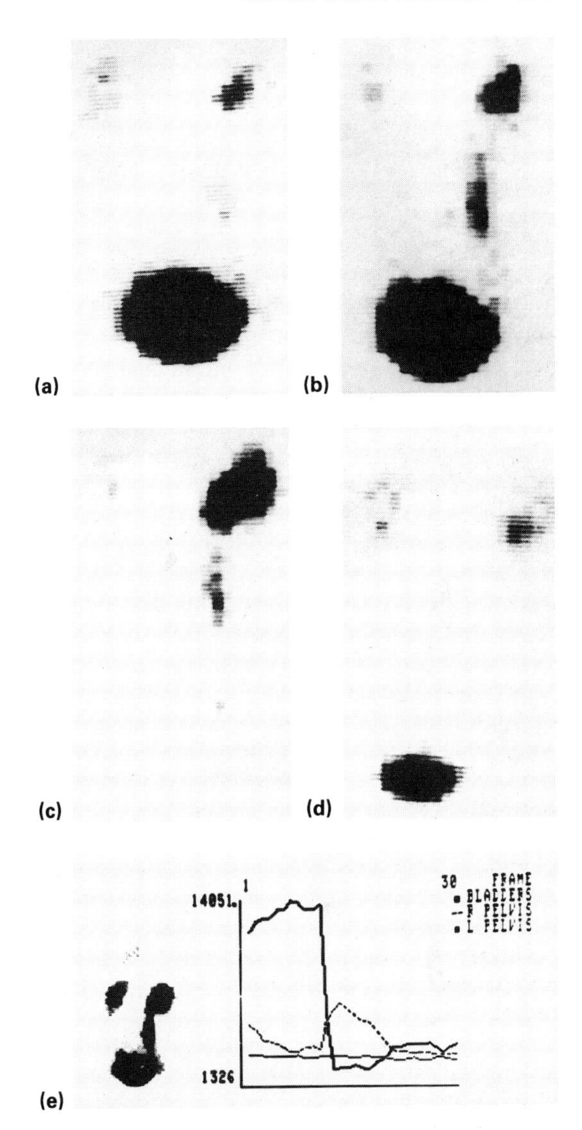

Figure 5.12 The indirect vesicoureteric reflex study shows positive reflux on the right side using ^{99m}Tc-labelled DTPA. (a) Pre-micturition; (b) right-sided reflux at the initiation of micturition; (c) further reflux as the bladder empties and (d) rapid drainage to partially refill the bladder; (e) activity–time curves from the two pelves and the bladder.

volume is large enough. The activity–time curves should always be correlated with the images during reflux to avoid false-positive reports. This method has been shown to be sensitive and accurate and can be used as a follow-up procedure in addition to being less traumatic; avoiding catheterization and having a lower radiation dose it has the added advantage of providing functional renal information from the early part of the DTPA scan. The disadvantage, apart from lack of anatomical detail, is that a true filling phase reflux is not seen unless it occurs spontaneously during the renogram phase, showing up as multiple spikes in the third phase (Figure 5.13). The correlation of reflux detection using these methods is good; Hedman *et al.* (1978) showed 90/102 renal units in agreement and Kogan *et al.* (1986) suggested that about 75% of MCUs could be dispensed with. Grading of the degree of reflux can also be achieved satisfactorily using this method. Zhang *et al.* (1987) showed an 80% correlation when all five grades were compared and 100% when grades IV and V were combined into one high-grade reflux grade. Measurement of the actual volume of refluxed urine is also possible and can be made very accurate when performed with careful attention to detail and quantification (Godley *et al.*, in press).

Further uses are in the screening of siblings with reflux and the screening of patients presenting with urinary tract infections.

5.9.2 RETROGRADE (DIRECT) METHOD

This method is used for children less than 3–4 years of age who are usually not able to cooperate with the indirect method. The bladder is catheterized and ^{99m}Tc-labelled DTPA diluted in saline is run into the bladder during imaging with the gamma camera. This is similar to an MCU investigation, but without the anatomical detail; on the other hand, there is a much lower radiation dose and it can be made more quantitative. A refinement of this method is to include ^{99m}Tc-labelled colloid in the radiopharmaceutical and image the kidney after 20 h, when residual radioactivity in the kidney indicates the presence of intrarenal reflux (Rizzoni *et al.*, 1986).

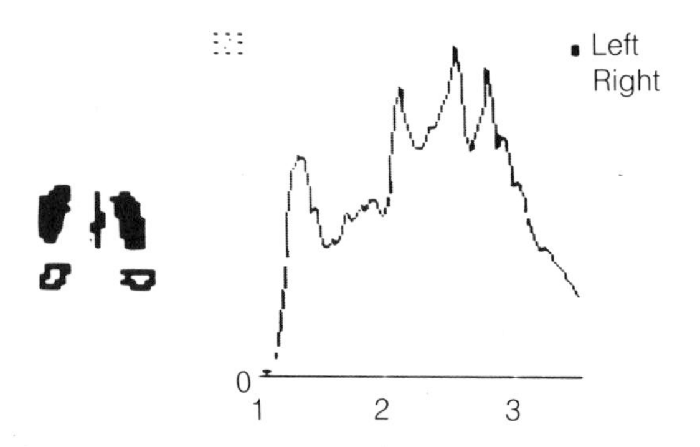

Figure 5.13 Activity–time curve from the third phase of the renogram curve showing intermittent reflux into the left renal area during bladder filling.

5.10 RENAL TRANSPLANTATION *BY A. J. W. HILSON*

5.10.1 ASSESSMENT OF THE DONOR

(a) The live-related donor

Once a suitable donor has been found for a patient with irreversible renal failure, it is necessary to ensure that the donor will not suffer any harm as a result of the donation. In particular it is necessary to ensure that the donor has two well-functioning kidneys.

Therefore, after a general medical examination with special attention to blood pressure and urinalysis, the laboratory work-up of the donor should start with estimation of serum creatinine to exclude major renal disease, followed by the measurement of GFR using ^{51}Cr-EDTA or ^{99m}Tc-DTPA. The divided function is then assessed using ^{99m}Tc-DPTA or DMSA to ensure that the renal function is evenly divided. At the same time the imaging study will exclude any major structural abnormality. Having confirmed that the prospective donor has two kidneys with normal function, radiographic procedures are necessary to confirm anatomical normality. Usually these will consist of an IVU to demonstrate renal and ureteric morphology, followed by a selective renal arteriogram with special attention to ensure that all renal vessels are demonstrated.

(b) Cadaver donors

Often the decision that a cadaver is suitable for use as a renal donor is taken urgently, and there is no time for investigation of renal function other than the measurement of serum creatinine. However, the tendency now is for more kidneys to be taken from patients who are diagnosed as 'brain-dead' whilst on cardiorespiratory support. Although it is not one of the accepted criteria for the diagnosis of brain death (Conference of Medical Royal Colleges, 1976), the demonstration of lack of cerebral blood flow is of value in screening possible donors (Ashwal, Smith, Torres, Loken and Chou, 1977), especially where a mobile gamma camera is used. Measurement of GFR may be of value where the previous renal status is not known.

5.10.2 THE NORMAL POST-OPERATIVE KIDNEY

On return from the operating theatre, the transplanted kidney should be forming urine freely, and the recipient should be having a brisk diuresis as the kidney is exposed to the high osmotic and fluid load of a recipient in renal failure. This is more likely to be the case where the kidney has been taken from a live donor or the period of ischaemia has been short. In these circumstances there is no need for urgent investigation, as the progress of the kidney can be monitored by following the fall in the serum creatinine. However, it is desirable to carry out an initial assessment of the kidney between 24 and 48 h after the operation to give the base line for further studies.

5.10.3 ACUTE TUBULAR NECROSIS (ATN)

The majority of transplanted kidneys show an element of ATN. This may manifest itself as severe oliguria from the time of return from the operating theatre especially when the period of ischaemia has been long. However, its onset may be delayed, and it is very common for the kidney to be passing reasonable quantities of urine immediately after the operation, but for this to fall off gradually over the next 24 h, even in response to an osmotic and fluid load and intravenous frusemide. During this period there may be a fall in renal perfusion, and it is therefore worth waiting 24–48 h before carrying out the first radionuclide study.

The findings on the ^{99m}Tc-DTPA dynamic study are diagnostic (Hilson, Maisey, Brown, Ogg and Bewick, 1978). The kidney is moderately well perfused, but there is little or no selective accumulation of the tracer, no activity is seen in the bladder, and the arterial and background curves show a rise in activity over 30 min. (Unless the bladder or catheter bag are routinely imaged the study may be misinterpreted. This image should always be recorded for future reference, even if no counts are obtained.) There is no functional peak in the renal curve. It is important to note that this picture may be seen even if the kidney is passing large volumes of urine. This corresponds to 'polyuric' ATN, and the urine will be found to contain little creatinine or urea. Imaging with ^{131}I or ^{123}I-hippuran at this stage shows uptake of tracer, but no excretion, this combination being suggestive, but not diagnostic, of ATN (Rodriguez-Antunex, Gill and Egleston, 1970). Imaging with ^{99m}Tc-sulphur colloid may show some uptake, but usually less than in bone marrow (George, Codd, Newton, Henry and Donati, 1975).

In uncomplicated ATN there is a recognizable sequence. The period of oliguria may last for several weeks (during which the patient is maintained on dialysis). During this time the ^{99m}Tc-DTPA study, which should be performed on alternate days, shows continuing perfusion of the kidney, with a perfusion index (Hilson *et al.*, 1978) which falls steadily towards the normal range (Figure 5.14). A rise in the perfusion index indicates some further complication superimposed on the ATN. As the kidney recovers, selective accumulation of tracer will be apparent, and this may allow prediction of return of function. Once the kidney starts passing urine, the functional

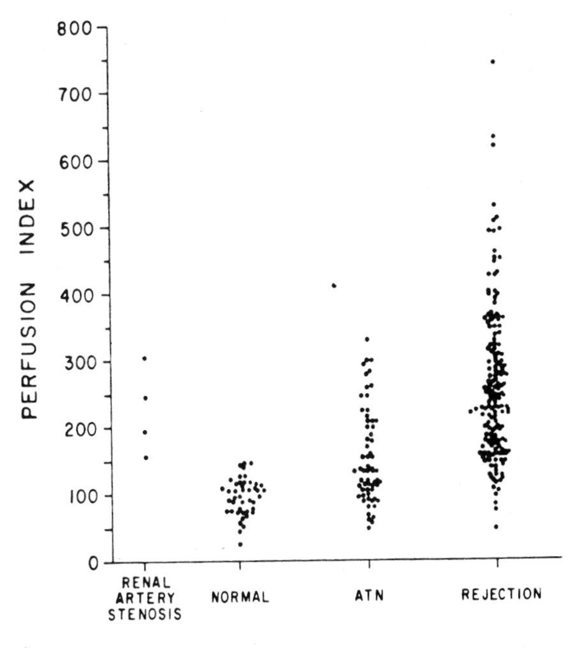

Figure 5.14 Values of perfusion index in 276 studies in patients known renal transplant status (after Hilson *et al.* 1978).

peak will appear, though it may be delayed (Pavel, Westerman, Bergan and Kahan, 1976).

During the phase of oliguric ATN, the only other diagnostic methods available are arteriography and renal biopsy, which are both invasive and somewhat hazardous.

5.10.4 THE ANURIC RENAL TRANSPLANT

Although the majority of kidneys are passing urine on return from the operating theatre, a proportion are anuric. This is particularly likely where there has been a long period of renal ischaemia or the operation has been difficult. In addition, complete anuria may develop at any time after the operation. In either case, a dynamic study with ^{99m}Tc-DTPA should be performed as a matter of urgency. Usually the kidney is seen to be perfused, and the study will show the findings of ATN. Less commonly, there will be no perfusion of the kidney, and it is not possible to differentiate between vascular occlusion and severe rejection (hyperacute rejection, although described, is unlikely if there has been a negative crossmatch before surgery). This appearance is an indication for urgent arteriography.

The anuric kidney is a source of great anxiety to all concerned, and it is important to be able to demonstrate the status of the graft non-invasively. Indeed in the series of Whitaker *et al.* (1973) the morbidity and graft loss of kidneys with delayed function was attributed totally to investigation. It should be remembered that there are two causes for the imaging appearance or non-visualization of the kidney in the patient who is forming urine. One cause is true vascular occlusion in a patient who still has his own kidneys, which may be producing the urine. The other cause is that the wrong side has been imaged! This latter is more common in the first post-operative study.

5.10.4 REJECTION

This is the most difficult problem for those concerned with the management of patients with renal transplants, who must navigate between the Scylla of undertreatment and consequent loss of the graft, and the Charybdis of overtreatment and loss of the patient from the complications of immunosuppression. In the full-blown rejection episode there is no problem, as the graft becomes tender and swollen, the urinary output falls off, the serum creatinine rises, the platelet count falls, and the patient feels unwell. However, the majority of rejection episodes are modified by the immunosuppressive therapy, and there may be no more than a minor rise in the serum creatinine as the only indicator. The generally accepted absolute indicator of rejection is the renal biopsy, but interpretation may be difficult in the early stages of rejection, the procedure is not without risk, and the indications for biopsy are not always clear cut, especially in the patient who is oliguric or anuric and on dialysis, where the serum creatinine is already showing gross fluctuation.

It is in this group that the radionuclide study comes into its own. The ^{99m}Tc-DTPA study shows a rise in the perfusion index, corresponding to the fall in renal blood flow which occurs as one of the earliest changes in rejection (Hollenberg, Remik, Rosen, Murray and Merrill, 1968). This may occur up to 48 h before any clinical features of rejection, and in our experience it is rare for it not to have occurred by the time clinical features raise the possibility of rejection. It is important to emphasize that it is the change of *perfusion* which is important, as the renal *function* may be improving at the same time, because of recovery from ATN. Similarly, it is the rise in the perfusion index, rather than any absolute value, which is important. At the same time, the whole study should be examined to see if there are any other features of rejection, such as prolongation of intrarenal transit or ureteric dilatation (see the section on Obstruction, section 5.10.7). However, any rise in the perfusion index should be considered to have a high probability of being due to rejection, even if no other features are present.

The ^{99m}Tc-sulphur colloid study may show increased uptake of colloid in the graft but this is also seen in ATN (Frick, Loken, Goldberg and Simmons, 1976), and is therefore of uncertain diagnostic value although it may be of value as a confirmatory investigation. Various measurements have been put forward to allow rejection to be diagnosed on the I-hippuran study, but none has achieved wide acceptance, and most rely on the formation of urine (Dubovsky *et al.*, 1975).

An interesting approach is the use of ^{111}In-labelled leucocytes (Frick *et al.*, 1979) or platelets (Smith, Chandler, Hawker, Hawker and Barnes, 1979; Senech, Nicholls and Smith, 1981; Hofer, Sinzinges, Leithnes, Schwarz and Bergman, 1981). Preliminary results suggest that these are taken up in rejecting transplants, but that the leucocytes are also taken up in infected kidneys. However, this is still in a very early stage, and further results are awaited.

Radiologically, the diagnosis of rejection is difficult. Although vascular changes may be seen on arteriography, they are not seen in all cases, or in early rejection, and most series conclude that it is often not possible to distinguish between ATN and rejection (Jones *et al.*, 1978). In addition, arteriography may cause deterioration in renal function. The visualization of the renal pelvis on IVU without visualization of the calyces is said to be specific for rejection (Seymour and Rittenberg, 1978; Küss, Poisson and Guillon, 1973), but it may be difficult to see any of the collecting system, or even the transplant, in the poorly functioning graft. It has been claimed that ultrasonography may detect changes in renal size and renal oedema and be able to differentiate between ATN and rejection, but the sensitivity and specificity of this method are not known (Maklad, Wright and Rosenthal, 1979; Hricak, Toledo, Pereyra, Eyler, Madrazo and Sy, 1979).

Many biochemical and serological tests have been described for the diagnosis of rejection, but these have not gained widespread acceptance, and many rely on the production of urine and/or complex assays. Following the decision that a graft is being rejected, and is to be treated, the question arises as to how often the patient should be studied. In our experience, it may take 5–7 d for the perfusion index to return to normal, and in the patient who is passing urine well, the study need not be repeated for about a week, or when the creatinine has returned to normal. The study is then repeated to obtain a 'base line' value, which is reproducible if the rejection has been fully treated. If the perfusion index has not returned to the base line, then the study should be repeated. If the patient is anuric or oliguric the studies should be performed on alternate days to follow the progress of the ATN, to confirm the response to anti-rejection therapy, and to allow the detection of further rejection episodes.

Very occasionally the patient may undergo rejection of such an extreme degree that no renal perfusion whatsoever is seen (a 'black hole'). When this occurs, the implication is that there is no blood supply to the kidney, and no kidney with this finding has ever been shown to recover function. This is, therefore, an indication for stopping anti-rejection therapy, and abandoning the graft.

5.10.5 EXTRAVASATION OF URINE

This is probably the commonest surgical complication of transplantation (although it is still uncommon) (Bewick *et al.*, 1974). The two common sites of leakage are at the vesico–ureteric anastomosis and from the cystotomy in the roof of the bladder which is performed to allow access to the bladder for this anastomosis. Very occasionally the entire ureter may necrose. This is usually ischaemic, often associated with damage to a lower polar artery, and so may develop over several days. The first indication of a leak may be the passage of urine through the wound. Alternatively, it may be suspected following the finding of an abdominal swelling or abdominal tenderness, especially in an 'anuric' patient. However, it is important to emphasize that extravasation of urine may be asymptomatic in the immunosuppressed patient.

Where the patient is having regular ^{99m}Tc-DTPA studies, the first clue may be the appearance of a perirenal collection (see below). When one is seen, or when there is a clinical suspicion, then it is essential to prolong the study, and record delayed images for up to 6 h, before and after emptying the bladder (Texter and Haden, 1975). This may show that activity passes into the perirenal collection, confirming the leak, and often shows the site of leakage. The definitive study for the demonstration of extravasation is a cystogram. If the graft is functioning well, then an IVP may demonstrate the leak. If the graft is functioning poorly, then percutaneous antegrade introduction of contrast may be necessary. Ultrasound will demonstrate the presence or absence of a collection, which may be of value where there is some doubt, but is not diagnostic.

5.10.6 PERIRENAL COLLECTIONS

Three types of perirenal collection may be seen. Immediately following operation, perirenal haematomas are relatively common, but are usually small and reabsorb spontaneously. Occasionally, they may be so large as to cause renal obstruction, or to cause clinical concern if bleeding continues. Urinary collections ('urinomas') are associated with extravasation of urine. The third type of collection is the lymphocele. This is composed of lymphatic fluid, and arises following disturbance of the lymphatic system at the time of operation (Bingham, Hilson and Maisey, 1978).

All three types of collection give rise to a similar appearance on the ^{99m}Tc-DTPA study of a photon-deficient area, which may take the form of a 'halo'. In the immediate post-operative period a similar appearance may be seen from oedema, but this usually resolves rapidly. The differentiation between a haematoma and a lymphocele may be difficult on the radionuclide study, but is usually easy clinically. The diagnosis of a urinoma has already been considered above (see Extravasation of urine, section 5.10.5).

Where the appearances on the radionuclide study are uncertain, ultrasound is often of value, particularly where the collection is perirenal. In addition to confirming the presence of a collection, ultrasound may give an indication as to its nature. Urinomas are relatively anechoic, whereas lymphoceles often show an irregular echo pattern (Marley, 1975).

5.10.7 OBSTRUCTION

The incidence of obstruction following transplant surgery depends on the surgical technique used. If the ureter is inserted through a 'tunnel' in the base of the bladder, the incidence of obstruction is higher than in the alternative technique where the ureter is inserted into the apex of the bladder. However, the latter technique has a higher incidence of reflux. Obstruction may also occur at other sites, such as the pelviureteric junction or where the ureter has to pass below other structures, such as the peritoneal reflection, and whenever obstruction appears possible it is essential to discuss the surgical method used in that patient with the surgeon concerned.

The diagnosis of obstruction in the transplanted kidney is no easier or more difficult than in the normal kidney. If the ureter appears prominent on the ^{99m}Tc-DTPA study, and no activity is seen in the bladder by 10 min, than a 'late' image at 30 min is indicated. If the ureter still seems prominent, a post-micturition image will show whether there is hold-up. If there is still doubt, a frusemide-diuresis study is indicated. Radiology may be of help in defining the level of obstruction, and confirming whether there is pelvicalyceal dilatation.

In our experience, ureteric obstruction is relatively uncommon. On the other hand, a prominent ureter is a common finding in association with acute rejection. This 'pseudo-obstruction' is associated with the oedema and loss of peristalsis of the ureter in rejection (Hasegawa, Smith, Lee and Hume, 1975) together with renal oedema (Seymour and Rittenburg, 1978). The dilated ureter washes out with frusemide. In addition, the deterioration in the renal perfusion index associated with rejection should also suggest the correct diagnosis.

5.10.8 RENAL VASCULAR COMPLICATIONS

These are all uncommon. The most severe vascular complication is complete occlusion of the renal artery or vein. As noted above this is seen in complete anuria, with no perfusion on the dynamic radionuclide study. Segmental renal artery occlusion may be asymptomatic, but is seen first as a wedge-shaped defect in the vascular phase of the ^{99m}Tc-DTPA study.

The commonest renal vascular problem is renal artery stenosis, which is more likely where there has been an end-to-end anastomosis (essential in live-related transplants) than where a patch of aorta has been used. The clinical suspicion may arise from persistent hypertension, but there are no definite features on the radionuclide imaging study. However, a strong suspicion may arise when the perfusion index shows continuing impairment of flow in the later post-operative period, which persists in spite of anti-rejection therapy, often combined with a renal biopsy showing little or no rejection. The definitive diagnosis of renal artery stenosis is made by radiology, which should be performed as soon as the suspicion arises.

5.10.9 EXTRARENAL COMPLICATIONS

The ever-present hazard of immunosuppression is infection, and ^{67}Ga imaging is often indicated for localization of possible sites. It is important to remember that ^{67}Ga is taken up in the transplanted kidney both during rejection and in infection. Avascular necrosis of bone is often a problem in transplanted patients, and bone imaging may be of value in diagnosis and in following its progress.

5.10.10 TECHNICAL METHODOLOGY

To assess the renal transplant adequately, the study should be carried out with a gamma camera and computer. The patient lies under the camera, which is positioned so that the aortic bifurcation is at the upper edge of the field, and the centre of the field is over the kidney (which can usually be felt). ^{99m}Tc-stannous-DTPA is injected as a bolus, in a dose of 10mCi (500 MBq) (corrected for body surface area in children). A 'vascular' image is recorded for 30 s following the injection. Starting at 2 min from the time of injection, an image is recorded for 300 000 counts (400 000 if a large-field camera is used). The time taken for this is noted, and further images are recorded for this same time at 5 and 10 min after injection. Ideally, further images should be recorded at 15, 20, 25 and 30 min, but it is sometimes necessary to compromise, in which case a full study should be performed when the patient is first seen, and a 10-min study thereafter, with just a 30-min image if there is any worry about obstruction.

At the same time, the study is recorded on the computer, using a frame rate of 1 frame per second for the first 30s, followed by 1 frame per minute for 10 or 30 min. A 64 × 64 matrix is used, using byte mode for the initial phase, then word mode for the second phase. For analysis, regions of interest are defined over the iliac artery (distal to the transplant), the transplant (excluding any portions overlying the artery) and a background area. Activity-time curves are generated, and a perfusion index obtained from the ratio of the areas under the arterial and renal curves, which changes with changes in relative renal blood flow (see Figure 5.14). For further details as to method and interpretation the reader is referred to Hilson *et al.* (1977) and Ayres, Hilson and Maisey (1980).

REFERENCES

Al-Nahhas, A. A., Jafri, R. A., Britton, K. E. *et al.* (1988) Clinical experience with 99m-Tc-MAG3, mercaptoacetyltriglycine and a comparison with 99mTc-DTPA. *Eur. J. Nucl. Med.*, **14**, 453–62.

Al-Nahhas, A., Marcus, A. J., Brinanji, J. *et al.* (1989) Validity of the mean parenchymal transit time as a screening test for the detection of functional renal artery stenosis in hypertensive patients. *Nucl. Med. Commun.*, **10**, 807–15.

Bricker, N. S. (1969) On the meaning of the intact nephron hypothesis. *Am. J. Med.*, **46**, 1–3.

Britton, K. E. and Brown, N. J. G. (1971) *Clinical Renography*, Lloyd Luke, London.

Britton, K. E., Nimmon, C. C., Whitfield, H. N. *et al.* (1979) Obstructive nephropathy: successful evaluation with radionuclides. *Lancet*, **i**, 905–7.

Britton, K. E., Bernardi, M., Wilkinson, S. P. *et al.* (1980) in *Radionuclides in Nephrology* (eds N. K. Hollenburg and S. Lange), Georg Thieme, Stuttgart, pp. 204–208.

Britton, K. E., Naura, M. K., Nimmon, C. C. *et al.* (1986) Total and intrarenal flow distribution in healthy subjects. *Nephron*, **43**, 265–73.

Britton, K. E., Nawaz, M. K., Whitfield, H. N. *et al.* (1987) Obstructive nephopathy: comparison between parenchymal transit time index and frusemide diuresis. *Br. J. Urol.*, **59**, 127–32.

Britton, K. E., Al-Nahhas, A., Nimmon, C. C. *et al.* (1990) The measurement of intrarenal plasma flow distribution, in *Radionuclides in Nephrology* (eds) M. D. Blanfox, N. K. Hollenburg and C. Raynaud) Karger, Basel, pp. 79, 186–9.

Brown, N. J. G. (1982) in *Radionuclides in Nephrology* (eds A. M. Joekes, A. R. Constable, N. J. G. Brown and W. N. Tauxe), Academic Press, London, pp. 113–18.

Carlsen, J. E., Moller, M. L., Lund, J. O. *et al.* (1980) Comparison of four commercial Tc-99m Sn DTPA preparations used for the measurement of glomerular filtration rate. *J. Nucl. Med.*, **21**, 126–9.

Davidson, A., Jones, A., Orvig, C. *et al.* (1981) A new class of oxo-technetium (+5) chelate complexes containing a Tc ON2S2 core. *Inorg. Chem.*, **20**, 1629–32.

Davies, E. R., Roberts, J. E. M., Heney, N. M. and Seadden, G. (1971) Renal scintigraphy in pyelonephritis. *Proc. R. Soc. Med.*, **64**, 63–4.

De Grazia, J. A., Scheibe P.O., Jackson, P. E. *et al.* (1974) Clinical application of a kinetic model of hippurate distribution and renal clearance. *J. Nucl. Med.*, **15**, 102–6.

Delcourt, E., Franken, P., Motte, S. *et al.* (1985) Measurement of glomerular filtration rate by means of a ^{99m}Tc DTPA complex and a scintillation camera: a method based on the kinetics of the distribution volume of the tracer in the kidney area. *Nucl. Med. Commun.*, **6**, 787–94.

Dondi, M., Franchi, R., Levorato, M. *et al.* (1989) Evaluation of hypertensive patients by means of Captopril enhanced renal scintigraphy with technetium-99m DTPA. *J. Nucl. Med.*, **30**, 615–21.

Duffy, G. J., Casey, M. and Barker, F. (1982) in *Radionuclides in Nephrology* (eds A. M. Joekes, A. R. Constable, N. J. G. Brown and W. N. Tauxe), Academic Press, London, 101–6.

Fritzberg, A. R., Sudhaker, K., Eshima, D. *et al.* (1986) Synthesis and biological evaluation of Tc-99m MAG3 as a hippuran replacement. *J. Nucl. Med.*, **27**, 111–16.

Gates, G. F. (1982) Glomerular filtration rate: estimation from functional renal accumulation of 99-Tcm DTPA. *Am. J. Roentgenol.*, **138**, 565–70.

Gates, G. F. (1984) Computation of glomerular filtration rate with 99-Tcm DTPA: an in-house computer programme. *J. Nucl. Med.*, **25**, 613–18.

Giese, J., Mogensen, P. and Munck, O. (1975) Diagnostic value of renography for detection of unilateral renal or renovascular disease in hypertensive patients. *Scand. Clin. Lab. Invest.*, **35**, 307–10.

Ginjaume, M., Casey, M., Barker, F. *et al.* (1985) Measurement of glomerular filtration rate using technetium 99m DTPA. *J. Nucl. Med.*, **26**, 1347–9.

Godley, M. L., Ransley, P. G., Parkhouse, H. F. *et al.* (in press) Quantitation of vesicoureteric reflux by radionuclide cystography and urodynamics. *Paediatr. Nephrol.*

Goris, M. L., Daspit, S. G., McLaughlin, R. and Kriss, J. P. (1976) Interpolative background subtraction. *J. Nucl. Med.*, **17**, 744–7.

Groshar, D., Frankel, A., Iosilevsky, G. *et al.* (1989) Quantitation of renal uptake of technetium-99m DMSA using SPECT. *J. Nucl. Med.*, **30**, 246–50.

Gruenewald, S. M., Nimmon, C. C., Nawaz, M. K. and Britton, K. E. (1981) A non-invasive Y camera technique for the measurement of intrarenal flow distribution in man. *Clin. Sci.*, **61**, 385–9.

Hauser, W., Atkins, H. L., Nelson, K. G. *et al.* (1970) Technetium-99m DTPA: a new radiopharmaceutical for brain and kidney scanning. *Radiology*, **94**, 679–84.

Hawkins, L. A., Elliott, A. T., Shields, R. *et al.* (1982) A rapid quantitative method for the production of ^{125}I iodo hippuric acid. *Eur. J. Nucl. Med.*, **7**, 58–61.

Hay, A. M., Norman, W. J. Rice, M. L. *et al.* (1984) A comparison between diuresis renography and the Whitaker test in 64 kidneys. *Br. J. Urol.*, **56**, 561–4.

Hedman, P. J. K., Kempi, V. and Voss, H. (1978) Measurement of vesicoureteral reflux with intravenous 99mTc-DTPA compared to radiographic cystography. *Radiology*, **126**, 205–8.

Hunter, G. J., Gordon, I., Sweeney, L. *et al.* (1987) 99mTc DTPA scanning with diuretic washout: is it useful in the investigation of obstruction in the presence of gross renal tract dilatation? *Br. J. Urol.*, **59**, 208–10.

Jafri, R. A., Britton, K. E., Nimmon, C. C. *et al.* (1988) 99m-Tc MAG3: a comparison with I-123 and I-131 orthoiodohippurate in patients with renal disorder. *J. Nucl. Med.*, **29**, 147–58.

Kawamura, J., Ifoh, H., Okeida, Y. *et al.* (1983) Preoperative and postoperative critical function of a kidney with staghorn calculus assessed by 99mTc DMSA scintigraphy. *J. Urol.*, **130**, 430–3.

Klingensmith, W. C., III, Fritzberger, A. R., Spitzer, V. M. *et al.* (1984) Clinical evaluation of Tc-99m *N,N*-bis (mercaptoacetyl)-2,3-diaminopropionate as a replacement for I-131 hippurate. *J. Nucl. Med.*, **25**, 42–48.

Koff, S. A., Thrall, J. H. and Keyes, J. W. J. R. (1978) Diuretic radionuclide urography. *J. Urol.*, **122**, 541–4.

Kogan, S. J., Sigler, L., Levitt, S. B. *et al.* (1986) Elusive vesicoureteral reflux in children with normal contrast cystograms. *J. Urol.*, **136**, 325–8.

Lee, T. Y., Constable, A. R. and Cranage, R. W. (1982) in *Radionuclides in Nephrology* (eds A. M. Joekes, A. R. Constable, N. J. G. Brown and W. N. Tauxe), Academic Press, London, pp. 107–12.

Luke, R. G., Briggs, J. D., Kennedy, A. C. and Barr Stirling, W. (1968a) The isotope renogram in the detection and assessment of renal artery stenosis. *Q. J. Med.*, **35**, 237–60.

Luke, R. G., Kennedy, A. C., Briggs, J. D. *et al.* (1968b) Results of nephrectomy in hypertension associated with unilateral renal disease. *Br. Med. J.*, **3**, 764–8.

Maxwell, M. H., Marks, L. S., Varady, P. D. *et al.* (1975) Renal vein renin in essential hypertension. *J. Lab. Clin. Med.*, **86**, 901–9.

Merrick, M. V., Uttley, W. S. and Wild, S. R. (1980) The detection of pylonephritic scarring in children by radioisotope imaging. *Br. J. Radiol.*, **53**, 544–56.

Mogensen, P., Munck, O. and Giese, J. (1975) ^{131}I-Hippuran renography in normal subjects and patients with essential hypertension. *Scand. J. Clin. Invest.*, **35**, 301–6.

Monsour, M., Azmy, A. F. and MacKenzie, J. R. (1987) Renal scarring secondary to vesicoureteric reflux: critical assessment and new grading. *Br. J. Urol.*, **70**, 320–4.

Nimmo, M. J., Merrick, M. V. and Allan, P. L. (1987) Measurement of relative renal function: a comparison of methods and assessment of reproducibility. *Br. J. Radiol.*, **60**, 861–4.

Nimmon, C. C., Britton, K. E., Gruenewald, S. *et al.* (1982) in *Radionuclides in Nephrology* (eds A. M. Joekes, A. R. Constable, N. J. E. Brown and W. N. Tauxe), Academic Press, London, pp. 55–63.

Nimmon, C. C., Britton, K. E., Bomanji, J. *et al.* (1988) in *Proceedings of the European Nuclear Medicine Congress* (eds M. A. E. Schmidt and L. Csernay), Schattauer Verlag, Stuttgart, pp. 472–6.

Nissen, O. I. (1968) The extraction fraction of *p*-amino hippurate in the superficial and deep venous drainage area of the cat kidney. *Acta Physiol. Scand.*, **73**, 329–38.

Nordyke, R. A., Tubis, M. and Blahd, W. (1960) Use of radioiodinated hippuran for individual kidney function tests. *J. Lab. Clin. Med.*, **56**, 438–45.

Oei, N. Y., Geyskes, G. G., Dorhout Mees, T. J. *et al.* (1984) Captopril induced renographic alteration in unilateral renal artery stenosis. *J. Nucl. Med.*, **25**, 36.

Oei, N. Y., Geyskes, G. G., Mees, E. J. D. *et al.* (1987) in *Radionuclides in Nephrology* (Contributions to Nephrology, Vol. 56) (eds A. Bischof-Delaloye and M. D. Blaufox), Karger, Basel, pp. 95–103.

Oppenheim, B. E. and Appledorn, C. R. (1981) Functional renal imaging through factor analysis. *J. Nucl. Med.*, **22**, 417–23.

O'Reilly, P. H., Shields, R. A. and Testa, H. J. (1987) *Nuclear Medicine in Urology and Nephrology* (2nd edn), Butterworths, London, pp. 91–108.

Pauwels, E. K. J., Lycklania, A. A. B., Nijeholt, A. *et al.* (1987) The determination of relative kidney function in obstructive uropathy with ^{99m}Tc DMSA. *Nucl. Med. Commun.*, **8**, 865–7.

Peters, A. M., Gordon, I., Evans, K. *et al.* (1987) Background in the 99mTc-DTPA renogram: analysis of intravascular and extravascular components. *Am. J. Physiol. Imaging*, **2**, 66–71.

Piepsz, A., Froideville, J. L., Kinhaert, J. *et al.* (1987) in *Radionuclides in Nephrology* (Contributions to Nephrology, Vol. 56) (eds A. Bischof-Delaloye and M. D. Blaufox), Karger, Basel, pp. 77–81.

Rizzoni, G., Perale, R., Bui, F. *et al.* (1986) Radionuclide voiding cystography in intrarenal reflux detection. *Ann. Radiol.*, **29**, 415–20.

Russell, C. D., Thorstad, B. L., Yester M. V. *et al.* (1988) Quantitation of renal function with technetium-99m MAG3. *J. Nucl. Med.*, **29**, 1931–3.

Rutland, M. D. (1983) Glomerular filtration rate without blood sampling. *Nucl. Med. Commun.*, **4**, 425–33.

Rutland, M. D. (1985) A comprehensive analysis of renal DTPA studies. I. Theory and normal values. *Nucl. Med. Commun.*, **6**, 11–20.

Rutland, M. D. and Stuart, R. A. (1986) A comprehensive analysis of renal DTPA studies. III. Renal artery stenosis. *Nucl. Med. Commun.*, **7**, 879–85.

Schlegel, J. V. and Hamway, S. A. (1979) Individual renal plasma flow determination in 2 minutes. *J. Urol.*, **122**, 447–50.

Sfakianakis, G. N., Bourgoignie, J. J., Jaffe, D. *et al.*

(1987) Single dose captopril scintigraphy in the diagnosis of renovascular hypertension. *J. Nucl. Med.*, **9**, 1383–92.

Shone, R. M., Koff, S. A., Mentser, M. *et al.* (1984) Glomerular filtration rate in children: determination from the TC-99m DTPA renogram. *Radiology*, **151**, 627–33.

Smellie, J. M., Shaw, P. J., Prescod, N. P. and Bantock, H. M. (1988) ^{99m}Tc dimercaptosuccinic acid (DMSA) scan in patients with established radiological renal scarring. *Arch. Dis. Child.*, **63**, 1315–19.

Smith H. W. (1956) Unilateral nephrectomy in hypertensive disease. *J. Urol.*, **76**, 685–701.

Sreenevasan, G. (1974) Bilateral renal calculi. *Ann. R. Coll. Surg. Engl.*, **55**, 3–12.

Taylor, A. (1982) Quantitation of renal function with static imaging agents. *Semin. Nucl. Med.*, **12**, 330–44.

Tonnesen, K. H., Munck, O., Hald, T. *et al.* (1975) in *Radionuclides in Nephrology* (eds K. Zum Winkel, M. D. Blaufox and J. L. F. Brentano), Georg Thieme, Stuttgart, pp. 79–86.

Verboven, M., Ham, H. R., Josephson, S. *et al.* (1987) ^{99m}Tc DMSA uptake in obstructed kidneys: how inaccurate are the 5-hour measurements? *Nucl. Med. Commun.*, **8**, 1–4.

Vivian, G. and Gordon, I. (1983) Comparison between individual kidney GFR estimation at 20 minutes with ^{99m}Tc DTPA plus 51-Cr EDTA GFR in children with a single kidney. *Nucl. Med. Commun.*, **4**, 108–17.

Wenting, G. J., Tan-Tjiong, H. L., Derkx, F. H. M. *et al.* (1984) Split renal function after captopril in unilateral renal artery stenosis. *Br. Med. J.*, **288**, 886–90.

Whitfield, H. N., Britton, K. E., Hendry, W. F. *et al.* (1979) Frusemide intravenous urography in the diagnosis of pelviureteric junction obstruction. *Br. J. Urol.*, **51**, 445–8.

Wilkinson, S. P., Smith, I. K., Clarke, M. *et al.* (1977) Intrarenal distribution of plasma flow in cirrhosis as measured by transit renography. *Clin. Sci. Mol. Med.*, **52**, 469–75.

Wilkinson, S. P., Bernardi, M., Pearce, P. C. *et al.* (1978) Validation of 'transit renography' for the determination of the intrarenal distribution of plasma flow. *Clin. Sci. Mol. Med.*, **54**, 277–83.

Williams, E., Parker, D. and Roy, R. (1986) Multiple-section radionuclide tomography of the kidney: a clinical evaluation. *Br. J. Radiol.*, **59**, 975–83.

Wujanto, R., Lawson, R. S., Prescott, M. *et al.* (1987) The importance of using anterior and posterior views in the calculation of differential renal function using ^{99m}Tc DMSA. *Br. J. Radiol.*, **60**, 869–72.

Yee, C. A., Lee, H. B. and Blaufox, M. D. (1981) ^{99m}Tc DMSA renal uptake: influence of biochemical and physiological factors. *J. Nucl. Med.*, **22**, 1054–8.

Zananin, M. C., Jarritt, P. H., Sarfarazi, M. *et al.* (1987) Relative and absolute ^{99m}Tc DMSA uptake measurements in normal and obstructed kidneys. *Nucl. Med. Commun.*, **8**, 869–80.

Zechmann, W. (1988) The experimental approach to explain some misinterpretations of diuresis renography. *Nucl. Med. Commun.*, **9**, 283–94.

Zhang, G., Day, D. L., Loken, M. *et al.* (1987) Grading of reflux by radionuclide cystography. *Clin. Nucl. Med.*, **12**, 106–9.

REFERENCES FOR SECTION ON RENAL TRANSPLANTATION

Ashwal, S., Smith, A. J. K., Torres, F., Loken, M. and Chou, S. N. (1977) Radionuclide bolus angiography: a technique for verification of brain death in infants and children. *J. Pediatr*, **91**, 722–8.

Ayres, J. G., Hilson, A. J. W. and Maisey, M. N. (1980) Complications of Renal Transplantation: Appearances using ^{99}7mTc-DTPA. *Clin. Nucl. Med.*, 5, 473–80.

Bewick, M., Collins, R. E. C., Saxton, H. M., Ellis, F. G., McColl, I. and Ogg, C. S., (1974) The surgery and problems of the ureter in renal transplantation. *Br. J. Urol.*, **46**, 493–510.

Bingham, J. B., Hilson, A. J. W. and Maisey, M. N. (1978) The appearances of renal transplant lymphocoele during dynamic renal scintigraphy. *Br. J. Radiol.*, **51**, 342–6.

Conference of Medical Royal Colleges and their Faculties (UK) (1976) Diagnosis of brain death. *Br. Med. J.*, **2**, 1187.

Dubovsky, E. V., Logic, J. R., Diethelm, A. G., Balch, C. M. and Tauxe, W. N. (1975) Comprehensive evaluation of renal function in the transplanted kidney. *J. Nucl. Med.*, **16**, 1115–20.

Frick, M. P., Henke, C. E., Forstrom, L. A., Simmons, R. A., McCullough, J. and Loken, M. K. (1979) Use of ^{111}In-labelled leukocytes in evaluation of renal transplant rejection. *Clin. Nucl. Med.*, **4**, 24–5.

Frick, M. P., Loken, M. K., Goldberg, M. E. and Simmons, R. L. (1976) Use of ^{99m}Tc-sulphur colloid in evaluation of renal transplant complications. *J. Nucl. Med.*, **17**, 181–3.

George, E. A., Codd, J. E., Newton, W. T., Henry, R. E. and Donat, R. M. (1975) Further evaluation of ^{99m}Tc-sulphur colloid in rejecting renal transplants and in a canine model. *Radiology*, **116**, 121–6.

Hasegawa, A., Smith, M. J. V., Lee, H. M. and Hume, D. M. (1975) Cinefluoroscopic studies of ureteral function in the human renal transplant. *J. Urol.*, **114**, 381–4.

Hilson, A. J. W., Maisey, M. N., Brown, C. B., Ogg, C. S. and Bewick, M. S. (1978) Dynamic renal transplant imaging with Tc-99m DTPA (Sn) supplemented by a transplant perfusion index in the management of renal transplants. *J. Nucl. Med.*, **19**, 994–1000.

Hofer, R., Sinzinger, H., Leithner, C., Schwartz, M. and Bergman, H. (1981) Experiences with ^{111}In-oxine labelling of autologous platelets in follow-up studies in human kidney transplants. *Nucl. Med. Commun.*, **2**, 120.

Hollenberg, N. K., Remik, A. B., Rosen, S. M., Murray, J. E. and Merrill, J. P. (1986) The role of vasoconstriction in the ischaemia of renal allograft rejection. *Transplantation*, **6**, 59–69.

Hricak, H., Toledo-Pereryra, L. H., Eyler, W. R., Madrazo, B. L. and Sy, G. S. (1979) Evaluation of acute post-transplant renal failure by ultrasound. *Radiology*, **133**, 443–7.

Jones, B. J., Palmer, F. J., Charlesworth, J. A., Shirley, D. V., MacDonald, G. J., Williams, R. M. and Robertson, M. R. (1978) Angiographyin the diagnosis of renal allograft dysfunction. *J. Urol.*, **119**, 461–2.

Küss, R., Poisson, J. and Le Guillon, M. (1973) L'Urographie intraveneuse au cours de la crise de reject du transplant. *J. d'Urol. Nephrol.*, **7–8**, 605.
Maklad, N. F., Wright, C. H. and Rosenthal, S. J. (1979) Gray scale ultrasonic appearances of renal transplant rejection. *Radiology*, **131**, 711–7.
Morley, P. (1975) Ultrasound in the diagnosis of fluid collections following renal transplantation. *Clin. Radiol.*, **26**, 199–207.
Pavel, D. G., Westerman, S. R., Bergan, J. J. and Kahan, B. D. (1976) Computer-processed ^{99m}Tc-DTPA studies of renal allotransplants. *Surgery*, **79**, 152–60.
Rodriguez-Antunex, A., Gill, W. M. and Egleston, T. A. (1970) Assessment of function in the transplanted kidney with ^{131}I-Hippuran. *J. Urol.*, **103**, 574–6.
Senech, A., Nicholls, A. and Smith, F. W. (1981) Indium (111)-labelled platelets in the diagnosis of renal transplant rejection: preliminary findings. *Br. J. Radiol.*, **54**, 325–7.
Seymour, E. Q. and Rittenberg, G. M. (1978) Non-visualization of renal calices during excreting urography as an indicator of renal transplant rejection. *J. Urol.*, **119**, 720–1.
Smith, N., Chandler, S., Hawker, S. J., Hawker, L. M. and Barnes, A. D. (1979) Indium-labelled autologous platelets as diagnostic aid after renal transplantation. *Lancet*, **ii**, 1241–2.
Texter, J. H., Jr and Haden, H. (1976) Scintiphotography in the early diagnosis of urine leakage following renal transplantation. *J. Urol.*, **116**, 547–8.
Whittaker, J. R., Veith, F. J., Soberman, R., Lalezari, P., Tellis, I., Freed, S. Z. and Gliedman, M. L. (1973) The fate of the renal transplant with delayed function. *Surg. Gynec. Obstet.*, **136**, 919–22.

GENERAL REVIEW AND FURTHER READING

Bischof-Delaloye, A. and Blaufox, M. D. (1987) Radionuclides in nephrology. *Contrib. Nephrol.*, **86**, 77–81.
Blaufox, M. D. (1987) The current status of renal radiopharmaceuticals. *Contrib. Nephrol.*, **56**, 31–7.
Dubovsky, E. V. and Russell, C. D. (1988) Radionuclide evaluation of renal transplants. *Semin. Nucl. Med.*, **18**, 181–98.
Fine, E. J. and Sarkar, S. (1989) Differential diagnosis and management of renovascular hypertension through nuclear medicine techniques. *Semin. Nucl. Med.*, **19**, 101–15.
Fogelman, I. and Maisey, M. N. (1988) *An Atlas of Clinical Nuclear Medicine*, Martin Dunitz, London.
Gordon, I. (1986) Use of TC-99m DMSA and Tc-99m DTPA in reflux. *Semin. Urol.*, **4**, 99–108.
Gordon, I. (1990) Urinary tract infection in paediatrics: the role of diagnostic imaging. *Br. J. Radiol.*, **63**, 507–11.
Heyman, S. (1989) An update of radionuclide renal studies in paediatrics. *Nucl. Med. Annual*, **1989**, 179.
O'Reilly, P. H., Shields, R. A. and Testa, H. J. (1987) in *Nuclear Medicine in Urology and Nephrology* (eds H. J. Testa, R. A. Shields and P. H. O'Reilly), Butterworths, London.
Russell, C. D. and Dubovsky, E. V. (1989) Measurement of renal function with radionuclides. *J. Nucl. Med.*, **30**, 2053–7.
Sfakianakis, G. N. and Sfakianaki, E. D. (1988) Nuclear-medicine in paediatric urology and nephrology. *J. Nucl. Med.*, **29**, 1287–1300.

CHAPTER SIX

Bone scanning

I. Fogelman

6.1 INTRODUCTION

The isotope bone scan was only performed on a limited scale prior to 1972, but since the introduction of the ^{99m}Tc-labelled phosphate and diphosphonate compounds (Subramanian *et al.*, 1972; Castronovo, 1972) the value of this investigation in clinical practice has become increasingly recognized and it is now the most important and frequently requested study in any nuclear medicine department. Nowadays the bone scan is almost exclusively performed with ^{99m}Tc-labelled diphosphonate (methylene diphosphonate being the most popular) and the technique shows exquisite sensitivity for the detection of skeletal abnormality. However, there is the major limitation that scan appearances are non-specific. Nevertheless, in many clinical situations recognizable patterns of bone scan abnormality may be seen, which can often suggest a specific diagnosis. In this chapter, the current status of bone scanning in metastatic and benign skeletal disease will be discussed.

6.2 PATHOPHYSIOLOGY OF BONE UPTAKE OF DIPHOSPHONATE

A skeletal X-ray indicates the net result of bone resorption and repair. For a destructive lesion in trabecular bone to be recognized on X-ray, it must be greater than 1–1.5 cm in diameter, with loss of approximately 50% of bone mineral content (Edelstyn *et al.*, 1967). The bone scan, however, provides quite different information, which reflects skeletal metabolic activity. While the exact mechanism of uptake of bone-seeking radiopharmaceuticals is incompletely understood, it is thought most likely that they react through the phosphorus group by chemisorption onto the calcium of hydroxyapatite in bone, i.e. the diphosphonate molecule is adsorbed onto the surface of bone (Fogelman, 1980). The major factors which affect this adsorption are believed to be osteoblastic activity and skeletal vascularity, and there is preferential uptake of tracer at sites of active bone formation. The bone scan therefore reflects the metabolic reaction of bone to a disease process, whether neoplastic, traumatic or inflammatory. When bone resorption occurs, there may not be sufficient bone destruction to be identified on X-ray, although the bone scan may be strongly positive. This ability to detect functional change, which occurs earlier than structural change, is the explanation why the bone scan is more sensitive than conventional radiology. Bone scan findings are, however, relatively non-specific because virtually all disease processes result in an alteration in osteoblastic activity and blood flow. Thus, to obtain optimal information, the bone scan will often require to be correlated with corresponding X-rays.

6.3 EQUIPMENT

Bone scanning is invariably performed using a wide field of view gamma camera. However, there is some variation in the policy of departments as to whether to obtain the study using a scanning gamma camera, or else with multiple overlapping images of the skeleton. Any scanning gamma camera producing a single image of the whole skeleton has lower resolution than the same camera used in the static mode (Figures 6.1 and 6.2). The reason for this is that resolution falls rapidly as the distance between the collimater face and the patient increases. Therefore 'spot' views will always show higher resolution than those obtained with a scanning mechanism. Most often the bone scan will be requested as a screening test for skeletal metastases because of its known high sensitivity. It is therefore important to obtain im-

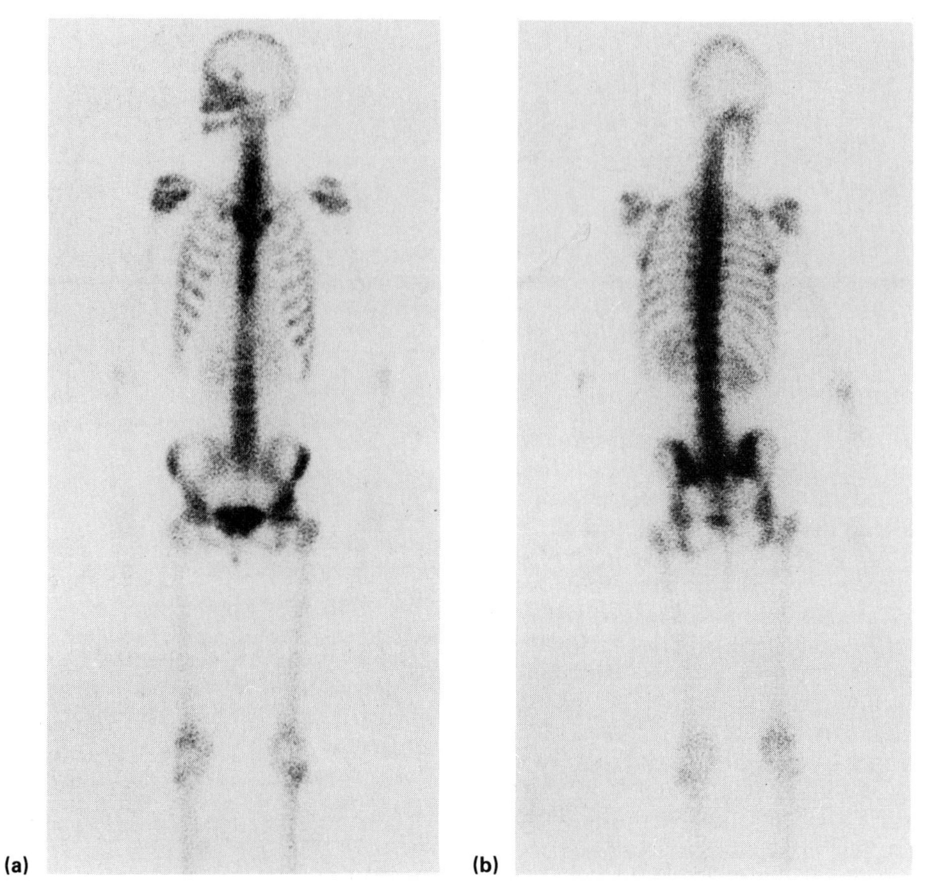

Figure 6.1 Normal whole body bone scan: (a) anterior view; (b) posterior view.

ages with the best possible resolution, and this is a powerful argument in favour of always obtaining overlapping views.

6.4 THE NORMAL BONE SCAN

The most important feature in a normal bone scan is symmetry about the mid-line in the sagittal plane. The left and right halves of the skeleton should be virtually mirror images of each other. There should be uniform uptake of tracer throughout most of the skeleton. Clear visualization of the whole skeleton should be obtained, with particular attention paid to ensure that, with overlapping views, there are no areas of omission such as the upper femur. The count rate is highest in those parts of the skeleton which are metabolically most active, and these areas generally contain a high percentage of trabecular bone and are subject to considerable stress, e.g. the axial skeleton. Diphosphonate which is not taken up by the skeleton is excreted via the urinary tract, and in a normal study the kidneys are clearly visualized.

The timing of bone scan images may depend upon the clinical problem under investigation. There is at present no complete agreement as to the optimal time interval between injection and static imaging, but it is customary to obtain images at 2–4 h. The longer the delay between injection and imaging, the greater the contrast between lesion and normal bone.

6.5 'THREE-PHASE' BONE SCAN

In certain circumstances a 'three-phase' bone scan will provide valuable additional information with regard to the vascularity of a lesion. This involves

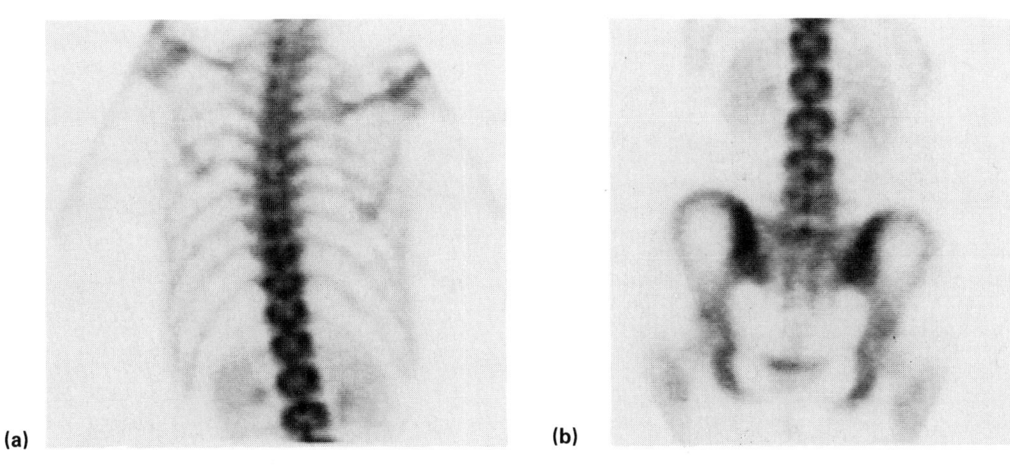

Figure 6.2 Spot views from normal subject: (a) thoracic spine; (b) posterior view of pelvis.

obtaining an initial dynamic flow study of the area of interest, with rapid sequential images being obtained every 2–3 s for 30 s. This is followed by a blood pool image at 5 min, when the radiopharmaceutical is still predominantly within the vascular compartment. A delayed static image or images will then be obtained 3 h later. An example of the use of 'three-phase' bone scan imaging is when osteomyelitis is suspected in a limb which is hot and swollen. If there is only increased vascularity, as demonstrated on the dynamic and blood pool images, but with no bone lesion seen, then this would support inflammation in the soft tissues, and would exclude osteomyelitis.

6.6 PATTERN RECOGNITION

To evaluate an abnormal bone scan fully one must be familiar with not only the normal bone scan appearances but also with the commonly seen variants (Figure 6.3) (Merrick, 1987). While the bone scan appearances are non-specific, recognizable patterns of abnormality are often seen, which may strongly suggest a specific diagnosis (Figures

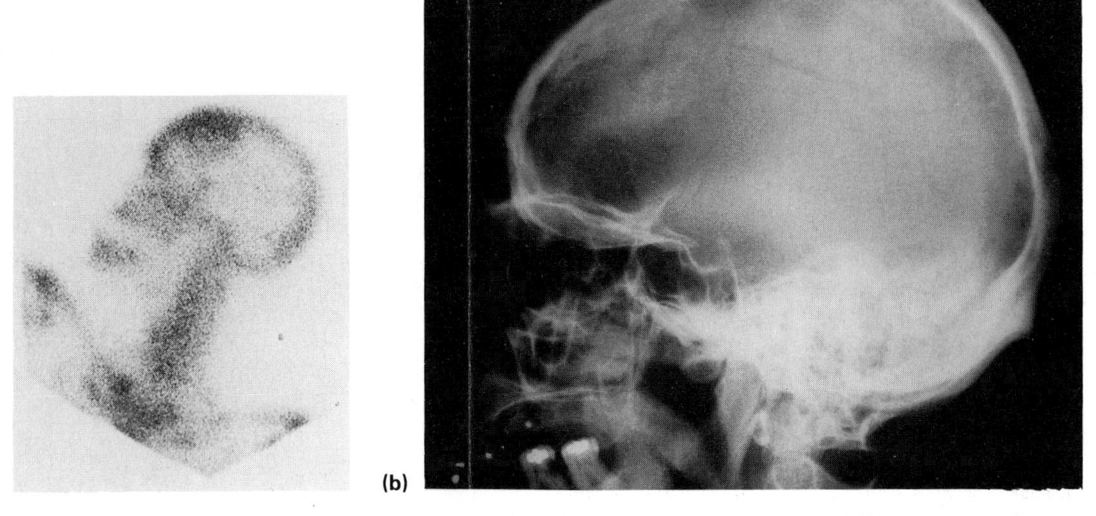

Figure 6.3 Bone scan: (a) left lateral skull; (b) skull X-ray. On bone scan study there is diffusely increased tracer uptake seen in the frontal region of the skull. Scan findings are those of hyperostosis frontalis, which is confirmed on X-ray.

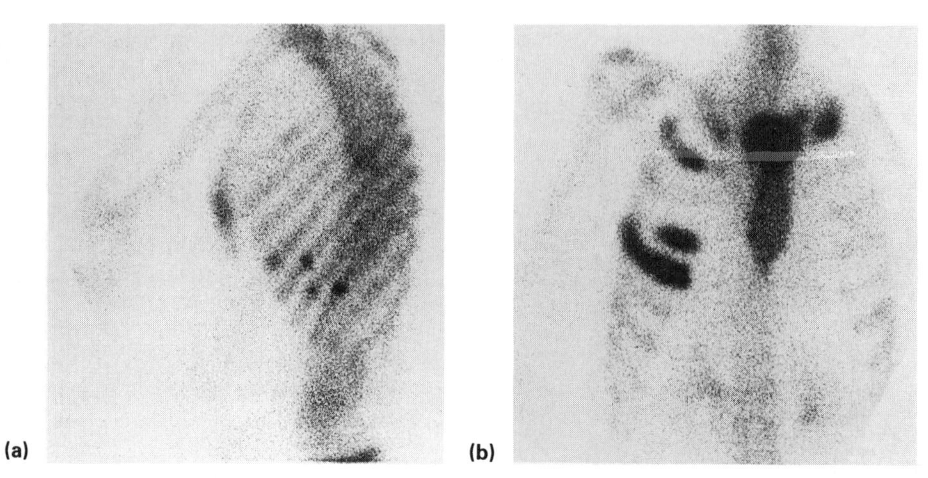

Figure 6.4 (a) Bone scan; lateral view of thorax. Focal lesions are seen in ribs in a relatively linear pattern. Appearances are characteristic of fracture due to trauma. (b) Bone scan view of anterior thorax. Increased tracer uptake is seen extending along first ribs bilaterally, right second, fourth and fifth ribs, and upper sternum. The right third rib is not clearly visualized in its anterior aspect. This patient had carcinoma of the breast with skeletal metastases. Note extension of disease along the rib, which is suggestive of metastatic involvement.

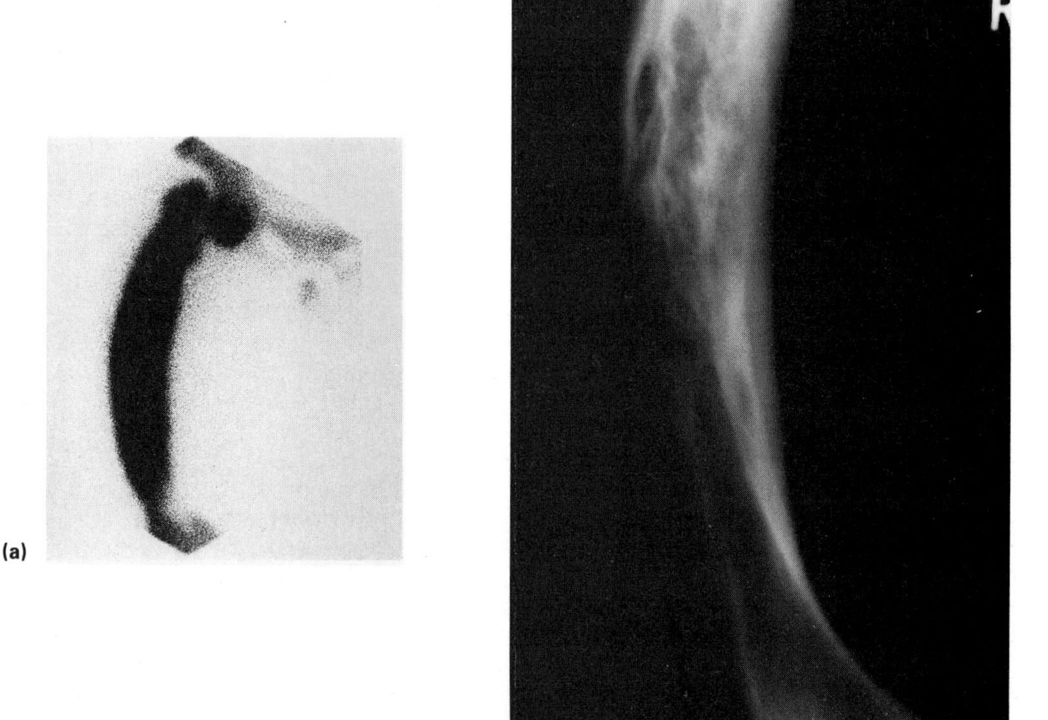

Figure 6.5 Bone scan view of right femur (a), and (b) X-ray. There is a striking increase in tracer uptake throughout the right femur, which is bowed. Appearances are typically those of Paget's disease. This is confirmed on X-ray.

6.4 and 6.5). An experienced observer will regularly be correct when suggesting that a specific diagnosis has a high probability of being present. Nevertheless, even an expert will be incorrect on occasion, and one should not consider the bone scan as a definitive investigation, but rather one that provides high sensitivity for lesion detection which, if present, will often require further investigation.

6.7 THE BONE SCAN IN MALIGNANCY

The detection of metastatic disease throughout the skeleton remains the most important indication for performing a bone scan. The common cancers are frequently associated with skeletal metastases and, in particular in carcinoma of the breast and prostate, there is autopsy evidence of an approximate 80% incidence of bone lesions (Abrams *et al.*, 1950; Gilbert and Kagan 1976). As previously discussed, the bone scan may identify metastases at an earlier stage than conventional radiology, and there is now extensive literature confirming this (Tofe *et al.*, 1975; Pistenma *et al.*, 1975; Citrin *et al.*, 1977). We have recently found in carcinoma of the breast that the bone scan may have up to an 18-month lead time over radiology, with the average being four months. The most characteristic feature of metastases is irregular focal lesions in a pattern that does not correspond to any single anatomical structure (Figure 6.6). The most common sites of involvement are the spine, pelvis, ribs, proximal humerus and femur, and the skull. Although uncommon, metastatic disease may involve the distal skeleton in approximately 7% of cases (Corcoran *et al.*, 1976; Rappaport *et al.*, 1978), and a survey of the entire skeleton is therefore advisable.

If a metastasis does not induce an osteoblastic response then the bone scan may be normal. False-negative results occur in less than 3% of cases (Pistenma *et al.*, 1975; Citrin and McKillop, 1978) and are seen on occasion in myeloma. Rarely a metastasis may be recognized on the bone scan as an area of decreased tracer uptake (cold spot or photopaenic lesion) (Stadalnik, 1979). Photopaenic metastases are most often seen in myeloma (Wahner *et al.*, 1980) and in renal carcinoma (Kim *et al.*, 1983). It is possible that such lesions will be identified more often as newer gamma cameras with increased resolution become available. One problem that may arise when interpreting a bone scan image is recognizing a superscan of malignancy (Constable and Cranage, 1981). This occurs when focal lesions are so extensive that they coalesce to produce a relatively diffuse image (Figure 6.7). Nevertheless, this is often apparent as one's initial impression is that the scan is too good to be true, due to very high uptake in the skeleton with heightened contrast between bone and soft tissue. The renal images are generally not visualized due to the increased contrast, and also because there is less tracer available to be excreted via the urinary tract. Very often irregularity of tracer uptake and some focal lesions will be apparent, particularly in the ribs (Fogelman *et al.*, 1977b). On the rare occasion that any doubt exists as to whether a bone scan is normal or represents a superscan of malignancy a single X-ray of the pelvis will clarify the issue as this is always abnormal in such cases. Where quantification of bone uptake is available, this will provide further diagnostic information. As noted above, an abnormal bone scan should be followed by more specific investigations, directed to the sites of scan abnormality. Figure 6.8 provides a suggested diagnostic pathway for the investigation of a patient with suspected metastatic disease. In those cases where a patient presents with X-ray evidence of bone metastases, the bone scan will often provide valuable additional information in demonstrating more accurately the extent of disease. This may have relevance when planning radiotherapy fields or to identify a more readily accessible site for biopsy.

6.8 INITIAL STAGING OF MALIGNANCY

The bone scan is important in the initial evaluation of patients with malignancy, as the knowledge that metastases are or are not present may alter subsequent management. It is not uncommon for a patient with a known malignancy to complain of bone pain, and this is a clear indication for a bone scan. However, the relationship between bone pain and metastases is complex. Although a patient may complain of a single site of bone pain, on further investigation multiple metastases are often identified, whereas others with extensive metastatic disease may be asymptomatic (Front *et al.*, 1979). Another feature which may indicate the presence of skeletal metastases is the identification of hypercalcaemia (Figure 6.9). However, this also correlates poorly with bone scan findings. While most patients with carcinoma of the breast have skeletal metastases with many other

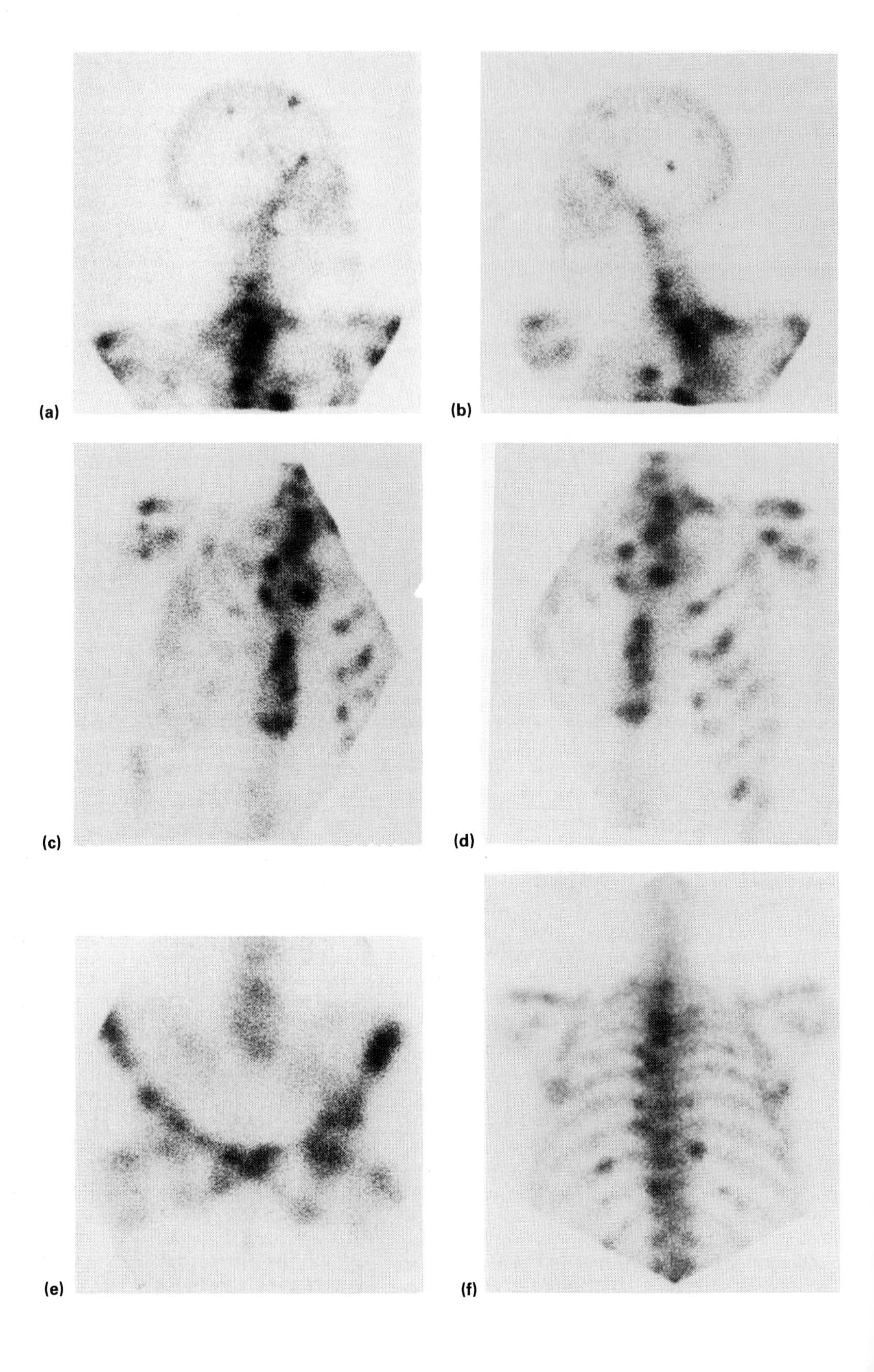
(a)
(b)
(c)
(d)
(e)
(f)

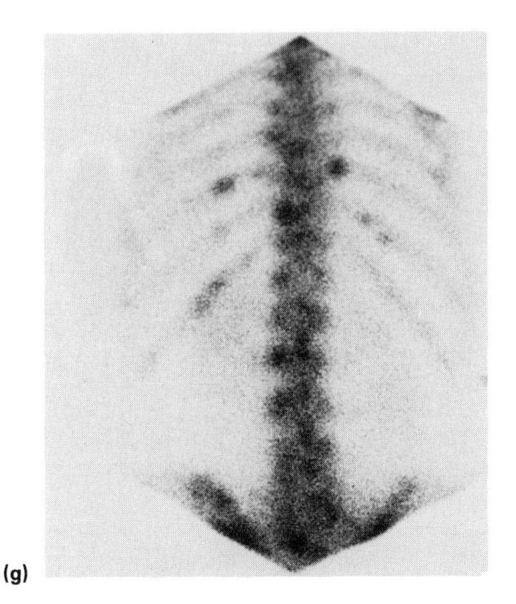

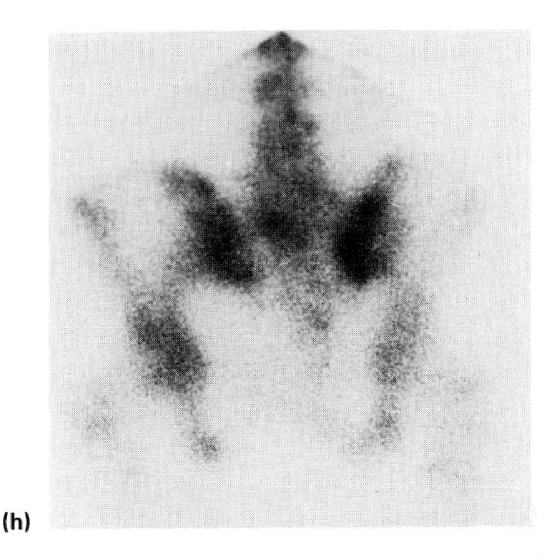

Figure 6.6 Bone scan views: (a) right lateral skull; (b) left lateral skull; (c) right anterior chest; (d) left anterior chest; (e) anterior pelvis; (f) posterior thoracic spine; (g) posterior lumbar spine; (h) posterior pelvis. This 45-year-old woman with carcinoma of the breast complained of back pain. Bone scan shows multiple focal abnormalities throughout the skull, spine, ribs, pelvis, both upper femora and upper humeri. Scan findings are those of widespread metastatic involvement of the skeleton.

tumours there may be no evidence of skeletal metastases (Ralston *et al.*, 1982), the hypercalcaemia being largely due to a humoral factor causing a generalized increase in skeletal metabolism and increased tubular reabsorption of calcium.

6.9 ASSESSMENT OF RESPONSE TO THERAPY

The bone scan may be used to monitor progression of disease and response to therapy (Figure 6.10), as reliance on symptoms alone can be misleading. Further, radiological evidence of healing is slow, and not possible in the presence of sclerotic metastases. The use of bone scans to assess the response of skeletal metastases to systemic therapy does, however, require some caution. Clearly, the reproducibility of scan technique is essential, particularly with regard to image contrast. While a reduction in the number of lesions on the bone scan and lessening of intensity indicates successful therapy and, conversely, a dramatic increase in the number of lesions suggests progression of metastatic disease it is now recognized, however, that transient worsening of scan findings may be seen in the initial few months following successful instigation of therapy. This is the so-called flare response (Figure 6.11) (Rossleigh *et al.*, 1982, 1984), and reflects the activation of osteoblasts as part of the healing process. Most often this is noted as an increase in intensity of individual lesions, but on occasion new lesions may also be seen. A flare response can be particularly misleading if a bone scan is obtained within a few months of change of therapy, but should not be a factor after six months.

6.10 ASSESSMENT OF RISK OF FRACTURE

Many orthopaedic surgeons are nowadays prepared to carry out prophylactic surgery in patients with extensive metastatic disease who are at high risk of sustaining a fracture of a long bone. This is performed to reduce morbidity, as patients with perhaps several months to live would have a particularly miserable existence if bed-bound following a fracture. If such a policy is pursued locally, it is of considerable importance to evaluate the bone scan in terms of metastatic involvement of the long bones. While the bone scan cannot identify risk of fracture, if there is long bone involvement then this should be noted and the appropriate X-rays obtained.

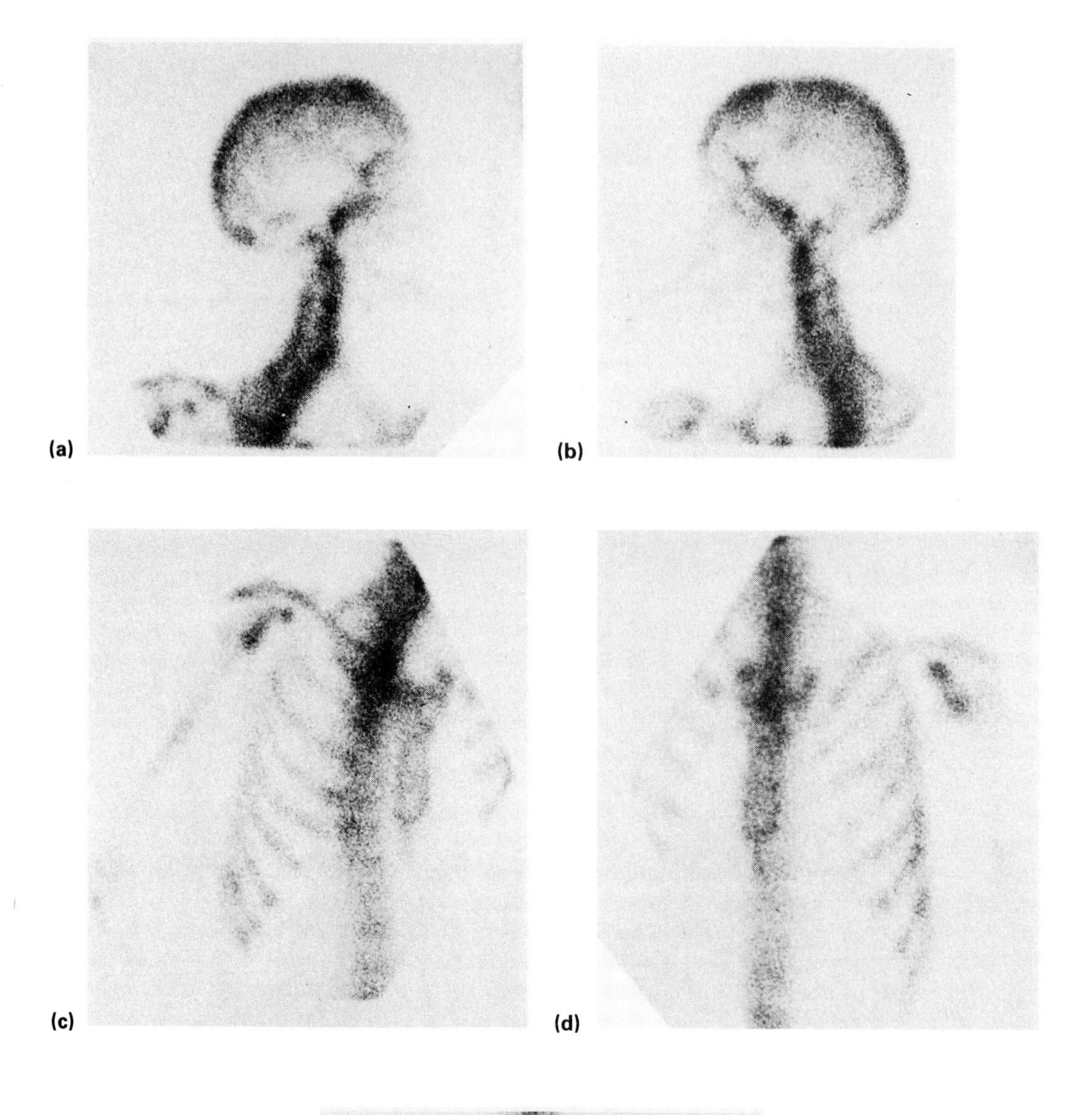
(a)
(b)
(c)
(d)

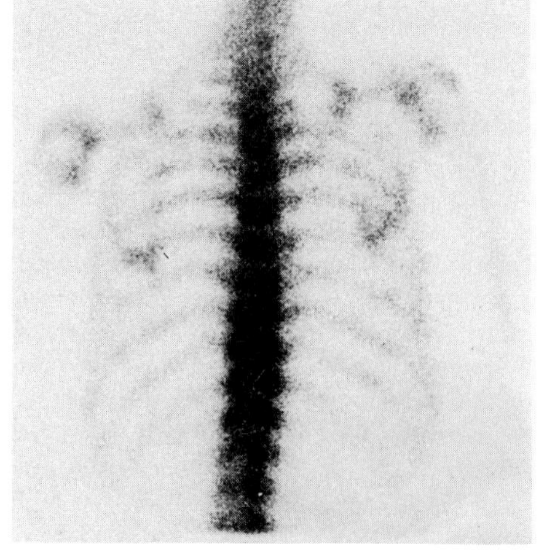
(e)

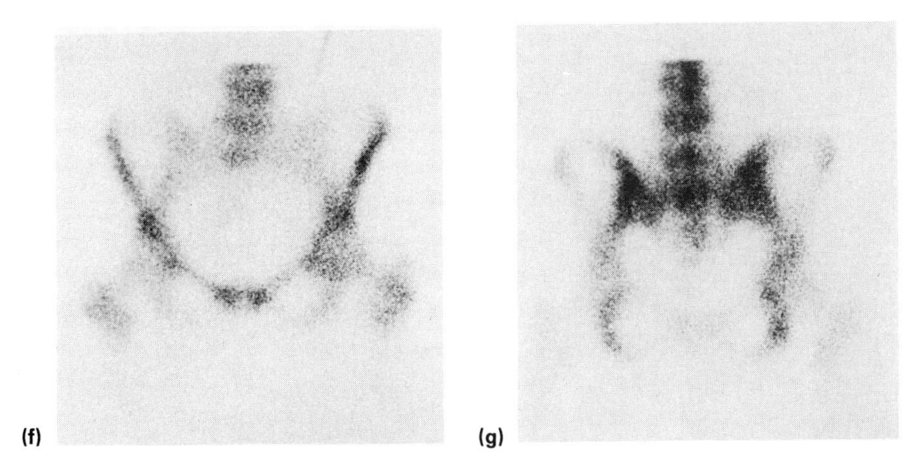

Figure 6.7 A 57-year-old woman with carcinoma of the breast. Bone scan views: (a, b) skull; (c, d) anterior chest; (e) posterior thoracic and lumbar spine; (f) anterior pelvis; (g) posterior pelvis. There is increased tracer uptake throughout the whole skeleton, with high contrast between bone and soft tissue. There is, however, slight irregularity of tracer uptake, particularly throughout the ribs and skull, but no clear discrete focal abnormality is seen. Renal images are not visualized. The scan appearances are those of 'superscan' of malignancy.

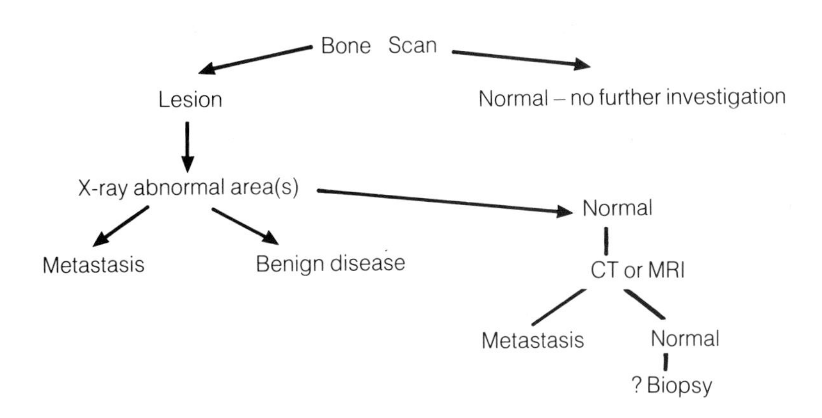

Figure 6.8 Evaluation of suspected skeletal metastases.

6.11 INDIVIDUAL TUMOURS

It is not possible to discuss all tumours, and a more full review can be obtained elsewhere (McKillop, 1987). Here the clinically most important tumours, i.e. breast, prostate and lung will be briefly commented upon.

6.11.1 BREAST CANCER

Bone scanning has been extensively evaluated in patients with carcinoma of the breast (El Domeiri and Shroff, 1976; Citrin *et al.*, 1976; Campbell *et al.*, 1976; Baker *et al.*, 1977; Gerber *et al.*, 1977; Davies *et al.*, 1977; McNeil *et al.*, 1978; O'Connell *et al.*, 1978; Hammond *et al.*, 1978; Clark *et al.*, 1978; Lindholm *et al.*, 1979; Komaki *et al.*, 1979; Burkett *et al.*, 1979; Wilson *et al.*, 1980; Kunkler *et al.*, 1985). Nevertheless, there remains considerable disagreement over the role of bone scanning, particularly in patients with clinically early breast cancer, and no symptoms of bone metastases. A wide variety of results has been published, with a reported positive incidence ranging between 0% and 18% in clinical stage I, with a mean value of 4.4%. In stage II the range is 0–32%, with a mean

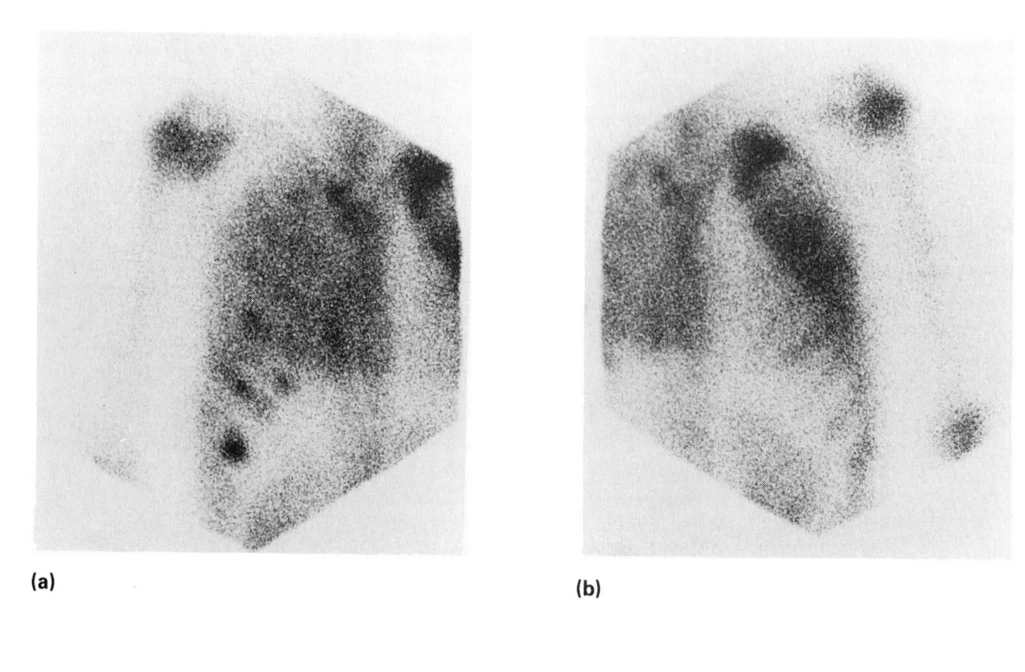

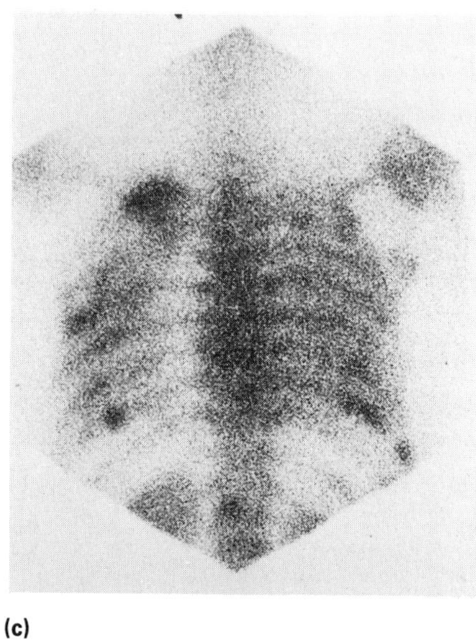

Figure 6.9 Bone scan views: (a) right anterior chest; (b) left anterior chest; (c) posterior thoracic spine. A 33-year-old woman with carcinoma of the breast and hypercalcaemia. Bone scan shows multiple metastases throughout the skeleton. In addition, there is extensive soft tissue uptake throughout both lung fields. Scan findings were due to microcalcification in lungs, reflecting hypercalcaemia.

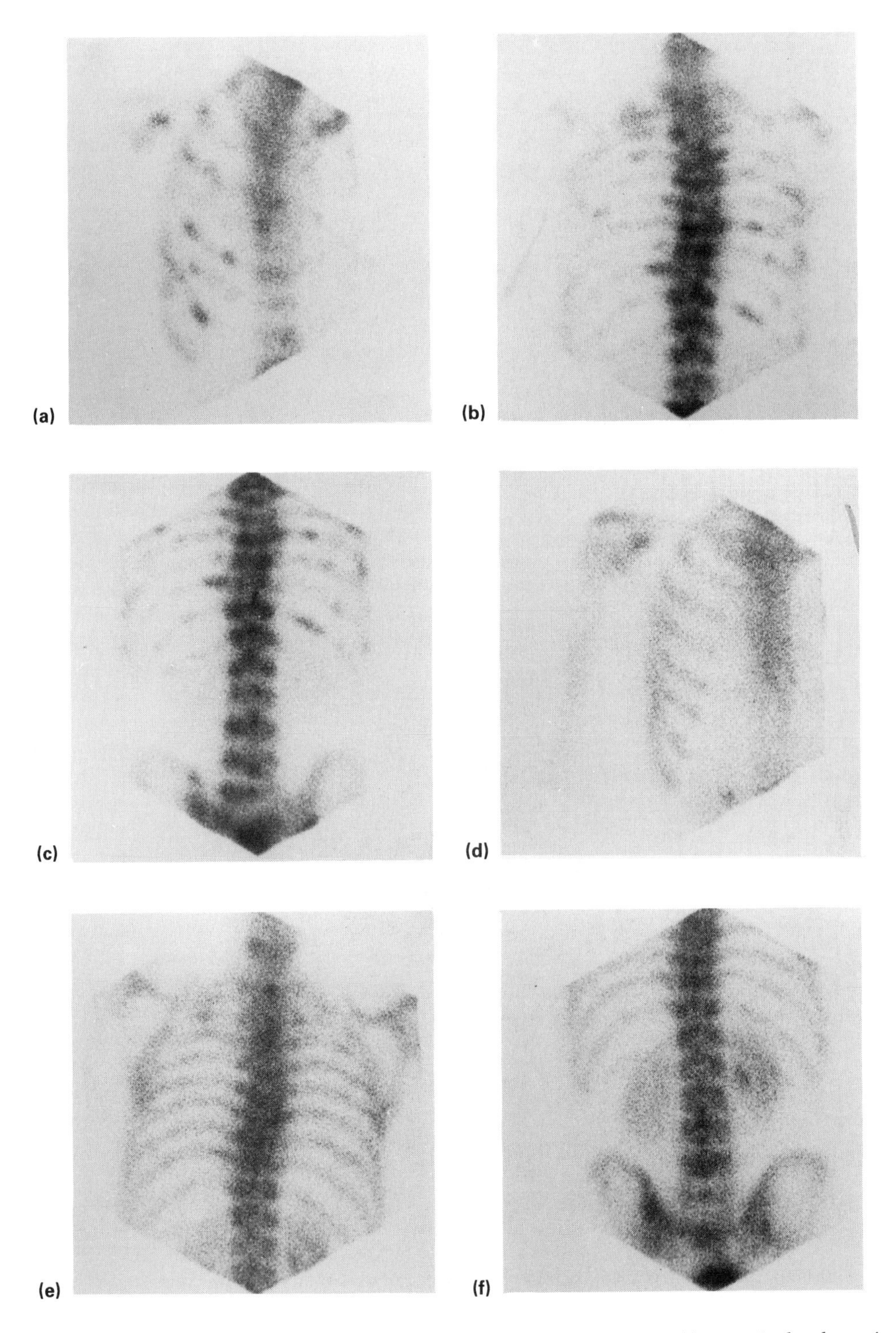

Figure 6.10 Bone scan views: (a) right anterior chest; (b) posterior thoracic spine; (c) posterior lumbar spine; (d–f) six months post-therapy. This male with carcinoma of the prostate had widespread metastatic involvement of the skeleton. Six months following therapy there has been almost complete resolution of widespread bony metastases. Note also that renal images are now clearly visualized.

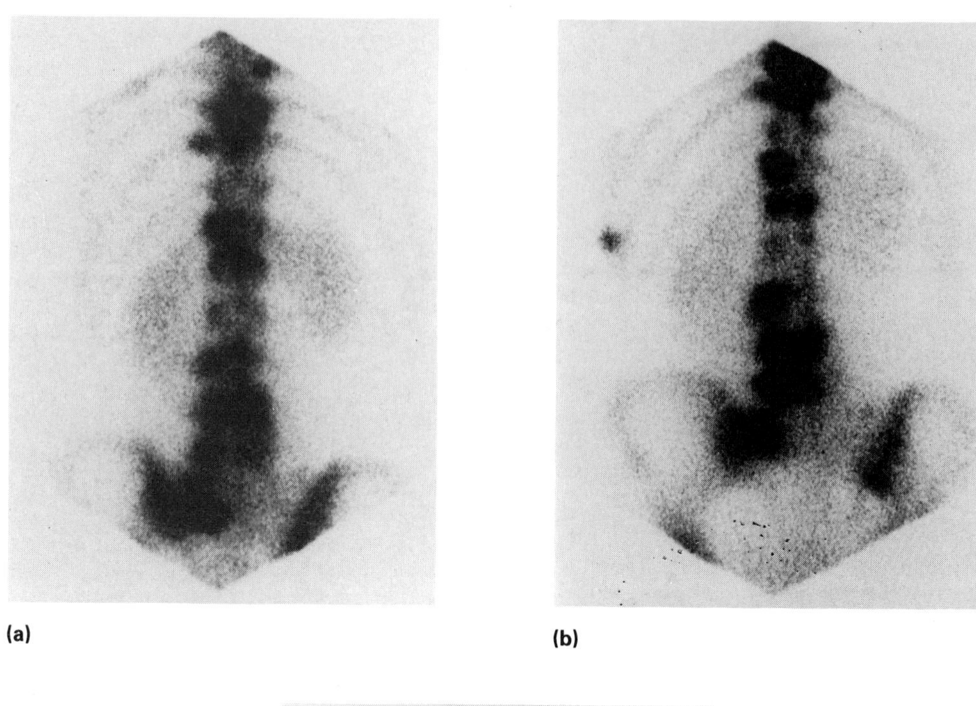

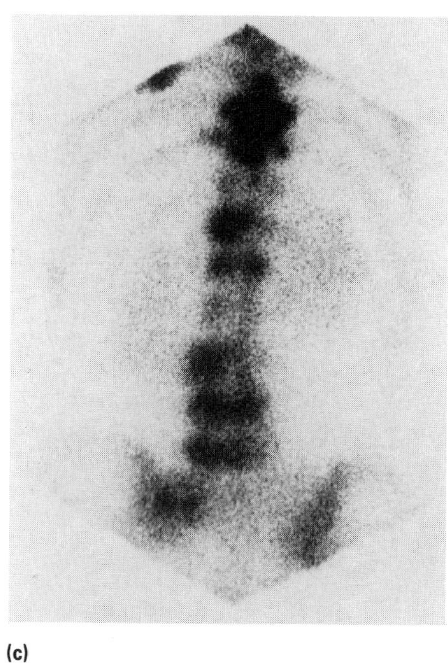

Figure 6.11 (a) Bone scan views of posterior lumbar spine from a woman with metastases from carcinoma o breast. (b) Scan three months later, after treatment with chemotherapy shows increased tracer uptake in previousl noted lesions and a new lesion in a rib. (c) Six months after start of treatment uptake in lesions is less. This series o scans demonstrate the flare phenomenon.

value of 7.2%. Why findings should be so discrepant is not known and, while there may be some differences in clinical staging, it is likely that much of the variation will be accounted for by differences in bone scan reporting. It is, nevertheless, apparent that the pick-up rate of a positive bone scan in patients with early breast cancer is low, probably of the order of 3% for clinical stage II disease (Coleman *et al.*, 1988). The question arises as to whether such screening is cost effective. Many surgeons nowadays perform radical mastectomy less often, and a positive bone scan may therefore no longer influence the primary operation. Further, it has not been shown that modern chemotherapeutic regimes have significantly altered patient mortality, and thus the clinical implications of a positive bone scan with regard to patient benefit are not certain. What is apparent is that the bone scan does provide the most sensitive means of evaluating the skeleton in carcinoma of the breast. It also provides a baseline for subsequent studies. Clearly, if patients have metastases, then they cannot be considered to have early disease and are stage IV. It would thus appear that, for many centres, routine bone scanning in early breast cancer is not appropriate but, for those with an academic interest in carcinoma of the breast and who wish full documentation of disease, then bone scanning remains essential. This situation would be completely transformed if an effective therapy became available for patients with evidence of early metastatic disease.

The frequency of abnormal bone scans at presentation in patients with more advanced breast cancer is accepted as being high (Gerber *et al.*, 1977; Clark *et al.*, 1978; Lindholm *et al.*, 1979; Komaki *et al.*, 1979), with a mean figure of the order of 28%. There is no doubt that an abnormal bone scan is a serious prognostic factor, with mean survival of between two and three years (McKillop *et al.*, 1978).

The role of bone scanning in serial studies of patients with carcinoma of the breast also presents conflicting data (McKillop, 1987). However, this again is now less often performed in many centres and at the present time I believe that routine serial bone scanning should be performed only in those units with an academic interest in monitoring the occurrence of skeletal metastases, or the effect of therapy (Fogelman and Coleman, 1988).

6.11.2 PROSTATIC CANCER

Patients with skeletal metastases from prostatic cancer may have prolonged remission with endocrine therapy and, even when this does not occur, such treatment may be of value in controlling symptoms or slowing progression of disease. The use of bone scanning in this situation has been less extensively studied, but it is apparent that there is a relatively high incidence of metastases at presentation at around 38% (Shafer and Reinke, 1977; O'Donoghue *et al.*, 1978; McGregor *et al.*, 1978; Paulson and the Uro-Oncology Research Group, 1979; Biersack *et al.*, 1980; Lund *et al.*, 1984). As expected, the frequency of metastases rises with more advanced clinical staging (Biersack *et al.*, 1980; O'Donoghue *et al.*, 1978).

It has been suggested that an abnormal bone scan at presentation has a mortality rate of around 45% at two years, compared with 20% for those with a normal scan (Lund *et al.*, 1984). In view of the relatively high pick-up rate at presentation, a strong case could be made for all patients with carcinoma of the prostate having a bone scan at this time. There is very little information available with regard to serial studies although some data do suggest that annual scans may be of value in detecting occult metastases, which will require endocrine therapy (Lund *et al.*, 1984).

6.11.3 LUNG CANCER

Patients with carcinoma of the lung have generally a poor prognosis, with multi-organ involvement at the time of presentation. While bone metastases are common, their identification will generally not provide information of clinical value unless palliation with radiotherapy is being considered. However, a certain percentage of patients will be considered for surgery, with a view to cure, but surgery is clearly inappropriate for those with disseminated disease, particularly as there is a relatively high operative mortality. Thus, bone scanning has an important role to play in the initial work-up of any patient who is considered to have a resectable tumour. The significance of a positive bone scan in carcinoma of the lung is dire, with an 87% mortality within six months (Gravenstein *et al.*, 1979). It is absolutely critical, however, that when a scan abnormality is identified its precise cause be confirmed by other methods to ensure that false-positive results do not exclude patients from potentially curative resection.

The bone scan will also show typical abnormalities in those with hypertrophic pulmonary osteoarthropathy (HPO) (Lopez-Majano and Sobti, 1984), with increased tracer uptake in the lateral aspect of long bones, i.e. pericortical activity, the so-called tramline sign. Scan evidence of HPO may resolve following successful therapy of the primary tumour (Freeman and Tonkin, 1976).

The other tumour that is worth commenting upon is multiple myeloma, as this is the classical situation where a false-negative bone scan may occur (Wahner *et al.*, 1980; Waxman *et al.*,1981). Such an occurrence is in fact uncommon, but arises when lesions are purely lytic, with no osteoblastic response. Nevertheless, it is certainly correct that the bone scan may underestimate the extent of skeletal disease but, as in other situations, may identify lesions which are not apparent on X-ray (Wollfenden *et al.*, 1980; Freeman *et al.*, 1984). Thus, radiology and bone scanning can be considered as complementary investigations, when accurate documentation of all skeletal disease is required.

6.12 PRIMARY BONE TUMOURS

The most common use of bone scanning in primary bone tumours is for the evaluation of the malignant tumours, osteogenic sarcoma and Ewing's sarcoma, or to diagnose the benign tumour osteoid osteoma. Osteogenic sarcoma is probably the more frequently encountered malignant tumour, and may arise at any site in the skeleton, but with 90% found in the long bones (Lichtenstein, 1977). While the bone scan is strikingly positive (Goldmann *et al.*, 1975; Papanicolaou *et al.*, 1982), initial evaluation requires X-ray and computed tomography (CT) to define the precise margins of the tumour. Further, the role of bone scanning becomes less important as skeletal metastases at the time of presentation are rare, with the lungs being the common primary site of spread. In Ewing's sarcoma the bone scan is also strikingly positive, but in this situation the incidence of bone metastases at presentation is much higher and there is therefore a clear case for bone scanning as part of the initial work-up of all patients (Goldstein *et al.*, 1980; Nair, 1985).

Osteoid osteoma is a relatively uncommon tumour, which accounts for approximately 10% of benign bone neoplasia. The lesion is found most often in adolescents and young adults, and it is generally not seen after the age of 30 (Lichtenstein, 1977). While the tibia (Figure 6.12) or femur accounts for 50% of cases, any bone can be involved. Patients usually present with pain, which characteristically is severe, worse at night, and relief is obtained with aspirin. Typical radiographic findings are of a small, round focus that is radiolucent, the central nidus surrounded by reactive sclerosis. However, X-ray may on occasion by negative (Swee *et al.*, 1979), and bone pain in an otherwise healthy young individual may lead to suspicion of a psychiatric disorder. The bone scan appearances are usually characteristic, and there is higher sensitivity for lesion detection than with X-ray (Smith and Gilday, 1980; Omjola *et al.*, 1981). Typically, a small intense focus of increased tracer uptake is seen. A normal bone scan virtually excludes the diagnosis of osteoid osteoma.

6.13 THE BONE SCAN IN METABOLIC BONE DISEASE

In contrast to metastatic disease and most other clinical situations where a bone scan is recognized as abnormal by the presence of focal lesions, in metabolic bone disease the whole skeleton is typically involved by the metabolic process, and there may be diffusely increased tracer uptake with no focal lesions identified. The problem which arises is that assessment of increased uptake of tracer is subjective and, when mild disease is present, may

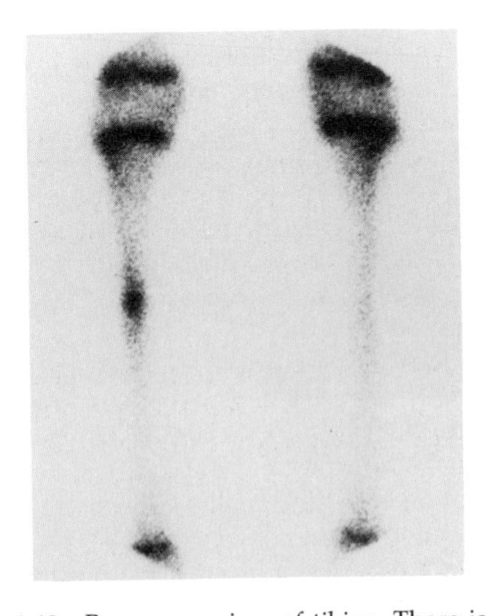

Figure 6.12 Bone scan view of tibiae. There is an intense focus of increased tracer uptake in the mid right tibia. Scan findings are typically those of osteoid osteoma, which was confirmed on X-ray and by surgery.

Table 6.1 Metabolic features

1. Increased tracer uptake in axial skeleton
2. Increased tracer uptake in long bones
3. Increased tracer uptake in periarticular areas
4. Faint or absent kidney images
5. Prominent calvaria and mandible
6. Beading of the costochondral junctions
7. 'Tie sternum'

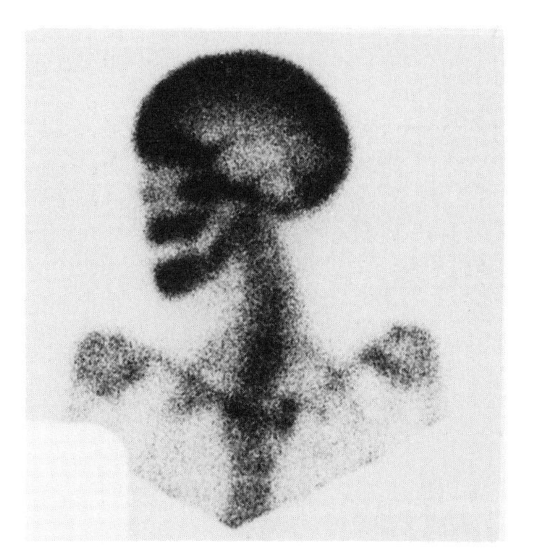

Figure 6.13 Bone scan view of left lateral skull. There is a striking increase in tracer uptake throughout the skull and mandible. Appearances are typically those of secondary hyperparathyroidism.

not be recognizable at all. However, in more severe cases, characteristic metabolic features may be seen (Fogelman *et al.*, 1979). Table 6.1 lists these features. An abnormal scan is most often found in renal osteodystrophy (Figure 6.13) and osteomalacia (Figure 6.14) (Fogelman, 1987) and in general the severity of disease reflects the degree of hyperparathyroidism that is present. Nevertheless, all the metabolic features are nonspecific, and with the exception of absent kidney images can be seen in normal individuals. Altered skeletal metabolism may be found wherever there is a stimulus to osteoblastic activity, and other examples of this would be thyroid hormone excess or active acromegaly. Focal lesions can be found in osteomalacia when pseudofractures are present (Figure 6.14) (Fogelman *et al.*, 1977). Much less commonly, focal lesions will be seen in hyperparathyroidism with brown tumours (Fogelman and Citrin, 1981).

6.13.1 OSTEOPOROSIS

In osteoporosis there is generally only a very gradual reduction in bone mass, which reflects minor abnormalities in skeletal metabolism occurring over many years. The measurement of bone mass is becoming increasingly important in clinical practice (Fogelman, 1989). The bone scan appearances of osteoporosis are usually normal and metabolic features are not seen (Fogelman and Carr, 1980). However, osteoporotic bones are abnormally brittle, and pathological fractures occur. These appear on the bone scan as focal abnormalities and, when vertebral collapse has occurred, the scan appearances are characteristic, with linearly increased tracer uptake corresponding to the whole of the collapsed vertebral body (Figure 6.15) (Martin, 1979). Generally this increased tracer activity fades over the following 9–24 months, and complementary information is obtained with both bone scan and X-ray, as the bone scan enables one to obtain some estimate of the time interval since vertebral collapse occurred (Fogelman and Carr, 1980a).

6.13.2 PAGET'S DISEASE

Paget's disease of bone is a common disorder which affects primarily the elderly, with a reported incidence of around 4% (Hamdy, 1981). The disease is characterized in its initial phase by excess resorption of bone, which is followed by an intense osteoblastic response and deposition of collagen in a mosaic pattern (woven bone) rather than the lamellar arrangement seen in normal bone (Alexandre *et al.*, 1981). There is thus an imbalance of bone remodelling in favour of formation, and overall the size of affected bones tends to increase. Paget's disease is usually polyostotic, but may be monostotic in approximately 20% of cases (Vellenga *et al.*, 1984). The bone scan appearances are usually striking, with lesions showing high avidity for bone-seeking radiopharmaceuticals (Figures 6.5 and 6.16). The amount of tracer uptake appears to be directly related to the degree of activity of the disease process (Shirazi *et al.*, 1974). The typical appearance is of markedly increased uptake of tracer, which is usually distributed evenly throughout most, or all, of the affected bone. A common exception to this general rule is osteoporosis circumscripta (lytic disease involving the skull) where tracer uptake is most intense at the margins of the lesion (Rausch *et al.*, 1977). Unlike most other skeletal disorders,

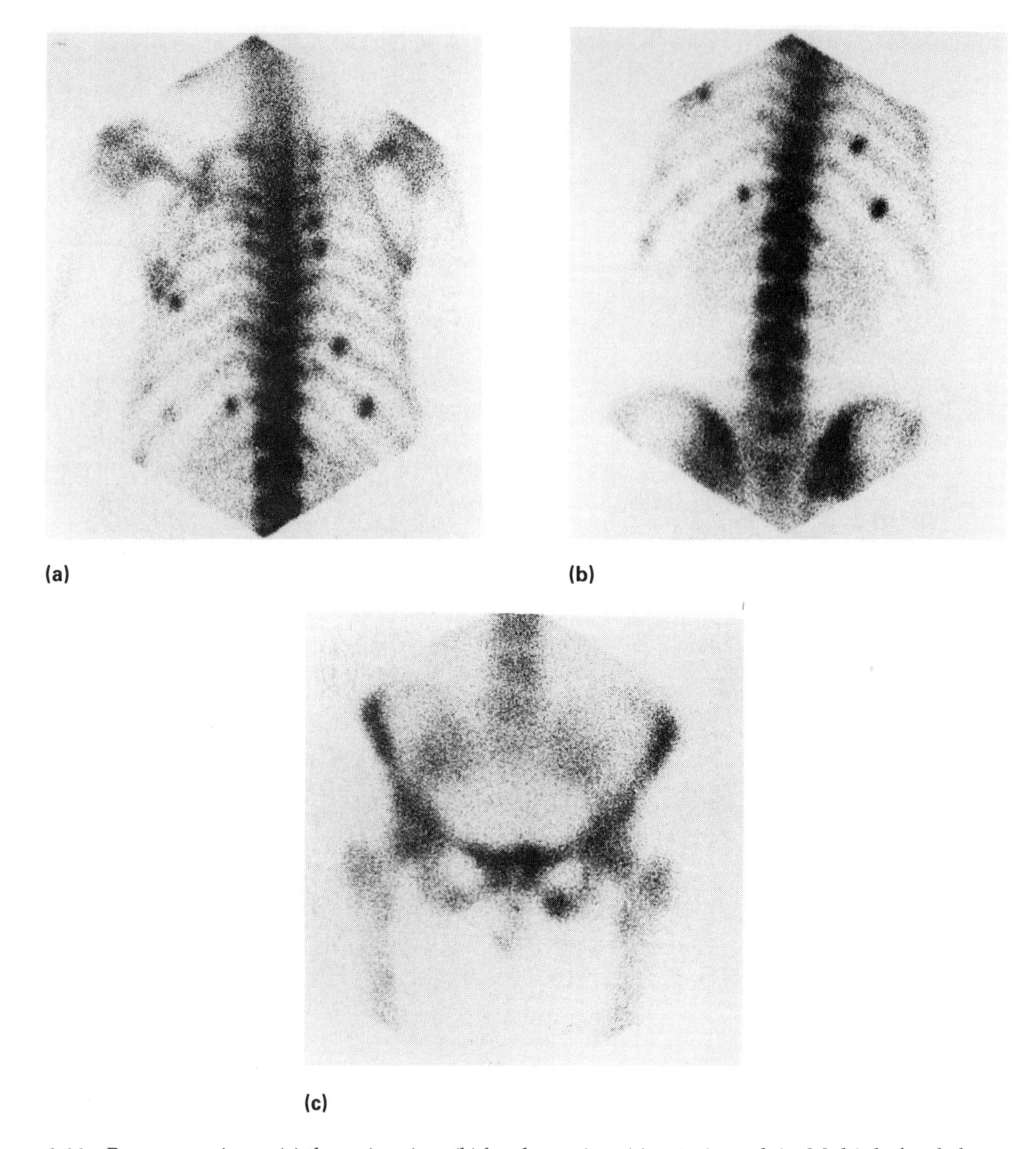

Figure 6.14 Bone scan views: (a) thoracic spine; (b) lumbar spine; (c) anterior pelvis. Multiple focal abnormalities are present throughout the ribs, and further lesions are present in both inferior pubic rami and the medial aspect of the upper third of right femur. Note also high uptake of tracer throughout axial skeleton and that renal images are only faintly visualized. This 44-year-old Asian woman had severe osteomalacia with multiple pseudofractures.

Paget's disease tends to preserve, and even enhance, the normal anatomical configuration of bone. Expansion, and on occasion distortion, of involved bones may be seen. Individual lesions appear to be 'picked out' on the bone scan, as the borders between normal and abnormal bone are well delineated. When the apendicular skeleton is involved, lesions generally commence at the articular end of the bone, and progress into the shaft. The distal aspect of the lesion may be seen to have a sharp edge, which corresponds to the flame-shaped resorption front seen on X-ray. Paget's disease confined to the diaphyseal area can occur, but is extremely uncommon (Frank, 1981; Schubert *et al.*, 1984).

Several studies have compared bone scanning and radiology in lesion detection, and it has now been convincingly shown that bone scanning is

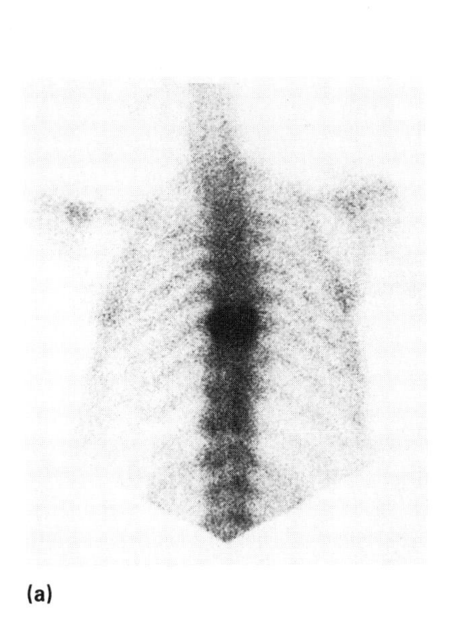

(a)

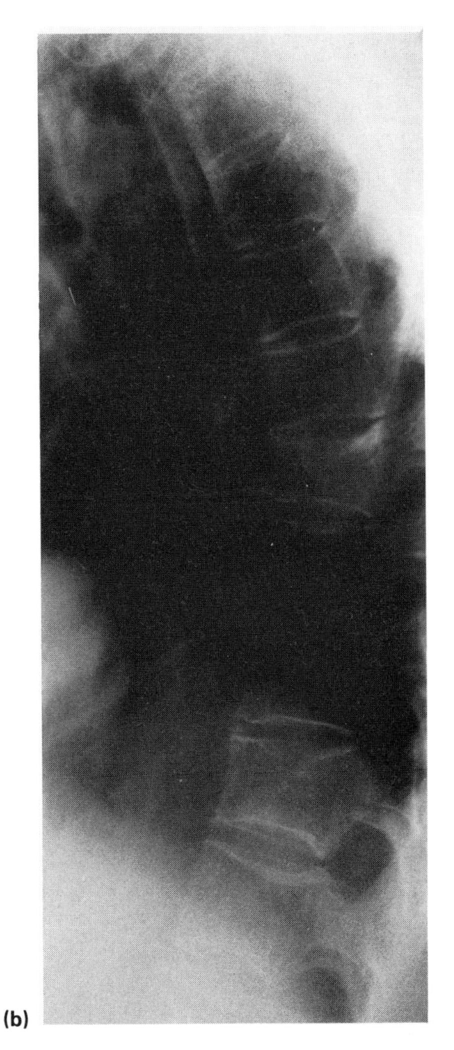

(b)

Figure 6.15 Vertebral collapse: (a) bone scan view of posterior thoracic spine; (b) lateral thoracic X-ray. On the bone scan there is a focal area of intensely increased tracer uptake involving the eighth thoracic vertebra. Scan findings were due to benign vertebral collapse.

the more sensitive for detecting sites of Paget's disease (Khairi *et al.*, 1974; Shirazi *et al.*, 1974; Serafini, 1976; Vellenga *et al.*, 1976). In addition, clear visualization of the whole skeleton is obtained, and those sites considered difficult with routine radiology, such as the ribs, scapula and sternum, are easily identifiable on the bone scan when disease involvement is present (Fogelman and Carr, 1980b).

6.14 INFECTION

As acute infections of bone are associated with increased metabolic bone activity, the bone scan is often the first, and certainly an important, early study in the evaluation of the skeleton in such cases. It is now generally accepted that the bone scan will be abnormal in patients with osteomyelitis, several days to weeks before conventional radiology shows changes (Handmaker and Leonards, 1976). The characteristic scan pattern of acute osteomyelitis is a focal area of intensely increased tracer uptake in bone (Figure 6.17). It is advisable to perform a three-phase study of the suspected area, as most acute bone infections have markedly increased blood flow. The entire skeleton should, however, be studied since the problem can be multifocal, and discovery of other

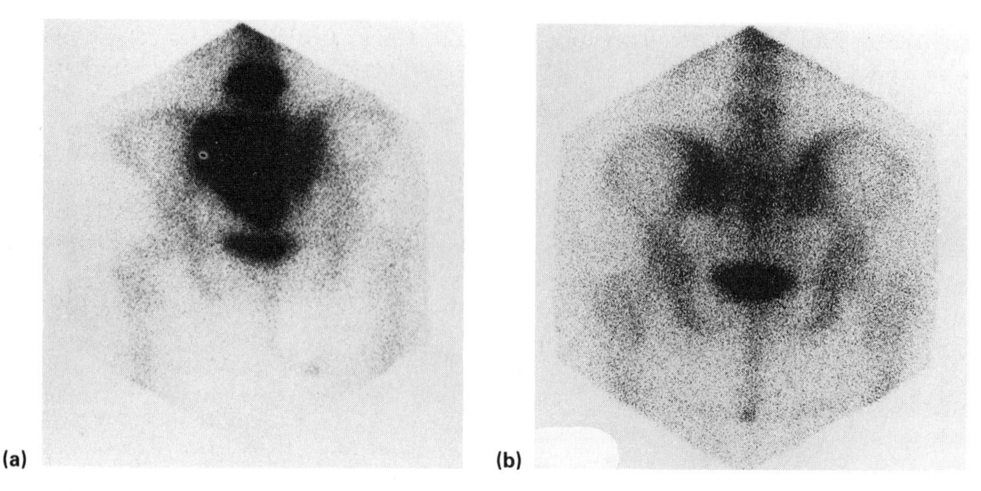

Figure 6.16 Bone scan view: (a) posterior pelvis; (b) after treatment. On original study there is increased tracer uptake in L4 and left sacrum due to Paget's disease. This patient received six months' therapy with oral diphosphonate, and there is marked resolution of disease.

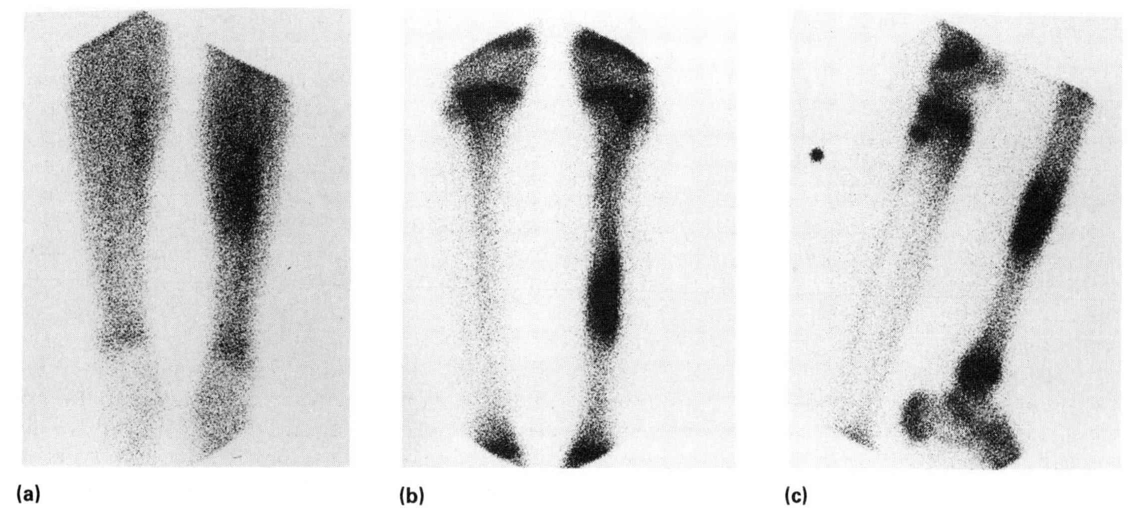

Figure 6.17 Bone scan views: (a) equilibrium, anterior tibiae; (b) delayed image, anterior tibiae; (c) lateral view. A 15-year-old Asian boy with pain in his left leg. Bone scan study shows an extensive, intensely active lesion in the mid-shaft of the left tibia. This is associated with increased blood flow. Scan findings were due to osteomyelitis.

lesions may eventually lead to a change in the final diagnosis. In children, the site of infection is often adjacent to an epiphysis, which normally appears 'hot' on the study. Lesions may thus be hidden if a whole body scan is obtained. Spot views and, on occasion, pinhole views will be required to clarify the problem. As pinhole views take a long time to acquire, it may be necessary to restrain the area of interest and sedation will be required in some cases. In the differential diagnosis of acute osteomyelitis, cellulitis may be a problem but, as discussed earlier, a three-phase bone scan should clarify this. The bone scan is generally abnormal in the great majority of cases after 48 h, and it should be noted that abnormality can persist for many months after clinical recovery. If clinically, relevant, further studies with ^{67}Ga (Burleson *et al.*, 1975) or ^{111}In-labelled white cells (McDougall *et al.*, 1979; Peters, 1990) may be necessary to assess activity. On occasion, if patients have had prior treatment with antibiotics or corticosteroids a false-negative image may be obtained.

6.15 ARTHRITIS

On the normal bone scan, there is some increase of tracer uptake seen immediately adjacent to joints, and in general this appears symmetrical. For a joint to appear positive on scanning, there thus requires to be increased tracer uptake relative to an uninvolved joint, or markedly higher uptake when compared with adjacent, non-articular bone.

6.15.1 RHEUMATOID ARTHRITIS

Inflammatory synovitis is associated with increased blood flow to the synovium and periarticular bones, and as hyperaemia is recognized as a cause of increased tracer uptake it is likely that this is an important contributory factor to a positive bone scan. However, the intensity of uptake of a bone-seeking radiopharmaceutical has been shown to be higher than that obtained with a blood pool imaging agent, suggesting that tracer uptake is not simply related to acute inflammation, and that there is increased uptake by periarticular bone, perhaps due to local remodelling following bone resorption (Beckerman *et al.*, 1975; Rosenthall and Hawkins, 1977). Whatever the precise mechanism, there is no doubt that in rheumatoid arthritis intense foci of increased tracer uptake are seen at sites of activity, but the appearances are non-specific and may be found in a wide variety of conditions, including psoriatic and gouty arthritis, ankylosing spondylitis, seronegative polyarthritis, hypertrophic osteoarthropathy, reflex sympathetic dystrophy syndrome and regional migratory osteoporosis (Rosenthall and Lisbona, 1980). However, the presence of symmetrical disease with peripheral joint activity greater than axial activity, uniform involvement of the wrists and proximal joints of the limbs and feet, and typical skeletal deformities would favour a diagnosis of rheumatoid arthritis (Weissberg *et al.*, 1978).

In rheumatoid arthritis, the bone scan has been found to antedate clinical and radiographic manifestation of inflammatory synovitis (Rosenthall and Lisbona, 1980; Weissberg *et al.*, 1978; Hoffer and Genant, 1976). Nevertheless, once this diagnosis has been established the bone scan will not provide any additional information, and therefore its role in the routine management of patients with rheumatoid arthritis is limited. While it has been suggested that the bone scan may provide an accurate means of monitoring a patient's response to therapy (Rosenthall and Lisbona, 1980), its advantage in clinical practice over simpler techniques remains to be established.

In children, the bone scan has proven to be disappointing in the detection of rheumatoid arthritis. This is thought to be due to the fact that tracer uptake in the growth plate obscures any increased uptake in periarticular bone (Rosenthall and Hawkins, 1977).

6.15.2 ANKYLOSING SPONDYLITIS

Acute sacroiliitis will produce a positive bone scan image, and it is now well established that bone scanning may identify radiologically negative sacroiliitis (Rosenthall and Lisbona, 1980; Lentle *et al.*, 1977b; Namey *et al.*, 1977). The difficulty which arises when assessing the sacroiliac joints on the bone scan is that they are usually hotter than the surrounding pelvis and sacrum in normal subjects, and even more so in young subjects in whom sacroiliitis is most frequently seen. Also, while sacroiliitis may be unilateral, it is commonly bilateral and abnormality may not be apparent on subjective evaluation of the scan. To overcome such difficulties, quantitative techniques have been developed whereby a ratio relating the uptake of tracer by each sacroiliac joint to that of the body of the sacrum or surrounding bone is obtained (Russell *et al.*, 1975; Davis *et al.*, 1984). This ratio is abnormally high early in the disease process, when X-ray findings are often minimal or absent, but tends to approach normality as end-stage fusion of the joints develops. In patients with ankylosing spondylitis, it may be possible to identify a diffuse increase in spinal uptake of tracer, most often present in the lower dorsal spine, and in addition more focal abnormalities can be seen in the apophyseal joints. As there is a tendency to bony ankylosis, the scan image will often fail to clearly illustrate the normal segmental anatomy of the spine. Ankylosing spondylitis may be associated with a peripheral arthropathy, which can be identified on the bone scan (Lentle *et al.*, 1977a).

6.15.3 OSTEOARTHRITIS

In osteoarthritis, the increased mechanical stresses occurring at altered joint surfaces lead to an osteoblastic reaction and reactive new bone formation, which is readily demonstrated by bone scanning. Typically, the scan appearances show increased tracer uptake at sites of involvement, which correspond to the weight-bearing joints and distal joints of the hands and feet. It is now apparent that osteoarthritis may have an inflammatory component, and in early disease increased vascularity can be seen.

Patchy tracer uptake with more focal lesions in the lower lumbar spine is a common scan finding in the presence of degenerative disease. As degerative disease of the spine is frequently present, such appearances may occasionally lead to confusion when metastatic disease is suspected. For this reason, it is always essential to X-ray any such area of abnormality to confirm the presence of degenerative change. In the assessment of osteoarthritis of the knee, the bone scan has been shown to be more sensitive than physical examination, radiography and double-contrast arthrography, and it was found that the scan provided important supplementary information in those patients in whom surgery was contemplated (Thomas *et al.*, 1975).

6.16 AVASCULAR NECROSIS AND BONE INFARCTION

The bone scan may be of value in the diagnosis of avascular necrosis and bone infarction in disorders such as Perthes' disease, sickle cell anaemia (Figure 6.18) and caisson disease (Rosenthall, 1987). The initial pathological process in each is bone ischaemia, and bone images obtained at an early stage will show a zone of decreased tracer uptake. As the pathological process continues, a peripheral zone of increased uptake develops, and slowly replaces the photon-deficient area. In practice, a hot lesion is almost always seen, and this represents the reaction of the surrounding normal bone to the presence of non-viable bone. As will be discussed later, SPECT imaging will on occasion reveal a central photon-deficient area, e.g. in the hip, even when planar imaging suggests diffusely increased tracer uptake.

The femoral head is susceptible to necrosis following fracture of the femoral neck, with displaced fractures having a higher incidence than undisplaced ones. Three-phase bone scanning may be of value in predicting avascular necrosis after femoral head fracture.

6.17 TRAUMA

Fractures remain the most common bone lesion, and a diagnosis is usually apparent from the clinical evidence and X-ray findings. However, it is becoming increasingly recognized that many small or incomplete fractures may not be seen on X-ray, and the bone scan can be of value in locating sites of suspected or unsuspected trauma. Bone scans may remain abnormal for some time after a fracture (Martin, 1979) but persistently positive scans beyond 18–24 months are usually associated with secondary degenerative disease or healing in poor alignment.

As the public becomes more aware of physical health, a rising incidence of sports-related bone and soft tissue injuries is seen. In some situations, such as shin splints, the diagnosis will not be apparent on routine X-ray but can be detected easily by nuclear medicine techniques (Martin, 1988).

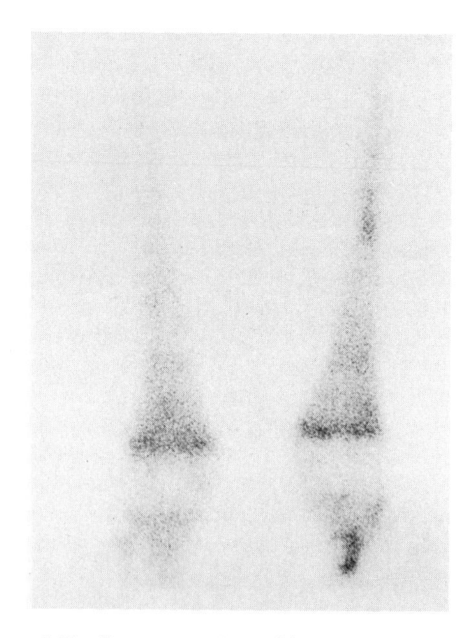

Figure 6.18 Bone scan view of femora. There is somewhat increased tracer uptake generally in mid and lower femora. More focal areas of uptake are seen in left mid-femur and left upper tibia. These appearances represent marrow hyperplasia and bone infarcts related to sickle cell disease.

6.17.1 STRESS FRACTURES

Stress fractures usually arise from repeated stresses to a bone, with a resultant injury where the skeletal reparative processes are unable to cope with the damage. Such injuries are often seen in athletes with excessively heavy training regimes, or else in untrained individuals who participate in new types of exercise. X-rays may be of limited value in detecting acute stress fractures, while the early diagnosis can be of practical relevance, as a stress fracture of the tibia will require immobilization for approximately six weeks. If the individual continues to exercise, then there is a significant risk of complete fracture.

6.17.2 SHIN SPLINTS

Shin splints are an important differential diagnosis of pain in a lower limb in a physically active individual. Typically the pain is in the posterior medial aspect of the tibia, and is due to a periosteal reaction at the site of insertion of the tibialis posterior and soleus muscle groups. On the bone scan, increased tracer uptake is seen in the posterior aspect of the lower third of the tibia, running along the cortical border (Figure 6.19) (Brill, 1983; Holder and Matthews, 1984). It should be noted that this appearance will not be detected if anterior or posterior views alone are obtained, and indeed any abnormality may be considered focal and thought to represent stress fracture. It is important to obtain lateral views, and the diagnosis will then be apparent.

6.17.3 OCCULT FRACTURE

On occasion, X-ray may not reveal a suspected fracture, although confirmation is usually found on a later, repeat examination. In such cases a bone scan may be of value in either confirming or excluding significant injury. The bone scan may also be useful in cases of suspected non-accidental injury of childhood where multiple lesions may be identified throughout the skeleton (Haase *et al.*, 1980). A skull X-ray should always be obtained in infants as a skull fracture may on occasion be missed on the scan. As a general rule, if a bone scan is normal at 24 h following injury, then this excludes significant bony injury. Even in the older patient the bone scan is almost always usually abnormal at the fracture site within 72 h (Martin, 1979).

6.18 SINGLE-PHOTON EMISSION COMPUTED TOMOGRAPHIC (SPECT) BONE SCANNING

To date there is only limited experience with SPECT imaging of the skeleton, and this has been largely in the orthopaedic field. Nevertheless, when compared with planar bone scanning, SPECT has the technical advantage that unwanted activity from superimposed structures

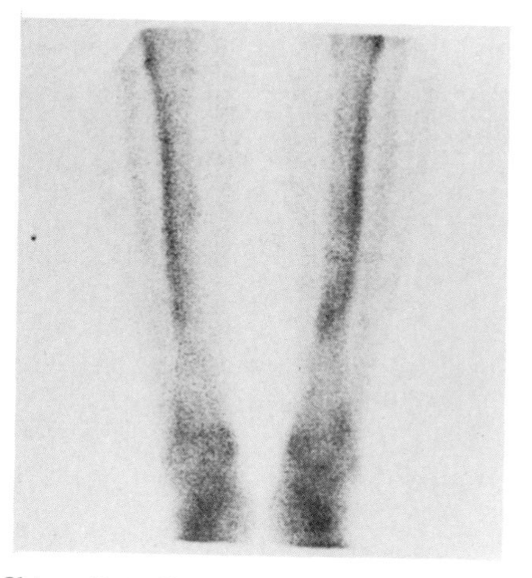

(a)

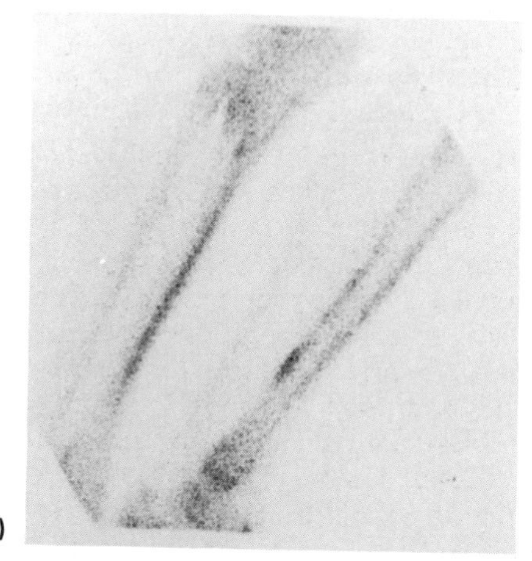

(b)

Figure 6.19 Shin splints. Bone scan views of lower limbs: (a) anterior; (b) left lateral. There is generally increased tracer uptake throughout both tibiae. In addition, there is increased tracer uptake seen in the lower third of the left tibia posteriorly. The appearances in both tibiae presumably reflect cortical hypertrophy. Appearances of posterior left tibia are typically those of shin splints. Appearances are not those of fracture.

can be removed. There is therefore heightened contrast between lesion and background (Figure 6.20). A further advantage of SPECT is improved anatomical positioning of a lesion. There are disadvantages, which include increased radiation exposure as doses of 20–30 mCi are often used, extended imaging time, and the possibility of introducing artefacts, e.g. from a full bladder when examining the hips and pelvis.

The most dramatic documented benefit of SPECT imaging is in avascular necrosis. In the hips, scan findings on planar imaging are invariably of increased tracer uptake due to the reaction of surrounding bone. However, with SPECT, on occasion it may be possible to clearly identify a central photon-deficient lesion (Collier *et al.*, 1985). Increasingly, SPECT is being used to evaluate the patient with low back pain. The detection lesions is more sensitive together with the accurate anatomical localization.

6.19 QUANTITATIVE TECHNETIUM DIPHOSPHONATE UPTAKE MEASUREMENTS

As previously discussed, diphosphonate uptake in the skeleton reflects metabolic activity. In situations of diffusely altered skeletal metabolism, slight increases of diphosphonate uptake will not be apparent when subjectively evaluating bone scan images. Nevertheless, diphosphonate uptake is a sensitive measure of altered skeletal metabolism, and if accurately quantified would potentially be of considerable clinical value. To date, such techniques have been most extensively applied in the field of metabolic bone disease. Although of limited value in the diagnosis of focal bone disease, some work has been carried out to assess therapeutic response (Vellenga *et al.*, 1984a; Espinasse *et al.*, 1981; Stevenson *et al.*, 1984).

6.19.1 LOCAL MEASUREMENT

To quantify uptake of diphosphonate in an area of focal disease, the count rate in the area is often obtained and compared to that in an adjacent site of normal bone or soft tissue. Thus, an uptake ratio is obtained rather than an absolute count rate. Uptake ratios are obtained from computerized bone scan images, most often by drawing a region of interest around the areas being studied, or by obtaining a profile across the region of interest. Profiles have been used, for example, to assess sacrioliac joint activity (Russell *et al.*, 1975; Davis *et al.*, 1984). The region of interest technique is often used to obtain ratios of activity between lesions and surrounding bone. This has been extensively used to diagnose, and more commonly monitor, focal skeletal abnormality.

6.19.2 WHOLE BODY MEASUREMENTS

The most commonly employed technique is to measure 24 h whole body retention (WBR) of technetium-labelled diphosphonate (Fogelman *et al.*, 1978). This undoubtedly provides the most sensitive method for assessing total skeletal metabolism, as the whole skeleton, rather than a small area, is used. The basic theory is that, while most of the injected diphosphonate is taken up by the skeleton, the remainder is excreted via the urinary tract and by 24 h after injection most of soft tissue activity has been excreted, and the great majority of diphosphonate remaining in the body is in the skeleton. Small amounts of ^{99m}Tc diphosphonate can be injected and, by using a whole body counter, the activity following injection and at 24 h is obtained. It should be noted that whole body retention is only valid as an index of skeletal metabolism if renal function is normal, and has therefore no role to play in the assessment of patients with renal osteodystrophy (Fogelman and Bessent, 1982). While an elevated WBR is diagnostic of altered skeletal metabolism, it is non-specific and can be found in osteomalacia, Paget's disease and the majority of patients with primary hyperparathyroidism.

An indirect method of quantification is provided by measuring the bone 'clearance' of diphosphonate by the ^{51}Cr-labelled ethylene diamine tetraacetic acid (EDTA)/technetium MDP ratio. This relies on the assumption that ^{51}Cr-labelled EDTA is cleared only by the kidneys, whereas ^{99m}Tc-labelled MDP is removed from the plasma both by renal excretion and bone uptake. Thus, by injecting the combination of radiopharmaceuticals and measuring the ratio of the two in a single plasma sample (e.g. at 4 h), an indirect measure of bone uptake can be obtained (Nisbet *et al.*, 1983, 1984).

6.20 SOFT TISSUE UPTAKE OF BONE-SEEKING AGENTS

^{99m}Tc-labelled diphosphonate which is not taken up by the skeleton is excreted via the urinary tract

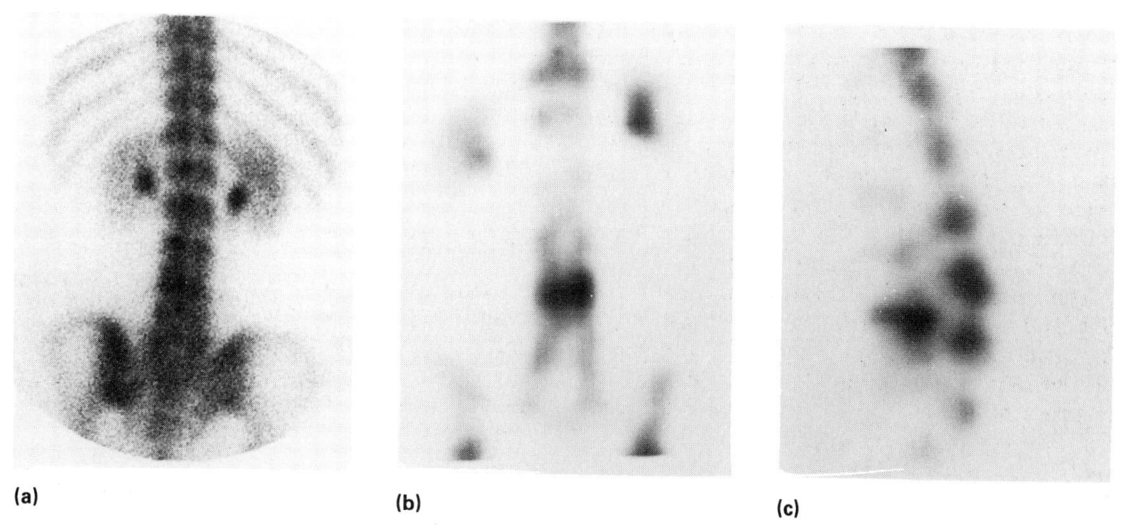

Figure 6.20 (a) Bone scan view of posterior lumbar spine. SPECT views: (b) coronal; (c) sagittal. This patient was complaining of low back pain. Planar views of the lumbar spine were unremarkable and interpreted as normal. However, SPECT study is clearly abnormal being due to lumbar articular facet disease. (Provided by Dr B. D. Collier.)

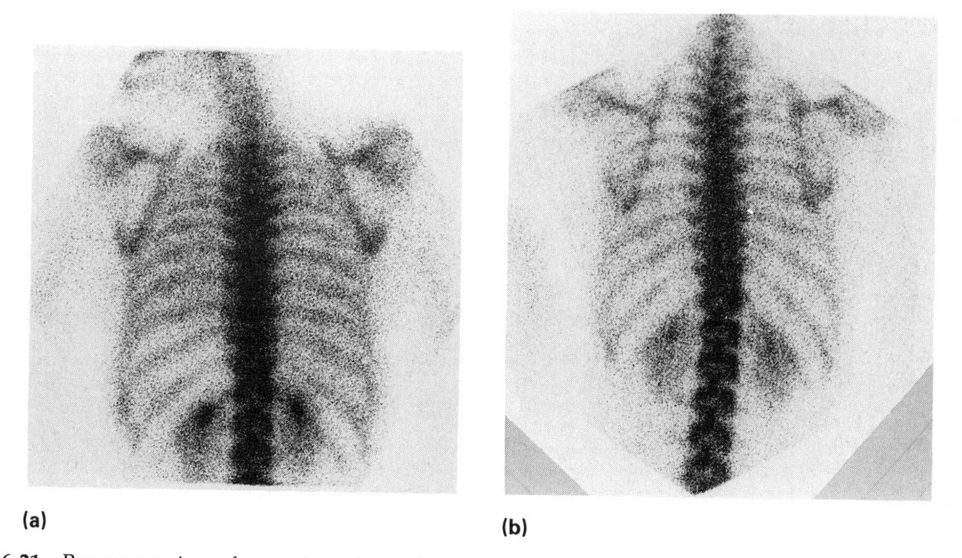

Figure 6.21 Bone scan view of posterior spine: (a) supine; (b) erect. Foci of increased tracer uptake are seen in the region of both twelfth ribs posteriorly. However, with change of position it is apparent that tracer accumulation is associated with slightly dilated renal calyces.

and renal images are normally seen on the bone scan and on occasion renal activity may mimic a bone lesion (Figure 6.21). The kidneys should be evaluated as part of the routine interpretation of any bone scan. It is quite common to detect renal pathology, which is otherwise unsuspected (Figure 6.22).

On occasion, tracer uptake is seen in soft tissue other than the kidneys (Figure 6.23), and the mechanism for this is uncertain, except for sites of

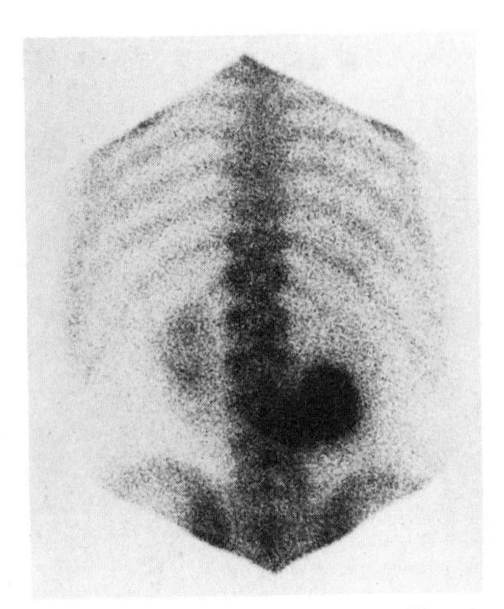

Figure 6.22 Posterior bone scan view of lumbar spine. This patient had horsehoe kidney, with an obstructed right-sided moiety.

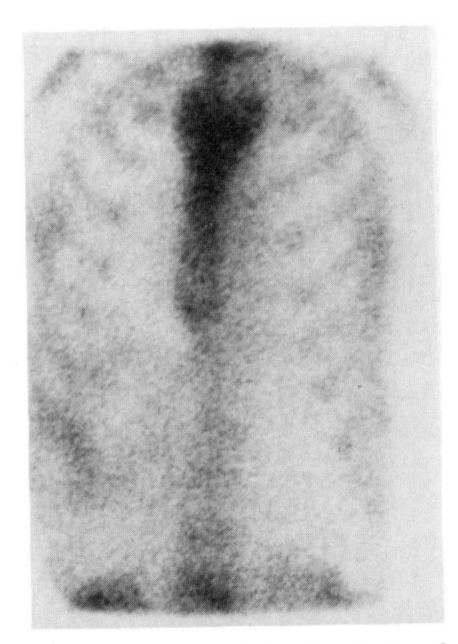

Figure 6.23 Bone scan view of anterior thorax. A patient with metastatic breast carcinoma. There is some abnormal tracer accumulation in the right upper abdomen in association with hepatic metastases.

heterotopic new bone formation, where clearly this is similar to that for the skeleton. In other situations, it is probable that the tracer binds to sites where microcalcification is present.

REFERENCES

Abrams, H. L., Spiro, R. and Goldstein, N. (1950) Mestastases in carcinoma: analysis of 1000 autopsied cases. *Cancer*, **3**, 74–85.

Alexandre, C., Meunier, P. J., Edouard, C. *et al.* (1981) Effects of EHDP (5 mg/kg/day dose) on quantitative bone histology in Paget's disease of bone. *Metab. Bone Dis. Relat. Res.*, **23**, 309–15.

Baker, F. R., Holmes, E. R., Alderson, P. O. *et al.* (1977) An evaluation of bone scans as screening procedures for occult metastases in primary breast cancer. *Ann. Surg.*, **186**, 363–8.

Beckerman, C., Genant, H. K., Hoffer, P. B. *et al.* (1976) Radionuclide imaging of the bones and joints of the hand. *Radiology*, **118**, 653.

Biersack, H. J., Wegner, G., Distelmaier, W. and Krause, U. (1980) Ossare Metastasierung des Prostatakerzinoms in Abhangigkeit von Tumorgrosse und Geschwulstdifferenzienung. *Nuklearmedizin*, **19**, 29–32.

Brill, D. R. (1983) Sports nuclear medicine: bone imaging for lower extremity pain in athletes. *Clin. Nucl. Med.*, **8**, 101–6.

Burkett, M. E. Scanlon, E. C., Garces, R. F. and Khandekar, J. D. (1979) The value of bone scans in the management of patients with carcinoma of the breast. *Surg. Gynecol. Obstet.*, **149**, 523–35.

Burleson, R. L., Holman, B. L. and Tow, D. E. (1975) Scintigraphic demonstration of abscesses with radioactive gallium labelled leukocytes. *Surg. Gynecol. Obstet.*, **141**, 379–82.

Campbell, D. J., Banks, A. J. and Davis, G. D. (1976) The value of preliminary bone scanning in staging and assessing the prognosis of breast cancer. *Br. J. Surg.*, **63**, 811–16.

Castronovo F. P. and Callahan, W. J. (1972) New bone scanning agent: 99m-Tc-labelled 1-hydroxyethylidene-1, 1-disodium phosphate. *J. Nucl. Med.*, **13**, 823–7.

Citrin, D. L. and McKillop, J. H. (1978) *Atlas of Technetium Bone Scans*. Saunders, Philadelphia.

Citrin, D. L., Furnival, C. M., Bessent, R. G. *et al.* (1976) Radioactive technetium phosphate bone scanning in preoperative assessment and follow up study of patients with primary cancer of the breast. *Surg. Gynecol. Obstet.*, **143**, 360–4.

Citrin, D. L., Bessent, R. G. and Greig, W. R. (1977) A comparison of the sensitivity and accuracy of the 99m-Tc-phosphate bone scan and skeletal radiography in the diagnosis of bone metastases. *Clin. Radiol.*, **28**, 107–17.

Clark, D. G., Painter, R. W. and Sziklas, J. J. (1978) Indications for bone scans in preoperative evaluation of breast cancer. *Am. J. Surg.*, **135**, 667–70.

Coleman, R. E., Rubens, R. D. and Fogelman, I. (1988) Reappraisal of the baseline bone scan in breast cancer. *J. Nucl. Med.*, **29** (6), 1045–9.

Collier, B. D., Carrera, G. F., Johnson, R. P. *et al.* (1985) Detection of femoral head avascular necrosis in adults by SPECT. *J. Nucl. Med.*, **26**, 979–87.

Constable, A. R. and Cranage, R. W. (1981) Recognition of the superscan in prostatic bone scintigraphy. *Br. J. Radiol.*, **54**, 122–5.

Corcoran, R. J., Thrall, J. H. and Kyle, R. W. (1976) Solitary abnormalities in bone scans of patients with extraosseous malignancies. *Radiology*, **121**, 663–7.

Davies, C. J., Griffiths, P. A., Preston, B. J. *et al.* (1977) Staging breast cancer: role of scanning. *Br. Med. J.*, **2**, 603–5.

Davis, M. C., Turner, D. A., Charters, J. R. *et al.* (1984) Quantitative sacroiliac scintigraphy: the effect of method of selection of region of interest. *Clin. Nucl. Med.*, **9**, 334–40.

Edelstyn, G. A., Gillespie, P. J. and Grebell, F. S. (1967) The radiological demonstration of osseous metastases: experimental observations. *Clin. Radiol.*, **18**, 158–62.

El Domeiri, A. A. and Shroff, S. (1976) Role of preoperative bone scan in carcinoma of the breast. *Surg. Gynecol. Obstet.*, **142**, 722–4.

Espinasse, D., Mathieu, L., Alexandre, C. *et al.* (1981) The kinetics of Tc99m labelled EHDP in Paget's disease before and after dichloromethylenediphosphonate treatment. *Metab. Bone Dis. Relat. Res.*, **2**, 321–4.

Fogelman, I. (1980) Skeletal uptake of diphosphonate: a review. *Eur. J. Nucl. Med.*, **3**, 224–5.

Fogelman, I. (ed) (1987) in *Bone Scanning in Clinical Practice*. Springer-Verlag, London, pp. 73–87.

Fogelman, I. (1989) An evaluation of the contribution of bone mass measurements to clinical practice. *Sem. Nucl. Med.*, **xix**, 62–8.

Fogelman, I. and Bessent, R. G. (1982) Age-related alterations in skeletal metabolism: 24 hour whole-body retention of diphosphonate in 250 normal subjects: concise communication. *J. Nucl. Med.*, **23**, 296–300.

Fogelman, I. and Carr, D. (1980a) A comparison of bone scanning and radiology in the evaluation of patients with metabolic bone disease. *Clin. Radiol.*, **31**, 321–6.

Fogelman, I. and Carr, D. (1980b) A comparison of bone scanning and radiology in the assessment of patients with symptomatic Paget's disease. *Eur. J. Nucl. Med.*, **5**, 417–21.

Fogelman, I. and Citrin, D. L. (1981) Bone scanning in metabolic bone disease: a review. *Appl. Radiol.*, **10**, 158–66.

Fogelman, I. and Coleman, R. E., (1988) Breast cancer and bone scanning, in *Nuclear Medicine Annual* (eds L. M. Freeman and H. S. Weissmann) Raven Press, New York.

Fogelman, I., McKillop, J. H., Greig, W. R. and Boyle, I. T. (1977a) Absent kidney sign associated with symmetrical and uniformly increased uptake of tracer by the skeleton. *Eur. J. Nucl. Med.*, **2**, 257–60.

Fogelman, I., McKillop, J. H., Greig, W. R. and Boyle, I. T. (1977b) Pseudo-fracture of the ribs detected by bone scanning. *J. Nucl. Med.*, **18**, 1236–7.

Fogelman, I., Citrin, D. L., Turner, J. G. *et al.* (1979) Semi-quantitative interpretation of the bone scan in metabolic bone disease. *Eur. J. Nucl. Med.*, **4**, 287–9.

Fogelman, I., Bessent, R. G., Turner, J. G. *et al.* (1978) The use of whole-body retention of Tc-99m diphosphonate in the diagnosis of metabolic bone disease. *J. Nucl. Med.*, **19**, 270–5.

Frank, J. W. (1981) The value of radionuclide bone imaging in atypical Paget's disease. *Nucl. Med. Comm.*, **2**, 302–6.

Freeman, M. H. and Tonkin, A. K. (1976) Manifestations of hyertrophic pulmonary osteoarthrophy in patients with carcinoma of the lung: demonstration by 99mTc pyrophosphate bone scans. *Radiology*, **120**, 363–5.

Freeman, M. L., Van Drunen, M., Gergans, G. and Kaplan, E. (1984) Accumulation of bone scanning agent in multiple myeloma. *Clin. Nucl. Med.*, **9**, 49.

Front, D., Schneck, S. O., Frankel, A. and Robinson, E. (1979) Bone metastases and bone pain in breast cancer. *JAMA*, **242**, 1747–8.

Gerber, F. H., Goodreau, J. J., Kirchner, P. T. and Fonty, W. J. (1977) Efficacy of preoperative and postoperative bone scanning in the management of breast carcinoma. *N. Engl. J. Med.*, **297**, 300–3.

Gilbert, H. A. and Kagan, A. R. (1976) in *Fundamental Aspects of Metastases* (ed. L. Weiss), Elsevier, Amsterdam, pp. 385–405.

Goldmann, A. B., Becker, M. H., Braunstein, P. *et al.* (1975) Bone scanning – osteogenic sarcoma: correlation with surgical pathology. *Radiology*, **124**, 83–90.

Goldstein, H., McNeil, B. J., Zufall, E. and Treves, S. (1980) Is there still a place for bone scanning in Ewing's sarcoma? *J. Nucl. Med.*, **21**, 10–12.

Gravenstein, S., Peltz, M. A. and Poreis, W. (1979) How ominous is an abnormal scan in bronchogenic carcinoma? *JAMA*, **241**, 2523–4.

Haase, G. M., Ovitz, V. N., Sfakianakis, G. N. and Morse, T. S. (1980) The value of radionuclide bone scanning in the early recognition of deliberate child abuse. *J. Trauma*, **20**, 873–5.

Hamdy, R. C. (1981) *Paget's Disease of Bone*. Praeger, Eastbourne, pp. 13–21, 37–46.

Hammond, N., Jones, S. E., Salmon, S. E. *et al.* (1978) Predictive value of bone scans in an adjuvant breast cancer program. *Cancer*, **41**, 138–42.

Handmaker, H. and Leonards, R. (1976) The bone scan in inflammatory osseous disease. *Semin. Nucl. Med.*, **6**, 95.

Hoffer, P. B. and Genant, H. K. (1976) Radionuclide joint imaging. *Semin. Nucl. Med.*, **6**, 121.

Holder, L. E. and Matthews, L. S. (1984) in *Nuclear Medicine Annual* (eds L. M. Freeman and H. S. Weissmann), Raven Press, New York, pp. 81–140.

Khairi, M. R. A., Robb, J. A., Wellman, H. N. and Johnston, C. C. (1974) Radiographs and scans in diagnosing symptomatic lesions of Paget's disease of bone (osteitis deformans). *Geriatrics*, **29**, 49–54.

Kim, E. E., Bledin, A. G., Gutierrez, C. and Haynie, T. P. (1983) Comparison of radionuclide images and radiographs for skeletal metastases from renal cell carcinoma. *Oncology*, **40**, 184–6.

Komaki, R. Donegan, W., Manoli, R. and Teh, E. L. (1979) Prognostic value of pretreatment bone scans in breast carcinoma. *Am. J. Roentgenol. Radium Ther. Nucl. Med.*, **132**, 877–81.

Kunkler, I. H., Merrick, M. V. and Rodger, A. (1985) Bone scintigraphy in breast cancer: a nine year follow up. *Clin. Radiol.*, **36**, 279–282.

Lentle, B. C., Russell, A. S., Percy, J. S. and Jackson, F. I. (1977a) Scintigraphic finding in ankylosing spondylitis. *J. Nucl. Med.*, **18**, 524–8.

Lentle, B. C., Russell, A. S., Percy, J. S. and Jackson, F. I. (1977b) The scintigraphic investigation of sacroiliac disease. *J. Nucl. Med.*, **18**, 529–33.

Lichtenstein, L. (1977) *Bone tumours* (5th edn), Mosby, St Louis.

Lindholm, A., Lundell, L., Martenson, B. and Thulin, A. (1979) Skeletal scintigraphy in the initial assessment of women with breast cancer. *Acta Chir. Scand.*, **145**, 65–71.

Lopez-Majano, V. and Sobti, P. (1984) Early diagnosis of pulmonary osteoarthropathy in neoplastic disease. *J. Nucl. Med. Allied Sci.* **28**, 69–76.

Lund, F., Smith, P. H. and Suciu, S. (1984) Do bone scans predict prognosis in prostatic cancer? *Br. J. Urol.*, **56**, 58–63.

Martin, P. (1979) The appearance of bone scans following fractures, including immediate and long-term studies. *J. Nucl. Med.*, **20**, 1227–31.

Martin, P. (1988) Basic principles of nuclear medicine techniques for detection and evaluation of trauma and sports medicine injuries, **18**, 90–112.

McDougall, I. R., Baumert, J. E. and Lantieri, R. L. (1979) Evaluation of In-111 leukocyte-whole body scanning. *Am. J. Roentgenol. Radium Ther. Nucl. Med.*, **133**, 849–54.

McGregor, B., Tulloh, A. G. S., Quinlin, M. F. and Lovegrove, F. (1978) The role of bone scanning in the assessment of prostatic carcinoma. *Br. J. Urol.*, **50**, 178–81.

McKillop, J. H. (1987) in *Bone Scanning in Clinical Practice* (ed. I. Fogelman), Springer-Verlag, London, pp. 41–60.

McKillop, J. H., Blumgart, L. H., Wood, C. B. *et al.* (1978) The prognostic and therapeutic implications of the positive radionuclide bone scan in clinically early breast cancer. *Br. J. Surg.*, **65**, 649–52.

McNeill, B. J., Pace, P. D., Gray, E. B. *et al.* (1978) Preoperative and follow up bone scans in patients with primary carcinoma of the breast. *Surg. Gynecol. Obstet.*, **147**, 745–8.

Merrick, M. V. (1987) in *Bone Scanning in Clinical Practice* (ed. I. Fogelman), Springer-Verlag, London, pp. 19–29.

Nair, N. (1985) Bone scanning Ewing's sarcoma. *J. Nucl. Med.*, **26**, 349–52.

Namey, T. C., McIntyre, J., Buse, M and Le Roy, E. C. (1977) Nucleographic studies of axial spondarthritides. I. Quantitative sacroiliac scintigraphy in early HLA-B27-associated sacroiliitis. *Arthritis Rheum.*, **20**, 1058.

Nisbet, A. P., Mashiter, G., Winn, P. *et al.* (1983) Quantitation of 99mTcMDP retention during routine bone scanning. *Nucl. Med. Comm.*, **4**, 67–71.

Nisbet, A. P., Edwards, S., Lazarus, C. R. *et al.* (1984) Chromium 51 EDTA/technetium 99m MDP plasma ratio to measure total skeletal function. *Br. J. Radiol.*, **57**, 677–80.

O'Connell, M. J. Wahner, H. J., Ahmann, D. L. *et al.* (1978) Value of preoperative radionuclide bone scans in suspected primary breast carcinoma. *Mayo Clin. Proc.*, **53**, 221–6.

O'Donoghue, E. P., Constable, A. R., Sherwood, T. *et al.* (1978) Bone scanning and plasma phosphatases in carcinoma of the prostate. *Br. J. Urol.*, **50**, 172–177.

Omjola, M. F., Cockshott, W. P. and Beatty, E. G. (1981) Osteoid osteoma: an evaluation of diagnostic modalities. *Clin. Radiol.*, **132**, 199–204.

Papanicolaou, N., Kozakewich, H., Treves, S. *et al.* (1982) Comparison of the extent of osteosarcoma between surgical pathology and skeletal scintigraphy. *J. Nucl. Med.*, **23**, P7 (abstract).

Paulson, D. F. and the Uro-Oncology Research Group (1979) The impact of current staging procedures in assessing disease extent of prostatic adenocarcinoma. *J. Urol.*, **121**, 300–2.

Peters, A. M. and Lavender, J. P. (1990) Diagnosis of bone infection. *Nucl. Med. Commun.*, **11**, 463–7.

Pistenma, D. A., McDougall, I. R. and Kriss, J. P. (1975) Screening for bone metastases: are only scans necessary? *JAMA*, **231**, 46–50.

Ralston, S., Fogelman, I., Gardner, M. D. and Boyle, I. T. (1982) Hypercalcaemia and metastatic bone disease: is there a causal link? *Lancet*, **ii**, 903–5.

Rappaport, A. H., Hoffer, P. B. and Genant, H. K. (1978) Unifocal bone findings by scintigraphy: clinical significance in patients with known primary cancer. *West. J. Med.*, **129**, 188–92.

Rausch, J. M., Resnick, D., Goergen, T. G. and Taylor, A. (1977) Bone scanning on osteolytic Paget's disease: case report. *J. Nucl. Med.*, **18**, 699–701.

Rosenthall, L. (1987) in *Bone Scanning in Clinical Practice* (ed. I. Fogelman), Springer-Verlag, London, pp. 151–74.

Rosenthall, L. and Hawkins, D. (1977) Radionuclide joint imaging in the diagnosis of synovial disease. *Semin. Arthr. Rheum.*, **7**, 49–61.

Rosenthall, L. and Lisbona, R. (1980) in *Nuclear Medicine Annual* (eds L. M. Freeman and H. S. Weissmann), Raven Press, New York.

Rossleigh, M. A., Lovegrove, F. T. A., Reynolds, P. M. and Byrne, M. J. (1982) Serial bone scans in the assessment of response to therapy in advanced breast carcinoma. *Clin. Nucl. Med.*, **7**, 397–402.

Rossleigh, M. A., Lovegrove, F. T. A., Reynolds, P. M. *et al.* (1984) The assessment of response to therapy of bone metastases in breast cancer. *Aust. NZ J. Med.*, **14**, 19–22.

Russell, A. S., Lentle, B. D. and Percy, J. S. (1975) Investigations of sacroiliac joint: comparative evaluation of radiological and radionuclide techniques. *J. Rheumatol.*, **2**, 45–51.

Schubert, F., Siddle, K. J. and Harper, J. S. (1984) Diaphyseal Paget's disease: an unusual finding in the tibia. *Clin. Radiol.*, **35**, 71–4.

Serafini, A. N. (1976) Paget's disease of the bone. *Semin. Nucl. Med.*, **6**, 47–58.

Shafer, R. B. and Reinke, D. B. (1977) Contribution of the bone scan, serum acid and alkaline phosphatase and radiographic bone survey to the management of newly diagnosed carcinoma of the prostate. *Clin. Nucl. Med.*, **2**, 200–3.

Shirazi, P. H., Ryan, W. G. and Fordham, E. W. (1974) Bone scanning in evaluation of Paget's disease of bone. *CRC Crit. Rev. Clin. Radiol. Nucl. Med.*, **5**, 523–58.

Smith, F. W. and Gilday, D. L. (1980) Scintigraphic appearances of osteoid osteoma. *Radiology*, **137**, 191–5.

Stadalnik, R. C. (1979) 'Cold spot': bone imaging. *Semin. Nucl. Med.*, **9**, 2–3.

Stevenson, J. S., Bright, R. W., Dunson, G. L. and Nelson, F. R. (1984) Technetium-99m phosphate bone imaging: a method of assessing bone graft healing. *Radiology*, **110**, 391–4.

Subramanian, G., McAfee, J. G., Blair, R. J. *et al.* (1972) 99m-Tc-EHDP: a potential radiopharmaceutical for skeletal imaging. *J. Nucl. Med.*, **13**, 947–50.

Swee, R. G., McLeod, R. A. and Beabout, J. W. (1979)

Osteoid osteoma: detection, diagnosis and localisation. *Radiology*, **132**, 117–23.
Thomas, R. H., Resnick, D., Alazraki, N. P. *et al.* (1975) Compartmental evaluation of osteoarthritis of the knee. *Radiology*, **116**, 585.
Tofe, A. J., Francis, M. A. and Harvey, W. J. (1975) Correlation of neoplasms with incidence and localisation of skeletal metastases: an analysis of 1355 diphosphonate bone scans. *J. Nucl. Med.*, **16**, 986.
Vellenga, C. J., Pauwels, E. K. J., Bijvoet, E. O. and Hosking, D. J. (1976) Evaluation of scintigraphic and roentgenologic studies in Paget's disease under treatment. *Radiol. Clin.*, **45**, 292–301.
Vellenga, C. J. L. R., Pauwels, E. K. J. and Bijvoet, O. L. M. (1984a) Comparison between visual assessment and quantitative measurement of radioactivity on the bone scintigram in Paget's disease of bone. *Eur. J. Nucl. Med.*, **9**, 533–7.
Vellenga, C. J. L. R., Pauwels, E. K. J., Bijvoet, O. L. M. *et al.* (1984b) Untreated Paget's disease of bone studied by scintigraphy. *Radiology*, **153**, 799–805.
Wahner, H. W., Kyle, R. A. and Beabout, J. W. (1980) Scintigraphic evaluation of the skeleton in multiple myeloma. *Mayo Clin. Proc.*, **55**, 739–46.
Waxman, A. D., Siemsen, J. K., Levine, A. M. *et al.* (1981) Radiographic and radionuclide imaging in multiple myeloma: the role of gallium scintigraphy. *J. Nucl. Med.*, **22**, 232–6.
Weissberg, D. L. *et al.* (1978) *Am. J. Roentgenol.*, **131**, 665.
Wilson, G. S., Rich, M. A. and Brennan, M. J. (1980) Evaluation of bone scan in preoperative clinical staging of breast cancer. *Arch. Surg.*, **115**, 415–19.
Wollfenden, J. M., Pitt, M. J., Durie, B. G. M. and Moon, T. E. (1980) Comparison of bone scintigraphy and radiology in multiple myeloma. *Radiology*, **134**, 723–8.

CHAPTER SEVEN

The brain

P. J. Ell and K. E. Britton

7.1 INTRODUCTION

It is interesting to reflect on the present growth of radionuclide brain scanning. Not so many years ago, and in particular in the mid-1970s, after the peak effect of X-ray computed tomography (CT) brain scanning, radionuclide brain studies significantly declined in frequency and clinical importance. Now, after a decade, radionuclide studies of the brain have gained renewed interest.

This reflects a growing awareness of the inadequacy of recording data of great anatomical detail without an adequate functional if not metabolic correlate, and it also corresponds to a need to provide insight into pathologies which primarily reflect a disturbance of the internal biochemical milieu rather than a significant change in the structure of the brain. Epilepsy, dementia, and early or transient ischaemia are typical examples of such conditions. The disturbing finding of the neurological manifestations of AIDS adds importance to the understanding of degenerative changes of the central nervous system (Riccio, 1987; Carne, 1987).

This new insight in the study of the neurological or psychiatric patient is a consequence of significant progress with the instrumentation available for the study of the brain, but perhaps more importantly the result of a new range of radiopharmaceuticals available for such studies (Ell *et al.*, 1987a). In this chapter, and because of the still ongoing interest in conventional brain scanning (more appropriately designated as blood–brain barrier (BBB) scanning), a brief review of such studies is given, but emphasis will be placed on the more recent applications of the radioactive tracer method to the brain, and in particular its application with single photon emission computed tomography (SPECT). A review of the present state of pharmaceuticals labelled with conventional radionuclides is included. Positron emission tomography (PET) is not discussed, as this aspect is beyond the aim of this review.

7.2 RELEVANT ANATOMY AND PHYSIOLOGY

One may consider the head anatomically from the outside, i.e. the hair and scalp to the deep midbrain (Figure 7.1) and physiologically from the inside outwards as the movement of nutrients pass from the arterial and capillary supply to the neuroglia and then to the functioning nerve cells. The whole may be considered strategically as a mechanical and functional protective system for the intellectual and regulatory centres of the brain.

The blood–brain barrier is the name given to the conjunction of capillary walls, neuroglia and nerve cells (Figure 7.2). It constitutes a barrier to the passage of compounds unnecessary to brain metabolism and limits the movement of potentially toxic substances from the blood to the brain. This is achieved by physical and physiological factors. The capillaries in the skin and muscles have pores and gaps between the cells that allow free diffusibility of crystalloids and, for example, an inert gas like xenon, but this is not true of capillaries in the brain. There is in effect no separation or channel between the endothelial cells and pinocytosis is rare. Instead, there are specific carrier systems across the capillary wall enabling active transport, for example, of sugars including fluorodeoxyglucose and amino acids. Pertechnetate ions are barred. The second method of entry is through lipid solubility. Lipid-soluble compounds diffuse through the double phospholipid lamellae to enter the capillary wall. The capillary wall is intimately linked to the neuroglia through their foot processes. The nutrients pass into these supporting and feeding cells of the brain which

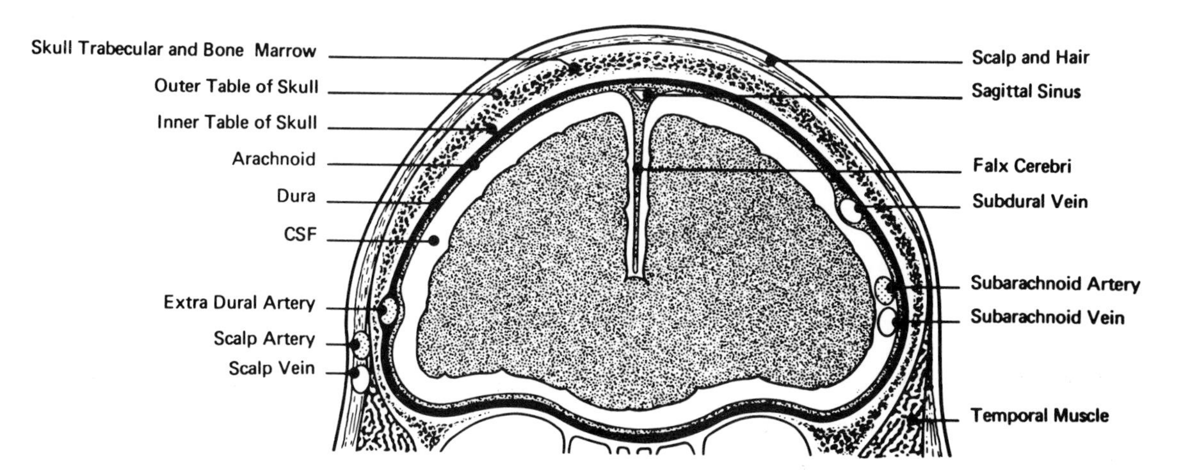

Figure 7.1 The layers around the brain and the distribution of vessels.

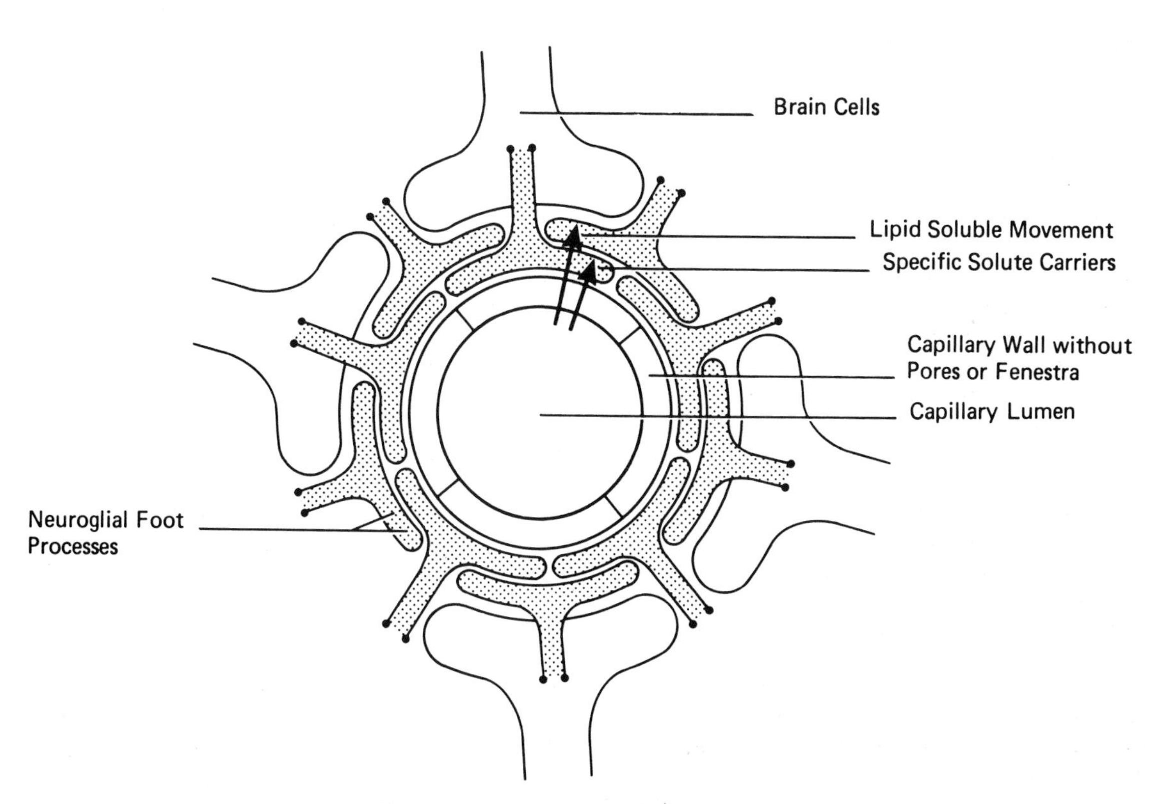

Figure 7.2 The blood–brain barrier (BBB).

appear to pass energy to the nerve cells through connecting processes. This close-packed arrangement leaves little room for extracellular fluid.

From the point of view of brain imaging, the importance of the layers around the brain is their relation to the main arteries and veins. Scalp contusions are common with arterial and venous bleeding, which is an easily palpated cause of a local increase in skull-related activity. Fracture of the skull may involve a branch of the extradural meningeal arteries. The high-pressure extradural haemorrhage is a surgical emergency in which brain imaging would waste valuable time. The low-pressure venous subdural bleed is another cause of a local increase in skull-related activity and chronic subdural haemorrhage is described later in this text. The cerebrospinal fluid between the layers of the arachnoid acts as an absorbent buffer to protect the brain during movement and a liquid environment from which materials and carbon dioxide diffuse through the pia arachnoid which clothes the cerebrum.

The major branches of the internal carotid and vertebral arteries pass through the arachnoid space and the point of branching is a common site for a developmental weakness, which may become an aneurysm whose rupture gives a subarachnoid haemorrhage.

It is necessary to distinguish between the volumes and flows of the brain and its extracerebral coverings. The brain acts almost as an arteriovenous fistula. The resistance to flow is very low and a volume flow rate of blood, about 1000 ml min^{-1}, rushes through a total cerebral blood volume of about 75 ml in the 1500 g of normal brain tissue, giving a mean transit time of 4.5 s. In the diseased brain the blood volume can vary considerably, for example between 50 ml and 100 ml which for the same flow would give a range of mean transit times of 3–6 s. Thus any technique that measures only an aspect of passage time or wash-out time as a representation of blood flow may lead to considerable error unless the total volume and the distribution of its volume is constant. Secondly, the resistance to flow through the scalp and extracerebral tissues is relatively high since blood passes through a normal arteriolar capillary bed and, for the same reason, their blood volume is relatively high, of the order of 25% of the cerebral volume, i.e. 20 ml. Considering an extracerebral volume flow of the order of 5% of cerebral blood flow, 50 ml min^{-1} gives a mean transit time of about 24 s. Thus extracerebral activity will interfere with the external monitoring of cerebral blood flow to a major extent when there is recirculation and equilibrium of a tracer in blood because its volume is of an important size relative to cerebral volume and because it is superficial. It is important to learn the usual vascular territories perfused by the anterior, middle and posterior cerebral arteries in each view of the brain (Figure 7.3). If in a patient with neurological signs an abnormality detected on the brain scan crosses over a vascular boundary, it is unlikely to have an acquired vascular cause, whereas if it is confined to one territory it may be due to a cerebrovascular accident (Figure 7.4).

There is no cerebral flow in brain death. This may be investigated using a mobile camera by undertaking a dynamic and static flow study (Nagle, 1980). However, recent work with a more specific agent for cellular integrity appears to offer a more promising alternative (Roine *et al.*, 1986).

7.3 RADIOPHARMACEUTICALS

The development of new radiopharmaceuticals for the study of brain function is leading to a complete rethink of the role of radionuclide brain

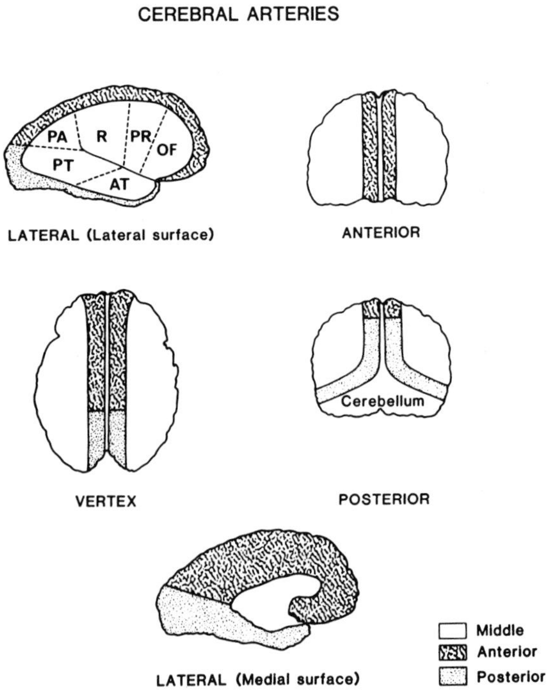

CEREBRAL ARTERIES

PA R PR OF PT AT

LATERAL (Lateral surface) ANTERIOR

Cerebellum

VERTEX POSTERIOR

LATERAL (Medial surface)

Middle
Anterior
Posterior

Figure 7.3 The vascular territories of the brain.

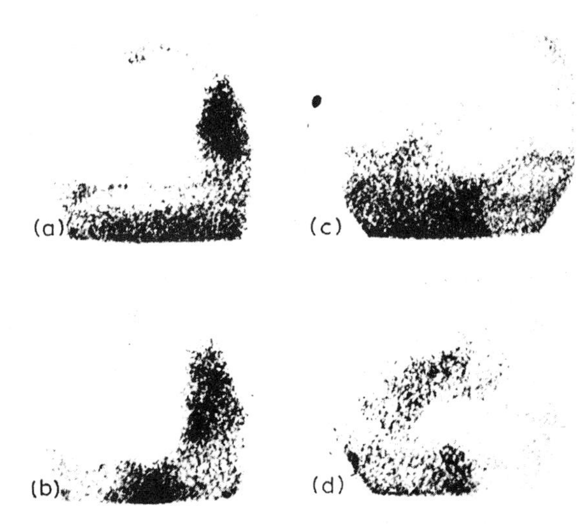

Figure 7.4 A right middle cerebral infarction. (a) Posterior view; (b) anterior view; (c) left lateral view; (d) right lateral view. The area of disrupted BBB is confined to one vascular territory only.

scanning. From this point of view, a similar phenomenon was only observed in nuclear medicine with the introduction of ^{99m}Tc-labelled phosphates and phosphonates for bone scintigraphy and the introduction of ^{201}Tl-labelled chloride as a routine agent in the investigation of myocardial perfusion. It is therefore important to consider these new developments, since they will colour the range and scope of the application of the radioactive tracer method to the study of the brain.

Different tracers are designed to investigate different aspects of brain function. In Table 7.1 these are grouped into four categories: blood–brain barrier (BBB) imaging, cerebral blood volume (CBV) imaging, cerebral blood flow (CBF) imaging and neuroreceptor (NR) imaging. In Table 7.2, for each of these four categories, radiation dosimetry estimates are given and compared with standard X-ray imaging procedures.

7.4 BBB RADIOPHARMACEUTICALS

A number of these tracers permit the investigation of the damaged BBB. From these, ^{99m}Tc as sodium pertechnetate and eluate of the ^{99}Mo/^{99m}Tc generator (Potchen and McCready, 1972) or ^{99m}Tc-labelled glucoheptonate (GH) (Boyd *et al.*, 1973) are most often utilized. ^{99m}Tc-labelled GH requires no patient preparation (no choroid plexus blockade) and gives superior or at least identical signal/noise ratios in the demonstration of alteration of the BBB, when compared with [^{99}Tc]-pertechnetate. It clears faster from blood than pertechnetate, and its distribution is not altered with the prior administration of tin-containing radiopharmaceuticals, as occurs with pertechnetate. Both tracers enjoy the advantages of being labelled with ^{99m}Tc.

^{99m}Tc-labelled diethylene triamine pentaacetic acid (DTPA) has been utilized (Hauser *et al.*, 1970), as well as ^{201}Tc-labelled chloride (Ancri *et al.*, 1978), the latter particularly in the detection of space-occupying disease. There are no significant

Table 7.1 Tracers for the brain

Non-lipophilic		*Lipophilic*	
^{99m}Tc		^{133}Xe gas*	
Pertechnetate		^{123}I	
Glucoheptonate		Iodoantipyrine*	
DTPA	BBB imaging	HIPDM	
^{201}Tl		IMP	
Chloride		^{99m}Tc*	
		PnAO	CBF imaging
^{99m}Tc		^{201}Tl	
RBC		DDC	
HSA		^{99m}Tc	
^{111}In	CBV imaging	HMPAO	
Transferrin		ECD	
^{113m}In		^{123}I	
Transferrin		Raclopride	
		QNB	Receptor imaging
		^{77}Br	
		Methylspiperone	

*Requires a fast SPECT tomograph (dynamic SPECT).

Table 7.2 Radiation dosimetry estimates: a comparison

	Dose (MBq)	*Eff. dose equiv. (mSv)*
^{123}I IMP	150	5.8
^{99m}Tc-labelled HMPAO	740	12.4
^{99m}Tc-labelled ECD	740	6.2
$^{99m}TcO_4$	740	7.4
^{133}Xe gas	400/L/90″	0.6
X-ray CT	—	3.5
Chest X-ray	—	0.1
Stable Xe-enhanced CT – CBF	—	15

advantages of these two tracers above the other radiopharmaceuticals just mentioned.

7.5 CBV RADIOPHARMACEUTICALS

^{99m}Tc-labelled red blood cells (RBC) (Gray *et al.*, 1979) or labelled serum albumin (HSA) (Schall *et al.*, 1971) are in most common use. These tracers are widely available, labelling is simple, high yields (85–95%) are obtained, and stability *in vivo* can be achieved with minimal elution from label to plasma (±3%).

7.6 CBF RADIOPHARMACEUTICALS

^{133}Xe is an inert and freely diffusible radioactive gas, with a half-life of 5.25 days and γ-energy of 81 keV. It is widely available, relatively cheap, and has been widely used for day-to-day measurements of CBF (Obrist *et al.*, 1975). Once given to the patient (intra-arterial and intravenous injection methods have been developed as well as inhalation techniques), there is rapid saturation of the brain, followed by wash-out. The rate of wash-out from the brain is proportional to CBF, and this proportionality has been the basis of the general methodology of CBF measurements with planar probe recording devices. Repeat studies, baseline and intervention studies are easily carried out (in view of the wash-out of the tracer) in a few minutes, and the dosimetry is the most favourable of all the tracers presently considered for CBF studies. Simple instrumentation has been developed for true bedside monitoring of CBF (Figure 7.5), this being of particular importance in the monitoring of acute conditions (subarachnoid haemorrhage, for example).

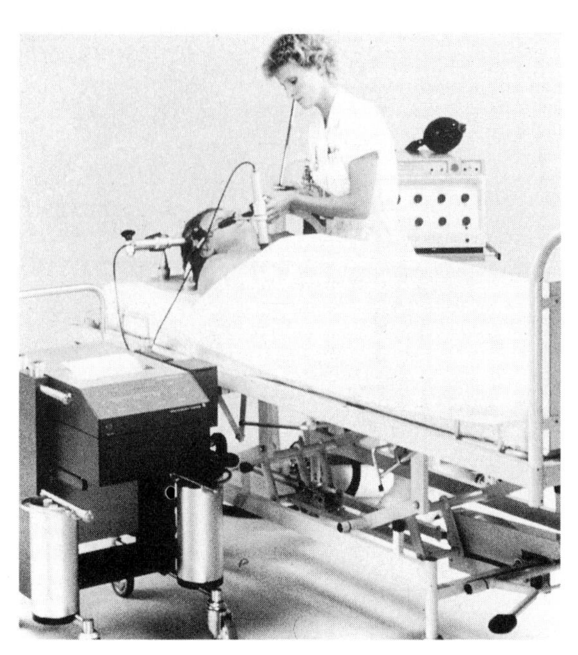

Figure 7.5 A portable ^{133}Xe CBF instrument.

More recently, dedicated instrumentation has also been manufactured in order to obtain tomographic maps of CBF (Plate 12). Multiple detectors are utilized; a sequence of four 1 min images is utilized to record a transaxial map of CBF. As with the planar probes, CBF is expressed in units of ml min^{-1} per 100 g of brain substance.

7.6.1 ^{123}I-4-IODOANTIPYRINE

This crosses the intact BBB, with flow-dependent cerebral uptake and very rapid wash-out. Over ^{133}Xe it has the distinct advantage of the physical properties of the labelling radionuclide, but it is much less available and significantly costlier to use.

7.6.2 ^{123}I-LABELLED AMINES (HIPDM AND IMP)

These compounds represent a first generation of lipid-soluble radiopharmaceuticals, capable of passage of the BBB, with uptake of compound closely in parallel with CBF, at least during the first hour of intravenous administration. Winchell *et al.* (1980), Tramposch *et al.* (1980), and Kuhl *et al.* (1983) extensively reported the main characteristics of the ^{131}I- and subsequently ^{123}I-labelled tracers and early clinical work was reported by Hill *et al.* (1982) and Ell *et al.* (1983).

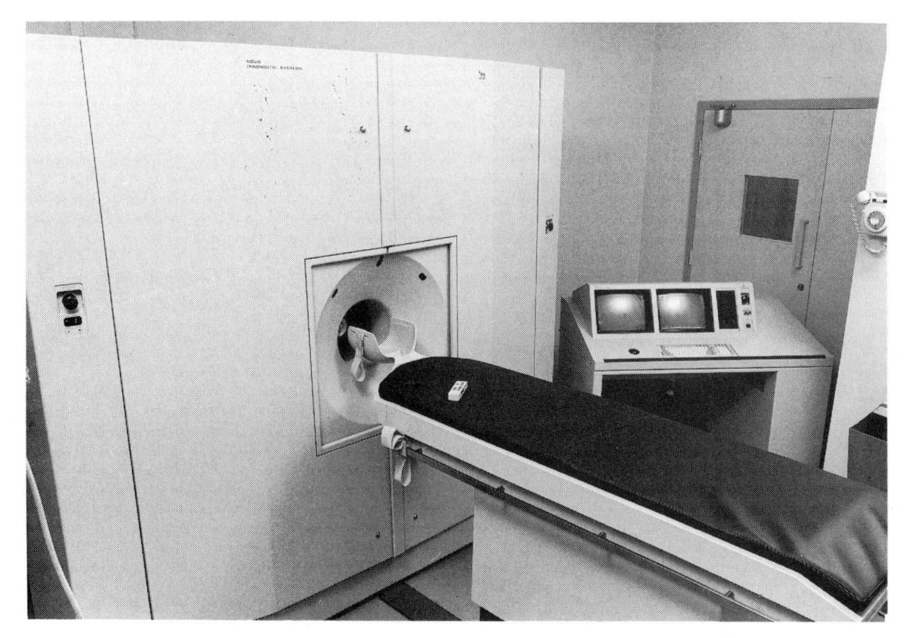

Figure 7.6 Rapid tomographic brain scanner optimized for ^{99m}Tc.

^{123}I-*N*,*N*,*N*′-trimethyl-*N*′(2-hydroxyl-3-methyl-5-iodo-benzyl)-1,3-propane diamine (HIPDM) (Figure 7.7) became available in 1981–2, preceded by ^{123}I-*n*-isopropyl-*p* iodoamphetamine (IMP) (Figure 7.8). Both these compounds have been extensively investigated in man, IMP being commercially available (Medi-Physics Inc., Emeryville, CA).

From the point of view of the physical properties of ^{123}I, this label is almost ideal. With a main energy γ-ray emission of 159 keV, most photons can be efficiently stopped and converted by the half-inch thick sodium iodide crystal of the gamma camera. Counting statistics are inferior, however, to those achievable with ^{99m}Tc. In the specific case of brain scanning, a factor of three will be gained if ^{99m}Tc can be utilized instead.

While ^{123}I-HIPDM and IMP have somewhat different pharmacokinetics (HIPDM reaches its peak brain activity at 10–15 min post-administration, IMP reaches maximum brain activity at 20–30 min post-injection (p.i.) with somewhat different uptake and wash-out properties from the lungs), brain uptake of these two tracers is proportional to blood flow, at least in the first hour after intravenous administration. An equilibrium period of the tracer in the brain is obtained, during which conventional SPECT can be carried out with routinely available machinery (such as the rotating gamma camera, Figure 7.9). HIPDM has slightly higher brain uptake than IMP, is more lipophylic, with both compounds exhibiting significant protein binding at equilibrium.

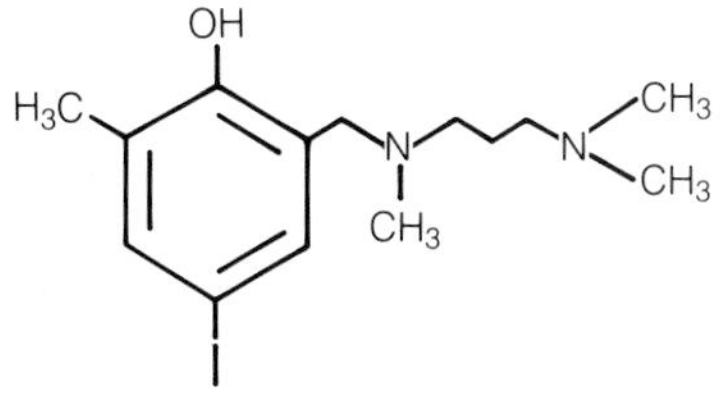

Figure 7.7 ^{123}I-HIPDM and ^{123}I-labelled antipyrine structure.

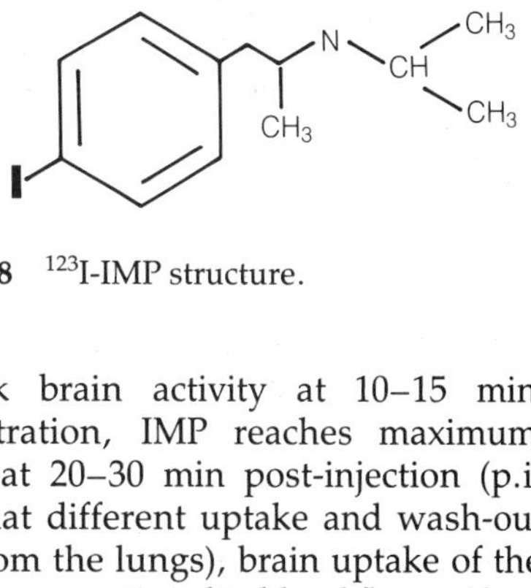

Figure 7.8 ^{123}I-IMP structure.

In contrast to other radiopharmaceuticals (such as hexamethylpropyleneamineoxime (HMPAO) and diethyldithiocarbamate (DDC)), these compounds do not behave like a chemical microsphere. There is rapid metabolism, incomplete extraction from the blood, and significant wash-out of tracer from the brain. With time, and significantly after one hour p.i., the compounds change their intracerebral distribution. While this phenomenon has been addressed (Moretti *et al.*, 1987), the nature and extent of this redistribution is still poorly understood. Cerebral ischaemia and stroke, when imaged early with these compounds, leads to the well-known pattern of reduced uptake and distribution of compound, whilst images taken 3–6 h p.i. demonstrate a progressive filling in of these abnormalities – more pronounced in acute than established stroke, and in reversible ischaemia rather than prolonged or non-reversible cerebral ischaemia (Figure 7.10).

7.6.3 ^{99m}Tc-LABELLED PnAO AND HMPAO

Over 90% of all nuclear medicine *in vivo* studies are carried out by radiopharmaceuticals labelled with ^{99m}Tc. This radionuclide, routinely available in most countries and in all continents, has become the true universal radionuclide. With an almost monoenergetic γ-ray emission of 141 keV, a physical half-life of 6 h, and obtainable from a most useful generator with a shelf life which permits daily availability throughout the week (^{99}Mo generator, half-life = 67 h), it can be made to react with a wide variety of hydrophilic compounds and, recently, with an increasing number of lipophilic compounds.

While Volkert *et al.* (1984) proposed ^{99m}Tc-labelled PnAO as the first ^{99m}Tc-labelled lipophilic compound available for rCBF studies, Amersham International (UK) has introduced a derivative of this tracer, namely ^{99m}Tc-labelled HMPAO (Ell *et al.*, 1985a). The *d,l* derivative of this compound was subsequently studied in man by Sharp *et al.* (1986) and by Ell *et al.* (1985b) and by Costa *et al.* (1986a) within a short period (Figure 7.11).

Should ^{99m}Tc-labelled PnAO (propyleneamineoxime) become available, it could (justifiably) replace ^{133}Xe as the more ideal compound for dynamic rCBF/SPECT. It has a high extraction efficiency, it is taken up in the brain in proportion to blood flow, and offers to dynamic SPECT the advantages of ^{99m}Tc as a radionuclide. Counting statistics, lower photon attenuation, costs and availability of ^{99m}Tc would all favour this compound over the ^{133}Xe gas. Holm *et al.* (1985) has reported first studies in man with a fast rotating brain tomograph. The major drawback of PnAO reflects its short residence time in the brain (as occurs with ^{133}Xe gas or ^{123}I iodoantipyrine). This is a significant drawback since it prevents SPECT being carried out without the specialized equipment required as for the xenon gas method. Since this type of equipment is unlikely to become available in large numbers, the 'marketability' of PnAO remains in doubt. Also, the dosimetry expected from PnAO will be significantly worse than that obtained from ^{133}Xe.

^{99m}Tc-labelled HMPAO is undergoing clinical trials in a number of countries and is commercially available in several of them, including the UK. Dedicated SPECT brain scanners have been designed to take advantage of this new development (Figure 7.6) (Jarritt *et al.*, 1979).

When ^{99m}Tc-labelled HMPAO is given intravenously, there is rapid binding to serum proteins. The lipophilic fraction which is available to extraction by the brain (supplied by the arterial input to the brain) is of the order of 60% of total compound administered. From this fraction, in the first circulation, approximately 85–90% is extracted by the cells of the brain. This high extraction fraction forms the basis of its distribution to the brain in proportion to CBF. Changes in cardiac output will, however, reflect the amount of compound offered to be extracted by the cerebrum, and hence the total amount taken up by this organ.

In dogs, the distribution of ^{99m}Tc-labelled HMPAO in the brain remains proportional to CBF up to approximately 150–200 ml min^{-1} per 100 g of tissue. Once trapped intracellularly, little redistribution or wash-out occurs with time; the compound behaves like a chemical microsphere (Costa *et al.*, 1986b). In this, ^{99m}Tc-labelled HMPAO is clearly different from IMP or xenon, and advantages can be gained from this behaviour. SPECT can be carried out by conventional equipment (slowly rotating Anger gamma cameras) and once injected imaging can be delayed for as long as statistically reliable information can be recorded (here the only constraint is the 6 h physical half-life of ^{99m}Tc).

The preparation of ^{99m}Tc-labelled HMPAO needs some attention, so that high yields and chemical purity can be obtained (see Table 7.3). For optimal results, ^{99m}Tc-labelled HMPAO should be administered to patients as soon as possible after preparation of this compound in the radiopharmacy.

It is still to be seen whether activation studies can be carried out with ^{99m}Tc-labelled HMPAO in a manner which correlates with the expected

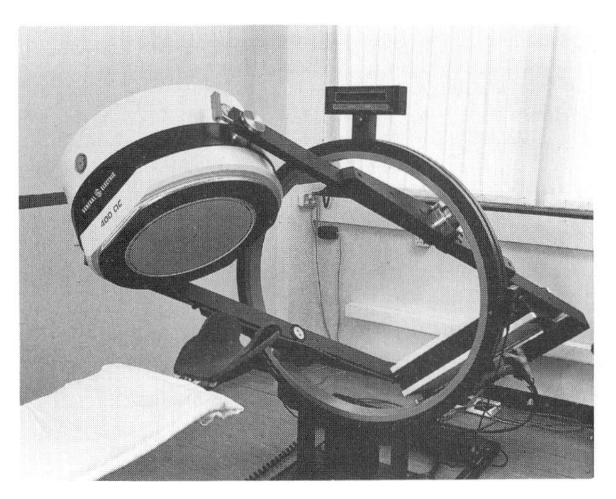

Figure 7.9 The standard single-head rotating Anger gamma camera computer system.

Figure 7.10 ^{123}I-IMP acute stroke study.

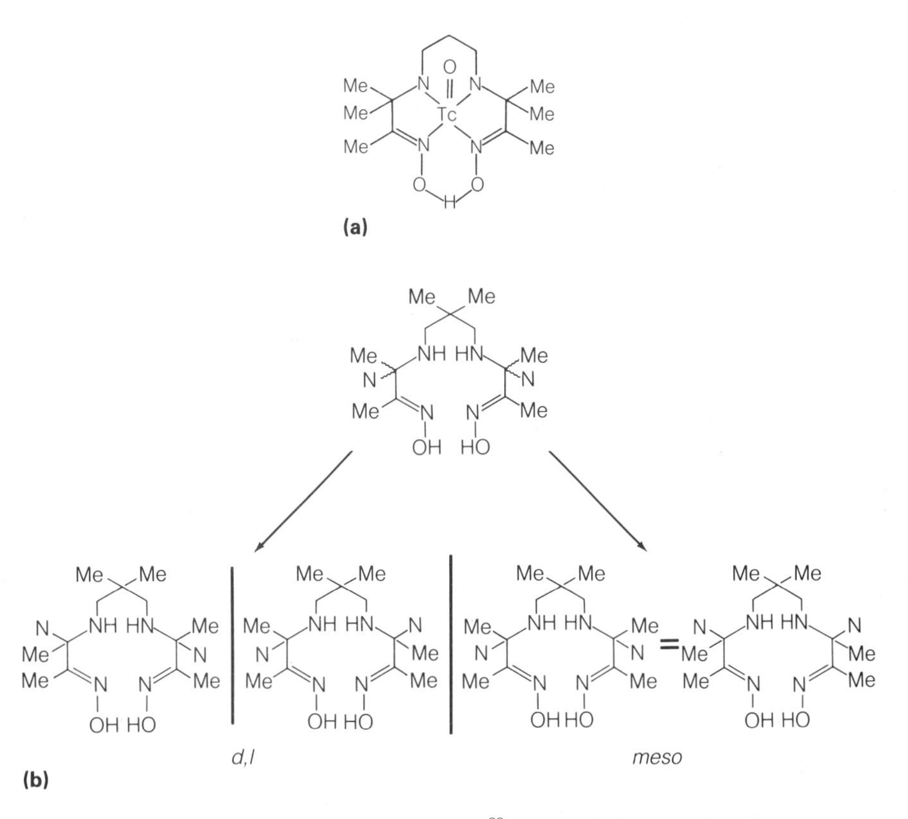

Figure 7.11 The structure of (a) PnAO and (b) ^{99m}Tc-labelled HMPAO and its isomers.

Table 7.3 Preparation of ^{99m}Tc-labelled HMPAO

	Notes
1. Place the vial in a shielding container and swab the closure with the sterilizing swab provided 2. Using a 10 ml syringe, inject into the shielded vial 5 ml of sterile eluate from a ^{99m}Tc generator (see notes 1–4). Before withdrawing the syringe from the vial withdraw 5 ml of gas from the space above the solution to normalize the pressure in the vial. Shake the shielded vial for 10 s to ensure complete dissolution of the powder 3. Assay the total activity and calculate the volume to be injected 4. Complete the label provided and attach to the vial 5. Use within a maximum of 30 min after reconstitution. Discard any unused material	1. For the highest radiochemical purity reconstitute with freshly eluted ^{99m}Tc generator eluate 2. Use only eluate which was eluted less than 2 h previously from a generator which was previously eluted within 24 h 3. 0.37–1.11 GBq (10–30 mCi) ^{99m}Tc may be added to the vial 4. Before reconstitution the generator eluate may be adjusted to the correct radioactive concentration (0.37–1.11 GBq in 5 ml) by dilution with saline for injection 5. The use of pertechnetate complying with the specifications prescribed by the USP and BP/EP monographs on sodium pertechnetate (^{99m}Tc) injection will yield a preparation of an appropriate quality 6. The pH of the prepared injection is in the range 9.0–9.8

changes of regional CBF. Bekier (unpublished) has shown that activation studies are possible, both with motor stimulation and with the administration of oxygen/gas mixture. In rats exposed to carbon dioxide, a barely statistically significant increase has been observed with ^{99m}Tc-labelled HMPAO (personal observation). In humans, carbon dioxide response is unpredictable and non-significant (personal observation).

^{99m}Tc-labelled HMPAO demonstrates the resulting alteration in blood flow in neoplasia of the brain. Metastatic disease is often the cause of cerebral focal ischaemia, clearly observable with the SPECT methodology. Primary brain tumours may take up the compound. High-grade glioma and a neuroblastoma (personal observation) have been seen to lead to positive images on SPECT. However, most gliomas and metastases lead to a fall in local CBF. Acute stroke is clearly demonstrated with ^{99m}Tc-labelled HMPAO/SPECT. In terms of its detection, the smallest cold and spherical volume which can be demonstrated is of the order of 1 ml; the smallest volume from which accurate uptake and CBF/CBV ratios can be derived will be of the order of 15 ml. Serial studies on the same patient are feasible at intervals of 24 h, whilst with background subtraction techniques studies at 12 h are technically feasible (the contribution from the first study being 20% of the total in the second study). The limiting aspect will be the radiation dosimetry of this technique (see Table 7.2). To reduce radiation exposure to patients, and in view of the excretion of ^{99m}Tc-labelled HMPAO from gut and kidneys, we recommend the administration of a mild laxative on the day after the SPECT study and the maintenance of a good urinary output, with hydration of the patient. The data in Table 7.2 represent a worst-case estimation, and significant reduction of radiation exposure can be achieved by the simple procedures outlined above.

Resting studies of patients with Jacksonian type or temporal lobe epilepsy may pinpoint the site of abnormality, with alterations of the CBF/CBV ratios (Buell *et al.*, 1987), while studies performed shortly after the crisis demonstrate the site of electric discharge as a focus of increased blood flow in man. This is supported by the evidence from PET studies, where there appears to be no decoupling between flow and glucose during the acute period of the epilepsy. Both Gemmell *et al.* (1984) and Shields *et al.* (1986) have shown 'typical' patterns of impaired CBF in patients with Alzheimer's disease, the group from Manchester having the benefit of biopsy-proven case histories. A drop in temporal and parietal blood flow was observed, similar to the studies recorded with PET methodology. Shields *et al.* (1986) have shown frontal hypoperfusion in Pick's disease, in the presence of normal X-ray CT methodology.

7.6.4 ^{201}Tl-LABELLED DIETHYLDITHIOCARBAMATE (DDC)

Bruine *et al.* (1985) proposed ^{201}Tl-labelled DDC as an alternative tracer to ^{123}I-isopropyl-*p*-iodoamphetamine for the study of rCBF in man (Figure 7.12). Following intravenous administra-

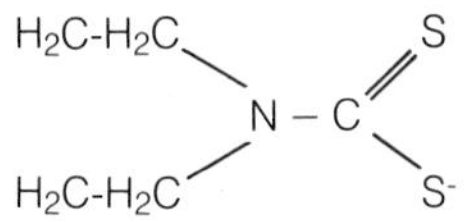

$H_2C\text{-}H_2C$ S
N – C
$H_2C\text{-}H_2C$ S^-

Figure 7.12 The structure of DDC.

tion, a plateau activity is obtained in the brain at 1 min, with no redistribution over many hours. There is good contrast between grey and white matter, and by now a number of clinical studies have shown the potential of this tracer. Typical patterns of rCBF abnormality have been seen in patients with stroke, Alzheimer's and Pick's dementia.

Since little or no redistribution of tracer occurs with time, and ^{201}Tl has a physical half-life of 73 h, ^{201}Tl-labelled DDC can be given to a patient in the immediate acute period of a manifestation, and imaging carried out the day after. The study will still reflect the distribution of rCBF at the time of tracer administration. This property may facilitate the study of acutely ill patients, suffering from acute but transient phenomena, such as stroke, transient ischaemic attacks (TIA), epilepsy and so on.

^{201}Tl-labelled DDC/SPECT has drawbacks: ^{201}Tl is not a radionuclide of choice (only 10% of its photons are emitted at energies suitable for imaging, the majority are emitted at lower energies around 80 keV, which is too soft), its dosimetry is not ideal and worse than ^{123}I, and the overall image quality is inferior to that obtained with ^{99m}Tc-labelled HMPAO.

When studying the subcellular localization of ^{99m}Tc-labelled HMPAO and ^{201}Tl-labelled DDC, significant differences can be found. An experiment was carried out in 51 unanaesthetized Wistar rats (180–200 g weight range). The animals were sacrificed 5 min p.i. and the brain was dissected into cerebellum (CER), paleocortex (PAL) and neocortex (NEO). Homogenates of these regions were obtained and differential centrifugation was performed to separate cytosol (free and protein-bound fractions) from organelles (e.g. myelin (M), lisosomes (L)). Centrifugation in discontinuous sucrose gradient was used to separate nuclei of neurons (N) from those of glial cells (G).

The total brain uptake (percentage of whole body) equalled 2.1 for the HMPAO and 2.8 for DDC ($p < 0.01$). The remaining activity in the brain at 24 h was, respectively, 92% (HMPAO) and 62% (DDC), $p < 0.001$. HMPAO appeared mainly in the organelles (>55%), whilst DDC was found mainly in the cytosol (>92% free, <8% protein bound). Table 7.4 shows the results (% counts mg^{-1} of protein) for M, L and N, G (Costa *et al.*, 1987a).

These data confirm a different subcellular distribution of the two lipophilic agents studied and suggest different pharmacokinetics in rat brains.

7.6.5 ^{99m}Tc-LABELLED ECD

^{99m}Tc-labelled *V*-oxo-1,2-*N*,N_1-ethylenedylbis-L-cysteine diethylester (ECD) is the most recent significant addition to these ^{99m}Tc-labelled radiopharmaceuticals designed to be taken up by the brain as a function of CBF. It is the second ^{99m}Tc-labelled tracer to be utilized in humans for rCBF SPECT studies (produced by DuPont de Nemours) (Figure 7.13) (Vallabhajosula *et al.*, 1989; Holman *et al.*, 1989).

The compound exhibits both animal specificity and stereo-isomer specificity. There is little uptake of the compound in the swine, rabbit and dog, but significant uptake in monkey. Whilst the L form of the compound shows long retention in monkey brain (with a half-life of 7.24 h), there is no significant retention with the D form. The compound is metabolized by monkey brain, and this metabolite (yet to be identified) is found in the cerebrospinal fluid of the rhesus monkey.

The uptake of the compound by the human brain is of the order of 5%, there is rapid clearance from the blood (with a half-life of 3.3 h), little lung

Table 7.4 Intracellular distribution of rCBF tracers in rat brains*

	CER				*PAL*				*NEO*			
	M	*L*	*N*	*G*	*M*	*L*	*N*	*G*	*M*	*L*	*N*	*G*
HMPAO	19	43	6	2	19	39	5	1	33	28	5	0.4
DDC	86	6	8	15	78	5	4	2	75	5	5	0.03

*See text for explanation of abbreviations.

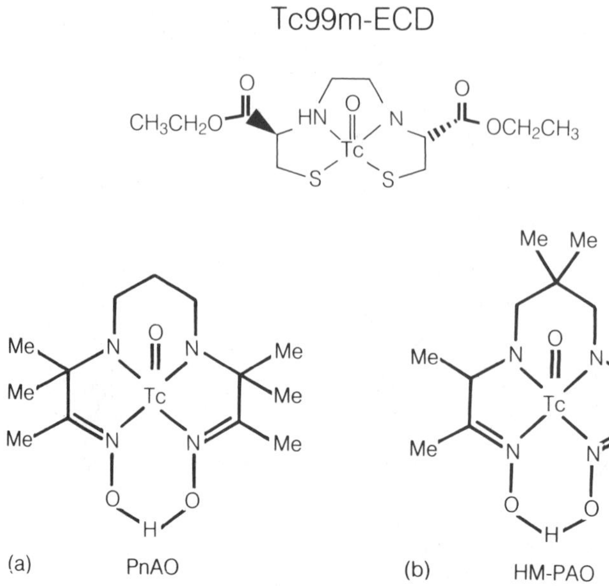

Tc99m-ECD

(a) PnAO

(b) HM-PAO

Figure 7.13 The structure of ^{99m}Tc-labelled ECD and the structure of ^{99m}Tc-Pn AO and ^{99m}Tc-HMPAO.

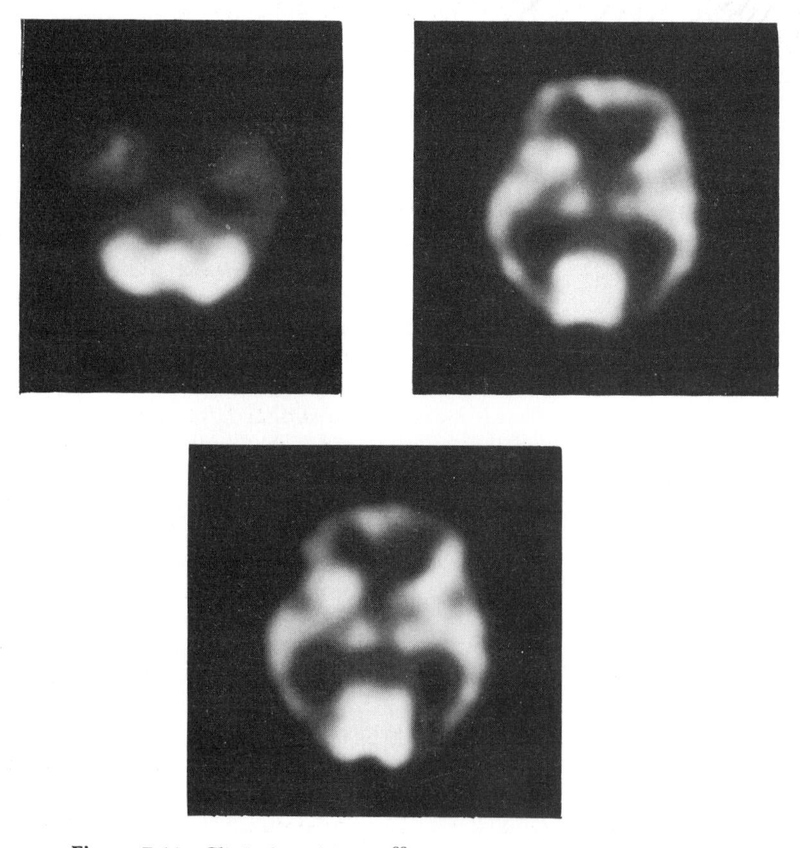

Figure 7.14 Clinical study with ^{99m}Tc-labelled ECD (normal).

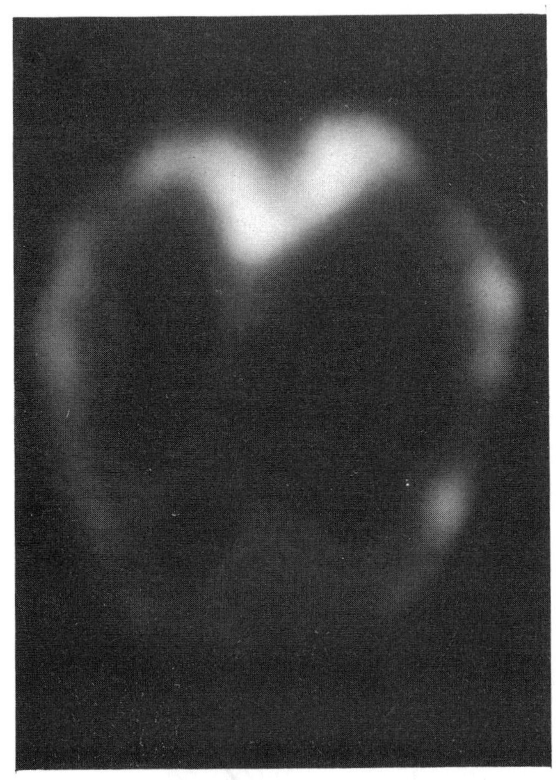

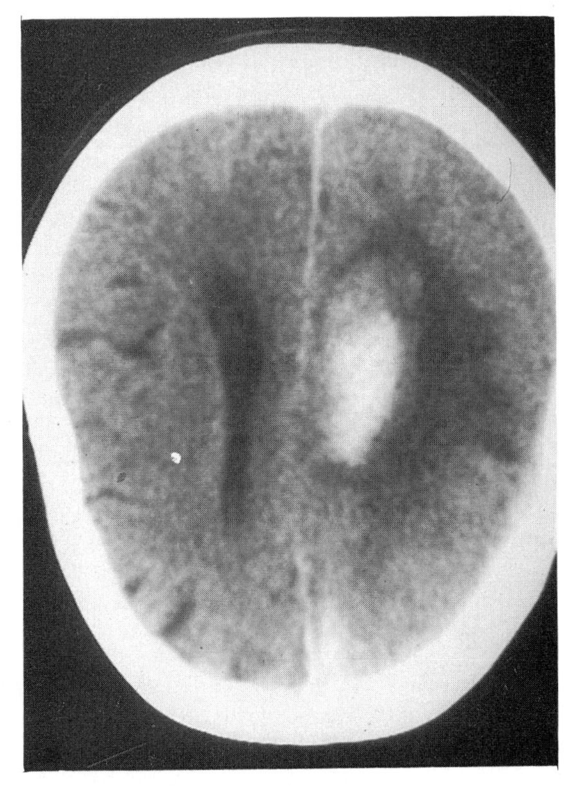

Figure 7.15 Clinical study with ^{99m}Tc-labelled ECD (cerebral haemorrhage).

uptake and significant urinary excretion. The compound is stable *in vitro* with a dosimetry more favourable than that of ^{99m}Tc-labelled HMPAO. The half-life of ECD in adult human brain is shorter than that of ^{99m}Tc-labelled HMPAO, and of the order of 24 h. Despite the more rapid wash-out from the brain, conventional gamma camera SPECT CBF can be carried out (Figures 7.14 and 7.15).

7.7 THE BLOOD–BRAIN BARRIER SCAN

7.7.1 PATIENT PREPARATION

Thirty minutes prior to a brain scan a patient is given orally 400 mg of sodium or potassium perchlorate. This will prevent ^{99m}Tc-pertechnetate from being taken up by the choroid plexus. Otherwise these normal intracerebral structures may be seen on the brain scan, leading to difficulties in image analysis. The effect of perchlorate is practically immediate, and no significant time interval is required between administration of perchlorate and of ^{99m}Tc-pertechnetate. Sodium perchlorate can be given intravenously (slowly) and may be mixed (in a single injection) with ^{99m}Tc-pertechnetate. This is not advisable whenever dynamic brain scanning is envisaged since the injected bolus is then diluted. Discharge of ^{99m}Tc-pertechnetate from normal salivary gland structures can be implemented by the administration of atropine. However, this is no longer in common practice and is restricted to scanning techniques where a vertex view is a routine projection in a complete study.

It is good practice to hydrate patients to increase urinary flow and reduce radiation exposure. Whenever possible, brain scanning should be performed prior to steroid therapy (which reduces tracer uptake in neoplasms and, by reducing oedema, in acute cardiovascular accidents). Visualization of the ventricles during routine brain scanning (apart from lack of administration of perchlorate) can be caused by anoxia, methotrexate administration, choroid plexus papilloma, tuberculosis or sometimes intraventricular haemorrhage.

7.7.2 TECHNIQUE

A brain scan should be performed in two stages: an initial gamma camera computer-processed dynamic study, followed by static imaging at appropriate time intervals after administration of the radioactive tracer.

7.7.3 DYNAMIC STUDY

Positioning of the patient must be optimized in accordance with the clinical problem. If frontal signs are present or the abnormality is thought to be anterior, then an anterior projection of the brain scan will be recorded. If the lesion is thought to be posterior (e.g. homonymous hemianopia), then a posterior projection is recorded. In cases of doubt, vertex views offer an alternative approach to this study (appropriate shielding of neck and shoulders is in this case mandatory) although the definition of neck vessels is lost. An attempt to give an intravenous bolus injection should be made. High specific activity ^{99m}Tc-pertechnetate is available today in most departments of nuclear medicine (eluted from fission ^{99m}Tc-generators) so that the volume of the radioactive tracer dose can be kept at or below 1 ml. The tracer is given in an antecubital vein (preferably in a basilic vein) and is rapidly flushed with 20–30 ml of saline. Alternatively, but less effectively, the Oldendorf injection technique can be used. A blood pressure cuff is inflated above the systolic arterial pressure and suddenly released. This will help the bolus to progress rapidly towards the right side of the heart; 15–20 mCi (555–740 MBq) of ^{99m}Tc-pertechnetate represents a commonly used dose. At the time of injection the gamma camera computer system is set up to record a 30 s to 1 min study. Two- or three-second images are usually recorded on transparent X-ray film. The computer can be set to take up any desirable frame rate (usually 0.5 s frames) and computer-processed images are chosen to correspond to the arterial phase of the dynamic brain study. Regions of interest are often chosen (for instance, over the middle cerebral arteries) and time–activity curves are recorded, providing information on cerebral perfusion. Separate carotid to brain transit times can be investigated and give useful complementary data (Figure 7.16).

7.7.4 STATIC BRAIN SCAN

For most purposes, one hour after the intravenous administration of the tracer static brain imaging is commenced. Routinely, four projections are recorded: anterior, posterior, right and left lateral views. Some institutions also record a vertex view. Usually 400 000 counts per view are collected. This takes between 4 min and 6 min per view, depending on the type of gamma camera collimation available. Often, the time to collect 400 000 counts is recorded in the first projection to be scanned. This time will then be applied to the exposure and counting of all remaining views (preset time imaging). This offers the advantage of comparability of scans recorded with slight variations in patient positioning. Modern instrumentation allows for setting up automatically information density (ID) per view and a statistically appropriate ID will be applied throughout the study (ID of 200–300 counts cm^{-2}).

In cases where image interpretation is doubtful, delayed scans are often taken. Improvement in the target to non-target distribution of the tracer will permit an improvement in lesion contrast. For a chronic subdural haemorrhage, static imaging should be performed late, preferably 4 h after intravenous administration of the tracer. Although large subdural haemorrhages may become visible on the scan earlier, it is advisable in cases of doubt to proceed with delayed imaging. Static images are recorded in a way that most of the counts collected in the scan represent photons emitted from the organ of interest. Masking of adjacent areas such as salivary structures, oropharynx and neck is sometimes performed. This, however, becomes unnecessary if preset time imaging or imaging based on information density per view is practised.

7.7.5 THE NORMAL BRAIN SCAN

In the dynamic gamma camera computer sequence, most often a series of anterior projections are recorded (Figure 7.17). Symmetrical arrival of the radioactive bolus is observed and both internal carotid arteries are defined. The middle cerebral arteries appear on either side of the brain, outlining the cerebral cortex. The anterior cerebral arteries, usually not individually resolved, appear as a single vascular structure in the mid-zone of the scan. After a brief capillary phase the venous structures become prominent with particular definition of the sagittal sinus. Often a symmetric and bilateral area of reduced intensity is seen in the lower third of both carotids, reflecting the absorption of ^{99m}Tc photons by the jaw.

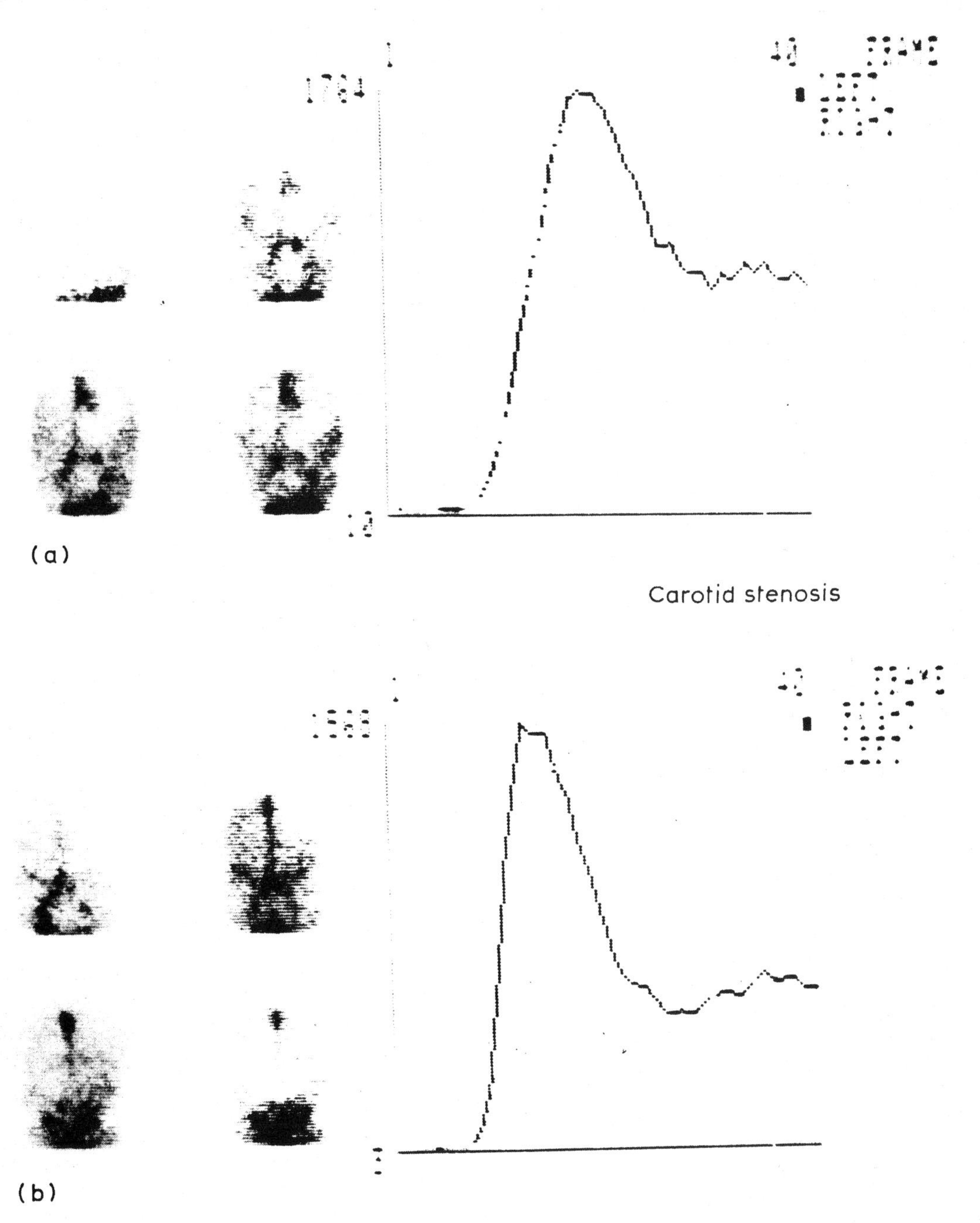

Figure 7.16 Dynamic brain study with $^{99m}TcO_4$.

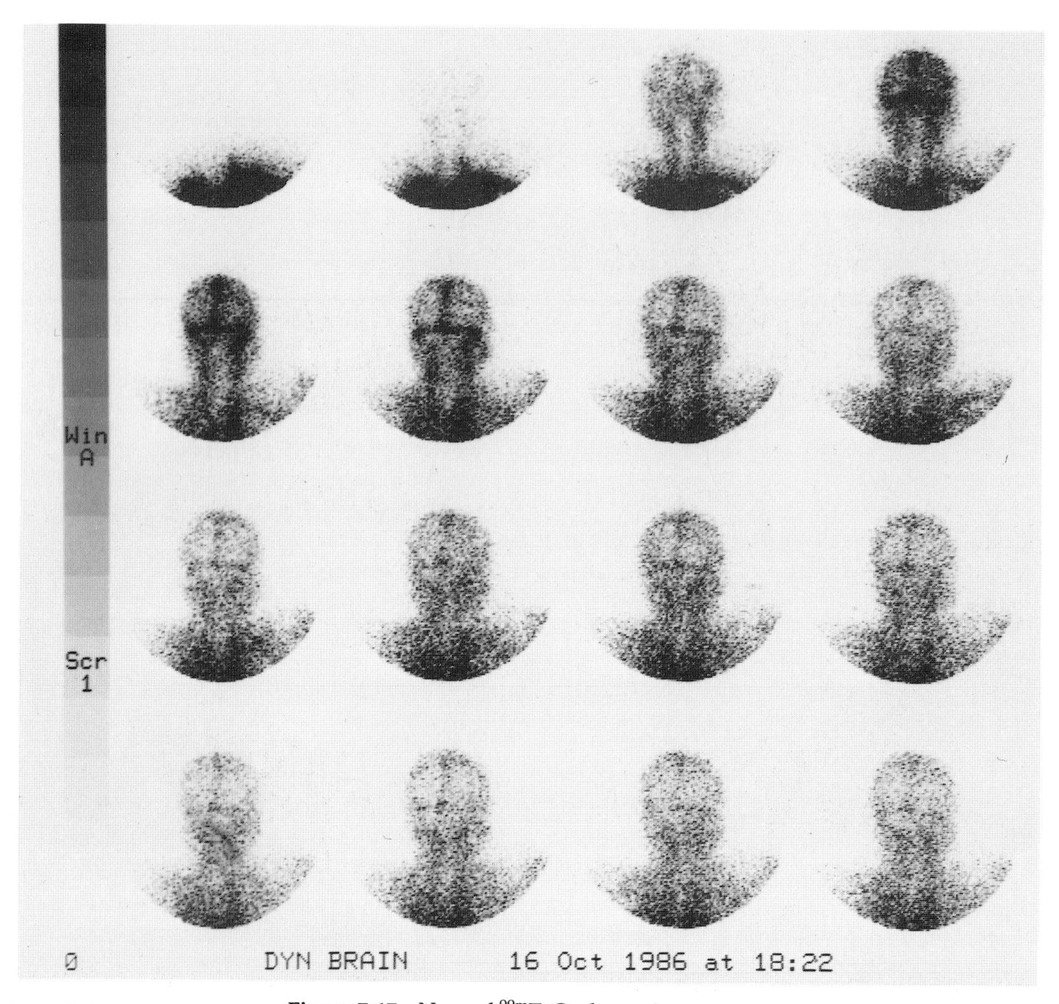

Figure 7.17 Normal $^{99m}TcO_4$ dynamic sequence.

At this stage of the recording of static brain scans the images mainly reflect the extracellular distribution of ^{99m}Tc-pertechnetate. The venous structures are prominent and are often the most important reference points for image interpretation: sagittal sinus, torcula, transverse sinus (Figure 7.18). Little radioactivity is seen in the brain cortex due to the integrity of the BBB, and the scan reflect the relative photon-free area of hemisphere and cerebellar tissue. The posterior and lateral projections show the posterior fossa and are most suited for the investigation of pathology in this area and in the cerebellopontine angle. Frontal, temporal and parietal lobes are best assessed in the anterior and lateral projections. Traditionally a number of areas in the brain scan are difficult for the observer. These include the base of the brain, the pituitary fossa, and often even the posterior fossa. Cross-sectional imaging of the brain by computerized emission tomography helps to interpret the pathology in these areas (Figure 7.19). A dominant transverse sinus may lead to asymmetric activity distribution in the posterior projection. Temporal muscle activity is sometimes difficult to distinguish from temporal lobe activity and care must be taken in reporting the pathology in these regions. Once again, emission tomography is of considerable help here.

7.7.6 THE ABNORMAL BRAIN SCAN

Breakdown in the BBB which accompanies space-occupying disease of the brain leads to hot-spot detection of lesions in brain scanning. From the

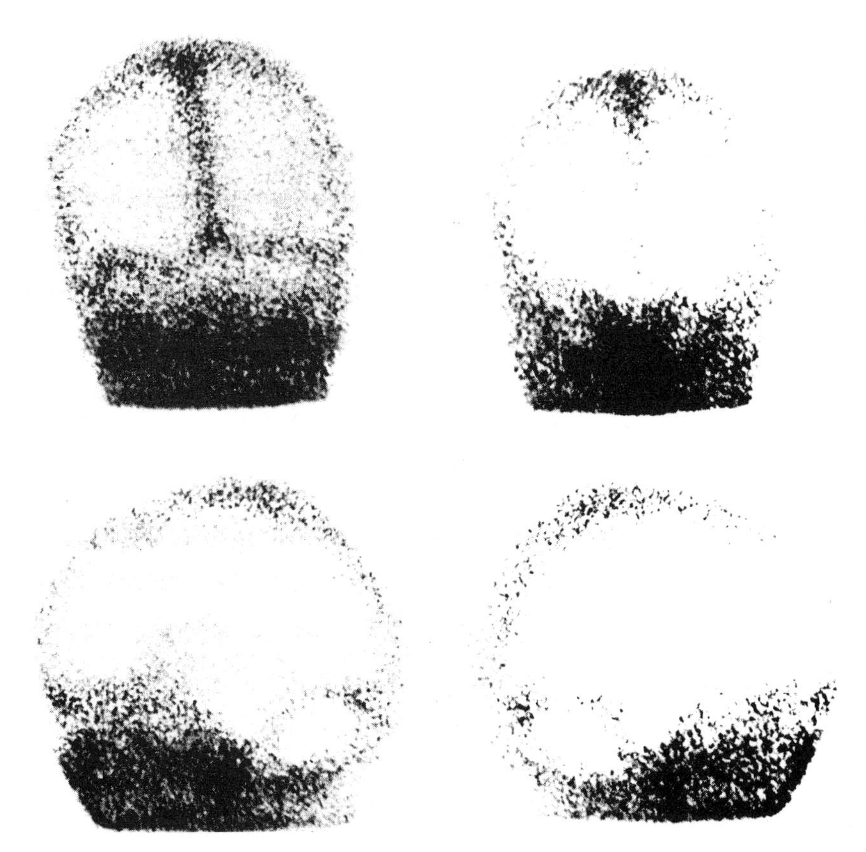

Figure 7.18 The normal $^{99m}TcO_4$ static brain scan.

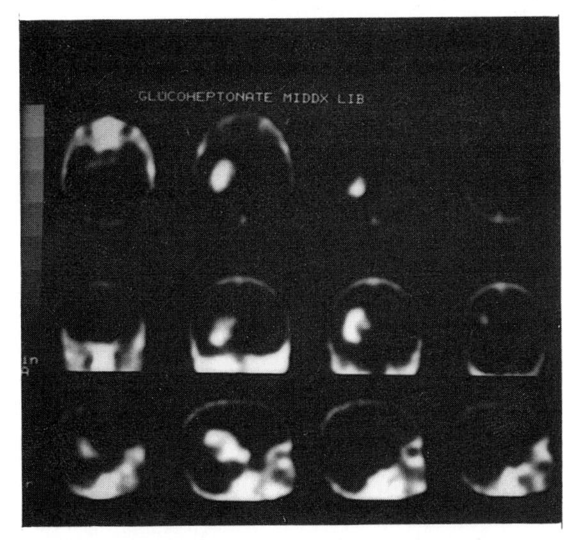

Figure 7.19 A $^{99m}TcO_4$ BBB/SPECT study. Transverse (top row), coronal (middle row) and sagittal (bottom row) sections. Malignant studies.

timing of tracer uptake in the lesions, shape and positioning of these, and their behaviour with time, progress has been made in the pattern recognition of pathology in this organ. It is, however, clear that the brain scan, although highly sensitive, loses specificity in the areas of finer differential diagnosis.

7.7.7 NEOPLASMS (PRIMARY OR SECONDARY BRAIN TUMOURS)

Breakdown of the BBB, increased neovascularity within neoplasms (e.g. meningiomas) increased protein binding (e.g. astrocytomas) and other mechanisms leading to increased tracer concentration of ^{99m}Tc-pertechnetate in the peritumoral extracellular fluid explain the high sensitivity of lesion detection of brain scanning. A number of neoplasms, however, are known to escape easy visualization by these techniques. They include the tumours of the pituitary, the ependymomas

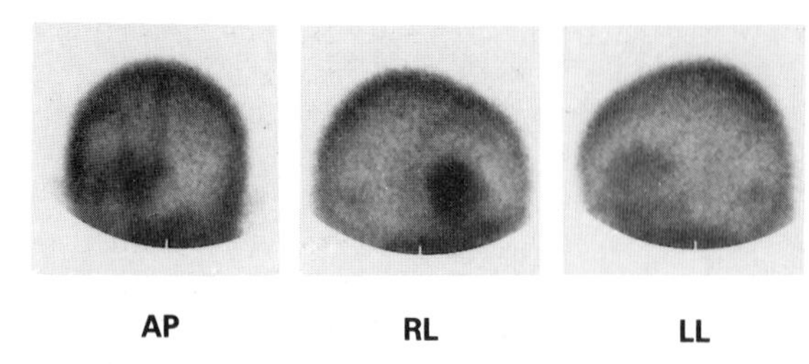

Figure 7.20 $^{99m}TcO_4$ BBB study: brain tumour.

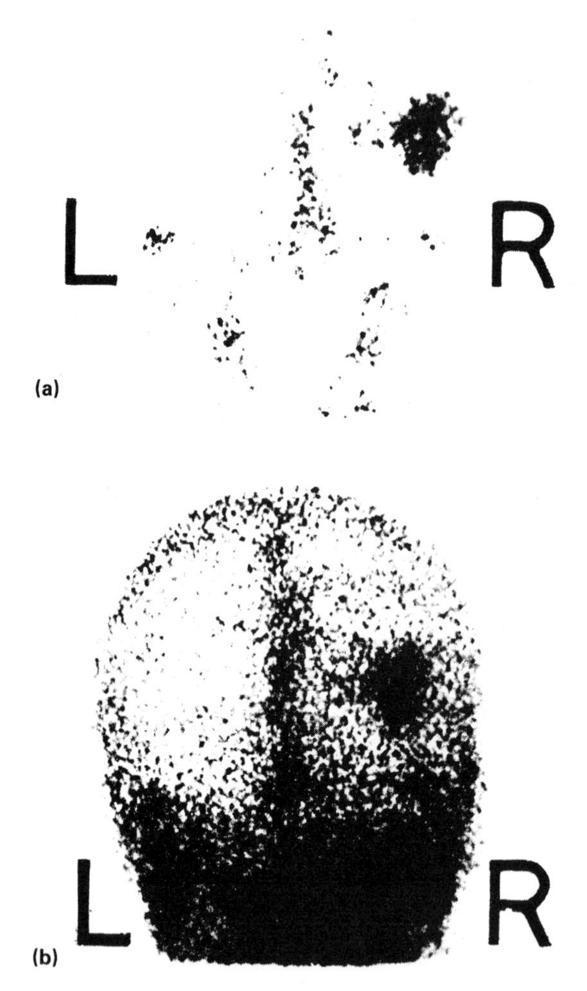

Figure 7.21 $^{99m}TcO_4$ BBB dynamic study: Brain tumour.

and craniopharyngiomas, and low-grade oligodendrogliomas, or even astrocytomas. Lesions with little cellular activity, such as cysts, will not be seen on the brain scan due to lack of tracer uptake.

A neoplasm appears on the brain scan as an area of increased concentration (hot spot), usually round in shape, with regular and defined borders (Figure 7.20). The distribution of the tracer does not follow any arterial distribution and the location of the abnormality may give indications as to the nature of the lesion (e.g. meningiomas classically in the vicinity of the meninges; falx, sphenoid wing, and brain secondaries, classically multiple and often in the posterior fossa). On the brain scan the differential diagnosis of cerebrovascular disease is facilitated by the negative image of the brain scan a few days after infarction. The degree of vascularity of a neoplasm can be assessed with the initial dynamic brain scan study (Figure 7.21), where an initial but persistent vascular flush usually indicates the presence of a meningioma. Classically, cerebral secondaries remain silent during the initial dynamic brain scan work-up. So-called doughnut signs, reflecting an area of reduced tracer uptake (cold spots) surrounded by increased tracer concentration (figure 7.22), are most often associated with tumours with central necrosis, or even with cerebral abscesses (it was once thought that the doughnut shape was characteristic of the latter). Low-grade and infiltrating tumours are often difficult to visualize on the brain scan. Skull and brain secondaries can be easily differentiated with SPECT/BBB imaging. The anatomy at the base of the brain and its normal structures are also better visualized by this means (Tables 7.5 and 7.6).

It is interesting to look back to conventional brain scanning in the era before radiographic CT, and this has been well documented by George and Wagner (1975), whose data are summarized in Table 7.7. These authors also showed that although brain imaging increased tenfold the mortality rate of patients diagnosed changed little. Nevertheless, they argued that the reduction in morbidity was important for the

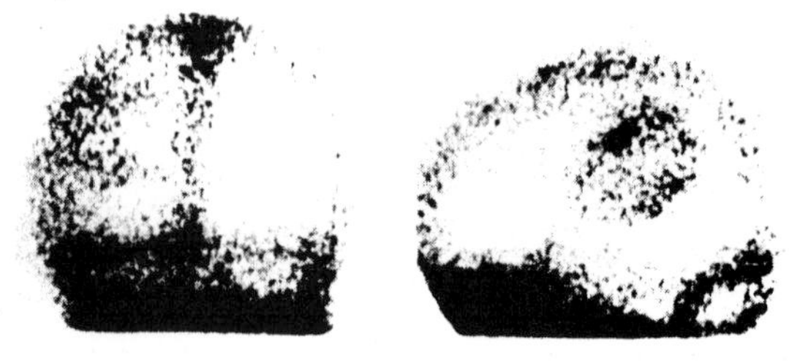

Figure 7.22 $^{99m}TcO_4$ BBB study: brain tumour and doughnut sign.

Table 7.5 A comparison of radiographic CT and ECAT

	CT	*ECAT*
Apparatus	Transmission	Emission
Result	Differential attenuation of X-rays by different tissues	Distribution, uptake and quantity of γ rays
Information	Structure	Distribution of function
Advantage	Good anatomical and pathological detail	Normal and abnormal distribution of function
Disadvantages	Poor estimate of function Reactions to contrast media High radiation Cost	Poor structural detail Requires radiopharmaceuticals Education gap

Table 7.6 Brain imaging: conventional scanner, gamma camera (GC), ECAT, and radiographic transmission tomography, (TCAT) compared

	True-positives		*True-negatives*	
Scanner	83/140	59%	363/372	98%
ECAT	107/140	76%	367/372	99%
			(Carril *et al.*, 1979)	
GC	42/62	68%	133/138	96%
ECAT	48/62	77%	137/138	99%
TCAT	26/35	74%	43/47	91%
		(Hill, Lovett and McNeil, 1980)		
ECAT	182/209	87%	37/37	100%
TCAT	196/209	94%	36/37	97%
		(Ell, Deacon and Jarritt, 1980)		

Diagnosis of subdural

	Present	*Equivocal*	*Missed*	*Total*	*Correct*
GC	22	1	2	25	92%
TCAT	13	7 (shift only)	5	25	80%

(Razzak, Mudarris and Christie, 1980)

following reasons: the earlier excision of benign tumours; the more accurate staging of cancer through the demonstration of metastases; the importance of a normal study reducing the need for invasive investigation especially in children; its accuracy in the detection of brain abscess; and the increased detection rate when serial scanning is undertaken. Since the advent of radiographic CT the accuracy of diagnosis of brain lesions has been further improved and in most cases the nature of the pathology is evident, particularly when contrast medium is given intravenously, although this latter addition gives a mortality rate to this otherwise non-invasive procedure.

The reliability of static rectilinear brain imaging for cerebral lesions has been reviewed by Boucher and Sear (1980) over a ten-year period. Out of 2120 scans, 2036 were correctly negative (96%). Carril *et al.* (1979) showed that 363 out of 372 brain scans were correctly negative (98%). The low false-negative rate is the basis of a cost-effective strategy using the brain scan to assess patients whose result is likely to be normal; and using radiographic CT scanning primarily for those patients likely to show brain pathology or who have had equivocal brain scans. The equivocal radiographic CT or when its result conflicts with the clinical findings are indications for brain scanning before more invasive procedures are undertaken.

The discrepancy between the accuracy of brain scanning and CT scanning was most evident shortly after the technique was introduced, when its results were compared with those of conventional brain scanning performed on low-performance gamma cameras (see, for example, De Boulay and Marshall, 1975). In that series the extra success was mainly in conditions in which no change in management follows diagnosis. The radiographic CT includes a computer and should

Table 7.7 Brain tumour scanning at Johns Hopkins 1962–72: comparative accuracy at presentation

	Brain scanning (%)	*Angiography (%)*	*Air studies (%)*
Frontal tumours	77	82	70
Temporal tumours	81	100	83
Parietal tumours	91	89	94
Occipital tumours	90	86	Not done
Cerebellopontine angle tumours	95	57	80
Thalamic, sellar and parasellar tumours	60	84	92
Cerebellar tumours	53	53	91
Pontine tumours	25	80	78
Metastases any site	74	75	65
Overall accuracy	77	84	88

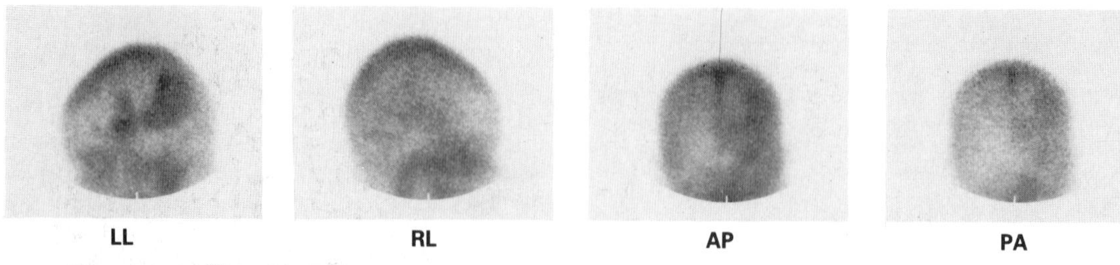

Figure 7.23 ^{99m}Tc-labelled GH study: acute stroke. Predominant posterior cerebral artery territory.

be compared with brain scanning with quantitative computer analysis. However, when brain scanning with SPECT is compared with radiographic CT, the accuracies of each are similar (Ell *et al.*, 1980).

7.7.8 CEREBROVASCULAR DISEASE

Following a stroke the characteristic appearance in the brain scan, due to cerebral infarction, is of an area of increased activity, usually wedge-shaped, with more or less well-defined borders and in the territory of one of the major vessels of arterial supply (usually the middle cerebral, followed by the anterior or posterior cerebral arteries) (Figure 7.23). It is important to understand the time relationship between the time of onset and appearance of a positive brain scan. For the first few days of a stroke (up to one week), the brain scan usually remains silent and this does help in the differential diagnosis between neoplasia or stroke.

Positive uptake, as described above, is seen for a period of one to two weeks, after which the brain scan tends to normalize again. This evolution with time is also helpful in differential diagnosis (serial scanning). In the dynamic brain scan typical appearances are usually seen. In the arterial phase a delay and/or reduction or absence of perfusion is seen leading to the site of the lesion, whereas in the venous phase excess perfusion of the site of the lesion may lead to an image with increased tracer uptake (flip-flop sign).

Watershed infarction also has typical appearances on the brain scan. The ^{99m}Tc-pertechnetate uptake is extensive, diffuse, and occupies large areas of the brain between the major supply vessels. Small areas of infarction (lacunar strokes and transient ischaemic attacks) often remain silent on the brain scan; the differential diagnosis between haemorrhage and infarction remains the domain of computerized X-ray transmission

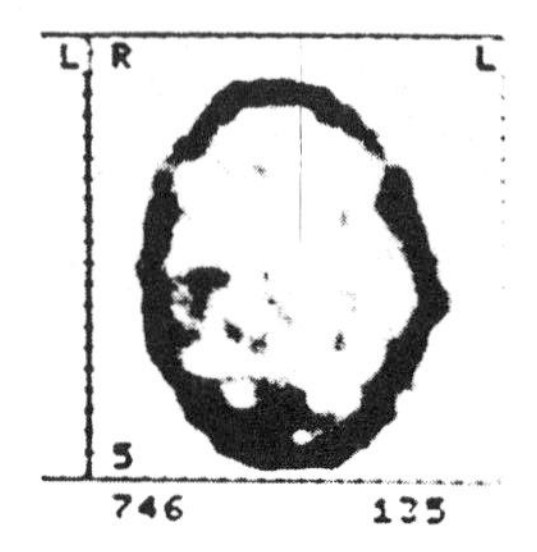

Figure 7.24 ^{99m}Tc-labelled GH SPECT study: acute stroke, light sided, wedge shaped area, in a typical vascular territory.

tomography. Figure 7.24 shows the typical appearance of a cerebrovascular accident on a SPECT/BBB brain scan.

7.7.9 CHRONIC SUBDURAL HAEMATOMA

The story of an old lady presenting with deteriorating mental and social behaviour who cannot remember the fall she had a few weeks before is well known, but still the diagnosis of chronic subdural haemorrhage may not be made and she be confined to an institution. Signs of local head injury and lateralizing neurological signs, the dilated pupil on the side of the subdural haemorrhage and contralateral hemiparesis may or may not be present. When bilateral subdural haemorrhage occurs the clinical signs may be of raised intracranial pressure, paticularly in children.

Investigation usually commences with a skull radiograph to seek for pineal shift from the midline and possible fracture. A brain scan should be undertaken starting with a dynamic study in the anterior view where a lens-shaped absence of flow will be seen peripherally demarcated by the skull activity and the flow in the compressed brain. This is followed by a static study at 20 min showing a crescent sign (Figure 7.25) which must be re-

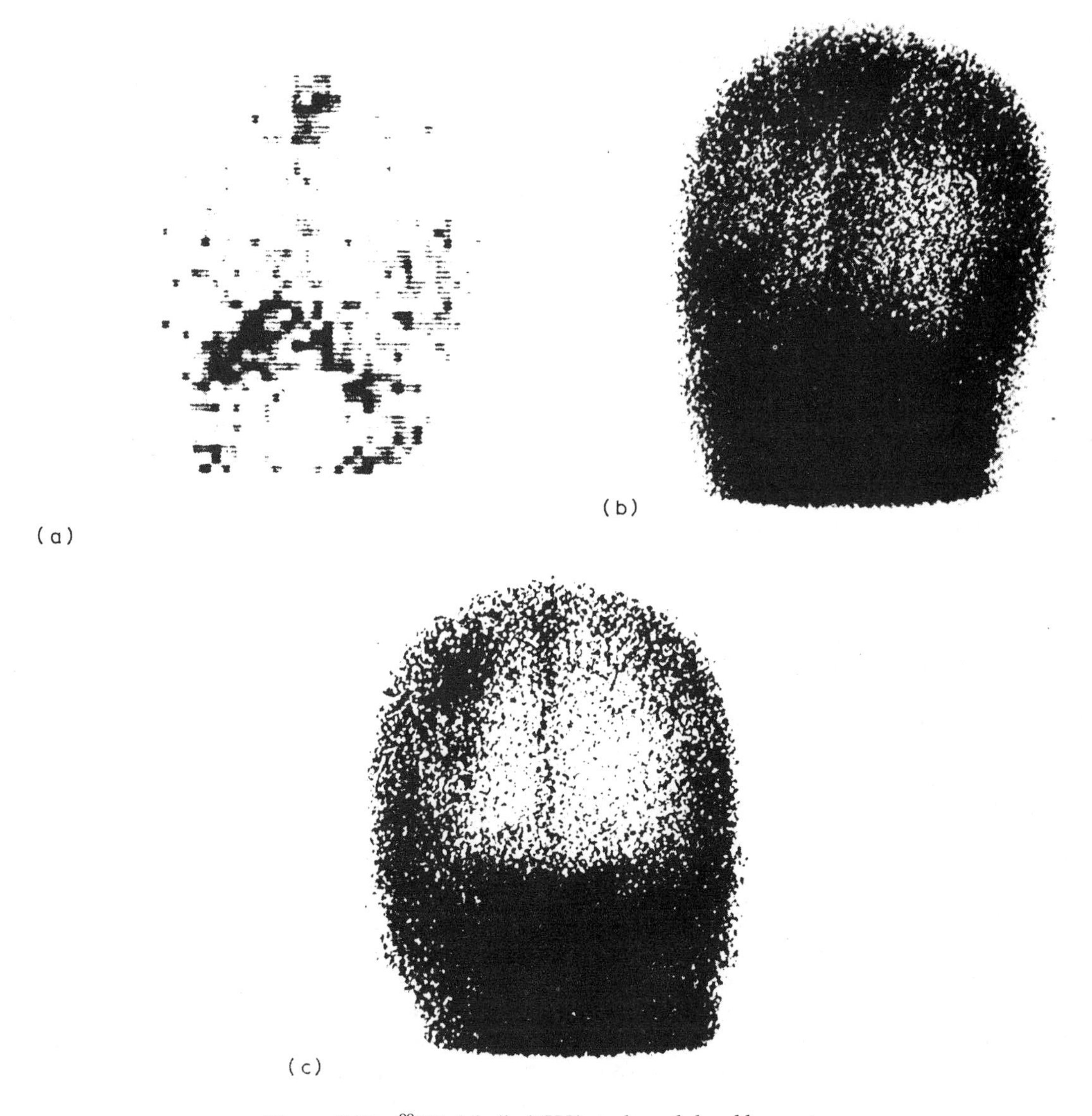

Figure 7.25 ^{99m}Tc-labelled GH* study: subdural haematoma.

peated after 4 h or more. The progressive filling of the crescent with time is strong evidence of subdural haemorrhage as the pertechnetate permeates into the subdural collection. SPECT is very helpful in confirming these findings. Radiographic CT should also be done in parallel, although some chronic subdural haemorrhages are missed because they contain liquid blood of similar attenuation properties to brain, but the combination is more accurate than either test alone (Razzak *et al.*, 1980). The brain scan is particularly difficult to interpret when there is lateral movement or rotation of the patient's head due to lack of cooperation.

Differential diagnosis of the image of a chronic subdural haemorrhage, although rarely in the demented, includes other subdural collections, in particular lymphoma or leukaemia en plaque, subdural pus complicating meningitis and rarely granuloma such as Wegener's. In the acute subdural a brain scan is difficult to interpret because of scalp oedema, blood clot and/or skull fracture and is not recommended. Radiographic CT is the investigation of choice in head injury.

7.7.10 CEREBRAL ABSCESSES

Infection of the brain leading to focal areas of abscess can be visualized with brain scanning techniques with high sensitivity of detection. The previously mentioned doughnut appearance of tracer uptake very frequently is associated with a cerebral abscess and remains a useful clinical sign. It is, however, not typical and may be associated with lesions other than infection (mainly tumours with central cellular necrosis).

7.7.11 THE FALSE-POSITIVE BRAIN SCAN

False-positive brain scans usually are readily recognized. Artefacts due to malposition, choroid plexus uptake, uptake in the vicinity of surgical flaps (usually less than six months old) and superficial trauma to the head all may lead to abnormal looking images. However, examination of the patient and knowledge of previous history and present symptoms permits the differential recognition of most of these image patterns.

7.7.12 THE ^{133}Xe CBF STUDY (PLANAR APPROACH)

Inert gases and an inhalation method were used by Kety and Schmidt (1945) to measure CBF. Nitrous oxide was used and blood sampling (arterial from a peripheral artery, and venous from an internal jugular vein) carried out. Lassen and Munck in 1955 used radioactive ^{85}Kr and Ingvar and Lassen (1961) introduced the intra-arterial carotid ^{133}Xe method. Mallet and Veall (1965) developed the practical application of this approach, using an intravenous or inhalation technique.

The patient is studied supine, or sitting on a chair, in an erect position. The detector pairs are placed in contact with the surface of the skull and, depending on their number, aimed at the frontal, temporal, parietal or occipital lobes. A gas mask is applied to the patient, and inhalation of ^{133}Xe for approximately 1 min is carried out. The ^{133}Xe supply is then switched off, and after the inhalation period the decreasing (wash-out) activity from the brain is recorded over a 10 min period. ^{133}Xe is also measured from the gas mask. A two-compartment model and a simple computer program will then permit the calculation of CBF values (see section on Methodology).

In baseline studies, the patient should be made to feel at ease, the simple procedure explained, and lighting and noise levels kept to a minimum (without sensory deprivation).

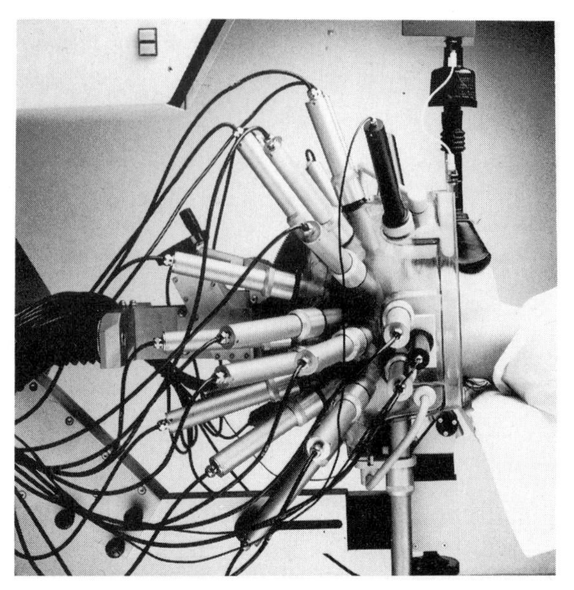

Figure 7.26 Helmet ^{133}Xe CBF approach.

From an instrumentation point of view, simple portable detectors have developed over the years. Systems with two detectors on one side of the spectrum and systems with 254 detectors on the other side of the spectrum have been assembled. The two- to ten-detector systems are eminently easy to use and crude bedside measurements can be carried out, and studies in the coronary care unit, intensive therapy unit and operating theatre have been applied to patients. More complex arrangements have included the helmet configuration, with close packing of detectors surrounding the brain and skull (Figure 7.26). The 254-detector system leads to the recording of ^{133}Xe CBF maps and appears promising as a method for intervention studies (Figure 7.27 and 7.28) (Risberg, 1987).

Whilst the intra-arterial (intracarotid) method is invasive and has been largely replaced by the inhalation method, several improvements have been carried out in order to improve the reliability of the method. This includes correction for scattered radiation from air passages, correction for background activity from previous studies and curve-fit indices (Risberg 1987). With these improvements, measurements can be made every 20 min, in view of the favourable dosimetry characteristics of ^{133}Xe. The inhalation approach to the measurement of CBF with ^{133}Xe remains non-

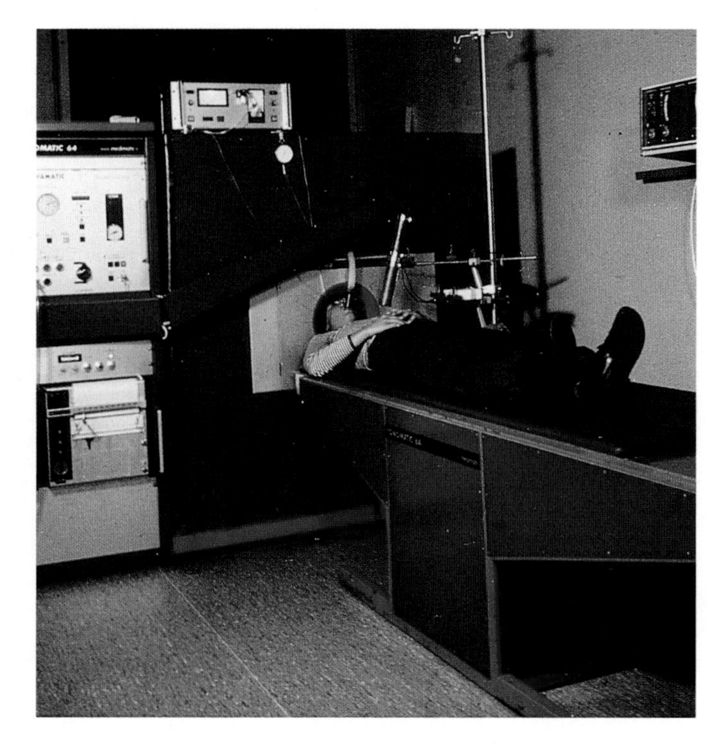

Plate 1 Rapid tomographic brain scanner optimized for ^{133}Xe.

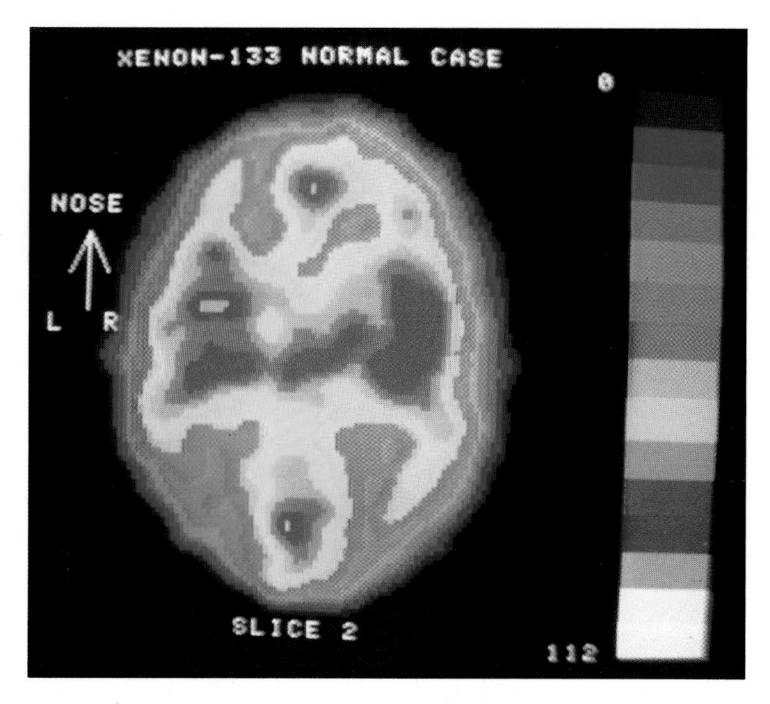

Plate 2 ^{133}Xe SPECT CBF study: normal.

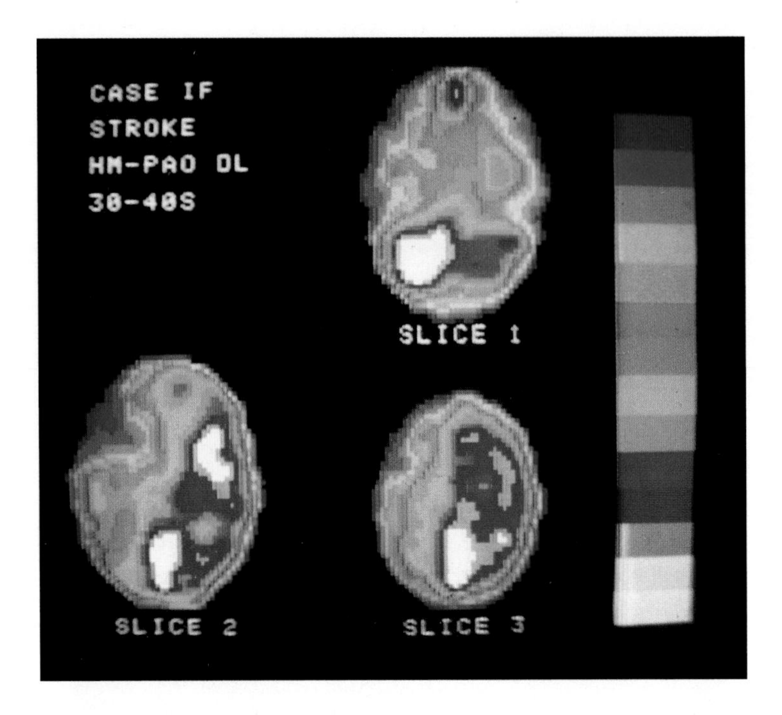

Plate 3 ^{133}Xe SPECT CBF study: stroke.

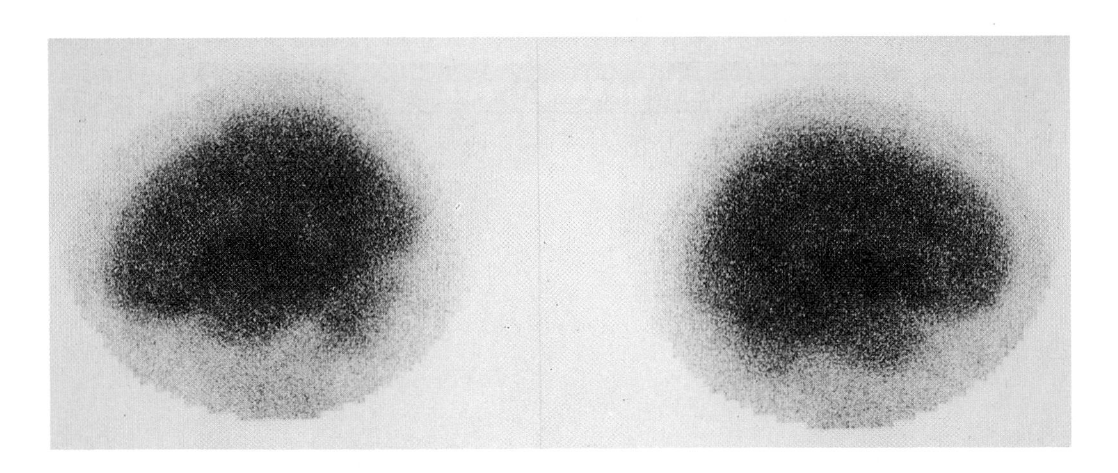

LT. Lateral **RT. Lateral**

Plate 4 Planar ^{123}I-IMP: normal study.

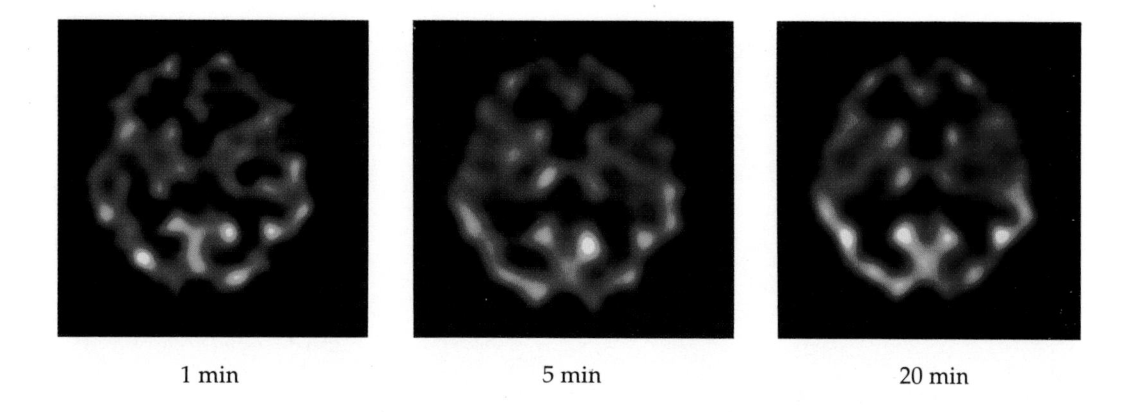

Plate 5 ^{99m}Tc-labelled HMPAO: 1 min, 5 min, 20 min study in subdural haematoma with dedicated scanner.

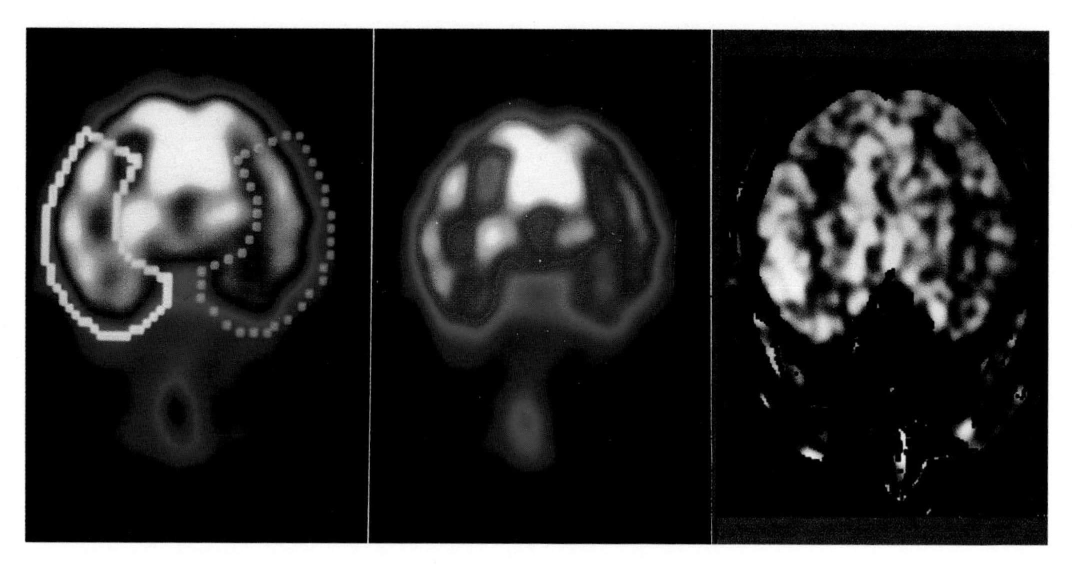

Plate 6 SPECT ^{99m}Tc-labelled HMPAO: epilepsy in optimal temporal lobe plane reconstruction. Comparative study with Xe-enhanced CT. Impaired CBF in left temporal lobe.

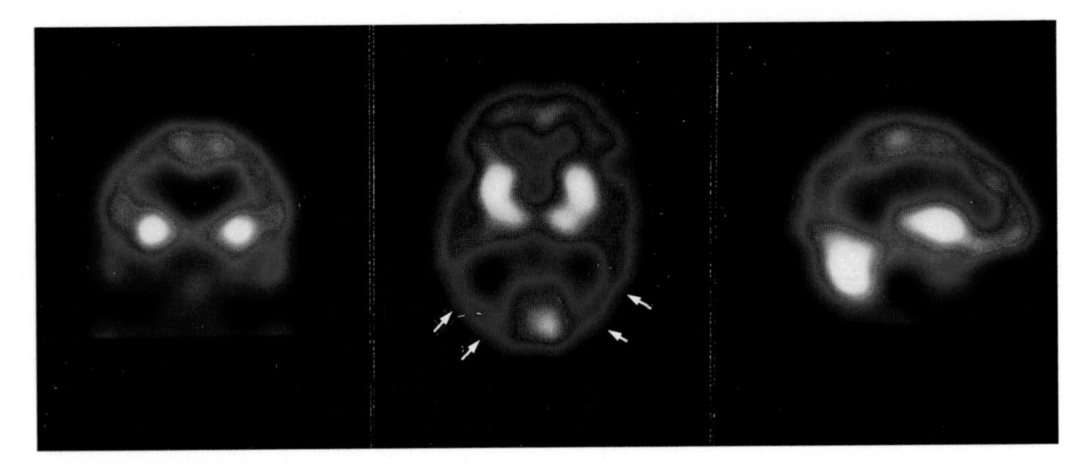

Plate 7 Typical SPECT ^{99m}Tc-labelled HMPAO SDAT. Bilateral temporoparietal loss of CBF (arrows).

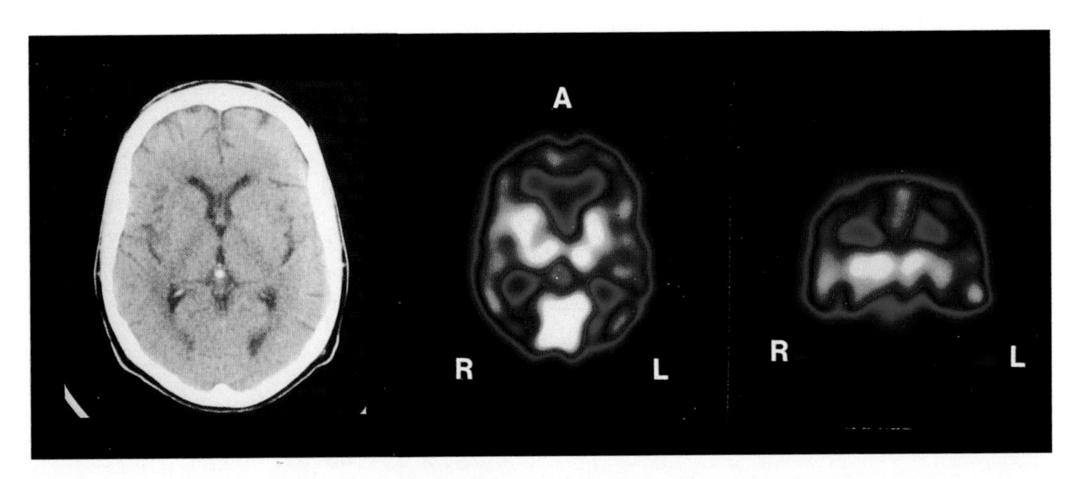

Plate 8 ^{99m}Tc-labelled HMPAO SPECT study in AIDS. Normal CT study. Impaired CBF in temporal and parietal lobes.

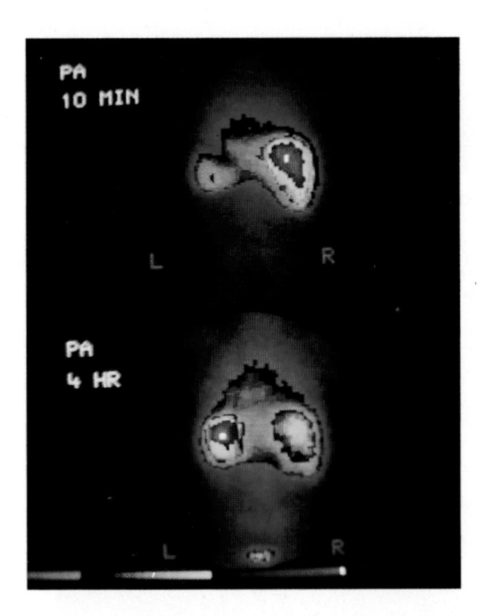

Plate 9 RIS of neuroblastoma using radioiodinated UJ13A in a 4-year-old child. Posterior abdominal images at 10 min and 4 h with ^{123}I-labelled UJ13A. At 4 h the tumour is evident as a focal area of high uptake (red) in contrast to the spleen and liver (green).

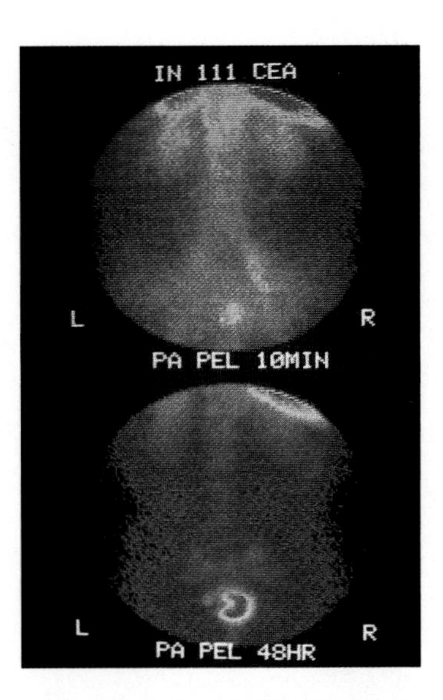

Plate 10 RIS with ^{111}In-labelled anti-CEA monoclonal antibody, in a rectal adenocarcinoma. Posterior abdominal views at top, 10 min; and bottom, 48 h. Slight vascularity is seen at 10 min in the pelvis while at 48 h shows uptake as a reverse 'C' in the pelvis with a small focal area of uptake to its left, probably in lymph nodes. Normal vascular activity is seen at 10 min, and renal but not urinary activity, high liver, spleen and marrow uptake on both views.

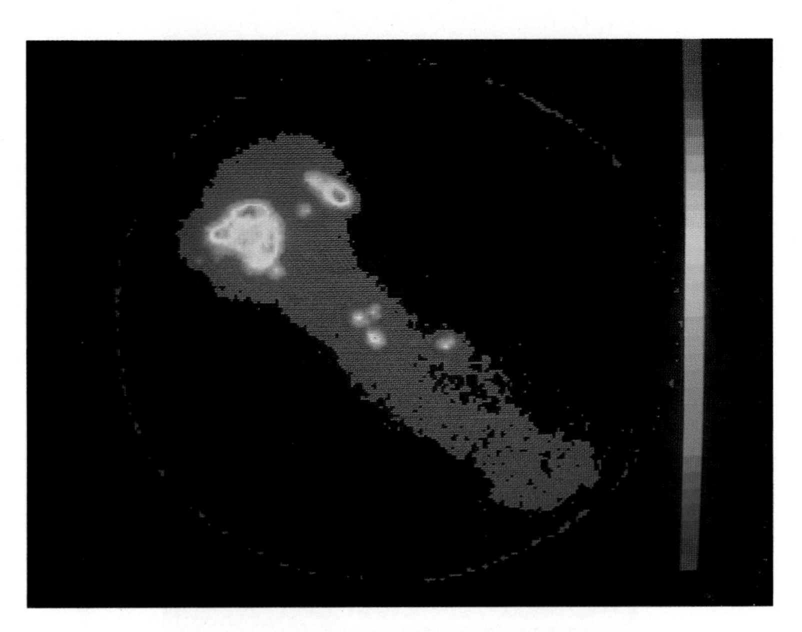

Plate 11 RIS with ^{111}In-labelled anti-CEA monoclonal antibody, in a rectal adenocarcinoma. Image of the surgical specimen taken at 72 h showing uptake in the tumour in red and yellow (the cut is made opposite to the mesentery to display the bowel lumen, hence the tumour has been divided) and uptake in lymph nodes. Note none of these lymph nodes contained tumour cells on histology (Dukes, B., see text).

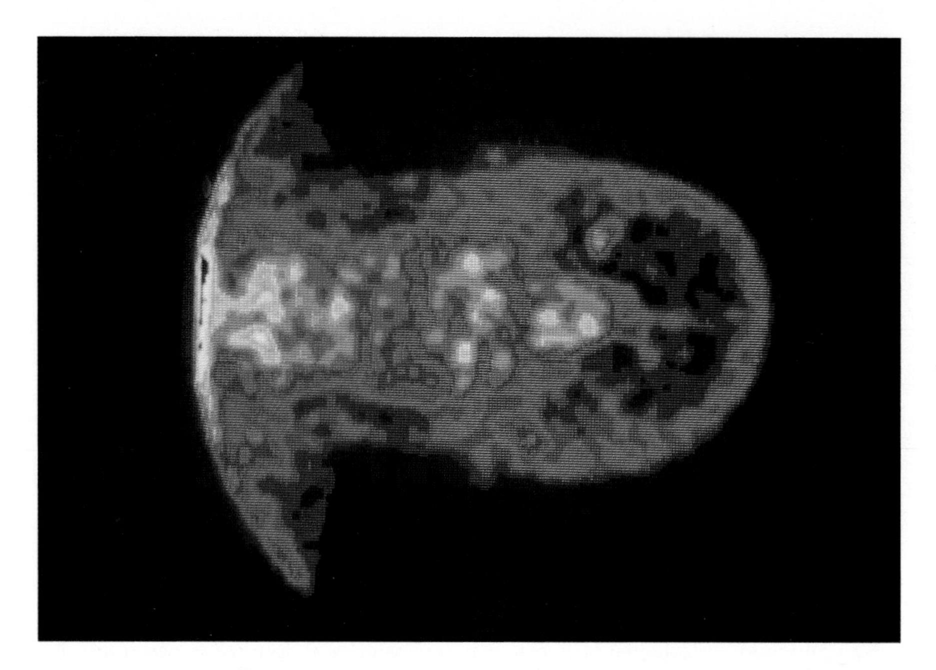

Plate 12 RIS with ^{99m}Tc-labelled $F(ab')_2$ anti-high-molecular-weight melanoma antigen, 225.22S monoclonal antibody. Tilted anterior view to show the orbits taken at 6 h after injection. A focal area of increased uptake is seen in the right orbit at the site of the 5 mm diameter ocular melanoma confirmed at operation. The left orbit is normal. Nasal and vascular activity is seen centrally. (Courtesy Dr Jamshed Bomarji.)

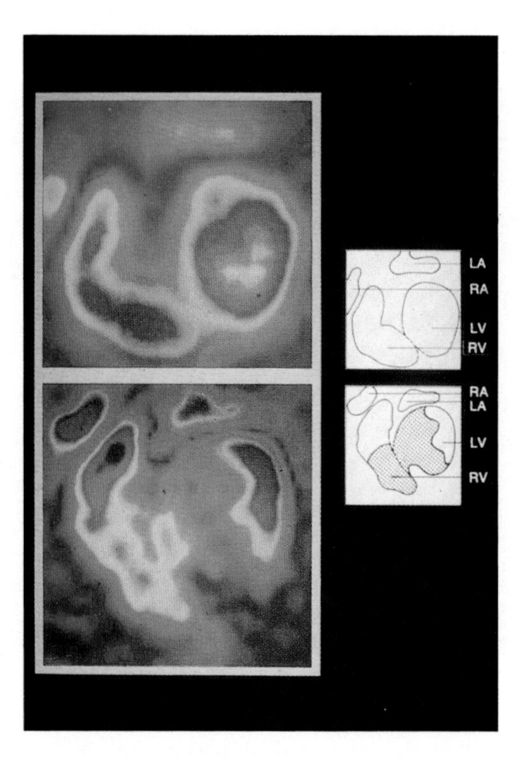

Plate 13 Amplitude image from gated myocardial study; upper panel is normal result, lower panel shows myocardial infarct affecting shaded portion of LV and RV. (courtesy Prof. P.J. Ell, UCMSM, London)

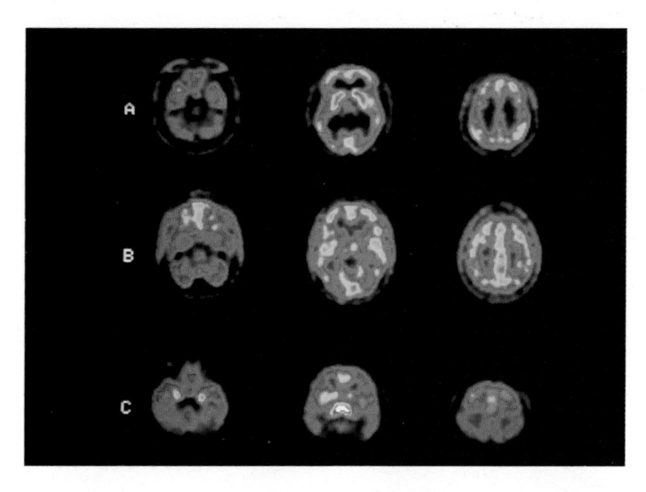

Plates 14A-C Receptor sites which have been imaged with PET include: A, dopamine D2 sites imaged with ^{11}C-N-methylspiperone; B, benzodiazepine sites with ^{11}C-suriclone; and C, opiate sites with ^{11}C-carfentanil. Each row of images shows three slices of the human brain. (Used with permission from J. James Frost (1986) *Trends in Pharmacological Sciences,* Elsevier Science Publishers, Amsterdam, December, pp. 490-6.)

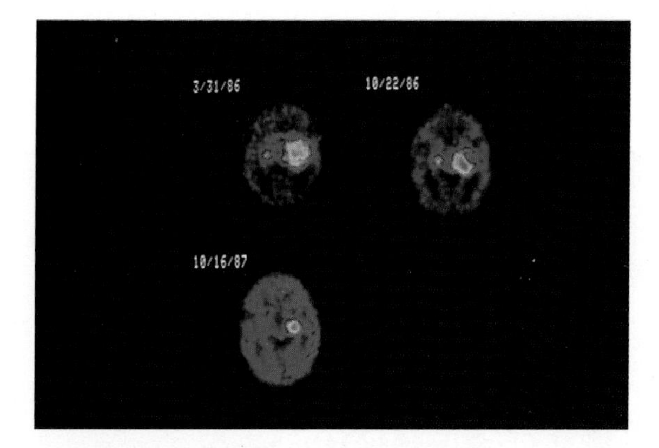

Plate 15 ^{11}C-Methionine concentrates in metabolically active brain tumours and was used in this patient to follow improvement during a course of chemotherapy.

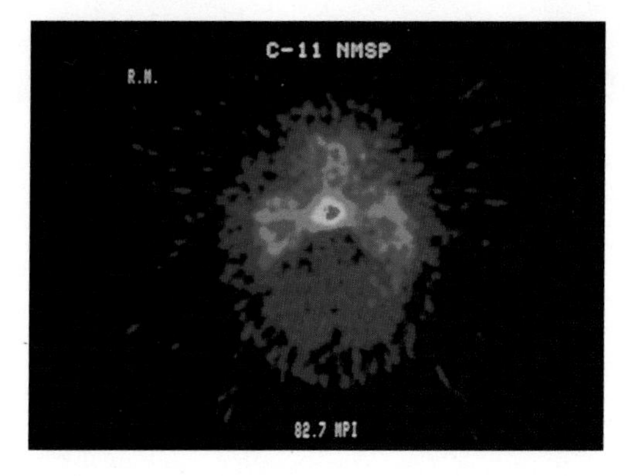

Plate 16 ^{11}C-N-Methylspiperone concentrates in a pituitary adenoma which contains dopamine receptors.

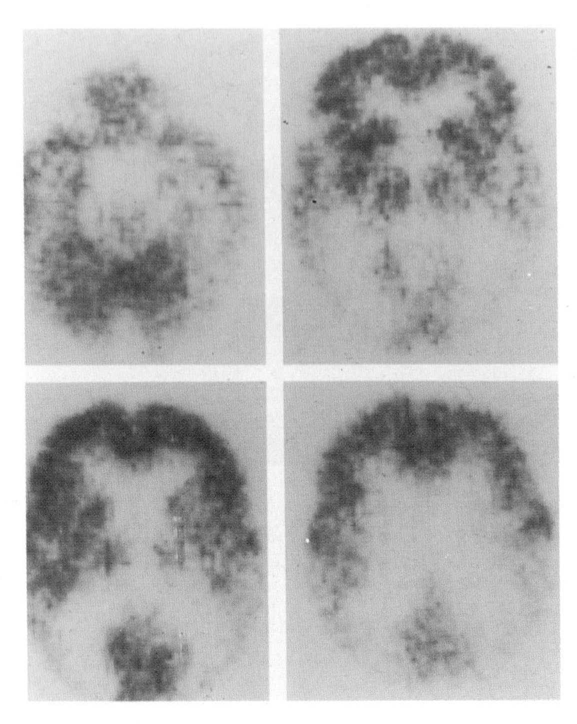

Plate 17 A ^{18}F-fluorodeoxy-D-glucose study in a patient with Alzheimer's disease.

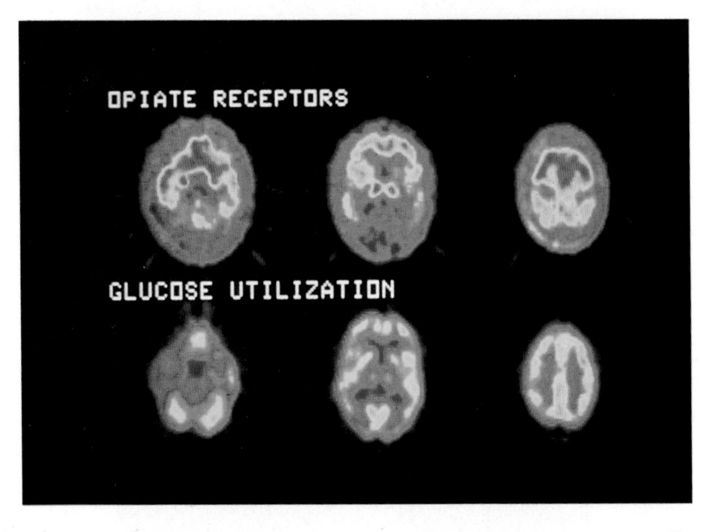

Plate 18 In a patient with epilepsy there is an increased concentration of ^{11}C-carfentanil, indicating increased opiate receptor binding, in the left temporal lobe and decreased utilization of ^{18}F-FDG in the same area, which is the seizure focus. (Used with permission from J. James Frost (1988) *Ann. Neurol.*, **23**, 231-7.)

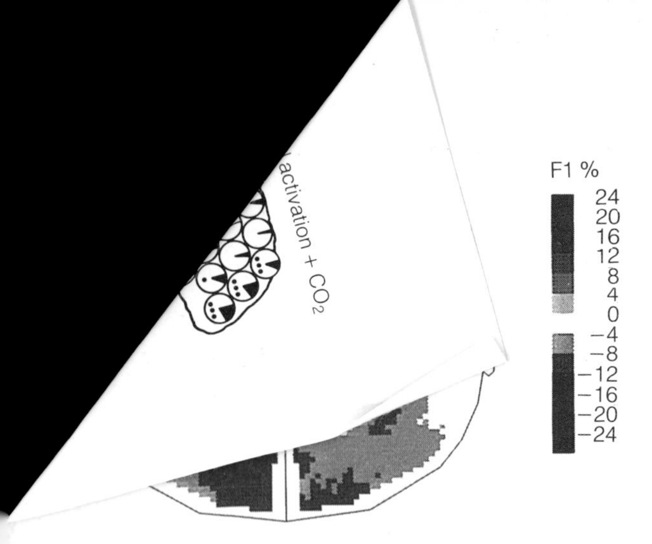

Figure 7.27 ^{133}Xe CBF maps with 254-detector system (resting).

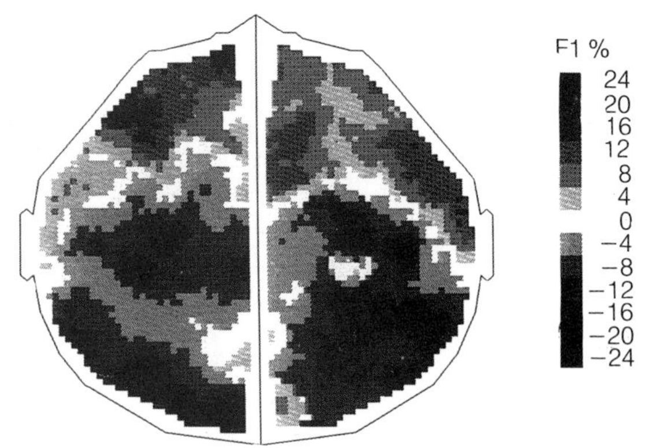

Figure 7.28 ^{133}Xe CBF maps with 254-detector system (talking).

invasive and simple, quantitative, portable and inexpensive. Relative disadvantages of the method include poor spatial resolution, absent depth discrimination and significant cross-talk from opposing areas of the brain.

With the ^{133}Xe planar approach to CBF analysis, a large body of data has emerged from the literature of the 1960s and 1970s. In general terms, the method appears more successful in the evaluation of dominant cortical flow than in the evaluation of the slower component of blood flow in white matter and deeper subcortical regions of the brain. The repeatability of the method allows a variety of intervention studies to be carried out (visual stimulation, mental activation, etc.), hence the extensive application in the areas of psychiatry, neuropsychology and comparative psychometric assessment of the individual patient. Resting values of CBF have been extensively investigated (Risberg *et al.*, 1977; Maximilian *et al.*, 1978; Prohovnik *et al.*, 1980). In normal subjects and with this planar method, there is a symmetrical distribution of CBF values (Figures 7.29–7.32).

Ingvar and Risberg (1965, 1967), using the intracarotid method, demonstrated increased CBF in response to mental stimulation. Still with the intra-arterial method, response to sensory, motor and complex mental activity with an increase in CBF has been documented by Olesen (1971), Ingvar (1975), Lassen *et al.* (1977), Risberg and Ingvar (1972). With the inhalation method, CBF changes in relation to mental activity were first demonstrated by Risberg *et al.* (1975).

The same group has led the application of this method to the investigation of dementia. With ^{133}Xe, it was first shown that there is a good correlation between areas of cortical atrophy and regions of reduced CBF (Gustafson *et al.*, 1977), that there is generalized reduction of CBF and localized parietal CBF impairment in Alzheimer's disease, and that the CBF abnormalities in Pick's disease (predominantly frontal) and in multi-infarction dementia (multi-focal) can be distinguished with reasonable sensitivity (Risberg, 1987). Impairment of the flow response to mental-activation in patients with dementia was also demonstrated (Ingvar *et al.*, 1975).

7.7.13 THE ^{133}Xe CBF SPECT SCAN

With a fast sampling (10 s) tomograph (Figure 7.6, Plate 1) with sufficient sensitivity, tomographic ^{133}Xe CBF studies can be carried out. As with the planar probe method, units of CBF are expressed in ml min^{-1} 100 g^{-1}. The spatial resolution of these CBF maps is somewhat inferior (full width half maximum (FWHM) of the order of 17 mm is achieved) with a slice thickness of 20 mm. Since the technique is based on ^{133}Xe, a constant partition coefficient of $\lambda = 0.85$ ml g^{-1} is assumed, for grey and white matter, and in normal and abnormal tissue. The partial volume effect is significant – spherical volumes below 40 ml will not be accurately measured, although smaller cold spherical volumes, down to 1 ml, may be detected (Lassen *et al.*, 1981; Buell *et al.*, 1984) (Plate 2 and 3).

The ^{133}Xe CBF/SPECT approach is less sensitive to activation studies than the planar ^{133}Xe method. For instance, hand movement activation studies lead to a change of about 15% in CBF, while the cortical planar probe measurements can

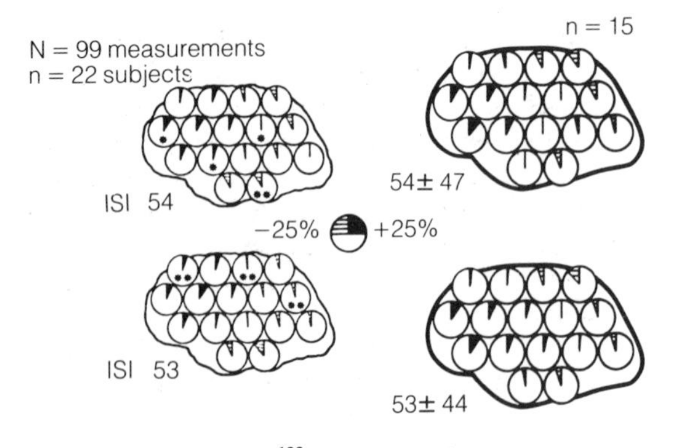

Figure 7.29 Resting ^{133}Xe rCBF study.

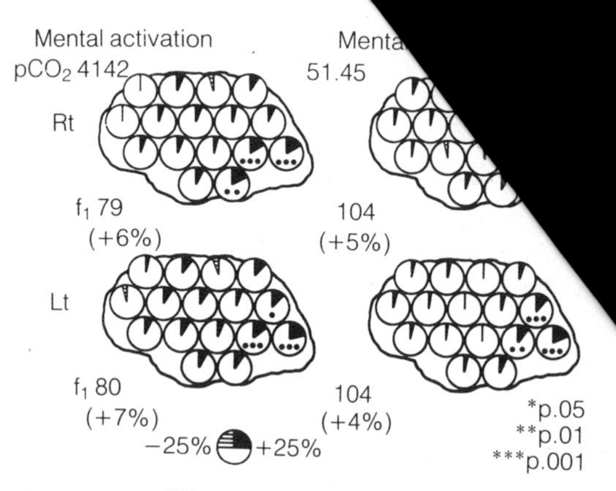

Figure 7.31 ^{133}Xe CBF activation study.

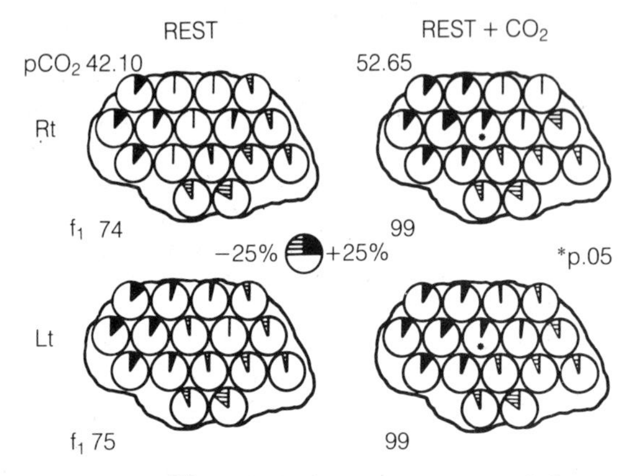

Figure 7.30 ^{133}Xe CBF during normo- and hypercapnia.

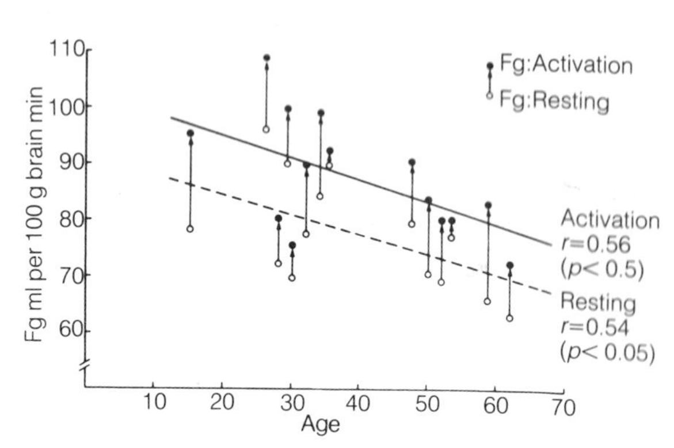

Figure 7.32 Mean grey matter CBF values with ^{133}Xe.

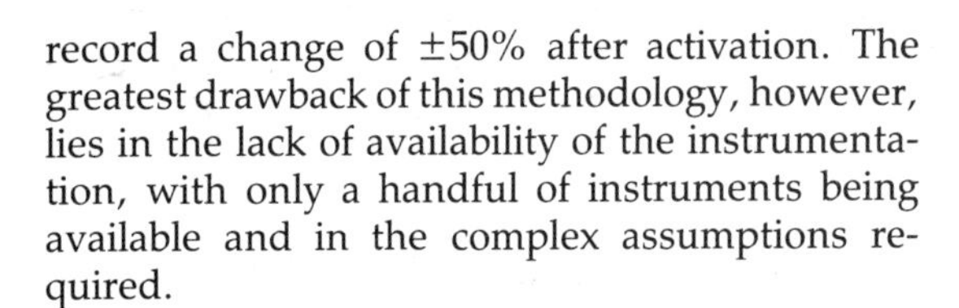

record a change of ±50% after activation. The greatest drawback of this methodology, however, lies in the lack of availability of the instrumentation, with only a handful of instruments being available and in the complex assumptions required.

7.7.14 THE ^{123}I-IMP CBF SCAN

The usual administered dose of ^{123}I-IMP or HIPDM is of the order of 4 mCi (185 MBq). After intravenous administration, the compound traverses the intact BBB and is then trapped intracellularly for a number of hours. Wash-out occurs and a degree of redistribution, between grey and white matter. However, for approximately 5–10 min, and for about 1 h post-administration, the distribution of the tracer closely follows the distribution of CBF.

7.7.15 PLANAR IMAGING

When planar imaging is undertaken, there is uniform distribution of tracer throughout the brain and cerebellum, with the ventricle space sometimes identified in the lateral images as a band of reduced activity. (Plate 4). Superposition of deeper structures onto the information received from more superficial anatomy prevents significant anatomical detail from being recorded. However, areas of reduced uptake can be demonstrated (as in acute stroke, cross-cerebellar diaschisis – best seen in the posterior projection) whilst it is more difficult to localize areas of increased tracer uptake (usually caused by a rise in CBF, as in ictal epilepsy). Interictal foci of reduced CBF cannot be demonstrated by planar imaging.

In normals, the relative quantification of the intracerebral distribution of these compounds is

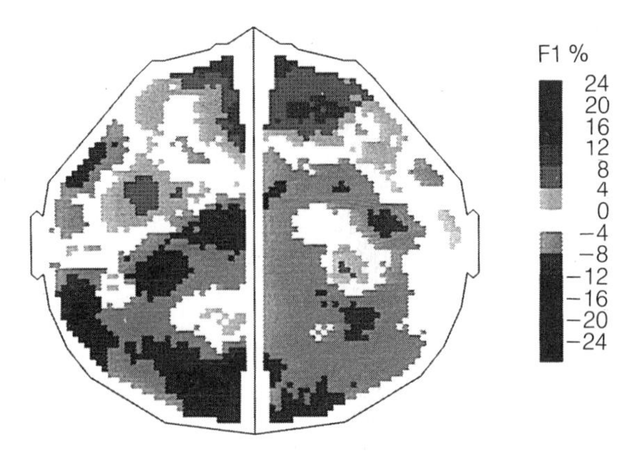

Figure 7.27 ^{133}Xe CBF maps with 254-detector system (resting).

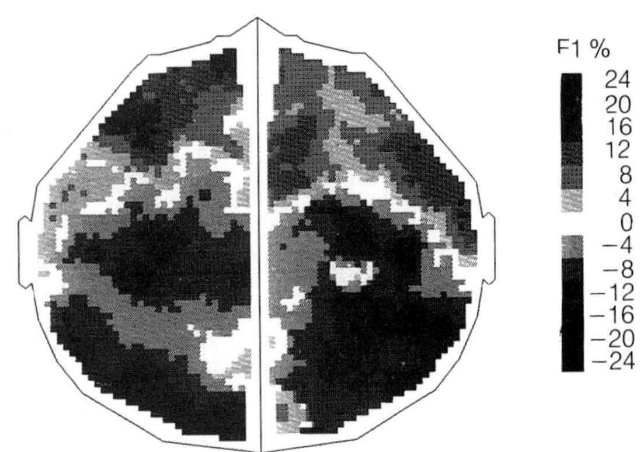

Figure 7.28 ^{133}Xe CBF maps with 254-detector system (talking).

invasive and simple, quantitative, portable and inexpensive. Relative disadvantages of the method include poor spatial resolution, absent depth discrimination and significant cross-talk from opposing areas of the brain.

With the ^{133}Xe planar approach to CBF analysis, a large body of data has emerged from the literature of the 1960s and 1970s. In general terms, the method appears more successful in the evaluation of dominant cortical flow than in the evaluation of the slower component of blood flow in white matter and deeper subcortical regions of the brain. The repeatability of the method allows a variety of intervention studies to be carried out (visual stimulation, mental activation, etc.), hence the extensive application in the areas of psychiatry, neuropsychology and comparative psychometric assessment of the individual patient. Resting values of CBF have been extensively investigated (Risberg *et al.*, 1977; Maximilian *et al.*, 1978; Prohovnik *et al.*, 1980). In normal subjects and with this planar method, there is a symmetrical distribution of CBF values (Figures 7.29–7.32).

Ingvar and Risberg (1965, 1967), using the intracarotid method, demonstrated increased CBF in response to mental stimulation. Still with the intra-arterial method, response to sensory, motor and complex mental activity with an increase in CBF has been documented by Olesen (1971), Ingvar (1975), Lassen *et al.* (1977), Risberg and Ingvar (1972). With the inhalation method, CBF changes in relation to mental activity were first demonstrated by Risberg *et al.* (1975).

The same group has led the application of this method to the investigation of dementia. With ^{133}Xe, it was first shown that there is a good correlation between areas of cortical atrophy and regions of reduced CBF (Gustafson *et al.*, 1977), that there is generalized reduction of CBF and localized parietal CBF impairment in Alzheimer's disease, and that the CBF abnormalities in Pick's disease (predominantly frontal) and in multi-infarction dementia (multi-focal) can be distinguished with reasonable sensitivity (Risberg, 1987). Impairment of the flow response to mental-activation in patients with dementia was also demonstrated (Ingvar *et al.*, 1975).

7.7.13 THE ^{133}Xe CBF SPECT SCAN

With a fast sampling (10 s) tomograph (Figure 7.6, Plate 1) with sufficient sensitivity, tomographic ^{133}Xe CBF studies can be carried out. As with the planar probe method, units of CBF are expressed in ml min^{-1} 100 g^{-1}. The spatial resolution of these CBF maps is somewhat inferior (full width half maximum (FWHM) of the order of 17 mm is achieved) with a slice thickness of 20 mm. Since the technique is based on ^{133}Xe, a constant partition coefficient of $\lambda = 0.85$ ml g^{-1} is assumed, for grey and white matter, and in normal and abnormal tissue. The partial volume effect is significant – spherical volumes below 40 ml will not be accurately measured, although smaller cold spherical volumes, down to 1 ml, may be detected (Lassen *et al.*, 1981; Buell *et al.*, 1984) (Plate 2 and 3).

The ^{133}Xe CBF/SPECT approach is less sensitive to activation studies than the planar ^{133}Xe method. For instance, hand movement activation studies lead to a change of about 15% in CBF, while the cortical planar probe measurements can

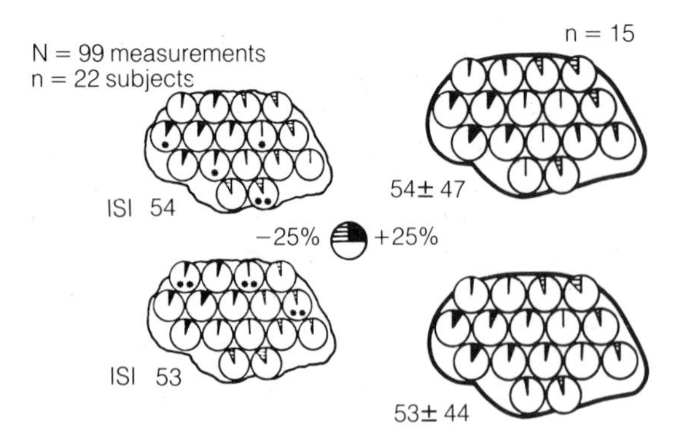

Figure 7.29 Resting ^{133}Xe rCBF study.

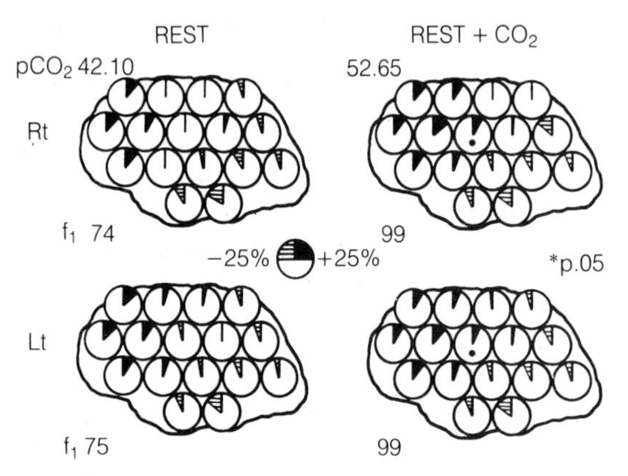

Figure 7.30 ^{133}Xe CBF during normo- and hypercapnia.

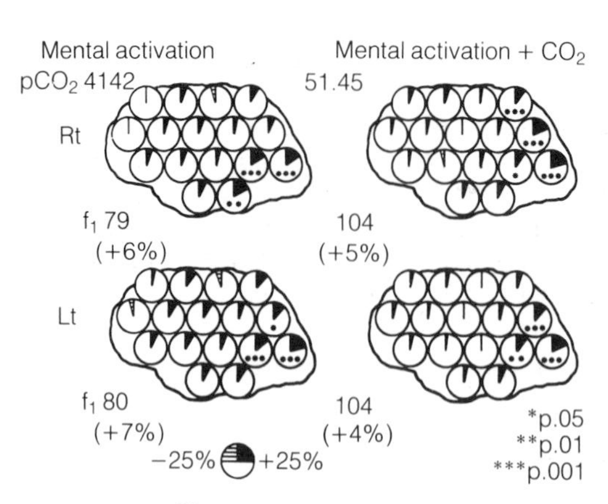

Figure 7.31 ^{133}Xe CBF activation study.

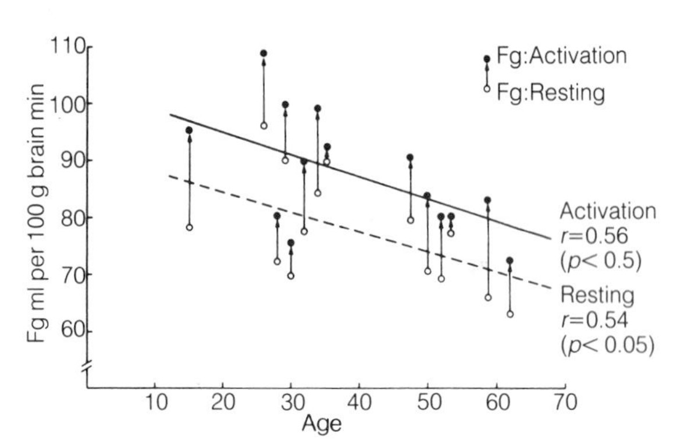

Figure 7.32 Mean grey matter CBF values with ^{133}Xe.

record a change of ±50% after activation. The greatest drawback of this methodology, however, lies in the lack of availability of the instrumentation, with only a handful of instruments being available and in the complex assumptions required.

7.7.14 THE ^{123}I-IMP CBF SCAN

The usual administered dose of ^{123}I-IMP or HIPDM is of the order of 4 mCi (185 MBq). After intravenous administration, the compound traverses the intact BBB and is then trapped intracellularly for a number of hours. Wash-out occurs and a degree of redistribution, between grey and white matter. However, for approximately 5–10 min, and for about 1 h post-administration, the distribution of the tracer closely follows the distribution of CBF.

7.7.15 PLANAR IMAGING

When planar imaging is undertaken, there is uniform distribution of tracer throughout the brain and cerebellum, with the ventricle space sometimes identified in the lateral images as a band of reduced activity. (Plate 4). Superposition of deeper structures onto the information received from more superficial anatomy prevents significant anatomical detail from being recorded. However, areas of reduced uptake can be demonstrated (as in acute stroke, cross-cerebellar diaschisis – best seen in the posterior projection) whilst it is more difficult to localize areas of increased tracer uptake (usually caused by a rise in CBF, as in ictal epilepsy). Interictal foci of reduced CBF cannot be demonstrated by planar imaging.

In normals, the relative quantification of the intracerebral distribution of these compounds is quite easy to achieve with data processing, and R/L ratios or interhemispheric ratios are usually very close to unity. These simple methods of quantification are, however, relatively sensitive in the demonstration of unilateral ischaemia, particularly if predominantly cortical in origin. This approach is also valid for other tracers, such as ^{99m}Tc-labelled HMPAO (Leonard *et al.*, 1987).

7.7.16 TOMOGRAPHIC IMAGING (SPECT)

Despite the inferior counting statistics when compared with ^{99m}Tc-labelled compounds, surprisingly good tomographic maps of CBF can be recorded (provided the data acquisition process is sufficiently quality controlled) (Figure 7.33). Attempts have been made to provide data expressed in ml min^{-1} 100 g^{-1} (Lucignani *et al.*, 1985; Matsuda *et al.*, 1986).

The deeper structures of grey matter (head of caudate nucleus, sometimes putamen, and thalamus), are often well identified, whilst the internal capsule is usually masked.

Acute stroke is typically seen as an area of wedge-shaped ischaemia, filling in with images taken as late as 6 h after administration of the tracer (Figure 7.10). This can also be seen in reversible ischaemia ((Transient ischaemic attack TIA), whilst in established stroke the ischaemia zone does not alter with time (after the administration of the tracer) (Moretti *et al.*, 1985).

Interictal scans have shown areas of ischaemia, whereas ictal episodes appear as focal areas of increased tracer uptake and flow, most tumours (but not all) and metastases, lead to an area of surrounding ischaemia and perturbation of CBF (often even seen in the contralateral hemisphere). Cross-cerebellar diaschisis accompanies cerebrovascular disease. Its incidence is variable ($\pm$50% of supratentorial stroke patients), and its significance is still uncertain. It appears to result in a reduction of glucose metabolism and flow in the contralateral cerebellar hemisphere. It is most often seen with large cortical infarcts of the frontal and temporal loves and is associated with subcortical lesions of the internal capsule (Baron, 1987a).

Typical patterns have been described in dementia. Multi-infarct dementia (Figure 7.34) causes (not surprisingly) multiple defects of tracer distribution, and Alzheimer's dementia a variety of flow patterns (described in more detail when ^{99m}Tc-labelled HMPAO studies are discussed) with predominant loss of flow to the temporal and particularly parietal lobes. Pick's dementia can be demonstrated with significant loss of flow to the frontal lobes – similar observations have been made in certain types of schizophrenia. Attempts are being made to link the degree of late redistribution of these compounds to cell viability and clinical prognosis (particularly in stroke). The outcome of such studies is awaited with interest (Royal *et al.*, 1985; Mueller *et al.*, 1986).

Hill *et al.* in 1984 compared CBF SPECT with ^{123}I-IMP with conventional X-ray CT methodology. Whilst small lacunar type of infarcts could not be detected by ^{123}I-IMP SPECT, there were also flow abnormalities present in patients with normal X-ray CT studies. Often, the low-density area on X-ray CT was smaller than the observed flow defect. Quantification of data appeared useful in the individual patient, but difficult to apply between groups of patients between normals and diseased individuals. The variation of tracer clearance from the lungs and formation of different lipophilic species, still with brain uptake properties, limit the accuracy with which more absolute determination of flow can be achieved with this compound.

The relative distribution of flow and volume with SPECT has been pioneered by Knapp *et al.* (1986), following the original PET approach of Gibbs *et al.* (1984). A method is hereby proposed which permits the haemodynamic assessment of cerebrovascular disease. CBV may precede changes in CBF and hence provide for a more sensitive parameter of circulatory impairment. Since with this approach only ratios of tracer distributions are calculated, the difficulties which arise from absolute quantification in SPECT are circumvented.

7.7.17 THE ^{99m}Tc-LABELLED HMPAO CBF SCAN

This is the first ^{99m}Tc-labelled lipophilic compound designed specifically to investigate CBF in man. In order to cross the BBB, the ^{99m}Tc complex has to be small (less than 500 daltons), be lipophilic and have a neutral charge (Neirinckx *et al.*, 1987). From the initial parent compound – ^{99m}Tc-labelled PnAO – a series of derivatives were tested in order to obtain a ligand that exhibited sufficient residence time in the brain such that CBF SPECT of the brain could be carried out with conventional instrumentation (rotating Anger gamma camera). The result of this research at

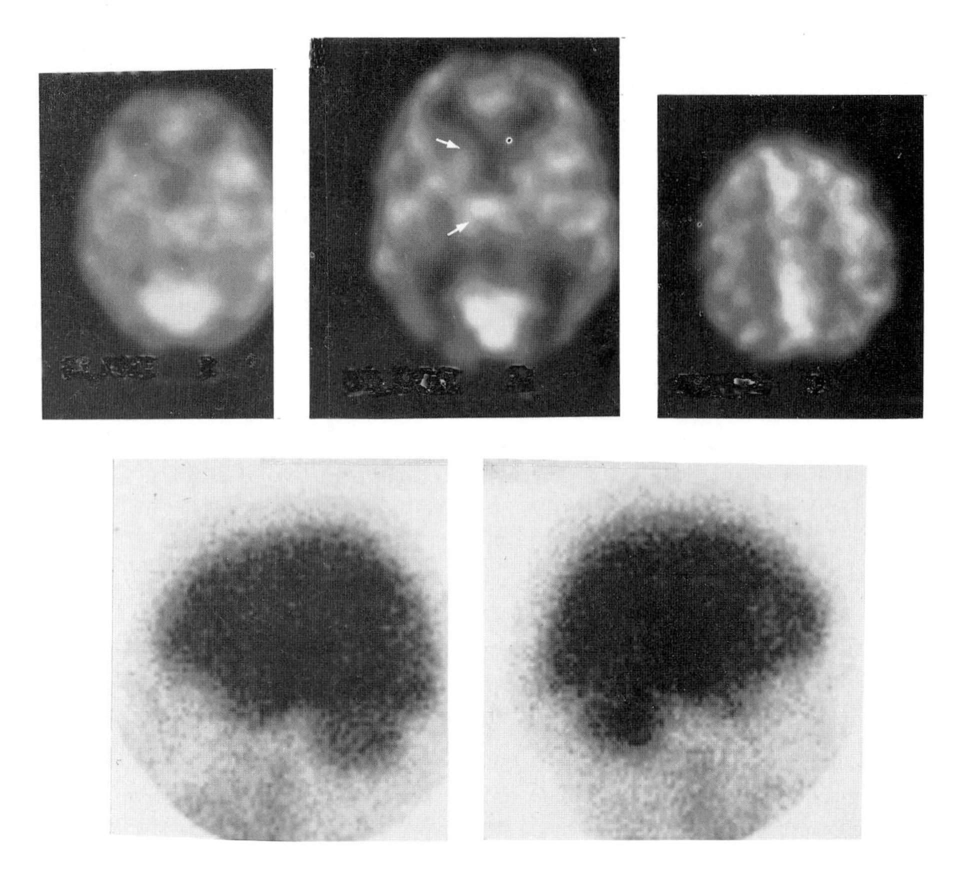

Figure 7.33 ^{123}I-IMP SPECT study: normal case.

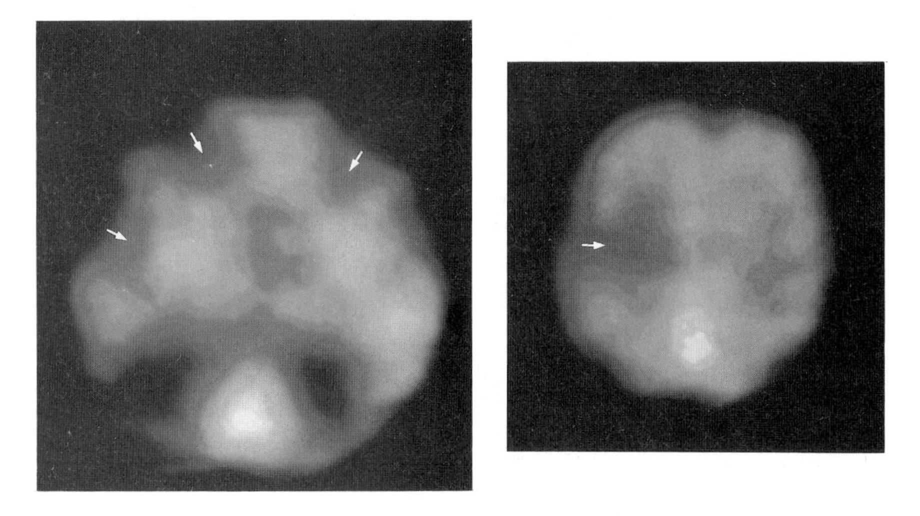

Figure 7.34 ^{123}I-IMP SPECT study: multi-infarct dementia.

Amersham International Laboratories led to ^{99m}Tc-labelled HMPAO, which exists in two diastereoisomeric forms (*d,l* and meso). The *d,l* form of HMPAO exhibits better properties of brain uptake and retention, and is the compound in clinical use today (Ell *et al.*, 1987b).

7.7.18 PLANAR IMAGING

Excellent images can be recorded. A conventional camera computer system is used, a high-resolution collimator and 15–20 mCi of tracer (555–740 MBq). The imaging protocol is conventional, with four to six planar views obtained (a vertex view is helpful), with 600 000 counts recorded per image.

The planar studies appear very similar to those recorded with ^{123}I-IMP, but the definition in these scans is slightly superior (Figure 7.35).

7.7.19 TOMOGRAPHIC IMAGING (SPECT)

With dedicated scanners, improved resolution is achieved. Rapid scanning times (1–5 min) permit a fast screen with a series of transaxial sections, such that a particular brain cut of interest can be identified, for improved data collection (a 10–15

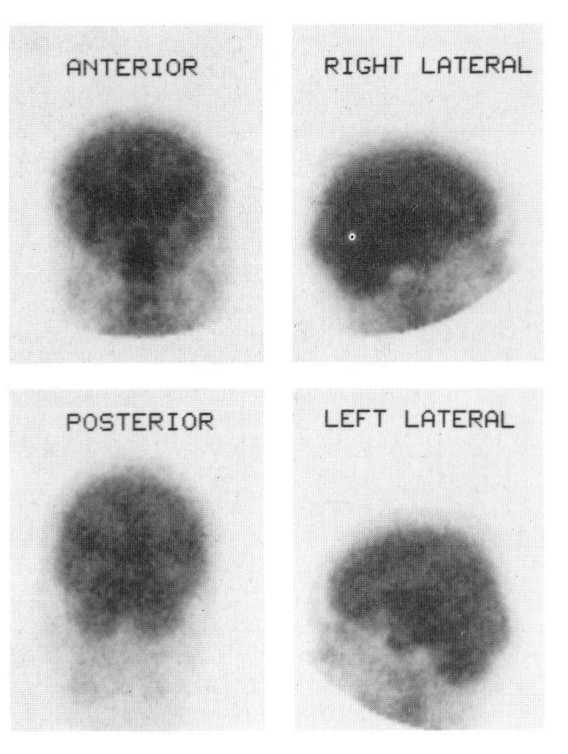

Figure 7.35 Planar ^{99m}Tc-labelled HMPAO: normal study.

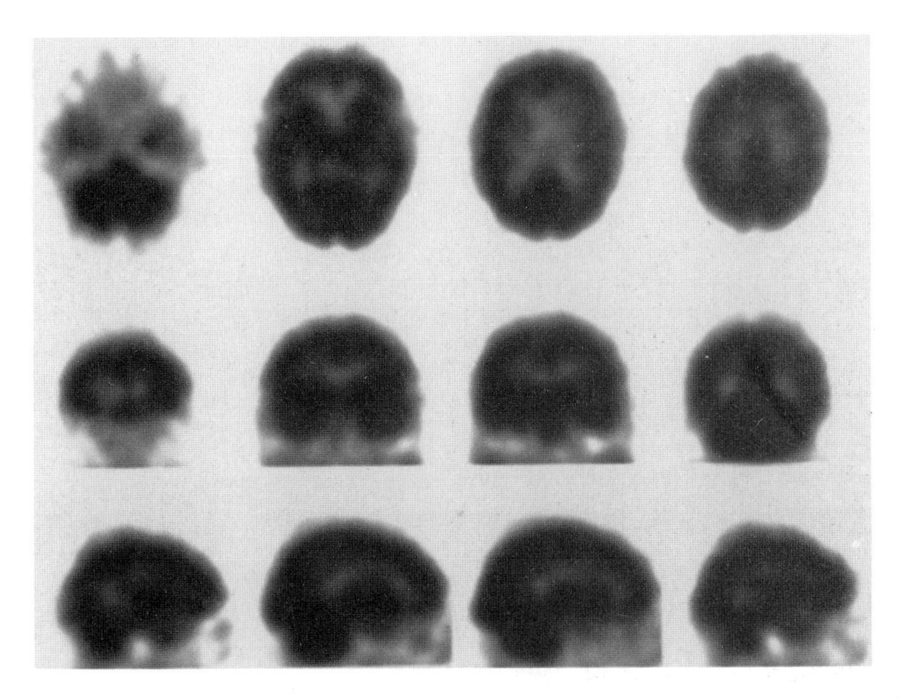

Figure 7.36 SPECT ^{99m}Tc-labelled HMPAO: normal study with IGE/400 A/T STARCAM: multiple planar reconstruction. Top row, transaxial; middle row, coronal; bottom row, sagittal sections.

min scan can then subsequently be recorded, and if required repeated with exact reproduction, after intervention – carbon dioxide Diamox, physiological stimulus etc.) (Plate 5).

With conventional Anger gamma camera/computer technology, good CBF maps of ^{99m}Tc-labelled HMPAO are also obtained, but data acquisition will take approximately 30 min (this can be shortened with more than single-headed gamma camera systems) (Figure 7.36). Repeat studies are therefore more difficult to achieve, particularly if repositioning of the patient is required. Since the whole organ volume is studied with this approach, all data for the whole brain are recorded simultaneously. This can be an important advantage, since data processing allows for all slices in several planes to be processed and displayed. Reorientation of slices after the initial study is possible and optimal planes of reconstruction can be chosen – parallel to the external auditory meatus line, optimized for temporal lobe analysis (Plate 6), etc. This process can also be disadvantageous, however, since movement of the patient at any point during the 30 min acquisition time will disrupt the whole test. Maximal patient cooperation is therefore required.

7.7.20 STROKE

The sudden onset of altered or loss of consciousness usually with lateralizing neurological signs due to vascular cause constitutes the syndrome of stroke. The syndrome may be classified by implied pathology – haemorrhage, embolism and infarction, or by duration – the transient ischaemic attack (TIA) lasting a few minutes or hours, the reversible progressive disorder lasting over 24 h and the completed stroke with long-lasting disability. Since there is no convincing evidence that the prognosis of the completed stroke can be altered by therapeutic intervention, the emphasis is on prevention. The key to prevention is by control of hypertension or polycythaemia but more specifically by the full evaluation of the transient ischaemic attack that so often forecasts a stroke to come.

7.7.21 THE TRANSIENT ISCHAEMIC ATTACK

That neurological control is interrupted transiently is taken as evidence of temporary loss of blood supply and this can come about either through embolism, occlusion or hypotension. The commonest cause is embolism for an irregular often ulcerated plaque of atheroma in the territory of the carotid or vertebral arteries from which turbulent flow excoriates a predominantly platelet- or cholesterol-containing fragment. Inherent in this event is the requirement that the vessel is sufficiently narrowed that the Reynolds number at which non-turbulent flow has turned to turbulent flow has been exceeded. But this occurs when the lumen has been narrowed by only about one-quarter of its radius – more so if the indentation is sharp rather than smooth. Thus the narrowing required to initiate turbulence and embolism is much less than that required to reduce the volume flow of blood significantly (Britton *et al.*, 1977b). The latter is called a 'critical' stenosis, and needs to exceed 85% of the lumen to cause a reduction in volume flow. Cerebral haemodynamic effects only occur when the flow in the circle of Willis cannot compensate because of disease of the other supplying vessels. Alternatively, the onset of a complete stroke may be associated with the final occlusion of a single critical stenosis.

The influence of the heart in the aetiology of transient ischaemia is well documented. The fibrillating atrium and the valvular vegetations of bacterial endocarditis are classical sources of emboli, but the clot overlying subendocardial infarct and the mitral valve distorted by prolapse are commonly cited contenders whose frequencies are difficult to assess.

With ^{99m}Tc-labelled HMPAO, acute stroke can be identified, and cortical as well as subcortical abnormalities defined. Interruption of flow distant from the primary site can be seen, reflecting the deafferentation/de-efferentation between cortical grey and white matter. This is observed with cerebellar diaschisis in stroke (Figure 7.37), with

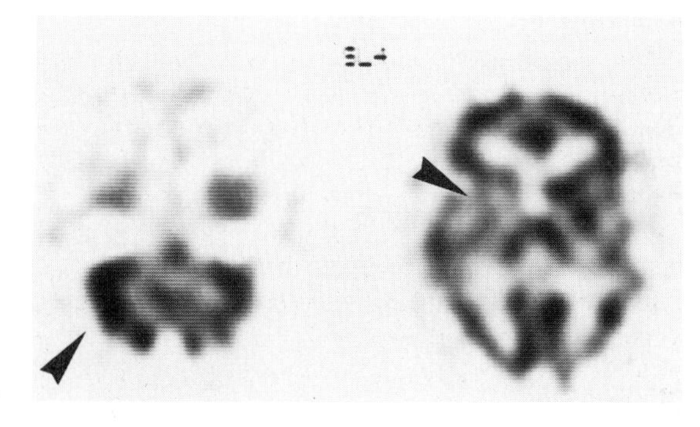

Figure 7.37 SPECT ^{99m}Tc-labelled HMPAO: acute stroke with cerebral diaschisis.

thalamic and lacunar infarctions, and with solid, primary or secondary malignancy of the brain.

At this stage, it is useful to define some of the haemodynamic changes which occur in acute stroke and can be observed with the application of SPECT. **Misery perfusion** is found when oxygen supply does not meet oxygen demand, oxygen extraction (OEF) is raised, and CBF is mildly or severely depressed. The cerebral metabolic rate for oxygen ($CMRO_2$) is, however, preserved. **Luxury perfusion** is found when oxygen supply is in excess of demand. OEF is reduced. CBF in this case can be increased, normal or decreased, but always in excess of $CMRO_2$ (Baron, 1987b; Lassen, 1966) (Figure 7.38).

Misery perfusion is seen in about half of all acute stroke cases studied within four days of this event. Luxury perfusion can be seen also in almost half of all cases in the first few days of stroke, but luxury perfusion is very often demonstrated after the second week of acute stroke (Ackerman *et al.*, 1981; Baron, 1985; Lenzi *et al.*, 1982; Wise *et al.*, 1983). Luxury perfusion is always associated with irreversible cellular damage and tissue necrosis.

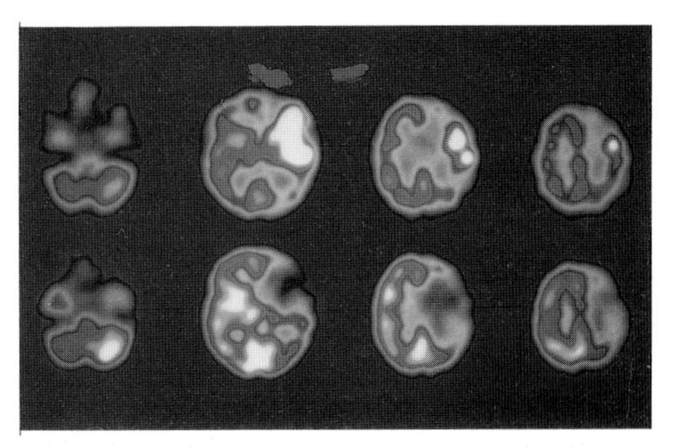

Figure 7.38 ^{99m}Tc-labelled HMPAO SPECT: luxury perfusion in stroke studied on day 13 and day 40 after acute event.

7.7.22 AUTOREGULATION

In normal man CBF, technically cerebral perfusion, varies between 50 and 60 ml min^{-1} per 100 g of brain substance. The flow in normal grey matter is higher (65–85 ml min^{-1} per 100 g) than in normal white matter 27–33 ml min^{-1} per 100 g). Normal cerebral function is still possible with mean CBF values as low as 20 ml min^{-1} per 100 g, the brain compensating with an increase in oxygen extraction ratio. Values below this threshold lead to positive electroencephalograph (EEG) changes. At 15 ml min^{-1} per 100 g critical ischaemia is reached, and if prolonged cellular necrosis occurs.

During autoregulation, CBV can increase (through vessel dilatation) in order to preserve flow, which in turn is dictated by metabolic demand. This occurs over a wide range of blood pressure. Systemic hypotension leads to vasodilatation in the brain, with a fall in the vascular resistance, maintenance of perfusion pressure and flow. Conversely, hypertension induces vasoconstriction in the brain, a rise in vascular resistance and maintenance of perfusion pressure and flow.

The ratio of CBF/CBV varies as a function of perfusion pressure, and has shown utility in the investigation of patients with bilateral carotid occlusive disease, unilateral disease and patent carotid vessels (Lenzi *et al.*, 1982; Gibbs *et al.*, 1984).

In view of this, there is a unique opportunity for the application of the radioactive tracer method to the investigation of cerebrovascular disease, the analysis of the treatment regime and the study of the normal history of stroke (as far as the underlying haemodynamic and pathophysiological changes are concerned). SPECT is a particularly promising methodology in the analysis of the CBF/CBV ratios. The tracers used, ^{99m}Tc-labelled HMPAO and ^{99m}Tc-labelled RBC are easy to prepare and widely available. Buell *et al.* (1987) have pioneered this approach with these tracers and have given details of methodology and results.

7.7.23 MIGRAINE

Migraine is a fashionable title for many a head pain but should be limited to the headache associated with nausea. Prodromal visual symptoms such as flashing lights are often noted. The headache is typically unilateral and accompanied by photophobia, nausea and a desire to lie down. The site of onset is usually around an orbit from which it spreads, and it is an important detail to confirm that in the past the headache has arisen on either side of the head.

The study of common and classical migraine includes the investigation of the possible role of changes in CBF during and after the acute attack. It is still not clear whether or not pain is always associated with a change in CBF (we have observed an increase in CBF in classical migraine

(Costa *et al.*, 1987b)), whether changes occur in common migraine, and whether they differ from those occurring in classical migraine. Biersack *et al.* (1987) reported on five patients with migraine where there was a reduction of CBF in three, and an increase of CBF in two studies. Vangelista *et al.* (1987) studied five patients with common migraine, in which no CBF changes could be detected (at rest) with ^{99m}Tc-labelled HMPAO. Suess *et al.* (1986) reported that in two of seven patients with migraine studied during the attack a regional reduction of CBF could be demonstrated.

Most of these findings are preliminary, and a controlled study of patients with classical or common migraine, investigated during or near to and after the acute event, is required, to throw light on the possible role of CBF and possibly CBV change in this condition (Lauritzen, 1987).

7.7.24 EPILEPSY

From PET studies, it has been established that metabolic (glucose) and flow changes remain coupled. In the interictal phase there is focal reduction in glucose and flow, whilst during the ictal period significant focal increases in glucose utilization and flow occur (Mazziotta and Phelps, 1986). This coupling between metabolism and flow form the basis for the application of the ^{99m}Tc-labelled HMPAO CBF SPECT to the identification of a focus of epilepsy, particularly in those patients with temporal lobe abnormality, where the disease appears refractory to medical treatment.

Suess *et al.* (1987) studied 22 patients suffering from partial complex seizures, all with normal X-ray CT studies; 78% of seizure patients could be discriminated correctly from normal controls. In two patients studied during the ictal phase, a pronounced rise in CBF was demonstrated. Biersack *et al.* (1987) demonstrate a change in CBF in 37 out of 45 patients studied. In a single personal observation, we demonstrated a change (rise) in CBF in a patient with partial facial seizures precipitated by speech alone (in the presence of a normal CT and EEG), which reverted to normal after two weeks of phenytoin treatment (this study was, however, carried out with ^{123}I-IMP). Buell et al. (1987) also reported high sensitivity in the detection of foci of reduced CBF in the interictal phase of epilepsy when ^{99m}Tc-labelled HMPAO SPECT was utilized.

7.7.25 NEOPLASIA

Keeling *et al.* (1986) have studied CBF with ^{99m}Tc-labelled HMPAO in various types of brain tumour before and after radiotherapy. Their studies confirmed, in general, the depression of CBF in the area of neoplasia, with changes of CBF occurring during the course of treatment. Langen *et al.* (1987) observed various degrees of ^{99m}Tc-labelled HMPAO uptake in eight out of 25 patients with glioma. In low malignant glioma, uptake was always reduced. Similar observations have been mostly recorded when CBF has been studied in patients with single or multiple intracerebral deposits.

7.7.26 DEMENTIA

Dementia describes a syndrome characterized by generalized cognitive impairment in an alert patient (Rossor, 1987). Many causes are recognized as leading to this syndrome (Van Horn, 1987). These include primary degeneration (as in the senile dementias of the Alzheimer's type (SDAT), Pick's disease, Parkinson's disease, Huntington's chorea), cerebrovascular disease (as in multi-infarct dementia (MID), Binswanger's disease, subdural haematoma), storage disorders, neoplasia, infective/inflammatory disease (as in acquired immunodeficiency syndrome (AIDS), Kreuzfeld–Jacob disease, multiple sclerosis), toxic (as with alcohol, poison, heavy metals) and metabolic.

Whilst some of the conditions mentioned above can be diagnosed on clinical grounds, and conventional laboratory and radiological investi-

Table 7.8 The ischaemia score of Hachinski *et al.* (1975)*

Abrupt onset	2
Stepwise deterioration	1
Fluctuating course	2
Nocturnal confusion	1
Relative preservation of personality	1
Depression	1
Complaint about somatic symptoms	1
Emotional incontinence	1
History of hypertension	1
History of stroke	2
Any other evidence of artherosclerosis	1
Focal neurological symptoms	2
Focal neurological signs	2

*Scores of less than 4 indicate a higher probability of Alzheimer's disease and scores of 7 and above a high probability of multi-infarct dementia.

Table 7.9 Clinical dementia rating (CDR) (Berg, USA)*

	Healthy CDR 0	*Questionable dementia* CDR 0.5	*Mild dementia* CDR 1	*Moderate dementia* CDR 2	*Severe dementia* CDR 3
Memory	No memory loss or slight inconsistent forgetfulness	Mild consistent forgetfulness; partial recollection of events; 'benign' forgetfulness	Moderate memory loss, more marked for recent events; defect interferes with everyday activities	Severe memory loss; only highly learned material retained; new material rapidly lost	Severe memory loss; only fragments remain
Orientation	Fully oriented		Some difficulty with time relationships; oriented for place and person at examination but may have geographic disorientation	Usually disoriented in time, often to place	Orientation to person only
Judgement + problem solving	Solves everyday problems well; judgement good in relation to past performance	Only doubtful impairment in solving problems, similarities, differences	Moderate difficulty in handling complex problems, social judgement usually maintained	Severely impaired in handling problems, similarities, differences; social judgement usually impaired	Unable to make judgements or solve problems
Community affairs	Independent function at usual level in job, shopping, business and financial affairs, volunteer and social groups	Only doubtful or mild impairment in these activities	Unable to function independently at these activities though may still be engaged in some; may still appear normal to casual inspection	No pretence of independent function outside home. Appears well enough to be taken to functions outside a family home	Appears too ill to be taken to functions outside a family home
Personal care	Fully capable of self-care		Needs prompting	Requires assistance in dressing, hygiene, keeping of personal effects	Requires much help with personal care; often incontinent

*Score only impairment due to cognitive loss, not impairment due to other factors.

gations, the differential diagnosis of some of the SDAT and MID remains controversial. These conditions may coexist, yet their prognosis is quite different. Auxiliary methods for diagnosis (such as the Hachinski score for ischaemia (Table 7.8) and Berg's scoring system (Table 7.9) can help, but remain insensitive and non-specific.

Alzheimer's disease is a relatively common condition. The UK dementia data show that one in 14 of the 8 million men and women over the age of 65 are demented, a total of 570 000 people. Of these, 210 000 are over the age of 80. As many as 30% of patients with dementia are in chronic care, at a cost of £2000 million per annum. An alarming trend is seen in the prevalence of dementia in patients with AIDS. Whilst the true incidence is so far unknown, it is important to realize that human immunodeficiency virus (HIV) has been found in stage I (acute seroconversion) of the disease, and that dementia may occur before the development of AIDS (Navia *et al.*, 1986a, 1986b) or without physical signs of HIV disease (Bach and Boothby, 1986; Riccio, 1987).

CBF/SPECT with ^{99m}Tc-labelled HMPAO has been recently applied to the study of Alzheimer's dementia (Shields *et al.*, 1986; De Roo *et al.*, 1987; Testa *et al.*, 1987). The findings are similar but not identical to those reported in the literature by groups utilizing PET (Frackowiak *et al.*, 1981; Chase *et al.*, 1984; Mazziotta and Phelps, 1986; Chawluk *et al.*, 1987). In advanced disease, a typical pattern of impaired CBF is demonstrated, mainly in the posterior parietal and temporo-parietal cortex, often with bilateral distribution (Plate 7).

However, in the early stages of SDAT, a more varying pattern can be found, often with asymmetric or unilateral distribution, affecting temporal lobes, sometimes the frontal lobe, and also the parietal lobe. The basal ganglia appear non-involved, and defects in CBF may not but often do match areas of cerebral atrophy as seen on X-ray CT. A pattern of impaired CBF as seen by ^{99m}Tc-labelled HMPAO SPECT has recently been described in patients with AIDS, which is similar to the CBF abnormalities seen in SDAT (Ell *et al.*, 1987c) (Plate 8). Treatment of Alzheimer's dementia is controversial and, so far, ineffective. However, new approaches with cholinergic drugs show cause for some optimism (Summers *et al.*, 1986; Davis and Mohs, 1987).

In Parkinson's disease, preliminary studies are in progress, studying patients in the on and the off phase of this condition when treated with L-dopa (Costa *et al.*, 1987c). There appears to be a different distribution of CBF in the basal ganglia, which reverses between the on and the off phases. The significance and ultimate specificity of this finding is still unclear. In Pick's disease the abnormalities of CBF are seen to involve predominantly the frontal cortex, sparing the parietal and temporal lobes.

Table 7.10 Requirements for routine CBF measurement in man

1. Non-invasive
2. Standard nuclear medicine equipment
3. Standard radiopharmaceutical
4. Total and regional flow
5. Quantitative as well as qualitative
6. Application to patients with cerebrovascular disease and the unconscious as well as the normal
7. Separate estimation of volume of tracer distribution as well as time globally and regionally to reduce assumptions
8. Avoidance of the need to assume tracer partition coefficients
9. Correction of extracerebral activity
10. Capable of adaptation to the estimation of cerebral metabolism as well as flow

7.8 METHODOLOGY: GENERAL COMMENTS ON THE MEASUREMENT OF CBF

The measurement of total and regional cerebral flow routinely in man requires certain criteria to be met (Table 7.10).

7.8.1 THE COMPARTMENTAL APPROACH

This approach considers the brain as a single- or two-compartment system. A diffusible lipid-soluble indicator such as ^{133}Xe is given intra-arterially, intravenously or by inhalation. It is assumed to diffuse rapidly through the whole volume of the brain, so that this is a constant factor during the study. It partitions between water and lipid and this partition coefficient differs in grey matter and white matter. The diffusion of the tracer out of the brain is considered to depend only on the rate of CBF.

By external counting techniques, the rapid rise and slow fall of ^{133}Xe in the head is recorded. If these data are plotted on semi-logarithmic paper, the graph is not a straight line but approaches linearity with time. By drawing or calculating the best fit of a straight line to the linear portion and extrapolating it back to cut the vertical axis at time zero, a 'slow component' is obtained and its slope is measured. Subtracting the values of the slow component from the composite curve, a 'fast component' is obtained whose slope is approximately linear. λ is measured from the slope of the fast component. Where the extrapolated slopes of the slow and fast components cut the vertical axis at time zero, the relative weights of grey and white matter are thought to be indicated. The 2 min initial slope method is an approximation to the fast component of the wash-out curve. It is obtained by recording for only 2 min. This systematic error has little effect on serial studies in the same patient. The analysis of flow may be simplified as follows:

$$\text{CBF (ml min}^{-1}) = VP\lambda \text{ (ml min}^{-1})$$

where V is the volume of distribution, λ is the rate of wash-out, and P is the partition coefficient for xenon.

For ^{133}Xe, the volume of distribution depends on its partition between brain and blood, but neither V nor P can be measured. A value for P is determined *in vitro* and substituted. The problem of V is reduced by converting V to weight by multiplying by density (unit weight of tissue, W/V) (g ml^{-1}) and then taking density as unity. Thus

$$\text{CBF} = V\,(W/V)\,P\lambda$$

then $$\text{CBF}/W = P\lambda \text{ (ml min}^{-1}\text{ g}^{-1})$$

CBF/W is called 'cerebral perfusion', CP, and is the flow per unit weight of tissue. Thus CP = $P\lambda$ (ml min^{-1} g^{-1}). In this way, a measurement of ^{133}Xe wash-out made in units of 'per minute' is aggrandised to one in ml min^{-1} per 100 g.

The assumptions of the ^{133}Xe wash-out technique include all those of the indicator dilution technique and many others. In the intracarotid injection technique a delay of 30 min after contrast injection is necessary for flow to resettle and full mixing of the indicator in the carotid arterial blood stream is unlikely. A detector does not view specifically grey or white matter but a combination of both. Due to Compton scattering about a quarter of the γ-rays from a particular detector, depending on its design, arise from outside its field of view (Potchen *et al.*, 1971).

The indicator should leave the bloodstream after the first circulation. Although ^{133}Xe is almost totally exhaled, the fact that, as Austin *et al.* (1973) showed, intravenous injection of ^{133}Xe has been used to estimate cerebral perfusion indicates that recirculation of ^{133}Xe does occur. This is more likely when there is impairment of ventilation, as in those with chronic obstructive disease of the airways.

The assumption required for ^{133}Xe wash-out is that the ^{133}Xe is diffused through the whole volume of the brain. For example, there is no evidence for the uptake of ^{133}Xe by neuroglia from capillary endothelium. The theory requires rapid influx of ^{133}Xe and rapid simultaneous efflux of ^{133}Xe in proportion to blood flow. This assumption was thought to be valid for the brain because it is valid for the wash-out of ^{133}Xe from muscle by capillary flow. This is because the capillaries in muscle are fenestrated with pores but, as Oldendorf (1975) showed, the capillaries of the brain have no such pores (Figure 7.2). ^{133}Xe, with its high lipid solubility, is likely to persist in the lipid membrane of the BBB, through which it must pass. To attempt to correct for some of these effects, the volume of distribution is multiplied by a partition coefficient, P, which has been shown to be different for white and grey matter but not measured for neuroglia. Usually a 'mean' partition coefficient set to a fixed value such as 1.1 is used. This may be satisfactory for normal brain with normal hemispheres but cannot be assumed to be appropriate for asymmetrical brain pathology such as symptomatic epilepsy or cerebrovascular disorder. Van Duyl and Volkers (1980) have demonstrated in pigs the non-validity of the relative weight of the first clearance component as an anatomical or functional parameter.

The assumptions of constancy of volume of distribution and constancy of partition coefficient are absolutely essential to the interpretation of the results of λ per minute in terms of cerebral perfusion. It can thus be appreciated that Xe wash-out does not measure regional CBF when a wash-out curve is obtained over a region of the brain. It should be noted further that since CP = $P\lambda$, and since P is not measured, there is no way of distinguishing the one from the other. It appears very likely that metabolic activity will affect P, which is approximated by the partition of ^{133}Xe between lipid and water. Metabolic activity in the capillary endothelium, BBB and brain cells burns sugar and creates water. Thus the lipid/water ratio intracellularly is likely to alter with metabolic activity. Evidence from the uptake of ^{18}F-labelled deoxyglucose has indicated that some of the interpretations of ^{133}Xe wash-out in terms of changes in flow are better interpreted as alterations of metabolism. Thus in conclusion ^{133}Xe wash-out is a reasonable approach to the study of flow plus 'metabolism' in the normal brain but its assumptions make it much less reliable when the brain is disordered.

7.8.2 THE LINEAR SYSTEM APPROACH

This considers the system under study as a black box and describes the fractions of activity that take various times to transit through the system. For the head, the system includes the root of the aorta, the common carotid, internal carotid, vertebral and cerebral arteries together with the venous sinuses and jugular viens. Moses *et al.* (1973) demonstrated that the vertex view best visualizes the distribution of the cerebral arteries. A non-diffusible indicator, ^{99m}Tc-labelled RBC, is confined to this vascular system.

A simplified account of the CBF measurement follows. To monitor the input to the system a probe with a short geometric focus collimator is set over the root of the aorta, its position being checked by a bolus of 1 mCi (37 MBq) ^{99m}Tc pertechnetate at the start of the study, after which a 'background' blood sample is taken. With the right arm abducted, a bolus of 15 mCi (555 MBq) ^{99m}TcRBC or albumin in less than 0.3 ml is given intravenously using a 20 ml saline flush. First pass and equilibrium data are recorded from the vertex camera, shielded from the body. Three regions of interest (ROI) are set on each hemisphere, avoiding the scalp edge and the sagittal sinus. These ROI are obtained in three ways: as anatomical regions related to the vessel distribution (Figure 7.3), as divisions of the hemisphere into thirds; and as divisions of the middle cerebral region only.

The first-pass activity is recorded from each ROI. By means of deconvolution analysis of the aortic input activity–time curve and those of each ROI, the transit times from aortic root through each region are calculated. These are corrected from the appearance times of arrival of activity from the aortic detector to the brain as shown on the vertex view, to give the mean transit time through each ROI. Since regional flow is given by regional volume divided by its mean transit time, it is necessary to measure the regional volumes. This is performed by determining the fraction of blood volume in each region. The equilibrium activity is recorded over the vertex between 2.5 and 3.5 min after injection and a blood sample is taken at 3 min to calibrate this activity in terms of volume. The volume of the blood sample is measured by weight difference and it is counted later on the face of the camera, the factor relating a blood sample to the volume of the brain having been determined previously from phantom studies.

The regional volume, V_R, is given by $(N_R/N_T) \times (Eq/S)$, where N_R is the first-pass activity of the region; S is the blood sample activity per unit volume; N_T is the total vertex first-pass activity; and Eq is the total vertex activity at equilibrium. Eq/N_T is in effect a factor relating the first-pass regional activity, N_R, to the 3 min blood sample, S. The activity at equilibrium has to be corrected for the extracerebral activity, whereas, for the reasons outlined earlier, the first-pass activity does not need this correction. The distribution of activity at the first pass in the brain should be the same as in the brain at equilibrium. By dividing the regional equilibrium activity, Eq, by the first-pass activity, N_T, a remainder, R_i, is obtained which gives the difference between the two and indicates the activity of the non-cerebral component. The value of Eq is then corrected for R_i to give the true cerebral equilibrium activity free of any extra-cerebral contribution (Britton *et al.*, 1979b). This corrected Eq is substituted for Eq in the calculation of the regional flow and thereby gives the true CBF. If V_R is in millilitres and the regional transit time is converted to minutes, regional flow is obtained (ml min^{-1}) and total flow as the sum of these. This flow is not a perfusion but in the same units as cardiac output and effective renal plasma flow. When this flow is combined with that of a diffusible or metabolic tracer, the difference between the cerebral red cell flow and that of the other tracer will give the 'metabolic flow'. Since regional volume and regional mean transit times are obtained independently, it is much more rigorous than the ^{133}Xe wash-out technique, requiring no assumptions about the volume of distribution or partition coefficients. It is thus applicable to patients with cerebrovascular disease (Britton *et al.*, 1981, 1985). This technique fulfils all the criteria given in Table 7.8. It has been used in bypass surgery (Britton *et al.*, 1979a), in subarachnoid haemorrhage (Granowska *et al.*, 1980) and in the evaluation of the hypotensive agent prazosin (Rutland *et al.*, 1980). The method is reproducible to within 6% for each region and 3% for total blood flow (Britton *et al.*, 1981). In these publications ^{99m}Tc-labelled HSA was used (normal range uncorrected flow > 1000 ml min^{-1}) and ^{99m}Tc-labelled RBC are used now, for example in studies into dementia (normal range > 870 ml min^{-1}, mild brain damage 650–870 ml min^{-1}, moderate 435–650 ml min^{-1}, severe < 435 ml min^{-1}).

7.9 HYDROCEPHALUS

A subgroup of patients with ventricular enlargement but usually without cerebral atrophy have a form of hydrocephalus that may be improved by shunting the CSF from the lateral ventricles to the

Table. 7.11 Adult hydrocephalus

Type	*Site of block*	*Pressure*	*Radiographic CT*	*CBF imaging*	*Shunting helpful*
Obstructive	In the ventricular system or at its exits	High	Dilated lateral ventricles and ventricular system beyond block	Lateral ventricles not seen; no ventricular filling beyond block	Yes
Communicating	No block; direct communication between ventricular system and subarachnoid space	Low, fluctuating	Dilated lateral IIIrd and IVth ventricles	Lateral ventricles retain activity over 48 h	Often
Intermediate	Block in basal cisterns or paracerebral	Moderate or low	Dilated lateral IIIrd, IVth ventricles; some cerebral atrophy	Lateral ventricles retain activity maximally at 24 h; subarachnoid para- and supracerebral activity diminished or absent	Sometimes
Atrophic	No block; dilatation due to cerebral atrophy	Low	Moderately dilated lateral ventricles; cerebral atrophy	No lateral ventricular uptake, normal paracerebral activity with dilated sulci	No

extracerebral cisterns. They typically have a moderate to severe dementia of onset over a few months with urinary incontinence and moderate disturbance of gait. They are not easily differentiated from other dements. The hydrocephalus may be obstructive or communicating (Table 7.11).

7.10 THE CEREBROSPINAL FLUID

The choroid plexuses in the lateral ventricles and the third and fourth ventricles secrete CSF and the fluid leaves the fourth ventricle to enter the subarachnoid space. Some descends around the spinal cord but most flows around and anterior to the brain stem and then between and over the hemispheres, entering the arachnoid villi, which act effectively as one-way valves to the venous sagittal sinus. The CSF volume is about 150 ml and is normally changed six times a day. Crystalloids may diffuse in or out of the CSF at any site, therefore radiopharmaceuticals need to be larger than simple crystalloids to trace the CSF pathways.

Two CSF radiopharmaceuticals are compared in Table 7.12. It is incredible that ^{131}I-labelled HSA, which cannot be prepared to pharmaceutical intrathecal standards, was ever sanctioned for CSF studies and its use almost amounts to negligence now that ^{111}In-labelled DTPA is readily available. An unopened bottle must always be used; its contents must never be diluted; and the only needle puncture of the bottle should be that of the neurosurgeon proceeding with the injection of the tracer into the CSF after the patient has been prepared to surgical aseptic standards. Introduction of CSF tracer into the cisterna magna is to be

Table 7.12 CSF imaging agents

	^{111}In-labelled DTPA	*^{131}I-labelled albumin*
Prepared and sterilized to standards essential for intrathecal use	Yes	No
Non-irritating	Yes	No
Reliably moves over the hemispheres with time	No	Yes
Low radiation dose	Yes	No

preferred. This is not only because a neurosurgeon is required who is therefore aware of the precautions, but also because this need for his presence will help to limit the use of the technique to patients in whom the neurosurgeon might contemplate surgery, and he would be aware of the sources of misinterpretation of the results.

The distinction between low-pressure hydrocephalus, as diagnosed by retention of tracer activity in the lateral ventricles for 48 h and more, and hydrocephalus not benefiting from surgery is not as simple as enthusiasts for CSF imaging would have us believe. Both failures of shunting in typical cases of low-pressure communicating hydrocephalus and successes in others without typical features occur. Pericranial pressure transducer measurements show big fluctuations in CSF pressure in all types of 'low'-pressure hydrocephalus and may be a more reliable indicator for likely surgical benefit than CSF imaging (Symon and Dorsch, 1975). The difference between an arachnoid cyst and a porencephalic cyst is that the former will take up ^{111}In-labelled DTPA whereas the latter is excluded from the CSF and does not. ECAT may be helpful in determining the extent of these cysts (Woolley *et al.*, 1977).

7.11 VENTRICULAR SHUNT PATENCY

Intraventricular injection of ^{111}In-labelled DTPA will be demonstrated by a detector over the ventriculoatrial shunt if it is patent. This can also be confirmed by serial blood sampling; the appearance and rise in activity should be rapid, within 30 min.

7.12 RHINORRHOEA

The leakage of CSF implies a break in the arachnoid and dural lining of the brain and is usually associated with a fracture, especially of the paranasal sinuses. Its presence acts as a possible site for infection to ascend into the brain and create a local abscess or meningitis. The diagnosis requires the demonstration that the fluid dripping from the nose is CSF. CSF contains glucose, but if nasal secretions which are without glucose are contaminated with tears which contain some glucose this test may not be reliable. CSF protein electrophoresis is advised (Meurman *et al.*, 1979). The fracture and the site of leak may be identifiable by plain radiography or radiographic CT, but intrathecal soluble tracer such as ^{99m}Tc-pertechnetate, preferably injected into the cisterna magna (Di Chiro *et al.*, 1968), is the simplest way. Pledgets of gauze may be placed strategically in the nose and at the outlets of the nasal sinus during the study and counted later to aid the localization of the leak, but their positioning is difficult and often not worthwhile. As well as the conventional anterior view, anterior views with the head flexed and head extended may be of help as well as the lateral views. Intrathecal contrast injection with radiographic CT is an alternative (Drayer *et al.*, 1977).

7.13 NEURORECEPTOR STUDIES

The most recent development in the radionuclide studies of the brain concerns the investigation of neuroceptor function and distribution. Positron Emission Topography has led the field, with a series of studies involving the central dopamine receptor. D2 receptor density or occupancy in treated and untreated psychotic patients has been studied with ^{76}Br-spiperone, ^{11}C-raclopride, and ^{11}C-methyl spiperone. The striatal/cerebellar distribution of these compounds has been applied to investigate responders and non-responders to treatment (for instance in patients with schizophrenia, see Figure 7.39) and to a sub-group of patients such as neuroleptic treated but resistant psychosis in comparison with therapy-responding patients.

The aim of such studies is clear – to characterize disease, investigate its responsiveness to treatment and identify possible improvements in therapeutic regimes. Other neuroreceptor systems are beginning to be studied, with the radioactive tracer method. Amongst these, one may mention the opiate receptor studied in man with ^{11}C-carfentanyl or ^{11}C-diprenorphine, the benzodiazepine receptor with ^{11}C-labelled flumazenil or indeed ^{123}I-labelled flumazenil, the serotonin receptor with ^{11}C or indeed ^{123}I-labelled ketanserin. The nicotonic receptor and the muscarinic receptor are being studied with appropriate radiolabelled ligands, and no doubt in the future many other receptor systems will be amenable to the investigation by the radionuclide tracer methodology.

Dopamine D2 receptors in the brain are located on terminals and cell bodies of nigrostriatal and mesolimbic dopamine neurons and possibly on terminals of the cortico-striate pathway. Altered states of central dopamine D2 receptor densities

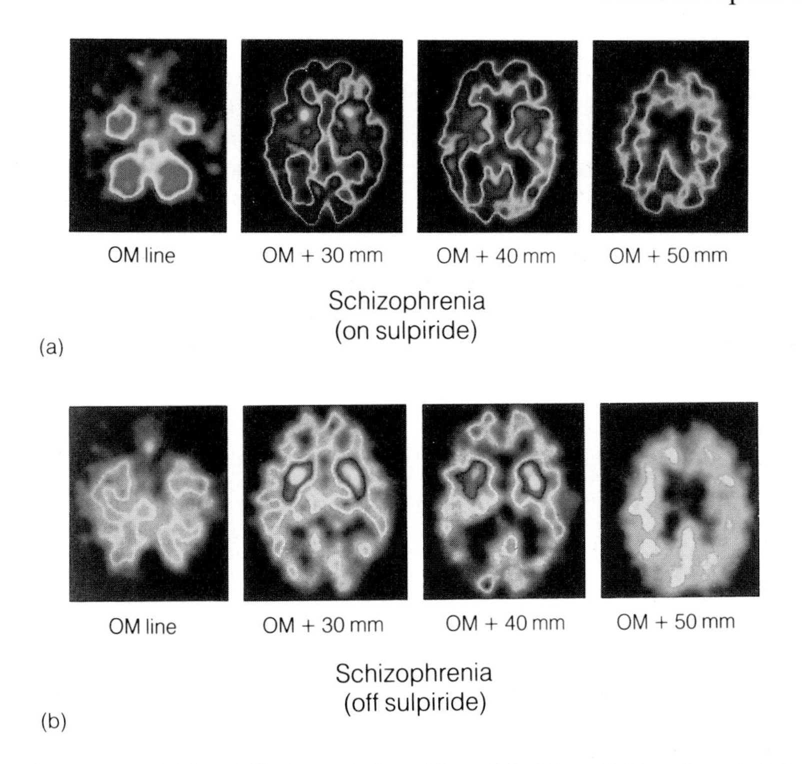

Figure 7.39 SPECT images at 1.5 h p.i. Horizontal slices (10mm/slice) from OML − 5mm to OML + 60mm. (a) A 52-year-old woman with schizophrenia using Sulpiride 200mg b.d. for 2 years; (b) the same patient 6 days after withdrawal of Sulpiride. It is clearly visible that there is increased uptake of ^{123}I-IBZM in striatal tissue after Sulpiride withdrawal.

are involved in a number of neurologic and psychiatric conditions, including Parkinsonism, Huntingdon's disease, tardive dyskinesia, and schizophrenia. In patients with Parkinsonism, dopamine neurons are markedly reduced and dopamine receptors may increase in the striatum as a compensatory response. In the treatment of psychosis, D2 receptors are known to mediate the antipsychotic and extrapyramidal motor effects of neuroleptics. Measurement of D2-dopamine receptor occupancy by SPECT with ^{123}I-labelled ligands may be a rapid and efficient procedure for defining the minimal effective dosage of neuroleptics that gives sufficient occupancy for antipsychotic efficacy with a minimum of side effects.

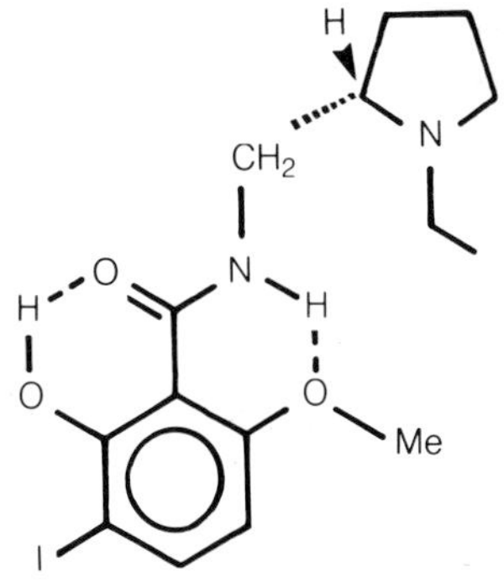

7.13.1 PROPERTIES OF ^{123}I-IBZM

IBZM belongs to the class of benzamide neuroleptics which are known to bind specifically to dopamine D2 receptors. Various *in vitro* studies have shown the high specificity and high affinity of IBZM to this receptor type (Kung *et al.*, 1989; Verhoeff *et al.*, 1989). Thus, IBZM is more specific in binding to the D2 receptor than spiperone which also binds to serotonine 5-HT2 receptors in the brain. The relative high affinity and uptake in the brain of IBZM are partially due to the incorporation of iodine in the molecule, causing in-

Figure 7.40 Structural formula of IBZM.

creased lipophilicity compared to other benzamides.

^{123}I-IBZM is supplied by Cygne in a sterile, isotonic solution. The activity concentration amounts to 75 MBq/mL. The production method for the radionuclide ^{123}I via ^{124}Xe results in an extremely high radionuclide purity. The labelling and quality control procedure applied for IBZM meets the specific activity and radiochemical purity specifications required for receptor imaging.

REFERENCES

Ackerman, R. H., Correia, J. A., Alpert, N. M. *et al.* (1981) Positron imaging in ischaemic stroke disease using compounds labelled with oxygen-15. *Arch. Neurol.*, **38**, 537–43.

Ancri, G., Basset, J.-Y., Leuchamp, Y. and Eavard, C. (1978) Diagnosis of cerebral lesions by thallium-201. *Radiology*, **128**, 417–22.

Austin, G., Laffin, D., Roche, S. *et al.* (1973) A non-invasive i.v. isotope method for measuring cerebral blood flow. *Stroke*, **4**, 362–3.

Bach, M. C. and Boothby, J. A. (1986) Dementia associated with human immunodeficiency virus with a negative ELISA. *N. Engl. J. Med.*, **315**, 891–2.

Baron, J. C. (1985) Positron tomography ischemia: a review. *Neuroradiology*, **27**, 509–16.

Baron, J. C. (1987a) in *Journal of Functional Imaging in Neurology and Psychiatry* (eds J. Wade, S. Knezevic, V. A. Maximilian *et al.*), J. Libbey, pp. 91–100.

Baron, J. C. (1987b) in *Clinical Efficacy of Positron Emission Tomography* (eds W. D. Heiss, G. Pawlik, K. Herholz and K. Wierhard), Martinus Nijhoff, Amsterdam.

Biersack, H. J., Reichmann, K., Stefan, H. *et al.* (1987) SPECT: Befunde bei Epilepsie und Migrane. *Nucl. Med.*, **26**, 100–4.

Boucher, B. J. and Sear, R. (1980) A summary of the results of radioisotope brain scans on a large series of patients. *Br. J. Radiol.*, **53**, 1174–6.

Boyd, R. E., Robson, J., Hunt, F. C. *et al.* (1973) ^{99m}Tc gluconate complexes for renal scintigraphy. *Br. J. Radiol.*, **46**, 604–12.

Britton, K. E., Nimmon, C. C., Jarritt, P. H., Granowska, M. *et al.* (1977) in *Advanced Medicine*, Vol. 13 (ed. G. M. Besser), Pitman Medical, London, pp. 444–61.

Britton, K. E., Granowska, M., Rutland, M. *et al.* (1979a) in *Progress in Stroke Research*, Vol. 1 (eds R. M. Greenhalgh and F. C. Rose), Pitman Medical, London, pp. 307–15.

Britton, K. E., Granowska, M., Nimmon, C. C. *et al.* (1985) Cerebral blood flow in hypertensive patients with cerebrovascular disease. *Nucl. Med. Commun.*, **6**, 251–61.

Britton, K. E., Nimmon, C. C., Granowska, M. and Lee, T. Y. (1979b) in *Information Processing in Medical Imaging*, INSERM, Paris, pp. 469–86.

Britton, K. E., Granowska, M. and Nimmon, C. C. (1981) in *Proceedings of the International Symposium on Medical Radionuclide Imaging, Heidelberg 1980*, International Atomic Agency, Vienna.

Bruine, J. F., van Royen, E. A., Vyth, A. *et al.* (1985) Thallium-201 diethyldithiocarbamate: an alternative to iodine-123 *N*-isopropyl-*p*-iodoamphetamine. *J. Nucl. Med.*, **26**, 925–30.

Buell, U., Moser, E. A., Schmiedek, P. *et al.* (1984) Dynamic SPECT with Xe-133: regional cerebral blood flow in patients with unilateral cerebrovascular disease: concise communication. *J. Nucl. Med.*, **25**, 441–6.

Buell, U., Stirner, H., Ferbert, D. *et al.* (1987) Cerebral blood flow/volume–SPECT with Tc-99m labelled hexamethylpropyleneamine oxime (HMPAO) and red blood cells in cerebrovascular disease (CVD) or epilepsy (E). *J. Nucl. Med.*, **28**, 600.

Carne, C. A. (1987) Neurological manifestations: ABC of AIDS. *Br. Med. J.*, **294**, 1399–402.

Carril, J. M., MacDonald, A. F., Dendy, P. P. *et al.* (1979) Cranial scintigraphy: value of adding emission computed tomographic sections to conventional pertechnetate images. *J. Nucl. Med.*, **20**, 117–23.

Chase, T. N., Foster, N. L., Fedio, P. *et al.* (1984) Regional cortical dysfunction in Alzheimer's disease as determined by positron emission tomography. *Ann. Neurol.*, **15** (Suppl. S), 170–4.

Chawluk, J. B., Alavi, A., Dann, R. *et al.*(1987) Positron emission tomography in aging and dementia: effect of cerebral atrophy. *J. Nucl. Med.*, **28**, 431–7.

Costa, D. C., Ell, P. J., Cullum, I. D. *et al.* (1986a) The *in vivo* ditribution of ^{99}Tc^{m}-HMPAO in normal man. *Nucl. Med. Commun.*, **7**, 647–58.

Costa, D. C., Jones, B. E., Steiner, T. J. *et al.* (1986b) Relative ^{99m}Tc-HMPAO and ^{113}Sn-microspheres distribution in dog brain. *Nuklearmedizin*, **25**, A53.

Costa, D. C., Lui, D., Sinha, A. K. *et al.* (1987a) Tc-99m-*d,l*-HMPAO vs. Tl-201-DDC: subcellular distribution in rat brain. *J. Nucl. Med.*, **28**, 593.

Costa, D. C., Davies, P. T. G., Jones, B. E. *et al.* (1987b) Cerebral blood flow imaging in migraine patients with ^{99m}Tc-HM-PAO and single photon emission tomography: preliminary findings and a report on its efficacy. *Adv. Headache Res.*, 75–80.

Costa, D. C. Ell, P. J., Stibe, C. M. A. *et al.* (1987c) Tc-99m-HMPAO rCBF/SPET in Parkinsonians with the 'on–off' syndrome: preliminary results. *Nuklearmedizin*, **26**, 111.

Davies, K. L. and Mohs, R. C. (1986) Cholinergic drugs in Alzheimer's disease. *N. Engl. J. Med.*, **315**, 1286–7.

DeBoulay, G. H. and Marshall, J. (1975) Comparison of E. M. I. and radioisotope imaging in neurological disease. *Lancet*, **ii**, 1294–7.

De Roo, M., Mortelmans, L., Devos, P. *et al.* (1987) Clinical experience with Tc-99m-HMPAO high resolution SPECT of the brain in patients with cerebrovascular disease. *Nuklearmedizin*, **26**, 148.

Di Chiro, G., Ommaya, A. K., Ashbvurn, W. L. and Briner, W. H. (1968) Isotope cisternography in the diagnosis and follow up of cerebrospinal fluid rhinorrhoea. *J. Neurosurg.*, **28**, 522–9.

Drayer, B. P., Wilkins, R. H., Boehnke, M. *et al.* (1977) Cerebrospinal fluid rhinorrhoea demonstrated by metrizamide CT cisternography. *Am. J. Roentgenol.*, **129**, 149–51.

Ell, P. J., Deacon, J. M. and Jarritt, P. H. (1980) *Atlas of Computerized Emission Tomography*, Churchill Livingstone, Edinburgh.

Ell, P. J., Harrison, M. and Lui, D. (1983) Cerebral blood flow with iodine-123 labelled amines. *Lancet*, **ii**, 1348–52.

Ell, P. J., Cullum, I., Costa, D. C. *et al.* (1985a) A new regional cerebral blood flow mapping with $^{99}Tc^m$-labelled compound. *Lancet*, **ii**, 50–1.

Ell, P. J., Hocknell, J. M. L., Jarritt, P. H. *et al.* (1985b) A $^{99}Tc^m$-labelled radiotracer for the investigation of cerebral vascular disease. *Nucl. Med. Commun.*, **6**, 437–41.

Ell, P. J., Cullum, I. D., Lui, D. *et al.* (1987a) in *Journal of Functional Imaging in Neurology and Psychiatry* (eds J. Wade, S. Knezevic, V. A. Maximilian *et al.*), John Libbey, pp. 54–70.

Ell, P. J., Costa, D. C., Cullum, I. *et al.* (1987b) *The Clinical Application of rCBF Imaging by SPECT. Amersham*, Little Chalfont, UK.

Ell, P. J., Costa, D. C. and Harrison, M. (1987c) Imaging cerebral damage in HIV infection. *Lancet*, **i**, 569–70.

Frackowiak, R. S. J., Pozzilli, C., Legg, N. J. *et al.* (1981) Regional cerebral oxygen supply and utilization in dementia: a clinical and physiological study with oxygen-15 and positron tomography. *Brain*, **104**, 753–78.

Gemmell, H. G., Sharp, P. F., Evans, N. T. S. *et al.* (1984) Single photon emission tomography with ^{123}I-isopropyleamphetamine in Alzheimer's disease and multi-infarct dementia. *Lancet*, **ii**, 1348.

George, R. O. and Wagner, H. N. (1975) in *Non-Invasive Brain Imaging* (eds H. J. DeBlanc and J. A. Sorenson), Society of Nuclear Medicine, New York, pp. 3–23.

Gibbs, J. M., Wise, R. J. S., Leeuders, K. L. and Jones, T. (1984) Evaluation of cerebral perfusion reserve in patients with carotid artery occlusion. *Lancet*, **i**, 310–14.

Granowska, M., Britton, K. E., Afshar, F. *et al.* (1980) Total and regional cerebral flow non-invasive quantitation in patients with subarachnoid haemorrhage. *J. Neurosurg.*, **53**, 153–9.

Gray, W. R., Hickey, D., Parkey, R. W. *et al.* (1979) *Clinical Nuclear Cardiology* (eds R. W. Parkey, F. J. Bonte, L. M. Buja and J. T. Willerson), Appleton Century Crofts, New York, pp. 297–308.

Gustafson, L., Brun, A. and Ingvar, D. H. (1977) in *Cerebral Vascular Disease* (eds J. D. Meyer, H. Lechner and M. Reivich), Excerpta Medica, Amsterdam, pp. 5–9.

Hackinski, V. (1978) Cerebral blood flow: differentiation of Alzheimer's disease and multi-infarct dementia, in *Alzheimer's Disease: Senile Dementia and related disorders* (eds R. Katzman, R. D. Terry and K. L. Bick) Raven Press, New York, pp. 97–103.

Hauser, W. *et al.* (1970) Technetium-99m DTPA: a new radiopharmaceutical for brain and kidney scanning. *Radiology*, **94**, 679.

Hill, T. C., Holman, L., Lovett, R. *et al.* (1982) Initial experience with SPECT (single photon computerised tomography) of the brain using *N*-isopropyl-I-123 *p*-iodoamphetamine: concise communication. *J. Nucl. Med.*, **23**, 3.

Hill, T. C., Magistretti, P. L. Holman, B. L. *et al.* (1984) Assessment of regional cerebral blood flow (rCBF) in stroke using SPECT and *N*-isopropyl-(I-123)-*p*-iodoamphetamine (IMP), *Stroke*, 40–5.

Holm, S., Andersen, A. R., Vorstrup, S. *et al.* (1985) Dynamic SPECT of the brain using a lipophilic technetium-99m complex, PnAO. *J. Nucl. Med.*, **26**, 1129–34.

Holman, B. L., Hellmon, R. S., Goldsmith, S. J. *et al.* (1989) Biodistribution, dosimetry and clinical evaluation of Technetium 99m ethyl cysteinate driver in normal subjects and in patients with chronic cerebral infarction. *J. Nucl. Med.*, **30**, 1018–24.

Ingvar, D. H. (1975) *Brain work: Alfred Benzon Symposium VIII* (eds D. H. Ingvar and N. A. Lassen), Munksgaard, Copenhagen, pp. 397–413.

Ingvar, D. H. and Lassen, N. A. (1961) Quantitative determination of regional cerebral blood flow in man. *Lancet*, **ii**, 806–7.

Ingvar, D. H. and Risberg, J. (1965) Influence of mental activity upon regional cerebral blood flow in man. *Acta Neurol. Scand.*, **41** (Suppl. 43), 42–73.

Ingvar, D. H. and Risberg, J. (1967) Increase of regional cerebral blood flow during mental effort in normals and in patients with focal brain disorders. *Exp. Brain Res.*, **3**, 195–211.

Ingvar, D. H., Risberg, J. and Schwartz, M. S. (1975) Evidence of subnormal function of association cortex in presenile dementia. *Neurology*, **10**, 964–74.

Jarritt, P. H., Ell, P. J., Myers, M. J. *et al.* (1979) A new transverse section brain imager for single gamma emitters. *J. Nucl. Med.*, **20**, 319–27.

Keeling, F., Babich, J., Flower, M. A. *et al.* (1986) Early experience with $^{99}Tc^m$HMPAO in patients with brain tumours. *Nucl. Med. Commun.*, **7**, 274.

Kety, S. S. and Schmidt, C. F. (1945) The determination of cerebral blood flow in man by use of nitrous oxide in low concentrations. *Am. J. Phys.*, **143**, 53–66.

Knapp, W. H., von Kummen, R. and Kubler, W. (1986) Imaging of cerebral blood flow to volume distribution using SPECT. *J. Nucl. Med.*, **27**, 465–70.

Kung, K. F., Pan, S., Kung, M. P., Billings, J., Kasliwal, R., Reilley, J., Alavi, A. (1989) *In vitro* and *In vivo* evaluation of ^{123}I-IBZM. A potential CNS D-2 dopamine receptor imaging agent. *J. Nucl. Med.*, **30**, 88–92.

Kung, H. F., Tramposch, K. M. and Blau, M. (1983) A new brain perfusion imaging agent: *N,N,N'*-trimethyl-*N'*-(2-hydroxy-3-methyl-5-iodobenzyl)-1,3 propanediamine (HIPDM). *J. Nucl. Med.*, **24**, 66–72.

Langen, K.-J., Roosen, N., Kuwert, T. *et al.* (1987) ^{99m}Tc-HMPAO SPECT in the study of cerebral tumours: results in 40 patients. *Nuklearmedizin*, **26**, 118.

Lassen, N. A. (1966) The luxury perfusion syndrome and its possible relation to acute metabolic acidosis localised within the brain. *Lancet*, **ii**, 1113–15.

Lassen, N. A. and Munck, O. (1955) The cerebral blood flow in man determined by the use of radioactive krypton. *Acta Phys. Scand.*, **33**, 30.

Lassen, N.A., Roland, P. E., Larsen, B. *et al.* (1977) Mapping of human cerebral functions: a study of the regional cerebral blood flow pattern during rest, its reproducibility and the activations seen during basic sensory and motor functions. *Acta Neurol. Scand.*, **56** (Suppl. 64), 262–3.

Lassen, N. A., Henriksen, L. and Paulson, O. (1981) Regional cerebral blood flow in stroke by ^{133}xenon inhalation and emission tomography. *Stroke*, **12**, 3.

Lauritzen, M. (1987) in *Journal of Functional Imaging of*

Neurology and Psychiatry (eds J. Wade, S. Knezevic, V. A. Maximilian *et al.*), John Libbey, London.

Lenzi, G. L., Frackowiak, R. S. J. and Jones, T. (1982) Cerebral oxygen metabolism and blood flow in human cerebral ischemic infarction. *J. Cereb. Blood Flow Metab.*, **2**, 321–35.

Leonard, J.-P., Nowotnik, D. P. and Neirinckx, R. D. (1987) Technetium-99m-*d,l*-HM-PAO: a new radiopharmaceutical for imaging regional brain perfusion using SPECT: a comparison with iodine-123 HIPDM. *J. Nucl. Med.*, **27**, 1819–1823.

Lucignani, C., Nehlig, A., Blasberg, R. *et al.* (1985) Metabolic and kinetic considerations in the use of ^{125}I-HIPDM for quantitative measurement of regional cerebral blood flow. *J. Cereb. Blood Flow Metab.*, **5**, 86–96.

Mallet, B. L. and Veall, N. (1965) The measurement of regional cerebral clearance rates in man using xenon-133 inhalation and extracranial recording. *Clin. Sci.*, **29**, 179–91.

Matsuda, H., Seki, H., Sumiya, H. *et al.* (1986) Quantitative cerebral blood flow measurements using *N*-isopropyl-(iodine-123)*p*-iodoamphetamine and single photon emission computed tomography with rotating gamma camera. *Am. J. Phys. Imaging*, **1**, 186–94.

Maximilian, V. A., Prohovnik, I., Risberg, J. and Hakansson, K. (1978) Regional blood flow changes in the left cerebral hemisphere during word pair learning and recall. *Brain Lang.*, **6**, 22–31.

Maziere, B. and Maziere, M. (1990) Where have we got to with neuroreceptor mapping of the human brain? *European Journal of Nuclear Medicine*, **16**, no. 11, 817–837.

Mazziotta, J. C. and Phelps, M. E. (1986) in *Positron Emission Tomography and Autoradiography: Principles and Applications for the Brain and Heart* (eds M. Phelps, J. Mazziotta and H. Schelbert), Raven Press, New York, pp. 493–570.

Meurman, O. H., Irjal, K., Suonpaa, J. and Laurent, B. (1979) A new method for the identification of cerebrospinal fluid leakage. *Acta Otolaryngol.*, **87**, 366–9.

Moretti, J. L., Defer, G., Cesaro, P. *et al.* (1985) Early and late SPECT with *n*-isopropyl-*p*-iodoamphetamine-I-123 (IAMP) in cerebral ischaemia. *Eur. J. Nucl. Med.*, **11** (suppl.): A24.

Moretti, J. L., Cinotti, L., Cesaro, P. *et al.* (1987) Amines for brain tomoscintigraphy. *Nucl. Med. Commun.*, **8**, 581–95.

Moses, D. C., Natarajan, T. K., Previosi, T. J. *et al.* (1973) Quantitative cerebral circulation studies with sodium pertechnetate. *J. Nucl. Med.*, **14**, 142–8.

Mueller, S. P., Johnson, K. A., Hamil, D. *et al.* (1986) Assessment of I-123 IMP SPECT in mild/moderate and severe Alzheimer's disease. *J. Nucl. Med.*, **27**, 889.

Nagle, C. E. (1980) Use of immediate static scans in combination with radionuclide cerebral angiography as a confirmatory test in the diagnosis of brain death. *Clin. Nucl. Med.*, **5**, 152–3.

Navia, B. A., Jordan, B. D. and Price, R. W. (1986a) The AIDS dementia complex: I. Clinical features. *Ann. Neurol.*, **19**, 517–24.

Navia, B. A., Cho, E.-S., Petito, C. K. *et al.* (1986b) The AIDS dementia complex: II. Neuropathology. *Ann. Neurol.*, **19**, 525–35.

Neirinckx, R. D., Canning, L. R., Piper, I. M. *et al.* (1987) Technetium-99m *d,l*-HM-PAO: a new radiopharmaceutical for SPEC imaging of regional cerebral blood perfusion. *J. Nucl. Med.*, **29**, 191–202.

Obrist, W. D., Thomson, H. K., Wang, H. S. and Wilkinson, W. E. (1975) Regional cerebral blood flow activated by ^{133}Xe-inhalation. *Stroke*, **6**, 245–56.

Oldendorf, W. H. (1975) in *Non-invasive Brain Imaging* (eds H. J. De Blanc and J. A. Sorenson), Society of Nuclear Medicine, New York, pp. 17–23.

Olesen, J. (1971) Contralateral focal increase of cerebral blood flow in man during arm work. *Brain*, **94**, 635–46.

Potchen, E. J. and McCready, V. R. (1972) Neuronuclear medicine. *Prog. Nucl. Med.*, **1**, 2.

Potchen, E. J., Holman, B. L. Evans, R. G. *et al.* (1971) in *Proceedings of the 4th International Symposium in Brain and Blood Flow* (ed. R. W. R. Russell), Pitman, London, pp. 94–7.

Prohovnik, I., Hakansson, K. and Risberg, J. (1980) Observations on the functional significance of regional blood flow in 'resting' normal subjects. *Neuropsychologia*, **18** (2), 203–17.

Razzak, M. A., Muddaris, F. and Christie, J. H. (1980) Sensitivity of radionuclide brain scan imaging and computerized axial tomography in detecting subdural haematoma. *Clin. Nucl. Med.*, **5**, 154–8.

Riccio, M. (1987) Aids and dementia. *Br. J. Hosp. Med.*, 11 July, **38**, 11.

Risberg, J. (1987) in *Journal of Functional Imaging in Neurology and Psychiatry* (eds J. Wade, S. Knezevic, V. A. Maximilian *et al.*), John Libbey, London, pp. 35–43.

Risberg, J. and Ingvar, D. H. (1972) Multibolus technique for measuring the distribution of cerebral blood flow over short intervals in man. *Circ. Res.*, **31**, 889–98.

Risberg, J., Halsey, J. H., Wills, E. L. and Wilson, E. M. (1975) Hemispheric specialization in normal man studied by bilateral measurements of the regional cerebral blood flow: a study with the 133-Xe inhalation technique. *Brain*, **98**, 511–24.

Risberg, J., Maximilian, A. V. and Prohovnik, I. (1977) Changes of cortical activity patterns during habituation to a reasoning test: a study with the ^{133}Xe inhalation technique for measurement of regional cerebral blood flow. *Neuropsychologia*, **15**, 793–8.

Roine, R. O., Launes, J., Lindroth, L. and Nikkinen, P. (1986) ^{99m}Tc-hexamethylpropyleneamine oxime scans to confirm brain death. *Lancet*, **ii**, 1223–4.

Rossor, M. (1987) Dementia. *Br. J. Hosp. Med.*, **38**, 46–50.

Royal, H. O., Hill, Th. C. and Holman, B. L. (1985) in *Seminars in Nuclear Medicine XV* (eds L. M. Freeman and M. D. Blaufox), Grune and Stratton, New York, pp. 357–76.

Rutland, M. D., Lee, T. Y., Nimmon, C. C. *et al.* (1980) Measurement of the effects of a single dose of Prazosin on the cerebral blood flow in hypertensive patients. *Postgrad. Med. J.*, **56**, 818–22.

Schall, G. L., Zeiger, L. S. and Di Chino, G. (1971) Clinical comparison of 2 ^{99m}Tc tracers for brain scanning: pertechnetate versus labelled albumin. *Radiology*, **99**, 361–8.

Sharp, P. F., Smith, F. W., Gemmell, H. G. *et al.* (1986)

Technetium-99m HMPAO stereoisomers as potential agents for imaging regional cerebral blood flow: human volunteer studies. *J. Nucl. Med.*, **27**, 171–7.

Shields, R. A., Burjon, A. W., Prescott, M. C. *et al.* (1986) Tc-99m-HMPAO: a new brain imaging agent: biodistribution studies and initial clinical trials in dementia. *Nucl. Med. Commun.*, **7**, 284–5.

Suess, E., Podreka, I., Goldenberg, G. *et al.* (1986) Initial experience with $^{99}Tc^{m}$-hexamethylpropyleneamineoxime brain SPECT. *Nucl. Med. Commun.*, **7**, 285.

Suess, E., Podreka, I., Baumgartner, Ch. *et al.* (1987) $^{99}Tc^{m}$-HMPAO brain SPECT in partial complex seizures. *Nucl. Med. Commun.*, **8**, 240.

Summers, W. K., Majovski, L. V., Marsh, G. M. *et al.* (1986) Oral tetrahydroaminoacridine in long term treatment of senile dementia, Alzheimer type. *N. Engl. J. Med.*, **315**, 1241–5.

Symon, L. and Dorsch, N. W. C. (1975) Use of long term intracranial pressure measurement to assess hydrocephalic patients prior to surgery. *J. Neurosurg.*, **42**, 258–73.

Testa, H. J., Shields, R. A., Burjan, A. W. I. *et al.* (1987) Investigation of dementia using $^{99}Tc^{m}$-HMPAO and single photon emission tomography. *Nucl. Med. Commun.*, **8**, 241.

Tramposch, K. M., Kung, H. F. and Blau, M. (1980) Brain imaging with I-123 labelled amines for brain studies: localisation of I-123 iodophenylakyl amines in rat brain. *J. Nucl. Med.*, **21**, 940–6.

Vallabhajosula, S., Zimmermon, R. E., Micord, M. *et al.* (1989) Technetium-99m ECD: A new brain imaging agent: *In vivo* kinetics and biodistribution studies in normal subjects. *J. Nucl. Med.*, **30**, 599–604.

Van Duyl, W. A. and Volkers, A. C. W. (1980) Measurement of cerebral blood flow in the pig by Xe-133 clearance technique: failure of the two compartmental clearance model. *Eur. J. Nucl. Med.*, **5**, 86–96.

Vangelista, R., Visentin, E., Dalla Pozza, F. *et al.* (1987) Brain SPECT with ^{99m}Tc-labelled hexamethyl propylene amine oxime (^{99m}Tc-HM-PAO): our experience. *J. Nucl. Med. Allied Sci.*, **31**, 166.

Van Horn, G. (1987) Dementia. *Am. J. Med.*, **83**, 101–10.

Verhoeff, N. P. L. G., Bobeldijk, M., Van Royen, E. A., Feenstra, M. G. P., Boer, G. J., Van Doremalen, P.A.P.M. (1989) In Vitro and In Vivo binding of dopamine D2 receptors with ^{123}I-Iodobenzamide in rat brain. *Pharmaceutisch Weekblad Scientific Edition*, **11**, *Suppl. J*: J13.

Verhoeff N. P. L. G., Van Royen, E. A., Costa, D. C., Cullum, I. D., Lui, D., Ell, P. J., Sved, G. M. S., Barrett, J. J., Toone, B. (1990) A study of the dopamine D2 receptor in human brain with ^{123}I-IBZM SPET. *Nucl. Med. Commun.*, **3**, 246.

Volkert, W. A., Hoffman, T. J., Seger, R. M. *et al.* (1984) Tc-99m propylene amine oxime (Tc-99m-PnAO): a potential brain radiopharmaceutical. *Eur. J. Nucl. Med.*, **9**, 511–16.

Winchell, H. S., Horst, W. D., Braun, L. *et al.* (1980) *N*-Isopropyl (iodine-123) *p*-iodoamphetamine: single pass brain uptake and washout: binding to brain synaptosomes and localisation in dog and monkey brain. *J. Nucl. Med.*, **21**, 947–52.

Wise, R. J. S., Bernardi, S., Frackowiak, R. S. J. *et al.* (1983) Serial observations on the pathophysiology of acute stroke: the transition from ischaemia to infarction as reflected in regional oxygen extraction. *Brain*, **106**, 197–222.

Woolley, J. L., Williams, B. and Ventakesh, S., (1977) Cranial isotope section scanning. *Clin. Radiol.*, **28**, 517–28.

FURTHER READING

Editorial (1989) SPECT and PET in epilepsy, *Lancet*, **i**, 135–7.

Kung, H. F. (1990) New technetium-99m labelled brain perfusion imaging agents, *Semin. Nucl. Med.*, **20**, 150–8.

Maziere, B. and Maziere, M. (1990) Where have we got to with neuroceptor mapping of the human brain?, *Eur. J. Nucl. Med.*, **16**, 817–35.

CHAPTER EIGHT

Thyroid disease

M. N. Maisey and I. Fogelman

8.1 INTRODUCTION

The prevalence of diseases of the thyroid is high although not always diagnosed clinically. In a population study of north-east England, Tunbridge *et al.* (1977) reported that the prevalence of hyperthyroidism in adult females was 1.9–2.7%, of overt hypothyroidism 1.4–1.9%, of subclinical hypothyroidism 7.5% and of non-toxic goitres 8.6%. The prevalence of each condition, however, was much lower in males. In 1956 Permlulter and Slater estimated that 4–12% of the population of the USA had palpable thyroid nodules of which 2–5% were probably malignant.

The correct management of thyroid diseases depends on an accurate diagnosis followed by appropriate treatment and follow-up. Radionuclides have always played a leading part in all aspects of the management of thyroid diseases: radioimmunoassay techniques have revolutionized the investigation of thyroid dysfunction while radionuclide scanning has long been the main method of investigating the thyroid *in vivo*. Over the last decade the potential role of thyroid scanning in clinical practice has been expanded by the introduction of new radiopharmaceuticals – ^{123}I, ^{99m}Tc-labelled pentavalent dimercapto succinic acid (DMSA), ^{131}I-*meta*-iodobenzylguanidine (MIBG), etc. (Table 8.1) – and in addition the development of other imaging techniques has altered the role of radionuclide scanning in the management of thyroid disease. For example, the use of ultrasound scanning of the thyroid and the more widespread application of fine needle aspiration cytology have both altered the way in which we investigate thyroid nodules. Since the introduction of routine screening programmes for the detection of neonatal hypothyroidism the part played by radionuclide thyroid scanning in babies with early thyroid failure has had to be revised. The increasing use of other diagnostic imaging techniques such as X-ray, computed tomography (CT) and nuclear magnetic resonance (NMR) will all have an impact on the way we use radioisotopes in the investigation of thyroid disease, but have not in any instance significantly detracted from the use of radionuclide scanning. Radioactive iodine has become established as a simple, cheap and effective method of treating thyrotoxicosis, and in many cases represents the treatment of choice. Fear that its use might result in an increased risk of cancer and other genetic complications has not been substantiated after worldwide experience for more than three decades.

Table 8.1 Radiopharmaceuticals used in the investigation of thyroid diseases

Radiopharmaceutical	*Applications*
^{99m}Tc-pertechnetate	Routine thyroid scanning
^{123}I	Thyroid scanning when a radioisotope of iodine is required
^{131}I	The investigation of thyroid cancer
^{127}I (stable)	Investigation of thyroid nodules and suppressed tissue
^{67}Ga citrate	Investigation of thyroid lymphoma, silent thyroiditis, thyroid infection and amyloid
^{201}Tl	Investigation of thyroid cancer, thyroid nodules, demonstration of suppressed thyroid tissue
^{99m}Tc-labelled pentavalent DMSA	Investigation of medullary thyroid carcinoma
^{131}I/^{123}I-MIBG	Investigation of medullary thyroid carcinoma
Monoclonal antithyroglobulin antibody	Investigation of thyroid cancer

Table 8.2 Classification of thyroid disease

I. Diseases primarily characterized by euthyroidism
A. Non-toxic diffuse goitre
  1. Sporadic
  2. Endemic
  3. Compensatory, following subtotal thyroidectomy
B. Non-toxic uninodular goitre
  1. Functional nodule
  2. Non-functional
C. Non-toxic multinodular goitre due to causes under IA
  1. Functional nodules
  2. Non-functional nodules
  3. Functional and non-functional nodules
D. Tumours
  1. Adenoma and teratoma
  2. Carcinoma
  3. Lymphoma
  4. Sarcoma
E. Acute thyroiditis
  1. Suppurative
  2. Subacute, non-suppurative
F. Chronic thyroiditis
  1. Lymphocytic (Hashimoto)
  2. Invasive fibrous (Riedel)
  3. Suppurative
  4. Non-suppurative
G. Degeneration or infiltration
  1. Haemorrhage or infarction
  2. Amyloid
  3. Haemochromatosis
H. Congenital anomaly

II. Diseases primarily characterized by hyperthyroidism
A. Toxic diffuse goitre (Graves', Basedow's disease)
  1. With eye changes (ophthalmopathy)
  2. With localized myxoedema (dermopathy)
  3. With acropachy
  4. Neonatal or congenital
  5. With incidental non-functional nodule or nodules
  6. With euthyroidism and eye changes
B. Toxic uninodular goitre
C. Toxic multinodular goitre
  1. Functional nodules, non-functional parenchyma
  2. Functional nodules, functional parenchyma
D. Nodular goitre with hyperthyroidism due to exogenous iodine (Jod–Basedow)
E. Exogenous thyroid hormone excess
  1. Thyrotoxicosis factitia
  2. Thyrotoxicosis medicamentosa
F. Tumours
  1. Adenoma of thyroid, follicular
  2. Carcinoma of thyroid, follicular
  3. Thyrotrophin-secreting tumours

III. Diseases primarily characterized by hypothyroidism
A. Idiopathic hypothyroidism
  1. Myxoedema
  2. Cretinism
B. Thyroid destruction due to
  1. Surgery
  2. Radioiodine
  3. X-ray
C. Thyrotrophin deficiency
  1. Isolated
  2. Panhypopituitarism
D. Thyrotrophin-releasing factor (TRF) deficiency due to hypothalamic injury or disease.

Classification of thyroid disease modified from Werner (1969).

Radioactive iodine is also important in the treatment and follow-up of differentiated thyroid cancer.

In this chapter we discuss systematic and practical approaches to the management of the most important clinical problems in thyroid disease with emphasis on the role of nuclear medicine techniques.

The classification of thyroid disease is shown in Table 8.2.

8.2 DIAGNOSIS OF THYROID DYSFUNCTION

8.2.1 PATHOPHYSIOLOGY

A knowledge of the changes that occur in hyperthyroidism and hypothyroidism is fundamental to an understanding of the laboratory investigations of these conditions.

The basic abnormality in hyperthyroidism and hypothyroidism is an increased or decreased concentration of circulating free thyroid hormones with a corresponding change in the total serum concentration of these hormones. The estimation of free serum thyroxine (fT4) and triiodothyronine (fT3) has been difficult because of the small absolute and relative concentrations with respect to total hormone concentrations; however, recent advances have now made them routinely available.

In hyperthyroidism both serum T3 and T4 are usually raised and therefore it is not necessary to measure both hormones routinely for diagnosis, but in a significant proportion of hyperthyroid patients (about 10%) serum total T3 concentration may be abnormally raised at presentation when serum T4 lies within the normal range (T3 toxicosis); elevated serum T4 with normal T3 (T4 toxicosis) has rarely been reported. These discrepancies occur less often with fT3 and fT4. Other factors beside hyperthyroidism such as a coexisting severe non-thyroidal illness which impairs peripheral conversion of T4 to T3 may account for disparities in hormone concentrations. For most patients with hyperthyroidism, the rise in serum T3 is much greater than that of serum T4. It is clear from these observations that measurement of serum T3 is a more sensitive and reliable investigation for hyperthyroidism than serum T4.

In hypothyroidism there is a greater and earlier fall in serum T4 compared to serum T3 which may often remain within the normal range when serum T4 is well below normal. Thus, while serum T3 is the investigation of choice for hyperthyroidism, serum T4 is a better screening test for hypothyroidism. Thyroid failure may be a primary abnormality of the thyroid gland or rarely may be secondary to impaired secretion of thyroid-stimulating hormone (TSH) by the pituitary gland. In primary hypothyroidism, the low serum T4 is accompanied by a rise of serum TSH whereas in secondary hypothyroidism the low serum T4 is associated with a low serum TSH. Measurement of serum TSH is therefore essential to distinguish between primary and secondary hypothyroidism. A low serum TSH is not always sufficient to confirm hypothyroidism due to pituitary failure and it may be necessary to show that serum TSH concentration is unresponsive to thyrotrophin-releasing hormone (TRH) stimulation. Recently the TSH assays have increased in sensitivity so that low suppressed levels of serum TSH that occur in hyperthyroidism can be distinguished from normal levels. These ultrasensitive TSH assays have consequently been used as a primary investigation of hyper- and hypothyroidism, but there is not universal agreement on the effectiveness of this approach to diagnosis.

Changes in serum total T3 and T4 levels may be due not only to altered thyroid function but also to altered concentrations of carrier proteins, especially thyroxine-binding globulin (TBG) in the absence of any thyroid dysfunction. Since over 99% of the total circulating thyroid hormones are bound to serum proteins an increase or decrease in serum TBG is accompanied by a corresponding increase or decrease in bound and total serum T3 and T4 in the presence of normal concentrations of free hormones. In such cases, serum total T3 and T4 levels may not reflect the patient's true thyroid status. Serum TBG should therefore be measured in any condition which is known to alter its concentration (Table 8.3) and whenever the serum tT3 or tT4 is close to the limits of the normal range or does not correspond to the clinical status of the patient. Artefactual changes in the total serum T3 and T4 concentrations can also occur if the binding of these hormones to TBG is interfered with by drugs such as salicylates, sulphonylureas and phenytoin in the absence of any change in the TBG concentration. However, with the more widespread use of free hormone measurements these considerations are of less importance.

Table 8.3 Factors that affect serum TBG concentration

Increased TBG	*Decreased TBG*
1. Contraceptive pill and other oestrogens	1. Androgens and anabolic steroids
2. Pregnancy	2. Severe illness
3. Hypothyroidism	3. Hyperthyroidism
4. Inherited disorders of TBG production	4. Inherited disorders of TBG production
	5. Chronic diseases especially liver disease, nephrotic syndrome, malnutrition/malabsorption

8.2.2 CLINICAL SITUATIONS

(a) Hyperthyroidism

The single most reliable test for hyperthyroidism is a sensitive TSH measurement which will show a TSH suppressed below the normal range (0.3–3 mU litre^{-1}). A serum total or free T3 level will provide increased diagnostic certainty and in the absence of an available sensitive TSH assay the T3 measurement will provide the primary test for hyperthyroidism. Rarely the serum T4 will be elevated when a T3 is normal but if the TSH is used and a T4 measured when a normal T3 is found with a suppressed TSH this should not be a problem. The TRH stimulation test remains a useful discriminating test when results are equivocal but is much less frequently used now that low levels of TSH can be routinely measured. If total hormone levels are being used the use of TBG measurements may be helpful when discrepantly high or low total hormone levels are discovered.

(b) Hyperthyroid patients receiving treatment

(i) β-Blockers Propranolol or other β-blocking drugs that are used for symptomatic treatment of hyperthyroidism may slightly lower serum T3 concentrations, probably by interfering with peripheral conversion of T4 to T3. However, quantitatively the fall is minimal and does not account for the main therapeutic effect of the drugs and is unlikely to cause confusion in the laboratory assessment of thyroid function.

(ii) Antithyroid drugs Patients having treatment with antithyroid drugs should have serum T3 and T4 levels measured regularly to assess whether they are being undertreated or overtreated because it is often difficult to assess their clinical status. There is a tendency for an earlier and greater fall in serum T4 compared to serum T3 during treatment and measurement of one hormone may be misleading. A persistently raised serum T3 and raised or normal serum T4 means the patient is still hyperthyroid. A normal serum T3 and T4 or a borderline high serum T3 with normal or borderline low T4 indicate that the patient is euthyroid. A low serum T4 with normal or low serum T3 means the patient is becoming hypothyroid. The dose of antithyroid drugs will be adjusted in the light of the thyroid function results and the patient's clinical state. The TSH level may be helpful in indicating excess treatment if it is elevated but the reverse does not apply – the patient may be euthyroid or hypothyroid with a persistently suppressed TSH level.

(iii) Radioiodine and subtotal thyroidectomy Both serum T3 and TSH should also be routinely measured during the first few months (usually at six-weekly intervals) following radioidine treatment or subtotal thyroidectomy to determine whether the patient remains hyperthyroid, or is becoming euthyroid or hypothyroid. When the T3 has become normal the TSH and T4 measurements are used to detect developing hypothyroidism. Hypothyroidism occurring within the first six months of radioiodine or surgical treatment may be transient and revert spontaneously, especially when the fall in T4 is not accompanied by a rise in TSH. On the other hand hypothyroidism developing later is usually permanent. Early asymptomatic or mild hypothyroidism is best left untreated and followed up regularly with serum TSH measurement to allow recovery to occur. If the patient is symptomatic, thyroid replacement should not be withheld but it is advisable to stop treatment for four to six weeks at the end of the first year to exclude transient hypothyroidism. All patients who have been treated with ^{131}I or had surgery for hyperthyroidism must have long-term follow-up to detect late hypothyroidism. An annual serum T4 estimation is the best and easiest routine follow-up investigation for screening in the absence of any specific symptoms or signs. If serum T4 is below normal, hypothyroidism can be confirmed by measurement of serum TSH on the same sample. If recurrent hyperthyroidism is suspected clinically, serum T3 should be estimated. The addition of a sensitive TSH measurement to the follow-up protocol improves the effectiveness of the assessment but increases the cost.

(iv) Block/replacement regime The best tests for assessing the effectiveness of this regime where antithyroid drugs and thyroid hormones are given together will depend on which thyroid hormone (T3 or T4) is given in combination with the antithyroid drug. The TSH level should ideally be maintained in the normal range during treatment. If T4 is given the T3 and T4 should be measured and maintained in the normal range; however, a better regime is to give T3 as the replacement hormone and keep the TSH, and T3 should be maintained in the normal range. The T4 level under these circumstances should be almost undetectable and will establish whether the antithyroid drug-blocking effect is complete.

(c) Hypothyroidism

When hypothyroidism is suspected clinically, laboratory investigations should be performed not only to confirm the diagnosis but also to differentiate between primary and secondary thyroid failure. The distinction is important as secondary hypothyroidism requires further investigation and management of the underlying cause such as a pituitary tumour in addition to thyroid replacement.

Serum T4 is usually the initial investigation of choice as it is a more sensitive and reliable test of hypothyroidism than serum T3; better results are obtained if this is combined with TSH, which should always be measured when T4 levels are found to be low.

(i) Normal serum T4 If the serum T4 is well within the normal range, the diagnosis of hypothyroidism is practically excluded and no further investigation is necessary unless the clinical suspicion of thyroid failure remains high, when further confirmatory investigations should be performed.

(ii) Low or borderline low serum T4 If the serum T4 is below or near the lower limit of the normal range, serum TSH concentration should be measured on serum stored from the same blood specimen. Raised serum TSH and low or borderline low serum T4 in the same patient confirms mild primary hypothyroidism. It is useful to measure thyroid microsomal autoantibodies in the serum of these patients as their presence in significant titres indicates primary hypothyroidism due to autoimmune thyroiditis (Hashimoto's disease), which usually requires life-long thyroid replacement. This should be distinguished from the transient hypothyroidism which may be associated with De Quervain's thyroiditis, radioiodine therapy or subtotal thyroidectomy.

If the serum TSH is not elevated in spite of a low serum T4, the patient may either have secondary hypothyroidism or, if total T4 has been measured, may be euthyroid and have a low serum TBG. A low TBG should be excluded by measuring serum TBG or T4. A TRH stimulation test should be performed to confirm or exclude pituitary hypothyroidism, when an absent TSH response to TRH with a low serum T4 will confirm pituitary hypothyroidism. Further investigations including full pituitary function tests and radiographs and CT of the pituitary fossa should be carried out to establish the nature and extent of the pituitary abnormality.

(d) Treatment of hypothyroidism

Thyroid function tests should be used to monitor thyroid hormone replacement in hypothyroid patients. L-Thyroxine (T4) is the usual preparation used and the normal replacement dose is 0.1–0.2 mg daily (100–200 μg). A low dose is used initially, (0.05 mg T4 daily), increasing gradually by small increments every two to four weeks until the full replacement dose is achieved. In elderly patients, those with prolonged hypothyroidism or associated heart disease, the starting dose should be even lower, 0.025 mg (25 μg) daily, and increased very slowly every four weeks otherwise tachycardia and myocardial ischaemia may be precipitated.

The dose of thyroid hormone is adjusted until the elevated serum TSH has fallen to normal levels but not suppressed below the normal range; it is important to realize that the TSH levels may continue to fall for several weeks after a change of dose. Thyroid function tests should not be performed until the patient has been on the same dose of thyroxine for at least four weeks. When the serum TSH has returned to normal, serum T4 is usually found to be in the upper normal range or slightly elevated, whereas the T3 is usually in the mid-normal range. It is advisable to check the serum TSH concentration once a year in all patients receiving thyroid replacement to ensure that their requirements do not change.

With pituitary hypothyroidism, since serum TSH is not elevated initially, serum T4 estimation is used to monitor the dose of thyroid replacement, which is increased until the serum T4 concentration is within the upper normal range.

It may necessary to assess whether thyroxine treatment need be continued in patients who were started on hormone replacement without a firm diagnosis of hypothyroidism. Thyroid medication is withheld for four to six weeks and serum T4 and TSH measured. If the patient is unwilling to withhold the full treatment dose for the test, the dose is halved for six weeks and serum T4 and TSH are measured. Unless the patient is biochemically hypothyroid on half doses, medication can then be withheld completely and the tests repeated.

(e) Neonatal hypothyroidism

Congenital hypothyroidism is an important cause of severe mental retardation, with an estimated incidence of one in every 3000–6000 live births in Europe and America. Early diagnosis and treatment can significantly improve the prognosis for mental development. Therefore biochemical screening of all newborn babies for congenital hypothyroidism is now considered essential for the early diagnosis and treatment of this condition.

Screening is carried out on capillary blood collected on filter paper on day 4–6 after birth at the same time that screening for phenylketonuria by the Guthrie test is carried out. This enables samples to be mailed by postal service to a central laboratory. Alternatively, cord blood collected at the time of delivery can be used but is less suitable for dispatch. Commercial radioimmunoassay kits are now available for T4 or TSH estimation on dried capillary blood collected on filter paper.

Measurement of serum T4 alone will miss 30% of cases of neonatal hypothyroidism (Delange *et al.*, 1979), including particularly those with 'compensated hypothyroidism', i.e. normal T4 and high TSH at or shortly after birth, which may occur with ectopic thyroids. Frank hypothyroidism and associated mental retardation may develop subsequently if the condition is undiagnosed and untreated. Measurement of serum TSH alone is a more sensitive screening test than serum T4 but will miss secondary hypothyroidism (normal TSH, low T4) but which contributes only 3–5% of all cases of congenital hypothyroidism

(Delange *et al.*, 1979). Measurement of both serum T4 and TSH will detect all cases but the increased workload and cost make it a less practical proposition, particularly since the detection rate is only improved by 3–5% over that of screening with serum TSH alone.

It is intended that the screening programme will permit the diagnosis of congenital hypothyroidism to be made as quickly as possible after birth, preferably within two weeks so that patients can be recalled for assessment and further testing if necessary and treatment started with minimum delay. It has also been shown that hypothyroidism may be transient in about 10% of cases, so that the need to continue permanent thyroid replacement should be reviewed at a suitable time when treatment may be safely withheld for a few weeks for repeat thyroid function tests.

(f) Pregnancy and oestrogen therapy

Due to high circulating oestrogen concentrations, pregnant women and those on the contraceptive pill or other oestrogen preparation have raised serum TBG concentrations which increase serum total T3 and T4 levels even when they are euthyroid; therefore free hormones should be used to assess thyroid function whenever possible. If total T3 and T4 are used, these patients should also have serum TBG measured and the serum T3 and T4 concentrations interpreted carefully in the light of the serum TBG value. A TRH test may be necessary to confirm or exclude hyperthyroidism if both serum T3 and TBG are raised, but should be avoided in pregnancy. However, sensitive serum TSH measurements are the most useful measurements together with the free hormones.

(g) Elderly sick patients

Serum T3 falls slightly but significantly in old age even in the absence of any thyroid dysfunction (Lipson *et al.*, 1979). Serum T4 decreases comparatively less or remains unchanged. The fall in serum T3 becomes more marked in elderly patients who are seriously ill for whatever reason, probably due to failure of peripheral conversion of T4 to T3. Consequently the serum concentration of these hormones, particularly serum T3, may not reflect the true thyroid status. Serum TSH estimation and its response to TRH are necessary to confirm or exclude thyroid dysfunction in elderly sick patients, particularly since clinical diagnosis is often difficult in this age group. Alternatively, serum T3 or T4 can be reassessed when the patient has recovered from the acute illness and compared with the normal range for this age group.

8.3. HYPERTHYROIDISM

The diagnosis of hyperthyroidism is incomplete unless its cause is also established, because the choice of management and prognosis will depend on the underlying cause. Table 8.4 lists the most important causes of hyperthyroidism and a brief discussion of the aetiology and mechanism of hyperthyroidism in these conditions is relevant to understand the method of investigation and diagnosis.

Most commonly, excess thyroid hormone secretion is associated with the presence of an abnormal 'thyroid-stimulating immunoglobulin' (TSI or TSab) directed against the TSH receptor. This thyroid stimulator is found in patients with a toxic diffuse goitre (Graves' disease) and results in diffuse hyperplasia with hyperfunction of all thyroid tissue capable of responding. If the gland contains pre-existing non-functioning nodular areas, cysts or scars, only the paranodular tissue will be stimulated and the gland may feel nodular. The cause of hyperthyroidism is then Graves' disease superimposed on a previous nodular goitre, i.e. Graves' disease with incidental non-functioning nodules.

Hyperthyroidism may also occur if a localized area of the thyroid has changed in such a way that the follicular cells secrete thyroid hormones independently of TSH control. This is an autonomous

Table 8.4 Causes of hyperthyroidism

1. Graves' disease (diffuse or nodular variants)
2. Solitary or multiple toxic autonomous nodules (toxic adenoma, Plummer's disease)
3. Thyroid hormone 'leakage'
   (a) Subacute (De Quervain's) thyroiditis
   (b) Painless (silent) thyroiditis
   (c) Hashimoto's thyroiditis
   (d) Post-partum thyroiditis
4. Iodide-induced hyperthyroidism (Jod–Basedow's phenomenon)
5. Excess thyroid hormone ingestion
6. Rare causes including:
   (a) Pituitary TSH-dependent hyperthyroidism
   (b) Ectopic TSH-secreting tumour
   (c) Extensive functioning differentiated thyroid cancer
   (d) Trophoblastic tumour
   (e) Struma ovarii

functioning nodule and, as the nodule grows in size, it may secret sufficient hormones to exceed the physiological requirements and the patient becomes hyperthyroid. The rest of the gland may be normal but have function suppressed due to secondary suppression of TSH. The gland may also contain pre-existing non-functioning nodules if the antonomous change has occurred in a pre-existing nodular goitre. Hyperthyroidism caused by one or more such autonomous functioning nodules is also referred to as single or multiple toxic adenomas, or Plummer's disease, and sometimes toxic nodular goitre. The last terminology is the least satisfactory and should be avoided as it is a descriptive clinical term for a nodular goitre associated with hyperthyroidism which may be due to either autonomous functioning nodules or non-functioning nodules in a diffuse toxic goitre as discussed above.

Hyperthyroidism may occur if stored hormones leak out of the thyroid due to an inflammatory process which damages the follicles. This may be related to recent viral infection, subacute De Quervain's thyroiditis or an autoimmune process, hashitoxicosis, post-partum thyroiditis or the cause may be unknown (painless thyroiditis). In each case, hyperthyroidism is usually mild and transient. Hyperthyroidism may be precipitated by excess iodide or thyroid hormone ingestion and very rarely may be due to extensive functioning papillary or follicular thyroid carcinoma or excess TSH production. In practice, Graves' disease and single or multiple autonomous toxic nodules (uninodular or multinodular Plummer's disease) account for the majority of cases of thyrotoxicosis. Nevertheless the remaining causes are clinically important and should always be borne in mind because their management and clinical course follow entirely different lines.

8.3.1 CLINICAL DIAGNOSIS OF THE CAUSE OF HYPERTHYROIDISM

The history and physical examination will often suggest the cause of hyperthyroidism in patients with Graves' disease but a clinical diagnosis can only be made with certainty in the presence of pathognomonic ocular or cutaneous signs, i.e. exophthalmos or other infiltrative eye signs, localized pretibial myxoedema and acropachy. However, this classical presentation of Graves' disease is less common and investigations are usually necessary to confirm or establish the aetiology. A diffuse goitre although most commonly associated with Graves' disease is not by itself diagnostic of the condition as it may occur in patients with subacute or painless thyroiditis or in those who are ingesting excessive thyroid hormones for a non-toxic goitre.

Similarly, the finding of a thyroid nodule or a multinodular goitre in a hyperthyroid patient does not establish the cause of hyperthyroidism since the diagnosis may be either Plummer's disease or variants of Graves' disease as discussed above. In a proportion of hyperthyroid patients the thyroid gland is not palpable and clinical diagnosis of the underlying cause may be even more difficult. The patient should be carefully questioned for the possibility of iodide or thyroid hormone-induced hyperthyroidism but most commonly the cause of hyperthyroidism is found on investigation to be a small diffuse toxic goitre.

Hyperthyroidism associated with subacute thyroiditis typically presents with a short history of painful tender goitre often accompanied by fever, anorexia and other constitutional symptoms. The clinical picture is often atypical and in most cases investigations are necessary to confirm or establish the diagnosis. Painless thyroiditis as a cause of hyperthyroidism can only be diagnosed by appropriate investigations, although a proportion of these occurring in epidemics have been shown to be due to the incorporation of beef thyroid into hamburger meat. It is thus apparent that investigations are usually necessary to establish the cause of hyperthyroidism.

8.3.2 THE DIAGNOSIS AND MANAGEMENT OF THYROTOXICOSIS

The appropriate management of patients with hyperthyroidism depends in many instances on an accurate initial diagnosis, and the value of the thyroid scan in thyrotoxicosis has been reviewed by us (Fogelman *et al.*, 1986a). The radionuclide scan has three main roles in managing hyperthyroidism: establishing the cause of thyrotoxicosis; the measurement of tracer uptake and gland size for the selection of appropriate ^{131}I therapy regimes; and for the follow-up of patients after treatment.

(a) Establishing the cause of thyrotoxicosis

There are a large number of patients in whom the diagnosis cannot be made clinically and, without the thyroid scan, an incorrect diagnosis may often

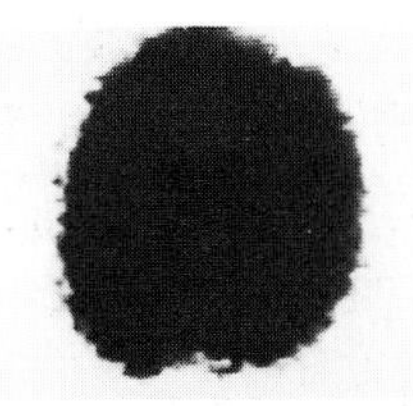

Figure 8.1 A typical left-sided thyroid toxic nodule with complete suppression of the right lobe.

be assumed. This can result in inappropriate treatment, and in a recent review (Cooke *et al.*, 1986) we found that 22% of patients with toxic nodules (Plummer's disease) had received long-term antithyroid medication before the correct diagnosis was established and appropriate treatment instituted.

(i) The solitary thyroid nodule and thyrotoxicosis When a patient with thyrotoxicosis is found to have a solitary thyroid nodule on clinical examination this is usually due to an autonomous toxic nodule (Figure 8.1). However, clinical examination may be unreliable, with 32% incorrectly diagnosed in one series (Fogelman *et al.*, 1986a). Other causes may be identified by subsequent investigations; a solitary non-functioning nodule in a patient with Graves' disease (Figure 8.2), an asymmetrically enlarged thyroid (Figure 8.3), or diffuse enlargement of a single lobe with agenesis of the other lobe may all simulate a toxic nodule. It may not always be possible to differentiate between these on the initial scan; for example, differentiating a large toxic nodule with complete suppression of the other lobe from agenesis of a lobe in a patient with Graves' disease will require further investigations; for example, repeating the scan after stimulation with exogenous TSH will demonstrate suppressed tissue;

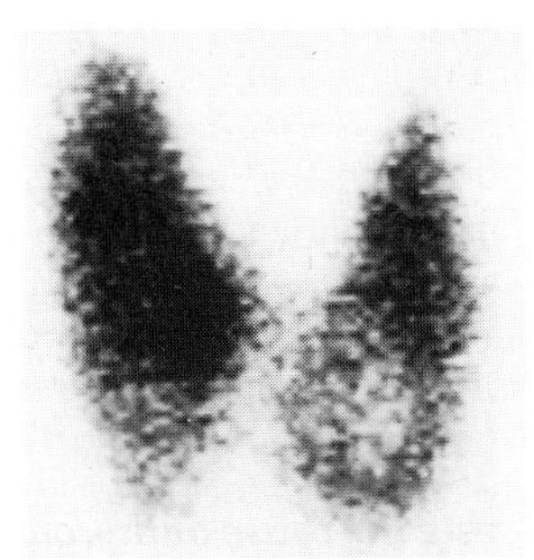

Figure 8.2 This scan shows a patient with a diffuse toxic goitre (Graves' disease) and an incidental cold nodule in the left lower pole.

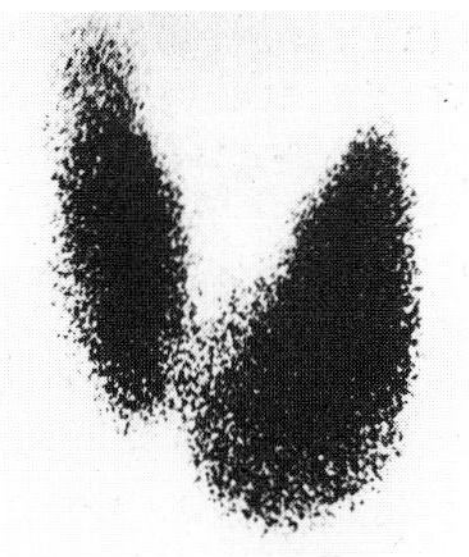

Figure 8.3 Graves' disease presenting with an asymmetrical goitre simulating a single nodule on clinical examination.

scanning with ^{201}Tl (Corstens *et al.*, 1988) will often show uptake in tissue which is not accumulating $^{99m}TcO_4$ or $^{123}I/^{131}I$ (Figure 8.4); ultrasound will demonstrate a lobe which is present, but not taking up tracer, or a hypoplastic or aplastic lobe; and the use of X-ray fluorescent measurements or scans (Jonckheer, 1987) will establish the presence of ^{127}I-containing tissue on the contralateral side. Even a simple method of shielding the active nodule with lead on routine thyroid scintigraphy may be sufficient to show the other lobe. The importance of making the correct diagnosis lies in the choice of treatment and subsequent follow-up. Patients with toxic nodules respond well to radioiodine treatment, and the nodule usually decreases in size to approximately 60% of the volume (Hegedus *et al.*, 1986), with complete cure being the normal outcome and hypothyroidism a rare sequel (Ratcliffe *et al.*, 1986). Whereas a single lobe with Graves' disease will be treated in a conventional manner usually with antithyroid drugs followed by ablative therapy only when a relapse occurs. Some centres prefer to treat these nodules surgically, but this now represents a minority view. Children with toxic nodules will usually be treated surgically (de Luca *et al.*, 1986). A patient with Graves' disease who has an incidental non-functioning nodule on the radionuclide scan is usually treated by subtotal thyroidectomy in order to detect possible malignancy, the incidence of which has been reported to be as high as 21% (Lividas *et al.*, 1976). Our own experience would, however, suggest that the true incidence of malignancy is very much lower. An alternative approach is fine needle aspiration cytology examination of the nodule followed by radioiodine treatment of the toxic diffuse goitre, after which some non-functioning nodules which are TSH dependent will function after resolution of disease (Marine–Lenhart syndrome) (Figure 8.5) (Marine

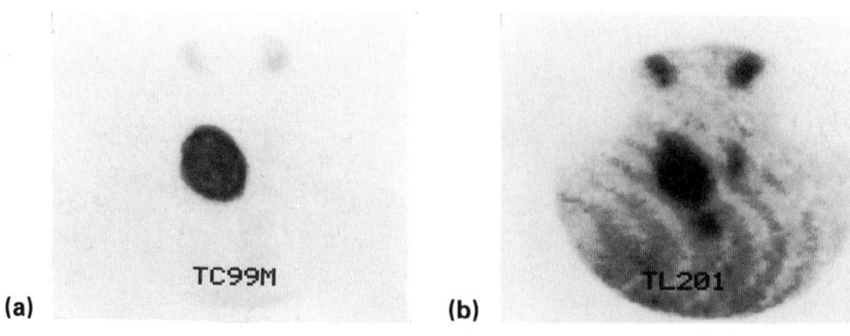

Figure 8.4 (a) ^{99m}Tc-pertechnetate scan with virtually no uptake on the left side. (b) ^{201}Tl scan shows the presence of metabolically active thyroid tissue on the left.

and Lenhart, 1911; Charkes, 1982). These nodules probably do not require surgical treatment, but a definitive study has not been carried out.

(ii) Nodular goitre associated with thyrotoxicosis When a thyrotoxic patient presents with a multinodular goitre they are often labelled as having a toxic nodular goitre. There are, however, three possible aetiologies: multiple toxic nodules developing in a long-standing multinodular goitre (Plummer's disease); Graves' disease supervening in a patient with a previous long-standing multinodular goitre; and a patient with Graves' disease in whom the enlarged gland becomes nodular. The latter two can only be differentiated by the presence or absence of a previous history of nodular goitre. The scan appearances of Plummer's disease may vary from that of a single toxic nodule to multiple clearly defined nodules throughout the gland. Occasionally the nodules appear almost confluent when the scan may be difficult to differentiate from Graves' disease in a multinodular gland (Figure 8.6). Most often the diagnosis can easily be made from the scan, although appearances do overlap and further investigations may be necessary. These include the

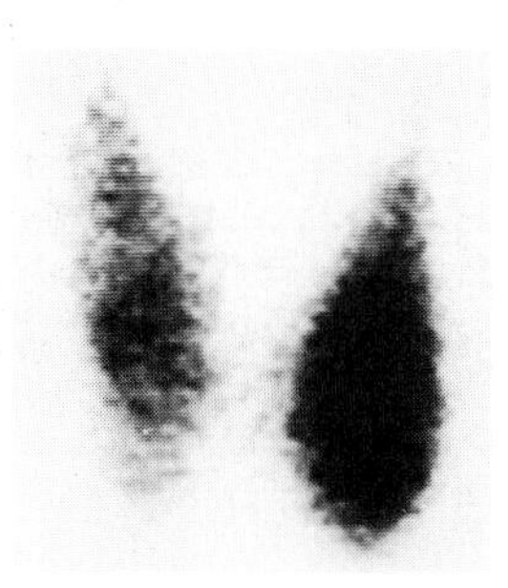

Figure 8.5 The non-functioning nodule in Figure 8.2 is now taking up the tracer: the Marine–Lenhart syndrome.

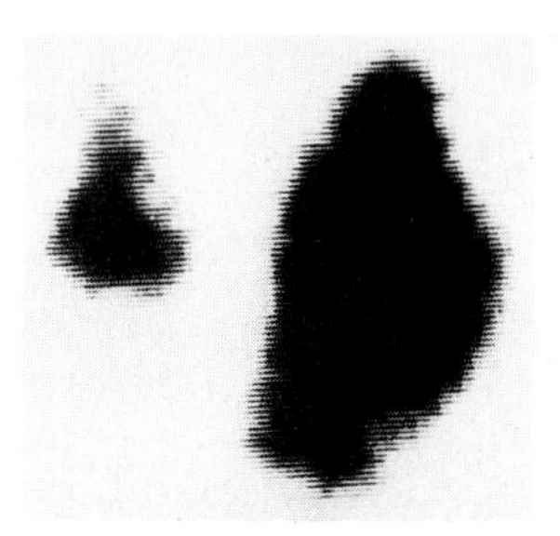

Figure 8.6 Confluent nodules in a patient with multiple autonomous toxic thyroid nodules.

measurement of serum thyroid-stimulating antibody, the use of repeat scans after TSH to demonstrate stimulation of suppressed tissue – this effect may also be achieved when the serum TSH rises if antithyroid drugs are given – alternatively a diagnosis may be established retrospectively when patients are scanned after radioiodine treatment (Figure 8.7). As mentioned previously for the single nodule ^{201}Tl can be used to demonstrate tissue in which the uptake function but not the metabolic activity is suppressed and may demonstrate the suppressed perinodular thyroid tissue.

(iii) The impalpable gland and thyrotoxicosis If the thyroid is small it may be difficult to palpate and when it is not obviously enlarged in thyrotoxicosis a thyroid scan should always be performed. The scan may demonstrate any of the recognized patterns associated with thyrotoxicosis, i.e. diffuse uptake, low uptake or functioning nodules. This is particularly important in elderly patients with atrial fibrillation, who should have a scan to detect toxic nodules which may not be producing obvious clinical disease as these can be easily treated with radioiodine. In a recent series of patients with toxic nodules, 10% were impalpable and some of these nodules could

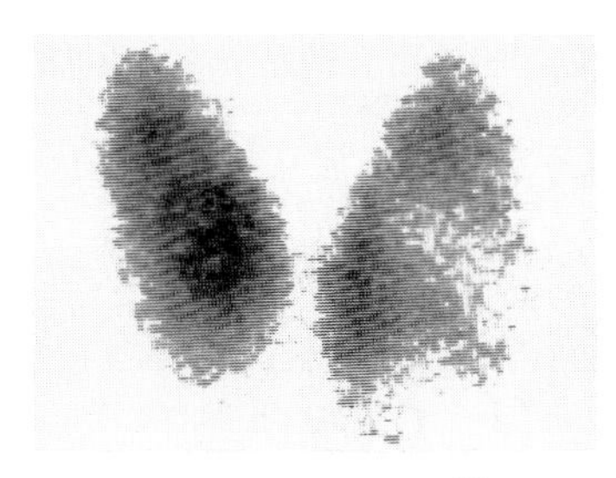

Figure 8.7 After treatment with ^{131}I of the patient whose scan is shown in Figure 8.6 there is a quite different distribution of uptake, confirming the original diagnosis.

not be palpated even after identification on the scan (Cooke *et al.*, 1986).

(iv) Low tracer uptake and thyrotoxicosis The thyroid scan in patients with thyrotoxicosis can have low tracer uptake. This finding may indicate a cause for thyrotoxicosis which could be self-limiting and will prevent the unnecessary administration of radioiodine, which would not be effective. These conditions are shown in Table 8.5.

Amiodarone, an iodine-rich drug, has recently been recognized to be a frequent cause of thyrotoxicosis through a number of mechanisms (Wiersinga and Trip, 1986; Gammage and Franklyn, 1987) and is almost always associated with low uptake of tracer and non-visualization of the thyroid on the scan. In a review of 35 patients with amiodarone-induced thyrotoxicosis (Martino *et al.*, 1985) 12 patients had no palpable abnormality and all had 24 h ^{131}I uptake (RAIU) less than 4%, but 17 with goitres had RAIU more than 8%.

Ectopic tissue may rarely cause hyperthyroidism and there will be non-visualization of the 'normal' thyroid on routine scanning. Ober *et al.* (1987) described a case of thyrotoxicosis due to metastatic follicular cancer which was resistant to conventional treatment, and in addition to drawing attention to the rarity of this case it again emphasizes the potential importance of a thyroid scan before therapy is undertaken. A retrosternal goitre may contain a toxic nodule, and Tang Fui *et al.* (1979) and Fogelfield *et al.* (1986b) have described patients with ectopic intrathoracic goitre causing thyrotoxicosis. In both cases the cervical uptake was low either due to suppression or absence of tissue. In females the scan in such cases should include the pelvis to identify the rare struma ovarii (March *et al.*, 1988). Post-partum thyroiditis is being increasingly recognized (Fung *et al.*, 1988) and may be associated with both hypo- and hyperthyroidism (or occasionally both) and is usually transient. The scan reveals low tracer uptake in both situations.

Table 8.5 Causes of low tracer uptake in hyperthyroidism

Subacute thyroiditis
Iodine-induced thyrotoxicosis (Jod–Basedow)
Amiodarone-induced thyrotoxicosis
Ectopic thyroid tissue
Thyrotoxicosis factitia (excess thyroid hormone administration)
Recent high iodine load (due to dilutional effects)

Subacute thyroiditis continues to be a regular cause of transient hyperthyroidism. This is usually diagnosed clinically in a patient with a painful thyroid and a low ^{99m}Tc or iodine uptake on the scan (Figure 8.8). Occasionally the diagnosis may be more difficult, and White *et al.* (1985) describe two cases of subacute thyroiditis being investigated for pyrexia of unknown origin (PUO) where intense ^{67}Ga uptake in the thyroid identified the cause of the PUO and hyperthyroidism. While subacute thyroiditis is occasionally painless, what was initially thought to be a mini-epidemic of such cases resulted from the addition of bovine thyroid tissue to hamburgers – 'hamburger thyrotoxicosis' (Hedberg *et al.*, 1987).

8.3.3 TREATMENT OF HYPERTHYROIDISM

The diagnosis of hyperthyroidism should be confirmed biochemically and its cause established, as discussed in preceding sections, before specific

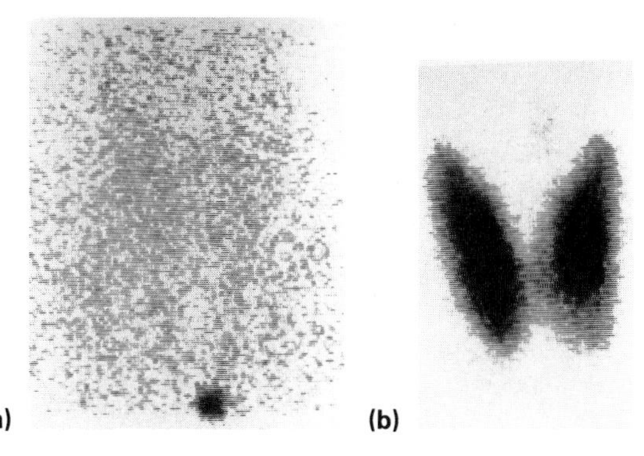

Figure 8.8 (a) Subacute thyroiditis causing thyrotoxicosis. (b) With resolution of the hyperthyroidism the scan returns to normal.

therapy is advised. While awaiting laboratory investigations, provided there are no contraindications such as asthma, a β-adrenergic blocking drug such as propranolol may be prescribed to relieve sympathetic symptoms such as sweating, tremor, palpitations or irritability. An adequate adult dose is 40 mg of propanolol two or three times daily or a single daily dose of 160 mg of a long-acting preparation. Specific treatment can subsequently be instituted when the diagnosis is confirmed.

The importance of diagnosing the cause of hyperthyroidism is stressed as it determines the choice of therapy, the clinical course of the condition and the likelihood of hypothyroidism or recurrent hyperthyroidism. The tendency of some physicians to initiate therapy with antithyroid drugs routinely in every patient with hyperthyroidism is open to criticism as they may be ineffective in certain types of hyperthyroidism, such as that associated with thyroiditis, or may not represent the treatment of choice in other cases, such as elderly patients or those with Plummer's disease.

(a) Graves' disease (toxic diffuse goitre)

The conventional treatments for hyperthyroidism due to Graves' disease include antithyroid drugs, subtotal thyroidectomy and radioactive iodine. The advantages and disadvantages of each form of therapy are summarized in Table 8.6 and should always be weighed against each other when selecting the most appropriate treatment for an individual patient. The treatment of choice for a particular patient depends on several factors: the patient's age; the presence of any associated cardiovascular problems such as atrial fibrillation, heart failure, ischaemic heart disease or other major medical problems; a previous history of hyperthyroidism and the type of treatment received; local medical facilities such as the availability of an experienced thyroid surgeon or an adequately equipped nuclear medicine department; the physician's personal experience and preference and the patient's willingness to the particular form of therapy advised.

For a young patient with uncomplicated Graves' disease the conventional treatment is a course of antithyroid drug therapy for six months to two years. Drugs such as propylthiouracil and carbimazole, which is widely used in Europe, or methimazole, which is more popular in America, are effective in reducing thyroid hormone production and release, but in at least 50% of patients (Hershman *et al.*, 1966) there is an early relapse or later recurrence of hyperthyroidism when treatment is stopped even after a prolonged course such as two years or more. It has been reported (Greer *et al.*, 1977) that the likelihood of recurrence or relapse is no worse after a shorter course of antithyroid drugs, e.g. six months. Side effects of antithyroid drugs are uncommon and usually become manifest within a few weeks of starting treatment. Allergic skin reactions are the commonest but the most serious is agranulocytosis, which has been reported in 0.2–0.3% of patients. One should immediately discontinue the drug as agranulocytosis is reversible in the early stages. The drug should not be resumed or replaced by another one of the same group. A different class of antithyroid drugs may be tried under close supervision or an alternative form of treatment advised.

Subtotal thyroidectomy offers a higher chance of cure in a much shorter time but requires

Table 8.6 Treatment of Graves' disease: advantages and disadvantages of each type of treatment

	Drugs	*Surgery*	*Radioiodine*
Relapse or recurrence	High	Low	Low (dose-related)
Hypothyroidism	Low	Intermediate	High (dose-related)
Complications	Rare	Low but significant mortality and morbidity	Rare
Ease of treatment and cost	Intermediate	Least favourable	Simple and cheap
Onset of therapeutic effect	Moderate (1 or 2 weeks)	Rapid after pre-op. preparation	Slow (few weeks)

admission, an experienced thyroid surgeon and the patient's fitness and willingness to undergo surgery. Complications of subtotal thyroidectomy depend on the surgeon's experience and the adequacy of the patient's pre-operative preparation. They include post-operative haemorrhage, recurrent laryngeal nerve palsy and transient or permanent hypoparathyroidism; the morbidity ranges between 0.2% and 1%. It is now used only for patients with very larger goitres where there is a suspicion of malignancy or when the patient is particularly keen to avoid radioiodine therapy.

Radioactive iodine provides the highest rate of cure, approaching 100%, although the effective dose is variable and more than one treatment dose may be necessary. Radioiodine has the advantage of being a very simple and cheap form of therapy. In the past radioiodine treatment has been confined entirely to hyperthyroid patients over the reproductive age, owing to the fear of radiation-induced cancer or genetic complications. There has been no evidence so far of an increased risk of thyroid or other malignancies or of genetic complications in patients who have now been followed up for twenty years or more after ^{131}I therapy for Graves' disease. As experience with radioiodine treatment has increased, many thyroidologists now feel that the use of ^{131}I need no longer be restricted but may be extended to younger adults. The therapeutic use of ^{131}I in hyperthyroid children is claimed to be safe but has not yet received widespread acceptance in view of the limited duration of follow-up. The major disadvantage of radioiodine therapy for Graves' disease is the high incidence of post-treatment hypothyroidism. With moderate doses of ^{131}I the incidence of hypothyroidism is about 20% in the first year of treatment, with an additional annual increase of 3% over subsequent years, so that by ten years up to 50% of treated patients may be hypothyroid. The risk of hypothyroidism is less with smaller doses of radioiodine but the chance of successful therapy is also reduced. Large single doses of radioiodine, e.g. 15 mCi ^{131}I, achieve a high cure rate of Graves' hyperthyroidism, with 70–90% requiring T4 replacement (Wise *et al.*, 1975).

(b) Choice of therapy for hyperthyroidism

(i) Children and adolescents Antithyroid drugs are the treatment of choice in very young patients with Graves' disease but the duration of therapy may be a problem. The aim of therapy is to continue with antithyroid drugs in yearly courses as necessary until the patient has reached the late teens or early twenties. Clinical and biochemical evidence of persistent or recurrent hyperthyroidism is sought at the end of each course of antithyroid drugs before resuming a new course of treatment.

(ii) Adults In general a course of antithyroid drugs for six months to two years is recommended for most adults with newly diagnosed Graves' disease. At the end of the course of treatment, if the disease is still active or if it recurs subsequently, they are referred for ^{131}I therapy. In a small proportion of patients, hyperthyroidism is not satisfactorily controlled with a regular maintenance dose of antithyroid drugs. The problem can usually be overcome by keeping these patients on a 'block-replace' regime which consists of a full dose of antithyroid drugs to completely block endogenous thyroid hormone production supplemented by a replacement dose of exogenous thyroid hormone, e.g. 20–40 μg of T3 or 0.1–0.2 mg of T4 daily. Replacement with exogenous T3 is preferred in this so that the block of endogenous hormone production can be assessed by measuring serum T4 which comes only from endogenous secretion and should be very low. Patients with associated disease such as cardiac disease or diabetes are best treated with ^{131}I.

(iii) Pregnancy and lactation Radioiodine treatment or investigation is absolutely contraindicated during pregnancy and lactation owing to irradiation of the fetus or newborn from radioiodine transferred across the placenta and in the milk, as well as indirect exposure from the radioiodine in the mother. The choice of treatment therefore lies between surgery and antithyroid drugs. Surgery should in any case be avoided during the first and third trimester of pregnancy owing to the risk of abortion or premature labour. The middle trimester is thus the safest period for thyroidectomy if considered necessary. Hypothyroidism after surgery should be detected and treated as soon as possible as it increases the risk of spontaneous abortion and fetal death. Many clinicians recommend that thyroxine therapy should routinely be given after surgery and the dose subsequently adjusted rather than wait until the patient is hypothyroid.

The preferred treatment during pregnancy is antithyroid drugs but it is essential to avoid overtreatment, which may increase fetal mortality from maternal hypothyroidism, and as antithyroid drugs cross the placenta they may induce fetal goitre and hypothyroidism particularly when used in larger doses. It is therefore safer to maintain the mother in a slightly hyperthyroid state using the smallest possible dose of antithyroid drugs. Thyroid function tests including serum fT3, fT4 and TSH should be carried out frequently.

Iodide treatment and propranolol should be avoided during pregnancy. The former crosses the placenta, blocks the fetal thyroid and may induce goitre or hypothyroidism; the latter increases uterine muscle tone, which may result in a small placenta and growth retardation of the fetus. Propranolol can also induce bradycardia in the newborn baby, hypoglycaemia and impaired response to anoxia.

As antithyroid drugs are secreted in breast milk, they should either be stopped whenever possible if the mother wishes to breast feed, or if treatment needs to be continued artificial feeding should be advised. It is essential to check babies born of mothers with Graves' disease for neonatal hyperthyroidism or hypothyroidism, which is usually transient (due to placental transfer of maternal thyroid-stimulating immunoglobulins) and may be prolonged. When treatment of the baby is indicated it usually involves antithyroid drugs and propranolol but great care should be taken to avoid hypothyroidism in the newborn child owing to the risk of subsequent mental and physical retardation.

(iv) Thyrotoxicosis in the elderly Hyperthyroidism in the elderly constitutes a more serious problem, with an increased mortality and morbidity rate, particularly due to cardiovascular complications such as heart failure and atrial fibrillation, with the added risk of arterial embolism. The aim of treatment in these patients is to cure hyperthyroidism promptly and permanently when they first present in order to avoid or reverse these cardiovascular problems and prevent recurrence of the hyperthyroid state, with associated complications. This is best achieved with radioiodine in view of the increased risk of surgery in this age group and the high relapse rate after antithyroid drugs. Elderly patients and all those with cardiac complications or other associated serious medical problems, irrespective of age, should be treated with a short course of antithyroid drugs in full dosage (usually four to eight weeks) until they are clinically and biochemically euthyroid. The drug is then stopped for 48–72 h, after which the patient is given a single large oral dose of radioiodine, such as 550 MBq of ^{131}I, which will result in a 70–90% cure rate of Graves' hyperthyroidism at the risk of permanent hypothyroidism. It is advisable to resume the antithyroid drug at a suitable dosage two to three days after the radioiodine drink for another four to six weeks to cover the period before the ^{131}I has its full therapeutic effect. Patients under the age of 65 years with atrial fibrillation may also be anticoagulated prophylactically against thromboembolism, but this remains controversial. Digoxin and/or β-blockers may be used to control the heart rate and diuretics may be needed to control heart failure. Treated in this way many patients with atrial fibrillation initially will revert to sinus rhythm spontaneously while being treated. Those who are still in atrial fibrillation after they have become euthyroid or hypothyroid should be advised DC cardioversion, which will often restore sinus rhythm. Anticoagulants and digoxin may be stopped if sinus rhythm is maintained for a few weeks when the patient is euthyroid or hypothyroid.

(c) The thyroid scan before ^{131}I treatment

One of the major factors involved in calculating the radiation from a therapeutic dose of ^{131}I is the measurement of thyroid mass. There have been a number of formulae proposed for calculating the thyroid mass derived from the thyroid scan which make assumptions about the geometry of the lobe (Becker and Hurley, 1982). Thyroid volume is best calculated using a combined radionuclide and ultrasound method. However, with regard to calculating the dose of ^{131}I for therapy the functional tissue volume as opposed to the total tissue volume is likely to be much more important. Positron emission tomography may be the optimal technique for this (Ott *et al.*, 1987) although single-photon emission computed tomography (SPECT) studies which will be more widely available may eventually be able to achieve this.

The second important factor in dose calculation is the peak uptake of ^{131}I. At the present time no careful studies have been performed comparing the early ^{99m}Tc uptake, which can be routinely obtained, with the 24 h ^{131}I uptake, although the diagnostic accuracy is equal (Maisey *et al.*, 1973) and ^{123}I uptake measured at 4–5 h using a gamma camera can replace the ^{131}I uptake (Floyd *et al.*, 1985). However, it is not certain that in the absence of detailed measurements of ^{131}I turnover and possibly some measure of tissue sensitivity the results from these measurements can significantly improve upon the results achieved using an arbitrary choice of dose which is much more convenient (Ratcliffe *et al.*, 1986a).

It has been suggested that the thyroid scan together with an uptake measurement may be used to assess the activity of the thyroid during antithyroid drug treatment to provide an indication as to the likelihood of a relapse when the patient discontinues treatment (Wilson *et al.*, 1985), and this has been found to be particularly valuable in children (Duck and Sty, 1985). However, others (Wilson *et al.*, 1985) found that the ^{99m}Tc uptake was a poor predictor of relapse in 49 patients with Graves' disease compared to the TSH receptor antibody, which was superior. Turner *et al.* (1985) in a detailed study of 76 patients with Graves' disease using 21 clinical, biochemical, scan and tracer-kinetic parameters concluded that no single or combination of treatment variables was able to predict outcome from ^{131}I treatment.

(d) Treatment of toxic autonomous nodules (Plummer's disease)

Treatment is similar for hyperthyroidism caused by single or multiple autonomous nodules but differs in several important aspects from that of Graves' disease. First, long-term antithyroid drugs should not be used to treat Plummer's disease as functioning nodules rarely go into spontaneous remission. Second, hyperthyroidism due to Plummer's disease is more resistant to radioiodine and usually requires larger therapeutic doses, but despite this post-radiation hypothyroidism is rarely observed (Ng Tang Fui and Maisey, 1979). This is explained on the basis that in Graves' disease the whole gland concentrates radioiodine and becomes irradiated and leads to hypothyroidism. In contrast, in Plummer's disease radioiodine concentrates only in the autonomous nodules, which are destroyed, while the suppressed extranodular tissue takes up little radioiodine and returns to normal function after the nodules have been destroyed. It is important to note that this is only true if at the time of radioiodine treatment the extranodular tissue has not been stimulated with exogenous TSH administered for diagnostic purposes or with endogenous TSH as a result of preceding antithyroid drug therapy.

It is important to obtain a thyroid scan before radioiodine is used to treat autonomous toxic nodules (Plummer's disease); in particular in those who have received antithyroid drug therapy, because it is necessary to be sure that the normal thyroid tissue is fully suppressed at the time of administration of ^{131}I to prevent subsequent hypothyroidism. When patients with toxic nodules are treated in this way the likelihood of hypothyroidism is very low. In a series of 48 patients treated with 500 MBq of ^{131}I no patient became hypothyroid in the follow-up period (mean 37 months) (Ratcliffe *et al.*, 1986b). The only patients who become hypothyroid have received antithyroid drugs before treatment without establishing that the normal tissue remained suppressed and the TSH was not elevated. If normal thyroid tissue is not fully suppressed because the TSH has risen during treatment then a further period of time off antithyroid drugs is required, or alternatively thyroid hormone may be given, if clinically acceptable, and the thyroid scan repeated before ^{131}I is given.

Treatment consists of a large single dose of ^{131}I, usually a standard dose of 400–500 MBq. Unless the patient is seriously ill with thyrocardiac complications such as heart failure or atrial fibrillation, preceding treatment with antithyroid drugs should be avoided as it increases the risk of post-radioiodine hypothyroidism. A course of propranolol for two to four weeks may be helpful for symptomatic treatment until the radioiodine starts to have a therapeutic effect. If the patient has received antithyroid drugs, these should be stopped and radioiodine treatment postponed for four weeks (Figure 8.9). Similarly, if exogenous TSH has been given, radioiodine administration is deferred for at least a week to restore suppression of the extranodular tissue.

After radioiodine treatment, patients are usually reviewed at one, three, six, nine and 12 months. A repeat thyroid scan is carried out after six months, at which time most patients with Plummer's disease will be clinically and biochemically euthyroid and have normal TSH response to TRH. The thyroid scan can be used to establish that radioiodine therapy has been completely successful in destroying an autonomous nodule or nodules (Figure 8.10). Successfully treated nodules will be non-functional on the scan by six months after treatment, but those with a liabil-

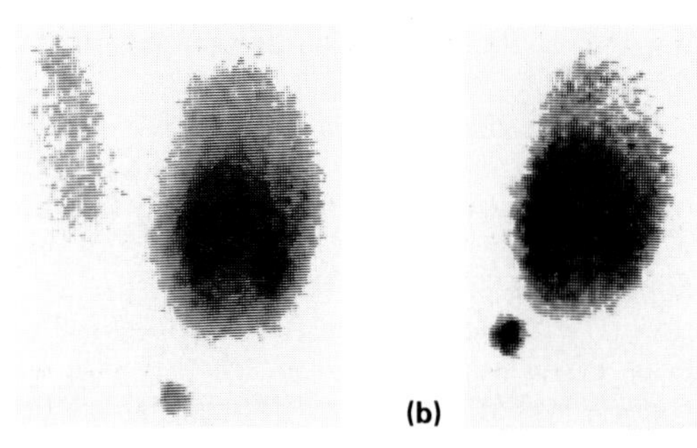

Figure 8.9 Patient with thyrotoxicosis who has received treatment with antithyroid drugs. (a) The use of these drugs has permitted some tracer uptake into the normally suppressed perinodular tissue. (b) After discontinuing the drugs for a few weeks there is a return to the suppressed state.

ity to relapse will retain some functional activity (Ratcliffe *et al.*, 1986). The scan at six months can thus be valuable as an indicator of prognosis as any residual activity in the nodule predisposes to a subsequent relapse of thyrotoxicosis and these patients should be followed. Those who are not cured at six months are given a second dose of 15 mCi of ^{131}I and followed as before. Once the patient is cured annual examination is sufficient, although post-radiation hypothyroidism is rare.

Patients who refuse ^{131}I may be treated with surgery. Radioiodine has the added advantage that it also destroys functioning micronodules and thus prevents recurrence of hyperthyroidism.

(e) Treatment of other types of hyperthyroidism

The management of hyperthyroidism due to causes other than Graves' disease and Plummer's disease depends on the underlying condition but in general treatment with antithyroid drugs, subtotal thyroidectomy or radioiodine is not applicable to these conditions.

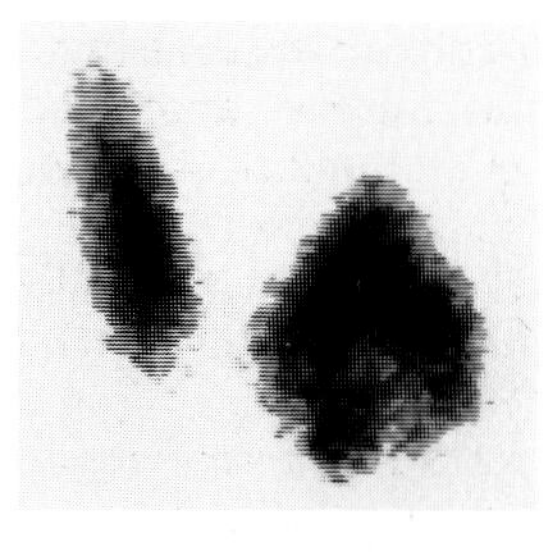

Figure 8.10 Complete destruction of toxic nodule shown in Figure 8.1 has resulted in a return to normal function of the previously suppressed tissue.

(i) Subacute thyroiditis and Hashimoto's thyroiditis Hyperthyroidism is usually mild, transient and requires no specific therapy except possibly symptomatic treatment with a β-sympathetic blocking drug such as propranolol. Since the raised serum hormones in these conditions are due to leakage of stored thyroid hormones accompanying the inflammatory process rather than excess production, the conventional treatment for Graves' disease is ineffective. In subacute thyroiditis and occasionally with Hashimoto's thyroiditis, pain and tenderness over the neck with or without constitutional symptoms may require symptomatic relief with an anti-inflammatory analgesic such as salicylate. In more severe cases, steroid treatment in moderate doses, e.g. prednisolone 30–40 mg daily for a few weeks, may be necessary. Subacute thyroiditis is a self-limiting condition and complete recovery after a few weeks or months is the rule. Mild hypothyroidism may occur in the recovery stage but this is usually transient. On the other hand permanent hypothyroidism is common with Hashimoto's thyroiditis and long-term thyroid replacement is usually necessary.

(ii) Hyperthyroidism associated with excess iodide Hyperthyroidism precipitated by acute excess iodide such as administration of radiological contrast media is also usually mild and remits spontaneously without any specific treatment. Rarely, if the condition is severe, a course of antithyroid drugs is necessary but surgery and radioiodine treatment are not used. The low radioiodine uptake in this condition as in thyroiditis precludes the use of radioiodine. In the case of chronic excess iodide ingestion, appropriate dietary advice should also be given to avoid persistence of the condition. One of the commonest causes of iodine-induced hyperthyroidism is now the anti-arrhythmic cardiac drug amiodarone. Initial treatment with antithyroid drugs together with withdrawal of amiodarone followed by ^{131}I when the uptake is high enough is generally advised. Ideally this will result in hypothyroidism, enabling the patient to restart amiodarone.

(iii) Hyperthyroidism associated with excess thyroid hormone If the patient is on an excessive dose of thyroid hormone for documented hypothyroidism, the dose should be adjusted until the patient is clinically and biochemically euthyroid. The usual therapeutic dose of thyroxine is 100–200 μg daily. Occasionally, a patient may have been put on thyroid replacement for unrecognized transient hypothyroidism and subsequently produces adequate or even excess endogenous hormone. Thyroid hormone medication should therefore be stopped and the patient's thyroid status and need to continue thyroid replacement reassesed. Patients taking excess thyroid hormones on their own accord should be advised to discontinue the drug and their thyroid status reassessed clinically and biochemically. Some of these patients may also need psychiatric assessment and advice.

(iv) Hyperthyroidism associated with thyroid cancer This is a rare complication of extensive metastatic functioning papillary or follicular thyroid cancer which may secrete excess endogenous thyroid hormones due to the large mass of functioning tumour. The management is essentially that of the underlying carcinoma, involving large doses of radioiodine. If hyperthyroidism is severe, treatment with antithyroid drugs and β-blockers may be necessary. Exogenous thyroid hormone medication should of course not be given while hyperthyroidism from tumour secretion persists.

Hyperthyroidism may also occur if patients with thyroid cancer are put on excess suppressive doses of thyroid hormone. The optimal dose is that which suppresses the TSH below normal and in the average patient this is 150–300 μg of thyroxine daily. Patients with functioning metastases producing significant amounts of endogenous hormones will of course need smaller doses of thyroid hormone.

Hyperthyroidism associated with pituitary or ectopic TSH hypersecretion, trophoblastic tumours and ectopic thyroid tissue in ovarian tumours is exceedingly rare and will be treated by removing the primary cause.

8.4 SOLITARY THYROID NODULES

8.4.1 INVESTIGATION AND MANAGEMENT OF SOLITARY NODULES

This is a common clinical problem because in the population there may be found as many as 15.5% with palpable nodules (Tunbridge *et al.*, 1977), with 3.2% solitary in women and 0.8% solitary in men in England, and it has been reported that in the USA 4–7% have thyroid nodules (Rojeski and Gharib, 1985). The causes of a thyroid nodule are shown in Table 8.7.

Table 8.7 Causes of solitary thyroid nodules

Thyroid cyst
Local subacute thyroiditis
Local Hashimoto's disease
Functioning adenoma (hot nodule)
Benign adenoma
Colloid nodule
Thyroid cancer
Metastatic deposit

The likelihood of malignancy occurring in a single nodule is between 5% and 10% (Rojeski and Gharib, 1985) but will vary considerably from series to series depending on selection criteria. The problem is compounded by the frequency with which nodules are found in normal adults – up to 50% in those over 50 years of age (Horlocker *et al.*, 1986). There is an increased risk of thyroid cancer associated with previous external radiation to the head or neck, although the clinical course of the cancer is the same as thyroid cancers found in other settings. Schneider *et al.* (1986) identified 318 cases of thyroid cancer in 5379 patients given radiotherapy for benign conditions of head, neck and upper thoracic area. Metastases frequently occur in the thyroid, but rarely present clinically as thyroid nodules.

The clinical problem is how to detect the 5–10% of solitary thyroid nodules with cancer without the need to perform unnecessary operations on the other 90%, and it has been this goal, i.e. to identify benign disease with a high degree of accuracy without loss of sensitivity in detecting cancer, that has driven the diagnostic developments in this area.

Certain clinical features increase the probability of malignancy in a solitary nodule.

1. The presence of an invasive tumour may cause hoarseness, fixation and hardness of the nodule, rapid or painful enlargement, cervical lymphadenopathy or distant metastases. These clinical features are usually absent at the time of presentation of most differentiated thyroid carcinomas.
2. A previous history of irradiation to the head or neck should be specifically enquired about, as this will increase the likelihood of a solitary nodule being malignant.
3. Symptoms and signs that are characteristic

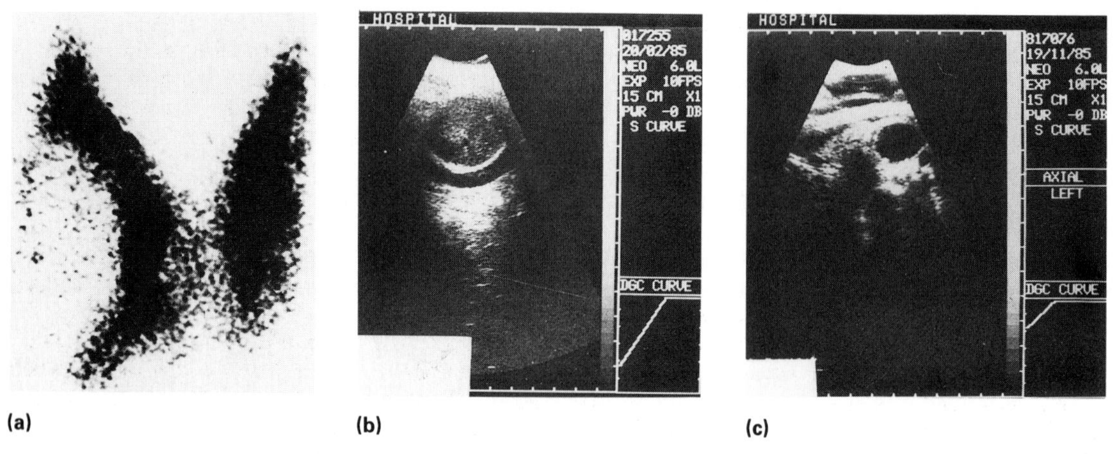

Figure 8.11 Non-functioning nodule in the right lobe (a) shown to be solid on ultrasound (b) compared to a cyst on ultrasound (c).

of a medullary thyroid carcinoma such as diarrhoea, mucosal neuromas, a marfanoid appearance, a history or suspicion of associated phaeochromocytoma or hyperparathyroidism, and a known family history of any of these conditions.

4. Age and sex of the patient; e.g. a solitary nodule in a man over 40 years has a higher probability of being malignant than in a young woman.

(a) Investigations

The thyroid scan (with ^{99m}Tc or ^{123}I) has been the most widely used method for investigating a thyroid nodule on the basis that finding a solitary cold nodule increases the probability of malignancy, whereas finding a functioning nodule or a simple multinodular goitre without a single dominant nodule decreases the chance of malignancy to very low levels.

(b) Solitary cold nodule

The probability of malignancy is increased if the scan demonstrates a solitary cold nodule but is very uncommon if it shows a hot nodule or a multinodulal goitre.

Ultrasound provides a valuable tool for demonstrating thyroid abnormalities and in particular to discriminate between solid and cystic lesions (Figure 8.11) (Simeone *et al.*, 1982). It can be used to measure thyroid volumes and to detect nodules. Most malignancies are echogenic but ultrasound cannot differentiate between functioning and non-functioning nodules, and even cystic lesions may occasionally be functional on a radionuclide scan. The role of ultrasound in the evaluation of thyroid disease has recently been well reviewed by Leisner (1987).

Probably the most important development as an adjunct to imaging is fine needle aspiration (FNA) of a nodule for cytological examination, and this is now becoming widely available. Lowhagen *et al.* (1981) in a review of the world literature of 3500 patients found a false-negative rate of less than 10% and a false-positive rate of less than 2%, although better results are possible. Anderson and Webb (1987) in a series of 373 patients found a false-negative rate of 6.3% and a false-positive rate of 0.6%. Several groups have shown a reduction in surgery rate for nodules as a consequence of routine FNA of cold nodules. For example Al Sayer *et al.* (1985) found a 25% reduction in surgery with an increased detection rate of malignancy from 31% to 50%. However, Reeve *et al.* (1986) found a 60% reduction with FNA and selective surgery. Christensen *et al.* (1984) in a prospective study of 100 consecutive patients selected for surgical treatment of a clinically solitary thyroid nodule who had FNA confirmed that all 12 cases which were hot on the scan were benign.

Westman-Naeser *et al.* (1986) in reviewing 860 patients where FNA was performed concluded that the scan is a supplement to physical examination and serves as a guide to FNA in pre-operative selection of patients. However, the problem of non-diagnostic/suspicious lesions remains. In a review of the Mayo Clinic experience it was found that non-diagnostic results constitute about 20% of all cases and follow-up of these indicates that about 20% of them are malignant (Gharib *et al.*, 1984).

It has been suggested that all patients with a solitary nodule should have FNA as their initial investigation and a thyroid scan is not required. However, clinical examination frequently fails to detect that the 'clinically solitary nodule' is the more easily palpable nodule of a multinodular goitre. It can be concluded that FNA is an efficient method for detecting cancer in patients who have a cold nodule on the thyroid scan.

The thyroid scan is of value in the follow-up of patients who have had thyroid cysts aspirated (Figure 8.12).

Other methods are used to reduce the surgical rate for thyroid nodules. X-ray fluorescence, which measures ^{127}I, is accurate for the identification of benign disease (Tang Fui and Maisey, 1983; Patton *et al.*, 1985) with a sensitivity of 63% and specificity of 99% in one series, but the technique is not widely available. More controversial is the use of ^{201}Tl for evaluating the thyroid nodule. It is well known that ^{201}Tl is taken up into the thyroid and may show thyroid tissue not identified by ^{99m}Tc or iodine isotopes, and also that malignant thyroid lesions take up ^{201}Tl preferentially. An early evaluation (Ochi *et al.*, 1982) obtained extraordinarily good results for differentiating between benign and malignant nodules, with a 94% sensitivity and 90% specificity, and if no fading of activity on a delayed image was a criterion of malignancy the specificity reached 100%. However, in further studies (Henze *et al.*, 1986; Hoschl *et al.*, 1984; Bleichrodt *et al.*, 1987) with semi-quantitative assessments of thallium uptake in cold nodules on ^{99m}Tc scans, all 37 patients with malignant lesions had equal or more tracer uptake than perinodular tissue, whereas benign lesions ranged from no uptake to uptakes well in excess of the perinodular tissue. Thus no uptake or uptake less than perinodular tissue confirmed benign disease and would allow a reduction in surgical rate. Thus while there may be a role for thallium in the evaluation of the thyroid nodule, the definitive study has not yet been performed and its routine use cannot be recommended.

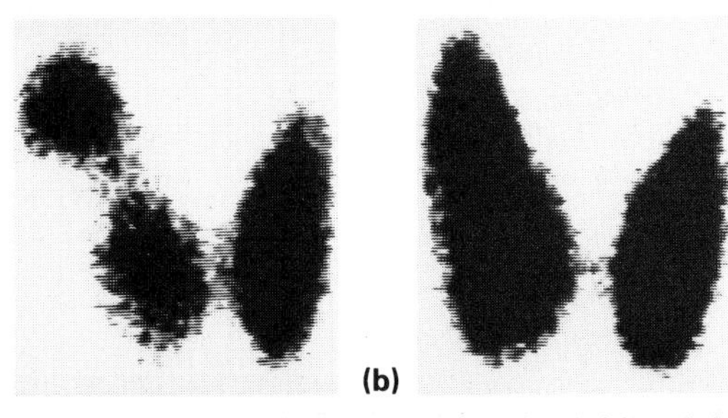

Figure 8.12 Patient who presented with a cold nodule in the right lobe (a) due to a cyst. Follow-up scan after aspiration (b) confirms complete aspiration with no recurrence.

It is generally agreed that the correct management of a non-functioning nodule is hemithyroidectomy as reviewed by Lennquist (1987) and not suppressive therapy with thyroxine as has been used in the past. Further, Gharib *et al.* (1987) have shown that there is no measurable decrease in size of these nodules with thyroxine therapy.

(c) Functioning 'hot' nodule

If the thyroid scan shows the solitary nodule to be functioning ('hot') the probability of malignancy is reduced to less than 1%, since most hot nodules are benign autonomously functioning adenomas; however, there have been occasional reports of malignancy. Ashcroft and Van Herle (1981) in their review of the literature reported 9% malignancy in warm and hot nodules. Nagai *et al.* (1987) reported three cases of malignancy in hot nodules on ^{123}I scans, and Evans (1987) found that 44% of patients with thyroid malignancy presented with warm nodules. Three problems can be identified in these reports. One is that some malignancies, while they do not organify the isotopes, do trap ^{99m}Tc and iodine, and appear as hot or warm nodules on ^{99m}Tc scans or early ^{123}I scans. If we only call 'functioning' those nodules that suppress TSH or cause a flat TRH test response or remain hot on a ^{123}I scan after a perchlorate discharge test or delayed imaging then the likelihood of malignancy remains very low. The second consideration is that nodules often occur in multinodular glands and the 'hot nodule' may be close to an 'incidentally' found malignancy which may behave differently from those cancers which present clinically. Third, many adenomas and carcinomas have a good blood supply and it is the blood volume which creates the 'warm' nodule and not true uptake of tracer.

Walfish *et al.* (1985) reviewed their experience of 12 FNA cases of functioning nodules to evaluate the consequences of not obtaining a radionuclide scan first. They concluded that not performing a scan to diagnose a functioning nodule could expose some unprepared patients with thyrotoxi-

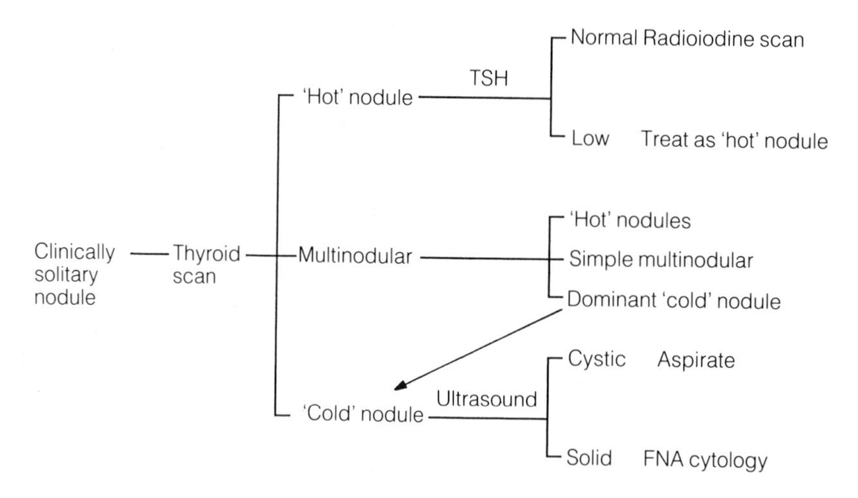

Figure 8.13 Scheme for the investigation of thyroid nodules.

cosis to surgical morbidity and could induce hyperthyroidism in patients with functioning nodules if they were treated with suppression therapy. FNA was not able to differentiate a functioning from a non-functioning adenoma.

There is as yet, therefore, no consensus on the investigation of this common clinical problem. Routine removal of all clinically apparent thyroid nodules no longer seems justified and results in a great deal of unnecessary surgery. A reasonable policy (Figure 8.13) would be a ^{99m}Tc or ^{123}I scan in the first instance, which is a cheap, accurate and widely available test. Functioning nodules will be identified and these patients should have a sensitive TSH or TRH test to confirm true biological function with subsequent follow-up and treatment for thyrotoxicosis as necessary. The evidence for any significant likelihood of malignancy in this group is not convincing. If reliable cytology is available (clinical decisions should not be made until at least 100 FNA have been undertaken and reviewed) then all non-functioning solitary nodules should have FNA cytology because of the well-documented reduction in unnecessary surgery. Ultrasound is only necessary as an adjunct to the scan when FNA is not available. Simple cysts can then be aspirated and recurrences may be considered for injection with sclerosants. ^{201}Tl can be used when there is a relative contraindication to surgery, when a negative or positive scan will help in making a decision, but it is probably not justified otherwise. The use of ^{127}I measurements by X-ray fluorescence justifies more widespread application, but at present is available in only a very few centres.

(d) Multinodular goitre

A proportion of patients who are thought to have a solitary nodule on palpation are shown to have a multinodular goitre on scanning. The frequency with which this is noted depends on the experience of the clinician in palpating the thyroid, the ease with which the patient's thyroid can be palpated and the technique of the scan. Alderson *et al.* (1976) reported that approximately 36% of clinically diagnosed solitary nodules were shown to be multiple on scan; an even higher percentage was found at operation or autopsy (Maisey *et al.*, 1973). It is often possible to palpate previously unsuspected nodules in the light of the scan findings.

The findings of a multinodular goitre when a solitary nodule was suspected clinically considerably decreased the probability of thyroid cancer in the absence of any clinical suspicion. Probably less than 1% of all multinodular goitres are malignant. Unless there are clinical suspicions of malignancy or local symptoms, a solitary nodule which is found to be part of a multinodular goitre on scanning does not need surgical excision.

The presence of a dominant cold nodule (Figure 8.14) in a gland with otherwise generally irregular uptake on scanning does not reduce the probability of malignancy to that of a typical multinodular goitre (Alderson *et al.*, 1976). Such dominant cold nodules should therefore be investigated with

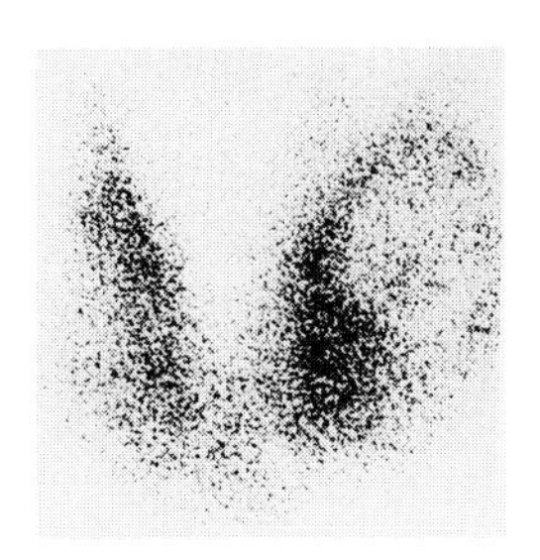

Figure 8.14 An example of a dominant non-functioning nodule in the left lobe of a multinodular gland.

ultrasound and aspiration cytology as for a solitary nodule and excised if indicated.

8.5 PAINFUL GOITRE

Pain originating from the thyroid associated with palpable enlargement may be due to one of the following conditions:

1. Subacute (De Quervain's) thyroiditis;
2. Subacute or acute onset of Hashimoto's thyroiditis;
3. Haemorrhage into a thyroid nodule or cyst;
4. Thyroid cancer, particularly anaplastic carcinoma;
5. Acute supurative thyroiditis (rare).

A careful history and clinical examination will often suggest the diagnosis, but should always be supplemented with appropriate investigations for confirmation. The most useful investigations include a full blood count and erythrocyte sedimentation rate (ESR), thyroid function tests, a radionuclide thyroid scan with ^{99m}Tc or ^{123}I, a perchlorate discharge test and serum thyroid microsomal antibodies. Rarely a biopsy may be necessary. Sudden onset of pain in the thyroid is most often caused by haemorrhage in a thyroid nodule or cyst which may either be solitary or part of a multinodular goitre. Thyroid function tests are normal; thyroid scan shows a solitary cold nodule or a multinodular goitre with one or more cold nodules. Pain due to haemorrhage into a thyroid nodule usually lasts only a few days and the nodule appears very rapidly, usually over a few hours. The nodule gets smaller and may disappear completely after a few weeks. The patient should therefore be reviewed after two or three months and the thyroid scan repeated to confirm resolution or reduction of the nodule. If symptoms persist, and the nodule enlarges, excision is advisable to exclude malignancy.

Subacute onset of pain over the neck, often described as a sore throat by the patient, associated with a recent upper respiratory infection, fever, malaise, anorexia and a tender diffuse goitre, are characteristic of subacute thyroiditis. However, similar features may sometimes be caused by subacute onset of Hashimoto's thyroiditis. Investigations will establish the correct diagnosis. A mild leukocytosis and moderately elevated ESR may occur in both conditions, but subacute thyroiditis is characterized by mild biochemical hyperthyroidism in the early stages, a diffusely low uptake on ^{99m}Tc scan and absence of thyroid antibodies or only a transient rise in low titre. On the other hand, in Hashimoto's thyroiditis, thyroid function tests usually show frank or compensated hypothyroidism (high TSH with low or low-normal serum T4); thyroid scan characteristically though not always shows a high ^{99m}Tc uptake, but a low radioiodine uptake indicating trapping of iodine without organic binding. This can also be shown by a perchlorate discharge test, which will have an increased discharge of radioiodine. Hashimoto's thyroiditis may occasionally be associated with a normal or raised radioiodine uptake. Thyroid microsomal antibodies are present in high titres and persist in Hashimoto's thyroiditis. The differential diagnosis of Hashimoto's and subacute thyroiditis is important because their clinical course is quite different. In subacute thyroiditis the thyroid usually recovers spontaneously after a few weeks or months without any sequelae, whereas Hashimoto's thyroiditis usually results in permanent hypothyroidism requiring long-term thyroid replacement.

Atypical cases of thyroiditis in which constitutional symptoms are minimal or absent and a painful goitre is the main feature may have to be distinguished from a rapidly enlarging anaplastic thyroid carcinoma. The latter condition usually affects older patients, and is often associated with evidence of local invasion such as hoarseness, Horner's syndrome, upper respiratory or oesophageal obstruction or distant metastases. The goitre is usually asymmetrical and hard and thyroid scan shows a focal area of low uptake with areas of normal uptake. Thyroid function tests are usually normal.

Acute suppurative thyroiditis due to bacterial or tuberculous infection is rare. The patient is very ill with marked constitutional symptoms, high fever and a very tender goitre. Biopsy may be necessary to establish the diagnosis and provide culture material for antibiotic sensitivity.

Confusion may be caused when subacute thyroiditis involves only one lobe with the characteristic low uptake in that lobe only on the scan. This may then resolve and the other lobe may be affected; this may occur in as many as 20% of cases.

8.6 NON-TOXIC GOITRES

8.6.1 INVESTIGATION AND TREATMENT OF NON-TOXIC GOITRES

The goitre may be diffuse or multinodular on examination although occasionally it may be difficult to describe it clearly as one type or the other. Outside endemic areas of iodine deficiency, the main causes of a non-toxic goitre are shown in Table 8.8 with the appearances on a thyroid scan.

Certain points in the history and clinical examination of the patient are helpful in the diagnosis. They include the age of onset and duration of the goitre, a family history of goitre (suggesting Hashimoto's thyroiditis or familial dyshormonogenesis), the regular ingestion of goitrogens or a low iodine intake, the presence of nerve deafness in the patient (Pendred's syndrome) and the type of goitre on palpation, for example a soft diffuse simple colloid goitre, a simple multinodular goitre with several discrete nodules, or a bosselated firm goitre of Hashimoto's thyroiditis. Recent rapid enlargement of a long-standing goitre should raise the suspicion of malignancy, especially lymphoma or anaplastic carcinoma.

The basic investigations of a non-toxic goitre consist of thyroid function tests, particularly serum T4 and TSH, estimation of serum thyroid microsomal or thyroglobulin antibodies and a thyroid scan with quantitative uptake. Further investigations which may be necessary include a perchlorate discharge test, studies of iodine kinetics *in vivo* and a thyroid biopsy.

(a) *Simple colloid goitre and simple multinodular goitre*

These are the commonest causes of a sporadic diffuse or nodular non-toxic goitre. The exact cause of these goitres is uncertain but they are thought to represent different stages of the same pathological process. Thyroid function tests including TSH are usually normal and thyroid antibodies are usually absent or in low titre. Uptake of ^{99m}Tc or radioiodine is normal. The distribution of uptake on the scan is diffuse in a simple colloid goitre, but markedly irregular often with discrete

Table 8.8 Role of the thyroid scan in the assessment of goitre

Scan findings	*Cause*	*Comment*
Diffuse, normal uptake of tracer	Diffuse non-toxic (simple) goitre	
Diffuse, with high uptake of tracer	Diffuse toxic goitre (Graves' disease)	May be first indication of hyperthyroidism
	Lymphocytic thyroiditis (Hashimoto's disease)	Occurs in early disease
	Iodine deficiency Organification defects (inherited or goitrogens)	May be difficult to distinguish
Diffuse, low uptake of tracer	Subacute thyroiditis (De Quervain's) Iodine-induced goitre Hashimoto's disease Lymphoma	May be indistinguishable on the scan but presentation is entirely different
Multifocal irregularity Normal uptake of tracer	Simple multinodular	Detection of autonomous nodule is important
	Hashimoto's disease	Diagnosis by antibodies
Irregular replacement of thyroid tissue	Diffuse cancer	Usually clinically apparent, but may be confused with multinodular goitre

From Fogelman and Maisey (1988).

areas of diminished uptake in a multinodular goitre. Oblique views may be helpful. Occasionally the goitre may contain one or more areas of increased uptake indicating developing autonomous functioning nodules. A TSH level will be suppressed and show impaired TSH response to TRH injection in spite of normal serum T3 and T4 concentration. These autonomous nodules may give rise to frank hyperthyroidism (Plummer's disease) as the disease progresses.

No specific treatment is usually necessary for asymptomatic simple colloid or multinodular goitres. A large multinodular goitre causing tracheal or oesophageal compression as shown by radiography of the thoracic inlet or a barium swallow should be resected. Thyroid hormone therapy in suppressive doses are rarely helpful in reducing goitre size but may be tried in moderate-sized goitres if serum TSH is elevated. Multinodular goitres with autonomous nodules should be followed up regularly for signs of developing hyperthyroidism, which should then be treated with radioiodine or surgery. Recent rapid enlargement of a long-standing multinodular goitre should raise the possibility of malignancy and an aspiration biopsy or ^{201}Tl scan should be performed, followed by surgical excision if indicated.

The appearance of two symmetrical solitary nodules in a goitre should raise the suspicion of a medullary thyroid cancer (Figure 8.15) (although this is an uncommon tumour) and will further increase the likelihood of it being the familial type which has arisen from symmetrically distributed C-cell hyperplasia. A calcitonin measurement in addition to FNA cytology may be helpful in making a pre-operative diagnosis as may uptake of ^{99m}Tc-labelled pentavalent DMSA or $^{123/131}$I MIBG (Clarke *et al.*, 1988). This will be of particular value in cases of multiple endocrine neoplasia, and

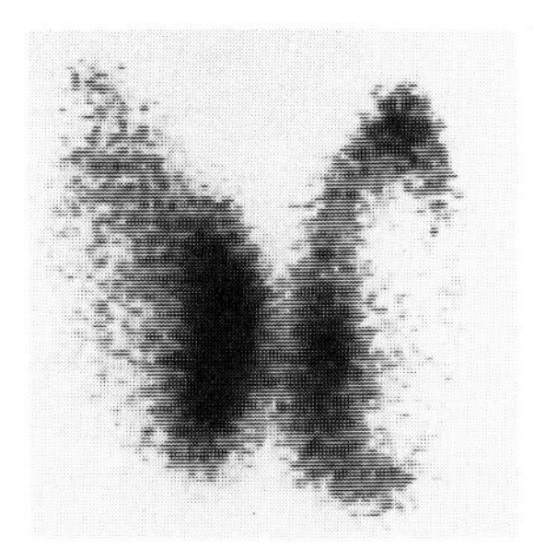

Figure 8.15 A patient discovered by family screening to have a medullary thyroid cancer showing the symmetrical cold areas due to bilateral medullary cancers.

clearly pheochromocytoma must be identified prior to initial surgery. First-degree family screening is undertaken in all patients with diagnosed medullary thyroid cancers to establish whether or not it is the inherited type. When an elevated calcitonin is detected in a relative of the patient investigation of the thyroid is necessary. Because most surgeons prefer to know if there is a nodule present rather than simply perform a prophylactic total thyroidectomy, it will also be necessary to use the radionuclide thyroid scan and ultrasound or CT.

A thyroid lymphoma may develop spontaneously, with the patient usually presenting with a rapidly enlarging diffuse goitre, or may occur in a patient with Hashimoto's disease where there is recognized to be an increased risk of lymphoma. A radionuclide thyroid scan is not helpful because in the latter situation the patient will be hypothyroid and receiving thyroxine treatment, and in the former case the scan will usually show diffuse enlargement with an overall low uptake due to the diffuse infiltration. In these instances it is usual to proceed directly to surgical biopsy but there are clinical circumstances, e.g. if the patient is too anxious or has other pathology, when this is not advised and then a gallium scan, which shows avid accumulation in lymphoma, may provide valuable information (Figure 8.16). Finally, De Quervain's subacute thyroiditis if it is localized or initially involves only one lobe may simulate a malignant lesion (Ramtoola and Maisey, 1988). Repeat thyroid scans show recovery of function in one area with appearance of the typical low uptake in the other lobe, confirming the diagnosis of thyroiditis and not malignancy.

(b) Hashimoto's thyroiditis

The diagnosis of this condition depends on three main features: first, the presence of a goitre which is typically bosselated and firm on palpation; second, subclinical or frank hypothyroidism, i.e. raised TSH with borderline low or low serum T4; and third, serum thyroid microsomal antibodies which are usually strongly positive although they have been reported to be negative in a small proportion of biopsy-proven Hashimoto's thyroiditis. Other investigations are of limited diagnostic value, e.g. thyroid scan may show high, normal or low uptake of radionuclide with varying distribution which may be uniform, irregular or nodular according to the degree of

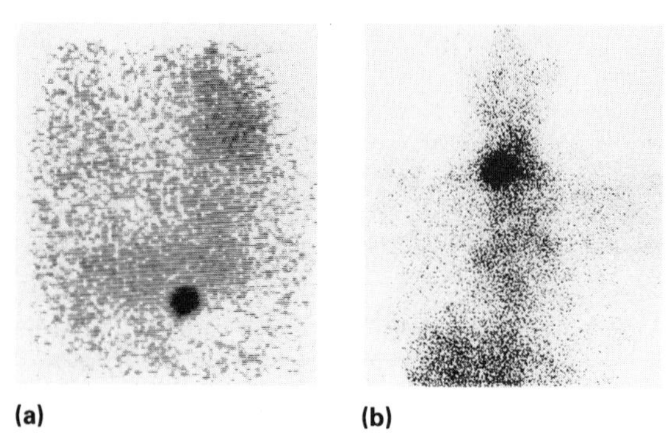

Figure 8.16 Scans of a patient with lymphoma (a) shows a large gland with low uptake ($^{99m}TcO_4$), but the ^{67}Ga scan (b) shows avid accumulation.

fibrosis. We have recently reviewed 32 cases, and a wide variety of scan patterns were obtained (Ramtoola *et al.*, 1988). The most common scan appearances were either of an enlarged gland with diffusely increased tracer uptake similar to Graves' disease or those of a multinodular gland. However, other scans appeared normal, or showed a focal defect or reduced tracer uptake throughout one lobe or generally low uptake by the whole gland. Perchlorate discharge test shows excess discharge of radioiodine in most of the cases. Cytology or biopsy may be helpful in equivocal cases.

Hashimoto's thyroiditis is treated with long-term suppressive doses of thyroid hormones, e.g. thyroxine 100–200 μg daily. If treatment is started in the early stages of the condition considerable reduction in size of the goitre can be expected, whereas if diagnosis is made late, when considerable fibrosis is present in the gland, little or no improvement in goitre size may occur.

(c) Dyshormonogenesis

This refers to a group of genetic abnormalities, each involving a specific enzyme defect in the metabolic pathway of thyroid hormones. Most are transmitted by autosomal recessive inheritance and are rare. The best known and least rare is Pendred's syndrome, in which a familial goitre is associated with nerve deafness. Familial dyshormonogenesis should be considered in the differential diagnosis of goitre in the younger patient with a family history of goitre, absent thyroid antibodies and subclinical or frank hypothyroidism.

From the point of view of clinical investigation, dyshormonogenesis may be divided into three groups.

(i) Abnormality of iodide transport into the thyroid cell This condition is characterized by a very low iodine uptake in the thyroid as well as in the salivary glands, which share the same iodide trapping mechanism. The salivary glands should therefore be included in the field of view when the thyroid scan is performed.

(ii) Abnormality of organification of iodine to tyrosine This defect is characterized by a normal iodine uptake in the gland but perchlorate discharge test reveals excess discharge of unorganified iodide. The best-known and commonest condition in this group is Pendred's syndrome. The organification defect is usually only partial, as indicated by normal or slightly low serum T4 with raised serum TSH and excess radioiodine discharge on perchlorate discharge test.

(iii) Other enzyme defects Familial goitres with a normal or high iodine uptake and normal perchlorate discharge may result from an abnormality in the metabolic pathway beyond the organification stage of iodine. Various types have been described, all of which are rare and depend on more detailed biochemical investigation for diagnosis.

8.7 ECTOPIC THYROID

Thyroid tissue may occur in anatomical positions other than the normal position, when it may constitute a diagnostic or therapeutic problem. The commonest places are at the back of the tongue (lingual thyroid), in the mid-line position of the upper neck (sublingual or subhyoid thyroid), inside the thoracic cavity (anterior or posterior mediastinal goitre) and in ovarian tumours (struma ovarii).

8.7.1 LINGUAL AND SUBLINGUAL THYROID

Failure or incomplete descent of the thyroid gland from its embryological mid-line position at the back of the tongue results in a lingual or sublingual thyroid. Either may contain the whole or only part of the patient's thyroid tissue. These ectopic thyroids usually present as a mid-line swelling at the back of the tongue or upper neck or as congenital hypothyroidism. Failure to recognize and diagnose a lingual or sublingual thyroid swelling may lead to inadvertent excision and permanent hypothyroidism requiring life-long thyroid replacement.

A midline swelling at the back of the tongue or upper neck should therefore always be investigated for the possibility of an ectopic thyroid before excision. The presence or absence of a normally situated thyroid gland should also be confirmed. The sublingual or subhyoid ectopic thyroid is particularly likely to be mistaken clinically for a thyroglossal cyst or other non-thyroid swelling.

Thyroid function tests are performed to assess the patient's thyroid status and a radionuclide scan is carried out. ^{123}I is better because of the higher uptake which avoids confusion with saliva and salivary glands on a ^{99m}Tc scan. The radiation dose with either radionuclide is small compared to ^{131}I and the scan can therefore be used in infants, children or adolescents. The whole area from the mouth to the sternal notch should be imaged and reference markers are placed on any palpable nodule and appropriate anatomical landmarks, e.g. the sternal notch. In the case of a lingual thyroid, a lateral view is important for accurate three-dimensional localization. Radionuclide uptake in the nodule confirms the presence of ectopic thyroid whereas other types of nodule, e.g. a thyroglossal cyst, appear cold. The presence or absence of a normal thyroid is also established at the same time. Rarely, if the normal thyroid is not visualized the scan should be repeated after TSH stimulation to exclude the possibility that its function may be suppressed.

A nodule which shows no uptake of ^{99m}Tc or ^{123}I can be excised. A functioning ectopic thyroid nodule can also be excised if the scan confirms the presence of a normal thyroid in addition in the normal site. However, a sublingual thyroid which contains the entire functioning thyroid tissue should be preserved. For cosmetic reasons the ectopic thyroid can be divided and relocated in the normal position.

In patients who have undergone previous thyroid surgery, congenital remnants of thyroid tissue along the thyroglossal tract may hypertrophy to produce a mid-line swelling in the upper neck, particularly with recurrence of Graves' disease. This can be confirmed on a thyroid scan.

8.7.2 INTRATHORACIC (MEDIASTINAL) GOITRES

A normally situated thyroid gland may enlarge downward into the anterior mediastinum to produce a retrosternal goitre, or less commonly it may extend behind the trachea and oesophagus downwards, as a posterior mediastinal goitre. These intrathoracic goitres are most commonly caused by non-toxic nodular goitres. Rarely they are congenitally ectopic glands which have migrated with the primitive heart into the mediastinum. They may be asymptomatic and come to light incidentally in the differential diagnosis of an upper mediastinal opacity noted on a routine chest radiography or they may cause symptoms due to compression of the trachea, oesophagus or superior vena cava. Occasionally a large diffuse toxic goitre or toxic nodule may extend retrosternally or in the posterior mediastinum and cause similar symptoms in addition to those of hyperthyroidism.

Most retrosternal goitres are associated with palpable enlargement of the cervical thyroid and the diagnosis of retrosternal goitre can be inferred if the lower border of the goitre cannot be felt in the neck.

To confirm the intrathoracic goitre and assess its extent a radiograph of the thoracic inlet and a thyroid scan with ^{123}I or ^{131}I should be performed. Although the presence of radioiodine uptake below the sternal notch confirms the diagnosis of intrathoracic goitre, its absence does not exclude a non-functioning intrathoracic goitre. In such cases, mediastinoscopy and tissue biopsy or a formal thoracotomy may be necessary to confirm the diagnosis. Mediastinal CT or MRI may be necessary to assess the extent and to evaluate tracheal compression.

Retrosternal or posterior intrathoracic goitres should be removed surgically if there is evidence of increasing tracheal or oesophageal compression as the goitre enlarges. If the patient is also thyrotoxic, initial treatment with antithyroid drugs until the patient is euthyroid, followed by surgery, is usually advised. However, if the patient is considered a poor surgical risk antithyroid drugs followed by radioiodine therapy under close supervision in hospital may be preferable.

8.8 NEONATAL HYPOTHYROIDISM

If congenital hypothyroidism remains undiscovered the neurological and skeletal sequelae can be irreversible and devastating. Over the past decade the usefulness of the introduction of widespread screening programmes for the detection of neonatal hypothyroidism has been confirmed. The incidence of disease in most countries is about 1 in 4000 (Fisher, 1983; Price *et al.*, 1982; LaFranchi, 1982), with a female preponderance of around 4:1. The diagnosis of primary congenital hypothyroidism is based on the finding of a low thyroxine together with an elevated TSH level. This, however, fails to distinguish between the presence of an ectopic or hypoplastic thyroid, athyreosis, dyshormonogenesis and transient hypothyroidism. Thus neonatal hypothyroidism represents a spectrum of disease ranging from transient underactivity to complete absence of a thyroid gland. It is in this context that the question of the role of the thyroid scan in the investigation and management of these patients continues to be discussed.

The thyroid scan accurately delineates the anatomy of infants with congenital hypothyroidism, but in addition provides functional information. A scan should be obtained before commencing treatment with thyroxine. Anatomical findings may be broadly characterized into four groups based on scan findings (Wells *et al.*, 1986):

1. A normal gland;
2. Ectopic location;
3. No detectable thyroid activity;
4. Normal location with increased size of gland or increased tracer uptake.

An ectopic thyroid gland is found in approximately 45% of cases and athyreosis in 35%. Some 10% will have a normal gland and 10% other abnormalities (Brooks *et al.*, 1988). In the latter cases it is presumed that there is a disorder of thyroid hormonogenesis and a number will have defects of thyroid hormone synthesis. A perchlorate discharge test will identify those cases with an organification defect. Two cases of a congenital defect in iodide trapping have been reported where the scan showed absence of not only thyroid but also gastric uptake (Leger *et al.*, 1987). There is some controversy as to the role of inhibitive immunoglobulins ('blocking' antibodies) as these may cause transient hypothyroidism (Connors and Styne, 1986). Further, the scan findings in isolation are misleading in terms of prognosis as there is no tracer uptake by the thyroid and will suggest athyreosis. The role of transplacental passage of maternal immunoglobulins may be important in the pathogenesis of sporadic congential hypothyroidism but it remains controversial.

The thyroid scan has prognostic significance as those with anatomical defects will have permanent hypothyroidism. Information obtained from a scan may also aid in genetic counselling as an ectopic thyroid or athyreosis occurs spontaneously while impaired biosynthesis of thyroid hormones implies an inherited defect. Further, thyroid scan data presented in a form patients find easy to understand and accept is important with long-term therapy as good patient compliance is required (Brooks *et al.*, 1988). Where an ectopic thyroid is present a scan may avoid an unnecessary operation for a base of tongue swelling.

While in the great majority of cases of neonatal hypothyroidism the disease is permanent some will have transient hypothyroidism and clearly it is desirable to identify these cases. It has, however, been found that those with an anatomical defect or a secondary rise in TSH after the TSH has been initially suppressed by throxine therapy have permanent hypothyroidism. Thus only approximately one-third of cases will qualify for a trial off therapy. Thyroxine should be discontinued for a three-week period after 3 years of age and this is adequate and safe to confirm that hypothyroidism is permanent. Only 1–2% of newborn cases of hypothyroidism identified on screening will have transient disease.

8.9 THYROID CANCER

8.9.1 TREATMENT AND FOLLOW-UP OF THYROID CANCER

The management of thyroid cancer depends chiefly on the histological type of tumour, which is usually classified as shown in Table 8.9.

(a) Papillary and follicular carcinomas

These account for at least 80% of all thyroid malignancies. By definition, follicular carcinomas consist entirely of neoplastic thyroid follicles, whereas papillary carcinomas contain cells in a papillary arrangement with a varying proportion of follicular structures. By virtue of their follicular components both these tumours have functioning endocrine properties which are similar to, but less efficient than, normal thyroid follicles. Thus under certain conditions which include total ablation of all normal thyroid tissue and excess TSH

Table 8.9 Pathological classification of thyroid tumours

Benign
Adenoma
Follicular
Papillary
Atypical
Teratoma
Malignant
Carcinoma
Papillary
Pure papillary
Mixed papillary and follicular
Follicular
Pure follicular
Clear cell
Oxyphil cell
Medullary
Undifferentiated
Small cell
Giant cell
Epidermoid
Other malignant tumours
Lymphoma (specify type)
Sarcoma (specify type)
Secondary tumour (specify site of origin, if determined)

stimulation these tumours are able to concentrate and organify small but significant amounts of iodine, an important property which can be exploited for their detection and treatment with radioiodine.

In general the management of papillary and follicular thyroid cancers follows closely similar lines. The management has been reviewed by Freitas *et al.* (1985).

(b) Early disease management

Most differentiated cancers are diagnosed when a hemithyroidectomy is performed for a solitary non-functioning thyroid nodule, although many other presentations are possible, such as a distant metastasis. In most instances a total thyroidectomy will be performed, whether at the time of the first operation or as a second procedure. This is necessary because of the high incidence of tumour in the other lobe and the possibility of recurrence. In addition total thyroidectomy enables subsequent follow-up of patients to be carried out with thyroglobulin estimations and whole body ^{131}I scans. In certain groups of patients – women under 40 years, with a small non-invasive tumour (less than 1.5 cm in diameter); when a small (0.75 mm or less) cancer is found incidentally during a thyroidectomy for another reason, e.g. multinodular goitre or Graves' disease; and when there is a relative contraindication to repeat surgery, e.g. a recurrent laryngeal nerve lesion – long-term suppressive therapy with thyroxine (TSH maintained <0.1 mIu/l or a flat TRH response) is an alternative approach. In all other cases a total thyroidectomy is performed.

Following total thyroidectomy a period for four weeks should elapse to permit serum TSH to rise before a scan is performed. If a subtotal operation has been done the scan and ^{131}I ablation therapy can be instituted immediately. Post-operatively the scan at four weeks will usually demonstrate some residual tissue in the neck which may be tumour or normal tissue (Figure 8.17), there being no reliable way to distinguish these two. The dose

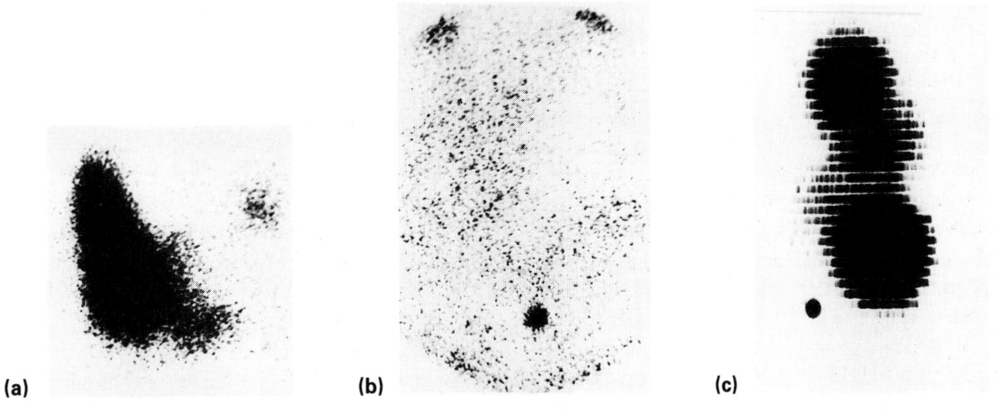

Figure 8.17 (a) A patient who presented with a left-sided cold nodule. (b) A few days after total thyroidectomy before there was a significant rise of TSH, there is no accumulation of ^{131}I. (c) However, after four weeks with no T4 replacement there is marked uptake, probably indicating residual tumour.

for ablation is somewhat controversial, but combining two series (Ramanna *et al.*, 1985a; Creutzig, 1987) it is apparent that only nine out of 29 cases were ablated with one 30 mCi dose, whereas 18/29 patients were ablated with a 100 mCi dose.

(c) Intermediate treatment

Subsequent follow-up ^{131}I scans are usually performed at six-monthly or yearly intervals with repeated ^{131}I therapy until tumour ablation is complete. These scans are performed after discontinuing thyroid hormone for four weeks (T4) or two weeks (T3) and establishing that the TSH is >30 Iu/l. These scans will identify most metastases which usually occur locally in the neck, in the lung and or in bone. Lung metastases are well shown on the ^{131}I scan, which is more sensitive than other imaging modalities (Figure 8.18). Piekarski *et al.* (1985) reviewed their experience with ^{131}I scans, CT and chest X-ray in 27 patients with micronodular metastases and showed that 19/27 had normal chest X-rays, while CT demonstrated micronodules in 14 of these 19 cases. CT also demonstrated micronodules in 7/13 patients with known previously treated metastases with no ^{131}I uptake, some of whom had detectable thyroglobulin levels. It was suggested that these nodules may be a result of fibrosis. They concluded that the ^{131}I scan was the most sensitive investigation, but CT was a valuable complementary procedure. There is no doubt about the clinical importance of pulmonary metastases. Samaan *et al.* (1985) reviewed 101 patients with lung metastases; of these 67 died of the disease, with the majority being over 40 years of age (16% survival). The prognosis was better when the ^{131}I scan was positive and X-ray negative, and it was found that pulmonary metastases occurred more frequently in patients who had not initially had a total thyroidectomy. De Groot and Reilly (1984) looked at the detectability of thyroid metastases in 108 patients using ^{131}I scan, chest X-ray, skeletal survey and bone scan. They found that physical examinations, chest X-ray and ^{131}I scans detected all metastases and skeletal surveys and bone scans did not contribute significantly. Occasionally metastases occur in the brain and it is important to identify them on the ^{131}I scan as cerebral oedema may occur following ^{131}I therapy. The choice of the maximum or optimal dose for ^{131}I therapy following a positive ^{131}I scan may be arbitrary (usually 150 or 200 mCi), or may be based on dosimetry, although there are problems in measuring the volume of residual tumour, the uptake and turnover of ^{131}I by the tumour, which cast doubt on its usefulness.

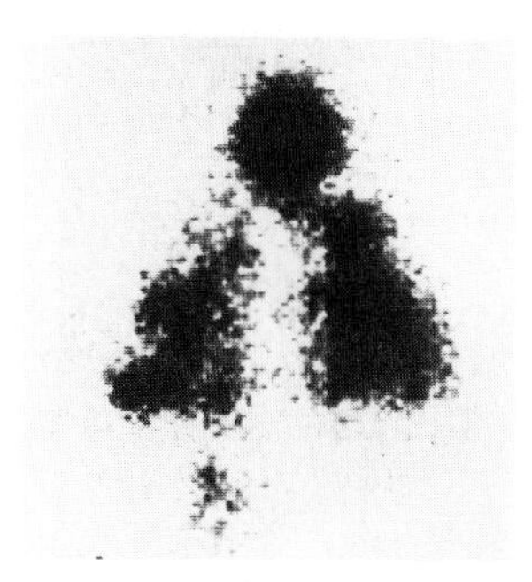

Figure 8.18 A patient having a scan of thyroid metastatic disease showing diffuse uptake of ^{131}I with a normal chest radiograph.

False positives on the ^{131}I scan, while uncommon, may occur. We have recently seen a patient with accumulation of trapped ^{131}I within a plaque of psoriasis and the lesion was originally considered to be in a lumbar vertebra. Wu *et al.* (1984) reported striking radioiodine and ^{99m}Tc localization in a disseminated gastric adenocarcinoma. Ziessman *et al.* (1987) looked at the frequency of hepatic uptake of ^{131}I, which may represent a possible false positive, and found hepatic visualization in 44% of cases which was related to the ^{131}I dose and functional activity of metastatic disease. Kim *et al.* (1984) reported ^{131}I uptake in a benign serous cystadenoma of the ovary and Hoschl *et al.* (1988) reported uptake in inflammatory lung disease as a potential pitfall.

The definition of ablation of tumour or thyroid tissue to some extent depends on the dose of ^{131}I used for scanning the patient. Ramanna *et al.* (1985b) found that some patients showed positive uptake at 10 mCi, but negative at 2 mCi dose levels. It is recognized that a scan performed after a therapeutic dose of ^{131}I may detect additional lesions. Doses used for scanning in different centres vary from 0.2 mCi to 30 mCi. However, some potentially treatable lesions will still be missed even at the higher dose level. Therefore the choice of dose is a balance between detecting treatable lesions and radiation dose to the patient. In practice we now use 400 MBq, which is the highest dose the patient can receive if returning home using public transport. The optimal scanning time is at 72 h. Lithium has been used as an adjunct to increase ^{131}I uptake by preventing its release from the thyroid. Pons *et al.* (1987) measured uptake in 14 metastatic lesions and 12 local remnants of normal thyroid tissue and showed a significant increase in metastases, but only a 50% increase in normal tissue.

8.9.2 THE USE OF THYROGLOBULIN

Thyroglobulin as an adjunt to the ^{131}I scan in the follow-up of thyroid cancer has been discussed extensively since initial publications showed its value (Black *et al.*, 1981; Maisey, 1981). There is no doubt that most well-differentiated tumours both take up ^{131}I and produce thyroglobulin, but in a few cases these aspects of cellular function appear to be separated (Sheppard, 1986). Ericsson *et al.* (1984) reviewed 262 patients with differentiated cancer and concluded that thyroglobulin can replace ^{131}I scans, while Ronga *et al.* (1986) reviewed 233 patients and found 43 thyroglobulin-positive cases without ^{131}I uptake and three with a positive scan and negative thyroglobulin, thus urging caution in replacing the ^{131}I scan, stressing the complementary role of the two tests. Girelli *et al.* (1985) reviewed 429 patients and found high thyroglobulin levels in 76% of patients with metastases detected by other diagnostic procedures which were unable to take up ^{131}I. Moser *et al.* (1988) reviewed 158 patients post-thyroidectomy and found a positive ^{131}I scan with negative thyroglobulin in 21% of patients, confirming that thyroglobulin could not replace the scan at this stage in the management. The incidence of positive scans with negative thyroglobulin is low (<4%) but may be strikingly important, as illustrated by a report of three cases with lung and bone metastases shown with ^{131}I, but with negative thyroglobulin levels (Arning *et al.*, 1987).

Some of the light microscopic and immunohistochemistry factors related to thyroglobulin secretion have been reviewed recently by Dralle *et al.* (1985). For management decisions it is probably wise to treat all patients with an elevated thyroglobulin and a negative scan with ^{131}I and scan following the treatment dose. Pacini *et al.* (1987) found 17 such patients of whom 16 showed a positive scan using the therapeutic dose of ^{131}I for imaging.

In summary the thyroglobulin level is of little value post-operatively, but is a valuable adjunct to the scan subsequently. When strongly positive in the face of a negative scan it will influence a decision to treat with ^{131}I and scan again following the therapeutic dose. Thyroglobulin probably cannot be relied on exclusively for follow-up on T4 suppression, but a reasonable compromise is annual physical examination, chest X-ray and thyroglobulin estimation after two whole body ^{131}I and thyroglobulin levels have been negative one year apart. Some centres would add a whole body ^{131}I scan at five-yearly intervals, which seems a sensible precaution in view of the occasional reported false-negative thyroglobulin measurements.

8.9.3 OTHER SCANNING TECHNIQUES

Khammash *et al.* (1988) evaluated the use of ^{99m}Tc-pertechnetate when compared with ^{131}I in 66 patients with thyroid carcinoma and found five false-negative ^{99m}Tc studies and one false-negative ^{131}I study, confirming as expected that ^{99m}Tc is less reliable than ^{131}I in the detection of thyroid cancer.

Other agents have been used to investigate and follow up patients with thyroid carcinoma, usually in an attempt to avoid having to discontinue thyroid hormone replacement treatment and the associated clinical hypothyroidism. The most widely used additional radiopharmaceutical is ^{201}Tl chloride (Figure 8.19). Hoefnagel *et al.* (1986) compared ^{201}Tl with ^{131}I in 620 scans in 303 patients and found positive thallium in 39 with negative ^{131}I (but eight medullary cases were included) and three negative thallium with positive ^{131}I, and concluded that thallium was superior. On the other hand Varma and Reba (1982) concluded that thallium was only of use in wide-

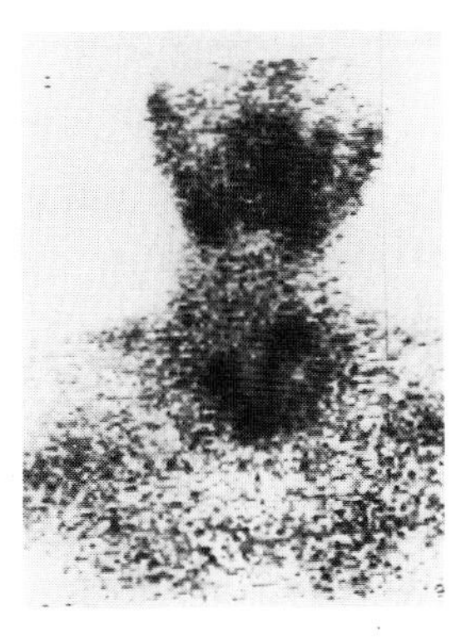

Figure 8.19 The ^{201}Tl scan of a patient with a suspected recurrence of follicular carcinoma while taking thyroxine. The ^{201}Tl scan shows uptake confirming the presence of tumour.

spread disease and could not replace ^{131}I for routine use. While there were differences in administered doses it was recommended that thallium should not be used for follow-up of patients with differentiated thyroid carcinoma. It was suggested that thallium may be helpful in localizing metastases in patients with a negative ^{131}I scan and abnormal levels of serum thyroglobulin.

8.9.4 MEDULLARY CARCINOMA

This is an uncommon tumour of the parafollicular or C-cell of the thyroid; the tumour may occur sporadically or may be inherited as an autosomal dominant condition in association with a phaeochromocytoma and parathyroid adenoma (multiple endocrine syndrome type II or Sipple's syndrome). The tumour secretes excessive calcitonin which can be measured using a radioimmunoassy. Patients who have a suspected medullary thyroid cancer can have a diagnosis made pre-operatively by showing elevated plasma calcitonin levels although low levels may be found in other unrelated conditions. Measurement of plasma calcitonin can be used to follow up patients who have been treated for medullary carcinoma and also to screen relatives of patients with the familial form of the tumour for early diagnosis. The tumour is associated with characteristic symptoms and signs which include diarrhoea, flushing with alcohol, mucosal neuromas and marfanoid appearance, which are useful clinical pointers.

The management of a patient who is suspected clinically to have a medullary carcinoma of the thyroid should include the following.

(a) Pre-operative diagnosis

Plasma calcitonin should be measured. A raised concentration would strongly support the diagnosis of medullary carcinoma, and a normal level, particularly if unchanged after pentagastrin or alcohol stimulation, would exclude the condition. A raised plasma calcitonin without any supportive clinical evidence is not in itself diagnostic of a medullary carcinoma.

Second, a radionuclide thyroid scan is carried out to localize the tumour. Magnified and oblique views should be performed if a thyroid nodule is not palpable. The tumour may not be detectable by palpation or scanning even though plasma calcitonin is raised, as the latter is a more sensitive investigation. In the presence of supportive evidence of a medullary carcinoma further investigations such as a chest radiography, bone and liver scans should be performed to exclude metastases.

(b) Exclusion of phaeochromocytoma and hyperparathyroidism

Before thyroidectomy is carried out, it is essential to exclude these associated endocrine conditions, particularly in patients with known family history of medullary thyroid carcinoma, phaeochromocytoma or hyperparathyroidism, as failure to do so may result in complicated or even fatal thyroidectomy. Screening investigations consist of estimation of urinary vanilmandelic acid (VMA) for phaeochromocytoma and plasma calcium for hyperparathyroidism. If either of these is raised further confirmatory investigations including urine or plasma cathecholamine concentration and plasma parathyroid hormone should be carried out. If a phaeochromocytoma is diagnosed from biochemical studies its management should precede that of the medullary carcinoma. Appropriate investigations to localize the adrenal tumour include ultrasound or CT scan of the abdomen and ^{123}I-MIBG and are followed by medical treatment with α- and β-sympathetic blocking drugs and surgical excision of the adrenal tumour(s).

(c) Surgical treatment and follow-up of medullary carcinoma

The specific treatment for medullary thyroid carcinoma is a total thyroidectomy as the tumour may be multicentric or may recur in the remaining thyroid tissue. Post-operatively, plasma calcitonin should be measured regularly as a marker for residual, metastatic or recurrent tumour. If significant levels are present, investigations such as chest radiograph, liver and bone scans or CT scan will help localize the lesions. Until recently there were no imaging techniques specifically for this tumour but there are now several possibilities. Ochi *et al.* (1984) showed uptake of pentavalent ^{99m}Tc-labelled DMSA and this has been confirmed by others (Clarke *et al.*, 1987), and its role is particularly valuable in relation to repeated surgical explorations (Figure 8.20). ^{201}Tl was evaluated by Arnstein *et al.* (1986), who presented two cases of recurrent medullary carcinoma, and Hoefnagel *et al.* (1986) reported eight positive uptakes. Finally, uptake of ^{131}I-MIBG in these tumours has been reported (Poston *et al.*,

1986; Von-Moll *et al.*, 1987; Itoh *et al.*, 1986; Coutris, *et al.*, 1986; Ansari *et al.*, 1986) but in general the frequency of uptake has been lower and less predictable than with ^{99m}Tc-labelled pentavalent DMSA, which has higher sensitivity (Clarke *et al.*, 1988). In animal studies (nude mice with medullary thyroid cancers) Guilloteau *et al.* (1985) showed good uptake of ^{131}I-MIBG but failed to find uptake using ^{131}I-labelled anticalcitonin antibody. Reiners *et al.*, (1986) evaluated the use of anti-chorioembryonic antigen (CEA) monoclonal antibody in nine patients but only showed uptake when there were very large secondaries. High-resolution ultra-sound or CT with iodine enhancement may also be useful. Rarely, venous sampling along the jugular veins or inferior vena cava for measurement of plasma calcitonin may be necessary to localize persistent tumour. Treatment of residual or recurrent tumour usually involves further surgery or radiotherapy. Diarrhoea may be difficult to control with persistent tumour.

(d) Screening of relatives

It should now be considered standard practice to screen the relatives of patients with medullary carcinoma, particularly those with a known family history of the condition, to detect the tumour at an early stage or in the pre-malignant phase of C-cell hyperplasia, when the chance of cure by total thyroidectomy is most likely. In those without a known family history initial screening at least is also probably justified to establish whether the disease is sporadic or familial.

The most sensitive screening method is the measurement of plasma calcitonin. However, while this is invariably raised in patients with macroscopic medullary carcinoma, those with microscopic tumours or the pre-malignant stage of C-cell hyperplasia may have normal basal plasma calcitonin but an exaggerated rise after provocation with pentagastrin or alcohol. Plasma calcitonin is measured in the fasting basal state and 2 and 5 min after intravenous pentagastrin or 5 and 10 min after 50 ml of sherry. If the test is negative it is repeated annually, but if the plasma calcitonin is elevated on the basal sample and/or after provocation, it should be repeated for confirmation. An abnormal plasma calcitonin at rest or after provocation on two separate occasions in a relative of a patient with medullary thyroid cancer is considered a positive screen for C-cell malignancy or pre-malignancy. A total thyroidectomy should then be advised after excluding an associated phaeochromocytoma. A thyroid scan with magnified views should also be carried out but often the tumour is too small to be identified on the scan. The ^{99m}Tc-labelled pentavalent DMSA scan may be helpful as is an iodine-enhanced CT scan of the neck. Some clinicians prefer to recommend a total thyroidectomy after the basal calcitonin level has been raised on two occasions, particularly if the level is rising.

8.9.5 ANAPLASTIC CARCINOMA

This type of thyroid cancer occurs most commonly in elderly patients and is fortunately rare, as the prognosis is extremely poor irrespective of the form of treatment. The majority of patients die within 6–12 months of diagnosis and no therapeutic measures have so far been shown to improve prognosis. Radioiodine has no part to play in the treatment of anaplastic thyroid carcinoma as the tumour does not concentrate iodine. The tumour is often fairly well advanced by the time the patient presents and evidence of metastatic spread is often observed clinically or on the chest radiograph, or liver and bone scans. Once the diagnosis is confirmed histologically on biopsy, management is palliative and supportive. Occasionally, some areas within the tumour may contain differentiated follicular structures which take up iodine and respond to radioiodine treatment. The overall prognosis is, however, unchanged and is determined by the anaplastic component of the tumour.

8.10 TECHNIQUES

In this section the technical details of the various investigation which involve radionuclides are described. These may be divided into tests which are carried out *in vitro* and those which are performed *in vivo*. The latter may be subdivided into imaging and non-imaging investigations. The various radionuclides which are used in the investigation or treatment of thyroid diseases and their main physical characteristics are summarized in Table 8.10.

Table 8.10 Radionuclides used in thyroid disease

	γ-rays	*β-particles*	*Half-life*	*Uses*
^{99m}Tc	140	0	6 h	Imaging
^{123}I	160	0	13 h	Imaging
^{125}I	27	0	57 d	Radioimmunoassay
^{131}I	364	Yes	8 d	Uptake measurements Whole body scanning Therapy

8.10.1 *IN VITRO* THYROID FUNCTION TESTS

(a) TRH test

This test, which measures the pituitary TSH response to TRH, is particularly useful under the following circumstances:

1. To confirm or exclude hyperthyroidism when serum T3 and T4 concentrations are equivocal;
2. To confirm secondary hypothyroidism when serum T4 is low but serum TSH is not elevated;
3. To assist in the diagnosis of non-toxic autonomous nodule or euthyroid ophthalmic Graves' disease when serum T3 and T4 are normal.

The original TRH test measures the TSH response to TRH after 20 and 60 min. However, the response at 60 min is only of diagnostic value in the rare cases of secondary hypothyroidism due to hypothalamic disorder and it is the response at 20 min which is important and therefore a shorter version of the original TRH test is sufficient.

(b) Short TRH test (20 min TRH test)

Blood is taken for serum TSH estimation immediately before (basal) and 20 min after an intravenous injection of 200 μg of TRH.

(c) Interpretation

Four types of TSH response to TRH are recognized.

(i) Normal response In euthyroid subjects, the basal serum TSH rises to a peak at 20 min and falls again by 60 min.

(ii) Impaired or absent response The basal serum TSH is normal or low and rises by less than 2 mIu/l above the upper normal range at 20 min after TRH. An impaired TSH response to TRH confirms hyperthyroidism and in the presence of normal serum T3 or T4 is characteristic of non-toxic autonomous nodules or euthyroid ophthalmic Graves' disease. In patients with low serum T4, an impaired TSH response confirms secondary hypothyroidism usually due to pituitary disorder.

(iii) Delayed response A delayed rise in serum TSH at 60 min may rarely occur in patients with secondary hypothyroidism due to a hypothalamic cause.

(iv) Exaggerated response A rise in serum TSH which exceeds the normal range is characteristic of primary hypothyroidism. However, such

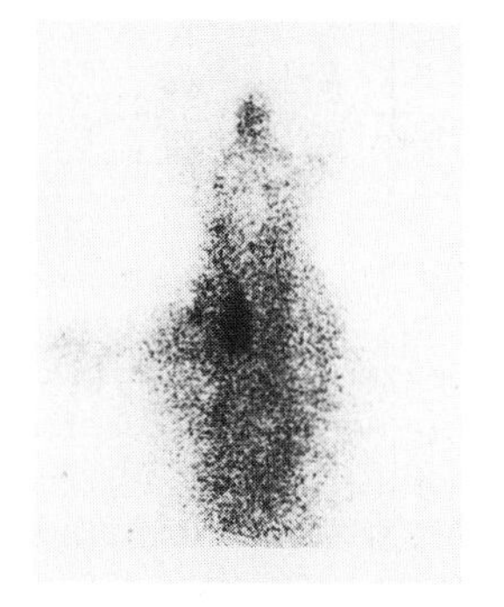
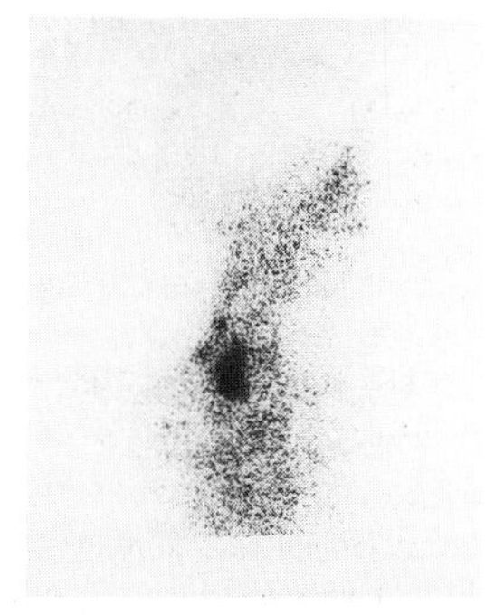

Figure 8.20 A patient with known medullary thyroid cancer and a persistently raised calcitonin level. The uptake of ^{99m}Tc-labelled pentavalent DMSA identified the site of tumour for surgical exploration.

patients usually have a raised basal serum TSH and a TRH test is therefore not usually required for diagnosis of primary hypothyroidism.

8.10.2 *IN VIVO* THYROID IMAGING

(a) Radionuclide thyroid scan

The thyroid scan is now most commonly performed with ^{99m}Tc and to a lesser extent with ^{123}I. ^{99m}Tc-pertechnetate is concentrated but not organified by the thyroid follicle, so that imaging with ^{99m}Tc is a reflection of the trapping property of the thyroid whereas the radioiodine scan reflects both the trapping and organification properties of the gland. Rarely, there may be a disparity between these two functions of the thyroid which results in dissimilar appearances of the image obtained with ^{99m}Tc and radioiodine.

In view of the emission of high-energy γ-rays and short-range β-particles and its long half-life (hence high radiation dose to the patient) ^{131}I has now been largely replaced by ^{99m}Tc or ^{123}I for routine thyroid scanning except when investigating intrathoracic goitre and metastatic differentiated thyroid cancer, when the better penetrating power of the 364 keV γ-photons of ^{131}I is an advantage. ^{123}I is the ideal scanning agent for physiological and physical reasons but unlike ^{99m}Tc it cannot be produced in the laboratory from 'generators' and at present its high cost and limited availability restrict its widespread clinical use. ^{99m}Tc is, therefore, probably the radionuclide most widely used for routine scanning.

Method The following technical points are important when performing a ^{99m}Tc thyroid scan.

1. Inject 1–5 mCi of ^{99m}Tc-pertechnetate intravenously.
2. Image after 20–30 min, when the thyroid/background count rate ratio is maximum.
3. Give the patient a drink of water immediately before imaging to flush away any secreted radionuclide in saliva which may pool in the pharynx or upper oesophagus.
4. Image with a gamma camera fitted with a pinhole or special parallel-holed collimator.
5. The patient should lie down comfortably with the head slightly extended and the collimator about 10 cm above the neck.
6. Image for a fixed count of 100 K with the gamma camera.
7. Whenever indicated, locate the position of anatomical landmarks such as the sternal notch, and any relevant palpable nodules with appropriate radionuclide markers for reference on the image.
8. Repeat images with oblique or magnified views are sometimes necessary.
9. Whenever possible, the percentage uptake by the thyroid should be measured by comparing the count rate over the thyroid against the total amount of radionuclide injected, allowance being made for background and decay.

(b) ^{123}I scan

The technique is similar but instead of giving intravenous ^{99m}Tc-200–500 μCi of ^{123}I-sodium iodide are administered orally and imaging is carried out after 4 h.

(c) Whole body radioiodine scan

This is the most sensitive investigation for detecting and localizing persistent or recurrent differentiated thyroid cancer after initial thyroid ablation. It is dependent on the ability of neoplastic thyroid follicles to concentrate sufficient radioiodine under optimal conditions and thus be detected as hot lesions when the whole body is imaged.

Technique

1. A high circulating TSH (30 mU/l) is essential for tumour uptake of radioiodine to take place. T4 or T3 therapy should therefore be discontinued for at least four weeks and two weeks, respectively, prior to scanning and the serum TSH checked.
2. A low-iodine diet reduces the stable iodide pool of the body, and improves radioactive iodine uptake and the visualization of the tumour.
3. An adequate dose, e.g. 5–15 mCi, of ^{131}I is given orally, as small scanning doses of ^{131}I may fail to produce sufficient uptake in some lesions which only become apparent after bigger doses.

4. The optimal time for imaging is 72 h after the dose of ^{131}I has been administered, when the target/background activity is maximal.
5. Imaging is carried out with either a rectilinear scanner incorporating paired detectors to image the front and back of the body simultaneously, or a gamma camera with multiple static views or one which can image in a scanning mode. A high-energy collimator for ^{131}I is essential.

8.10.3 *IN VIVO* NON-IMAGING INVESTIGATIONS

(a) Radioiodine uptake test

This test, which measures the percentage uptake by the thyroid of a measured dose of radioiodine, was one of the earliest *in vivo* methods of diagnosing thyroid dysfunction but has been superseded by direct measurement of serum thyroid hormones. It is now sometimes used as a guide to radioiodine dosimetry in the treatment of hyperthyroidism, in a modified form in the perchlorate discharge test and to predict relapse or remission of Graves' hyperthyroidism after a course of antithyroid drugs. The test is invalidated by several factors, of which the most important is the presence of excess circulating iodide from iodine-containing medication or radiological contrast media.

Method A tracer dose of ^{131}I (20 μCi) or ^{123}I (100–500 μCi) is given to the patient orally and an equal dose is measured and saved for reference counting.

The count rate over the neck is measured after a suitable time varying from 2 h to 24 h by means of a simple gamma counter placed at a standard distance in front of the neck. The extrathyroidal 'background' activity is assessed by measuring the count rate over the thigh at the same distance and subtracted from the total neck count.

The reference tracer dose is then counted in a phantom neck placed in the same geometrical position as the patient's neck. The percentage uptake is the ratio of the corrected thyroid count rate to that of the reference tracer dose injected.

(b) Perchlorate discharge test

This test is used to assess what proportion of the radioiodine uptake into the thyroid is organified and is therefore useful in the diagnosis of organification defects in the thyroid. Its principle is based on the ability of perchlorate to block further thyroidal uptake of a previously administered dose of radioiodine, allowing free radioiodine but not organified iodine to be discharged from the gland. In normal subjects less than 10% of radioiodine activity is discharged from the thyroid after perchlorate.

Method A tracer dose of ^{131}I or ^{123}I is given orally and the count rate over the thyroid region at a standard distance from the detector is measured at intervals for 2 h. One gram of potassium perchlorate (10 mg kg^{-1} in children) is then given orally and measurement of the count rate is continued at 15 min intervals for 1 h. A fall in count rate of 10% or more 1 h after perchlorate (allowing for decay) indicates an organification defect.

A quicker variant of the test has also been described. The tracer dose of ^{131}I or ^{123}I is given intravenously and the count rate is measured regularly for 10 min. Sodium perchlorate (200 mg) is then given intravenously and counting is continued for another 10 min. The test may also be performed using a gamma camera. The test is considered abnormal if the count rate 10 min after perchlorate has fallen by more than 5% of its value before.

The sensitivity of either test can be improved by giving 0.5–1 mg of stable iodide at the time the radioiodide tracer is given.

An abnormal perchlorate discharge test is seen in patients with congenital organification defect (e.g. Pendred's syndrome), in Hashimoto's thyroiditis, and in patients on antithyroid drugs which block organification, e.g. carbimazole, or after treatment with radioiodine.

REFERENCES

Alderson, P. O., Summer, H. W. and Siegel, B. A. (1976) The single palpable thyroid nodule. *Cancer*, **37**, 258–65.

Al Sayer, H. M., Krukowsi, Z. H., Williams, V. M. M. *et al.* (1985) Fine needle aspiration cytology in isolated thyroid swellings: a prospective two year evaluation. *Br. Med. J.*, **290**, 1490–2.

Anderson, J. B. and Webb. A. J. (1987) Fine needle aspiration biopsy and the diagnosis of thyroid cancer. *Br. J. Surg.*, **74**, 292–6.

Ansari, A. N., Siegel, M. E., De Quattro, V. and Gazarian, L. H. (1986) Imaging of medullary thyroid carcinoma and hyperfunctioning adrenal medulla using iodine-131 metaiodobenzylguanidine. *J. Nucl. Med.*, **27**, 1858–60.

Arning, G., Ehrenheim, C., Schober, O. and Hundeshagen, H. (1987) 131I-accumulating pulmonary and bone metastases of differentiated thyroid cancer with low serum thyroglobulin levels: an exception in tumor follow-up? *Nuklearmedizin*, **26**, 139–42.

Arnstein, N. B., Juni, J. E., Sisson, J. C. *et al.* (1986) Recurrent medullary carcinoma of the thyroid demonstrated by thallium-201 scintigraphy. *J. Nucl. Med.*, **27**, 1564–8.

Ashcroft, M. W. and Van Herle, A. J. (1981) Management of thyroid nodules 11: scanning techniques, 64 thyroid suppressive therapy and fine needle aspiration. *Head Neck Surg.*, **3**, 297–322.

Becker, D. V. and Hurley, J. R. (1982) Current status of radioiodine treatment of hyperthyroidism. *Nucl. Med. Annual*, 265–290.

Black, E. G., Cassoni, A., Gimlette, T. M. D *et al.* (1981) Serum thyroglobulin in thyroid cancer. *Lancet*, **ii**, 443–5.

Bleichrodt, R. P., Vermey, A., Piers, D. A. and Langen, Z. J. (1987) Early and delayed thallium 201 imaging: diagnosis of patients with cold nodules. *Cancer*, **60**, 2621–3.

Brooks, P. T., Archard, N. D. and Carty, H. M. L. (1988) Thyroid screening in congenital hypothyroidism: a review of 41 cases. *Nucl. Med. Commun.*, **9**, 613–17.

Charkes, N. D. (1982) Graves' disease with functioning nodules (Marine–Lenhart syndrome). *J. Nucl. Med.*, **13**, 885–92.

Christensen, S. B., Bondeson, L., Ericsson, U. B. and Lindholm, K. (1984) Prediction of malignancy in the solitary thyroid nodule by physical examination, thyroid scan, fine-needle biopsy and serum thyroglobulin: a prospective study of 100 surgically treated patients. *Acta Chir. Scand.*, **150**, 433–9.

Clarke, S. E. M., Lazarus, C. R., Fogelman, I. and Maisey, M. N. (1987) Technetium-99m(V)-DMSA in the imaging of medullary thyroid carcinoma. *J. Nucl. med.*, **25**, 252–3.

Clarke, S. E. M., Lazarus, C. R., Wraight, P. *et al.* (1988) Pentavalent (^{99m}Tc)DMSA, (^{131}I)MIBG, and (^{99m}Tc)MDP: an evaluation of three imaging techniques in patients with medullary carcinoma of the thyroid. *J. Nucl. Med.*, **29**, 33–38.

Connors, M. H. and Styne, D. M. (1986) Transient neonatal 'athyreosis' resulting from thyrotropin-binding inhibitory immunoglobulins. *Pediatrics*, **78**, 287–90.

Cooke, S. G., Ratcliffe, G. E., Fogelman, I. and Maisey, M. N. (1986) Prevalence of inappropriate drug treatment in patients with hyperthyroidism. *Br. Med. J.*, **291**, 1491–2.

Corstens, F., Huysmans, D. and Kloppenborg, P. (1988) Thallium-201 scintigraphy of the suppressed thyroid: an alternative for iodine-123 scanning after TSH stimulation. *J. Nucl. Med.*, **29**, 1360–3.

Coutris, G., Talbot, J. N., Kabla, G. *et al.* (1986) Uptake of 131-I MGIB by medullary carcinoma of thyroid in familial cases. *Eur. J. Nucl. Med.*, **12**, 77–9.

Creutzig, H. (1987) High or low dose radioiodine ablation of thyroid remnants. *Eur. J. Nucl. Med.*, **12**, 500–2.

De Groot, L. J. and Reilly, M. (1984) Use of isotope bone scans and skeletal survey X-rays in the follow-up of patients with thyroid carcinoma. *J. Endocrinol. Invest.*, **7**, 175–9.

Delange, F., Beckers, C., Hofer, R. *et al.* (1979) Neonatal screening for congenital hypothyroidism in Europe. Report of the Newborn Committee of The European Thyroid Association. *Acta Endocrinol.*, **90** (suppl.), 223.

de Luca, F., Chaussain, J. L. and Job, J. C. (1986) Hyperfunctioning thyroid nodules in children and adolescents. *Acta Paediatr. Scand.*, **75**, 118–23.

Dralle, H., Schwarzrock, R., Lang, W. *et al.* (1985) Comparison of history and immunohistochemistry with thyroglobulin serum levels of radioiodine uptake in recurrences and metastases of differentiated thyroid carcinomas. *Acta Endocrinol. (Copenh.)*, **108**, 504–10.

Duck, S. C. and Sty, J. (1985) Technetium thyroid uptake ratios in pediatric Graves' disease. *J. Pediatr.*, **107**, 905–9.

Ericsson, U. B., Tegler, L., Lennquist, S. *et al.* (1984) Serum thyroglobulin in differentiated thyroid carcinoma. *Acta Chir. Scand.*, **150**, 367–75.

Evans, D. M. (1987) Diagnostic discriminants of thyroid cancer. *Am. Surg.*, **153**, 569–70.

Fisher, D. A. (1983) Second international conference on neonatal thyroid screening: progress report. *J. Pediatr.*, **102**, 653.

Floyd, J. L., Rosen, P. R., Borchert, R. D. *et al.* (1985) Thyroid uptake and imaging with iodine-123 at 4–5 hours: replacement of the 24-hour iodine-131 standard. *J. Nucl. Med.*, **26**, 884–7.

Fogelman, F. and Maisey, M. N. (1988) in *An Atlas of Clinical Nuclear Medicine*, Martin Dunitz, London, p. 190.

Fogelman, I., Cooke, S. G. and Maisey, M. N. (1968a) The role of thyroid scanning in hyperthyroidism. *Eur. J. Nucl. Med.*, **11**, 397–400.

Fogelfeld, L., Rubinstein, U., Bar On, J. and Feigl, D. (1986b) Severe thyrotoxicosis caused by an ectopic intrathoracic goiter. *Clin. Nucl. Med.*, **11**, 20–2.

Freitas, J. E., Gross, M. D., Ripley, S. and Shapiro, B. (1985) Radionuclide diagnosis and therapy of thyroid cancer: current status report. *Semin. Nucl. Med.*, **15**, 106–31.

Fung, H. Y. M., Kologlu, M., Collison, K. *et al.* (1988) Postpartum thyroid dysfunction in Mid Glamorgan. *Br. Med. J.*, **296**, 241–4.

Gammage, M. D. and Franklyn, J. A. (1987) Amiodarone and the thyroid. *Q. J. Med.*, **62**, 83–6.

Gharib, H., Goellner, J. R., Zunsmeister, A. R. *et al.* (1984) Fine needle aspiration biopsy of the thyroid: the problem of suspicious cytological finding. *Ann. Intern. Med.*, **10**, 25–8.

Gharib, H., James, E. M., Charboneau, J. W. *et al.* (1987) Suppressive therapy with levothyroxine for solitary thyroid nodules: a double-blind controlled clinical study. *N. Engl. J. Med.*, **317**, 70–5.

Girelli, M. E., Busnardo, B., Amerio, R. *et al.* (1985) Serum thyroglobulin levels in patients with well-differentiated thyroid cancer during suppression therapy: study on 429 patients. *Eur. J. Nucl. Med.*, **10**, 252–4.

Greer, M. A., Kammer, K. and Bouma, D. J. (1977) Short term antithyroid drug therapy for the thyrotoxicosis of Graves' disease. *N. Engl. J. Med.*, **297**, 173–6.

Guilloteau, D., Baulieu, J. L. and Besnard, J. C. (1985) Medullary-thyroid carcinoma imaging in an animal model: use of radiolabelled anticalcitonin F(ab')2 and *meta*-iodobenzylguanidine. *Eur. J. Nucl. Med.*, **11**, 198–200.

Hedberg, C. W., Fishbem, D. B., Janssen, R. S. *et al.* (1987) An outbreak of thyrotoxicosis caused by the consumption of bovine thyroid gland in ground beef. *N. Engl. J. Med.*, **316**, 993–8.

Hegedus, L., Veiergang, D., Karstrup, S. and Hansen, J. M. (1986) Compensated 131I-therapy of solitary autonomous thyroid nodules: effect on thyroid size and early hyothyroidism. *Acta Endocrinol. (Copenh.)*, **113**, 226–32.

Henze, E., Roth, J., Boerer, H. and Adam, W. E. (1986) Diagnostic value of early and delayed 201Tl thyroid scintigraphy in the evaluation of cold nodules for malignancy. *Eur. J. Nucl. Med.*, **11**, 413–6.

Hershman, J. M., Givens, J. R., Cassidy, C. E. and Astwood, E. B. (1966) Long term outcome of hyperthyroidism treated with antithyroid drugs. *J. Clin. Endocrinol. Metab.*, **26**, 803.

Hoefnagel, C. A., Delprat, C. C., Marcuse, H. R. and Vijlder, J. M. M. (1986) Role of thallium-201 total-body scintigraphy in follow-up of thyroid carcinoma. *J. Nucl. Med.*, **27**, 1854–7.

Horlocker, T. T., Hay, I. D., James, E. M. *et al.* (1986) in *Frontiers in Thyroidology*, Vol. 1 (eds G. Neto and E. Gaitan), Plenum Press, New York, pp. 1309–12.

Hoschl, R., Murray, P. C. and McClean, R. G. (1984) Radio thallium scintigraphy in solitary non functioning thyroid nodules. *World J. Surg.*, **8**, 956–62.

Hoschl, R., Choy, D. H. L. and Gandevia, B. (1988) Iodine-131 uptake in inflammatory lung disease: a potential pitfall in treatment of thyroid carcinoma. *J. Nucl. Med.*, **29**, 701–6.

Itoh, H., Sugie, K., Toyooka, S., Kawase, M. *et al.* (1986) Detection of metastatic medullary thyroid cancer with 131-I MIBG scans in Sipple's syndrome. *Eur. J. Nucl. Med.*, **11**, 502–4.

Jonckheer, M. N. (1987) Clinical usefulness of thyroid imaging by means of X-ray fluorescence. *Horm. Res.*, **26**, 42–7.

Khammash, N. F., Halkar, R. K. and Dayem-Abdel, H. M. (1988) The use of technetium-99m pertechnetate in post operative thyroid carcinoma: Comparative study with iodine-131. *Clin. Nucl. Med.*, **13**, 17–22.

Kim, E. E., Pjura, G., Gobuty, A. and Verani, R. (1984) 131-I uptake in a benign serous cystadenoma of the ovary. *Eur. J. Nucl. Med.*, **9**, 433–5.

LaFranchi, S. (1982) in *Clinical Pediatric and Adolescent Endocrinology* (ed. S. A. Kaplan), Saunders, Philadelphia, p. 82.

Leger, F. A., Doumith, R., Courpotin, C. *et al.* (1987) Complete iodine trapping defect in two cases with congenital hypothyroidism: adaptation of thyroid to huge iodine supplementation. *Eur. J. Clin. Invest.*, **17**, 249–55.

Leisner, B. (1987) Ultrasound evaluation of thyroid disease. *Horm. Res.*, **26**, 33–41.

Lennquist, S. (1987) The thyroid nodule: diagnosis and surgical treatment. *Surg. Clin. North Am.*, **67**, 213–32.

Lipson, A., Nickoloff, E. L., Hsiung Hsu, T. *et al.* (1979) A study of age dependent changes in thyroid function tests in adults. *J. Nucl. Med.*, **20**, 1124–30.

Livadas, D., Psarvas, A. and Koutras, D A. (1976) Malignant cold nodules in hyperthyroidism. *Br. J. Surg.*, **63**, 726–8.

Lowhagen, T., Willems, J. S., Lundell, G. *et al.* (1981) Aspiration biopsy cytology in the diagnosis of thyroid cancer. *World J. Surg.*, **5**, 61–73.

Maisey, M. N. (1981) Methods of investigation in the diagnosis and management of thyroid carcinoma. *World J. Surg.*, **5**, 49–59.

Maisey, M. N., Moses, D C., Hurley, P. J. and Wagner, N. H., Jr (1973) Improved methods for thyroid scanning. *JAMA*, **223**, 761–3.

Maisey, M. N., Natorajam, T. K., Harley, P. J. and Wagner, H. N. (1973) Validation of a rapid computerised method of measuring ^{99m}Tc-pertechnetate uptake for routine assessment of thyroid structure and function. *J. Clin. Endocrinol. Metab.*, **36**, 317–22.

March, D. E., Desai, A. G., Park, C. H. *et al.* (1988) Struma ovarii: hyperthyroidism in a postmenopausal woman. *J. Nucl. Med.*, **29**, 263–5.

Marine, D. and Lenhart, C. H. (1911) Pathological anatomy of exophthalmic goiter. *Arch. Intern. Med.*, **8**, 265–316.

Martino, E., Aghini Lombardi, F., Lippi, F. *et al.* (1985) Twenty-four hour radioactive iodine uptake in 35 patients with amiodarone associated thyrotoxicosis. *J. Nucl. Med.*, **26**, 1402–7.

Moser, E., Fritsch, S. and Braun, S. (1988) Thyroglobulin and I-131 uptake of remaining tissue in patients with differentiated carcinoma after thyroidectomy. *Nucl. Med. Commun.*, **9**, 262–6.

Nagai, G. R., Pitts, W. C., Basso, L. *et al.* (1987) Scintigraphic hot nodules and thyroid carcinoma. *Clin. Nucl. Med.*, **12**, 123–7.

Ng Tang Fui, S. C. and Maisey, M. N. (1979) Standard dose I-131 therapy for hyperthyroidism caused by autonomously functioning thyroid nodules. *Clin. Endocrinol.*, **10**, 69–77.

Ober, K. P., Cowan, R. J., Sevier, R. E. and Poole, G. J. (1987) Thyrotoxicosis caused by functioning metastatic thyroid carcinoma: a rare and elusive cause of hyperthyroidism with low radioactive iodine uptake. *Clin. Nucl. Med.*, **12**, 345–8.

Ochi, H., Sawa, H., Fakuda, T. *et al.* (1982) ^{201}Thallium chloride thyroid scintigraphy to evaluate benign and malignant thyroid nodules. *Cancer*, **50**, 236–40.

Ochi, H., Yamamoto, K., Endo, K. *et al.* (1984) A new imaging agent for medullary carcinoma of the thyroid. *J. Nucl. Med.*, **25**, 323–5.

Ott, R. J., Batty, V., Webb, S. *et al.* (1987) Measurement of radiation dose to the thyroid using positron emission tomography. *J. Radiol.*, **60**, 245–51.

Pacini, F., Lippi, F., Formica, N. *et al.* (1987) Therapeutic doses of iodine-131 reveal undiagnosed metastases in thyroid cancer patients with detectable serum thyroglobulin levels. *J. Nucl. Med.*, **28**, 1888–91.

Patton, J. A. Sandler, M. P. and Partain, C. L. (1985)

Prediction of benignancy of the solitary 'cold' thyroid nodule by fluorescent scanning. *J. Nucl. Med.*, **26**, 461–4.

Perlmutter, M. and Slater, S. L. (1956) Which nodular goiters should be removed? A physiologic plan for the diagnosis and treatment of nodular goiter. *N. Engl. J. Med.*, **255**, 65–71.

Piekarski, J. D., Schlumberger, M., Leclere, J. *et al.* (1985) Chest computed tomography (CT) in patients with micronodular lung metastases of differentiated thyroid carcinoma. *Int. J. Radiat. Oncol. Biol. Phys.*, **11**, 1023–7.

Pons, F., Carrio, I., Estorch, M. *et al.* (1987) Lithium as an adjuvant of iodine-131 uptake when treating patients with well differentiated thyroid carcinoma. *Clin. Nucl. Med.*, **12**, 644–7.

Poston, G. J., Thomas, A. M., MacDonald, D. W. *et al.* (1986) Imaging of metastatic medullary carcinoma of the thyroid with 131-I-*meta*-iodobenzyl guanidine. *Nucl. Med. Commun.*, **7**, 215–21.

Price, D. A., Ehrlich, R. M. and Walfish, P. G. (1982) Congenital hypothyroidism: clinical and laboratory characteristics in infants detected by neonatal screening. *Arch. Dis. Child.*, **56**, 845.

Ramanna, L., Waxman, A. D., Brachman, M. B. *et al.* (1985a) Evaluation of low-dose radioiodine ablation therapy in post-surgical thyroid cancer patients. *Clin. Nucl. Med.*, **10**, 791–5.

Ramanna, L., Waxman, A. D., Brachman, M. B. *et al.* (1985b) Treatment rationale in thyroid carcinoma: effect of scan dose. *Clin. Nucl. Med.*, **10**, 687–9.

Ramtoola, S. and Maisey, M. N. (1988) Subacute (De Quervain's) thyroiditis. *Br. J. Radiol.*, **61**, 515–16.

Ramtoola, S., Maisey, M. N., Clarke, S. E. M. and Fogelman, I. (1988) The thyroid scan in Hashimoto's thyroiditis: the great mimic. *Nucl. Med. Commun.*, **9**, 639–45.

Ratcliffe, G. E., Fogelman, I. and Maisey, M. N. (1986a) The evaluation of radioiodine therapy for thyroid patients using a fixed dose regime. *Br. J. Radiol.*, **59**, 1105–7.

Ratcliffe, G. E., Cooke, S., Fogelman, I. and Maisey, M. N. (1986b) Radioiodine treatment of solitary functioning thyroid nodules. *Br. J. Radiol.*, **5**, 385–7.

Reeve, T. S., Delbridge, L., Sloan, D. and Crummer, P. (1986) The impact of fine needle aspiration biopsy on surgery for single thyroid nodules. *Med. J. Aust.*, **145**, 308–11.

Reiners, C., Eilles, C., Spiegel, W. *et al.* (1986) Immunoscintigraphy in medullary thyroid cancer using an 123-I or 111In-labelled monoclonal anti-CEA antibody fragment. *Nuklearmedizin*, **25**, 227–31.

Rojeski, M. T. and Gharib, H. (1985) Nodular thyroid disease evaluation and management. *N. Engl. J. Med.*, **313**, 428–36.

Ronga, G., Fiorentino, A., Fragasso, G. *et al.* (1986) Complementary role of whole body scan and serum thyroglobulin determination in the follow-up of differentiated thyroid carcinoma. *Ital. J. Surg. Sci.*, **16**, 11–15.

Samaan, N. A., Schultz, P. N., Naynie, T. P. and Ordonez, N. G. (1985) Pulmonary metastases of differentiated thyroid carcinoma treatment results in 101 patients. *J. Clin. Endocrinol. Metab.*, **65**, 376–80.

Schneider, A. B., Recant, W., Pinsky, S. M. *et al.* (1986) Radiation-induced thyroid carcinoma: clinical course and results of therapy in 296 patients. *Ann. Intern. Med.*, **105**, 405–12.

Sheppard, M. C. (1986) Serum thyroglobulin and thyroid cancer. *Q. J. Med.*, **59**, 429–33.

Simeone, J. F., Daniels, G. H., Mueller, R. P. *et al.* (1982) High resolution real time sonography of the thyroid. *Radiology*, **145**, 431–5.

Tang Fui, S. C. and Maisey, M. N. (1983) in *X-ray Fluorescent Scanning of the Thyroid* (eds M. H. Jonckheer and F. Deconinck), Martinus Nijhoff, Amsterdam.

Tang Fui, S., Prior, J., Saunders, A. J. and Maisey, M. N. (1979) Posterior intrathoracic goitre as a cause of thyrotoxicosis. *Br. J. Radiol.*, **52**, 995–7.

Tunbridge, W. M. G., Evered, D. C., Hall, R. *et al.* (1977) The spectrum of thyroid disease in a community: the Wickham survey. *Clin. Endocrinol.*, **7**, 481–93.

Turner, J., Sadler, W., Brownlie, B. and Rogers, T. (1985) Radioiodine therapy for Graves' disease: multivariate analysis of pre-treatment parameters and early outcome. *Eur. J. Nucl. Med.*, **11**, 191–3.

Varma, V. and Reba, R. (1982) in *Nuclear Medicine and Biology* (ed. C. Raynaud), Pergamon Press, Oxford, pp. 103–4.

Von-Moll, L., McEwan, A. J. Shapiro, B. *et al.* (1987) Iodine-131 MIBG scintigraphy of neuroendocrine tumors other than pheochromocytoma and neuroblastoma. *J. Nucl. Med.*, **28**, 979–88.

Walfish, P. G., Strawbridge, H. T. and Rosen, I. B. (1985) Management implications from routine needle biopsy of hyperfunctioning thyroid nodules. *Surgery*, **98**, 1179–88.

Wells, R. G., Sty, J. R. and Duck, S. C. (1986) Technetium 99m pertechnetate thyroid scintigraphy: congenital hypothyroid screening. *Pediatr. Radiol.*, **16**, 368–73.

Werner, S. C. J. (1969) Classification of thyroid disease. Report of the Committee on Nomenclature: American Thyroid Association. *J. Clin. Endocrinol.*, **29**, 860–2.

Westman-Naeser, S., Grimelius, L., Johansson, H. and Malmaeu, J. (1986) Fine needle biopsy and scintigram in the preoperative diagnosis of thyroid lesions. *Ups. J. Med. Sci.*, **91**, 67–76.

White, W. B., Spencer, R. P., Sziklas, J. J. and Rosenberg, R. J. (1985) Incidental finding of intense thyroid radiogallium activity during febrile illness. *Clin. Nucl. Med.*, **10**, 71–4.

Wiersinga, W. M. and Trip, M. D. (1986) Amiodarone and thyroid hormone metabolism. *Postgrad. Med. J.*, **62**, 909–14.

Wilson, R., McKillop, J. H., Pearson, D. W. M. *et al.* (1985) Relapse of Graves' disease after medical therapy: predictive value of thyroidal technetium-99m uptake and serum thyroid stimulating hormone receptor antibody levels. *J. Nucl. Med.*, **26**, 1024–8.

Wise, P. H., Burnet, R. B., Ahmad, A. and Harding, P. E. (1975) Intentional radioiodine ablation in Graves' disease. *Lancet*, **ii**, 1231–3.

Wu, S. Y., Kollin, J., Coodley, E. *et al.* (1984) I-131 total body scan: localization of disseminated gastric adenocarcinoma. Case report and survey of the literature. *J. Nucl. Med.*, **25**, 1204–9.

Ziessman, H. A., Bahar, H., Fahey, F. H. and Dubiansky, V. (1987) Hepatic visualization on iodine-131 whole-body thyroid cancer scans. *J. Nucl. Med.*, **28**, 1408–11.

FURTHER READING

Fogelman, I. and Maisey, M. N. (1989) The thyroid scan in the management of thyroid disease, in *Nuclear Medicine Annual*, Raven Press, New York, pp. 1–48.

CHAPTER NINE

In vitro thyroid function tests

N. J. Marshall, A. Sheldrake and M. G. Prentice

9.1 INTRODUCTION

Immunoassays of circulating thyroid hormones and thyroid-stimulating hormone (TSH) in serum are the major *in vitro* methods for assessing the thyroid status of a patient. Since their inception in the 1960s, immunoassays in a variety of forms have gained widespread usage in both nuclear medicine and clinical biochemistry. Four main attributes account for their successful application in diagnostic services, these being their sensitivity, specificity, precision and convenience. The first three are inherent consequences of the fundamental properties of the interactions between antibodies and their antigens which, as explained later, form the basis of immunoassay systems.

Nowadays these assays take one of two different forms, both of which are utilized for *in vitro* thyroid function tests. Although the two forms are collectively referred to as immunoassays, a somewhat confusing convention has arisen whereby one of the two alternative forms is itself referred to as the 'immunoassay' system, as in radioimmunoassays (RIAs). The other form is the 'immunometric' assay system as encountered in immunoradiometric assays (IRMAs). As suggested by this terminology, both RIAs and IRMAs employ a radioactive isotope as a 'label' or 'tracer', the radiation from which generates the final quantitative signal for the assay. Alternative non-isotopic labelling systems are being increasingly used. The names of the assays which employ these other systems have been derived accordingly (Table 9.1). It is important to realize that these many different assays are all based upon one of the two alternative systems, as should be reflected by the corresponding terminology.

As a starting point for the understanding of the basic principles of these two assay systems it is helpful to outline the methodology of each one separately, as we do below.

9.2 ASSAY PRINCIPLES

Both forms of assay are based upon the interaction between an antibody and its appropriate antigen. The latter, sometimes referred to as the analyte, is the substance being measured in the assay. For example, for an assay for TSH, the basic reaction can be represented as

$$\text{TSH} + \text{anti-TSH} \rightarrow \text{antibody-bound TSH} \quad (9.1)$$

In other words, if TSH is incubated with anti-TSH antibodies, the latter will bind to TSH and form the complex shown on the right-hand side of Equation (9.1). As will be explained later, this is a

Table 9.1 Commonly encountered alternative labelling systems for immunoassays and immunometric assays. The corresponding names of the assays derived from these different systems are shown together with commonly used abbreviations. For further details of the non-isotopic methods see Voller *et al.* (1981); Albertini and Ekins (1982); Butt (1984); Edwards(1985)

Label	*Immunoassay*	*Immunometric assays*
Radioactive isotope, e.g. ^{125}I, ^{3}H, ^{67}Co	Radioimmunoassays (RIA)	Immunoradiometric assays (IRMA)
Pulsed fluorescence	Fluoroimmunoassays (FIA)	Immunofluorometric assays (IFMA)
Enzymes	Enzyme immunoassays (EIA)	Immunoenzymometric assays (IEMA)
Chemiluminescence	Chemiluminescent immunoassays (CIA)	Immunochemiluminescent-metric assays (ICMA)

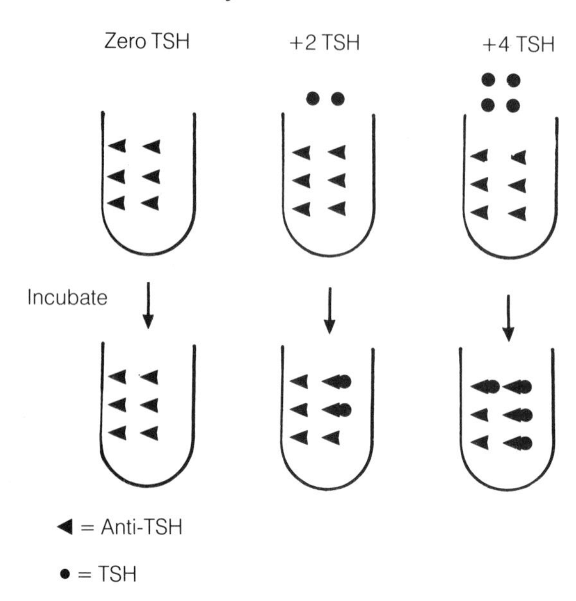

Figure 9.1 Diagrammatic representation of the basic assay system for TSH (see text for details).

simplification of the reaction, but it forms a useful approximation when explaining the principles in the first instance.

To set up the standard curve for an assay for TSH a constant amount of antibody is added to a series of tubes, whilst increasing and known amounts of TSH are added to each tube in succession (Figure 9.1). After a suitable incubation period the reaction depicted in Equation (9.1) will have occurred, and the tubes with the greater amount of TSH will form more bound complex. Clearly, by measuring the amount of complex formed, this can be related to the quantity of TSH which was originally added and one has an assay system for TSH. For immunometric assays the amount of complex formed is measured directly, but for immunoassays this is achieved in a more subtle and indirect manner, as will be explained later.

Some antibodies are capable of binding the antigen very tightly, and are referred to as high-affinity antibodies. In addition the binding site on the antigen can be highly restricted. These two properties of antigen–antibody interactions are responsible for the extreme sensitivity and specificity of the assay systems. Thus in the example used above (TSH), assays are available which will measure the circulating levels of TSH, which are of the order of 10^{-12} M. These assays should be specific for TSH such that they are not influenced by the presence of structurally similar glycoprotein hormones such as luteinizing hormone (LH), follicle-stimulating hormone (FSH) or human chorionic gonadotrophin (HCG), even when the latter are present in relatively higher concentrations.

9.3 IMMUNOMETRIC ASSAYS

The principle of an immunometric assay for TSH is shown in Figure 9.2, where we illustrate the setting up of a simple, two-tube standard curve. As described for Figure 9.1, a constant amount of anti-TSH antibody is added to each tube, together with increasing amounts of TSH in each successive tube (see tubes 1 and 2 in Figure 9.2). After incubation to allow the reaction shown in Equation (9.1) to take place, the amount of TSH bound to the antibody is detected by adding a labelled second anti-TSH antibody to all the tubes. This second antibody is directed against an antigenic site on TSH which is stearically remote from the binding site of the first antibody. Thus a triple complex is formed, whereby the TSH is 'sandwiched' between the two separate antibodies. The second antibody is also added as a constant amount to each tube, and is added as an excess. Since it carries a label (e.g. ^{125}I), the amount of complex formed can be measured by separating the complex from the excess unbound labelled second antibody and quantifying the label present in each tube, e.g. counting the radiation emitted by the ^{125}I associated with the separated complex, which is retained in the tubes. Consequently, if this radioactivity is measured and plotted against the increasing but known standard amount of TSH initially added, a standard curve can be generated, as is illustrated (Figure 9.2). In practice this curve is not a straight line passing through the origin as might be expected from equation (9.1), but is of the form shown in Figure 9.2. The reason for this will be explained later. In addition, to obtain this curve, clearly more than two standards are required. Usually between six and eight different concentrations of TSH will be used.

Clearly, if a sample tube is also run which contains an unknown amount of TSH, but is identical to the other tubes in all other respects, the amount of TSH which was present in the sample tube can be measured by interpolating from the standard curve in the manner shown (Figure 9.2).

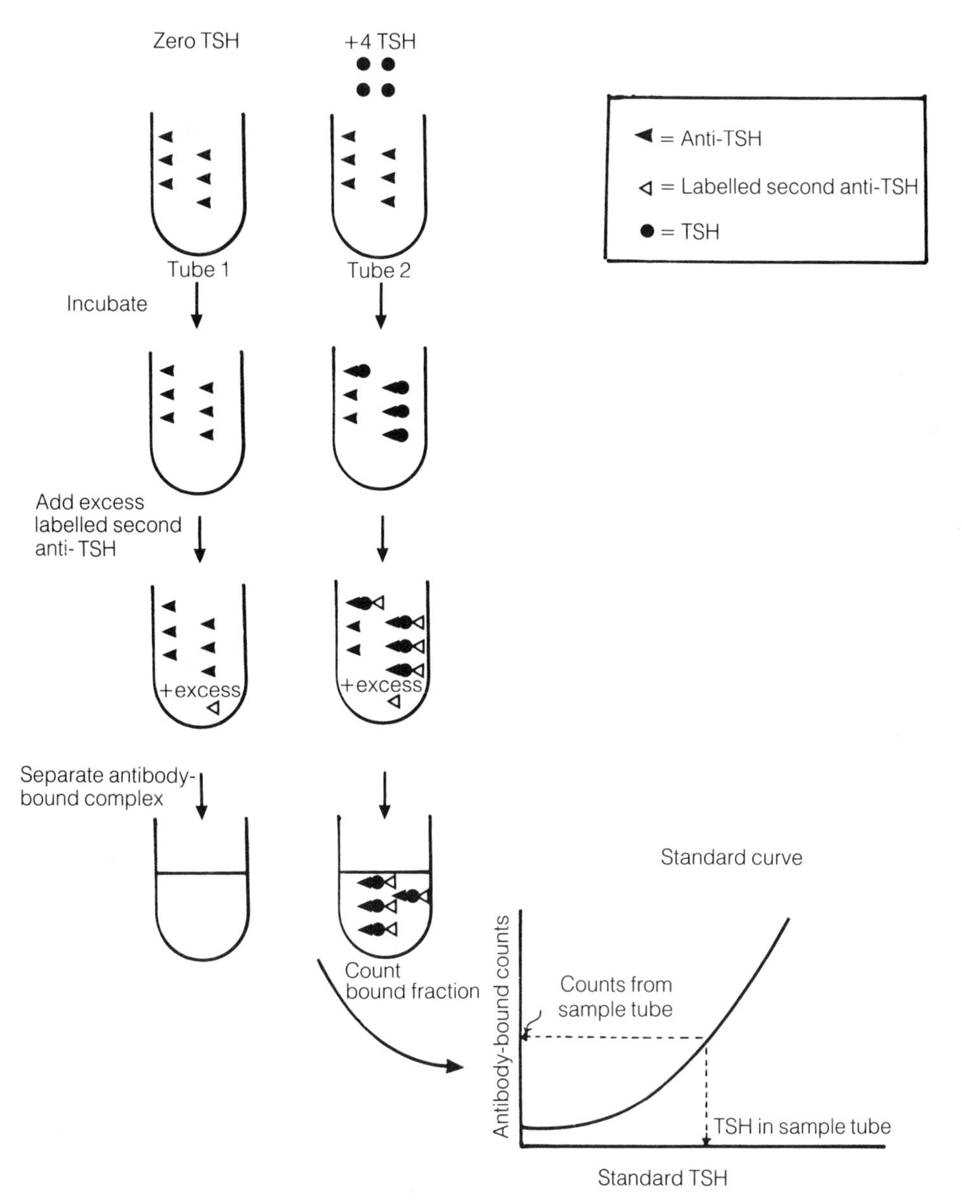

Figure 9.2 Diagrammatic representation of how a two-point standard curve for a TSH IRMA is set up. In practice the incubation steps with the first and second antibodies are usually combined, with both antibodies being added simultaneously. They are shown separately here to aid the visual representation. This is the two-site assay technology, which is the most commonly encountered design for IRMA nowadays. In its original form, the first antibody was labelled, doing away with the requirement for a second antibody (Miles and Hales, 1968a, 1968b).

9.4 IMMUNOASSAYS

9.4.1 BASIC PRINCIPLES: RIA OF TSH

The principle underlying the alternative immunoassay system for TSH is shown in Figure 9.3, which diagrammatically illustrates how a two-point standard curve is generated for a TSH RIA. As with the immunometric assay (Figure 9.2), constant amounts of anti-TSH are added to each tube. In addition, a constant amount of labelled antigen is also added to each tube; for this RIA this would be ^{125}I-labelled TSH. In the example shown, a 'zero' tube is set up, i.e. that containing zero unlabelled standard TSH, and also one containing a known amount of standard TSH (selected for the purpose of illustration to be). After a suitable incubation, to allow the reaction shown in Equation (9.1) to occur, since tube 1 contains twice as much ^{125}I-labelled TSH as anti-TSH antibody, according to our simple model, half the ^{125}I-labelled TSH will be bound by the antibody, but the other half will be unable to bind and be present as an 'excess'. In tube 2, unlabelled, standard TSH has also been added, which will compete with the ^{125}I-labelled TSH for the limited number of antibody binding sites available. In this way, the radioactivity bound to the antibody will be reduced. This reduction in bound radioactivity is the usual assay signal which is measured in response to the added unlabelled TSH. The bound TSH (both labelled and un-

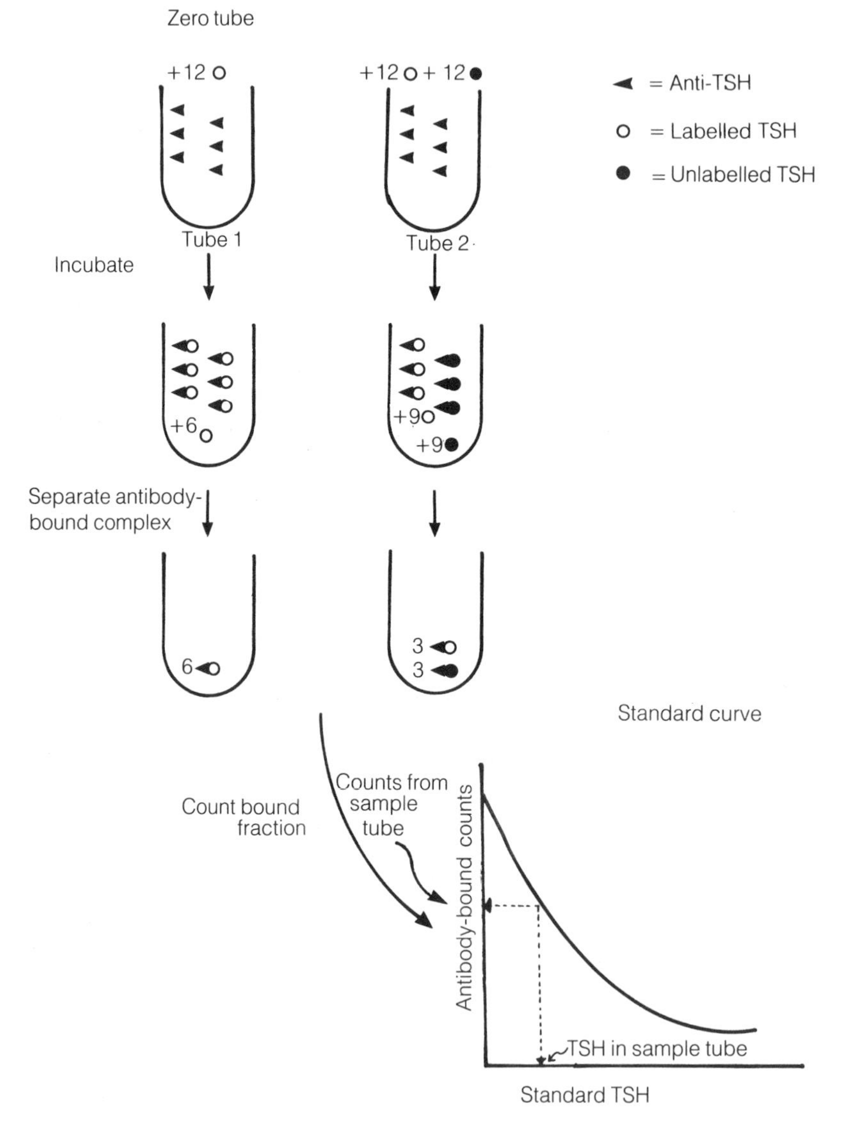

Figure 9.3 Diagrammatic representation of how a two-point standard curve for a TSH RIA is set up. Note: only small numbers are shown for added reagents for both Figures 9.2 and 9.3; in practice the numbers of molecules of each reagent present in a given tube will be of the order of 10^6–10^9. Under these conditions the competition between labelled and unlabelled TSH in tube 2 in this figure will be such that on 'average', in statistical terms, 50% of the antibody binding sites will be occupied by labelled TSH when competing with an equal amount of unlabelled TSH.

labelled) is separated, e.g. by precipitation, and the radioactivity associated with the bound fraction is counted. If this radioactivity is plotted against the increasing but known standard amounts of TSH initially added, a standard curve can be generated as is illustrated (Figure 9.3). It should be noted that in contrast to Figure 9.2, which represents the radioimmunometric system, for an RIA the antibody-bound radioactivity decreases with increasing amounts of unlabelled, standard TSH. As explained for the previous section describing immunometric assays, clearly more than two standard concentrations are required to define this curve, and in practice a total of between six and eight will be used.

To measure the TSH in a sample it is merely necessary to replace the standard TSH added with the sample, but otherwise add amounts of antibody and labelled TSH which are identical to those used for the standard curve and carefully process all the tubes in precisely the same manner through the assay. The TSH present in the sample can be interpolated from the standard curve in the manner shown (Figure 9.3). It is helpful at this stage to contrast the characteristics of the RIA and IRMA just described in Figures 9.2 and 9.3, as we do in Table 9.2.

Table 9.2 Comparison of RIA and IRMA systems as described in Figures 9.2 and 9.3

Reagents	*RIA*	*IRMA**
Standards	As for IRMA	As for RIA
Label	Labelled antigen	Labelled second antibody
First antibody	Added in limiting amounts	Added in relatively large amounts
Second antibody to 'sandwich' the antigen	Not added	Added as an excess
Assay response	Decreased binding of label	Increased binding of label

Relative performance characteristics
(1) IRMAs tend to be faster, more specific and sensitive than RIAs
(2) For *in vitro* thyroid function tests, TSH but not T3 or T4 is usually measured by IRMA. TSH (molecular weight ~30 000) is sufficiently large a glycoprotein to provide well-separated antigenic sites for the two antibodies

*As designed for the commonly encountered 'two-site' version.

9.4.2 RIA OF THYROID HORMONES

Thyroid hormones circulate in blood largely bound to specific binding proteins, and this presents an additional problem in their determination by RIA. One can adapt the methodology described above (a) to assay their total concentration or (b) to directly measure the concentration of free hormones present in serum. The methods for this are outlined below. In the past a group of indirect methods was also used, which yielded so-called 'free thyroxine indices'. These were derived from a combination of two independent parameters such as a determination of the total hormone concentration and an estimate of the binding capacity of the circulating binding proteins. Due to recent improvements in techniques for the direct measurement of free thyroid hormones, the use of the indirect methods has declined greatly, and will not be further discussed.

(a) Total thyroxine (T4) and triiodothyronine (T3)

To measure the total concentration of either T4 and T3, the bound hormone is displaced from the binding proteins and an RIA is then used to determine the total concentration of the hormone, which is now entirely present in a free form. There are three binding proteins, namely thyroxine-binding globulin (TBG), which is the dominant of the three, thyroxine-binding prealbumin (TBPA) and albumin. Hormone binding to these, which is non-covalent and reversible (see later), can be effectively inhibited by the addition of organic compounds such as anilino-naphthaline sulphonic acid (ANS). In practice the optimal concentration of ANS is added together with the other reagents for the RIA, i.e. no pre-incubation with ANS is required prior to the assay.

(b) Free T4 and T3

The measurement of the concentration of the minute fractions (0.03% and 0.3% for T4 and T3 respectively) of each hormone in the non-protein bound or 'free' form presents a much more substantial problem. One early difficulty, now resolved, was that additional sensitivity was required to measure the free thyroid hormones since they circulate at picomolar as opposed to the nanomolar concentrations of the total hormones. Antisera with sufficiently high affinities (see later) are now available which provide the requisite sensitivity.

Table 9.3 Examples of methods available for the direct measurement of free thyroid hormones

Method
Equilibrium dialysis (Ellis and Ekins, 1973)
Resin adsorption (Romelli *et al.*, 1979)
'Two-step' back-titration (Ekins *et al.*, 1980)
Labelled hormone analogue (Midgley and Wilkins, 1981)
Corning immunophase* (Odstrchel, 1982)
Damon microencapsulated antibody 'Liquisol' method (Buehler, 1982)

*Not strictly a 'direct' method.

Using the high-affinity antisera there are a number of different approaches to the measurement of free hormones (see Table 9.3). They all aim to measure the free hormone concentration without significantly shifting a 'dynamic equilibrium' which exists between the thyroid hormone and its binding proteins. The term 'dynamic equilibrium' is defined in the next section, when this concept is explained further. In the equilibrium dialysis method, for example, serum is dialysed against a relatively small volume of a buffer solution, and the concentration of the thyroid hormone in the dialysate is subsequently determined by conventional RIA as depicted in Figure 9.3. Provided the assay system is designed with care, the free hormone concentration in the dialysate closely approximates to that originally present in the serum before dialysis. This method is widely regarded as the reference method, but unfortunately it has proved technically difficult and laborious to run on a large-scale routine basis. Other methods such as the labelled hormone analogue method, which are as attractively convenient as routine RIAs, have consequently been more widely used. The basis of this method is the use of ^{125}I-labelled derivatives of T4 or T3 which have been chemically modified to drastically inhibit their binding to the endogenous serum binding proteins (Midgley and Wilkins, 1982a, 1982b). Thus the presence of the serum binding proteins is virtually 'irrelevant' to the labelled analogue. However, the anti-T4 or anti-T3 antibodies selected for use in the RIAs do not distinguish between the analogue and the appropriate endogenous hormone. Consequently the RIA of the free thyroid hormone is essentially as depicted in Figure 9.3, in which the free hormone and the ^{125}I-labelled analogue compete for a limited number of antibody binding sites. Once again, the assay must be carefully designed to ensure minimal disturbance of the equilibrium between the free and protien-bound thyroid hormones originally present in the serum.

There is general agreement that the measurement of the concentrations of the free circulating hormones is more relevant than the total levels, as an indicator of patient thyroid status. However, there are reservations about the detailed interpretation of results from these assays (Ekins, 1984; Pearce and Byfield, 1986) since the presence of grossly abnormal levels of normal binding proteins, aberrant proteins, or excessive levels of other serum constituents such as non-esterified fatty acids may introduce artefacts which distort the results. Such considerations have inhibited the more widespread use of these techniques in the diagnostic services and caused some laboratories to place greater emphasis on, for example, the measurement of TSH by sensitive IRMA techniques as 'front line' tests of thyroid function (see later). The latter practice is encouraged by the view that generally pituitary TSH secretion is a reliable guide to thyroid hormone sufficiency.

9.5 ADDITIONAL CONSIDERATIONS

As mentioned above, Equation (9.1) is a simplification of the true situation. In practice the reaction is reversible and should more properly be represented as follows:

$$\text{TSH} + \text{anti-TSH} \rightleftharpoons \text{antibody bound TSH} \quad (9.2)$$

which indicates that at any given time the antibody and its antigen TSH are both associating and dissociating. During the incubation period the reaction is reaching an equilibrium whereby the rate of association becomes equal to the rate of dissociation, and a steady-state position of equilibrium is reached, termed a dynamic equilibrium.*

*A useful analogy for didactic purposes is the dynamic equilibrium which exists in society between marriage (association) and divorce (dissociation). This may be represented as $M + F \rightleftharpoons MF$. When trying to visualize the various transformations of the law of mass action as discussed in this section, it can be helpful to apply this analogy; the results can be quite provocative! The binding of thyroid hormones to their binding proteins can also be described in this way, e.g. $T4 + TBG \rightleftharpoons T4.TBG$. The aim of free thyroid hormone assays is the measurement of free T4 without disturbing the 'dynamic equilibrium' which exists between the thyroid hormone and its binding proteins. Thus using this analogy this aim becomes the measurement of the 'concentration' of unmarried men without disturbing the dynamic equilibrium, i.e. causing more divorce. Clearly, the latter might occur if during their measurement an excessive number of unmarried men were removed from circulation.

This reversible reaction is governed by the law of mass action, so that the rate of the forward reaction (complex formation) and backward reaction (complex dissociation) will be as follows:

$$\text{Rate of forward reaction} = K_{+1} . [\text{TSH}] . [\text{anti-TSH}] \quad (9.3)$$

$$\text{Rate of backward reaction} = K_{-1} . [\text{antibody-bound TSH}] \quad (9.4)$$

where K_{+1} = association rate constant and K_{-1} = dissociation rate constant; both are physical constants which are a unique characteristic of each antigen–antibody reaction; and square brackets denote concentration.

At equilibrium, the rates of these two reactions will be equal, and the situation can be represented as

$$K_{+1} . [\text{TSH}] . [\text{anti-TSH}] = K_{-1} . [\text{antibody-bound TSH}]$$

$$\therefore \frac{K_{+1}}{K_{-1}} = \frac{[\text{antibody-bound TSH}]}{[\text{TSH}] . [\text{anti-TSH}]} \quad (9.5)$$

$$= \text{affinity constant } K_A$$

The affinity constant, which can also be termed the association constant, is a ratio of the two rate constants, and hence is also a physical constant which is a unique characteristic of each antigen–antibody reaction. Immunoassays, as opposed to immunometric assays, are particularly dependent upon a given antigen–antibody interaction having a high value for K_A, i.e. being high-affinity antibodies, if maximum sensitivity is required. The affinity constant is commonly determined by transforming the results presented as a standard curve for an RIA into a Scatchard plot (Figure 9.4). It is beyond the scope of this text to detail this procedure further, but some RIA data-processing packages may automatically carry out this transformation and provide this additional information if required.

This is only a brief outline of the underlying principles of these assay systems, but it should prove useful as a somewhat intuitive base for understanding some of the problems which will be encountered in running and controlling immunoassay and immunometric assay systems, as is explained in the next section.

A final word on assay terminology would be appropriate. The reaction represented in Equation (9.2) can be described as a saturation system. This is because if the anti-TSH concentration is kept constant – as it is in both assay systems – increas-

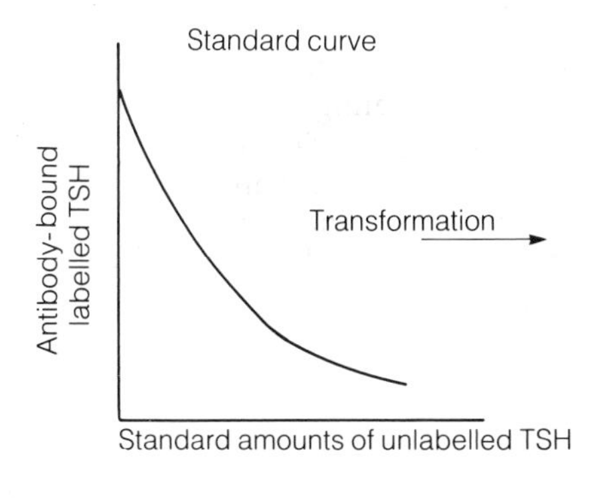

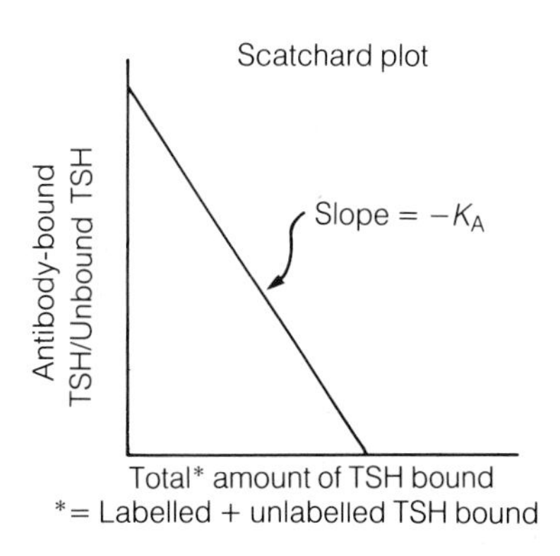

Figure 9.4 Diagram illustrating the relationship between the standard curve for a TSH RIA (see Figure 9.3) and the Scatchard plot which may be obtained by a simple transformation. To do this one should also know the specific radioactivity of the labelled TSH used for the standard curve and apply Scatchard's transformation of Equation (9.5), which is

$$\frac{[\text{antibody-bound TSH}]}{[\text{unbound TSH}]} = K_A . [\text{Ab}]_T - K_A . [\text{antibody-bound TSH}]$$

where $[\text{Ab}]_T$ = concentration of total antibody added to each tube, which is of course kept constant for all tubes. Clearly $[\text{Ab}]_T$ = [anti-TSH] + [antibody-bound TSH], and the transformation is achieved by using this to substitute for [anti-TSH] in Equation (9.5).

ing amounts of TSH will tend to 'saturate' the antibody. Because of the reversible nature of the reaction, all the antibody binding sites will never be occupied, even in the presence of exceedingly high TSH concentrations; at any given time dissociation will take place although reoccupancy will recur faster with the higher TSH concentrations. Consequently these assay systems are also referred to as saturation assays, and the kinetic systems described by Equations (9.2)–(9.5) are referred to as saturation kinetics. Immunoassays such as that described for the TSH RIA (Figure 9.3) are also referred to as competitive binding assays, the name being derived from the type of 'competitive model' represented in Figure 9.3. However, the term 'competition' has a very precise definition in biochemistry, and on these grounds this terminology can be criticized. Moreover, to the rigorous analyst the concept of 'competition' between the unlabelled and labelled TSH as depicted in Figure 9.3 is limited in its usefulness. It is more helpful to visualize the label as merely acting as a tracer which allows one to measure the distribution of the TSH as a whole between the antibody-bound and -unbound fractions. Thus in Figure 9.3, in tube 1 50% of the total TSH added is bound, whereas in tube 2 only 25% is bound. The latter is measured as $3/12$ of the label although it is also $3/12$ of the unlabelled or $6/24$ of the total [labelled + unlabelled TSH], i.e. the label is distributing itself in the same proportional manner as the unlabelled TSH. Thus the RIA system is seen to rely upon the decrease of the *proportion* of all the TSH which is bound with increasing added TSH, as its primary response system; this decreased proportion is revealed and measured by the decreased proportion of the label which is bound. In contrast, the IRMA system relies upon a measure of the increased *amount* of TSH bound (see Figure 9.2). In reality by using the law of mass action (equation (9.5)) it can easily be shown that one is merely a transformation of the other. Such an understanding can be helpful when one is, for example, interpreting the plot of another commonly encountered transformation, namely the Scatchard plot. Finally yet another alternative general description for these assay systems is in use, that of ligand binding assays. This terminology can be applied since the binding reagent need not be an antibody, but can be any one of a number of alternatives such as target cell-associated hormone receptors or even circulating binding proteins. For example, as is described later, the TSH receptor derived from the thyroid epithelial cell is utilized as the binding reagent in the TSH receptor assay which is employed to detect anti-TSH receptor antibodies.

9.6 THE PRACTICE OF IMMUNOASSAY

The effectiveness of an immunoassay laboratory will depend upon the understanding of the principles underlying the systems which were outlined in the previous section, and also the adherence to well-defined laboratory practices derived from these theoretical considerations. Recognition of these factors is essential if clinical confidence in the final results is to be achieved.

In this section we will outline the critical characteristics of the reagents and their subsequent use in immunoassays. We will also recommend control procedures and briefly mention commonly encountered problems which the quality-control programmes are designed to reveal. The control of the quality of results emerging from immunoassay laboratories has provided a significant challenge to clinical biochemists and, as will be discussed, many problems have yet to be resolved in this area. Finally there is a brief description of the essential requirements for an immunoassay laboratory.

9.6.1 REAGENTS

As explained in the first section, only three basic reagents are required for RIAs and IRMAs. These are the standard hormone preparations, the labelled material (antigen or antibody) and the specific antibody. In addition a separation procedure, to separate the antibody bound from the free hormone, is required. Each of these will be discussed in sequence, below:

9.6.2 STANDARDS

Hormones with simple and well-defined structures such as T3 and T4 can be readily purchased in a suitably purified form for use in RIAs. The absolute concentrations of the stock solutions from which the serial dilutions of the standards can be prepared are usually determined spectrophotometrically.

In contrast, for a complex glycoprotein such as TSH (molecular weight ~30 000) highly purified standard preparations from human pituitaries can only be obtained and calibrated with difficulty.

Nowadays this would virtually never be done *de novo* by an RIA laboratory. It is possible either to purchase good-quality material, or perhaps utilize the stocks of international reference preparations which are held by international agencies such as the National Pituitary Agency in the USA or the National Institute for Biological Standards and Control (NIBSC) in the UK. The standard TSH should be supplied with accompany data describing its evaluation. During the establishment of an international reference preparation, NIBSC will organize the determination of the potencies of a given preparation in specialist laboratories worldwide. These laboratories will utilize both immunoassays and several bioassays for this calibration. The difficulties associated with the establishment of these reference preparations, including the uncertainties of the structural forms of a hormone such as TSH, and the conflicting results which can be obtained in different bioassays, are reflected in the final expression of the quantity of TSH in terms of 'units' rather than in absolute molecular terms (e.g. nmoles T4 per litre). The 'unit' will refer to the potency of the preparation in a specific reference assay as will be stated in the evaluation report.

These standards will be used as a series of dilutions for a standard curve. They will be handled in solution, and the solvent in which they are dissolved is referred to as the 'standard matrix'. Ideally the series of standard solutions should be prepared to resemble the patient samples as clearly as possible, and this would apparently be achieved most simply by using human serum which is free of the hormone in question. However, this requires an adequate supply of human serum which has been certified to fulfil several stringent requirements. First, it must be free from potentially infective pathogens. In addition, it must itself ressemble the patient sera. For example, the procedures which have rendered the serum 'hormone free', and must not have inadvertently removed other relevant components from the serum. These might influence the basic kinetics of the reaction between the antigen and its antibody in the assay, or the efficiency of the separation system (see later).

If the latter requirement has not been fulfilled, anomalous results will occur in the final assay (see later under 'standard Matrix Effects' Table 9.5). Because of these difficulties in preparing hormone-free serum, synthetic 'cocktails' using various fractions of serum proteins in buffer solutions are sometimes substituted. However, these can be difficult to formulate, requiring substantial empirical experimentation.

9.6.3 LABELLED MATERIAL

Despite the various alternative labelling systems now available, which were discussed in the first section, radioisotopes and in particular ^{125}I at present predominate in immunoassay laboratories. The comments in this section will therefore emphasize the laboratory usage of ^{125}I.

^{125}I-labelled T3 or ^{125}I-labelled T4 may be purchased quite readily in a suitably purified quality for immediate use in RIA from radiochemical manufacturers. They are intrinsically relatively stable, and if suitably stored their shelf-life is largely governed by the decay of the ^{125}I.

Iodination of TSH or antibodies is still quite frequently carried out in the 'hot-labs' of RIA laboratories although satisfactory commercial preparations are also widely available. The basic reaction mimics the oxidative iodination of thyroglobulin in the thyroid gland. TSH or the antibody to be labelled is exposed to iodide under oxidizing conditions, and ^{125}I substitutes in exposed phenolic groups of tyrosine, as is illustrated in Figure 9.5. A number of different oxidizing agents are available for use in iodinations as are listed in Table 9.4. The different reagents and incubation conditions can produce widely differing labelled products, both in terms of ^{125}I incorporation, retention of the structural integrity of the hormone or antibody, and its stability on long-term storage. Inappropriate iodination conditions can result in labelled preparations with very short shelf-lives.

A flow diagram of a typical iodination and purification procedure is shown in Figure 9.6. The

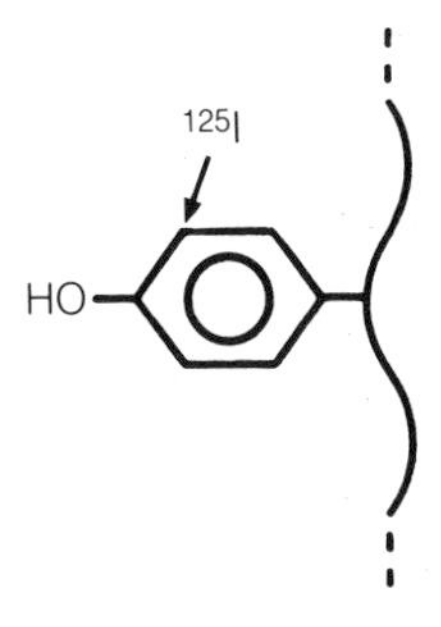

Figure 9.5 Iodination of the phenolic groups of tyrosine residues in proteins such as TSH.

Table 9.4 Examples of different reagents used in the iodination of TSH or antibodies. For further details see Bolton 1977 and Bolton 1981

Oxidizing reagents
Chloramine T (*N*-chloro-*p*-toluene sulphonamide)
Lactoperoxidase (liquid and solid phase)
Glucose oxidase (liquid and solid phase)
Iodogen (1,3,4,6-tetrachloro-3α,6α-diphenylglycoluril)
Preiodinated material for conjugation to amino groups
Bolton Hunter Reagent (N-Succinimidyl 3-(4-hydroxyphenyl) proprionate

purification process, subsequent to the iodination reaction, during which both excess ^{125}I and damaged hormone or antibody are removed, is essential for good-quality label for the final immunoassay. The ideal is to obtain ^{125}I-labelled hormone or antibody which is stable and immunologically indistinguishable from the unlabelled hormone in the final immunoassay reaction.

9.6.4 SPECIFIC ANTISERA

The widespread use of monoclonal antisera has contributed in many ways to recent improvements in immunoassay performance. Monoclonal techniques make available virtually unrestricted quantities of well-characterized, specific antibodies of the appropriate affinity. These are available commercially.

Anti-T3 and T4 antisera can now be routinely obtained with affinity constants (see Figure 9.4), which are sufficiently high to permit the measurement of circulating free T3 and free T4, i.e. picomolar concentrations, by RIA. They are clearly also required to be sufficiently specific to distinguish between the structures of T3 and T4.

The availability of relatively large quantities of anti-TSH antisera by monoclonal production techniques has been a major factor in the adoption of IRMAs as opposed to RIAs for the measurement of TSH. The former are more extravagant in their use of antisera compared with RIAs which use only limited amounts (see Table 9.2). These IRMAs have proved more rapid, precise and in particular more sensitive than RIAs for TSH. They make it possible to measure levels of TSH which are below the euthyroid reference range. As mentioned elsewhere in this chapter, this has had a profound effect on the thyroid testing strategies of many laboratories, with TSH becoming a 'front-line' test rather than a secondary, confirmatory test of thyroid status. An additional advantage of the use of the IRMA systems is that pairs of monoclonal antibodies may be selected to confer greater hormonal specificity than was achieved with most RIAs. By using two antibodies in the 'sandwich' system (see Figure 9.2), two discriminating probes are being used to distinguish TSH from closely related glycoproteins such as the gonadotrophins, which share common α-subunits with TSH.

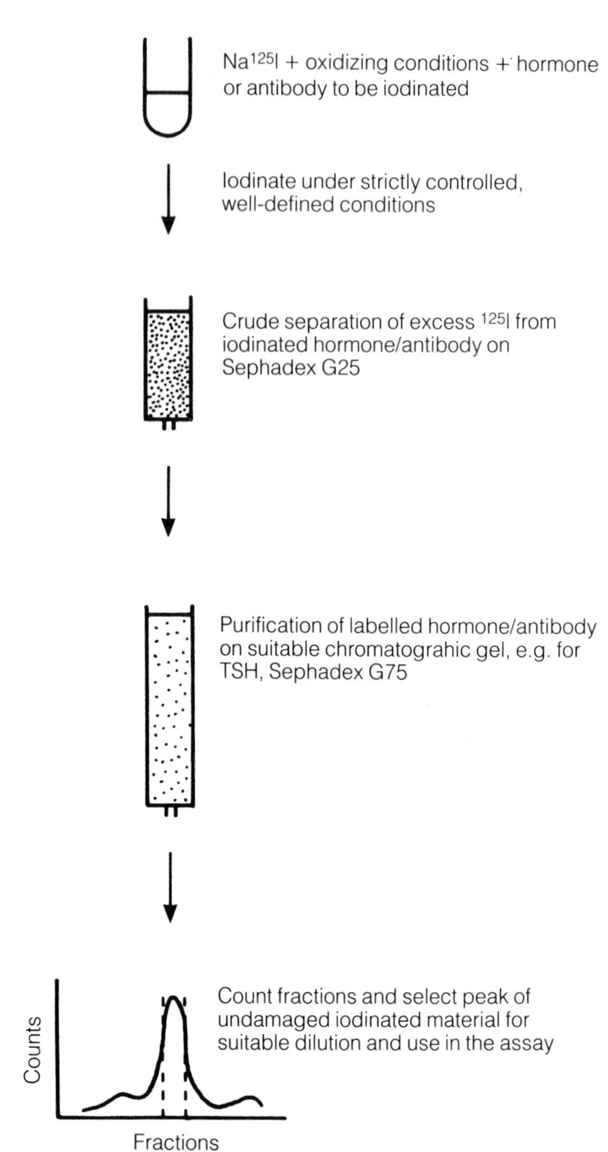

Figure 9.6 Flow diagram of a typical procedure for preparing iodinated TSH or antibodies.

9.6.5 SEPARATION SYSTEMS

Both RIAs and IRMAs depend upon separation processes which will efficiently separate antibody bound from unbound moieties (see Figures 9.2 and 9.3). A variety of techniques have been used and some which are in common usage at present are listed in Table 9.5.

When assaying small molecules such as T3 or T4, the unbound fraction may be adsorbed to charcoal which has been pretreated to prevent the antibody-bound fraction from binding. The charcoal may then be precipitated by centrifugation, and either the pellet or the supernatant counted for ^{125}I.

Conversely, and more commonly, the antibody-bound fraction may be precipitated by centrifugation. This can be achieved by adding a second antibody which is directed against the first antibody. For example, in a T3 assay, if the first specific anti-T3 antibody is raised in a rabbit, the second antibody would be an anti-rabbit IgG antiserum. Alternatively, precipitation of the antibody-bound fraction can be obtained by adding an appropriate concentration of a protein precipitant such as polyethylene glycol (PEG). Sometimes a combination of these two methods, referred to as 'PEG-assisted second (or double) antibody precipitation', is used.

Linkage of the antibody to solid phases, such as inert plastics, has led to elegant and exceptionally

Table 9.5 Examples of separation systems used in RIAs and IRMAs

Principle	*Reagent*
Adsorption of free hormone	Fine charcoal suspension
Precipitation of antibody–antigen complex	1. Second antibody 2. Protein precipitants, e.g. polyethylene glycol (PEG)
Solid-phase techniques	1. 'Solid-phase' antibody, i.e. linking antibody to inert particulate matter 2. Coating techniques, i.e. linking antibody to the inner surface of plastic tubes or microtitre wells, or to the surface of spheres

Table 9.6 Examples of commonly encountered problems in immunoassay performance

1. *Gross problems due to reagent deterioration*
Symptoms: Loss of assay sensitivity and precision
– flattened response curve
– increased differences between replicates
Gradual changes in absolute values of controls and samples

2. *Disturbance of the equilibrium of the reversible reaction (Equation (9.2)) by the separation system, e.g. charcoal absorption of the free fraction causing subsequent dissociation of the antibody-bound hormone*
Symptoms: Assay 'drift'
– values for a sample change when they are tested at the beginning and end of the assay

3. *Inefficient separation systems; due to contamination of, for example, the bound fraction with the free fraction, sometimes referred to as 'misclassification errors'*
Symptoms: poor within-assay precision

4. *'Batch-specific' effects with new batches of reagents*
Symptoms: Acute changes in absolute values of controls or samples. There may also be changes in precision, sensitivity or drift

5. *Standard 'matrix effects', e.g. due to differences in the 'milieu' of standards as opposed to samples*, e.g. complete serum of a patient sample as opposed to hormone-free serum used to dissolve the standard preparation.
Symptoms: Inappropriate values obtained for a sample, e.g. negative values. Non-parallel dilution of a sample and the standards, when the sample is diluted with the 'milieu' used for the standards
Excessive or low recoveries when a sample is 'spiked' with a known amount of standard material

6. *'Hook effect'*
Symptoms: The value of a sample *increases* when it is diluted with the hormone-free 'milieu' used for the standards. The best example is the pronounced bell-shaped standard curve which can be obtained with an IRMA when tested at very high hormone concentrations

7. *Incorrect determinations due to inappropriate curve fitting by automatic data-processing systems*
Symptoms: Aberrant curve fits when manual plots are compared with the computer-generated fit. This can lead to 'dose-related bias'

efficient separation systems. The solid phases may be used as suspensions of microspheres, which can be handled with conventional pipetting devices, and pelleted by centrifugation. Alternatively they can be of a form which does not require the final centrifugation, such as a surface coating on large spheres, or on the inner surfaces of plastic test tubes or microtitre plate wells. One great advantage of these systems is that they can be sufficiently stable to allow washing of the solid phase. This minimizes the contamination of the bound fraction with the free, which can be a major source of error. This type of error is frequently referred to as 'misclassification' error, since it is due to misclassification of the free fraction as the bound or vice versa.

The separation system selected can greatly influence the final quality of the assay, both in terms of convenience, ruggednes, sensitivity and precision. For further comment see Table 9.6.

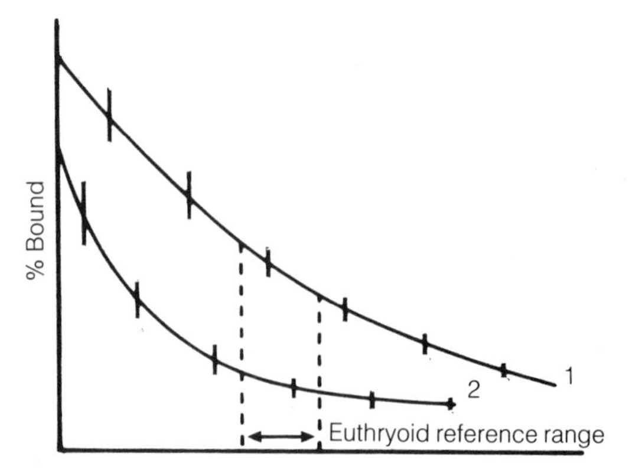

Figure 9.7 Contrasting two RIAs for total T4. RIA 1 is targeted for maximum precision of measurement over the euthyroid reference range, whereas RIA 2 is targeted to measure hypothyroid T4 levels most precisely.

9.7 IMMUNOASSAY DESIGN

Even though there are only three basic reagents required for immunoassays (see previous section), given the availability of two different basic systems (see Table 9.2), a variety of labels (see Table 9.1) and a range of contrasting separation systems (see Table 9.5) there is considerable flexibility in the design of a given immunoassay. The reader is referred to more detailed texts (Ekins, 1975; Thorell and Larson, 1978; Ekins, 1979; Jeffcoate, 1981; Hunter and Corrie, 1983; Butt, 1984; Edwards, 1985) for a thorough understanding, and only a few guidelines can be mentioned here. However, it is important that these points are appreciated, even if one is only trying to select different commercial kits.

Table 9.7 Equipment required for a typical RIA laboratory

Essential for all laboratories
1. Adequate supply of micropipettes dispensing liquid in volumes of 10–1000 μl
2. Suitable assay tubes: note that glass should be avoided due to its variable absorption of radiation from ^{125}I
3. Tube-mixing devices
4. Reliable temperature-controlled centrifuge
5. Gamma counter which is either multi-channel or with automatic sample changer
6. Manual data-processing facilities
7. Deep-freezer for storage of reagents

Essential for laboratories with large throughput (in addition to the above)
1. Automatic sample-processing stations, probably microprocessor driven
2. Multiple tube-mixing devices, e.g. a Multivortex
3. Gamma counter linked to a microprocessor for automated data processing, and cumulative quality control

First, the assay should be targeted on the appropriate range of clinical interest. This is illustrated in Figure 9.7, where it can be seen that within-assay reproducibility of T4 measurement (i.e. within-assay precision) for RIA 2 is optimal at hypothyroid levels, whereas RIA 1 is designed such that precision is better at the more usual clinical decision points, namely the upper and lower ends of the euthyroid reference range. It may be possible to establish both these assays using the same reagents, but combining them at different dilutions and varying assay conditions such as incubation times. The targeting of assays over the appropriate ranges is an important part of assay optimization.

In addition the assay should be designed to give reproducible results both for replicates within an assay and upon repeated assay of a given sample in different assays. Such optimal within- and between-assay precision should usually be accompanied by close agreement with other assays, such that there is not a large bias associated with a given assay. Agreement between different assays of different designs has proved difficult to achieve as is shown by the records of external quality-control schemes (see later). Any such disagreement is not customarily highlighted in commercial promotional literature, but when selecting from a number of kits on offer an important factor to consider is their performance on such quality-control programmes. Assay bias is usually less of a problem for simple structures such as T3 and T4, when the main differences will probably be due to differential behaviour of the standards and samples in assays with contrasting designs and matrices. But for complex structures, such as TSH, which may even exist in multiple forms which differ from each other in their detailed structure, the problem of assay bias may well be greater. Different assays, each employing antibodies which will recognize different epitopes on the hormone, may give different absolute values of hormone measurement. In addition different designs of assay will be subject to different degrees of interference from agents which might cause artefacts in certain patient sera. Examples of the latter are autoantibodies against thyroid hormones and possibly TSH, and abnormal levels of albumin or free fatty acids in some assays for free thyroid hormones (see previously).

9.8 ASSAY CONTROL

Since immunoassays are based upon a simple reaction (see Equation (9.2)), and require only three relatively robust reagents, the view is sometimes expressed that good control of the results must be readily achievable. However, this has not proved to be so in practice, and the maintenance of good assay precision together with minimal changes in absolute values is only possible if samples from well-designed quality-control schemes are included as a matter of routine.

Some potential pitfalls and commonly encountered problems are outlined in Table 9.6. This is by no means an exhaustive account, and it is difficult to generalize on problems and their solution. However, these problems should be continually monitored for by running appropriate quality-control samples, preferably at several positions in an assay.

In its simplest form, quality control requires the repeated running of the same samples in each assay. This is usually organized in three ways.

(a) Internal quality-control samples

A complex internal quality-control scheme is more difficult to apply and there is a tendency for it to be disregarded. As a consequence it is preferable to keep to a simple scheme that can be easily adhered to.

Typically, three internal quality controls should be included in all assays, having 'low', 'medium' and 'high' values. They should be human based, and can generally be obtained commercially. They should be run at least at the beginning and the end of all assays, to check for assay drift (See Table 9.6). New batches of quality-control material should be established with care, the values assigned to them being meaned from multiple assays, and quality-control charts constructed to show both the absolute mean value, and the between-assay variation normally expected.

Since large batches of commercially available quality-control material can be different from the average patient sample – for example the former are often reconstituted after lyophilization – they may not give a totally reliable indication of the performance of the assay. We therefore find it advisable to reassay randomly selected patient samples from previous assays, to check against this eventuality. To do this one has to store the patient samples under the appropriate conditions.

(b) External quality-control samples

When possible, it is essential to participate in external quality-control schemes, whereby samples which are distributed by national or international coordinating laboratories are assayed. This allows comparisons between values obtained not only by different laboratories, but also by different methods and commercially available kits. Such schemes generally reveal that whereas there can be good agreement of absolute values for the analysis of simple structures such as total T4 or T3 (currently a coefficient of variation (CV) of ±10% is achieved in the UK for the measurement of T4), this performance is more difficult to achieve for complex structures such as TSH. Moreover they demonstrate that the assay of free thyroid hormones can be greatly influenced by method-related artefacts. The performance of a given commercial kit in such external quality-control schemes should be an important criterion in its selection for further purchase and use in the laboratory.

(c) On-going records of assay performance

When trying to solve problems such as those

listed in Table 9.6, it is essential to have recourse to a cumulative record of the characteristics of a given assay, both in terms of internal and external quality-control schemes.

Assay characteristics which should also be routinely determined include the binding of the label at the zero hormone concentration (B_0), and the non-specific binding of the label, i.e. that obtained in the absence of the specific antiserum. Degradation of the label is frequently accompanied by a decrease of the B_0 in an RIA, and the increase in non-specific binding. Further information can be obtained by Scatchard analysis (Figure 9.4). Another useful parameter is the concentration of standard hormone required to reduce the B_0 by 50% in an RIA, or give 50% of maximal binding in an IRMA.

The precision of an assay is governed by two components, namely the slope of the response curve and also the error in the response as revealed by the scatter of replicate determinations (ΔR). This is illustrated in Figure 9.8, in which it can be seen that there are two ways in which the original assay can lose precision. Either, as in the case of inferior assay 1, by a decrease in the slope of the response curve, or, as for inferior assay 2, by an increase in the error of response. In practice, the deterioration in the precision of an assay is often due to a subtle combination of these two. Consequently an additional plot, referred to as a precision profile, can be a useful quality-control assessor for a given assay, since it monitors the combined effects of both of these components.

The precision of an assay from a given hormone concentration, e.g. H_1, can either be expressed as ΔH_1, or as a coefficient of variation (CV), when the precision is $(\Delta H_1/H_1)$ expressed as a percentage.

The precision profile (Figure 9.9) is a plot of either form of precision, i.e. ΔH or $(\Delta H/H)$% over the entire range of standard hormone concentration used (H); for Figure 9.8, in order to illustrate the concept of ΔH, only one concentration ($H_1 \pm \Delta H_1$) was shown. The precision profile usually has the form shown in Figure 9.9. It is shown here

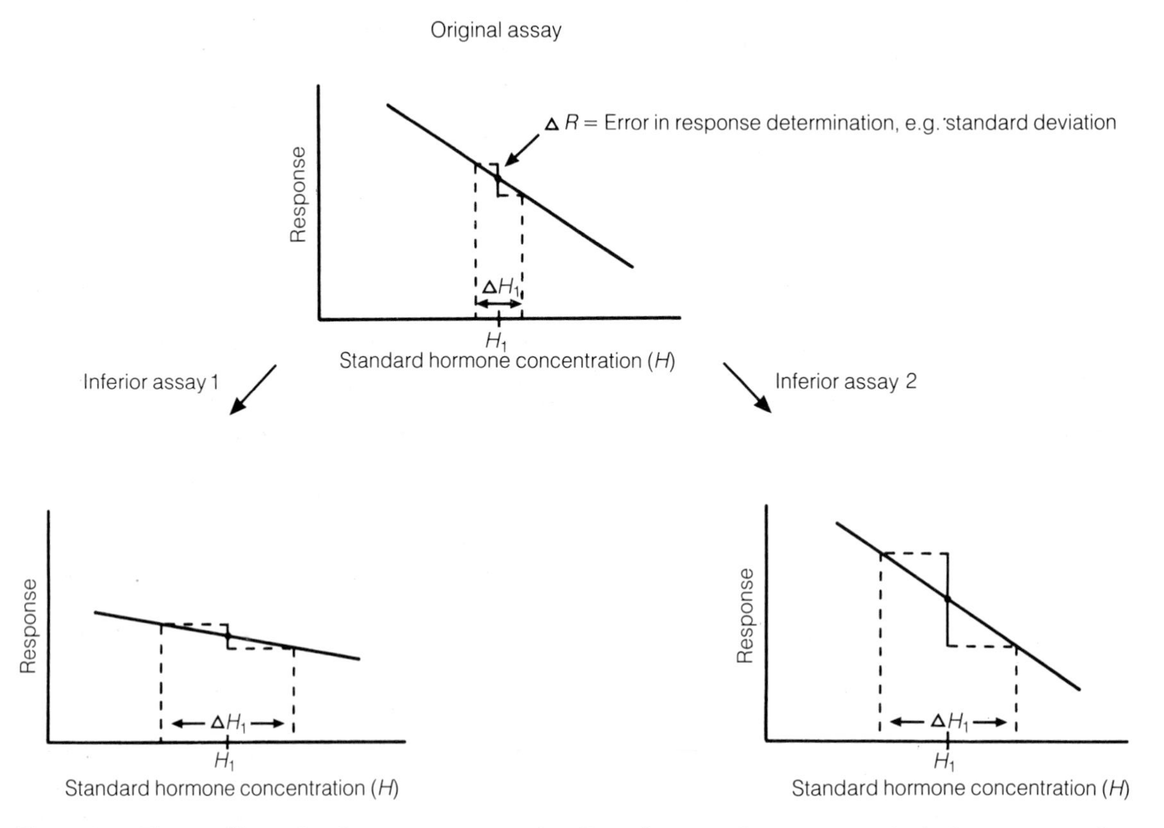

Figure 9.8 Diagram illustrating the two components (gradient of curve and response error) which may account for deterioration of assay precision.

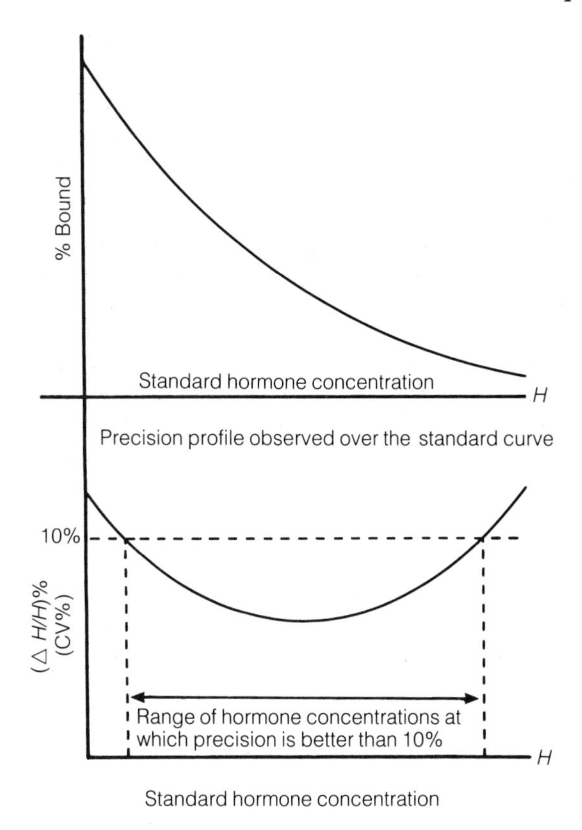

Figure 9.9 Standard curve for an RIA.

for an RIA, but is clearly a useful and valid plot for any assay system. Most immunoassays can be expected to achieve a within-assay precision of better than 10% over their target hormone range. A deterioration in assay performance in terms of within-assay precision would be revealed by an upward shift in the precision profile. Most good immunoassay data-processing programmes should include the automatic determination of the precision profile of an assay.

9.8.1 LABORATORY REQUIREMENTS

The equipment routinely required by an immunoassay laboratory is listed in Table 9.7. At present it remains a relatively labour-intensive area of the clinical chemistry laboratory, since full automation of the processing of the assay tubes has yet to be achieved. Wherever possible, automated equipment should be employed to minimize repetitive tasks which can lead to increased risk of human error. As is shown in Table 9.7, a considerable range of semi-automated devices are now available.

The laboratories should be designed to comply with the local codes of practice for handling radioisotopes, if isotopic labels are used. In typical RIAs isotope usage is usually restricted to a few microcuries; however, for IRMAs larger quantities may be required. If iodinations are to be carried out, millicurie amounts of ^{125}I will be handled, and it is essential to ensure that the 'hot-lab' used is of the standard required and in particular that adequate fume exhaust cabinets are provided, due to the volatility of iodine.

9.9 CLINICAL APPLICATIONS OF THYROID HORMONE ASSAYS

9.9.1 TSH

(a) Introduction

The fast, specific and highly sensitive IRMA assays for TSH have expanded the clinical use of TSH measurement in thyroid disease (Seth and Beckett, 1985). It has become routine laboratory practice to run TSH assays with detection limits of 0.2 mu/l or lower. RIAs used previously were generally about tenfold less sensitive. The major advantage of these more sensitive IRMAs is that it is now possible to separate out the population of presenting hyperthyroid as well as hypothyroid patients by TSH assay alone.

The TRH test, however, is still of value both in the diagnosis of hyperthyroidism, especially in sick patients (see later), and also in the diagnosis of pituitary and hypothalamic disease. Blood is taken for TSH before and 20 and 60 min after a bolus intravenous injection of 200 μg of TRH. The normal response is a TSH rise to a maximum at around 20 min (Ormston *et al.*, 1971).

(b) TSH in hypothyroidism

(i) Adults A basal TSH is clinically the most useful test to confirm primary hypothyroidism. Levels may vary from 40 to >60 mu/l and no particular level is diagnostic. The upper limit of normal TSH values is probably between 2 and 5 mu/l.

When thyroxine levels are within the normal reference range but TSH values are greater than 5 mu/l subclinical hypothyroidism should be suspected. Controversy still exists as to whether this condition should be treated with thyroxine, or whether these patients should be observed and allowed to become hypothyroid before therapy (Lancet, 1986; Pearce and Himsworth, 1984; Tibald and Barzel, 1985).

Replacement therapy with thyroxine can also be monitored easily using a single TSH assay. Opinions differ as to whether full suppression, i.e. undetectable, or suppression into the normal range (0.5–5 mu/l) should be aimed for (Pearce and Himsworth, 1984; Jennings *et al.*, 1984). Full suppression of TSH can usually only be achieved by allowing the free T4 to rise to the upper end of the normal range using thyroxine therapy. This may not be suitable for patients with cardiac conditions such as angina.

(ii) Neonatal hypothyroidism Because of the high incidence of neonatal hypothyroidism (one in 3000–6900 births) and the ease of diagnosis it is routine practice for blood spot TSH measurements to be made within the first week of life. At birth there is a fetal TSH surge which tails off over the second and third weeks, but a TSH of greater than 100 mu/l is highly suggestive of neonatal hypothyroidism. The TSH assay will fail to pick up hypothyroidism which is secondary to hypothalamic or pituitary disease but this only occurs in 3–5% of hypothyroid neonates (Delange *et al.*, 1979) and usually other signs of hypopituitarism are also present.

(iii) Hypothalamic pituitary function Even with the new IRMA TSH assay, a single baseline TSH is less useful for the estimation of hypothalamic pituitary function than a TRH test. An absent TSH response with undetectable levels after TRH is seen in:

1. Hyperthyroidism of all types except for the very rare cases which are due to excess TSH production;
2. Some euthyroid patients, in whom thyroid-stimulating antibodies are still active, who may have had Graves' disease previously; for further discussion of thyroid stimulating antibodies, see later;
3. Euthyroid patients with ophthalmic Graves' disease;
4. Euthyroid patients with Plummer's disease or toxic nodular goitre who are in the pre-toxic phase in which thyroid autonomy has been sufficient to suppress TSH but not quite sufficient to produce hyperthyroidism;
5. Patients with anterior pituitary failure.

An abnormal response is seen in patients with:

1. Hypothyroidism in which an excessive rise at 20 min is seen with a relative fall remaining above normal at 60 minutes;
2. Hypothalamic disease in which a peak level is reached only after 60 min and even then is usually below the peak value normally seen at 20 min.

Therefore a TRH test is useful to detect patients with subclinical hypothyroidism, pituitary and hypothalamic hypothyroidism and in certain doubtful cases for the determination of hyperthyroidism. A normal response excludes primary hyperthyroidism.

There is no indication for TRH testing in patients requiring thyroxine therapy since a basal TSH value will give adequate evidence of pituitary TSH suppression.

9.9.2 TRIIODOTHYRONINE AND THYROXINE

(a) Introduction

The main advance in thyroid hormone measurements has been the increasing use of the measurement of free hormones. It has now become clear that it is the small percentage of free hormones (0.3% for T3 and 0.03% for T4) which is the active moiety in thyroid hormone action. Measurements of total T3 or T4 are both subject to significant variation in plasma levels in those clinical conditions which result in changes in concentrations of binding proteins, particularly thyroxine-binding globulin (TBG) and thyroxine-binding prealbumin (PA). Consequently the measurement of the free hormones is likely to be a more direct reflection of thyroid hormone sufficiency.

Because serum T4 is 99.97% bound to the circulating transport proteins, any elevation of TBG can result in high levels of total T4 which do not necessary reflect the concentration of free hormones. This occurs in pregnancy, some patients with chronic hepatic disease or nephrotic syndrome and patients taking oral oestrogens. Other drugs can displace T4 from the binding proteins by competitive binding, e.g. diphenyl hydantoin on TBG and salicylates on PA. In general compounds and situations causing changes in TBG concentrations or its hormone binding capacity are associated with parallel alteration in total T4 and T3 while the free hormone levels remain normal. However, one exception to this may be the third trimester of pregnancy. Using several different free hormone assay systems, both free T3 and T4 are found to fall by the third trimester, and in some patients they may decrease to beneath the normal reference range. Due to the importance of thyroid sufficiency on fetal development a TSH estimation should be made a priority in this situation. For a fuller discussion of problems in the interpretation of results from assays for free thyroid hormones, particularly in unusual clinical circumstances, the reader is referred to the review article by Pearce and Byfield, 1986.

(b) Thyroid hormones in hypothyroidism

T4 is the first hormone to fall in primary hypothyroidism. It is unusual for T3 to fall out of the normal range before T4, and T3 is recognized as a poor discriminator of hypothyroidism.

Low free or total thyroid hormones, particularly T3, in a patient without other signs of hypothyroidism or a raised TSH is, however, a frequent finding in a wide variety of systemic illnesses. In such patients with non-thyroid illness, this condition is referred to as the 'sick' euthyroid syndrome. Although the thyroid hormones are low there is a normal TSH response to TRH. This can be interpreted to indicate a euthyroid state with adaptation to illness, rather than tissue hypothyroidism. Although not routinely performed, an assay for the alternative deiodination product of T4, namely rT3, would probably reveal raised levels. rT3 is apparently bioinactive, and its full significance is not understood. The cause of this syndrome is unknown and it is in particular not known whether this is a compensatory mechanism to protect the body in time of illness or is a toxic effect of illness on the hypothalamic pituitary thyroid axis (Utiger, 1980; Wehman *et al.*, 1985).

In most instances the finding of low thyroid hormones indicates primary hypothyroidism which can be confirmed with a TSH assay, which if raised will exclude the 'sick' euthyroid syndrome.

(c) Thyroid hormones in hyperthyroidism

In hyperthyroidism the thyroid gland synthesizes and secretes increased amounts of both T4 and T3. Usually it is the T3 which rises first. In a few patients, T3 alone can be persistently elevated ('T3-toxicosis'), but this condition is rare and usually associated with nodular goitre as opposed to Graves' disease.

Elevated T4 and T3 levels are therefore sensitive indicators of hyperthyroidism in the majority of patients. Confirmation should be sought, however, with a sensitive TSH assay which should show full suppression of TSH. If thyroid hormone levels are within the upper range of normal, but hyperthyroidism is nevertheless suspected, then an intravenous TRH test is probably the best discriminator between hyperthyroidism (full suppression) and the euthyroid state. Such a situation could arise, for example, with the combination of the 'sick' euthyroid state in an ill patient with concomitant hyperthyroidism. In addition, there appears to be a small but significant group of asymptomatic patients with subclinical hyperthyroidism.

Thyroid hormones will also need to be monitored during antithyroid drug therapy. After the thyroid hormones have fallen into the normal range for a period, a delayed rise in TSH from its suppressed levels will then be observed. More frequent monitoring of thyroid function is necessary for patients receiving graduated doses of antithyroid medication than for those receiving the 'block-replace regime' of full antithyroid drug therapy and simultaneous thyroid hormone replacement.

(d) Thyroxine-binding globulin (TBG)

As discussed previously (Section 9.2), the routine measurement of TBG as a secondary test to 'adjust' the total thyroid hormone levels indirectly by relating them to the TBG value has now become obsolete. This is due to the development of convenient free hormone assays. The use of TBG assays is now largely confined to confirming the diagnosis of congenital TBG deficiency, and for investigating abnormal thyroid function tests which result from changes in TBG concentrations. TBG estimation is also used for evidence of remaining thyroid follicular activity after ablation of the thyroid for carcinoma.

9.9.3 THYROID AUTOANTIBODIES

(a) Antimicrosomal and antithyroglobulin antibodies

Roitt *et al.* (1956) first described autoantibodies to the different components of the thyroid cell. These antibodies are detectable in about 10% of the normal population and their frequency is greater in females and increases with age. They are good autoimmune markers which contribute additional evidence as to the cause of thyroid dysfunction. Antimicrosomal and antithyroglobulin antibodies are positive in high titres in Hashimoto's thyroiditis. In Graves' disease about 80% of patients are antimicrosomal antibody positive, but at lower titres, and 30% have antithyroglobulin antibodies. In multinodular goitre without other superimposed thyroid disease, the frequency is no different from the normal population.

More recently antimicrosomal antibodies have been shown to be a marker of continuing thyroid dysfunction in patients who develop transient hypothyroidism and hyperthyroidism postpartum (Amino, 1983).

(b) Anti-TSH receptor antibodies

Autoantibodies which bind to the TSH receptor on the surface of thyroid follicular cells are well recognized. They can be tested for by radioreceptor assays (Southgate *et al.*, 1984). These are based upon the RIA system depicted in Figure 9.3, but in which the binding reagent is a preparation of TSH receptors, as opposed to the anti-TSH antibody. The TSH receptors are incubated with the test serum containing the autoantibodies, or an IgG preparation from this serum, together with ^{125}I-labelled TSH. The presence of the anti-TSH receptor antibody is detected by the decreased binding of ^{125}I-labelled TSH to its receptor. Usually about 90% of patients with untreated Graves' disease inhibit the ^{125}I-labelled TSH binding, and this is interpreted by many to indicate the presence of thyroid-stimulating antibodies. However, although this assay is attractively convenient to run, it cannot distinguish between antibodies which block the TSH receptor and those which interact with the receptor and subsequently activate the follicular cell. Moreover, there is not necessarily a direct relationship between the ability of stimulating antibody to inhibit TSH binding to its receptor, and its potency as a stimulator.

Thyroid-stimulating antibodies can, however, be measured by bioassays. Originally, stimulating antibodies were detected by *in vivo* bioassays, and were referred to as long-acting thyroid stimulators (LATS). A number of alternative *in vitro* assay systems have been developed, which are more convenient, sensitive and precise. The most recent rely upon stimulation of thyroid cell lines which can be maintained as stable TSH-responsive cells in culture indefinitely, and thereby provide reliable and rugged assays for thyroid-stimulating antibodies (Marshall and Ealey, 1986; Whitley *et al.*, 1987). These systems can also be adapted to measure 'thyroid growth-stimulating antibodies' and 'TSH-blocking antibodies'. Drexhage and coworkers have suggested that these may form part of a 'spectrum' of anti-TSH receptor autoantibodies (Drexhage and van der Gaag, 1986). At present, however, these bioassays are restricted to specialized laboratories and do not currently form part of a routine thyroid diagnostic service.

One of the major clinical uses of the measurement of thyroid-stimulating antibodies is for the pregnant patient with a personal or family history of thyroid disease, particularly Graves' disease, or other organ-specific autoimmune disease. This is because thyroid-stimulating antibodies may cross the placenta (Munro *et al.*, 1978). Intrauterine hyperthyroidism and transient neonatal hyperthyroidism can both occur due to transplacental passage of this autoantibody. It is therefore important that if the stimulator is present the fetal heart should be monitored, especially in the latter part of pregnancy, and the neonate should be carefully observed for post-partum symptoms of hyperthyroidism. Thyroid-stimulating antibodies may persist in patients after effective treatment for Graves' disease. In addition they may be present after hypothyroidism, either autoimmune or induced, e.g. by radioactive iodine, which has been treated by thyroxine replacement.

REFERENCES

Albertini, A. and Ekins, R. P. (eds) 1982) *Free Hormones in Blood*, Elsevier, Amsterdam.

Amino, N. (1983) in *Autoimmune Endocrine Disease* (ed. T. F. Davies), Wiley, New York, pp. 242–72.

Bolton, A. E. (1977) *Radioiodination Techniques*, Review 18, Radiochemical Centre, Amersham, UK.

Bolton, A. E. (1981) in *Immunoassays for the 80's* (eds A. Voller, A. Bartlett and D. Bidwell), MTP Press, Lancaster, Ch. 6, pp. 69–83.

Buehler, R. J. (1982) in *Free Hormones in Blood* (eds A. Albertini and R. P. Ekins), Elsevier, Amsterdam, pp. 91–99.

Butt, W. R. (ed.) (1984) *Practical Immunoassay: The State of the art* (Clinical and Biochemical Analysis, Vol. 14), (ed. W. R. Butt).

Delange, F., Beckers, C., Hofer, R. *et al.* (1979) Neonatal screening for congenital hypothyroidism in Europe:

report of the Newborn Committee of the ETA. *Acta Endocrinol. (Copenh.)* **90** (Suppl. 223).

Drexhage, H. A. and van der Gaag, R. D. (1986) in *Immunology of Endocrine Diseases* (ed. A. M. McGregor), MTP Press, Lancaster, pp. 51–72.

Edwards, R. (1985) *Immunoassay: An Introduction*, Heinemann, London.

Ekins, R. P. (1975) in *Clinical Biochemistry* (ed. C. H. Pasternak), Heyden, London, pp. 4–13.

Ekins, R. P. (1979) in *Radioimmunoassay and Saturation Analysis*, *Br. Med. J. Bull.*, **30**, 3–20.

Ekins, R. P. (1984) in *Practical Immunoassay: The State of the Art* (Clinical and Biochemical Analysis, Vol. **14**), (ed. W. R. Butt), pp. 217–51.

Ekins, R. P., Filetti, S., Kurtz, A. B. and Dwyer, K. (1980) A simple general method for the assay of free hormones (and drugs); its application to the measurement of serum free thyroxine levels and the bearing of assay results on the 'free thyroxine' concept. *J. Endocrinol.*, **85**, 29.

Ellis, S. and Ekins, R. P. (1973) Direct measurement by radioimmunoassay of the free hormone concentration in serum. *Acta Endocrinol. (Copenh.)*, Suppl. 177: 106–10.

Hunter, W. M. and Corrie, J. E. T. (eds) (1983) *Immunoassays for Clinical Chemistry*, 2nd edn, Churchill Livingstone, Edinburgh.

Jeffcoate, S. L. (1981) *Efficiency and Effectivenes in the Endocrine Laboratory*, Academic Press, London.

Jennings, P. E., O'Malley, B. P., Griffin, K. E. *et al.* (1984) Relevance of increased serum thyroxine concentrations associated with normal serum triiodothyronine values in hypothyroid patients receiving thyroxine: a case for 'tissue thyrotoxicosis'. *Br. Med. J.*, **289**, 1645–7.

Lancet (1986) Subclinical hypothyroidism: conflict (editorial). *Lancet*, **i**, 251–2.

Marshall, N. J. and Ealey, P. A. (1986) in *Immunology of Endocrine Diseases* (ed A. M. McGregor), MTP Press, Lancaster, pp. 25–50.

Midgley, J. E. M. and Wilkins, T. A. (1981) The direct estimation of free hormones by a simple equilibrium radioimmunoassay. Technical literature, Amersham International, Amersham, UK.

Midgley, J. E. M. and Wilkins, T. A. (1982a) An improved method for the estimation of relative binding constants of T4 and its analogues with serum proteins, *Clin. Endocrinol.*, **17**, 523–8.

Midgley, J. E. M. and Wilkins, T. A. (1982b) A defense of the Amerlex free thyroxine kit. *Clin. Chem.*, **28**, 2183–4.

Miles, L. E. M. and Hales, C. N. (1968a) The preparation and properties of purified ^{125}I-labelled antibodies to insulin. *Biochem. J.*, **108**, 611–15.

Miles, L. E. M. and Hales, C. N. (1968b) Labelled antibodies and immunological assay systems, *Nature*, **219**, 186–7.

Munro, D. S., Dirmikis, S. M., Humphries, H. and Smith, T. (1978) The role of thyroid stimulating immunoglobulins of Graves' disease in neonatal thyrotoxicosis, *Br. J. Obstet. Gynaecol.*, **85**, 837–42.

Odstrchel, G. (1982) in *Free Hormones in Blood* (eds A. Albertini and R. P. Ekins), Elsevier, Amsterdam, pp. 91–9.

Ormston, B. J., Garry, R., Cryer, R. J. *et al.* (1971) Thyrotrophin-releasing hormone as a thyroid function test. *Lancet*, **ii**, 3–4.

Pearce, C. J. and Byfield, P. G. H. (1986) Free thyroid hormone assays and thyroid function: review article. *Ann. Clin. Biochem.*, **23**, 230–7.

Pearce, C. J. and Himsworth, R. L. (1984) Total and free thyroid hormone concentrations in patients receiving maintenance replacement treatment with thyroxine. *Br. Med. J.*, **288**, 693–5.

Roitt, I. M., Doniach, D., Campbell, P. N. and Hudson, R. V. (1956) Autoantibodies in Hashimoto's disease. *Lancet*, **ii**, 820–1.

Romelli, P. B., Pennisi, F. and Vancheri, L. (1979) Measurement of free thyroid hormones in serum by column adsorption chromatography and radioimmunoassay. *J. Endocrinol. Invest.*, **2**, 25–32.

Seth, J. and Beckett, G. (1985) Diagnosis of hyperthyroidism: the newer biochemical tests. *Clin. Endocrinol. Metab.*, **14**, 373–96.

Southgate, K., Creagh, F., Teece, M. *et al.* (1984) A receptor assay for the measurement of TSH receptor antibodies in unextracted serum. *Clin. Endocrinol.*, **20**, 539–43.

Thorell, J. I. and Larson, S. M. (1978) *Radioimmunoassay and Related Techniques: Methodology and Clinical Applications*, Mosby, St Louis.

Tibald, J. and Barzell, U. S. (1985) Thyroxine supplementation: method for the prevention of clinical hypothyroidism. *Am. J. Med.*, **79**, 241–4.

Utiger. R. D. (1980) Decreased extrathyroidal triiodothyronine production in nonthyroidal illness: benefit or harm? *Am. J. Med.*, **69**, 807–81.

Voller, A., Bartlett, A. and Bidwell, D. (eds) (1981) *Immunoassays for the 80s*, MTP Press, Lancaster.

Wehmann, R. E., Gregerman, R. I., Burns, W. H. *et al.* (1985) Suppression thyrotrophin in the low-thyroxine state of severe non thyroidal illness. *N. Engl. J. Med.*, **312**, 546–52.

Whitley, G., Nussey, S. S. and Johnstone, A. P. (1987) SGHTL-34, a thyrotrophin responsive immortalised human thyroid cell line generated by transfection. *Mol. Cell. Endocrinol.*, **52**, 279–84.

CHAPTER TEN

Parathyroid scanning

A. J. Coakley and C. P. Wells

10.1 INTRODUCTION

The parathyroid glands are endocrine glands which produce parathormone (PTH), a hormone essential for the control of calcium metabolism. Clinical parathyroid disease occurs as a result of over-production or under-production of PTH, or from parathyroid cancer which may also result in hyperparathyroidism.

There is no pharmacological treatment for hyperparathyroidism, active treatment being surgical by the removal of the hyperfunctioning gland(s). There is debate as to whether all patients with hyperparathyroidism need surgery, particularly as the increased use of biochemical profiles is identifying more patients with asymptomatic disease. When surgery is undertaken a skilled parathyroid surgeon will cure over 90% of patients. Surgery in less skilled hands produces inferior results and there is an increased risk of morbidity and a lower chance of establishing normocalcaemia at subsequent re-operation.

In order to help the correct localization of abnormal parathyroid glands a number of diagnostic techniques have been employed. The potential of nuclear medicine in identifying hyperfunctioning tissue has been recognized for many years, but only recently has a radionuclide technique been established which appears sufficiently reliable to be widely adopted. The aim of this chapter is to give a brief account of the anatomy and pathophysiology of hyperparathyroidism, of radionuclides which have been used to localize abnormal glands, and of the place of localizing procedures in general in the management of hyperparathyroidism.

10.2 CLINICAL ASPECTS

10.2.1 ANATOMY

There are usually two pairs of parathyroid glands. The upper pair are normally found in close proximity to the dorsal side of the thyroid gland (or occasionally embedded in it), cephalic to the point where the recurrent laryngeal nerve crosses the inferior thyroid artery. The lower parathyroids are usually found at the lower pole of the thyroid, lateral to the trachea. The average total weight is 120–140 mg for the four glands.

More than four glands occur in 6% of normal individuals, probably arising as a result of division of one or more of the main glands during development. The lower glands develop, together with the thymus, from the third branchial pouch. They migrate caudally with the thymus and then separate, finishing in their usual position at the lower poles of the thyroid. Variation in the migration accounts for the wide range of locations of ectopic glands, these being found in the thymus, carotid sheath, pharyngeal submucosa and anterior mediastinum. The upper parathyroids are formed in the fourth branchial pouch but show little migration during development. Ectopic locations include the tracheo-oesophageal groove and retro-oesophageal space.

10.2.2 PHYSIOLOGY

The parathyroid glands secrete PTH which raises the level of ionized calcium in the blood by increasing calcium release from bone, promoting calcium reabsorption from the renal tubules and by increasing renal synthesis of 1,25-dihydroxycholecalciferol. Under normal conditions, increase in serum ionic calcium results in reduced PTH production, and falling levels stimulate PTH production.

10.2.3 HYPERPARATHYROIDISM

(a) Primary hyperparathyroidism

This occurs when there is endogenous hypersecretion of PTH. This may be due to:

1. Parathyroid adenoma – over 80% of cases are caused by a solitary parathyroid adenoma;
2. Hyperplasia of more than one gland, commonly all four glands being involved. This occurs in 10–15% of primary cases;
3. Carcinoma, occurring in 3–4% of cases.

(b) Secondary hyperparathyroidism

This is defined as a state of compensatory hypersecretion of PTH in any clinical condition in which there is a tendency to hypocalcaemia. The most common association is with chronic renal failure, but the condition has been described with rickets and osteomalacia, malabsorption syndrome and renal tubular disorders (Aurbach *et al.*, 1981). As a result of long-standing secondary hyperparathyroidism some glands may develop autonomous function, and correction of the underlying cause (e.g. by renal transplantation) may still leave the patient with hyperparathyroidism. This is called tertiary hyperparathyroidism, although there remains debate about the frequency and pathophysiology of this condition.

10.2.4 CLINICAL FEATURES OF HYPERPARATHYROIDISM

The most common presenting features are associated with calcium deposition in the urological tract, particularly renal stones. A wide variety of other presentations can be seen, including bone disease, gastrointestinal symptoms, thirst and polyuria, psychiatric presentations, myopathy or arthropathy. There is an association with hypertension and occasionally hyperparathyroidism may be part of multiple endocrine abnormalities. The more widespread use of automated biochemical profiles has resulted in increased recognition of asymptomatic cases.

10.2.5 DIAGNOSIS

Diagnosis of the condition is by exclusion of other causes of hypercalcaemia, e.g. malignancy, sarcoidosis, myelomatosis, and by the confirmation of persistent hypercalcaemia with inappropriate elevation of serum PTH (PTH is suppressed in other causes of hypercalcaemia). Radiological and bone scan changes are present in some cases (McAfee, 1987).

10.2.6 MANAGEMENT

Hyperparathyroidism can be corrected by surgical removal of the abnormal gland(s). There remains debate over which patients to select for surgery (van't Hoff *et al.*, 1983). Most endocrinologists advocate surgery for symptomatic patients and asymptomatic ones with high calcium levels, and in younger patients. Conservative management is practised in asymptomatic patients with milder disease or when there are contraindications to surgery, e.g. age, cardiopulmonary disease.

10.3 RADIONUCLIDE LOCALIZING TECHNIQUES

10.3.1 HISTORY

^{57}Co-labelled vitamin B12 is concentrated in the parathyroids (Beierwaltes *et al.*, 1964) but early attempts at imaging with this agent were unsuccessful. Potchen (1963) demonstrated that methionine is selectively concentrated in the parathyroids and ^{75}Se-selenomethionine has been used with varying degrees of success (Beierwaltes *et al.*, 1964; Potchen *et al.*, 1965; Bartelheimer *et al.*, 1965; Quinn, 1966; Di Giulio and Morales, 1966; McGeown *et al.*, 1968). Improved results were reported with ^{75}Se scanning when combined with a thyroid subtraction technique using iodine or pertechnetate (Ell *et al.*, 1975; Robinson, 1982). Many have found this technique unsatisfactory (Waldorf *et al.*, 1984) and it is now rarely used.

Cann and Prussin (1980) reported on the use of ^{67}Ga, ^{46}Sc and ^{177}Lu for localizing hyperactive parathyroid tissue. Used in rats ^{67}Ga showed much higher uptakes than selenomethionine and the data suggested that it may be useful in specific cases. However, Iwase *et al.* (1986) reported negative uptake of ^{67}Ga in nine patients with parathyroid adenomas and positive uptake in one patient with parathyroid carcinoma. Zwas *et al.*

(1981) reported some success using ^{131}I-labelled toluidine blue. Ferlin and coworkers (1981a) studied parathyroids using ^{131}Cs and ^{201}Tl. They concluded that ^{201}Tl would be of use if it was developed into a dual tracer technique using image subtraction. They presented their results with ^{201}Tl/^{99m}Tc at the Fifth Congress of the European Nuclear Medicine Society at Pisa (Ferlin *et al.*, 1981b). Young (1983) confirmed the value of the technique and this method is now the most widely adopted radionuclide procedure and is described in detail below.

10.3.2 CURRENT SCANNING TECHNIQUES

The ^{201}Tl/^{99m}Tc imaging method relies on the fact that thallium is taken up by the thyroid and by hyperactive parathyroid tissue whereas pertechnetate is taken up by the thyroid. Abnormal parathyroid tissue can be demonstrated by scanning with both radiopharmaceuticals and by subtracting the pertechnetate image from the thallium image using a gamma camera with an on-line computer.

There has been much debate about whether ^{201}Tl-thallous chloride or ^{99m}Tc-pertechnetate should be administered first (Fogelman *et al.*, 1984). From the physical properties of the radionuclides it can be seen (Figure 10.1) that ^{201}Tl should be given first as it produces the lower energy emissions, thus avoiding the problem of ^{99m}Tc emissions scattered in the patient and camera crystal into the ^{201}Tl energy window. However, from the biokinetics of the two radiopharmaceuticals (Figure 10.2) it can be seen that peak uptake of the tracers are at 4 min (Wells *et al.*, 1983) and 22 min (MIRD, 1976) for the ^{201}Tl and ^{99m}Tc respectively. To image at or around the time of peak uptake these data would point to the administration of the ^{99m}Tc first, which gives the added benefit of being able to see the thyroid outline when positioning the patient.

Despite these differing points of view there has been no discernible difference in the diagnostic sensitivity of the two techniques. Some centres image after injecting both radiopharmaceuticals together (Percival *et al.*, 1985a).

There are several theoretical advantages in using a converging collimator as it produces less distortion and higher sensitivity than pinhole collimators and can normally image a larger anatomical area of the patient. However, no reduction in diagnostic sensitivity has been shown by centres using pinhole collimators.

Particular attention must be paid to reducing patient movement during the procedure. Careful

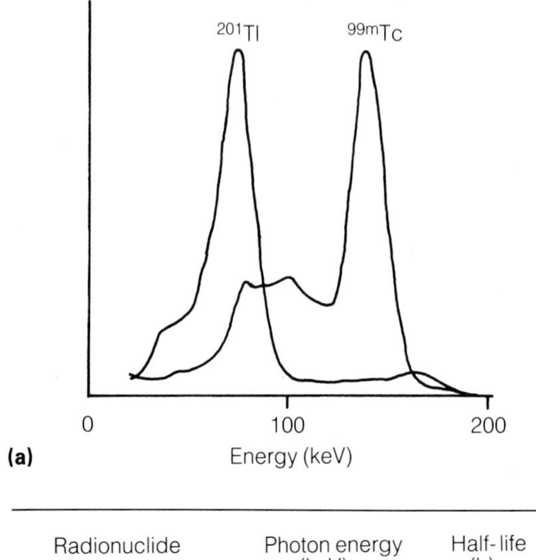

Radionuclide	Photon energy (keV)	Half-life (h)
^{201}Tl	69–83 (Gh K X-rays)	73.1
^{99m}Tc	142	6.0

(b)

Figure 10.1 (a) Spectra and (b) physical data for ^{201}Tl and ^{99m}Tc. (Spectra obtained using sources in a neck phantom.)

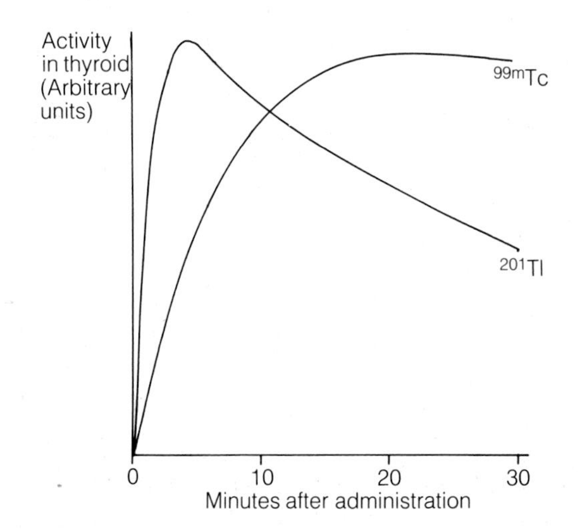

Figure 10.2 Uptake and clearance curves for ^{201}Tl and ^{99m}Tc in the thyroid: ^{201}Tl curve, own data (Wells *et al.*, 1983); ^{99m}Tc curve from MIRD data (MIRD, 1976).

explanation should be given to the patient prior to the test, which should be carried out in a quiet room on a comfortable imaging trolley. Head moulds or restraints are often useful.

Because of the wide variation in protocols used we include the procedure commonly used in our department.

1. Administer 75 MBq ^{99m}Tc-sodium pertechnetate intravenously. Wait 20 min.
2. Position patient under the camera with the neck extended and the thyroid towards the top of the field of view. The upper mediastinum must be in the field of view (most ectopics are inferiorly displaced).
3. Acquire one 5 min image in ^{99m}Tc window 64 × 64 static matrix.
4. Acquire one 5 min image in ^{201}Tl window 64 × 64 static matrix (scatter image). Administer 75 MBq ^{201}Tl-thallous chloride intravenously. Acquire in ^{201}Tl window 10 × 2 min 64 × 64 dynamic images.

10.3.3 PROCESSING

Prior to processing the images it is essential to ensure that the patient has not moved between pertechnetate and thallium imaging by examining the alignment of the thyroid outline in the two sets of images. If movement is apparent then it may be possible to re-align the images to match the thyroid outlines using standard computer software.

Figure 10.3 shows an example of the early thallium images. It can be seen that during the first frame (0–2 min) there is a blush of activity in the region of the subclavian vein and carotid artery on the injection side. This is a potential source of a false-positive result and therefore the first frame should be discarded prior to subtraction and the second frame inspected for any residual venous activity.

The first stage is to inspect the ^{99m}Tc and the summed, scatter-corrected ^{201}Tl images. In many cases the site of an adenoma is obvious (Figure 10.4) and a subtraction technique not essential (Winzelberg and Hydovitz, 1985). In the subtraction technique a series of images is usually produced with varying weighted proportions of the technetium image being subtracted from the thallium image. The weighting factors may vary widely, particularly in cases where iodine skin preparations or other agents are used which block uptake of the pertechnetate by the thyroid gland. A series of subtraction images are shown in Figure 10.5. The parathyroid gland can be seen both with thyroid uptake present (i.e. under-subtraction) and with a negative thyroid outline. After subtraction, if residual localized thallium uptake is present when the thyroid outline has just been eliminated then this is strongly suggestive of

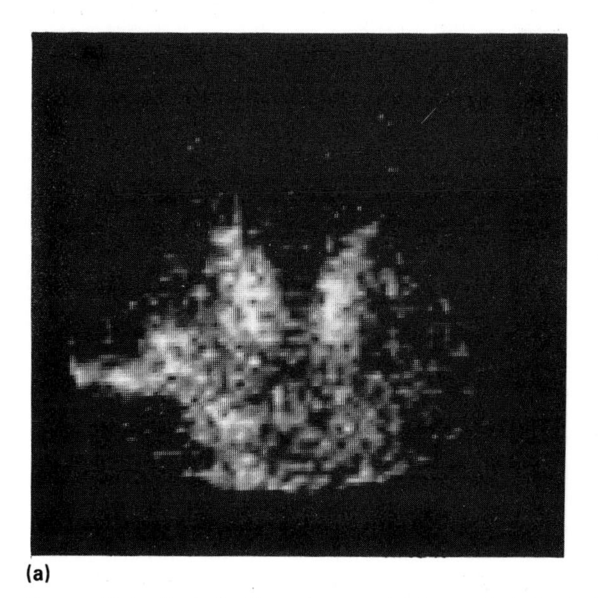
(a)

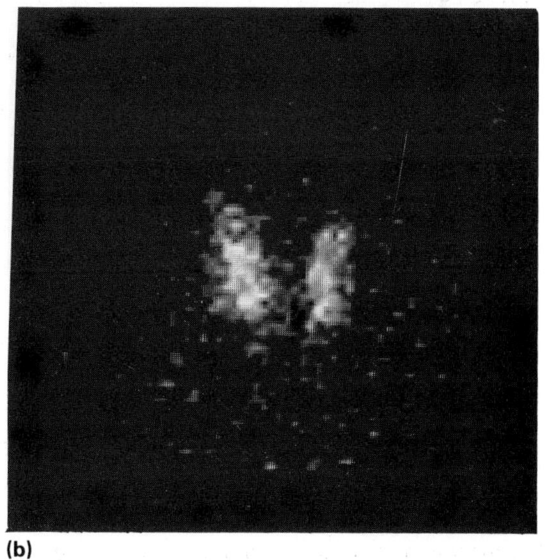
(b)

Figure 10.3 Early thallium images. (a) Frame 1: 0–2 min following ^{201}Tl injection. (b) Frame 2: 2–4 min following ^{201}Tl injection.

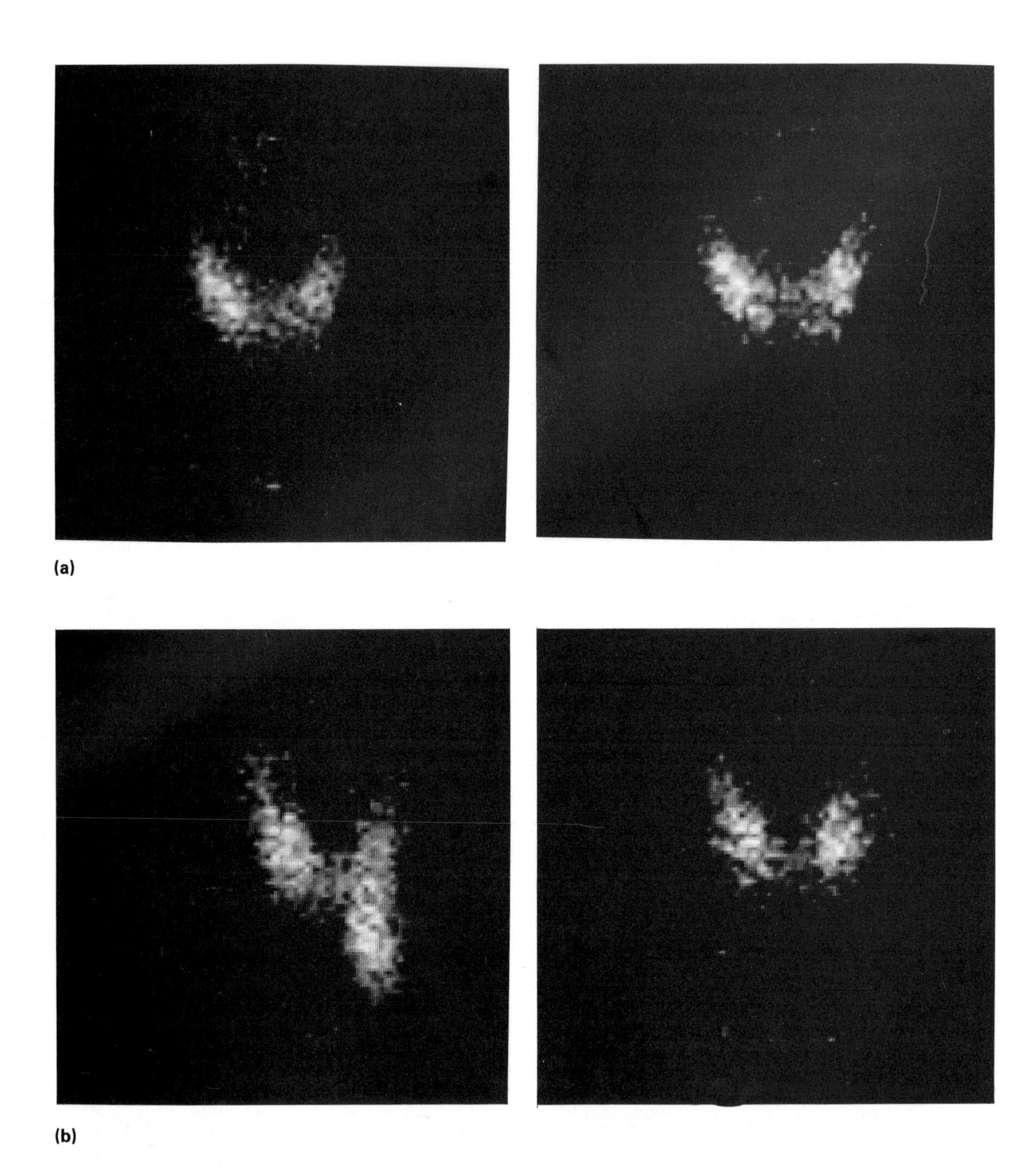

Figure 10.4 (a) Normal scan: ^{201}Tl and ^{99m}Tc images. (b) Adenoma: ^{201}Tl and ^{99m}Tc images.

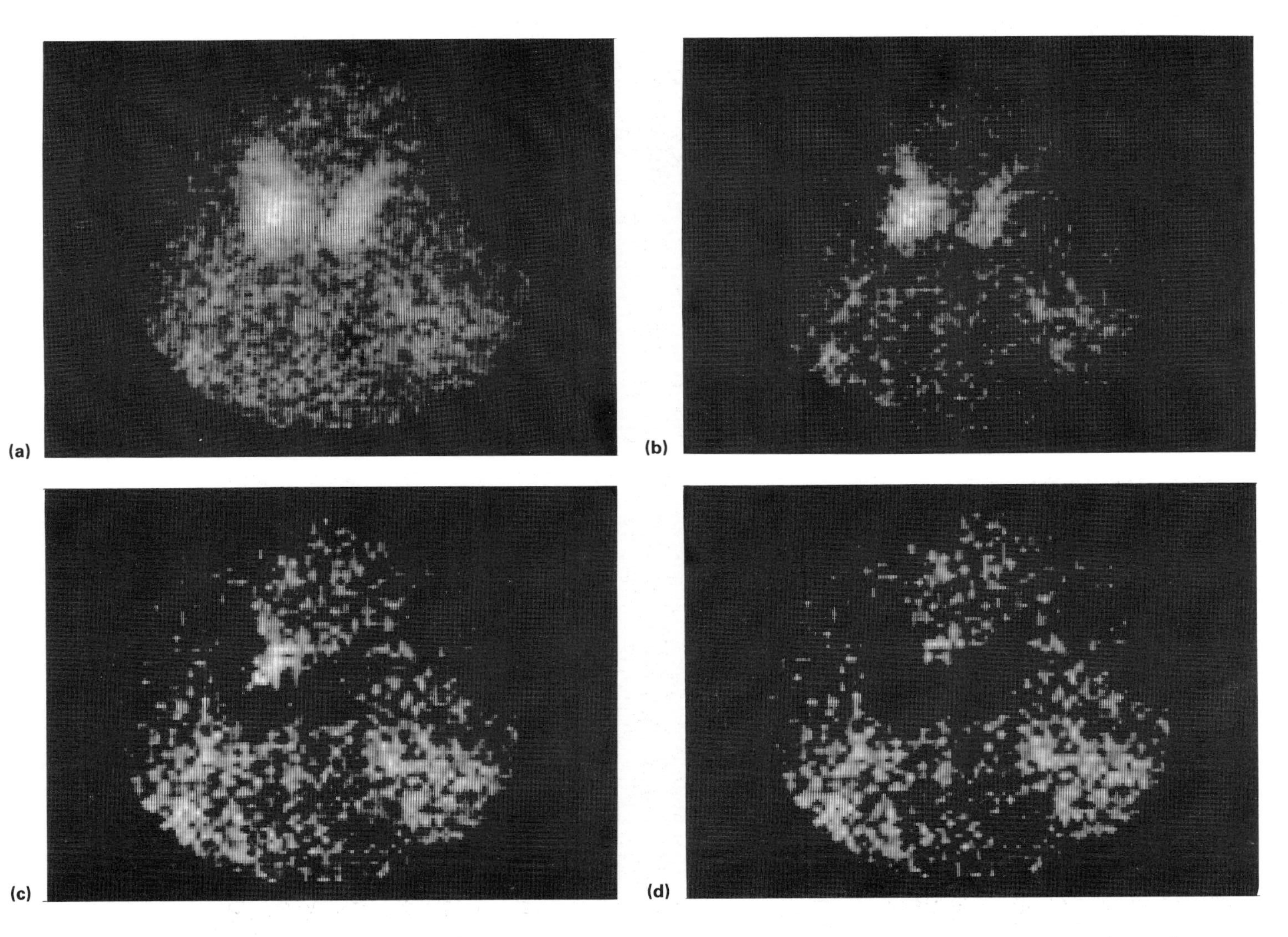

Figure 10.5 Subtraction images: (a) unsubtracted; (b) under-subtracted; (c) correct subtraction; (d) over-subtracted.

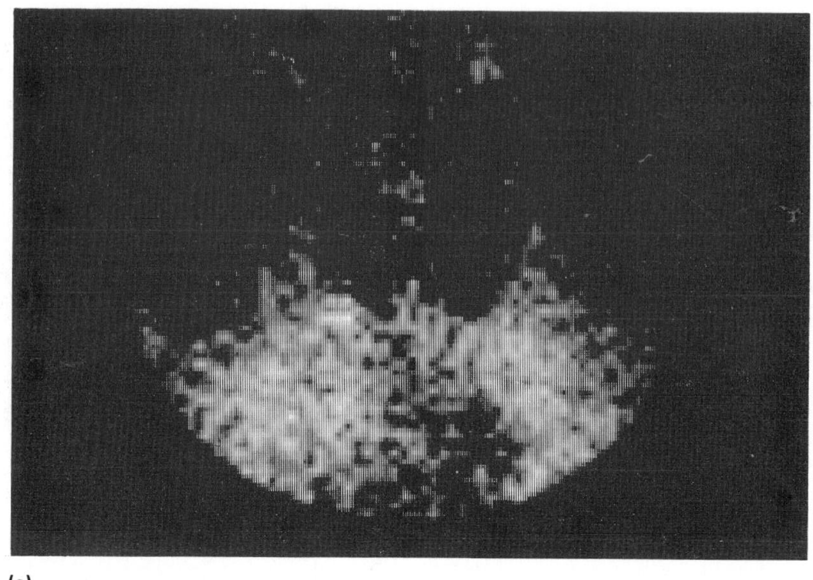

(a)

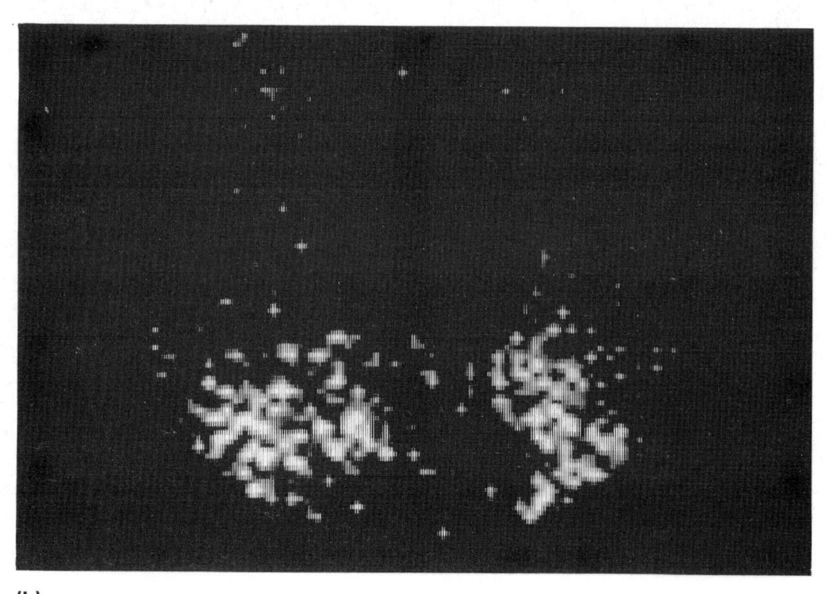

(b)

Figure 10.6 Scan of a normal patient with correct subtraction (a) and over-subtraction (b).

hyperactive parathyroid tissue. However, when there is no evidence of thallium localization in the subtracted image (Figure 10.6) further subtraction may cause artefacts to appear which could be mistaken for parathyroid glands. Over-subtraction in these situations can be a source of false positives.

In some patients, the uptake of ^{99m}Tc in the thyroid may be suppressed by, for example, iodine skin preparations. It may be of use in these patients to consider the use of oral ^{123}I and administering ^{201}Tl several hours later (Figure 10.7).

One problem with the ^{201}Tl/^{99m}Tc technique is that it is technically difficult to obtain depth information as the clearance of ^{201}Tl is fairly rapid.

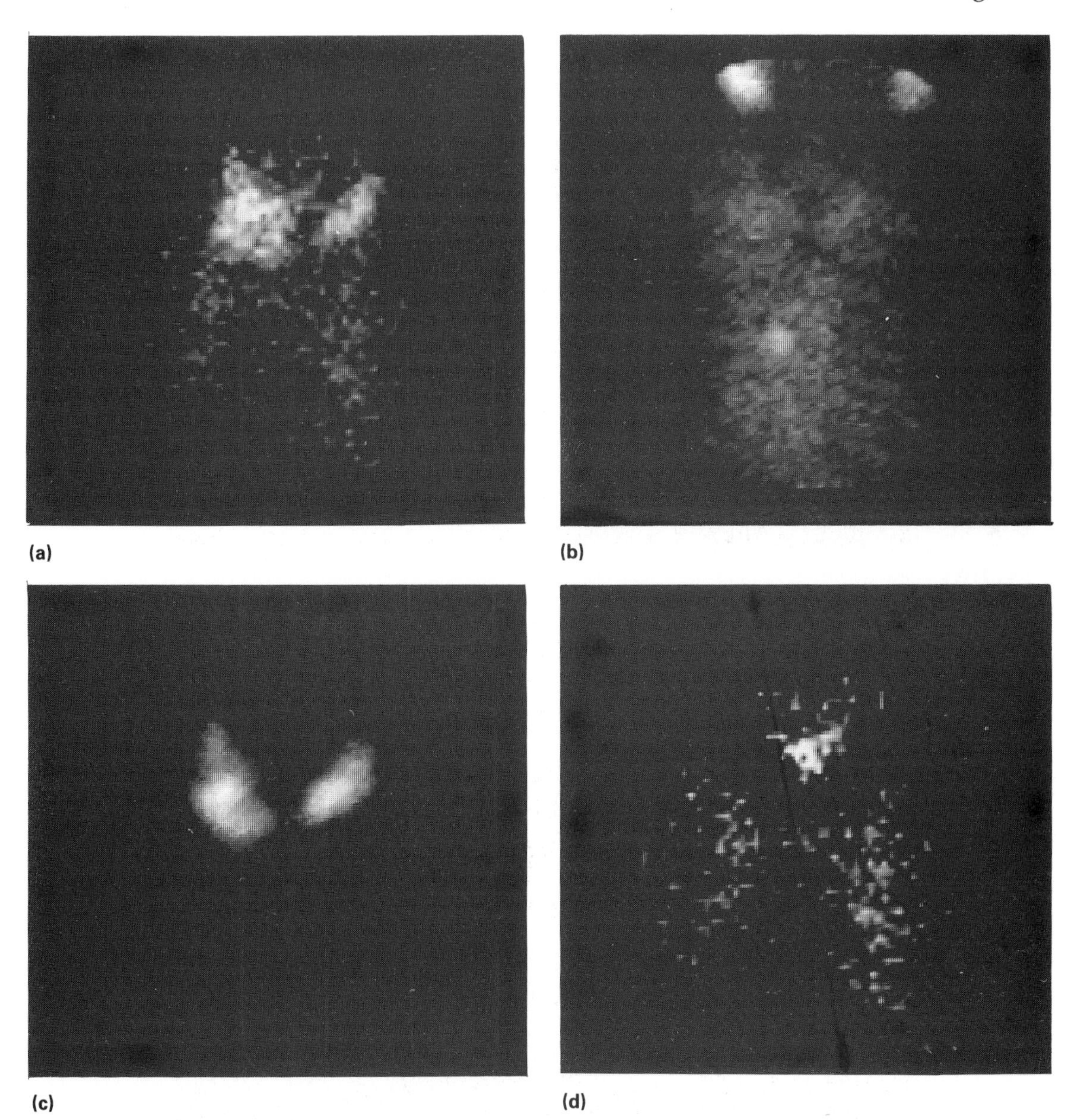

Figure 10.7 Use of ^{123}I in patient having received an iodine skin preparation: (a) ^{201}Tl image; (b) ^{99m}Tc image; (c) ^{123}I image; (d) ^{201}Tl/^{123} subtraction image showing adenoma.

Figure 10.8 shows the highly positive scan of a patient but, at surgery, only four normal parathyroid glands were found. The patient was re-imaged and a high thallium uptake was still apparent. The patient was given a bolus injection of ^{99m}Tc and it could be seen that the abnormal area was overlaid by the carotid artery. Lateral views confirmed the gland to be posterior to the thyroid. Upon re-exploration a parathyroid adenoma (i.e. a fifth ectopic gland) was found inside the carotid sheath.

The precise method of processing will affect the sensitivity and specificity of the technique (Liehn *et al.*, 1988). A combination of factors (imaging statistics, time/activity changes of ^{201}Tl in the thyroid and parathyroid and collimation problems) make emission computer-assisted tomography (ECAT) difficult.

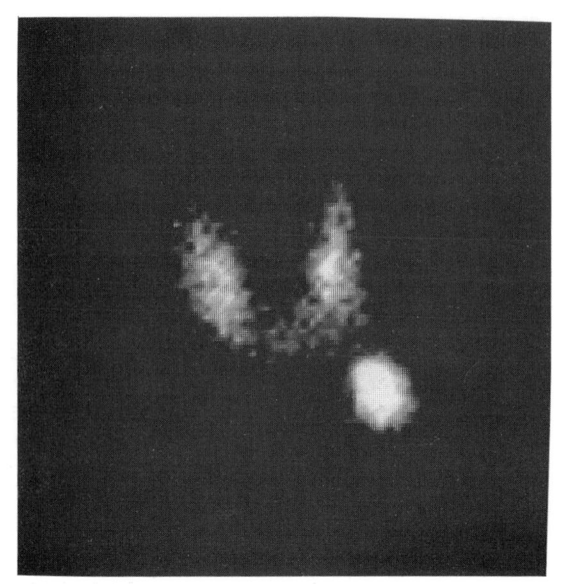

Figure 10.8 Thallium image of parathyroid adenoma found inside the carotid sheath.

10.3.4 ACCURACY OF THALLIUM/TECHNETIUM TECHNIQUE

(a) Primary hyperparathyroidism

Increasing evidence from a number of centres has confirmed the sensitivity of the technique for localizing parathyroid adenomas. Variation in sensitivity from 60% to 100% have been reported (Ferlin *et al.*, 1983; Young *et al.*, 1983; Gimlette *et al.*, 1985; Winzelberg and Hydovitz, 1985; Tindale *et al.*, 1987), with most studies having a sensitivity and specificity rate of between 85% and 95% (Gupta *et al.*, 1985; Basarab *et al.*, 1985). The main factors causing false-positive results is coexistent thyroid disease (see below).

Hypercalcaemia is caused by hyperfunctioning of more than one gland in 10–15% of cases of primary hyperparathyroidism. Series with large numbers in this subgroup have not been reported. The sensitivity of detection in this group is lower than with adenomas and appears similar to that seen in secondary hyperparathyroidism (Blake *et al.*, 1986).

Parathyroid carcinoma is rare and reports suggest the scan appearances may be indistinguishable from parathyroid adenomas (Ferlin *et al.*, 1983; Okerlund *et al.*, 1984). Experience in four cases at the time of presentation showed identical appearances to adenomas (Coakley and Wells, unpublished data). However, two of these patients redeveloped hypercalcaemia after their first operation and the technique failed to show multiple, small metastatic deposits in the neck.

(b) Secondary hyperparathyroidism

Most centres have reported inferior results in localizing glands in secondary hyperparathyroidism with sensitivity ranging from 30% to 83% (Nunan *et al.* 1984; Blake *et al.*, 1986; Takagi *et al.*, 1983; Okerlund *et al.*, 1984; Gupta *et al.*, 1985). Occasionally it is possible to locate all four glands (Figure 10.9). As all four glands are usually involved, there is little predictive value of the test for this group, and unless ectopically sited tissue is identified the technique is of little value to the surgeon.

(c) Scanning after failed parathyroidectomy

The sensitivity in patients who have undergone an unsuccessful parathyroidectomy varies from 26% to 100%, the sensitivity in general being lower in the reported series with larger numbers of patients (Table 10.1). It is inappropriate to estimate specificity in such a group since there are no true negatives and, with the exception of the report of Clark *et al.* (1985a), there are only a small number of false-positive scans reported in this group.

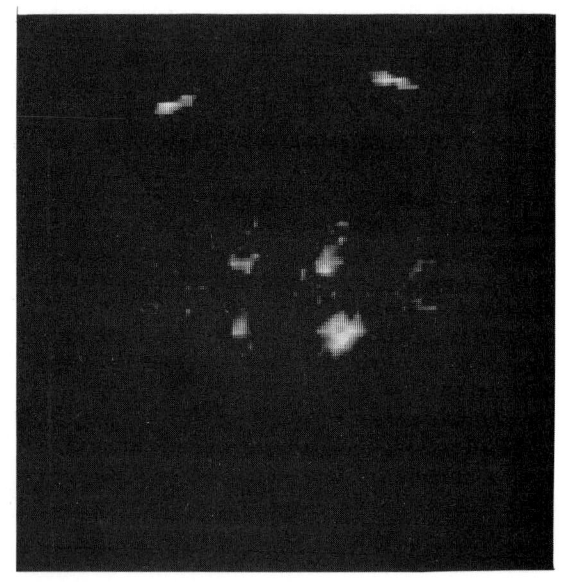

Figure 10.9 Subtracted image showing four-gland hyperplasia.

Table 10.1 $^{201}Tl/^{99m}Tc$ pertechnetate scans: re-operation

Number of patients	*Sensitivity (%)*	*Number false positive*	*Reference*
7	100	0	Basarab *et al.* (1985)
22	36	6	Clark *et al.* (1985a)
9	67	1	Percival *et al.* (1985a)
23	52	0	Skibber *et al.* (1985)
11	72	2	Gooding *et al.* (1986)
34	26	2	Miller *et al.* (1987)

10.3.5 FACTORS LIMITING ACCURACY OF $^{201}Tl/^{99m}Tc$ SUBTRACTION SCANNING

The precise mechanism of ^{201}Tl uptake by the parathyroids has not been defined. Blood flow is probably important although the gland does not have an increased blood pool, as demonstrated by scanning with labelled erythrocytes (Figure 10.10). Thallium is a potassium analogue and uptake by parathyroid cells is probably by means of the sodium/potassium pump.

In the absence of precise knowledge of the mechanism of thallium uptake by parathyroid glands, several factors have been postulated as being important in explaining the variations in sensitivity reported between different series and the lower sensitivity of detection in secondary hyperparathyroidism (Young *et al.*, 1983). In one small series measurements on excised parathyroid glands showed qualitative differences of thallium uptake between glands although there was little difference in uptake per gram of tissue between adenomas and hyperplastic glands (Gimlette *et al.*, 1986). There is only moderate correlation between sensitivity of detection and serum PTH levels (Percival *et al.*, 1985a; Gimlette *et al.*, 1986). The single factor which correlates best with sensitivity is size as described by gland mass. Several workers have shown this correlation (Okerlund *et al.*, 1984; Percival *et al.*, 1985b; Winzelberg and Hydovitz, 1985; Gimlette and Taylor, 1985) and below 300–400 mg it is unlikely that glands will be localized reliably. This fact is likely to account for the failure to visualize normal glands which rarely weigh more than 50 mg. Correlation between size and sensitivity of detection appears true in adenomas, primary hyperplastic glands and in secondary hyper-

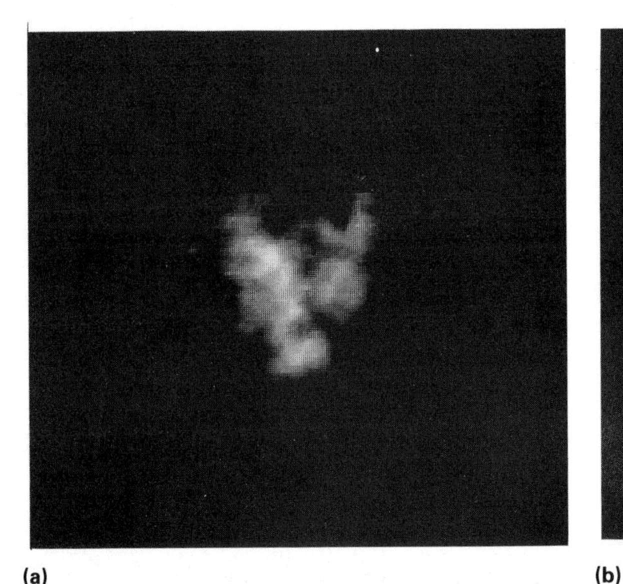
(a)

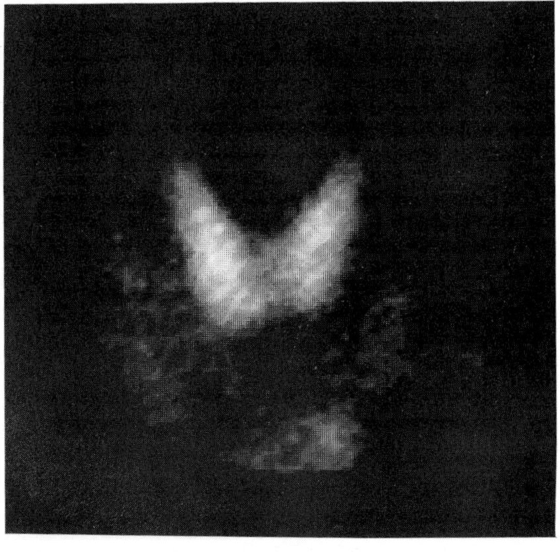
(b)

Figure 10.10 (a) ^{201}Tl image showing adenoma at right lower lobe. (b) ^{99m}Tc-labelled erythrocyte image showing absence of blood pool in region of adenoma.

plasia. Variations in surgical referral patterns result in differences in size of glands found at operation and this is likely to account for some of the differences in sensitivity in the reported literature.

Ectopic glands have been identified in a wide range of locations and, provided the gland lies within the field of view of the camera, it is unclear whether the sensitivity of the technique varies with gland location. One report describes a lower sensitivity of detection for upper pole adenomas when compared with lower pole ones (Tindale *et al.*, 1987), although others have not observed this finding (Okerlund *et al.*, 1984).

The lower overall sensitivity in secondary hyperparathyroidism is probably explained by the glands frequently being smaller than those seen with primary adenomas. High sensitivity was reported in renal hyperparathyroidism in a series of patients with mostly large glands and a threshold of detection of 500 mg described, below which accuracy of localization rapidly fell off (Takagi *et al.*, 1983). Renal failure has been shown to impair trapping mechanisms of the thyroid (Mooradian *et al.*, 1983). Uptake of iodide and pertechnetate is reduced and frequently uptake of thallium in this group is lower than in non-renal patients. There are insufficient data to exclude the possibility of similar qualitative differences in parathyroid trapping mechanisms. Counting statistics are important and it is more difficult to demonstrate four separate areas of functioning tissue than a single one of similar total function, and the higher background and lower trapping by the thyroid seen in renal failure result in poorer imaging statistics and increase errors in subtraction methods.

The most important factor limiting specificity is from false positives in patients with coexistent thyroid disease. Most thyroid adenomas show reduced trapping of pertechnetate and avid trapping of thallium (Figure 10.11) and this pattern cannot be distinguished from parathyroid adenomas. False positives have also been described with sarcoidosis (Young *et al.*, 1983) thyroid carcinoma (Intenzo and Park, 1985), lymphoma (Winzelberg and Hydovitz, 1985) and metastases (Punt *et al.*, 1985). As thallium is known to localize in a number of malignant and inflammatory disorders, false-positive results may be predicted in a wide range of conditions. This underlines the importance of using the technique not as a primary investigation as to whether a hypercalcaemic patient has hyperparathyroidism but as a technique useful for localizing abnormal parathyroid glands prior to surgery in cases where hyperparathyroidism has been proven biochemically.

10.4 FUTURE DEVELOPMENTS

The ideal radiopharmaceutical for parathyroid imaging is selectively taken up by parathyroid glands with a long residence time in these so delayed images can be performed with reduced background activity from adjacent vascular structures. This tracer should not be taken up by adjacent tissues, particularly the thyroid (normal or adenomas) or by bone, bone marrow, or myocardium. The pharmaceutical should have the other characteristics desirable of any potential radiopharmaceutical (low toxicity, ability to label easily with ^{99m}Tc with stability of radiolabelling etc). Such an ideal radiopharmaceutical does not exist, but two lines of research may improve the situation.

First, for some years surgeons have used phenothiazinium dyes for peroperative localization of parathyroid glands. Methylene blue is most commonly used in the UK, and is injected intravenously one hour before operation, and this stains parathyroid tissue making it easier to identify at surgery. Some dye is also taken up by thyroid and other soft tissues in the neck. Until recently radiolabelling of these dyes has proven difficult. Success in localizing parathyroid glands using toluidine blue labelled with ^{131}I has been reported (Zwas *et al.*, 1987), but the radiolabelling of the agent involved an incubation time of 24 hours and ^{131}I is an unsuitable radiolabel for routine diagnostic work. An improved labelling technique with an incubation time of 30 minutes has been described which allows ^{123}I to be used as a radiolabel (Blower *et al.*, 1989). Clinical studies are awaited.

The other promising development is being brought about by the introduction of a new range of ^{99m}Tc cationic complexes with similarities in biological behaviour to thallium. Most of these have been introduced as agents for assessing myocardial perfusion, but is has been shown that at least one such agent, ^{99m}Tc sestamibi (Cardiolite Du Pont) also localizes parathyroid adenomas (Coakley *et al.*, 1989) Figure 10.12. The preliminary work on these agents suggest they may prove suitable technetium labelled alternatives to ^{201}Tl. False positive localization in a thyroid adenoma was reported, as occurred with ^{201}Tl. Full

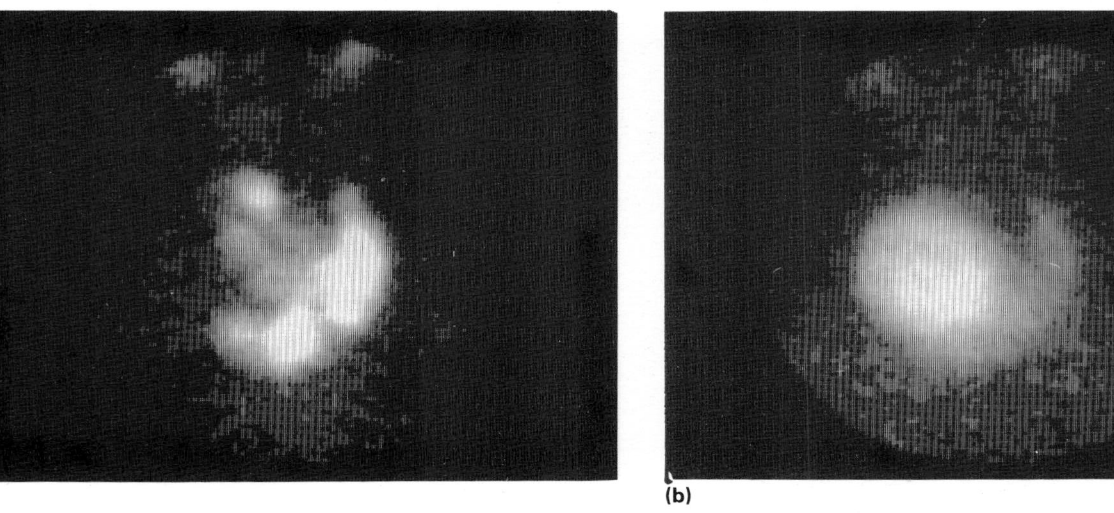

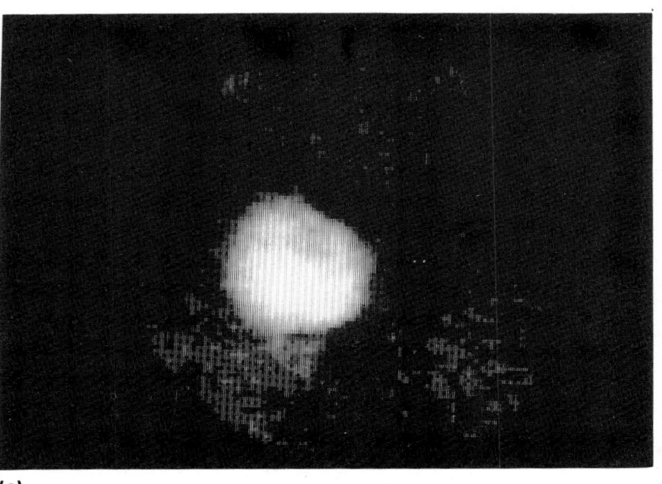

(a) (b) (c)

Figure 10.11 Thyroid adenoma. Scan shows cold nodule in the right lobe of the thyroid (a) with avid uptake of thallium (b), and subtracted image (c). Surgery confirmed a thyroid adenoma with a parathyroid adenoma situated posteriorly to this.

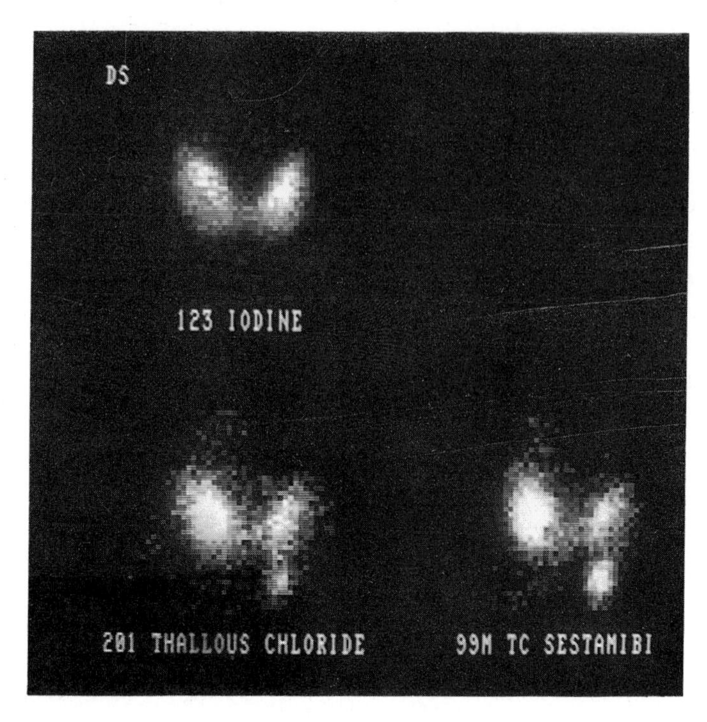

Figure 10.12 Scan showing ^{123}I thyroid image (top left) scatter subtracted ^{201}Tl image (bottom left) ^{99m}Tc sestamibi image (bottom right). Parathyroid adenoma sited below lower pole of left lobe of thyroid correctly localized with both thallium and sestamibi.

evaluation is necessary to see whether the sensitivity of detection improves with the new agent.

10.5 OTHER TECHNIQUES FOR LOCALIZING ABNORMAL PARATHYROID GLANDS

Advances in technology have resulted in a number of imaging modalities which have been employed to localize abnormal parathyroid glands. All of the techniques described have limitations.

10.5.1 SELECTIVE VENOUS SAMPLING

This technique involves introducing a catheter into veins in the neck and upper mediastinum (usually via the internal jugular vein catheterized by the transfemoral route). Venous samples obtained from various sites are analysed for PTH levels to localize the parathyroid gland. Reported accuracy of the technique varies, but for primary hyperparathyroidism is usually in the range 70–80% (Bilezikian *et al.*, 1973; McMillan *et al.*, 1983). For re-operation the accuracy is lower, and some have advocated arteriography (Edis *et al.*, 1978) or digital subtraction angiography (Miller *et al.*, 1987) prior to venous sampling. The technique has the advantage of maintaining its accuracy in the presence of coexisting thyroid disease. However, it is a highly skilled, operator-dependent technique and its invasiveness means it is only available in a small number of specialized referral centres and is expensive.

10.5.2 ARTERIOGRAPHY

Arteriography is also invasive and is associated with a significant morbidity (Edis *et al.*, 1978). It is occasionally employed in investigating patients who have had a failed parathyroidectomy and has been advocated in this situation for demonstrating vascular anatomy prior to selective venous sampling.

10.5.3 ULTRASOUND

Improvement in ultrasound techniques has resulted in its increased utilization for a number of cervical investigations. The technique is highly operator dependent but as ultrasound is now widely practised expertise is becoming increasingly available. In primary hyperparathyroidism sensitivity of detection for high-resolution ultrasound is between 60% and 80% (Buchwach *et al.*, 1987; Gooding *et al.* 1986; Winzelberg *et al.*, 1985). Predictably the sensitivity is higher for adenomas than diffuse hyperplasia and low for parathymic glands (Doppman *et al.*, 1985). The technique is cheap and widely available. Its accuracy is reduced with coexisting nodular thyroid disease (Karstrup and Hegedus, 1986) or after previous surgery when fascial planes and the vascular anatomy in the neck have been affected (Clark *et al.*, 1985b; Miller *et al.*, 1987).

10.5.4 CT SCANNING

In spite of the high resolution available with CT scanning, the results of parathyroid localization have been disappointing, with an accuracy of localization varying from 35% to 70% for adenomas (Roza *et al.*, 1984; McMillan *et al.* 1983; Jarhult *et al.*, 1985) and even lower accuracy for hyperplastic glands and following failed parathyroidectomy. The problems are mainly technical and caused by small-density differences between anatomical structures and by distortion from artefacts. These problems are particularly marked in the neck and the technique appears more accurate for upper mediastinal glands (Clark *et al.*, 1985b).

10.5.5 DIGITAL SUBTRACTION ANGIOGRAPHY (DSA)

This requires introduction of intra-arterial contrast material usually by injections into the carotid or subclavian arteries. A preliminary report shows a sensitivity of detection of 40% (Obley *et al.*, 1984). The invasiveness of the procedure and the limited availability of equipment mean it has not been widely used to assess primary disease. However, when available, it may have a role in failed parathyroidectomies (Miller *et al.*, 1987).

10.5.6 MAGNETIC RESONANCE IMAGING (MRI)

While spatial resolution with MRI is inferior to CT, there are no streak artefacts and tumours and lymph nodes are more easily differentiated from muscle and blood vessels because of superior soft tissue contrasts (Stark *et al.*, 1984). This factor may be particularly important in re-operative cases, and in one report eight out of 16 glands were successfully located by this technique (Miller *et al.*, 1987).

Peck (1987) reported marginally higher detection rates using MRI than obtained with scintigraphy, but with a greater number of false positive scans. The expense and its limited availability means MRI is unlikely to be used routinely for parathyroid localization, and its role after failed parathyroidectomy needs further evaluation.

10.6 USE OF LOCALIZING TESTS PRIOR TO SURGERY

Of the tests described only selective venous sampling can be regarded as specific, all the other tests showing anatomical or pathophysiological similarities with other cervical disorders which can be mistaken for abnormal parathyroid glands. For this reason it should again be stressed that the investigations described are localizing procedures for use in establishing hyperparathyroidism prior to surgery and not as part of the routine work-up of hypercalcaemic patients.

There is no consensus amongst surgeons as to the precise role of localizing tests prior to neck exploration in primary hyperparathyroidism. A major consideration is that experienced parathyroid surgeons will localize up to 95% of adenomas at the initial exploration without prior localizing procedures. Existing localizing tests are unlikely to exceed this degree of accuracy. The majority of failed parathyroidectomies at first time of exploration in primary disease occur in the hands of surgeons who undertake only occasional parathyroidectomies. When the glands are ultimately localized many are, in fact, in the neck or readily accessible from the neck (Figure 10.13). The main advantage of a non-invasive localizing procedure prior to the first exploration would seem to be that if the gland can be reliably localized then it will help reduce the time of neck exploration, which may be particularly valuable in elderly patients and those with cardiovascular or other risk factors. On some occasions it will allow a more appropriate incision, particularly if the gland is ectopic. Failure to localize the gland preoperatively will give the surgeon the opportunity of allowing more time for neck exploration when organizing his operating list.

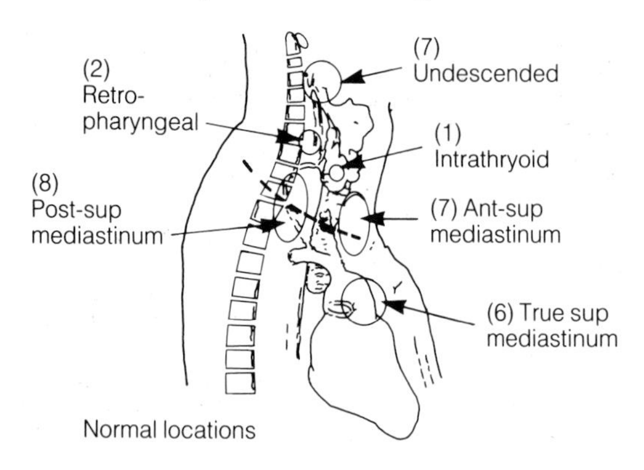

Figure 10.13 Location of pathological glands removed at re-operation in 40 patients (Edis, 1978).

While some surgeons do not request localization procedures prior to first exploration, an increasing number value a non-invasive localizing procedure. Technetium/thallium subtraction scanning is generally considered to be the single method of choice in this circumstance, although increasingly ultrasound is requested in addition (Gooding *et al.*, 1986). The main limitation of both of these techniques is the presence of coexisting thyroid nodules. In the absence of thyroid disease, it seems inappropriate to pursue other more costly and invasive investigations prior to first neck exploration.

With secondary hyperparathyroidism when four-gland disease is anticipated, the surgeon will be required to carefully explore all four parathyroid glands, and as a fifth gland occurs in 6% of cases he must also search for additional ectopic tissue. Because of this more extensive surgical exploration and a lower sensitivity of localizing abnormal glands with all techniques, the case for routine pre-operative localizing tests is less well established and we do not recommend routine localizing procedures in this subgroup.

The situation following a failed parathyroidectomy (whether in experienced or non-experienced surgical hands) is different (Brennan and Wells 1983). Re-operation is technically very much more difficult, has a significantly higher morbidity and there is a lower likelihood of establishing normocalcaemia. For these reasons any technique which can localize the abnormal parathyroid gland prior to re-operation is of value. All imaging techniques which have been described have a lower success rate in the post-surgical group and thallium/technetium scanning and ultrasound are the minimum appropriate investigations. CT of the upper mediastinum should be undertaken if these are negative. If these techniques fail there is an argument for going on to more invasive techniques. Of these selective venous sampling (possibly preceded by arteriography or DSA) appears the most appropriate and MRI may find a role in this situation.

REFERENCES

Aurbach, G. D., Marx, S. J. and Spiegel, A. M. (1981) in *Textbook of Endocrinology*, 6th edn, (ed. R. H. Williams), Saunders, Philadelphia, pp. 922–1031.

Bartelheimer, H., Fritcsche, H., Kuhlencordt, F. *et al.* (1965) Auffindung eines Nebenschilddrussen-Adenoms erst nach Szintigraphischer Darstellung mit 75Se-Methionin. *Klin. Wschr.*, **43**, 854 (Abstract).

Basarab, R. M., Manni, A. and Harrison, T. S. (1985) Dual isotope subtraction parathyroid scintigraphy in the preoperative evaluation of suspected hyperparathyroidism. *Clin. Nucl. Med.*, **10**, 300–14.

Beierwaltes, W. H., di Giulio, W. and Sisson, J. C. (1964) in *Scintillation Scanning in Clinical Medicine*, (ed. J. L. Quinn, III), Saunders, Philadelphia, p. 55.

Bilezikian, J. P., Doppman, J. L. and Shimkin, P. M. (1973) Pre-operative localization of abnormal parathyroid tissue. *Am. J. Med.*, **55**, 505–513.

Blake, G. M., Percival, R. C. and Kanis, J. A. (1986) Thallium-pertechnetate subtraction scintigraphy: a quantitative comparison between adenomatous and hyperplastic parathyroid glands. *Eur. J. Nucl. Med.*, **12**, 31–6.

Brennan, M. F. and Wells, S. A. (1983) in *Endocrine Surgery 2* (eds I. D. Johnston and N. W. Thompson), Butterworths, London.

Buchwach, K. A., Mangum, W. B. and Hahn, F. W. (1987) Preoperative localisation of parathyroid adenomas. *Laryngoscope*, **97**, 13–15.

Cann, C. E. and Prussin, S. G. (1980) Possible parathyroid imaging using Ga-67 and other aluminium analogs. *J. Nucl. Med.*, **21**, 471–4.

Clark, O. H., Okerlund, M. D., Moss, A. A. *et al.* (1985a) Localization studies in patients with persistent or recurrent hyperparathyroidism. *Surgery*, **98**, 1083–94.

Clark, O. H., Stark, D. A., Duh, Q. *et al.* (1985b) Value of high resolution real-time ultrasonography in secondary hyperparathyroidism. *Am. J. Surg.*, **150**, 9–17.

Di Giulio, W. and Morales, J. (1966) An evaluation of parathyroid scanning using selenium-75-methionine. *J. Nucl. Med.*, **7**, 380.

Doppman, J. L., Shawker, T. H., Krudy, A. G. *et al.* (1985) Parathymic parathyroid: CT, US, and angiographic findings. *Radiology*, **157**, 419–23.

Edis, A. J., Sheedy, P. F., Beahrs, O. H. and van Heerden, J. A. (1978) Results of reoperation for hyperparathyroidism, with evaluation of preoperative localization studies. *Surgery*, **84**, 384–93.

Ell, P. J., Todd-Pokropek, A. and Britton, K. E. (1975) Localization of parathyroid adenomas by computer-assisted parathyroid scanning. *Br. J. Surg.*, **62**, 553–5.

Ferlin, G., Conte N., Borsato, N. *et al.* (1981a) Parathyroid scintigraphy with 131-Cs and 201-Tl. *J. Nucl. Med. Allied Sci.*, **25**, 119–23.
Ferlin, G., Borsato, N., Perelli, R. *et al.* (1981b) Technetium-thallium subtraction scan: a new method in the pre-operative localization of parathyroid enlargement. *Eur. J. Nucl. Med.*, **6**, A13 (Abstract).
Ferlin, G., Borsato, N., Camerani, M. *et al.* (1983) New perspectives in localizing enlarged parathyroids by technetium-thallium subtraction scan. *J. Nucl. Med.*, **24**, 438–41.
Fogelman, I., McKillop, J. H., Bessent, R. G. *et al.* (1984) Successful localisation of parathyroid adenomata by thallium-201 and technetium-99m subtraction scintigraphy: description of an improved technique. *Eur. J. Nucl. Med.*, **9**, 545–7.
Gimlette, T. M. D. and Taylor, W. H. (1985) Localization of enlarged parathyroid glands by thallium-201 and technetium-99m subtraction imaging. *Clin. Nucl. Med.*, **10**, 235–9.
Gimlette, T. M. D., Brownless, S. M., Taylor, W. H. *et al.* (1986) Limits to parathyroid imaging with thallium-201 confirmed by tissue uptake and phantom studies. *J. Nucl. Med.*, **27**, 1262–5.
Gooding, G. A. W., Okerlund, M. D., Stark, D. D. and Clark, O. H. (1986) Parathyroid imaging: comparison of double-tracer (Tl-201, Tc-99m) scintigraphy and high-resolution US. *Radiology*, **161**, 57–64.
Gupta, S. M., Belsky, J. L., Spencer, R. P. *et al.* (1985) Parathyroid adenomas and hyperplasia. *Clin. Nucl. Med.*, **10**, 243–7.
Intenzo, C. and Park, C. H. (1985) Co-existent parathyroid adenoma and thyroid carcinoma. *Clin. Nucl. Med.*, **10**, 560–1.
Iwase, M., Shimizu, Y., Kitahara, H., Tobioka, N. and Takatsuki, K., (1986) Parathyroid carcinoma visualized by gallium-67 citrate scintigraphy. *J. Nucl. Med.*, **27**, 63–5.
Jarhult, J., Kristoffersson, A., Lundstrom, B. and Oberg, L. (1985) Comparison of ultrasonography and computer tomography in preoperative location of parathyroid adenomas. *Acta Chir. Scand.*, **151**, 583–7.
Karstrup S. and Hegedus L. (1986) Concomitant thyroid disease in hyperparathyroidism. *Eur. J. Radiol.*, **6**, 149–52.
McGeown, M. G., Bell, T. K., Soyannwo, M. A. O. *et al.* (1968) Parathyroid scanning in the human with seleno-methionine-75 Se. *Br. J. Radiol.*, **41**, 300.
McMillan, N. C., Smith, L., McKellar, N. J. *et al.* (1983) The localisation of parathyroid tumours: a comparison of computed tomography with cervical vein hormone assay. *Scott. Med. J.*, **28**, 153–6.
Miller, D. L., Doppman, J. L., Shawker, T. H. *et al.* (1987) Localization of parathyroid adenomas in patients who have undergone surgery. *Radiology*, **162**, 133–41.
MIRD Dose Estimate Report No. 8 (1976) Summary of current radiation dose estimates to normal humans from 99m-Tc as sodium pertechnetate. *J. Nucl. Med.*, **17**, 74–7.
Mooradian, A. D., Morley, J. E., Korchick, W. K. *et al.* (1983) Iodine trapping and organification in patients with chronic renal failure. *Eur. J. Nucl. Med.*, **8**, 495–8.
Nunan, T. O., Wolfe, J., Gaunt, J. I. *et al.* (1984) Thallium-201 and technetium-99m subtraction scanning of the parathyroid glands in patients with hyperparathyroidism due to renal osteodystrophy. *Nucl. Med. Commun.*, **5**, 254 (Abstract).
Obley, D., Winzelberg, G. G., Wholey, M. H. *et al.* (1984) Parathyroid adenomas studied by digital subtraction angiography. *Radiology*, **153**, 449–51.
Okerlund, M. D., Sheldon, K., Corpuz, S. *et al.* (1984) A new method with high sensitivity and specificity for localization of abnormal parathyroid glands. *Ann. Surg.*, **200**, 381–8.
Percival, R. C., Blake, G. M., Urwin, G. H. *et al.* (1985a) Assessment of thallium-pertechnetate subtraction scintigraphy in hyperparathyroidism. *Br. J. Radiol.*, **58**, 131–5.
Percival, R. C., Blake, G. M., Urwin, G. H. *et al.* (1985b) Thallium-technetium subtraction scintigraphy as an aid to parathyroid surgery. *Br. J. Urol.*, **57**, 133–136.
Potchen, E. J. (1963) Isotopic labeling of the rat parathyroid as demonstrated by autoradiography. *J. Nucl. Med.*, **4**, 480.
Potchen, E. J., Wilson, R. E. and Dealy, J. B. (1965) External parathyroid scanning with Se-75 selenomethionine. *Ann. Surg.*, **162**, 492.
Punt, J. A., De Hooge, P. and Hoekstra J. B. L. (1985) False-positive subtraction scintigram of the parathyroid glands due to metastatic tumor. *J. Nucl. Med.*, **26**, 155–6.
Quinn, J. L., III (ed.) (1966) in *Year Book of Nuclear Medicine*, Vol. 1, Year Book Publishers, Chicago, p. 172.
Robinson, R. J. (1982) Parathyroid scintigraphy revisited. *Clin. Radiol.*, **33**, 37–41.
Roza, A. M., Wexler, M. J., Stein, L. and Goltzman, D. (1984) Value of high-resolution computerized tomography in localizing diseased parathyroid glands. *Can. J. Surg.*, **27**, 334–6.
Skibber, J. M., Reynolds, J. C., Spiegel, A. M. *et al.* (1985) Computerized technetium/thallium scans and parathyroid reoperation. *Surgery*, **98**, 1077–82.
Stark, D. D., Clark, O. H. and Moss, A. A. (1984) Magnetic resonance imaging of the thyroid, thymus, and parathyroid glands. *Surgery*, **96**, 1083–91.
Takagi, H., Tominaga, Y., Uchida, K. *et al.* (1983) Image diagnosis of parathyroid glands in chronic renal failure. *Ann. Surg.*, **198**, 74–9.
Tindale, W. B., Everett, K. and Harding, L. K. (1987) Upper pole parathyroid adenomas: a problem for nuclear medicine. *Nucl. Med. Commun.*, **8**, 251 (Abstract).
van't Hoff, W., Ballardie, F. W. and Bicknell, E. J. (1983) Primary hyperparathyroidism: the case for medical management. *Med. Practise*, **287**, 1605–8.
Waldorf, J. C., van Heerden, J. A., Gorman, C. A. and Wahner, H. W. (1984) [75-Se] Selenomethionine scanning for parathyroid localization should be abandoned. *Mayo Clin. Proc.*, **59**, 534–7.
Wells, C. P., Gaunt, J. I., Coakley, A. J. *et al.* (1983) Technical aspects of technetium-thallium parathyroid adenoma localisation. *Nucl. Med. Commun.*, **4**, 144 (Abstract).
Winzelberg, G. G. and Hydovitz, J. D. (1985a) Radionuclide imaging of parathyroid tumours: historical

perspectives and newer techniques. *Semin. Nucl. Med.*, **15**, 161–70.
Winzelberg, G. G., Hydovitz, J. D., O'Hara, K. R. *et al.* (1985b) Parathyroid adenomas evaluated by Tl-201/Tc-99m pertechnetate subtraction scintigraphy and high-resolution ultrasonography. *Radiology*, **155**, 231–5.
Young, A. E., Gaunt, J. I., Croft, D. N. *et al.* (1983) Location of parathyroid adenomas by thallium-201 and technetium-99m subtraction scanning. *Br. Med. J.*, **286**, 1384–6.
Zwas, S. T., Czerniak, A., Avigad, I. and Wolfstein, I. (1981) Preoperative parathyroid localization using radioactive toluidine blue (RTB). *J. Nucl. Med.*, **6**, P5 (Abstract).

FURTHER READING

Anatomy, physiology and clinical parathyroid disease, in *Textbook of Endocrinology*, Ch. 19, pp. 922–1031 by G. D. Aurbach, S. J. Marx and A. M. Spiegel (ed. R. H. Williams), Saunders, Philadelphia (1981).
Reoperation for suspected hyperparathyroidism, in *Endocrine Surgery 2* (eds I. D. Johnson and N. W. Thompson), Butterworths, London (1983).
Radionuclide imaging of parathyroid tumors: historical perspectives and newer techniques, in *Seminars in Nuclear Medicine*, Vol. XV, No. 2 (eds G. G. Winzelberg and J. D. Hydovitz), *Grune & Stratton*, New York (1985).
Hypercalcaemia: localization of parathyroid glands. A. E. Young, *Br. J. Hosp. Med.*, 188, 198–203 (1984).
Presidential address: hyperparathyroidism, hypergraphia, and just plain hype. L. Rosoff, *Surgery*, 989–94 (1985).
Preoperative localisation of parathyroid adenomas. J. H. McKillop, I. T. Boyle, I. G. Gunn and J. S. F. Hutchinson, *Scott. Med. J.*, 10–14 (1986).
Parathyroid gland localisation. Editorial, *Lancet*, 726–7 (1986).

CHAPTER ELEVEN

The adrenal gland

F. A. Khafagi, B. Shapiro and M. D. Gross

11.1 INTRODUCTION

The adrenal glands are paired retroperitoneal organs lying superomedial to each kidney. Each adrenal gland consists of an outer **cortex** and an embryologically, histologically and functionally distinct **medulla**. The cortex is derived from the posterior coelomic mesoderm (the urogenital ridge). It is responsible for the synthesis of glucocorticoids (principally cortisol), mineralocorticoids (principally aldosterone) and weak androgens (dehydroepiandrosterone (DHEA), its sulphate (DHEA-S) and androstenedione). The adrenal medulla shares its origin from the neural crest with the sympathetic ganglia and paraganglia and other adrenergic tissues. Like those organs, it synthesizes and stores noradrenaline, but it is unique in its ability to convert noradrenaline to adrenaline.

Excess secretion of any of the adrenal cortical or medullary hormones gives rise to a number of well-known clinical syndromes (Table 11.1). They may result from benign or malignant adrenal tumours, adrenal hyperplasia or, least frequently, from extra-adrenal disease. Differentiating among these possibilities is often impossible on clinical or biochemical grounds alone. Location of the site(s) of excess hormone production in the past depended upon relatively insensitive or invasive radiological methods (e.g. nephrotomography, retroperitoneal air insufflation, adrenal arteriography and venography). The non-invasive evaluation of adrenal anatomy was revolutionized by the advent of X-ray computed tomography (CT), which can reliably detect tumours greater than 1 cm in diameter. However, CT is relatively insensitive for lesions less than 1 cm in diameter, for recognizing significant contour changes in bilateral hyperplasia, and for localizing extra-adrenal disease; it may be difficult to interpret post-operatively, particularly in the presence of surgical clips. Moreover, the functional significance of anatomical abnormalities cannot be determined from the CT scan. In patients with established clinical and biochemical diagnoses of adrenal cortical or medullary hyperfunction, incorporation of specific radiopharmaceuticals into the abnormal tissues allows scintigraphic localization of functional abnormalities with a high degree of efficacy. Adrenal scintigraphy can direct and complement anatomical studies with CT and magnetic resonance imaging (MRI), and the combination of scintigraphy and CT or MRI should in most cases obviate the need for more invasive procedures.

Table 11.1 Syndromes of adrenal hormone excess

Organ	*Zone*	*Hormone*	*Syndrome*
Cortex	Glomerulosa	Aldosterone	Primary hyperaldosteronism
	Fasciculata or reticularis	Cortisol	Cushing's syndrome
		Androgens	Virilism
			Congenital adrenal hyperplasia
Medulla		Adrenaline	Phaeochromocytoma
		Noradrenaline	Phaeochromocytoma
Paraganglia		Noradrenaline	Phaeochromocytoma

11.2 ADRENAL CORTEX

11.2.1 PHYSIOLOGY AND RADIOPHARMACOLOGY

Cholesterol is the precursor for steroid hormone biosynthesis. The major source of adrenal cholesterol is circulating cholesterol carried by low-density lipoprotein (LDL). In common with virtually all cell types, adrenal cortical cells bear specific, high-affinity cell membrane receptors for LDL. After the receptor–LDL complex is internalized, cholesterol is liberated, and that which is surplus to requirements for cell membrane maintenance is re-esterified by acyl-CoA:cholesterol acyltransferase (ACAT) and stored. An increase in the size of this intracellular storage pool inhibits endogenous cholesterol synthesis and results in a reduction or 'down-regulation' in the number of LDL receptors on the cell surface.

Adrenocortical cholesterol uptake is further modified by the major regulators of steroid hormone synthesis. Functionally, each adrenal cortex can be considered as two organs: the subcapsular **zona glomerulosa** which synthesizes aldosterone primarily under the control of the renin–angiotensin system; and the deeper **zonae fasciculata et reticularis** which elaborate glucocorticoids and androgens under the control of adrenocorticotrophic hormone (ACTH) from the anterior pituitary (Figure 11.1).

Cholesterol labelled with ^{131}I (^{131}I-19-iodocholesterol) was the first clinically successful adrenocortical scintigraphic agent (Beierwaltes *et al.*, 1971). It has been superseded by the cholesterol analogues ^{131}I-6β-iodomethyl-19-norcholesterol (NP-59) (Sarkar *et al.*, 1977) and ^{75}Se-6β-selenomethyl-19-norcholesterol (SMC, 'Scintadren') (Hawkins *et al.*, 1980), both of which have greater affinity for the adrenal cortex than ^{131}I-19-iodocholesterol and provide more favourable target-to-background ratios of activity. After intravenous injection, approximately 20% of the dose of labelled analogue is carried in the LDL fraction. Normal adrenal cortical uptake of the radiopharmaceutical is roughly symmetrical – the normal right : left adrenal uptake ratio on the posterior scintiscan (corrected for background) is 0.9–1.2, the slight right dominance being due to the slightly more posterior (superficial) location of the right gland. For both NP-59 and SMC, the normal uptake per adrenal ranges from 0.07% to 0.3% of the injected dose, with a mean of 0.16% for NP-59 and 0.19% for SMC. Following uptake, the radiocholesterol analogues may be esterified

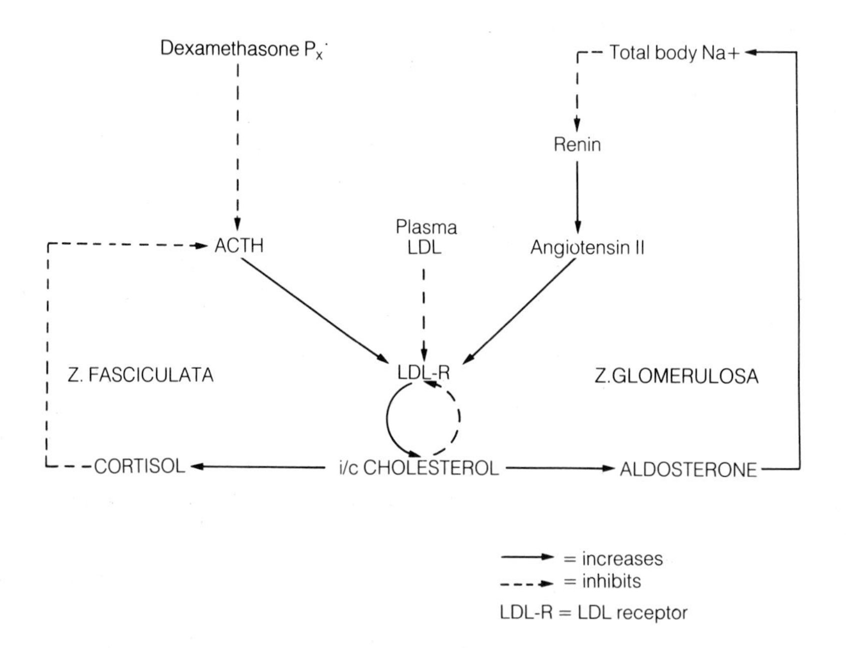

Figure 11.1 Regulation of the adrenal cortical intracellular (i/c) cholesterol pool and hormone biosynthesis.

Table 11.2 Characteristics of NP-59 and SMC

	^{131}I-6β-iodomethyl-19-norcholesterol (NP-59)	*^{75}Se-6β-selenomethyl-19-norcholesterol (SMC)*
Dose (adult)	37 MBq (1 mCi)	9.25 MBq (250 μCi)
% uptake (per adrenal)	0.07–0.26%	0.07–0.30%
Dosimetry (cGy/dose)		
Adrenals	28	6.1
Ovaries	8.0	1.9
Liver	2.4	3.5
Whole body	1.2	1.4
Photopeaks (principal)	364 keV (81.2%)	136 keV (61.0%) 265 keV (59.0%) 280 keV (25.2%)
β-Emission	Yes	No
Thyroid blockade required	Yes	No
Shelf-life	2 weeks, frozen	6 weeks room temp.
Imaging interval	3–7 d post-injection	7 and 14 d post-injection (earlier imaging also possible)

by ACAT but are not significantly metabolized further. The major pathway of radiocholesterol excretion is hepatobiliary, a small fraction being excreted as radiolabelled bile acid analogues.

Both NP-59 and SMC appear to behave virtually identically *in vivo*, as might be expected from their structural similarity; it has been suggested that SMC has marginally greater *in vivo* stability. Unlike ^{131}I, which is a β-emitter, ^{75}Se is a pure γ-emitter. This potential advantage is offset somewhat by the long physical half-life (119 days) and complex γ-spectrum of ^{75}Se. Thus dosimetry for both NP-59 and SMC is similar (Table 11.2) (Carey *et al.*, 1979; Hawkins *et al.*, 1980). Nevertheless, SMC does offer other advantages over NP-59: the principal photopeaks of ^{75}Se are more efficiently detected by current gamma cameras, allowing better counting statistics and the potential for single-photon emission CT (SPECT); SMC undergoes less autoradiolysis and can therefore be stored at room temperature; its longer physical half-life confers both a longer shelf-life and the potential for delayed imaging if required; and its use does not require concurrent thyroid blockade with stable iodide (Table 11.2).

Adrenocortical uptake of the radiocholesterol analogues parallels that of cholesterol and is modified by the same physiological influences (Figure 11.1). Thus ACTH stimulation enhances radiocholesterol uptake; conversely, complete suppression of endogenous ACTH secretion by dexamethasone has been shown to reduce adrenal radiocholesterol uptake by 50% (Gross *et al.*, 1981a). Similarly, sodium loading with resultant extracellular volume expansion inhibits renin secretion and angiotensin II production, and reduces adrenal radiocholesterol uptake by a further 10%. Thus 40% of adrenocortical radiocholesterol uptake is independent of either ACTH or angiotensin II stimulation. Hypercholesterolaemia, by diluting radiocholesterols in the expanded extracellular cholesterol pool and down-regulating LDL receptors, reduces adrenal radiocholesterol uptake and enhances hepatobiliary excretion (Lynn *et al.*, 1986).

It follows that several drugs may modify the uptake of adrenocortical scintigraphic agents (Table 11.3). In most cases, the drug effect can be predicted from its known actions on the simplified schema in Figure 11.1. Important exceptions are spironolactone (the mainstay of therapy for primary hyperaldosteronism) and the combination oral contraceptive pill (OCP). Spironolactone, in addition to its well-known aldosterone antagonism, inhibits aldosterone biosynthesis, at least in the first month of therapy (Conn and Hinerman, 1977). The combination OCP also has dual effects: the oestrogen increases hepatic synthesis of the renin substrate angiotensinogen, and increases plasma renin, while the progestagen induces a natriuresis which further promotes renin secretion; the net result is an increase in angiotensin II levels (Cain *et al.*, 1971). Clearly, proper interpretation of adrenal cortical scintiscans is critically dependent not only on a secure biochemical diagnosis of the syndrome in question but also on

Table 11.3 Clinically important modifiers of adrenocortical uptake of radiocholesterol analogues

Drug	*Effect on uptake*	*Mechanism*
Dexamethasone	Decrease (z. fasciculata/reticularis)	ACTH suppression
Spironolactone	Increase (z. glomerulosa)	Natriuresis + decr. aldosterone secretion and action = increased PRA*
Diuretics	Increase (z. glomerulosa)	Natriuresis = increased PRA
Oral contraceptives	Increase (z. glomerulosa)	Incr. angiotensinogen; increased PRA
Cholestyramine	Increase (all zones)	Decr. plasma cholesterol; Incr. LDL receptors

*PRA = plasma renin activity.

a careful drug history and exclusion of potential modifiers of radiocholesterol uptake.

11.2.2 CUSHING'S SYNDROME

Cushing's syndrome (CS) is due to excessive glucocorticoid secretion, usually associated to a greater or lesser extent with androgen excess. Pathogenetically, the syndrome may arise from one of several possible disorders: bilateral, symmetrical adrenocortical hyperplasia due to stimulation by ACTH from the anterior pituitary (Cushing's disease) or from an extrapituitary benign or malignant neoplasm (ectopic ACTH syndrome); or it may be due to a benign or malignant adrenal cortical tumour autonomously secreting excess cortisol. Rarely, CS results from autonomous cortical nodular hyperplasia (CNH) which, although bilateral, is typically asymmetrical. ACTH-secreting pituitary tumours are responsible for two-thirds of cases of CS. Ectopic ACTH secretion accounts for about 15% of cases, half of which are due to small-cell lung carcinoma. Adrenal cortical adenomas account for a further 10% of cases, and adrenal carcinomas and CNH each for approximately 5%.

The typical clinical features of CS include central obesity, facial plethora, hirsutism, acne, skin striae, easy bruising, proximal myopathy, menstrual disorders, psychological disturbance, hypertension, osteopenia, and varying degrees of carbohydrate intolerance. The ectopic ACTH syndrome, particularly if due to an underlying malignancy, may present atypically with cachexia, marked hyperpigmentation (due to the melanocyte-stimulating effects of the very high levels of ACTH and related peptides), severe diabetes and myopathy (due to the marked glucocorticoid excess), and hypokalaemic alkalosis (due to the high levels of the normally insignificant zona fasciculata/reticularis mineralocorticoids). Adrenal carcinomas synthesize steroids inefficiently, are usually large (greater than 5 cm in diameter) and have frequently spread locally by the time of presentation, and tend to produce more marked virilization than is usual in CS.

Irrespective of its pathogenesis, CS is characterized biochemically by excess cortisol secretion with loss of the diurnal variation in plasma cortisol levels. Integrated daily cortisol secretion is evaluated by measuring 24 h urinary free cortisol (UFC) levels. The response of UFC and plasma cortisol to attempted suppression with low (2 mg per day) and high (8 mg per day) doses of dexamethasone helps determine the aetiology of CS. Suppression to less than 50% of baseline values after the low dose effectively excludes CS. Suppression after high-dose but not low-dose dexamethasone is characteristic of Cushing's disease. Failure to suppress on either dose indicates either ACTH-independent CS (adrenal adenoma, carcinoma or CNH) or ectopic ACTH secretion. Specific assays for ACTH will distinguish between the last two possibilities: serum levels will be suppressed in ACTH-independent CS, whereas they will be high in the ectopic ACTH syndrome.

The scintigraphic patterns of radiocholesterol uptake in the various forms of CS reflect the underlying pathophysiology (Figure 11.2). In ACTH-dependent adrenal hyperplasia, radiocholesterol uptake is bilaterally increased, and the degree of uptake correlates closely with the 24 h UFC excretion (Gross *et al.*, 1981b); thus uptake in the ectopic ACTH syndrome is generally higher than in Cushing's disease. An autonomous adrenal cortical adenoma will demonstrate avid unilateral uptake; the suppression of pituitary ACTH secretion inhibits tracer uptake by the contralateral adrenal cortex (and the ipsilateral normal cortical tissue). Similarly, inhibition of contralateral

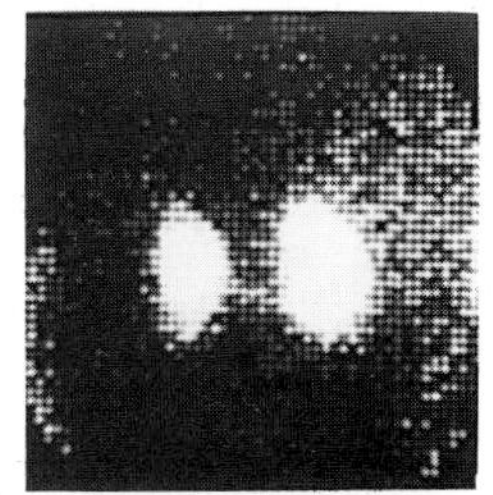

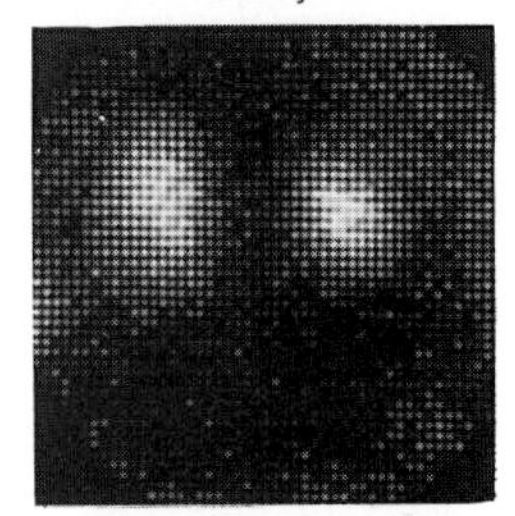

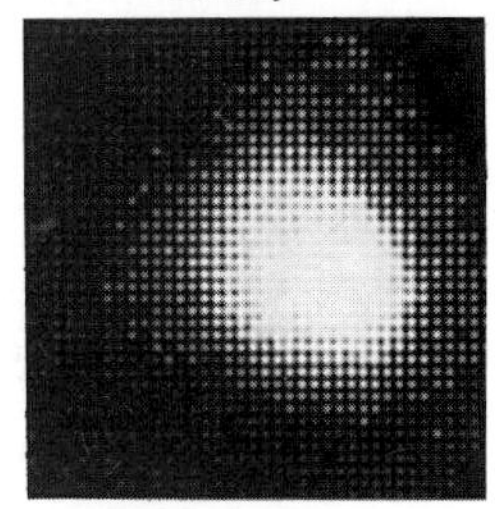

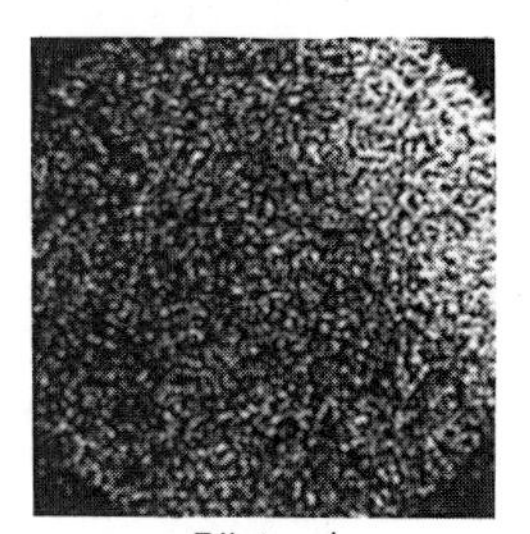

Figure 11.2 Patterns of adrenocortical scintigraphy in CS (NP-59, posterior scintiscans, no dexamethasone suppression). (Reproduced from Gross *et al.* (1982), with permission.)

radiocholesterol uptake occurs with functioning adrenal carcinomas; however, because cholesterol uptake per gram of tissue in these tumours is usually very low (Seabold *et al.*, 1977), the primary tumour is typically not visualized. Other causes of 'bilateral non-visualization' such as hypercholesterolaemia (a variable feature of CS) must be excluded in such cases. Radiocholesterol uptake by both primary and metastatic adrenocortical carcinoma has been reported rarely. Finally,

ACTH-independent CNH produces bilaterally but asymmetrically increased radiocholesterol uptake.

In clinical practice, adrenal cortical scintigraphy for CS is indicated only in patients with primary adrenal disease (Fig *et al.*, 1988). Once the biochemical diagnosis of ACTH-independent CS is made, abdominal CT is usually performed to locate the disease and define the surgical anatomy. CT will usually identify tumours larger than 1 cm, and will often demonstrate evidence of extra-adrenal spread by adrenal carcinomas. The larger the tumour, the greater the probability of malignancy; in large tumours without clear-cut CT signs of malignancy, scintigraphy will be helpful since 'bilateral non-visualization' will indicate the malignant nature of the tumour and allow appropriate surgical planning. Scintigraphy will reliably distinguish between adenoma and CNH; it is clearly indicated whenever the question of CNH arises – if CT has only identified a small tumour, if there appears to be more than one tumour, if there is any suggestion of a contralateral adrenal abnormality, in young patients, or in the very rare patient with intermittent or cyclical CS. Finally, in patients whose CS has relapsed after bilateral adrenalectomy for primary or secondary adrenocortical hyperplasia, scintigraphy is valuable for locating the functioning remnant(s) (Shapiro *et al.*, 1981).

11.2.3 PRIMARY HYPERALDOSTERONISM (CONN'S SYNDROME)

Excess aldosterone secretion by an adrenal cortical tumour (almost invariably benign) or by diffuse or nodular hyperplasia of the zona glomerulosa is characterized clinically by hypertension associated with hypokalaemia. Adenomas (aldosteronomas) account for 70% of cases. High circulating aldosterone levels result in kaliuresis, sodium retention and expansion of extracellular fluid volume with secondary inhibtion of renin release. It is essential to exclude more common causes of hypokalaemia among hypertensive patients, such as overt or covert use of diuretics and aperients. The diagnosis of primary hyperaldosteronism (PHA) rests on the demonstration of suppressed plasma renin activity (PRA) which cannot be stimulated by upright posture or frusemide administration, as well as elevated plasma or urinary aldosterone levels which cannot be suppressed by saline loading or exogenous mineralocorticoid administration. Adherence to these diagnostic criteria (viz. hypertension, unexplained hypokalaemia, suppressed PRA, non-suppressible aldosterone) will exclude the much more common cases of 'low-renin essential hypertension' (in whom K^+ and aldosterone levels are normal) and secondary hyperaldosteronism (in whom PRA is elevated), and the much rarer cases of desoxycorticosterone (DOC) excess and pseudohyperaldosteronism (in whom aldosterone levels are low).

The distinction between adenoma and hyperplasia as the cause of PHA is important, since the treatment is surgical in the former and medical in the latter. Biochemical clues in favour of an adenoma include: higher recumbent plasma aldosterone levels; no change (or a slight fall) in aldosterone levels after 2–4 h ambulation; and increased plasma levels of aldosterone precursors (DOC, corticosterone and 18-hydroxycorticosterone). However, the distinction ultimately depends upon localization studies. The standard has been selective adrenal vein sampling with comparison of the aldosterone : cortisol ratio in the effluent from each adrenal with the ratio in the peripheral circulation. In the case of an adenoma, the ratio is high on the affected side and aldosterone production is suppressed contralaterally. The technique is invasive, technically demanding, and associated with adrenal haemorrhage or infarction in 5% of cases.

As anticipated from the pathophysiology of PHA, patients with aldosteronoma have increased radiocholesterol uptake in the affected adrenal and normal uptake on the unaffected side, since ACTH-dependent uptake by the zona fasciculata/reticularis is unaffected. In bilateral hyperplasia, radiocholesterol uptake is increased bilaterally, often asymmetrically. However, since ACTH-dependent tissue normally accounts for 50% of adrenal radiocholesterol uptake (see above) and the normal range of radiocholesterol uptake is broad, there is a significant overlap between uptake in normals and in patients with PHA due to hyperplasia (Gross *et al.*, 1981a). The dexamethasone suppression (DS) adrenal scan was introduced to suppress the ACTH-dependent component of radiocholesterol uptake. In normal individuals, oral dexamethasone 1 mg every 6 h for seven days prior to injection of NP-59 and throughout the scanning period inhibits visualization of the adrenals until at least five days after injection (Gross *et al.*, 1979). Visualization at or

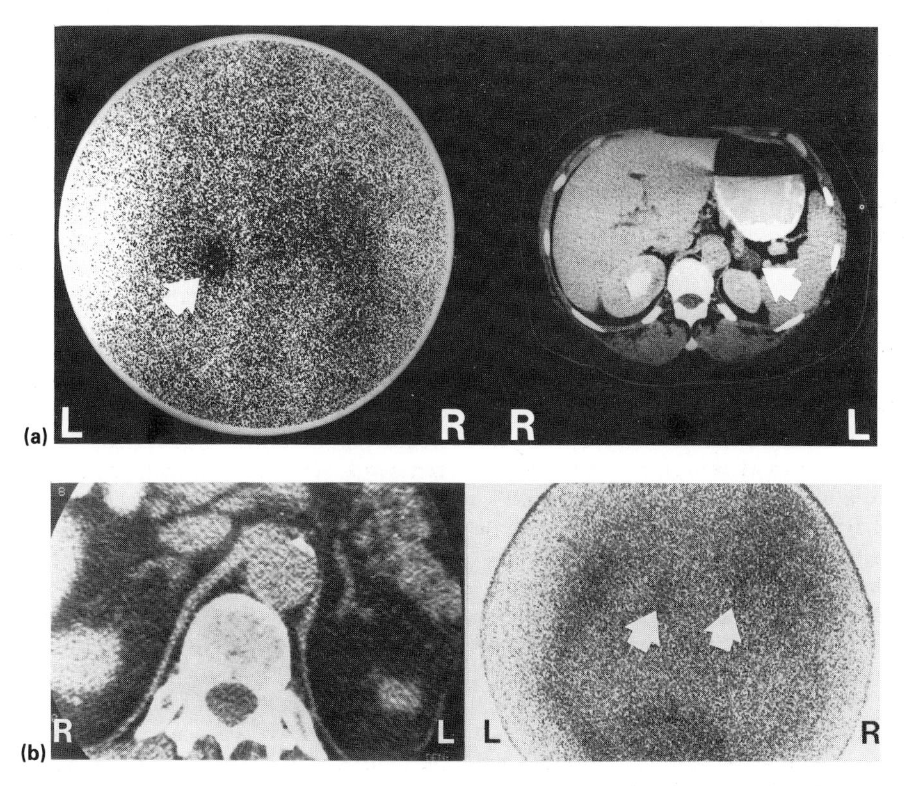

Figure 11.3 Dexamethasone-suppression adrenocortical scans in PHA (NP-59, 4 days after injection). (a) 2 cm left aldosteronoma (arrows). Right adrenal NP-59 uptake suppressed by dexamethasone. (b) Zona glomerulosa hyperplasia. The adrenals appeared morphologically normal on CT (left panel). Bilateral early uptake of NP-59 (left panel, arrows) despite dexamethasone.

beyond five days presumably reflects the 50% of normal radiocholesterol uptake that is ACTH independent. Unilateral or bilateral visualization earlier than five days after injection in patients with proven PHA indicates adenoma or hyperplasia, respectively (Figure 11.3). While quantification of NP-59 uptake on the DS adrenal scan has been shown to correlate with 24 h urinary aldosterone excretion (Gross *et al.*, 1983), the qualitative endpoint of early unilateral or bilateral visualization better separates adenoma from hyperplasia, since hyperplasia can produce such marked asymmetry of quantitative uptake as to suggest unilateral disease (Gross *et al.*, 1985). It should be noted that in the rare autosomal dominant variant, dexamethasone-suppressible PHA, early adrenal visualization will not occur. If it has not already been excluded during the patient's work-up, this possibility should be considered when the biochemical diagnosis of PHA appears secure but early radiocholesterol uptake is not seen on the DS scan.

Spironolactone should be withdrawn for three to four weeks prior to scintigraphy, since the spironolactone-induced increase in uptake by the contralateral zona glomerulosa in patients with unilateral adenoma may lead to a false diagnosis of hyperplasia (Fischer *et al.*, 1982). The same strictures apply to diuretics and the OCP (Table 11.3).

Since aldosteronomas are usually small (less than 2 cm) and have similar X-ray attenuation characteristics to normal adrenal cortical tissue, they are less readily detected on CT scans than the adenomas producing CS. Moreover, CT may not be able to distinguish between a solitary adenoma and a dominant hyperplastic nodule, and cannot reliably detect bilateral hyperplasia. Thus radiocholesterol scintigraphy plays an essential role in the non-invasive evaluation of PHA. If both

CT and scintigraphy demonstrate a unilateral adenoma, adrenalectomy can proceed without recourse to adrenal vein sampling. Since the diagnosis of adrenocortical hyperplasia implies a commitment to lifelong spironolactone therapy, adrenal vein sampling is indicated to confirm a scintigraphic diagnosis of hyperplasia, or when scintigraphy and CT disagree as to the side of unilateral disease (Gross *et al.*, 1984a).

11.2.4 VIRILISM (HYPERANDROGENISM)

Excessive ovarian or adrenal production of androgens in women causes hirsutism, menstrual disturbances or, in more severe cases, frank virilization. The major ovarian androgen is androstenedione, whereas the adrenal cortex secretes both androstenedione and DHEA-S. These weak androgens are converted to testosterone in the peripheral tissues. Measurement of circulating levels of all three androgens is required to establish the presence and the likely source(s) of hyperandrogenism in hirsute women. In general, the more marked the clinical degree of virilization, the higher the levels of testosterone and/or androstenedione and the greater the likelihood of an underlying ovarian or adrenal tumour; elevated DHEA-S levels point to an adrenal cause. The 24 h urinary excretion of 17-ketosteroids (17KS) provides an integrated measure of daily androgen secretion, but does not distinguish between ovarian and adrenal androgens. Clearly, CS must be ruled out if an adrenal cause is suspected.

In hirsute women with adrenal hyperandrogenism, DS adrenocortical scintigraphy (employing the same suppression regimen as described for PHA) demonstrates unilateral early visualization in patients with androgen-secreting adenomas and bilateral early visualization in patients with adrenal cortical hyperplasia (Gross *et al.*, 1985). In both cases, total adrenal uptake of radiocholesterol correlates with 24 h urinary 17KS excretion (Gross *et al.*, 1984b).

The combination OCP is frequently used to manage women with hirustism and menstrual disturbances, and should be stopped for one month prior to DS adrenocortical scintigraphy. Failure to recognize this may result in OCP-induced early visualization of the zona glomerulosa and an erroneous diagnosis of adrenal disease.

Ovarian causes of hyperandrogenism are more common than primary adrenal causes. The ovaries also take up radiocholesterols, and the ratio of ovarian to adrenal uptake is increased by dexamethasone suppression of adrenal cortical uptake. DS scintigraphy has been useful for defining the functional significance of ovarian enlargement discovered by ultrasonography or CT during the evaluation of hyperandrogenism. Indeed, the limited comparative data available indicate that DS scintigraphy is more accurate then either CT or selective adrenal/ovarian vein sampling in the differential diagnosis of hyperandrogenism (Taylor *et al.*, 1986).

The most common identifiable disorder in hirsute, oligomenorrhoeic or amenorrhoeic women is the polycystic ovary (Stein–Leventhal) syndrome (PCOS). The pathogenesis of PCOS is obscure, but abnormal adrenal androgen metabolism has frequently been demonstrated, probably as a secondary phenomenon. Adrenal radiocholesterol uptake (without prior dexamethasone suppression) tends to be bilaterally increased in these patients, with the mean uptake being similar to that found in patients with Cushing's disease (Gross *et al.*, 1986).

A rare adrenal cause of hyperandrogenism is **congenital adrenal hyperplasia** (CAH). The term refers to at least six autosomal recessive enzyme deficiencies, all of which involve the cortisol biosynthetic pathway and some of which also affect the synthesis of aldosterone and adrenal and gonadal sex steroids. The failure of cortisol synthesis results in ACTH-induced bilateral adrenal hyperplasia with overproduction of precursor steroids proximal to the synthetic block. The least rare variant is 21α-hydroxylase deficiency of the zona fasciculata/reticularis (Type I CAH) which is characterized biochemically by increased plasma 17-hydroxyprogesterone (17OHP) levels as well as increased DHEA-S. The classical clinical manifestations are pseudohermaphroditism with ambiguous external genitalia in female infants and precocious pseudopuberty in affected boys, as well as the sequelae of cortisol deficiency. However, Type I CAH appears to have several allelic variants; a late-onset form of the disease has recently been recognized in some hirsute women among whom 17OHP levels are elevated either spontaneously or in response to exogenous ACTH. As might be expected, adrenal radiocholesterol uptake is increased bilaterally in untreated or under-treated CAH, but is normal in patients who have received adequate long-term glucocorticoid replacement. 'Accessory' adrenal tissue in the broad ligament near the ovary and in the epididymis have been found scintigraphically in patients with CAH. While adrenocortical scintigraphy has no place in the routine diagnosis of CAH, it is likely that women with hyperandrogenism who demonstrate bilateral early adrenal visualization on the DS scan have a 'cryptic' variant of CAH.

One recommended approach to investigating virilized women with elevated basal DHEA-S levels is to measure the response of DHEA-S and 17OHP to ACTH stimulation and dexamethasone suppression. Positive results of these pharmacological tests indicate a variant of CAH and therapy with dexamethasone is advised. All other patients or patients with clinically impressive virilization should undergo a DS radiocholesterol study and confirmatory CT scans. Selective venous sampling studies should be reserved for those cases with equivocal findings on these non-invasive tests (Taylor *et al.*, 1986).

11.2.5 THE 'INCIDENTAL' ADRENAL MASS

The widespread availability of abdominal CT has resulted in the discovery of asymptomatic abnormalities of adrenal morphology in approximately 1% of examinations (Copeland, 1983). The frequency is considerably higher in CT scans performed in patients with known primary extra-adrenal malignancies, since the adrenal is a frequent site of metastasis, particularly for carcinomas of the lung, breast, stomach and kidney. However, over 50% of adrenal abnormalities in patients with known malignancies do *not* represent adrenal metastases. The CT appearance is usually non-specific and, unless there is clear evidence of spread beyond the adrenal indicating

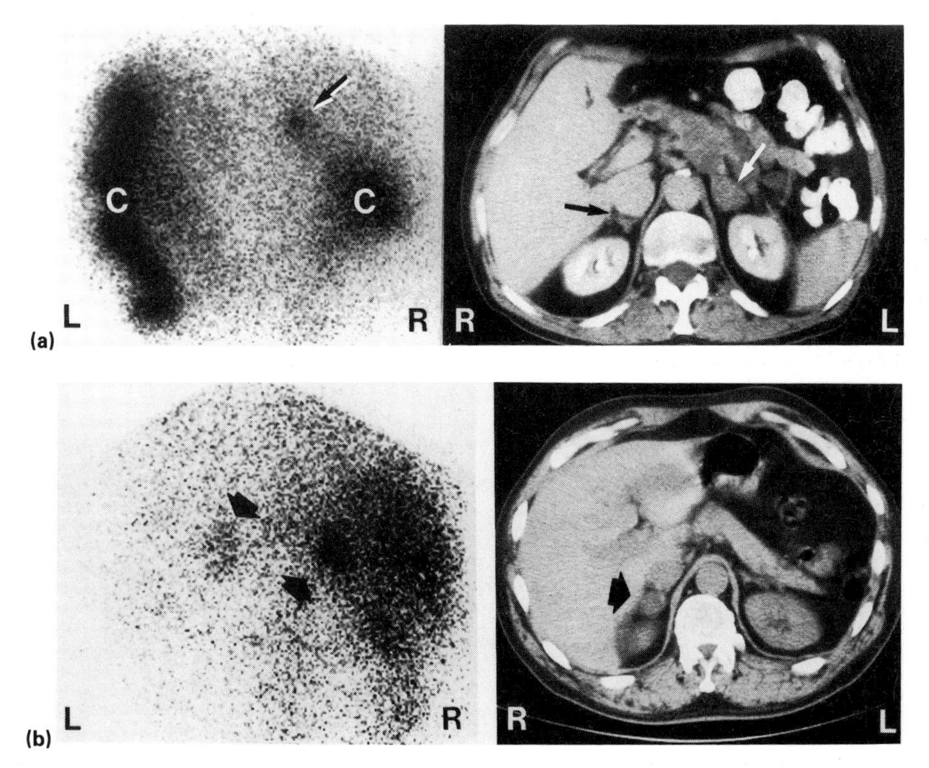

Figure 11.4 'Incidental' adrenal masses (NP-59, 5 days after injection, no dexamethasone suppression). (a) Discordant scintigraphy (left) and CT (right) left adrenal mass (right panel, white arrow) which failed to take up NP-59: metastatic adenocarcinoma on CT-guided biopsy. The right adrenal was morphologically and scintigraphically normal (black arrows). (C, NP-59 in colon.) (b) Concordant studies: 2 cm right adrenal mass (right panel, arrow) demonstrating higher uptake of NP-59 than the morphologically normal left adrenal. No biochemical evidence of adrenal cortical dysfunction (including adrenal vein sampling). (Reproduced from Gross *et al.* (1978), with permission.)

the mass to be malignant, the functional significance of the abnormality must be evaluated further.

Adrenal cortical or medullary hyperfunction needs to be excluded biochemically. Appropriate screening tests include plasma K^+ and DHEA-S, 24 h UFC, 24 h urinary excretion of vanillylmandelic acid (VMA) and/or metanephrines (see below), and an overnight dexamethasone suppression test. If these tests are negative, then the significance of the mass is best evaluated by quantitative radiocholesterol scintigraphy without dexamethasone suppression (Gross *et al.*, 1987). Absent or reduced tracer uptake on the side of the mass (discordant scintigraphy and CT, Figure 11.4(a)) indicates a non-functioning space-occupying lesion which merits further evaluation, usually by CT-guided needle biopsy. Depending on the patient population examined, 25–60% of these functionless lesions will prove to be adrenal metastases. Functioning masses (concordant studies, Figure 11.4(b)) have invariably been found to consist of benign adrenocortical tissue – no further intervention beyond periodic re-evaluation seems warranted in these cases. Whether this biochemically 'non-hyperfunctioning' adenomatous tissue will ultimately become autonomous is currently under investigation.

11.2.6 SUMMARY

The limited range of pathology responsible for adrenal cortical hyperfunction (viz. adenoma, carcinoma, bilateral hyperplasia) is reflected in the narrow repertoire of possible findings on radiocholesterol scintigraphy (Table 11.4). It is therefore essential to the intelligent performance and interpretation of these studies that the clinical, biochemical and anatomical findings be reviewed before the scan is done.

Adrenocortical scintigraphy is of proven value in the evaluation of ACTH-independent CS, PHA and the incidental adrenal mass. It is helpful in the differential diagnosis of virilism. Yet it remains an underutilized technique. The need for several visits by the patient is inconvenient, and the dosimetry, although by no means unacceptable, is less favourable than is usual for nuclear medicine studies. However, time and effort devoted to the proper evaluation of the patient is well spent. To perform a unilateral adrenalectomy mistakenly in a patient with bilateral disease is to do a gross disservice, and it is precisely this type of patient who is most likely to benefit from adrenocortical scintigraphy.

Nevertheless, the search continues for agents which can be labelled with ^{123}I or ^{99m}Tc in order to improve dosimetry and imaging characteristics. Because of the shorter physical half-lives of these radionuclides, such an agent would need to achieve adequate target-to-background ratios of activity within 12–24 h of injection. Radioiodinated 11β-hydroxylase inhibitors (metyrapol and SKF-12185) and pregnenolone esters have shown promise in animal studies but have not been used clinically.

11.3 ADRENAL MEDULLA

11.3.1 PHYSIOLOGY

Catecholamines are derived from the amino acid L-tyrosine. The first committed (and rate-

Table 11.4 Summary of scintigraphic findings in adrenocortical disorders

Disorder	*Pathology*	*Scintigraphy*
Cushing's syndrome	Adenoma	Ipsilateral incr. uptake, contralateral suppression
	Hyperplasia	Bilateral incr. uptake (may be asymmetrical)
	Carcinoma	Bilateral non-visualization
Primary hyperaldosteronism	Adenoma	Unilateral early visualization*
	Hyperplasia	Bilateral early visualization*
Virilism	Adenoma	Unilateral early visualization*
	Hyperplasia	Bilateral early visualization*
	(Ovarian)	(Ovarian visualization)*
'Incidental' mass	Space-occupying lesion	Ipsilateral decr. uptake
	'Non-hyperfunctioning' adenoma	Ipsilateral incr. uptake

*Dexamethasone-suppression scans.

determining) step in the catecholamine biosynthetic pathway is the hydroxylation of tyrosine to dihydroxyphenylalanine (dopa), catalysed by tyrosine hydroxylase. Dopa is decarboxylated in the cytosol to dopamine, which is taken up into the catecholamine storage vesicles, where it is hydroxylated to noradrenaline.

The above pathway is common to both adrenergic neurones and the adrenal medulla. The major blood supply to the adrenal medulla is via an adrenal portal system derived from the cortical sinusoidal plexus. The resulting high medullary level of cortisol induces and maintains the activity of the enzyme phenylethanolamine-*N*-methyltransferase (PNMT), which catalyses the methylation of noradrenaline to adrenaline.

Noradrenaline and adrenaline are stored in membrane-bounded storage vesicles in association with soluble proteins (chromogranins) and nucleotides (mainly ATP). Stimulation of the adrenal medulla by the preganglionic, cholinergic splanchnic nerves or by other secretagogues (angiotensin, serotonin, histamine, bradykinin) causes release of the vesicle contents by exocytosis. Some of the released catecholamines diffuse from the medullary interstitium (or, in the case of adrenergic neurones, from the synaptic cleft) into the general circulation. However, most of the catecholamines are inactivated locally simply by reuptake via a stereospecific, sodium- and energy-dependent, saturable pathway (*uptake-1*). This process is inhibited by reserpine, tricyclic antidepressants, cocaine and sympathomimetics such as amphetamines and phenylpropanolamine. Following re-uptake, the catecholamines are stored or, if unstored, are rapidly degraded by monoamine oxidase (MAO) to dihydroxymandelic acid. Circulating catecholamines are inactivated predominantly in extraneuronal, extra-adrenal tissues by uptake via a non-specific, sodium-independent mechanism (*uptake-2*), rapidly followed by metabolism by catechol-*o*-methyltransferase (COMT) to metanephrines (normetadrenaline and metadrenaline). Dihydroxymandelic acid and the metanephrines are both metabolized further (by COMT and MAO, respectively) to 3-methoxy-4-hydroxymandelic acid (Vanillylmandelic acid, VMA). Dopamine undergoes a similar metabolic sequence to homovanillic acid (HVA).

11.3.2 PHAEOCHROMOCYTOMA

Phaeochromocytomas are neoplasms arising from mature adrenal medullary cells (phaeochromocytes). They produce a well-known syndrome of hypertension associated with a classical triad of paroxysmal headache, palpitation and sweating attributable to episodic hypersecretion of catecholamines. The same syndrome can be produced by catecholamine-secreting tumours arising from the extra-adrenal paraganglia (functioning paragangliomas, 'extra-adrenal phaeochromocytomas') which include the organ of Zuckerkandl (caudal to the origin of the inferior mesenteric artery) and the 'chemoreceptor' organs such as the carotid bodies.

While hypertension is virtually a constant feature of this syndrome, it is paroxysmal in fewer than half of the cases. Most patients have sustained hypertension with or without further paroxysmal increases. The syndrome is rare, affecting only an estimated 0.1% of the hypertensive population. However, a high index of suspicion is essential, since these tumours have potentially life-threatening cardiovascular effects and their successful resection is curative. Important clinical clues include the presence of orthostatic hypotension in an untreated hypertensive, resistance of the hypertension to standard therapy (including possible exacerbation by β-blockers due to unopposed α-adrenergic peripheral vasoconstriction), and failure of the blood pressure to fall at night.

In most cases, the diagnosis can be established by demonstrating high urinary levels of free catecholamines and their metabolites (metanephrines and VMA). Adjustment of the excretion rates for creatinine excretion will correct for individual differences in body mass and renal function, and for incomplete urine collections. The use of specific assays has significantly remedied earlier problems with dietary and drug interferences. When the diagnosis is still strongly suspected in the face of equivocal urinary chemistry results, measurement of plasma catecholamines basally in the fasting, unstressed, recumbent state and again 2–3 h after a single 300 μg oral dose of clonidine may be diagnostic (Bravo and Gifford, 1984). In normal subjects and essential hypertensives, central α-stimulation by clonidine will produce a reflex reduction in peripheral neuronal catecholamine release; in patients with phaeochromocytoma, whose catecholamine levels reflect uncontrolled diffusion of excess hormone from the autonomous tumour into the circulation, levels will not be suppressed by clonidine.

Most phaeochromocytomas arise in the adrenal medulla. However, this condition has been referred to as 'the ten per cent disease' since approximately 10% of patients have bilateral adrenal tumours, 10% have extra-adrenal tumours, and 10% have malignant tumours (defined by local invasion or distant metastases). Ten per cent of cases are associated with one or other of the following autosomal dominant syndromes: multiple endocrine neoplasia (MEN) type 2a Sipple's syndrome) or 2b (the mucosal neuroma syndrome); neurofibromatosis (von Recklinghausen's disease); Lindau-von Hippel disease; or the syndrome of familial phaeochromocytomas with or without paragangliomas. Finally, 10% of phaeochromocytomas occur in children, among whom bilaterality, multiplicity and malignancy of tumours are more frequent than in adults. The finding of bilateral phaeochromocytomas should always raise the strong suspicion of a familial syndrome and should prompt a search for medullary thyroid carcinoma (MTC), characteristic of MEN-2a and 2b, as well as screening of family members for both phaeochromocytoma and MTC.

The first successful scintigraphic demonstration of phaeochromocytomas in man was reported in 1981, using a new radiopharmaceutical, ^{131}I-*meta*-iodobenzylguanidine (MIBG) (Sisson *et al.*, 1981). Since that report, extensive worldwide experience with this agent in large series of patients has shown uniformly high sensitivity (87%) and specificity (97%) of ^{131}I-MIBG for locating adrenal (Figure 11.5) and extra-adrenal (Figure 11.6)

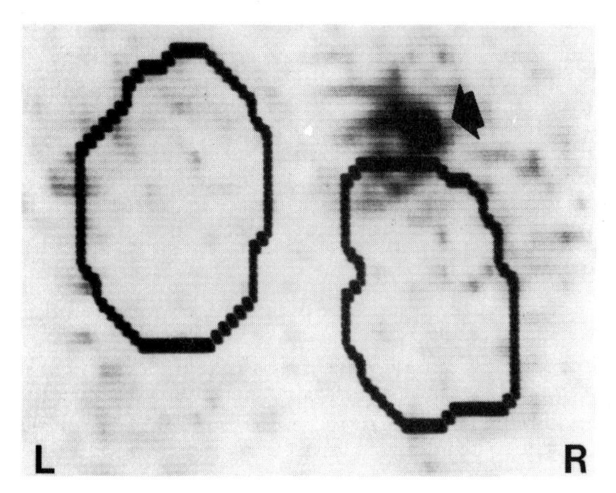

Figure 11.5 Right adrenal phaeochromocytoma (^{131}I-MIBG, posterior scintiscan, 48 h after injection). The renal outlines had been defined with ^{99m}Tc-labelled DTPA. Note reduced MIBG uptake by the partially necrotic inferomedial part of the tumour.

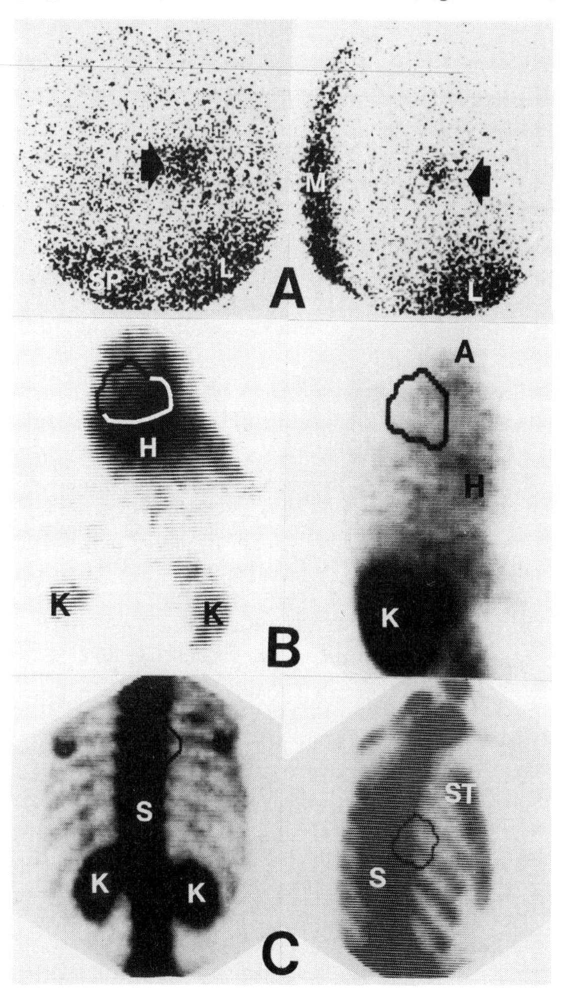

Figure 11.6 Left atrial phaeochromocytoma. Previous thoracic CT and exploratory thoracotomy had been negative. (a) Posterior (left) and right lateral (right) ^{131}I-MIBG scintiscans of chest, with area of abnormal uptake (arrow). (M, marker on spine; L, liver and SP, splenic uptake.) (b) ^{99m}Tc-labelled red cell blood pool images (anterior (left) and right lateral (right) views), with region of abnormal ^{131}I-MIBG uptake superimposed. (A, aortic arch; H, cardiac blood pool; K, kidney.) (c) ^{99m}Tc-labelled MDP bone scan (posterior (left) and right posterior oblique (right) views), with region of abnormal ^{131}I-MIBG uptake superimposed. (K, kidney; S, spine; ST, sternum.) (Reproduced from Shapiro *et al.* (1984a), with permission.)

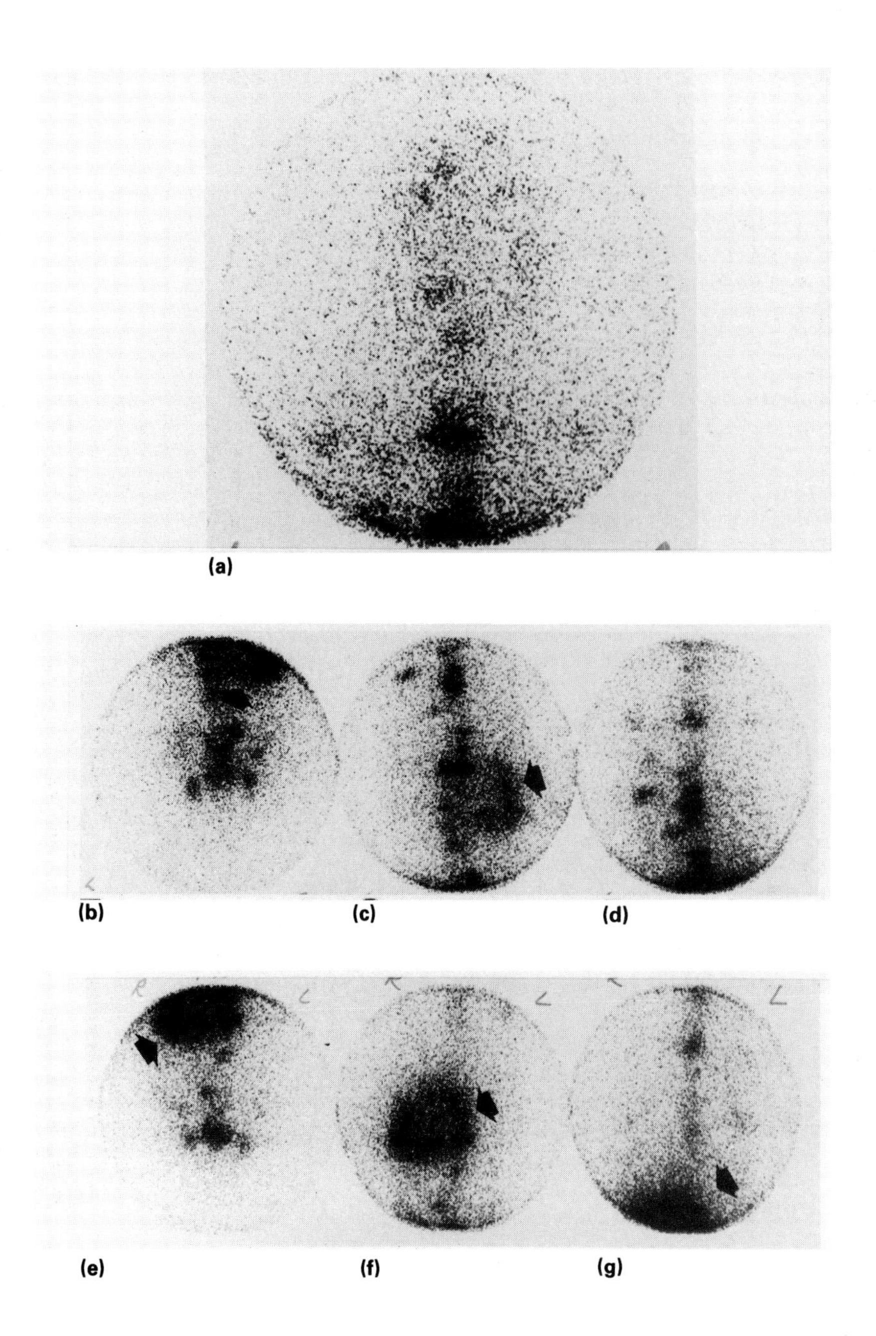

Figure 11.7 Malignant phaeochromocytoma. Widespread skeletal metastases demonstrated with ^{131}I-MIBG. (a) anterior head and neck; (b) posterior pelvis; (c) posterior abdomen; (d) posterior chest; (e) anterior pelvis; (f) anterior abdomen; (g) anterior chest. Arrows (c, e, f, g) indicate right adrenal primary – note photopenic, necrotic centre. (Reproduced from Shapiro *et al.* (1984b), with permission.)

tumour sites and metastases of malignant phaeochromocytoma (Figure 11.7) (Ackery *et al.*, 1984; Fischer *et al.*, 1984a; Shapiro *et al.*, 1984a, 1984b; Chatal and Charbonnel, 1985; Shapiro *et al.*, 1985; Swensen *et al.*, 1985). Whereas the sensitivity of CT approaches 100% for adrenal tumours greater than 2 cm in diameter, ^{131}I-MIBG has greater specificity for adrenal disease and has clearly superior sensitivity for smaller tumours and extra-adrenal sites. It can also detect preneoplastic adrenal medullary hyperplasia in asymptomatic affected relatives of patients with MEN-2a or 2b (Valk *et al.*, 1981).

11.3.3 RADIOPHARMACOLOGY

MIBG is an aralkylguanidine which structurally resembles noradrenaline sufficiently to be recognized by the uptake-1 mechanism and to be stored in the catecholamine storage vesicles (Tobes *et al.*, 1985). Whereas unstored noradrenaline is rapidly degraded, the halogenated benzyl ring of MIBG confers resistance to COMT while its guanidino side-chain is resistant to MAO. After the intravenous injection of ^{131}I-MIBG, approximately 50% of the administered radioactivity appears in the urine by 24 h and 70–90% is recovered within four days; 75–90% of the urinary activity is in the form of unaltered MIBG, with *meta*-iodohippuric acid and free iodide accounting for most of the remainder. There is thus little *in vivo* metabolism of MIBG (Mangner *et al.*, 1986).

Uptake of MIBG is inhibited both *in vitro* and *in vivo* by the uptake-1 inhibitors listed above (Table 11.5) (Tobes *et al.*, 1985). Phenylpropanolamine and other sympathomimetics are frequent constituents of non-prescription 'decongestants', cough remedies, and anorectic 'diet aids', the use of which should be specifically ruled out. Preliminary experience *in vivo* indicates that the combined α- and β-adrenergic blocking drug labetalol reduces uptake and/or retention of MIBG by phaeochromocytomas and adrenergic tissues (Khafagi *et al.*, 1989); this remains to be confirmed *in vitro*. However, other α- and β-blockers do not affect MIBG uptake and should *not* be discontinued in preparation for scintigraphy. There is evidence that concurrent calcium channel blockade, particularly with verapamil, inhibits MIBG uptake, but that the introduction of calcium channel blockers after MIBG injection prolongs the retention of MIBG (Jaques *et al.*, 1987).

Table 11.5 Drugs which interfere with MIBG uptake

Reserpine
Tricyclic antidepressants
Cocaine
Amphetamines
Phenylpropanolamine
Labetalol
Calcium-channel blockers

^{131}I-MIBG is normally taken up by liver, spleen, myocardium and the salivary glands (Nakajo *et al.*, 1983a; Shapiro *et al.*, 1985). Thyroid uptake of liberated radioiodide will also occur unless the thyroid is blocked with stable iodide. The normal adrenal glands are usually not seen, but faint uptake may be visible 48–72 h after injection in up to 16% of cases. Hepatic uptake is maximal at 24 h, declining to very low levels by 72 h; the rate of decline may be even more rapid in patients with phaeochromocytoma. Intraluminal colonic uptake is seen in 15–20% of cases and may mimic or obscure tumour activity. Splenic, myocardial and salivary gland uptake reflect the rich sympathetic innervation of these organs – thus salivary gland uptake cannot be blocked by perchlorate or iodide, but is reduced on the affected side in patients with Horner's syndrome or stellate ganglion blockade. The degree of

Table 11.6 Dosimetry of MIBG

	^{131}I-MIBG	*^{123}I-MIBG*
Dose (adult)	18.5 MBq (0.5 mCi)	370 MBq (10 mCi)
Dosimetry (cGy/dose)		
Adrenal	50	8–28*
thyroid†	18	22–26*
ovaries	0.5	0.6–0.7*
liver	0.2	0.5
whole body	0.05	0.2

*0–1.4% ^{125}I contamination.
†No thyroid blockade.

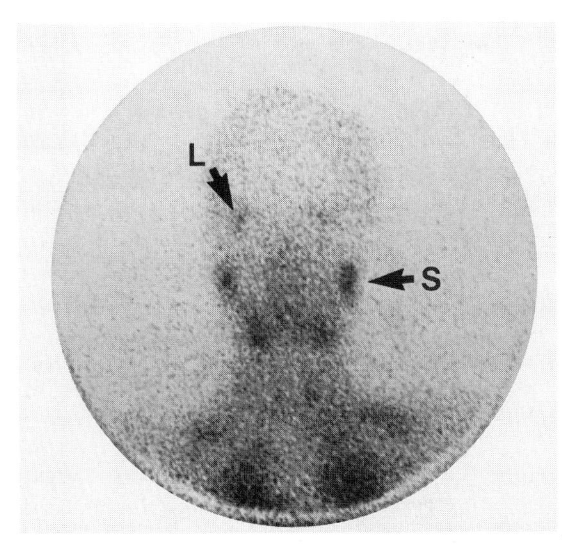

Figure 11.10 Anterior skull image of 400 000 counts, 4 h post-injection. (L) indicates uptake of ^{123}I-MIBG by the lacrimal glands, (S) indicates salivary gland uptake.

bladder activity may obscure pelvic or bladder tumour foci. Thus pelvic views are best obtained immediately after the patient has voided. Alternatively, simultaneous dual-window data acquisition following the injection of 74 MBq of ^{99m}Tc-labelled DTPA with subsequent computer-assisted subtraction of urinary tract activity may be used. The same principle, using the appropriate ^{99m}Tc-labelled radiopharmaceutical, has been used to clarify the relationship of abnormal MIBG uptake to bone, the liver or the cardiac blood pool (Figure 11.6).

Other radiolabelled aralkylamines have been investigated as potential adrenal medullary scintigraphic agents. None has demonstrated superiority over MIBG in animal or limited human studies so far.

11.3.4 NEUROBLASTOMA AND OTHER 'NEUROENDOCRINE' TUMOURS

Neuroblastomas are highly malignant neural crest tumours. They are the second most common solid malignancy of childhood, and 90% of cases occur before the age of 10 years. Approximately 50% of the primary tumours arise in the adrenals, 25% in the abdominal sympathetic ganglia and 15% in the posterior mediastinum. They are locally invasive and metastasize to liver, skin, bone and bone marow. Although they secrete catecholamines (mainly dopamine), these are extensively metabolized within the tumour itself, so that urinary levels of VMA and HVA are disproportionately elevated and hypertension is unusual. More common presentations are with an abdominal mass, fever of unknown origin, anaemia, haematuria, cord compression or pathological fracture. Other circulating biochemical markers of disease activity include carcinofetal isoferritins (detected as high serum ferritin) and neurone-specific enolase.

Prognosis and correct treatment are critically dependent on accurate staging, which should include abdominal and thoracic CT scans to assess the extent of primary disease, bone scans and bone marrow examinations. Neuroblastomas and their metastases have now been shown regularly to take up ^{131}I-MIBG (Kimmig *et al.*, 1984; Geatti *et al.*, 1985; Munkner, 1985; Hoefnagel *et al.*, 1987). MIBG uptake in the extremities may be a more sensitive index of skeletal involvement than conventional ^{99m}Tc-labelled MDP bone scans, in which the distinction between metastatic disease and normal childhood epiphyseal uptake is often difficult (Figure 11.9).

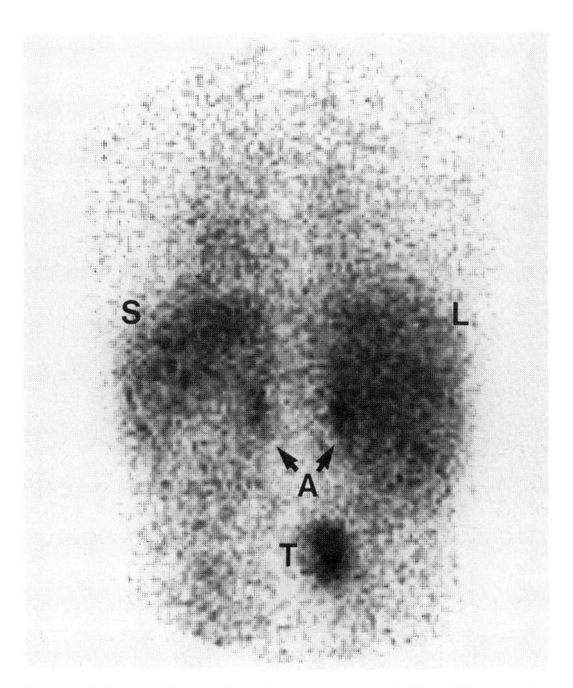

Figure 11.11 Posterior chest image of 400 000 counts, 22 h post-injection. (A) = normal adrenal medulla, (L) = liver, (S) = spleen, (T) = tumour (paraganglioma).

A number of tumours other than phaeochromocytomas and neuroblastomas have been shown sporadically to take up MIBG. They include non-functioning paragangliomas, MTC, carcinoid tumours, Merkel cell tumour of the skin, and metastases from these tumours (Hoefnagel *et al.*, 1987; Von Moll *et al.*, 1987). Although these tumours do not actively secrete catecholamines, they are all thought to originate from the neural crest – they retain the mechanisms for Amine Precursor Uptake and Decarboxylation (hence, 'APUDomas') and have typical dense-core neurosecretory granules on electron microscopy. Uptake of MIBG by these tumours is likely to be via a mechanism similar or identical to uptake-1.

11.3.5 THERAPY WITH ^{131}I-MIBG

Following the demonstration of ^{131}I-MIBG uptake by metastases of malignant phaeochromocytoma and neuroblastoma, it was hoped that MIBG would prove to be a useful therapeutic agent for these conditions. The cautious optimism raised by early reports (Sisson *et al.*, 1984; Fischer *et al.*, 1984b) has been borne out for only a small minority of malignant phaeochromocytomas, which are relatively radioresistant tumours. Currently, therapy with high doses (7.4 GBq per dose) of ^{131}I-MIBG is indicated only in patients with progressive disease who have failed conventional therapy or with intractable bone pain from skeletal metastases, and only if a previous dosimetric study has predicted a delivered tumour dose of over 0.5 cGy/MBq. An improved method for calculating tumour dosimetry has recently been described (Shulkin *et al.*, 1988). Total tumour doses in excess of 200 Gy are probably necessary to achieve a therapeutic effect; bone marrow toxicity is the limiting factor. Such therapy should be considered palliative only. It must be emphasized that the degree of MIBG uptake cannot be predicted from the biochemical activity of the tumour as assessed by plasma or urinary levels of catecholamines or their metabolites.

Neuroblastomas are inherently more radiosensitive than malignant phaeochromocytomas. Encouraging reports of successful palliative therapy of neuroblastoma with ^{131}I-MIBG following the failure of chemotherapy and conventional teleradiotherapy (Munkner, 1985; Hoefnagel *et al.*, 1987) have prompted a multicentre evaluation of the role of radiopharmacotherapy in this disease. This study is currently under way.

11.3.6 SUMMARY

In the relatively brief period since its development, MIBG has proved to be a safe, sensitive and highly specific agent for the location of phaeochromocytoma and neuroblastoma. Its use is clearly indicated in the evaluation of patients with these diseases, whether or not CT scanning has been positive. ^{123}I-MIBG should always be considered the radiopharmaceutical of choice for imaging purposes if it is available. Although MIBG uptake has been demonstrated by a variety of other tumours of presumed neural crest origin, its routine use in these situations is not warranted. The role of ^{131}I-MIBG in the therapy of malignant phaeochromocytoma and neuroblastoma remains to be clarified.

11.4 TECHNIQUES OF ADRENAL SCINTIGRAPHY

The technical aspects of adrenal cortical and medullary scintigraphy are summarized in Table 11.7.

As has already been emphasized, drugs known to interfere with the behaviour of the radiopharmaceutical to be used must be identified and withdrawn; in the case of cortical scintigraphy, this should be done several weeks beforehand. The biochemical diagnosis must be reviewed.

If DS cortical scintigraphy is indicated, the patient should take 1 mg dexamethasone orally every 6 h, beginning seven days before tracer injection and continuing for the duration of the study.

In order to minimize colonic retention of radiocholesterols, bisacodyl 5–10 mg at night should be prescribed, to start two nights before the first scan and to continue throughout the study period. Bisacodyl does not affect the enterohepatic circulation of cholesterol or bile salts (Shapiro *et al.*, 1983). In the case of suspected ovarian radiocholesterol uptake, colonic activity must be rigorously excluded and enemata may be required to ensure adequate bowel cleansing. Bisacodyl is also useful in the small proportion of patients who have potentially confusing bowel uptake on MIBG scans.

Patients receiving radioiodinated tracers require thyroid blockade with stable iodide during

Table 11.7 Techniques of adrenal scintigraphy

Radiopharmaceutical	*NP-59*	*SMC*	*^{131}I-MIBG*	*^{123}I-MIBG*
Thyroid blockade	2 d before to 14 d p.i.*	Not required	2 d before to 6 d p.i.	2 d before to 4 d p.i.
Dose (i.v.)	37 MBq per 1.7 m^2	9.25 MBq (0.12 MBq kg^{-1})	18.5 MBq per 1.7 m^2 (max. 37 MBq)	74–370 MBq (adult)
Imaging interval	Non-DS: 5 (7)† d p.i. DS: 3, 4 (5) d p.i.	7 (14) d p.i.‡	24, 48 (72) h p.i.	2–3, 24 (48) h p.i.
Camera	Wide field of view, interfaced with a computer			
Collimator	High-energy	Med.-energy	High-energy	Med.-energy
Photopeak, window	364 keV, 30%	137 keV, 20% (265 keV, 20%)	364 keV, 20%	159 keV, 20%
Views§	Posterior abdomen; lateral abdomen with thoracolumbar spine marker		Posterior abdomen; overlapping anterior views from pubis to skull vertex. Markers on iliac crests, lateral costal margins, axillae. Other localization procedures (e.g. ^{99m}Tc-labelled DTPA)	
Counting time/ counts (per view)	20 min/100 K	20 min/200 K (±SPECT)	20 min/100 K	10 min (3 h p.i.); 20 min/1 M (±SPECT)

*Abbreviations: p.i. = post-injection; DS = dexamethasone suppression; K = thousand counts; M = million counts.
†Numbers in parentheses indicate optional additional imaging times.
‡There is no published experience of use of DS scans with SMC.
§Minimum recommended views; additional views as clinically indicated.

the intervals indicated in Table 11.7. This is administered as one drop of SSKI or two of Lugol's solution thrice daily – SSKI is more palatable. Patients allergic to iodine may be given potassium perchlorate 200 mg every 8 h after meals or triiodothyronine 20 μg every 8 h.

Radiocholesterols are dissolved in an alcoholic vehicle containing Tween-80 and should be injected slowly, over 3 min, to avoid extremity pain or discomfort. MIBG could theoretically displace noradrenaline from storage vesicles; phentolamine should therefore be on hand, and the tracer should be injected slowly, over 2–3 min, with monitoring of vital signs before and 15 min and 60 min after injection. It is worth emphasizing that no significant adverse reactions have yet been reported.

The activity in the injection syringe should be measured before and after injection for accurate calculation of the administered dose. This step is essential if tracer uptake is to be quantified.

The patient should be imaged supine to minimize differences in adrenal depth, although the adrenals are far more constant in position than the kidneys.

Adrenal tracer uptake is calculated using an operator-semi-independent computer algorithm (Koral and Sarkar, 1977). The sensitivity and efficiency of the camera–collimator system for known activities at different depths in tissue-equivalent material must first be determined from phantom studies. From the posterior scintiscan, the computer locates the *XY* co-ordinates of the centre of each adrenal and determines the edge of gland activity. A two-pixel background region then circumscribes this edge. Adrenal depth (in pixels) is determined from the lateral (marker) view. Counts from each adrenal region of interest are then corrected for background activity and depth attenuation. Given the precise dose administered, the time interval since injection, and the sensitivity of the camera–collimator system, the net adrenal counts are decay-corrected and translated into actual uptake, expressed as a percentage of the administered dose.

REFERENCES

Ackery, D. M. *et al.* (1984) New approach to the localisation of phaeochromocytoma: imaging with iodine-

131-*meta*-iodobenzylguanidine. *Br. Med. J.*, **288**, 1587–91.

Beierwaltes, W. H. *et al.* (1971), Visualization of human adrenal glands *in vivo* by scintillation scanning. *JAMA*, **216**, 275–7.

Bomanji, J. and Britton, K. E. (1987) Uterine uptake of iodine-123 metaiodobenzylguanidine during the menstrual phase of uterine cycle. *Clin. Nucl. Med.*, **12**, 601–3.

Bomanji, J. *et al.* (1987a) Quantitation of *meta* (I-123) iodobenzylguanidine uptake by normal adrenal medulla in hypertensive patients. *J. Nucl. Med.*, **28**, 319–24.

Bomanji, J. *et al.* (1987b) Uptake of I-123 metaiodobenzylguanidine by phaeochromocytomas, other paragangliomas and neuroblastomas: a histopathological comparison. *J. Nucl. Med.*, **28**, 973–8.

Bomanji, J. *et al.* (1987c) Observations on the function of normal adrenomedullary tissue in phaeochromocytomas and paragangliomas. *Eur. J. Nucl. Med.*, **13**, 86–9.

Bomanji, J. *et al.* (1988) Imaging neural crest tumours with I-123 metaiodobenzylguanidine and X-ray computed tomography: a comparative study. *Clin. Rad.*, **39**, 502–6.

Bravo, E. L. and Gifford, R. W. (1984) Pheochromocytoma: diagnosis, localization and management. *N. Engl. J. Med.*, **311**, 1298–303.

Cain, M. D. *et al.* (1971) Effects of oral contraceptive therapy on the renin–angiotensin system. *J. Clin. Endocrinol. Metab.*, **33**, 671–6.

Carey, J. E. *et al.* (1979) Absorbed dose to the human adrenals from iodomethyl-norcholesterol (I-131), 'NP-59'. *J. Nucl. Med.*, **20**, 60–1.

Chatal, J. F. and Charbonnel, B. (1985) Comparison of iodobenzylguanidine imaging with computed tomography in locating pheochromocytoma. *J. Clin. Endocrinol. Metab.*, **61**, 769–72.

Conn, J. W. and Hinerman, D. L. (1977) Spironolactone-induced inhibition of aldosterone biosynthesis in primary hyperaldosteronism: morphological and functional studies. *Metabolism*, **26**, 1293–307.

Copeland, P. M. (1983) The incidentally discovered adrenal mass. *Ann. Intern. Med.*, **98**, 940–5.

Fig. L. M. *et al.* (1988). Adrenal localization in ACTH-independent Cushing's syndrome. *Ann. Intern. Med.*, **109**, 547–53.

Fischer, M. *et al.* (1982) Adrenal scintigraphy in primary aldosteronism: spironolactone as a cause of incorrect classification between adenoma and hyperplasia. *Eur. J. Nucl. Med.*, **7**, 222–4.

Fischer, M. *et al.* (1984a) 131I-metaiodobenzylguanidine: a new agent for scintigraphic imaging and treatment of pheochromocytoma. *Nuklearmedizin*, **23**, 77–9.

Fischer, M. *et al.* (1984b) Nuclear medical therapy of pheochromocytoma. *Schweiz. Med. Wochenschr.*, **114**, 1841–3.

Geatti, O. *et al.* (1985), ^{131}I-metaiodobenzylguanidine (131I-MIBG) scintigraphy for the localization of neuroblastoma: preliminary experience in 10 cases. *J. Nucl. Med.*, **26**, 736–42.

Gross, M. D. *et al.* (1979) The normal dexamethasone-suppression adrenal scan. *J. Nucl. Med.*, **20**, 1131–5.

Gross, M. D. *et al.* (1981a) The role of pharmacologic manipulation in adrenal cortical scintigraphy. *Semin. Nucl. Med.*, **9**, 128–48.

Gross, M. D. *et al.* (1981b) The relationship of adrenal iodomethylnorcholesterol uptake to indices of adrenal cortical function in Cushing's syndrome. *J. Clin. Endocrinol. Metab.*, **52**, 1062–6.

Gross, M. D. *et al.* (1982) Scintigraphic approach to the localization of adrenal lesions causing hypertension. *Urol. Radiol.*, **3**, 241–4.

Gross, M. D. *et al.* (1983) The relationship of adrenal gland iodomethylnorcholesterol uptake to zona glomerulosa function in primary aldosteronism. *J. Clin. Endocrinol. Metab.*, **57**, 477–81.

Gross, M. D. *et al.* (1984a) Scintigraphic localization of adrenal lesions in primary aldosteronism. *Am. J. Med.*, **77**, 839–44.

Gross, M. D. *et al.* (1984b) The relationship of I-131 6beta-iodomethyl-19-norcholesterol (NP-59) adrenal cortical uptake to indices of androgen secretion in women with hyperandrogenism. *Clin. Nucl. Med.*, **9**, 264–70.

Gross, M. D. *et al.* (1985) Limited significance of asymmetric adrenal visualization on dexamethasone-suppression scintigraphy. *J. Nucl. Med.*, **26**, 43–8.

Gross, M. D. *et al.* (1986) Scintigraphic evidence of adrenal cortical dysfunction in the polycystic ovary syndrome. *J. Clin. Endocrinol. Metab.*, **62**, 197–201.

Gross, M. D. *et al.* (1988) Distinguishing benign from malignant enadrenal masses. *Ann. Intern. Med.*, **109**, 613–18.

Hawkins, L. A. *et al.* (1980) ^{75}Se selenomethyl cholesterol: a new agent for quantitative functional scintigraphy of the adrenals: physical aspects. *Br. J. Radiol.*, **53**, 883–9.

Hoefnagel, C. A. *et al.* (1987) Radionuclide diagnosis and therapy of neural crest tumors using iodine-131-metaiodobenzylguanidine. *J. Nucl. Med.*, **28**, 308–14.

Jaques, S. *et al.* (1987) Effect of calcium channel blockers on acetylcholine stimulated and basal release of metaiodobenzylguanidine and norepinephrine in cultured bovine adrenomedullary cells. *J. Nucl. Med.*, **28**, 639–40 (Abstract).

Khafagi, F. A. *et al.* (1989) Labetalol reduces iodine-131-MIBG uptake by pheochromocytoma and normal tissues. *J. Nucl. Med.*, **30**, 481–9.

Kimmig, B. *et al.* (1984) Scintigraphy of neuroblastoma with ^{131}I-MIBG. *J. Nucl. Med.*, **25**, 773–5.

Koral, K. F. and Sarkar, S. D. (1977) An operator-independent method for background subtraction in adrenal uptake measurements: Concise communication. *J. Nucl. Med.*, **18**, 925–8.

Lynn, M. D. *et al.* (1985) Pheochromocytoma and the normal adrenal medulla: improved visualization with I-123 MIBG scintigraphy. *Radiology*, **155**, 789–92.

Lynn, M. D. *et al.* (1986) The influence of hypercholesterolaemia on the adrenal uptake and metabolic handling of 131I-6 beta-iodomethyl-19-norcholesterol (NP-59). *Nucl. Med. Commun.*, **7**, 631–7.

Mangner, T. J. *et al.* (1986) Metabolism of iodine-131 metaiodobenzylguanidine in patients with metastatic pheochromocytoma. *J. Nucl. Med.*, **27**, 37–44.

Munkner, T. (1985) ^{131}I-metaiodobenzylguanidine

scintigraphy of neuroblastoma. *Semin. Nucl. Med.*, **15**, 154–60.

Nakajo, M. *et al.* (1983a) The normal and abnormal distribution of the adrenomedullary imaging agent *m* [I-131]iodobenzylguanidine (131-I-MIBG) in man: evaluation by scintigraphy. *J. Nucl. Med.*, **24**, 672–82.

Nakajo, M. *et al.* (1983b) Inverse relationship between cardiac accumulation of meta-(131I)-iodobenzylguanidine (I-131 MIBG) and circulating catecholamines in suspected pheochromocytoma. *J. Nucl. Med.*, **24**, 1127–34.

Nakajo, M. *et al.* (1985) Rapid clearance of iodine-131 MIBG from the heart, and liver of patients with adrenergic dysfunction and phaeochromocytoma. *J. Nucl. Med.*, **26**, 357–65.

Sarkar, S. D. *et al.* (1977) A new and superior adrenal imaging agent ^{131}I-6β-iodomethyl-19-norcholesterol (NP-59): evaluation in humans. *J. Clin. Endocrinol. Metab.*, **45**, 353–62.

Seabold, J. E. *et al.* (1977) Detection of metastatic adrenal carcinoma using ^{131}I-6β-iodomethyl-19-norcholesterol total body scans. *J. Clin. Endocrinol. Metab.*, **45**, 788–97.

Shapiro, B. *et al.* (1981) Clinical experience with ^{75}Se selenomethyl cholesterol adrenal imaging. *Clin. Endocrinol.*, **15**, 19–27.

Shapiro, B. *et al.* (1983) Value of bowel preparation in adrenocortical scintigraphy with NP-59. *J. Nucl. Med.*, **24**, 732–4.

Shapiro, B. *et al.* (1984a) The location of middle mediastinal pheochromocytomas. *J. Thorac. Cardiovasc. Surg.*, **87**, 814–20.

Shapiro, B. *et al.* (1984b) Malignant phaeochromocytoma: clinical, biochemical and scintigraphic characterisation. *Clin. Endocrinol.*, **20**, 189–203.

Shapiro, B. *et al.* (1985) Iodine-131 metaiodobenzylguanidine for the locating of suspected pheochromocytomas: experience in 400 cases. *J. Nucl. Med.*, **26**, 576–85.

Shulkin, B. *et al.* (1988) Conjugate-view gamma camera method for estimating tumour uptake of iodine-131-metaiodobenzylguanidine. *J. Nucl. Med.*, **29**, 542–8.

Sisson, J. C. *et al.* (1981) Scintigraphic localization of pheochromocytoma. *N. Engl. J. Med.*, **305**, 12–17.

Sisson, J. C. *et al.* (1984) Radiopharmaceutical treatment of malignant pheochromocytoma. *J. Nucl. Med.*, **25**, 197–206.

Sisson, J. C. *et al.* (1987) Metaiodobenzylguanidine to map scintigraphically the adrenergic nervous system in man. *J. Nucl. Med.*, **28**, 1625–36.

Swensen, S. J. *et al.* (1985) Use of 131I-MIBG scintigraphy in the evaluation of suspected pheochromocytoma. *Mayo Clin. Proc.*, **60**, 299–304.

Taylor, L. *et al.* (1986) Diagnostic considerations in virilization: iodomethyl-norcholesterol scanning in the localization of androgen secreting tumors. *Fertil. Steril.*, **46**, 1005–10.

Tobes, M. C. *et al.* (1985) Effect of uptake-one inhibitors on the uptake of norepinephrine and metaiodobenzylguanidine. *J. Nucl. Med.*, **26**, 897–907.

Valk, T. W. *et al.* (1981) Spectrum of pheochromocytoma in multiple endocrine neoplasia: a scintigraphic portrayal using 131I-metaiodobenzylguanidine. *Ann. Intern. Med.*, **94**, 762–7.

Von Moll, L. *et al.* (1987) Iodine-131 MIBG scintigraphy of neuroendocrine tumors other than pheochromocytoma and neuroblastoma. *J. Nucl. Med.*, **28**, 979–88.

FURTHER READING

Gross, M. D. *et al.* (1984) The scintigraphic imaging of endocrine organs. *Endocr. Rev.*, **5**, 221–81.

McEwan, A. J. *et al.* (1985) Radioiodobenzylguanidine for the scintigraphic location and therapy of adrenergic tumors. *Semin. Nucl. Med.*, **15**, 132–53.

Mulrow, P. J. (ed.) (1986) *The Adrenal Gland*, Elsevier, New York.

CHAPTER TWELVE

The gastrointestinal tract

D. N. Croft and J. G. Williams

12.1 ANATOMY AND PHYSIOLOGY

The oesophagus extends from the pharynx at the level of the sixth cervical vertebra to the stomach at the level of T10. It lies in close relation to the aorta from T3 downwards and is behind the heart in the anterior/posterior plane from T5 to T10. It is lined by squamous epithelium.

The oesophagus joins the stomach at the cardia, which lies behind the seventh costal cartilage just to the left of the sternum. The stomach extends as a J-shaped loop to end in the duodenum just to the right of L1. The left kidney lies behind the body of the stomach and the aorta passes behind the antrum.

These relations are important as persisting circulating pertechnetate or enhanced renal activity may lead to errors in interpretation when assessing for Barrett's oesophagus, retained antrum or even Meckel's diverticulum.

The oesophageal mucosa is squamous. The stomach is lined by columnar mucus-secreting cells. The cardia forms a transitional zone between the squamous mucosa of the oesophagus and the columnar, glandular mucosa of the fundus and body of the stomach. In the cardiac region the glands beneath the columnar epithelium are predominantly simple mucus secreting, but a few acid- and pepsinogen-secreting cells may be present. In the fundus and body, mucus-secreting surface epithelium dips down to form crypts which extend downward as tubules lined by columnar parietal (acid-secreting) and chief (pepsin-secreting) cells. The antral mucosa is lined by a columnar mucus-secreting epithelium deep to which are coiled tubules lined with mucus-secreting cells. Acid-and pepsinogen-secreting cells are not present in this region.

Meckel's diverticulum is a remnant of the vitello-intestinal duct. It arises from the antemesenteric border of the ileum, usually 30–50 cm from the ileocaecal valve. It is present in 1–2% of the population and clinical symptoms only occur in 25–30% of those in whom the anomaly is present. Ectopic gastric mucosa is present in 5–6% overall and in all patients who present with rectal bleeding.

12.1.1 OESOPHAGEAL FUNCTION

The act of swallowing initiates a primary peristaltic wave which travels down the oesophagus at 3–4 cm s^{-1}, though this is much dependent on the size and consistency of the swallowed bolus. A liquid bolus induces slower peristalsis than a dry swallow. Secondary peristaltic waves occur in response to a local stimulus to the oesophageal wall such as residual food incompletely cleared by primary peristalsis, or regurgitated gastric contents. Tertiary contractions are non-peristaltic. They are seen occasionally as a normal phenomenon in the young, and are more common in the elderly. They are seen frequently in many dysmotility disorders. In achalasia all peristaltic activity is lost. The lower oesophageal sphincter is a high-pressure zone, about 4 cm long, at the lower end of the oesophagus. Pressure in the sphincter is normally about 20 mmHg above gastric fundal pressure. It relaxes at initiation of a swallow. Failure of sphincter relaxation is characteristic of achalasia.

12.1.2 GASTRIC EMPTYING

The emptying of the stomach is achieved by peristaltic waves which begin in the lower body and push food towards the pylorus. These regular waves are not always accompanied by dilation of the pylorus and therefore achieve substantial mixing of gastric contents as well as intermittent emptying. The fundus and upper body of the stomach act as a reservoir to accommodate swallowed food. From here the food is passed to the antrum by regular slow contractions. Simultaneous radioisotope and manometric studies have defined a correlation between antral motor activity and liquid emptying (Camilleri *et al.*, 1985).

The control of gastric emptying is multifactorial. It is influenced by the pH, osmolarity, volume and chemical composition and size of the meal (Davenport, 1971; Sandhu, *et al.*, 1987). Larger meals empty slower than the smaller ones and carbohydrate empties faster than protein, which empties faster than fat. Water drunk with meals, apart from its effect on volume and osmotic pressure, has no special influence. The osmotic pressure of gastric contents emptied into the duodenum affects the rate of emptying via the enterogastric reflex. The exact effect is complicated but fluids of higher osmotic pressure tend to empty more slowly. The pH of the gastric contents influences the rate of emptying as an indirect function of the neutralizing ability of the duodenum. The more acid the contents the slower the rate of emptying. There is marked individual variation and emptying is also influenced by position and by certain drugs.

12.1.3 GASTRIC ACID SECRETION

Gastric acid is secreted by the parietal cells. The sight, smell, thought or taste of food, and hypoglycaemia stimulate acid secretion via the vagus nerve. This excites the parietal cell direct and also indirectly via the G-cells of the gastric antrum, which are stimulated to release gastrin, which in turn acts on the parietal cells. Gastrin is also released in response to food in the stomach.

12.1.4 GASTRIC MUCUS SECRETION

Mucus is a complex structure, comprised of a number of glycoproteins. Gastric output of the mucus is stimulated by local irritation, cholinergic drugs or vagal stimulation. Mucus secretion is copious during the digestion of a meal.

12.1.5 SMALL INTESTINAL ABSORPTION

Fat, proteins, glucose, iron, most vitamins, water and electrolytes are absorbed in the upper small intestine. Vitamin B12 and bile salts are absorbed at specific sites in the distal ileum. Significant absorption of B12 does not occur unless it is complexed with intrinsic factor, secreted by the stomach.

Bile salts are necessary for the absorption of fats (except medium-chain triglycerides). Bile salt deficiency results in steatorrhoea. Bile salts undergo an enterohepatic circulation in which about 75% are absorbed unchanged in the terminal ileum, to be re-excreted into the bile by the liver. The remaining 25% pass into the large bowel to be deconjugated by bacteria and excreted in the stool. Unconjugated bile salts are ineffective in aiding fat absorption and are irritant to the large bowel, causing diarrhoea.

Carbohydrates tend to be absorbed only as monosaccharides (glucose, galactose and fructose). Disaccharides are not absorbed unless reduced to monosaccharides by the appropriate disaccharidase. If not digested in the small bowel, disaccharides tend to be irritant when fermented by bacteria in the colon, causing diarrhoea.

12.2 OESOPHAGEAL PAIN

The most common cause of oesophageal pain is gastro-oesophageal reflux. Typically, this presents with postural and post-prandial heartburn, perhaps associated with regurgitation of gastric contents and occasional dysphagia. Such a history does not present a diagnostic problem and where there is doubt the diagnosis can be confirmed by intraoesophageal pH monitoring, which is now established as an acceptable, practical and reliable investigation for the detection of reflux (Donald *et al.*, 1987). Radionuclide techniques are available (Fisher *et al.*, 1976; Velasco *et al.*, 1984) but not widely used. The difficulties lie in detecting other causes of oesophageal pain, in particular disorders of motility, which may mimic cardiac angina.

Oesophageal motility disorders can be broadly classified into four groups, as shown in Table 12.1.

All these dysmotility disorders may present with angina-like chest pain, though in some, especially achalasia, dysphagia is more common. They may be asymptomatic for much of the time, with symptoms precipitated at times of stress. Gastro-oesophageal reflux will induce dysmotility (Kjellen and Tibbling, 1985, van Trappen *et al.*, 1987) but it is often spontaneous.

Non-cardiac chest pain is due to oesophageal disease in 15–45% of cases presenting to a coronary care unit (Alban Davies *et al.*, 1982; Chobanian

Table 12.1 Disorders of oesophageal motility

Disorder	*Manometric characterization*
Diffuse spasm (DOS)	Repetitive, spontaneous, non-progressive contractions, usually distal; lower oesphageal sphincter (LOS) is normal
Nutcracker	High-pressure, long-duration peristalsic contractions
Achalasia	Absent peristalsis; high-pressure LOS
Non-specific	Various abnormalities, e.g. hypertensive, normally relaxing LOS; increased spontaneous contractions; multipeaked waves; decreased peristalsis

et al., 1986). About half of these patients will have oesophageal reflux disease which can be confidently diagnosed on clinical grounds. Half will have dysmotility. The history will identify some of these patients (Alban Davies *et al.*, 1985) but is not always reliable (Reidel and Clouse, 1985), and further investigation will be required (de Caesteker *et al.*, 1986). Endoscopy, radiology and/or pH monitoring will identify those with significant reflux disease but miss many with dysmotility, for which the gold-standard test is manometry. However, this requires sophisticated equipment and is difficult to perform and interpret. Measurement of the speed and pattern of transit down the oesophagus of a swallowed bolus offers a simple non-invasive alternative (Russell *et al.*, 1981). Dysmotility is manifest not only as prolongation of the normal mouth to stomach transit time, but also as failure of smooth progression of the swallowed bolus as shown on activity–time curves generated from regions of interest drawn over the oesophagus. Absence of smooth antegrade movement of the bolus implies hold-up due to a stricture (which will have been excluded by barium swallow or endoscopy), spasm (usually seen as to and fro movement) or atony (i.e. absence of primary or secondary contractions which may occur in achalasia or scleroderma). If the oesophagus is anatomically normal the finding of hold-up in the lower oesophagus when the study is repeated standing implies cardiospasm typical of achalasia (Rozen *et al.*, 1982).

There is reasonable concordance between radionuclide transit studies (RT) and manometry in the detection of dysmotility. De Caesteker and colleagues (1986) applied both techniques prospectively to 150 patients referred for motility studies and found agreement in 106 (71%), with a sensitivity of 75% for the RT and 83%. for manometry. Mughal *et al.* (1986) found less concordance – a sensitivity of 44% and specificity of 71% – when minimal manometric abnormalities were included. The RT is measuring movement, not pressure, and false negatives tend to occur with the nutcracker oesophagus, some non-specific disorders and occasionally in diffuse spasm (Blackwell *et al.*, 1983; Mughal *et al.*, 1986; Richter *et al.*, 1987). The abnormalities are often intermittent and as the technique is more rapid than manometry this may also lead to false-negative results. False positives will occur for technical reasons (e.g. double swallows, gastric scatter), anatomical abnormalities such as stricture or hiatus hernia (hence endoscopy or barium swallow should always be performed first) or interpretation difficulties due to reflux (Blackwell *et al.*, 1983).

The RT and manometry are essentially complementary but the former is simpler, quicker, more acceptable to the patient and requires less technical expertise. It is reliable in the diagnosis of disorders such as achalasia where early diagnosis is highly desirable and treatment is effective, and it is of use in the identification of other causes of oesophageal chest pain or dysphagia. It is potentially much more widely available than manometry and should follow endoscopy (or radiology), and 24 h pH monitoring in the evaluation of suspected oesophageal disease.

12.3 SALIVARY GLAND

Dry mouth can be a difficult symptom to assess clinically. Until radionuclide techniques became available it was not possible to measure it by objective methods. Radionuclide salivary gland scanning with ^{99m}Tc-pertechnetate is useful in assessing patients with this symptom and may be diagnostic in distinguishing genuine xerostomia from psychosomatic dry mouth.

A radionuclide salivary scan is performed after intravenous injection of ^{99m}Tc-pertechnetate, which is trapped and excreted by the gland in the same way as it does other anions such as iodide. Normal parotid and submaxillary glands concentrate the radiopharmaceutical, which is discharged into the mouth following a secretory stimulus (Schall *et al.*, 1981; Ohrt and Scafer,

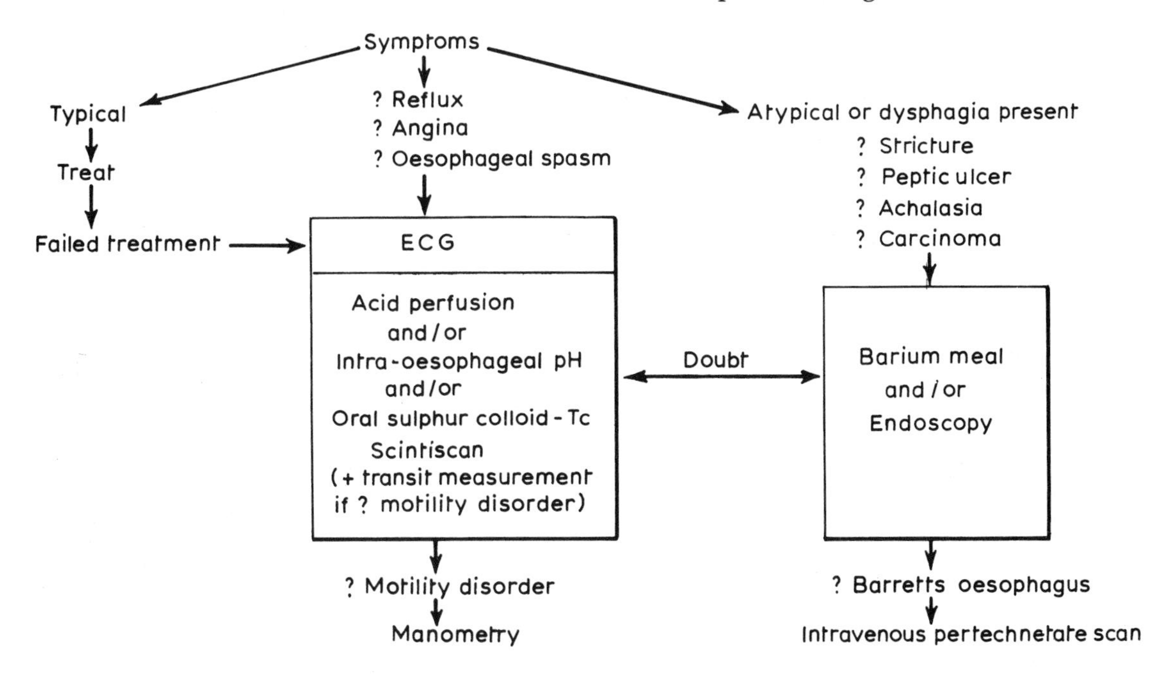

Figure 12.1 Clinical strategy for the evaluation of oesophageal symptoms.

1982). This is readily apparent on the images, but, in addition, activity–time curves of uptake and discharge after stimulation (Parret and Peyrin, 1979) may be obtained and analysed. For clinical purpose this is not necessary.

In genuine xerostomia due to sicca or Sjogren's syndrome there is no uptake into the four glands and no discharge into the mouth. Both these phases of salivary function are normal in psychosomatic xerostomia.

Radionuclide salivary scanning is also of some clinical value in other diseases of the salivary system. Usually, it is not difficult to determine which gland is affected on the clinical grounds of pain or swelling. A sialogram will usually be necessary if an ordinary radiograph does not demonstrate a stone in the salivary duct. However, there are occasions when salivary scanning will help to define the affected gland by demonstrating duct blockage with retention of radiopharmaceutical proximal to the obstruction.

12.4 ASPIRATION OF GASTRIC CONTENTS

Pulmonary aspiration of gastric contents may occur with or without clinical symptoms of reflux. It is a cause of severe morbidity in debilitated patients and in those undergoing emergency anaesthesia, particularly for Caesarean section. It has been implicated in the aetiology of asthma and of pulmonary fibrosis. When silent, gastropulmonary aspiration may be suspected but difficult to prove. Radiology of the chest will demonstrate the consequences but not the cause. In this situation pulmonary imaging the morning after oral ^{99m}Tc-labelled sulphur colloid may demonstrate aspiration into the lungs (Reich *et al.*, 1977). The technique is simple and non-invasive but may need to be repeated on several occasions to detect intermittent nocturnal aspiration, particularly in patients with chronic lung disease. It is of particular value in infants (Bronyaprara *et al.*, 1980; Guillet *et al.*, 1984).

12.5 GASTROINTESTINAL BLEEDING

12.5.1 ACUTE BLEEDING

Gastrointestinal bleeding presents a clinical problem when conventional techniques fail to demonstrate the cause. In the patient presenting with haematemesis and melaena, early endoscopy is the investigation of choice and will demonstrate the lesion in 92% of patients if performed within 24 h (Katon and Smith, 1973). In adults presenting with melaena only, diagnosis may be more difficult. If upper gastrointestinal endoscopy does not demonstrate a cause, bleeding from lower down the bowel must be considered. Colorectal bleeding is often dark red, and may mimic melaena if from the right colon, and upper gastrointestinal bleeding may appear as fresh blood per rectum if profuse. If sigmoidoscopy does not reveal the source, consideration must be given to radionuclide imaging, colonoscopy, arteriography and barium contrast studies in an attempt to make a diagnosis prior to laparotomy. Which is performed will depend upon the clinical situation. Life-threatening bleeding may well require emergency laparotomy before further investigations can be undertaken. Colonoscopy is often useful if bleeding has stopped, but is less likely to be helpful if bleeding is active and profuse, except possibly if done in the theatre at the time of laparotomy. It is effective in detecting inflammatory bowel disease, colonic polyps (Swarbrick *et al.*, 1978) and angiodysplasia (Wolff *et al.*, 1977). Arteriography in expert hands is highly effective.

In children, Meckel's diverticulum is a well-documented cause of acute gastrointestinal bleeding (Brayton, 1964), and may also cause abdominal pain. The anomaly is present in 1–2% of the population, but bleeding only occurs in those with ectopic gastric mucosa in the diverticulum (5–6% overall). Radiology is unhelpful in diagnosis (Meguid *et al.*, 1974). The radionuclide scan is a simple, safe investigation that has now been extensively used and reported. It can be used easily and early in the illness and has a 75–100% sensitivity in the detection of Meckel's diverticulum, (Berquist *et al.*, 1976; Gelfand *et al.*, 1978).

The pathophysiology, indications and methods for scintiscanning for Meckel's diverticulum have been reviewed by Shakianakis and Conway (1981). Pertechnetate is concentrated by gastric mucosa whether or not parietal cells are present. Positive scans show a persistent area of uptake in the mid-abdomen, usually between a hot stomach and bladder (Figure 12.2). The false-negative rate may be high. False positives or uninterpretable pertechnetate scans may occur due to gastric emptying into the small bowel (Berquist *et al.*, 1976). To avoid this excessive time between injection and scanning must be avoided. Gastric emptying can be rapid and scans may become uninterpretable due to activity in the small bowel as early as 25 min after the injection. If this happens the scan should be repeated with nasogastric aspiration (Feggi and Bighi, 1979). Perchlorate should not be used as this will inhibit uptake by the diverticulum as well as the stomach. Pentagastrin given subcutaneously 15 min before pertechnetate has been reported as enhancing uptake by the diverticulum in a patient within a previously equivocal scan (Treves *et al.*, 1978).

Apart from gastric emptying other possible causes of false-positive scans include localized

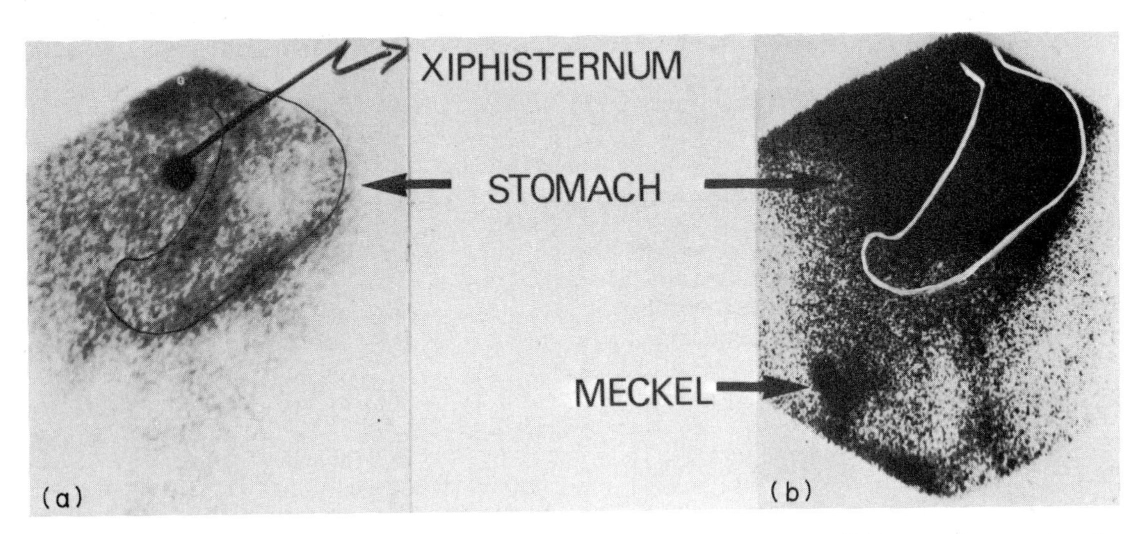

Figure 12.2 Meckel's diverticulum. (a) A normal abdominal scan after intravenous ^{99m}Tc pertechnetate showing the stomach. (b) The scan of a ten-year-old boy with rectal bleeding shows a dense area of activity in the right lower abdomen. A bleeding Meckel's diverticulum was confirmed surgically.

activity in the renal tract from ureteric obstruction or hydropelvis (Chaudhuri *et al.*, 1972). The bladder can also cause confusion and should be emptied before imaging is undertaken. Positive pertechnetate scans have also been reported in intestinal duplication (Schwesinger *et al.*, 1975), jejunal intersussception (Duszynski *et al.*, 1971) malignant lymphoma (Tauscher *et al.*, 1978), vascular ectasia of the caecum if actively bleeding (Tavormina *et al.*, 1978) and Crohn's disease. Lunia *et al.* (1979) suggested that prior medication with bowel irritants will enhance uptake by the lower small bowel (Duszynski *et al.*, 1971), but this is speculative and the reported cases may well have been due to rapid intestinal transit from the stomach.

Meckel's diverticulum is an uncommon cause of acute gastrointestinal bleeding in adults, and although abdominal imaging with pertechnetate will detect lesions unrelated to gastric mucosa (Tavormina *et al.*, 1978) active, even profuse bleeding must be occurring and gastric and renal tract activity can cause confusion. The same limitations apply to imaging with other tracers that are rapidly cleared from the circulation, such as ^{99m}Tc-labelled sulphur colloid (Alavi, 1982) (cleared from the circulation into the liver, spleen and possibly marrow) and ^{99m}Tc-labelled diethylenetriaminepentaacetic acid (DTPA) (Abdel–Dayem *et al.*, 1984; Elwan, 1984) (cleared through the urinary tract). These methods have the advantages of ease of use, ready availability and rapid result but are only applicable where bleeding is continuing actively (approximately 2–3 ml min^{-1}; Barry and Engle, 1978). Where bleeding is less rapid a method using a tracer which remains in the circulation is more applicable. The radionuclide therefore accumulates at the bleeding site over a period of time. Such methods use ^{99m}Tc *in vivo* labelled red cells (Panel *et al.*, 1977; Wakat *et al.*, 1981) or albumin (Miskowiak *et al.*, 1977, 1983). Serial abdominal images can be taken for 24 h at a time that the patient is bleeding. Labelled red cells will pick up the site of bleeding at blood loss rates as low as 0.35–1.25 ml min^{-1} (500–1800 ml over 24 h) (Winzelberg *et al.*, 1979) but radiolabelled albumin is less sensitive (Miskowiak *et al.*, 1977), possibly because of excretion of free pertechnetate into the gut (Hattner and Engelstad, 1983).

Because imaging can be performed rapidly, without preparation, and non-invasively, scintiscanning should be undertaken as an early investigation in the management of gastrointestinal bleeding. A clinical strategy is suggested in Figure 12.3. The sequence of investigations will be modified by local expertise and preference.

12.5.2 CHRONIC BLEEDING

Iron deficiency anaemia is common in women of childbearing age and is usually due to menorrhagia. In men and post-menopausal women it is often due to slow bleeding from the gastrointestinal tract. Up to 500 ml of blood per day may be lost in the faeces without the patient noticing any gastrointestinal or other symptoms (Cuddigan *et al.*, 1971). Intermittent bleeding may occur from lesions such as hiatus hernia which can make the diagnosis of the source of bleeding difficult.

If occult gastrointestinal bleeding is seriously suspected and there is no clinical indication of the site, it is usual to perform sigmoidoscopy, barium enema, and then barium meal or gastroscopy. This course may not resolve the problem and proof may be needed that the patient is bleeding continuously. Chemical tests of occult blood in the stool are unreliable if performed on only one sample (Goulston and Skyring, 1964) but may be of some help if they are repeatedly positive or repeatedly negative. The most accurate method of measuring gut bleeding is by the ^{51}Cr-chromate-labelled red cell technique (Croft and Wood, 1967). The method, which is described below, is accurate to 1–2 ml per day in routine clinical practice. Not only can gastrointestinal bleeding be substantiated but the rate of blood loss can be measured, and if heavy (such as 20–100 ml min^{-1}), may indicate the need for angiography and laparotomy.

Patients with chronic rheumatic disorders, in particular rheumatoid arthritis, are commonly anaemic. The anaemia is often due to chronic disease but iron deficiency may also be caused by bleeding due to ingestion of salicylates and other antirheumatic drugs. With continuous aspirin ingestion many bleed insignificantly but 10–15% lose more than 10 ml of blood per day (Croft and Wood, 1967). Thus in an individual patient with rheumatoid arthritis and persisting anaemia it is useful to look for bleeding due to antirheumatic drugs. The ^{51}Cr-labelled red cell technique is also helpful in assessing new antirheumatic drugs (Croft *et al.*, 1972).

^{59}Fe and a whole-body counter have been used to measure chronic gastrointestinal bleeding (Saito *et al.*, 1964; Holt *et al.*, 1967; Holt *et al.*, 1968;

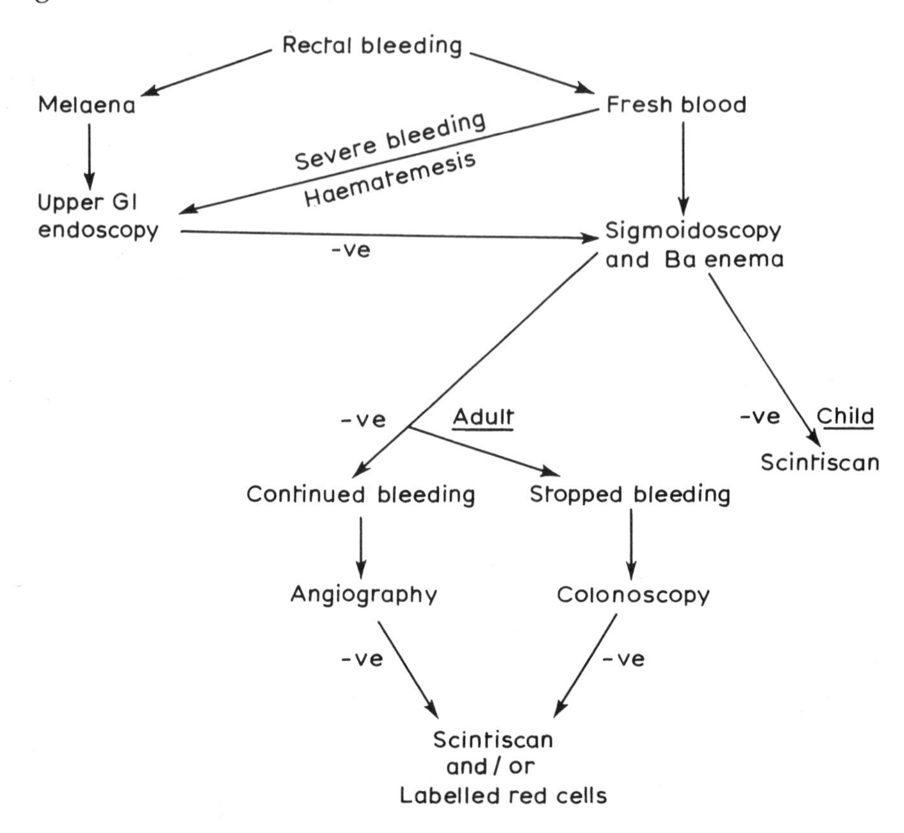

Figure 12.3 The clinical strategy for the medical investigation of the patient with acute rectal bleeding.

Callender, 1970). It is less accurate but has the advantage that bleeding can be measured for a matter of weeks or months. This is of particular value if bleeding is intermittent such as may occur from oesophagitis and hiatus hernia (Holt *et al.*, 1968).

12.5.3 RECURRENT ULCERATION

Recurrent ulceration follows gastric surgery for duodenal ulcer in up to 10% of patients (Stabile and Panaro, 1976). The diagnosis is most reliably made by endoscopy, but this will not reveal the cause. Acid secretion studies will demonstrate the completeness of vagotomy (insulin test) and may suggest hypergastrinaemia if a high basal secretion is not further increased by subcutaneous pentagastrin (pentagastrin test) (Baron, 1978).

If fasting gastrin assay confirms hypergastrinaemia, the source must be sought. The Zollinger–Ellison syndrome is a rare combination of severe recurrent ulceration and diarrhoea secondary to a gastrinoma, usually in the pancreas, but sometimes in the gut. The diagnosis rests on the finding of excessively high circulating gastrin and the subsequent localization of the tumour by arteriography, microsampling of mesenteric venous blood for gastrin and/or laparotomy. This disease may be very difficult to differentiate from the retained gastric antrum syndrome (RGAS), another rare cause of hypergastrinaemia, which occurs following Polya (Billroth II) gastrectomy. In this syndrome a cuff of mucosa from the gastric antrum is inadvertently left at the duodenal stump at gastrectomy (see Figure 12.4). No longer inhibited by gastric acid, the gastrin cells in the antral mucosa secrete high levels of gastrin. The prevalence of this syndrome is about 9% of all Polya gastrectomies (Stabile and Panaro, 1976).

Differential diagnosis between the two syndromes is difficult. Tests include serum gastrin assay in response to certain pharmacological stimuli such as secretin or calcium (which cause a further increase in gastrin in patients with gastrinoma, but a fall in normals and those with RGAS) or bombesin (which increases gastrin

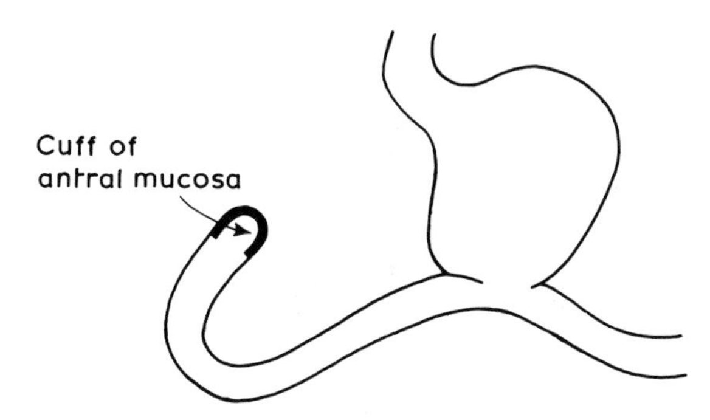

Figure 12.4 Retained gastric antrum at the duodenal stump following Polya partial gastrectomy.

secretion from normal antral mucosa) (Sciaretta *et al.*, 1978). Endoscopic biopsy is helpful if the duodenal stump can be reached, but this is often difficult and in some cases a diagnosis is not made until laparotomy.

Intravenous ^{99m}Tc-pertechnetate is taken up by the gastric mucosa. The cellular site of uptake is controversial, with evidence for both the parietal and the mucous cells (Williams, 1983). However, non-parietal cell containing antral mucosa will concentrate pertechnetate whereas small bowel or squamous (oesophageal mucosa) will not, and this is therefore a useful test for the detection of ectopic gastric mucosa as occurs in RGAS and also in Barrett's oesophagus and Meckel's diverticulum.

The technique for performing gastric scans in this situation is described later. Positive scans will show a small area of activity to the right of the larger area of gastric activity in the anteroposterior view. Such activity should start appearing by 20 min and be clearly visible by 30 min. If there is doubt, later frames should be taken as early liver and aortic activity may obscure poor uptake at the duodenal stump. The technique is sensitive. For instance, in a study in dogs, retained antral tissue as small as 1 cm could be detected (Safaie-Shirazi *et al.*, 1973). It has a low false-positive rate (Sciarretta *et al.*, 1978), but no data on false-negative scans have been reported.

A clinical strategy for the assessment of patients with recurrent ulcer is shown in Figure 12.5.

12.5.4 DIARRHOEA

Diarrhoea after gastric surgery is not uncommon, some looseness of stools occurring in up to 30% of patients in the early post-operative period. In most patients the symptom is not troublesome, but in less than 5% there is profuse watery intractable diarrhoea which presents a problem both to the patient and to the clinician. There are a number of possible causes (Shearman and Finlayson, 1982). Uncoordinated gastric emptying may allow large quantities of hypertonic foodstuff to arrive in the jejunum soon after a meal, and the osmotic effect of this will be cathartic; similarly relative lactose intolerance may develop. Enteric infections or bacterial overgrowth in a redundant loop of small bowel will be encouraged by hypochlorhydria and may cause malabsorption. The Zollinger–Ellison syndrome itself may be implicated. Intestinal motility is increased after truncal vagotomy.

12.5.5 DUMPING

The predominant symptom of the dumping syndrome is a feeling of faintness after meals. This may be associated with dizziness, pallor, palpitation and/or sweating and there may also be epigastric fullness and discomfort, borborygmi or cramps. The symptoms usually occur within 30 min of eating.

The mechanism of dumping is not clear, but it is often associated with rapid transit of at least part of the meal from the stomach into the small bowel, with either a sudden fall in plasma volume (early dumping) or reactive hypoglycaemia (late dumping).

12.5.6 EPIGASTRIC FULLNESS AND VOMITING

Gastric stasis may occur after gastric surgery, particularly vagotomy. The patient complains of

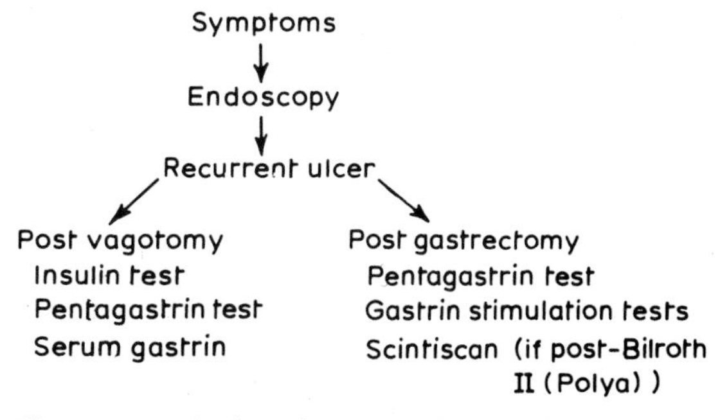

Figure 12.5 A clinical strategy for the assessment of patients with recurrent ulceration following gastric surgery.

epigastric fullness and vomiting. A sensation of epigastric fullness following partial gastrectomy may also occur due to jejunal distension as a result of rapid gastric emptying.

In all these conditions, information about the rate of gastric emptying is of value. Such information is unlikely to alter the clinical diagnosis, but may well be of great help in deciding the correct course of action. Historically, three types of emptying tests have been used: intubation, radiological and radioactive tracer techniques. These have been reviewed in detail by Sheiner (1975). More recently ultrasonography (Bolondi *et al.*, 1985) has been used.

Intubation tests require the passage of a nasogastric tube, through which the meal is aspirated to determine the volume left in the stomach. The emptying rate of liquid meals only can be assessed and repeated testing over a number of days is required to obtain sufficient points to be able to plot the pattern of emptying. This is time consuming and often uncomfortable to the patient, but nevertheless the test is reliable and reproducible. Many refinements have been described to reduce the errors and to maximize the information gained, and some of these involve radionuclide markers.

Radiological tests use the barium meal and only estimate the total emptying time. This measurement is crude and open to wide error. The test is little used. Cross-sectional area of the gastric antrum as measured by real-time ultrasound can give a measure of total emptying time (when the measurement returns to basal value). Measurement of gastric impedance is non-invasive, inexpensive, simple and quick, and early results suggest good correlation with scintigraphic measurements.

Radionuclide tests for gastric emptying were first introduced in 1966. The principle provides for great flexibility and allows the emptying of more than one component of the meal, including solids, to be assessed (Heading *et al.*, 1976). Many labelling techniques, from impregnated Perspex-sealed filter-paper squares to *in vivo* labelled chicken liver, have been described (Williams, 1986), and at present there is no consensus of agreement on standardization of method and interpretation of results. More work is required before this can be achieved. It is clear that in normals, liquids empty faster than solids and liquid emptying tends to be linear, but rates of emptying vary with different radionuclides used, probably as a result of varying affinity of the different labels for the meal. Whatever labels are used, it is most important to ensure that there is no transfer of label from liquid to solid or vice versa, either as a result of inadequate labelling or digestion (Wright *et al.*, 1981).

Results are expressed as $T_{1/2}$, i.e. the time taken for the volume of the meal remaining in the stomach to diminish by half. This is not entirely satisfactory (Elashoff *et al.*, 1982) as the emptying curve is not adequately described by a single exponential because of differences at the beginning and end of the meal, which tend to be more marked for solid than for liquid measurement. Nevertheless, $T_{1/2}$ is convenient and simple, and at present the advantages tend to outweigh the disadvantages.

The changes observed in gastric emptying following surgery can only be generalizations and the value of the technique lies in the assessment of the individual patient, particularly in relation to his own symptoms. Following vagotomy and pyloroplasty, the $T_{1/2}$ of the liquid component of the meal tends to be little changed by operation except in those who experience dumping symptoms or diarrhoea where the early rate of emptying is significantly faster than before the operation (Ralphs *et al.*, 1978; Colmer *et al.*, 1973). The type of operation performed is of importance. Proximal gastric vagotomy has little or no effect on emptying, whereas truncal vagotomy with pyloroplasty or antrectomy tends to result in rapid early emptying of solids, though this is variable and some patients display very slow emptying of solid food (Mayer *et al.*, 1984). This tends to improve with time (Cowley *et al.*, 1972). Clinically, if post-operative vomiting is persistent, and delayed gastric emptying persists for many weeks, a further drainage procedure should be considered.

12.5.7 GASTRITIS

Duodenogastric reflux commonly occurs after gastric surgery and has been implicated in the aetiology of gastritis (both post-surgical and in the non-operated stomach).

If duodenogastric reflux is suspected it can be quantified by nasogastric aspiration and measurement of bile (Hoare *et al.*, 1978), or using radionuclides. The first reported study used a duodenal tube to deposit ^{99m}Tc-labelled antimony sulphide colloid in the duodenum, followed by quantification of reflux using a gamma camera and computerized region of interest analysis (Rokkjaer *et al.*, 1977). Subsequently, to obviate the need for a nasogastric tube ^{99m}Tc-labelled HIDA compounds have been used (Muhammed *et al.*, 1980; Shaffer *et al.*, 1980). A refinement uses a dual-isotope technique to delineate clearly the position of the stomach (Baulieu *et al.*, 1986). Nasogastric aspiration after intravenous HIDA allows accurate measurement of small amounts of reflux, together with gastric secretion and emptying, but is invasive (Muller-Lissner *et al.*, 1983).

Although these techniques can be used non-invasively to detect and quantify duodenogastric reflux, the clinical and therapeutic value of such measurements has not yet been established (Rhodes, 1981), except in the assessment of patients after gastric surgery (Svensson, 1983), particularly with a view to a possible bile diversion procedure (Wickremesinghe *et al.*, 1983).

12.5.8 UPPER GASTROINTESTINAL SYMPTOMS IN OTHER CONDITIONS

Conditions such as scleroderma, uraemia and spinal cord transection may be associated with diverse gastrointestinal symptoms of a variety of possible causes, and a confident diagnosis is necessary if treatment is to be offered with confidence. Thus in scleroderma regurgitation, vomiting or dyspepsia may be due to impaired oesophageal or gastric motility or both (Maddern *et al.*, 1984); delayed gastric emptying is a factor in the nausea and vomiting of uraemia (McNamee *et al.*, 1985) and antral–duodenal motor incoordination occurs after high spinal cord transection (Fealey *et al.*, 1984) which may lead to vomiting, although other factors such as constipation or occult urinary tract infection are common. In all these conditions measurement of oesophagogastric function may be of clinical use.

12.6 MALABSORPTION AND GUT LOSS

Nutritional deficiencies are caused by inadequate intake of food, absorptive defects in the gut (Permun *et al.*, 1960) or by increased loss from the gastrointestinal tract (or other organs such as kidney or skin). As a global problem deficient intake is the commonest cause. In Western countries malnutrition is uncommon but does occur in the elderly living alone (who may develop scurvy), vegans (who may become B12 deficient) and immigrant children removed from sunshine (who may develop rickets). Failure to absorb nutrients occurs as a result of maldigestion from bile salt or digestive enzyme deficiencies, or small bowel intestinal disease causing an absorptive defect. Many intestinal diseases may also result in continuous loss of protein leading to hypoproteinaemia, and anaemia from bleeding may occur from lesions such as cancer or Crohn's disease at any site from mouth to anus. Thus malabsorption is not the only, or even the commonest, cause of nutritional deficiencies. Furthermore, weight loss may occur as a result of chronic continuous diarrhoea from any cause, including systemic diseases such as thyrotoxicosis. However, profound weight loss occurs in particular if the diarrhoea is associated with anorexia or with malabsorption. In the latter, the appetite is sometimes good, which may be an important clue to an absorptive defect. Steatorrhoea or fatty stools may be due to pancreatic exocrine insufficiency, bile salt deficiency or to lesions of the small bowel mucosa.

12.6.1 STEATORRHOEA

The usual way of proceeding to the diagnosis of malabsorption is to perform haematological and biochemical investigations and then to investigate the gastrointestinal tract. Sigmoidoscopy is followed by barium enema, small bowel meal and jejunal mucosal biopsy and, if necessary, pancreatic function tests. Breath tests of fat absorption have been devised and can be useful as a screening test for steatorrhoea, superior and simpler than the measurement of faecal fat (Newcomer *et al.*, 1979). ^{14}C-triolein is used and measurements are required for 6 h, the test being abnormal if less than 3.5% of the administered dose is exhaled per hour. In two groups of patients with proven steatorrhoea and irritable bowel syndrome, there were no false negatives and only one false positive, which represented 100% sensitivity and 96% specificity. This reliability has been confirmed subsequently (West *et al.*, 1981) and the method has been shown to be a useful out-patient screening test for steatorrhoea (Avgerinos *et al.*, 1981; Einarsson *et al.*, 1983; Mylvaganam *et al.*, 1986; Butler, 1987). Elevated breath ^{14}C activity after ^{14}C-triolein will confirm steatorrhoea but not indicate the cause. A dual isotope method using ^{14}C-triolein (digested by pancreatic lipase) and ^{3}H-oleic acid (absorbed directly without prior digestion) has been developed by Pedersen and Halgreen (1985) and has proved useful to differentiate fat maldigestion from malabsorption. Pancreatic scanning for chronic pancreatitis as a cause of steatorrhoea using selenomethionine is of limited value; a normal scan makes pancreatic pathology unlikely, but an abnormal scan is unhelpful as false positives are common. No reliable distinction can be made between chronic pancreatitis and carcinoma by means of pancreatic scanning (Cotton *et al.*, 1978).

12.6.2 BACTERIAL OVERGROWTH OF THE SMALL BOWEL

When bacterial overgrowth of the small intestine is suspected, the ^{14}C-glycine-labelled bile salt breath test is useful. This was first reported in 1971 by Fromm and Hofmann and has been reviewed by Hepner (1974) and by Thaysen (1977). ^{14}C-glycoholic acid is given by mouth. In normals this passes unchanged through the stomach and small bowel to be absorbed in the terminal ileum and re-excreted in the bile (enterohepatic circulation). A small proportion will pass on into the large bowel to be split by bacteria and excreted in the faeces. In the presence of bacterial overgrowth in the small bowel, as may occur following gastrointestinal surgery (blind loop syndrome), in jejunal diverticula, or as a result of stasis in diseases such as Crohn's or scleroderma, deconjugation of the bile acid occurs with liberation of the ^{14}C-glycine moiety of the labelled glycoholic acid. This is rapidly absorbed and metabolized and $^{14}CO_2$ is exhaled in the breath, where it can be trapped in solution and detected by a suitable counter.

The test will also be positive in the presence of terminal ileal bypass and resection or disease severe enough to cause bile acid malabsorption. In this situation, the labelled bile acid reaches the large bowel in significant quantities, where it is deconjugated by colonic bacteria. The liberated free $^{14}CO_2$ is absorbed and exhaled, to be detected in the breath.

False-negative results can occur in patients with bile acid malabsorption who have profuse diarrhoea. In this situation there is not time for the bile acid to be deconjugated by colonic bacteria. False-positive results can occur if there is intestinal hurry through the terminal ileum, preventing adequate absorption of conjugated bile salts. Excretion of $^{14}CO_2$ may also be increased in patients who have a cholecystectomy. This is due to an increase in the rate of enterohepatic cycling, with an increased proportion of unconjugated bile salts. These various sources of error result in this test having both poor specificity and low sensitivity.

Alternative methods for diagnosing infected small intestine include intubation studies to collect and culture jejunal juice or to detect deconjugated bile salts, and the detection of urinary indican (produced by the bacterial hydrolysis of tryptophan).

Exhaled non-radioactive hydrogen (H_2) has been shown to correlate well with hydrogen produced in the intestinal lumen (Levitt, 1969). This is released when carbohydrates are broken down by bacteria, and the test is therefore also of value in detecting jejunal bacterial overgrowth and also disaccharidase deficiency (see below). The H_2 breath test has the advantage of being non-radioactive, but has been reported as less sensitive than a ^{14}C breath test using ^{14}C-xylose as the test substrate (King and Toskes, 1986).

12.6.3 OTHER BREATH TESTS

^{14}C-urea has been proposed as a breath test for the detection of colonization of the stomach by *Campylobacter pylori* (Graham *et al.*, 1987). This organism has been implicated in the pathogenesis of gastritis and peptic ulceration (Marshall *et al.*, 1985), and treatment which eradicates the infection prevents relapse of duodenal ulcers (Marshall *et al.*, 1988).

Alactasia causes diarrhoea due to deficiency of the small intestinal mucosal enzyme lactase. It can be diagnosed by a ^{14}C-lactose breath test (Newcomer *et al.*, 1975). In the absence of lactase the labelled lactose is not absorbed and little $^{14}CO_2$ appears in the breath. The converse occurs if lactase is present to split the disaccharide to monosaccharides, which are absorbed. Sampling at 1 h is satisfactory and gives good separation between normals and alactasia. In units where the apparatus is available, hydrogen (non-adioactive) in the breath is as good, if not better, for screening for alactasia.

12.6.4 VITAMIN B12 MALABSORPTION

The Schilling test combined with the test with intrinsic factor is of use for diagnosing the site of malabsorption of B12. This can be due to gastric disease and lack of intrinsic factor, or to disease of the terminal ileum which is the site of B12 absorption.

^{58}Co-labelled B12 is given orally and it links with intrinsic factor from the stomach and is absorbed by the terminal ileum. A flushing dose of non-radioactive B12 is given by intramuscular injection. In normals, more than 8% of the labelled B12 given orally appears in the urine. Impaired absorption results in less than 8% appearing and in pernicious anaemia it is usually less than 3%. Falsely, low values occur with renal failure and incomplete urine saves. In renal impairment, urine should be collected for 48 h.

It is important to remember that it may take weeks or months for the intestinal epithelium to recover from B12 deficiency. Thus a Schilling test, even if repeated with intrinsic factor, may remain abnormal during this time. The test is therefore best done after the B12-deficient patient has been treated with B12 for two or three months.

A dual radionuclide modification of the Dicopac test (Bell and Lee, 1969; Bayley *et al.*, 1971) distinguishes malabsorption of B12 due to lack of intrinsic factor (caused by atrophic gastritis, pernicious anaemia or gastrectomy) and that due to a lesion of small intestine such as Crohn's disease of the terminal ileum. ^{58}Co-labelled B12 and ^{57}Co-labelled B12 attached to intrinsic factor are given together orally 2 h apart, and 24 h after a flushing dose of B12 the amount of each isotope in the urine is measured (Table 12.2) and also expressed as a ratio of ^{57}Co-labelled B12 + intrinsic factor to ^{58}Co-labelled B12. In the presence of low serum B12, if the ratio is greater than 1.8, lack of intrinsic factor due to pernicious anaemia or gastric surgery is the cause; if not, a small bowel lesion is suspected. This ratio is unaffected by incomplete urine saves.

B12 absorption can also be measured by the hepatic uptake of ^{58}Co-labelled B12 and by measuring the whole-body retention of ^{58}Co-labelled B12 using a whole-body counter. In general the Schilling or Dicopac tests have proved to be the better methods as they are clinically robust, and inexpensive.

12.6.5 HYPOPROTEINAEMIA AND PROTEIN-LOSING ENTEROPATHY

Like iron deficiency anaemia, hypoproteinaemia may occur as a result of a considerable variety of conditions, including protein-deficient diet, hepatic or renal disease. In the gut virtually any disease process may give rise to protein-losing enteropathy and hypoproteinaemia. Thus, in a patient with an unexplained low serum albumin, measurement of the gut loss of protein may reveal the cause of the low serum albumin (Jones *et al.*, 1966). In other conditions, such as lymphangiectasis, a gut lesion can be demonstrated by the ^{51}Cr-labelled chloride technique before the serum albumin level falls below normal (Eustace *et al.*, 1975). Recently transient protein-losing enteropathy in children has been shown by nuclear medicine techniques to be due to gastric infection with *Campylobacter pylori* (Hill *et al.*, 1987).

A number of techniques have been described for measuring intestinal protein loss. In clinical terms the one that has proved most reliable utilizes ^{51}Cr-labelled chloride (Walker-Smith *et al.*, 1967). When given intravenously, this radiopharmaceutical becomes non-specifically attached to plasma proteins. If there is a gut leak, more than 2% appears in the stool in five days. It is essential that the stool is not contaminated with urine as the isotope is excreted by the kidney. This makes this technique unreliable in babies and young children.

As a clinical test the ^{51}Cr-labelled chloride method is robust and reliable. It is of value not only in the diagnosis of protein-losing enteropathy but also in assessing the response to surgical or other treatment (Kinmonth and Cox, 1974).

12.7 DIARRHOEA

Diarrhoea which defies diagnosis on history, examination, sigmoidoscopy, rectal biopsy, stool culture, routine blood tests and barium enema is uncommon. Most cases will be attributed to the irritable bowel syndrome, and treatment is often unsatisfactory. A small proportion of patients may have terminal ileal malabsorption of bile salts which can be simply diagnosed using ^{75}Se-labelled homocholic acid taurine (SeHCAT) (Nyhlin *et al.*, 1983; Ferraris *et al.*, 1986; Sciarretta *et al.*, 1987; Schiller *et al.*, 1987), though it has been argued that it is simpler and cheaper to use a trial of treatment with cholestyramine (Heaton, 1986).

12.7.1 SeHCAT RETENTION

SeHCAT is a synthetic bile acid, the absorption and excretion of which are virtually identical to those of taurocholate. It contains ^{75}Se, a γ-emitter, which allows its retention after oral administration to be measured using a whole-body counter or a gamma camera (Merrick *et al.*, 1982). Using a gamma camera, anterior and posterior projections are obtained and compared with a phantom. The results are usually expressed as a seven-day retention which is a measurement of function in the terminal ileum (Nyhlin *et al.*, 1983; Merrick, 1986).

The test is useful for investigation of diarrhoea, particularly after surgical removal of ileum or radiotherapy to the lower abdomen. Damage or removal of as little as 20 cm of ileum can result in bile salt malabsorption by the ileum. As a result, toxic quantities of bile salts reach the large bowel and cause diarrhoea. Treatment with cholestyramine, a bile acid sequestering agent, will help these patients. If 1 m of ileum is damaged or removed, bile acids are lost at a rate that cannot be replaced by synthesis in the liver. Steatorrhoea will result, as fats in the small bowel lumen will not form micelles and thus they will not be absorbed. Treatment with short-chain fatty acids may help these patients.

SeHCAT retention can be combined with B12 absorption to elucidate ileal dysfunction (Smith and Bjarnason, 1990). Malabsorption of B12 alone usually indicates small bowel bacterial colonization in disorders such as blind loop and jejunal diverticulosis. This diarrhoea often responds to antibiotics. Malabsorption of SeHCAT alone, or both B12 and SeHCAT, indicates mucosal damage by diseases such as Crohn's. Cholestyramine treatment that sequesters bile salts often improves the diarrhoea. If both compounds are absorbed normally, one should look elsewhere, in the large bowel etc., for the cause.

SeHCAT retention is thus a useful technique in elucidating the cause of diarrhoea, particularly following gut resection or radiotherapy and in patients with Crohn's disease.

12.8 ABDOMINAL INFECTION AND INFLAMMATION

Labelled white cell and ^{67}Ga scanning of the abdomen is useful in two clinical situations: to find an intra-abdominal abscess and to determine the extent of inflammatory bowl disease in patients with ulcerative colitis or Crohn's disease. The technique for preparing labelled white cells requires experience and training, and takes a few hours. This is a limitation in the clinical usefulness of labelled white cells in the urgent investigation of seriously ill patients and in busy departments unable to spare staff for the lengthy labelling procedure. Recently ^{99m}Tc-HMPAO has been used as an alternative radiopharmaceutical citrate. ^{67}Ga has also been used for evaluation of AIDS-related intestinal infections (Tatsch *et al.*, 1990).

12.8.1 ^{67}Ga SCANNING FOR ABSCESS

^{67}Ga scanning is still used in some departments as it has the advantage in acutely ill patients that the detection of intra-abdominal abscesses can usually be made the same day by scanning at 6–8 h after the injection (Hopkins *et al.*, 1975, 1976). It also avoids the time it takes and the training and facilities required to label white cells.

Early scanning using ^{67}Ga reduces patient morbidity as the diagnosis is made sooner, thus allowing treatment to be started earlier. Early scanning also reduces the problems caused by bowel excretion of the ^{67}Ga and thus avoids the need for thorough bowel preparation as is needed when performing late scans.

Accurate localization of small subphrenic abscesses is usually impossible with conventional liver–lung ^{99m}Tc scans. However, a ^{67}Ga scan with a combined ^{99m}Tc-labelled sulphur colloid liver scan and computer-assisted subtraction technique will allow identification of about 95% of such abscesses (Damron *et al.*, 1974). Further information about the exact anatomical location of the abscess may be obtained by taking views from different angles and from the use of ^{99m}Tc-labelled sulphur colloid administered either orally or rectally to delineate the gastrointestinal tract in order to show the relation between the abscess and the gut.

Comparisons between ^{67}Ga scans and either ultrasound or CT scans have shown that, if anything, ^{67}Ga scans are more accurate than either of these other modes of investigation for intra-abdominal abscesses (Kumar *et al.*, 1977; Levitt *et al.*, 1979). However, the best results may be obtained by the combined use of two or more of these techniques. ^{67}Ga scanning has one distinct advantage over the others in that it may demonstrate inflammatory foci elsewhere than in the abdomen, thus enabling the cause of the patient's fever to be detected.

^{67}Ga scans have also been used to determine inflammatory bowel disease such as Crohn's disease of the terminal ileum (Goldenberg *et al.*, 1979). ^{67}Ga has also been shown to collect in recent surgical wounds. Although this should not cause confusion in the interpretation of abdominal scans, the possibility that an area of increased uptake may represent the wound must be borne in mind.

12.8.2 LABELLED WHITE CELL SCANNING (Saverymuttu, 1990)

Autologous ^{111}In-labelled leucocytes have been used for the evaluation of occult intra-abdominal spesis and are proving to be superior to ^{67}Ga especially for the detection of acute rather than chronic inflammation (Sfakianakis *et al.*, 1982; Barletti *et al.*, 1990). The technique can also be used to assess the distribution and extent of inflammatory bowel disease (Saverymuttu *et al.*, 1982, 1983, 1986), though the reliability in this context has been questioned (Buxton-Thomas *et al.*, 1984; Park *et al.*, 1988). Disease activity can also be quantified by faecal counting (Saverymuttu *et al.*, 1983), excretion of labelled cells correlating well with conventional indicators of activity such as C-reactive protein, ESR or the Crohn's disease activity index. External scintiscanning can also be used to quantify disease activity and response to treatment (Stein *et al.*, 1983) but recent data indicate that the correlation with disease extent is only 58% (Park *et al.*, 1988). The technique has the great advantage over radiological and colonoscopic assessment that bowel preparation is not required, and both the small and large bowel can be imaged in one examination. Furthermore it is safe, and can be used even in severely ill patients, where barium enema or colonoscopy might be contraindicated. The labelling procedure is difficult but effective (Zakhireh *et al.*, 1979) and the test may become more widely used if initial claims for easier labelling using ^{99m}Tc and hexamethylpropyleneamineoxime (HMPAO) are substantiated (Peters *et al.*, 1986; Mountford *et al.*, 1990; Hebbard *et al.*, 1990). ^{99m}Tc-labelled porphyrin may also prove to be a simpler alternative for the detection of occult inflammation (Zanelli *et al.*, 1986). ^{99m}Tc-labelled sucralfate has also been reported to localize in ulcerated inflammatory bowel disease (Dawson *et al.*, 1985) though this has not been confirmed by others (George *et al.*, 1987; Cramp *et al.*, 1987).

Ultrasound scanning and computed tomography are also used to localize abdominal sepsis and are probably preferable to leucocyte imaging when localizing signs are present or a rapid result is required (Knochel *et al.*, 1980; Coakley and Mountford, 1986). If an abscess with pus is present this is quickly and cheaply delineated by ultrasound scanning, which should be the initial imaging technique so long as there is experienced staff available.

12.8.3 OTHER ABDOMINAL SCANNING TECHNIQUES

Other radionuclide scanning techniques that have been reported but not fully evaluated for the investigation of intra-abdominal pathology include: ^{99m}Tc-labelled All Bran for irritable bowel syndrome (Trottman and Price, 1986); ^{111}In-labelled monoclonal antibodies and ^{125}I-labelled anti-carcino-embryonic antigen (CEA) for recurrent colonic cancer (Ballantyne *et al.*, 1988; Blair *et al.*, 1988); ^{99m}Tc labelled PRIA3 (Granowska *et al.*, 1990); and ^{111}In-labelled white blood cell scanning for pancreatitis (Anderson *et al.*, 1983). Further investigations are required to determine their place in clinical practice.

12.9 TECHNIQUES

12.9.1 SALIVARY RADIOISOTOPE SCANNING

Intravenous ^{99m}Tc-pertechnetate (1–2 mCi) is given and anterior and lateral images are taken with the patient in the supine position using a gamma camera and a low-energy parallel hole collimator. The neck is hyperextended and a lead shield is placed over the thyroid, and images of 300 000 counts are taken every 10 min for 45 min. A secretory stimulus such as a lemon drop or 500 mg of ascorbic acid is given and views are taken for a further 45 min. The procedure may be computerized in order to obtain curves of uptake and discharge (Parret and Peyrin, 1979).

12.9.2 OESOPHAGEAL REFLUX

^{99m}Tc-labelled sulphur colloid (300 μCi) is used, swallowed in 300 ml of saline. A nasogastric tube is not necessary. Provocation of reflux is produced with an inflatable abdominal binder, which when pressurized up to 100 mmHg raises the pressure across the lower oesophageal sphincter from 10 to 35 mmHg. Provocation is important; the test is considerably less sensitive under resting conditions. Reflux is measured using a gamma camera and computer. A radionuclide scan is obtained for a 30 s exposure at each 20 mmHg pressure gradient up to 100 mmHg. Reflux is measured using regions of interest over the lower oesophagus and stomach and expressed as a percentage of gastric counts, which allows for losses due to distal gastric emptying. In practice, reflux greater than 4% is visible without data processing and is considered abnormal (Malmud *et al.*, 1976; Fisher *et al.*, 1976). In infants the radiotracer is given in milk and abdominal compression is not required (Guillet *et al.*, 1984).

12.9.3 OESOPHAGEAL TRANSIT

The patient is positioned supine under a large field of view gamma camera, and the passage of a radiolabelled swallowed bolus from mouth to stomach is recorded. The bolus is usually liquid, but may be semi-solid or solid (Holloway *et al.*, 1983; Kjellen *et al.*, 1984; Richter *et al.*, 1987). ^{99m}Tc-labelled sulphur colloid (1 mCi swallowed in 20 ml water) is usually used, but studies with a very short half-life tracer (^{81m}Kr) have also been described (Ham *et al.*, 1984). A dry swallow is made at 30 s. Hard copy images are recorded at 3 s intervals, with computer aquisition in 0.5 s frames over 60 s. The generated data can be analysed in various ways. Arrival transit time is the time from swallowing to first arrival of activity in the stomach (normal 7.15 s ± 0.62 SEM; Williams *et al.*, 1986). Oesophageal retention measures residual activity in the gullet at 60 s as a percentage of peak activity after swallowing. Clearance measures the time taken to clear 90% of the swallowed activity (normal 9.8 s ± 0.7 SEM; Williams *et al.*, 1986). Segmental oesophageal emptying can be calculated, and generation of time–activity curves from regions of interest drawn over the oesophagus and stomach will allow visual inspection of transit patterns (Russell *et al.*, 1981; Blackwell *et al.*, 1983; Taillefer and Beauchamp, 1984) and sophisticated computer analysis (Klein and Wald, 1984). Parametric imaging can be used (Gibson and Bateson, 1985). Transit times are longer in the supine rather than the sitting position (Lamki, 1985; Kjellen and Svedberg, 1983), and in obese patients (Mercer *et al.*, 1985).

12.9.4 DETECTION OF BARRETT'S OESOPHAGUS

The patient attends fasted. ^{99m}Tc-pertechnetate (5–15 mCi) is given intravenously. No perchlorate is used and the patient is instructed not to swallow saliva. Gamma camera pictures are taken at 20 and 30 min after the injection, with the patient erect in front of the camera. Anterior, posterior and lateral views should be taken. For each image 300 000 –600 000 counts are accumulated. It should be possible to delineate clearly the stomach on such scans but if the gastro-oesophageal junction is difficult to localize a single radiograph following a small barium swallow may be taken.

12.9.5 GASTROPULMONARY ASPIRATION

^{99m}Tc-labelled sulphur colloid (10 mCi) is drunk with water last thing at night. If it is the patient's habit to take a snack or hot drink on retiring, this is also allowed. The following morning the chest is imaged in the anterior, posterior and right lateral positions using a gamma camera, accumulating 100 000 counts for each image. It is important to exclude counts from the upper abdomen. The localization of aspirated activity will depend on the position in which the patient sleeps.

12.9.6 RETAINED ANTRUM SYNDROME

The patient attends starved. ^{99m}Tc-pertechnetate (1 mCi) is given intravenously with the patient supine under the gamma camera. Scinti-photos are obtained over a period of 60 s at 20 and 30 min after the injection. No blocking agent such as perchlorate should be given as this will inhibit both antral and body mucosal uptake of pertechnetate.

12.9.7 GASTRIC EMPTYING

(Tothill *et al.*, 1978; Malmud *et al.*, 1982)

(a) Choice of preparations

There is no consensus of opinion on the ideal meal or label for the measurement of gastric emptying. Early studies used ^{51}Cr-sodium chromate incorporated into cornflakes and milk and in scrambled eggs. ^{113}In and ^{99m}Tc have been used and tend to demonstrate a shorter emptying time than with chromium (Heading *et al.*, 1971). Indium is now most commonly used as a marker of the liquid phase of emptying when labelled to diethylenetriamine pentaacetic acid (DPTA). For the solid phase ^{99m}Tc is used, whether as sulphur colloid which is aborbed on to pieces of filter paper, sometimes sealed in Perspex (Heading *et al.*, 1976), or mixed into a solid food such as mashed potatoes or liver. A refinement has been to feed ^{99m}Tc-pertechnetate to live chickens and use the fresh liver as the solid component of the meal (Meyer *et al.*, 1976). Recent evidence suggests that this refinement may not be required (Corinaldesi *et al.*, 1987) and injection of the marker into the liver before cooking (Wright *et al.*, 1981), or homogenization with liver pâté (Christian *et al.*, 1984) may be sufficient to ensure adequate labelling. ^{99m}Tc-labelled DPTA can also be used as a measure of the liquid phase of emptying if data on emptying of solids are not required.

(b) Imaging

Subjects are usually imaged supine and images obtained over a period of up to 1 h. With low-energy nuclides such as ^{99m}Tc, imaging with a double-headed scanner will minimize errors due to varying depth of the stomach (Tothill *et al.*, 1978), but in practice imaging with a gamma camera positioned posteriorly with correction for depth using a lateral image will yield accurate and reproducible results (Collins *et al.*, 1983; Collins *et al.*, 1984). Ideally, dynamic radionuclide scans are obtained continuously in 10–30 s frames according to the activity used. If intermittent scans are obtained the patient sits in a chair between recordings. If comparative scans are to be obtained in a single patient, it is important that conditions such as position during the scan, are reproduced as nearly as possible, as emptying is faster in the erect than in the supine position.

Region of interest analysis is used to obtain the number of counts in the stomach for each scan. Correction must be made for background and physical decay. The results are plotted as counts per unit area against time, and a single measurement of the time taken for the gastric contents to reduce by half is the most commonly used estimate of gastric emptying time, though more sophisticated analysis is more accurate and preferable (Elashoff *et al.*, 1982).

12.9.8 MECKEL'S DIVERTICULUM

The patient is studied and fasting. ^{99m}Tc-pertechnetate (1–5 mCi) is used, depending upon the size of the patient. No perchlorate is given but the results may be enhanced by pentagastrin (6 μg kg^{-1} subcutaneously) (Treves *et al.*, 1978) together with nasogastric aspiration, though these refinements are not always used (Feggi and Bighi, 1979). The pertechnetate is given intravenously and the patient is imaged supine with the gamma camera positioned over the abdomen. Multiple views (anterior, posterior and laterals) are taken at 10, 20 and 30 min after the injection. If taken too early blood background will not have decreased sufficiently and if taken too late gastric emptying will obscure the field of view. It is important that the subject empties his bladder prior to imaging. Cimetidine may improve detection rates, possibly by increasing retention of pertechnetate within gastric mucosa (Sagar and Piccone, 1981; Williams, 1983).

12.9.9 ^{51}Cr-LABELLED RED CELL BLEEDING (Cuddigan *et al.*, 1971)

The method adopted for labelling blood with ^{51}Cr is based on that used by Mollison (1961). A sample of 15 ml of blood is taken from each patient, placed in a sterile heparinized bottle, and centrifuged at 2000 rev min^{-1} for 10 min. The plasma is removed and 20 ml of citrate buffer is added to the red cells, which are then mixed thoroughly and recentrifuged. Most of the supernatant is removed and 200 μCi ^{51}Cr as sodium chromate added. This mixture is incubated at 37 °C for 15 min. After thorough washing sufficient saline is added to constitute a total volume of 20 ml, and 15 ml of this total is reinjected intravenously into the patient. Blood samples are then taken at 15 min and at one and two weeks. From these samples the percentage per litre of the administered dose remaining in the blood can be determined for any day in the trial.

Faeces are collected in waxed cartons, and radioactivity is measured in a large-volume scintillation counter (Clapham and Hayter, 1962). This contains two large plastic scintillators, and the top one can be removed to reveal a central well designed to give 4π counting geometry. By comparing each specimen with a known standard, the percentage of the administered dose can be determined, and hence the volume of blood in each sample:

$$\text{Blood in sample} = \frac{\text{\% administered dose in faeces} \times 100}{\text{\% litre administered dose in food}}$$

12.9.10 VITAMIN B12 ABSORPTION

(a) Schilling test

^{58}Co-labelled B12 (0.5 μCi) is given orally after an overnight fast. An intramuscular injection of 1 mg of non-radioactive cyanocobalamin (vitamin B12) is given within 2 h. Urine is saved for 24 h and its content of ^{58}Co is measured.

(b) Dicopac test

The Dicopac kit – a dual-isotope test for vitamin B12 malabsorption – with standards is obtainable from Amersham International, Amersham, UK. Each unit contains two capsules: one capsule (red/ivory) containing 1 ng ^{57}Co-cyanocobalamin (0.25 μg, nominal activity 0.5 μCi) bound to human gastric juice, and one capsule of ^{58}Co-cyanocobalamin. The patient fasts overnight. Both capsules are given to the patient orally at the same time and cyanocobalamin injection BP (1 mg) is given immediately following this or within the next 2 h. Urine is collected for 24 h and the ^{57}Co and ^{58}Co content measured by comparison with the standard provided. Incomplete urine saves should not be abandoned as the ratio can still be useful for diagnosis. The amount of ^{57}Co and ^{58}Co in the sample present no difficulty as the energy of the γ-emissions of the two radionuclides is substantially different.

12.9.11 ^{51}Cr-CHROMIUM CHLORIDE FOR PROTEIN-LOSING ENTEROPATHY

^{51}Cr-chromium chloride is obtainable from Amersham International. It has a long shelf-life and can be kept for two to three months. Various doses have been recommended, but in adults 30 μCi and in infants and children 5–10 μCi have been found satisfactory. The radiopharmaceutical is given intravenously and stools are saved (free of urine) for five days. It is convenient to count the whole stool sample within its container in a large-sample scintillation counter (Clapham and Hayter, 1962). Excretion of more than 2% of the administered dose in five days indicates significant protein loss.

12.9.12 $^{14}CO_2$ BREATH TESTS (Hepner, 1974)

Carbon dioxide is produced as a waste product of many metabolic processes, including absorption and gut function. This has led to the development of a number of tests of metabolism that depend on the measurement of the specific activity of $^{14}CO_2$ in the breath (Figure 12.6). In these tests the patient exhales (every 30–60 min for 4–8 h) into a solution containing a known amount of alkali and a drop of phenolphthalein as an indicator. The

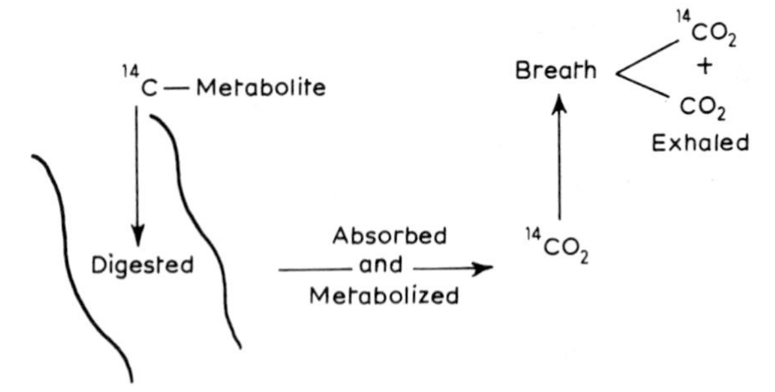

Figure 12.6 $^{14}CO_2$ breath tests.

carbon dioxide (both CO_2 and $^{14}CO_2$) is trapped and the solution changes from pink to clear when it is saturated. This change of pH occurs when there is a particular (and known) amount of carbon dioxide in the alkali. A scintillation liquid is added to the vial and the amount of $^{14}CO_2$ is measured using a liquid scintillation counter. As a known amount of CO_2 is trapped by the measured volume of alkali, the amount of $^{14}CO_2$ in the vial is a reflection of the total CO_2. Thus if there is more (or less) $^{14}CO_2$ produced this will be reflected by the amount of $^{14}CO_2$ in each vial. A curve of $^{14}CO_2$ over a period of 4–8 h can be obtained, or readings at a specific time such as 1 and 3 h.

(a) ^{14}C-glycocholic acid tests

The ^{14}C-glycocholic acid (bile acid) test is of established value in proving bile acid deconjugation (Hofmann and Thomas, 1973; James *et al.*, 1973). This usually results from bacterial overgrowth in the small intestine due to stagnation of contents in blind loops, diverticula, etc. (Scarpello and Sladen, 1977a). The test is also positive if there is ileal malabsorption of bile acids as a result of resection of Crohn's disease of the ileum (Scarpello and Sladen, 1977b).

The examination is performed after an overnight fast. ^{14}C-glycocholic acid (5 μCi) (Amersham International) is given orally with unlabelled glycocholate (0.1 mmol) as a carrier. The patient is then allowed to eat. Expired breath samples are collected over silica gel and trapped in counting vials containing hyamine hydrochloride (1 mmol) in 2 ml of ethanol with phenolphthalein ($20\ g\ l^{-1}$ in ethanolic solution) as indicator. Hourly samples are obtained in duplicate from 4 to 8 h. This mean hourly ^{14}C output in the breath is calculated as described by Fromm and Hofmann (1971) and expressed as a total accumulated output over 6 h. This is normally less than 4%.

(b) ^{14}C-triolein breath test (Newcomer *et al.*, 1979)

After an overnight fast 5 μCi ^{14}C-triolein is given by mouth, dissolved in 30 ml of high-calorie dietary supplement. Hourly $^{14}CO_2$ breath collections are made for 6 h and $^{14}CO_2$ is calculated as percentage dose per hour (Fromm and Hofmann, 1971).

(c) ^{14}C-lactose breath test (Newcomer *et al.*, 1975)

The fasting patient is given 5 μCi ^{14}C-lactose orally and $^{14}CO_2$ in the breath is measured for 4 h. The trapping solution is 2 mEq of hyamine hydrochloride with thymolphthalein as indicator (Fromm and Hofmann, 1971). $^{14}CO_2$ is expressed as the percentage of administered dose exhaled per hour.

The full potential of ^{14}C breath tests has not yet been reached. The technique is likely to be useful in other metabolic processes than gut function. For instance the ^{14}C-aminopyrine breath test is being used to evaluate hepatic microsomal function in relation to demethylation of aminopyrine (Hepner and Vesell, 1974; Bircher *et al.*, 1976; Galizzi *et al.*, 1978).

REFERENCES

Abdel-Dayem, H. M., Ziada, G., Owuawanne, A. *et al.* (1984) Scintigraphic detection of acute gastrointestinal bleeding using 99mTc DTPA. *Nucl. Med. Commun.*, **5**, 633–9.

Alavi, A. (1982) Detection of gastrointestinal bleeding with 99mTc sulphur colloid. *Semin. Nucl. Med.*, **12**, 126–38.

Albàn Davies, H., Jones, D. B. and Rhodes, J. (1982) Esophageal angina as the cause of chest pain. *JAMA*, **248**, 2274–8.

Alban Davies, H., Jones, D. B., Rhodes, J. and Newcombe, R. G. (1985) Angina-like esophageal pain: differentiation from cardiac pain by history. *J. Clin. Gastroenterol.*, **7**, 477–81.

Anderson, J. R., Spence, R. A. J., Laird, J. D. *et al.* (1983) ^{111}Indium autologous leucocyte scanning in acute pancreatitis. *Gut*, **24**, A490.

Avgerinos, A., Beavis, A. K., Misiewicz, J. J. and Silk, D. B. A. (1981) ^{14}C-triolein breath test as an outpatient screening test for detecting steatorrhoea. *Gut*, **22**, A442.

Ballantyne, K. C., Perkins, A. C., Pimm, M. V. *et al.* (1988) Detection of recurrent colorectal cancer by indium-111-791T/36 monoclonal antibody imaging. *Gut*, **29**, A740.

Baretti, C., Baccega, M., Rocsa, R. *et al.* (1990) The value of ^{111}Indium scintigraphy in the assessment of inflammatory bowel disease, in *Abstracts of the World Congress of Gastroenterology, Sydney 1990*. The Medicine Group, Abingdon, p. 781.

Baron, J. H. (1978) *Clinical Tests of Gastric Secretion*, Macmillan, London.

Barry, J. W. and Engle, C. V. (1978) Detection of haemorrhage in a patient with caecal varices using 99mTc-sulphur colloid. *Radiology*, **129**, 489–90.

Baulieu, F., Baulieu, J. L., Dorval, E. *et al.* (1986) Scintigraphy in duodeno-gastric reflux: a new method of quantification. *Nucl. Med. Commun.*, **7**, 747–54.

Bayley, J. H., Bell, T. K. and Waters, A. (1971) A dual isotope modification of the Schilling test. *Ergenbuisse klin. Nuklearmed.* Suppl. 9, 911–15.

Bell, T. K. and Lee, D. (1969) Evaluation of a dual radioisotope urinary excretion test in the diagnosis of pernicious anaemia. *Acta Haematol.*, **42**, 183–7.

Berquist, T. H., Nolan, N. G., Stephens, D. H. and Carlson, H. C. (1976) Specificity of 99mTc pertechnetate in scintigraphy diagnosis of Meckel's diverticulum: review of 100 cases. *J. Nucl. Med.*, **17**, 465–9.

Bircher, J., Kupfer, A., Gikalov, I. and Presig, R. (1976) Aminopyrine demethylation measured by breath analysis in cirrhosis. *Clin. Pharmacol. Ther.*, **20**, 484–92.

Blackwell, J. N., Hannan, W. J., Adam, R. D. and Heading, R. C. (1983) Radionuclide transit studies in the detection of oesophageal dysmotility. *Gut*, **24**, 421–6.

Blair, S. D., Riggs, S., Lloyd-Davies, E. R. V. *et al.* (1988) Peroperative scanning ^{125}I labelled anti-CEA monoclonal antibody to detect the extent of colorectal carcinoma. *Gut*, **29**, A731.

Bolondi, L., Bortolotti, M., Santi, V. *et al.* (1985) Measurement of gastric emptying time by real time ultrasonography. *Gastroenterology*, **89**, 752–9.

Brayton, D. (1964) Gastrointestinal bleeding of unknown origin. *Am. J. Dis. Child.*, **107**, 287–92.

Bronyaprara, S., Alderson, P. O., Garfunkel, O. G. *et al.* (1980) Detection of pulmonary aspiration in infants and children with respiratory disease. *J. Nucl. Med.* **21**, 314–18.

Butler, R. (1987) ^{14}C triolein breath test. *Gut*, **27**, 1320.

Buxton-Thomas, M. S., Dickinson, R. J., Maltby, P. *et al.* (1984) Evaluation of indium scintigraphy in patients with active inflammatory bowel disease. *Gut*, **25**, 1372–5.

Callender, S. T. (1970) The diagnostic uses of radioactive isotopes in haematology. *J. R. Coll. Phys. London*, **4**, 114–24.

Camilleri, M., Malagelade, J. R., Brown, M. L. *et al.* (1985) Relation between antral motility and gastric emptying of solids and liquids in humans. *Am. J. Physiol.*, **249**, 580–5.

Chaudhuri, T. K., Chaudhuri, T. K. and Christie, J. H. (1972) False positive Meckel's diverticulum scan. *Surgery*, **71**, 313.

Chobanian, S. J., Benjamin, S. B., Curtis, D. J. and Cattau, E. L. (1986) Systematic esophageal evaluation of patients with noncardiac chest pain. *Arch. Int. Med.*, **146**, 1505–8.

Christian, P. E., Moore, J. G. and Datz, F. L. (1984) Comparison of Tc-99m labelled liver and liver pate as markers for solid-phase gastric emptying. *J. Nucl. Med.*, **25**, 364–6.

Clapham, W. F. and Hayter, D. J. (1962) The measurement of gamma emitting isotopes in faeces. *Phys. Med. Biol.*, **7**, 313–17.

Coakley A. J. and Mountford P. J. (1986) Indium-111 leucocyte scanning – underused? *Br. Med. J.*, **293**, 973–4.

Collins, P. J., Horowitz, M., Cook, D. J. *et al.* (1983) Gastric emptying in normal subjects: a reproducible technique using a single scintillation camera and computer system. *Gut*, **24**, 1117–25.

Collins, P. J., Horowitz, M., Shearman, D. J. C. and Chatterton, B. E. (1984) Correction for tissue attenuation in radionuclide gastric emptying studies: a comparison of a lateral image method and a geometric mean method. *Br. J. Radiol.*, **57**, 689–95.

Colmer, M. R., Owen, G. M. and Shields, R. (1973) The pattern of gastric emptying after vagotomy and pyloroplasty. *Br. Med. J.*, **2**, 448–50.

Corinaldesi, R., Stanghellini, V., Raiti, C. *et al.* (1987) Validation of radioisotopic labelling techniques in gastric emptying studies. *J. Nucl. Med. Allied Sci.*, **31**, 207–12.

Cotton, P. B., Britton, K. E., Hazra, D. K. *et al.* (1978) Is pancreatic isotopye scanning worthwhile? *Br. Med. J.*, **1**, 282–83.

Cowley, D. J., Vernon, P., Jones, T. *et al.* (1972) Gastric emptying of solid meals after truncal vagotomy and pyloroplasty in human subjects. *Gut*, **13**, 176–81.

Croft, D. N. and Wood, P. H. N. (1967) Gastric mucosa and susceptibility to occult gastrointestinal bleeding caused by aspirin. *Br. Med. J.*, **1**, 137–41.

Croft, D. N., Cuddingan, J. H. P. and Sweetland, C. (1972) Gastric bleeding and benorylate, a new aspirin. *Br. Med. J.*, **3**, 545–7.

Cramp B. J., Kettle A. G., Field S. *et al.* (1987) 99mTc-scintigraphy and colonic disease. *Br. Med. J.*, **295**, 1134–5.

Cuddigan, J. H. P., Sweetland, C. and Croft, D. N. (1971) Assessment of drug-induced occult bleeding. *Rheumat. Phys. Med.*, **11**, 36–9.

Damron, J. R., Beihn, R. M., Selby, J. B. and Rosenbaum, H. D. (1974) Gallium–technetium subtraction scanning for the localisation of subphrenic abscess. *Radiology*, **113**, 117–22.

Dawson, D. J., Khan A. N., Miller V. *et al.* (1985) Detection of inflammatory bowel disease in adults and children: evaluation of a new isotopic technique. *Br. Med. J.*, **291**, 1227–30.

de Caesteker, J. S., Blackwell, J. N., Adam, R. D. *et al.* (1986) Clinical value of radionuclide oesophageal transit measurement. *Gut*, **27**, 659–66.

Donald, I. P., Ford, G. A. and Wilkinson, S. P. (1987) Is ambulatory esophageal pH monitoring useful in a district general hospital? *Lancet*, **ii**, 89–92.

Duszynski, D. O., Jewett, T. C. and Allen, J. E. (1971) Tc99m Na pertechnetate scanning of the abdomen with particular reference to small bowel pathology. *Am. J. Roentgenol. Rad. Ther. Nucl. Med.*, **113**, 258–62.

Einarsson, K., Bjorkhem, I., Eklof, R. and Blomstrand, R. (1983) ^{14}C-Triolein breath test as a rapid and convenient screening test for fat malabsorption. *Scand. J. Gastroentero.*, **18**, 9–12.

Elashoff, J. D., Reedy, T. J. and Meyer, J. H. (1982) Analysis of gastric emptying data. *Gastroenterology*, **83**, 1306–12.

Elwan, M. (1984) Scintigraphic detection of acute gastrointestinal bleeding using 99mTc-DTPA. *Nucl. Med. Commun.*, **5**, 633–9.

Eustace, P. W., Gaunt, J. I. and Croft, D. N. (1975) Incidence of protein-losing enteropathy in primary lymphoedema using chromium-51 chloride technique. *Br. Med. J.*, **4**, 737–8.

Fealey, R. D., Szurszewski, J. H., Merritt, J. L. and DiMagno, E. P. (1984) Effect of traumatic spinal cord transection on human upper gastrointestinal motility and gastric emptying. *Gastroenterology*, **87**, 69–75.

Feggi, L. M. and Bighi, S. M. (1979) Technical notes for scintigraphy of Meckel's diverticulum. *J. Nucl. Med.*, **20**, 888–9.

Ferraris, R., Jazrawi, R., Bridges, C. and Northfield, T. C. (1986) Use of a γ-labelled bile acid (75SeHCAT) as a test of ileal function. *Gastroenterology*, **90**, 1129–36.

Fisher, R. S., Malmud, L. S., Roberts, G. S. and Lobis, I. F. (1976) Gastroesophageal (GE) scintiscanning to detect and quantitate GE reflux. *Gastroenterology*, **70**, 301–8.

Fromm, H. and Hofmann, A. F. (1971) Breath test for altered bile acid metabolism. *Lancet*, **ii**, 621–5.

Galizzi, J., Lory, R. G., Billing, B. H. and Sherlock, S. (1978) Assessment of the (^{14}C) aminopyrine breath test in liver disease. *Gut*, **19**, 40–5.

Gelfand, M. J., Silberstein, E. B. and Cox, J. (1978) Radionuclide imaging of Meckel's diverticulum in children. *Clin. Nucl. Med.*, **3**, 4–8.

George, A., Merrick M. V., Palmer K. R. and Miller A. M. (1987) 99mTc sucralfate scintigraphy and colonic disease. *Br. Med. J.*, **295**, 578.

Gibson, C. J. and Bateson, M. C. (1985) A parametric image technique for the assessment of oesophageal function. *Nucl. Med. Commun.*, **6**, 83–9.

Goldenberg, D. J., Russell, C. D. Mihas, A. A. *et al.* (1979) Gallium for Crohn's disease. *J. Nucl. Med.*, **20**, 215.

Goulston, K. and Skyring, A. (1964) Effect of paracetamol (*N*-acetyl-*p*-aminophenol) on gastrointestinal bleeding. *Gut*, **5**, 463–6.

Graham, D. Y., Klein, P. D., Evans, D. J. *et al.* ((1987) *Campylobacter pylori* detected noninvasively by the ^{13}C-urea breath test. *Lancet*, **i**, 1174–7.

Granowska, M., Mather, S. J., Britton, K. E. *et al.* (1990) ^{99m}Tc radioimmunoscintigraphy of colorectal cancer. *Br. J. Cancer*, **62**, Suppl. X, 30–3.

Guillet, J., Basse-Cathalinat, B., Christophe, E. *et al.* (1984) Routine studies of swallowed radionuclide transit in paediatrics: experience with 400 patients. *Eur. J. Nucl. Med.*, **9**, 86–90.

Halter, F. (1981) Therapeutic implications of duodenogastric reflux. *Eur. J. Nucl. Med.*, 257–9.

Ham, H. R., Piepsz, A., Georges, B. *et al.*, (1984) Quantitation of esophageal transit by means of ^{81m}Kr. *Eur. J. Nucl. Med.*, **9**, 362–5.

Hattner, R. S. and Engelstad, B. L. (1983) An advance in identification and localisation of gastrointestinal haemorrhage. *Gastroenterology*, **83**, 484–5.

Heading, R. C., Tothill, P., Laidlaw, A. J. and Shearman, D. J. C (1971) Evaluation of 113m indium DTPA chelate in the measurement of gastric emptying by scintiscanning. *Gut*, **12**, 611–15.

Heading, R. C., Tothill, P., McLoughlin, G. P. and Shearman, D. J. C. (1976) Gastric emptying rate measurement in man. *Gastroenterology*, **71**, 45–50.

Heaton, K. W. (1986) Staying cool with a hot test: gastroenterologists and 75SeHCAT. *Br. Med. J.*, **292**, 1480–1.

Hebbard, G., Gibson, P. R., Lichtenstein, M. *et al.* (1990) The value of positive ^{99m}Tc-leucocyte scans in predicting intestinal inflammation, in *Abstracts of the World Congress of Gastroenterology, Sydney 1990*. The Medicine Group (UK), Abingdon, p. 737.

Hepner, G. W. (1974) Breath analysis: gastroenterological applications. *Gastroenterology*, **67**, 1250–6.

Hepner, G. W. and Vesell, E. S. (1974) Assessment of aminopyrine metabolism in man by breath analysis after oral administration of 14C-aminopyrine. *New Engl. J. Med.*, **291**, 1384–8.

Hill, I. D., Sinclair-Smith, C., Lastovica, A. J. *et al.* (1987) Transient protein losing enteropathy associated with acute gastritis and *Campylobacter pylori*. *Arch. Dis. Child.*, **62**, 1215–20.

Hoare, A. M., McLeish A., Thompson H. and Alexander-Williams, J. (1978) Selection of patients for bile diversion surgery: use of bile acid measurement in fasting gastric aspirates. *Gut*, **191**, 163–5.

Hofmann, A. F. and Thomas, P. J. (1973) Bile acid breath test: extremely simple, moderately useful. *Ann. Intern. Med.*, **79**, 734–4.

Holloway, R. H., Krosin, G., Lange, R. C. *et al.* (1983) Radionuclide esophageal emptying of a solid meal to quantitate results of therapy in achalasia. *Gastroenterology*, **84**, 771–776.

Holt, J. M., Mayet, F. G. H., Warner, G. T. and Callendar, S. T. (1967) Measurement of blood loss by means of a whole-body counter. *Br. Med. J.*, **4**, 86–8.

Holt, J. M., Mayet, F. G. H., Warner, G. T. *et al.* (1968) Iron absorption and blood loss in patients with hiatus hernia. *Br. Med. J.*, **3**, 22–5.

Hopkins, G. B., Kan, M. and Mende, C. W. (1975) Early ^{67}Ga scintigraphy for the localisation of abdominal abscess. *J. Nucl. Med.*, **16**, 990–2.

Hopkins, G. B., Kan, M. and Mende, C. W. (1976) Gallium-67 scintigraphy and intraabdominal sepsis. *West. J. Med.*, **125**, 425–30.

James, O. F. W., Agnew, J. E. and Bouchier, I. A. D. (1973) Assessment of the ^{14}C glycocholic acid breath test. *Br. Med. J.*, **3**, 191–5.

Jones, N. F., Creamer, B. and Gimlette, T. M. D. (1966) Hypoproteinaemia in anaphylactoid purpura. *Br. Med. J.*, **2**, 1166–8.

Katon, R. M. and Smith, F. W. (1973) Panendoscopy in the early diagnosis of acute upper gastrointestinal bleeding. *Gastroenterology*, **65**, 728–34.

King C. E. and Toskes P. P. (1983) The use of breath tests in the study of malabsorption. *Clin. Gastroenterol.*, **12**, 591–610.

Kinmonth, J. B. and Cox, S. J. (1974) Protein-losing enteropathy in primary lymphoedema: mesenteric lymphography and gut resection. *Br. J. Surg.*, **61**, 589–93.

Kjellen, G. and Svedberg, J. S. (1983) Oesophageal transit of radionuclide solid bolus in normals. *Clin. Physiol.*, **3**, 69–74.

Kjellen, G., Svedberg, J. B. and Tibbing, L. (1984) Solid bolus transit by esophageal scintigraphy in patients with dysphagia and normal manometry and radiography. *Dig. Dis. Sci.*, **29**, 1–5.

Kjellen, G. and Tibbling, L. (1985) Oesophageal motility during acid-provoked heartburn and chest pain. *Scand. J. Gastroenterol.*, **20**, 937–40.

Klein, H. A. and Wald, A. (1984) Computer analysis of radionuclide esophageal transit studies. *J. Nucl. Med.*, **25**, 957–964.

Knochel, J. Q., Keohler P. R., Lee T. G. and Welch D. M. (1980) Diagnosis of abdominal abscesses with computed tomography, ultrasound and ^{111}In-leucocyte scans. *Radiography*, **137**, 425.

Kumar, B., Alderson, P. O. and Geisse, G. (1977) The role of Ga-67 citrate imaging and diagnostic ultrasound in patients with suspected abdominal abscesses. *J. Nucl. Med.*, **18**, 534–7.

Lamki, L. (1985) Radionuclide esophageal transit (RET) study: the effect of body posture. *Clin. Nucl. Med.*, **10**, 108–10.

Levitt, M. D. (1969) Production and excretion of hydrogen gas in man. *N. Engl. J. Med.*, **281**, 122–7.

Levitt, R. G., Biello, D. R., Sagel, S. S. *et al.* (1979) Computed tomography and ^{67}Ca citrate radionuclide imaging for evaluating suspected abdominal abscess. *Am. J. Roentgenol.*, **132**, 529–34.

Lunia, S., Lunia, C., Chandramouly, B. and Chodos, R. B. (1979) Radionuclide Meckelogram with particular reference to false-positive results. *Clin. Nucl. Med.*, **4**, 285–8.

Malmud, L. S., Fisher, R. S., Lobis, I. and Mainer, W. (1976) Quantitation of gastroesophageal reflux (GE) reflux before and after therapy using the GE scintiscan. *J. Nucl. Med.*, **17**, 559–60.

Malmud, L. S., Fisher, R. S., Knight, L. C. and Rock, E. (1982) Scintigraphic evaluation of gastric emptying. *Semin Nucl. Med.*, **12**, 116–25.

Maddern, G. J., Horowitz, M., Jamieson, G. G. *et al.* (1984) Abnormalities of esophageal and gastric emptying in progressive systemic sclerosis. *Gastroenterology*, **87**, 922–6.

Marshall, B. J., McGechie, D. B., Rogers, P. A. *et al.* (1985) Pyloric campylobacter infection and gastrointestinal disease. *Med. J. Aust.*, **142**, 439–44.

Marshall, B. J., Goodwin C. S., Warren J. R. *et al.* (1988) Prospective double blind trial of duodenal ulcer relapse after eradication of *Campylobacter pylori*. *Lancet*, **ii**, 1437–41.

Mayer, E. A., Thompson, J. B., Jehn, D. *et al.* (1984) Gastric emptying and sieving of solid food and pancreatic and biliary secretions after solid meals in patients with nonresective ulcer surgery. *Gastroenterology*, **87**, 1264–71.

Mcnamee, P. T., Moore, G. W., McGeown, M. G. and Doherty, C. C. (1985) Gastric emptying in chronic renal failure. *Br. Med. J.*, **291**, 310–1.

Meguid, M. M., Wilkinson, R. H., Canty, T. *et al.* (1974) Futility of barium sulphate in diagnosis of Meckel's diverticulum. *Arch. Surg.*, **108**, 361–2.

Mercer, C. D., Rue, C., Hanelin, L and Hill, L. D. (1985) Effect of obesity on esophageal transit. *Am. J. Surg.*, **149**, 177–81.

Merrick, M. V. (1986) in *Nuclear Gastroenterology* (ed.

P. J. A. Robinson), Churchill Livingstone, Edinburgh, pp. 157–69.
Merrick, M. V., Eastwood, M. A., Anderson, J. R. and Ross, H. M. (1982) Enterohepatic circulation in man of a gamma emitting bile acid conjugate ^{75}Selena-25-homotaurocholic acid (SeHCAT). *J. Nucl. Med.*, **23**, 126–30.
Meyer, J. H., MacGregor, I. L., Martin, P. and Cavalier, I. R. (1976) 99mTc-tagged chicken liver as a marker of solid food in the human stomach. *Dig. Dis. Sci.*, **21**, 296–304.
Miskowiak, J., Nielson, S. L., Munck, Q. and Anderson, B. (1977) Abdominal scintophotography with 99mTc labelled albumin in acute gastrointestinal bleeding. *Lancet*, **ii**, 853–4.
Miskowiak, J., Munck, Q., Nielsen, S. L. *et al.* (1983) An advance in identification and localisation of gastrointestinal haemorrhage. *Gastroenterology*, **84**, 668–9.
Mollison, P. L. (1961) The further observations on the normal survival curve of ^{51}Cr-labelled red cells. *Clin. Sci.*, **21**, 21–36.
Mountford, P. J., Kettle, A. G., O'Doherty, M. J. *et al.* (1990) Comparison of Technatium ^{99m}leukocytes with Indium ^{111}oxime leukocytes for localising intrabdominal sepsis, *J. Nucl. Med.*, **31**, 311–15.
Mughal, M. M., Marples, M. and Bancewicz, J. (1986) Scintigraphic assessment of oesophageal motility: what does it show and how reliable is it? *Gut*, **27**, 946–53.
Muhammed, I., McLoughlin, G. P., Holt, S. and Taylor, T. V. (1980) Non-invasive estimation of duodeno-gastric reflux using Technetium 99m *p*-butyliminodiacetic acid. *Lancet*, **ii**, 1162.
Muller-Lissner, S. A., Fimmel, C. J., Sonnenberg, A. *et al.* (1983) Novel approach to quantify duodeno-gastric reflux in patients with Type I gastric ulcer. *Gut*, **24**, 510–18.
Mylvaganam, K., Hudson, P. R., Ross, A. and Williams, C. P. (1986) ^{14}C Triolein breath test: a routine test in the gastroenterology clinic. *Gut*, **27**, 1347–52.
Newcomer, A. D., McGill, D. B., Thomas, P. J. and Hofmann, A. F. (1975) Prospective comparison of indirect methods for detecting lactase deficiency. *New Engl. J. Med.*, **293**, 1232–5.
Newcomer, A. D., Hofmann, A. F., Dimago, E. O. *et al.* (1979) Triolein breath test: a sensitive and specific test for fat malabsorption. *Gastroenterology*, **76**, 6–13.
Nyhlin, H., Merrick, H. V., Eastwood, M. A. and Bryton, W. G. (1983) Evaluation of ileal function using ^{75}selena-25-homotaurocholate, a gamma labelled conjugated bile acid. *Gastroenterology*, **84**, 63–8.
Ohrt, H. J. and Scafer, R. B. (1982) An atlas of salivary gland disorders. *Clin. Nucl. Med.*, **7**, 370–6.
Panel, P., Kimmer, A. M. and Patterson, V. N. (1977) *In vivo* labelling of red blood cells with 99mTc: a new approach to blood pool visualisation. *J. Nucl. Med.*, **18**, 305–8.
Park, R. H. R., McKillop, J. H., Duncan, A. *et al.* (1988) Can ^{111}Indium autologous mixed leucocyte scanning accurately assess disease extent and activity in Crohn's disease? *Gut*, **29**, 821–5.
Parret, J. and Peyrin, J. O. (1979) Radioisotopic investigations in salivary pathology. *Clin. Nucl. Med.*, **4**, 250–61.
Pederson, N. T. and Halgreen, H. (1985) Simultaneous assessment of fat maldigestion and fat malabsorption by a double-isotope method using fecal radioactivity. *Gastroenterology*, **88**, 47–54.
Perman, G., Gullberg, R., Reizenstein, P. G. *et al.* (1960) A study of absorption patterns in malabsorption syndromes. *Acta Med. Scand.*, **168**, 117–25.
Peters, A. M., Danpure, H. J., Osman, S. *et al.* (1986) Clinical experience with 99mTc-hexamethylpropylene-amineoxime for labelling leucocytes and imaging inflammation. *Lancet*, **ii**, 946–9.
Ralphs, D. N. L., Thomson, J. P. S., Haynes, S. *et al.* (1978) The relationship between the rate of gastric emptying and the dumping syndrome. *Br. J. Surg.*, **65**, 637–41.
Reich, S. B., Earley, W. C., Ravin, T. H. *et al.* (1977) Evaluation of gastropulmonary aspiration by a radioactive technique. *J. Nucl. Med.*, **18**, 1079–81.
Reidel, W. L. and Clouse, R. E. (1985) Variations in clinical presentation patients with esophageal contraction abnormalities. *Dig. Dis. Sci.*, **30**, 1065–71.
Rhodes, J. (1981) The clinical significance of bile reflux. *Scand. J. Gastroenterol.*, **16** (Suppl. 67), 173–5.
Richter, J. E., Blackwell, J. N., Wu, W. C. *et al.* (1987) Relationship of radionuclide liquid bolus transport and esophageal manometry. *J. Lab. Clin. Med.*, **109**, 217–24.
Rokkjaer, M., Marqverson, J., Kraglund, K. and Brunn-petersen, J. (1977) Quantitative determination of pyloric regurgitation in response to intra duodenal bolus injection. *Scand. J. Gastroenterol.*, **12**, 827–32.
Rozen, P., Gelfond, M., Zaltzman, S. *et al.* (1982) Dynamic, diagnostic and pharmacological radionuclide studies of the esophagus in achalasia. *Radiology*, **144**, 587–90.
Russell, C. O. H., Hill, L. D., Holmes, E. R. *et al.* (1981) Radionuclide transit: a sensitive screening test for esophageal dysfunction. *Gastroenterology*, **80**, 887–92.
Safaie-Shirazi, S., Chandhuri, T. K., Chandhuri, T. K. and Condon, R. E. (1973) Visualisation of isolated retained antrum by using technetium 99m. *Surgery*, **73**, 278–83.
Sagar, W. and Piccone, J. M. (1981) The effect of cimetidine on blood clearance, gastric uptake, and secretion of 99mTc-pertechnetate in dogs. *Radiology*, **139**, 429–431.
Saito, H., Sargent, T. and Parker, H. G. (1964) Whole body iron in normal man measured with gamma spectrometer. *J. Nucl. Med.*, **5**, 571.
Sandhu, K. P., el Samahi, M. M., I Mena, C. P. and Dooley, J. E. (1987) Effect of pectin on gastric emptying and gastroduodenal motility in normal subjects. *Gastroenterology*, **92**, 486–92.
Saverymuttu, S. H. (1990) Leucocyte Scanning, in *Topics in Gastroenterology*, (eds D. P. Jewell and J. A. Snook) Blackwell, Oxford, pp. 165–74.
Saverymuttu, S. H., Peters, A. M., Hodgson, H. J. *et al.* (1982) Indium-111 autologous leucocyte scanning: comparison with radiology for imaging the colon in inflammatory bowel disease. *Br. Med. J.*, **285**, 255–7.
Saverymuttu, S. H., Peters, A. M., Lavender, J. P. *et al.*

(1983) ^{111}Indium autologous leucocytes in inflammatory bowel disease. *Gut*, **24**, 293–299.

Saverymuttu, S. H., Camilleri, M., Rees, H. *et al.* (1986) Indium-111 granulocyte scanning in the assessment of disease extent and disease activity in inflammatory bowel disease. *Gastroenterology*, **90**, 1121–8.

Scarpello, J. H. B. and Sladen, G. E. (1977a) Appraisal of the ^{14}C glycoholate acid test with special reference to the measurement of faecal ^{14}C excretion, *Gut*, **18**, 742–8.

Scarpello, J. H. B. and Sladen, G. E. (1977b) ^{14}C-glycocholate test in Crohn's disease: its value in assessment and treatment. *Gut*, **18**, 736–41.

Schall, G. L., Smith, R. R. and Barsocchini, L. M. (1981) Radionuclide salivery imaging usefulness in a private otolaryngology practice. *Arch. Otolaryngol.*, **107**, 40–44.

Schiller, L. R., Hogan, R. B., Morawski, S. G. *et al.* (1987) Studies of the prevalence and significance of radiolabelled bile acid malabsorption in a group of patients with idiopathic chronic diarrhoea. *Gastroenterology*, **92**, 151–60.

Schwesinger, W. H., Croom, R. D. and Habibian, M. R. (1975) Diagnosis of an enteric duplication with pertechnetate 99mTc scanning. *Ann. Surg.*, **181**, 428–30.

Sciaretta, G., Malaguti, P., Turba, E. *et al.* (1978) Retained gastric antrum syndrome diagnosed by (99mTc) pertechnetate scintiphotography in man: hormonal and radioisotopic study of two cases. *J. Nucl. Med.*, **19**, 377–80.

Sciarretta, G., Fagioli, G., Furno, A. *et al.* (1987) ^{75}Se HCAT test in the detection of bile acid malabsorption in functional diarrhoea and its correlation with small bowel transit. *Gut*, **28**, 970–5.

Sfakianakis, G. N., Al-Shekh, W., Heal, A. *et al.* (1982) Comparisons of scintigraphy with In-111 leukocytes and Ga-67 in the diagnosis of occult sepsis. *J. Nucl. Med.*, **23**, 618–26.

Shaffer, E. A., McOrmond, P. and Duggan, H. (1980) Quantitative cholescintigraphy: assessment of gall bladder filling and emptying and duodeno-gastric reflux. *Gastroenterology*, **79**, 899–906.

Shakianakis, G. W. and Conway, J. J. (1981) Detection of ectopic gastric mucosa in Meckel's diverticulum and in other aberrations by scintigraphy. *J. Nucl. Med.*, **22**, 647–54.

Shearman, D. J. C. and Finlayson, N. D. C. (1982) *Diseases of the Gastrointestinal Tract and Liver*, Churchill Livingstone, Edinburgh, pp. 169–91.

Sheiner, H. J. (1975) Gastric emptying tests in man. *Gut*, **16**, 235–47.

Smith, T. and Bjarnason, I. (1990) Experience with a gastrointestinal marker ($^{51}CrCl_3$) in a combined study of ileal function using ^{75}Se HCAT and $^{58}CoB_{12}$ measured by whole body counting, *Gut*, **31**, 1120–5.

Stabile, B. E. and Panaro, E. (1976) Recurrent peptic ulcer. *Gastroenterology*, **70**, 124–35.

Stein, D. T., Gray, G. M., Gregory, P. B. *et al.* (1983) Location and activity of ulcerative and Crohn's colitis by Indium-111 leukocyte scan. *Gastroenterology*, **84**, 388–93.

Svensson, J. O. (1983) Duodenic gastric reflux after gastric surgery. *Scand. J. Gastroenterol.*, **18**, 729–34.

Swarbrick, E. T., Feurde, D. I., Hunt, R. H. *et al.* (1978) Colonoscopy for unexplained rectal bleeding. *Br. Med. J.*, **2**, 1685–7.

Taillefer, R. and Beauchamp, G. (1984) Radionuclide esophogram. *Clin. Nucl. Med.*, **9**, 465–83.

Tatsck, K., Knesewitsch, P., Matuschke, A. *et al.* (1990) ^{67}Ga-scintigraphy for evaluation of AIDS-related intestinal infections. *Nucl. Med. Commun.*, **11**, 649–55.

Tauscher, J. W., Bryant, D. R. and Gruenther, R. C. (1978) False positive scan for Meckel's diverticulum. *J. Pediatr.*, **92**, 1022–3.

Tavormina, A., Mousave, A., Gordon, D. H. and Solomon, N. A. (1978) Extravasation of contrast material from vascular ectasia of the caecum detected with 99mTc pertechnetate. *Radiology*, **128**, 168.

Thaysen, E. H. (1977) Diagnostic value of the ^{14}C-cholyglycine breath test. *Clin. Gastroenterol.*, **6**, 227–45.

Tothill, P., McLoughlin, G. P. and Heading, R. C. (1978) Techniques and errors in scintigraphic measurements of gastric emptying. *J. Nucl. Med.*, **19**, 256–61.

Treves, S., Grant, R. J. and Eraklis, A. J. (1978) Pentagastrin stimulation of technetium 99mTc uptake by ectopic gastric mucosa in Meckel's diverticulum. *Radiology*, **128**, 711–12.

Trottman, I. F. and Price, C. C. (1986) Bloated irritable bowel syndrome defined by dynamic 'All Bran' Scan. *Gut*, **27**, A619.

van Trappen, G., Janssens, J. and Ghillebert, G. (1987) The irritable oesophagus: a frequent cause of angina-like pain. *Lancet*, **i**, 1232–4.

Velasco, N., Pope, C. E., Gannan, R. M. *et al.* (1984) Measurement of esophageal reflux by scintigraphy. *Dig. Dis. Sci.*, **29**, 977–82.

Wakat, M. A., Mustol, J. S., Baird, B. and Berry, R. E. (1981) Localisation of gastrointestinal bleeding using Tc-99m pyrophosphate in vivo labelled red cells. *Nucl. Med. Commun.*, **2**, 102.

Walker-Smith, J. A., Skyring, A. P. and Mistilis, S. P. (1967) Use of $^{51}Cr\ Cl_3$ in the diagnosis of protein-losing enteropathy. *Gut*, **8**, 166–8.

West, P. S., Levin, G. E., Griffin, G. E. and Maxwell, J. D. (1981) Comparison of simple screening tests for fat malabsorption. *Br. Med. J.*, **282**, 1501–4.

Wickremesinghe, P. C., Dayrit, P. Q., Manfredi, O. L. *et al.* (1983) Quantitative evaluation of bile diversion surgery utilising 99mTc HIDA scintigraphy. *Gastroenterology*, **84**, 354–63.

Williams, J. G. (1983) Pertechnetate and the stomach: a continuing controversy. *J. Nucl. Med.*, **24**, 633–6.

Williams, J. G. (1986) in *Recent Advances in Gastroenterology* (ed. R. E. Pounder), Churchill Livingstone, Edinburgh, pp. 181–209.

Williams, J. G., Turner, J. R. and Beckley, D. (1986) Does sclerotherapy affect oesophageal function? *J. R. Nav. Serv.*, **72**, 80–3.

Winzelberg, G. S., McKusick, K. A., Strauss, H. W. *et al.* (1979) Evaluation of gastrointestinal bleeding by red blood cells labelled in vivo with technetium-99m. *J. Nucl. Med.*, **20**, 1080–6.

Wolff, W. I., Crossman, M. B. and Shinya, H. (1977) Angiogysplasia of the colon: diagnosis and treatment. *Gastroenterology*, **72**, 329–33.

Wright, R. A., Thompson, D. and Syed, I. (1981) Simultaneous markers for fluid and solid gastric emptying: new variations on an old theme. *J. Nucl. Med.*, **22**, 722–76.

Zakhireh, B., Thakur, M. L., Malech, H. L. *et al.* (1979), Indium-111-labelled human polymorphonuclear leukocytes, viability, random migration, chemotaxis, bactericidal capacity and ultrastructure. *J. Nucl. Med.*, **20**, 741–7.

Zanelli, G. D., Bjarnason, I., Smith, T. *et al.* (1986) Technetium 99m labelled porphyrin as an imaging agent for occult infections and inflammation. *Nucl. Med. Commun.*, **7**, 17–24.

CHAPTER THIRTEEN

Abdominal trauma

D. L. Gilday and J. M. Ash

The triage of patients with blunt abdominal trauma is as follows. Life-threatening conditions must be corrected first. Often severe skeletal injuries have to be immobilized to prevent further damage. In the course of the patient's management, plain radiographs may be taken that can help evaluate the abdomen. If head or spinal injuries are present they must be evaluated and treated before the abdomen. If computed tomography (CT) or magnetic resonance imaging (MRI) is being carried out for this purpose, the sections of the abdomen can be used to screen the major organs for injury. If CT or MRI is not being performed, then usually radionuclide kidney and liver and spleen single-photon emission computed tomography (SPECT) imaging can be used to evaluate these organs. Ultrasound may be substituted but in some cases is not as reliable (Froelich, 1982). Ultrasound's main asset is its ability to detect fluid collections where SPECT imaging has proved to be more sensitive and descriptive of the injury to the liver, spleen or kidneys.

In the 1970s nuclear medicine techniques became useful in the evaluation of patients with abdominal trauma (Freedman, 1973; Gilday and Alderson, 1974). Usually such injuries manifest typical physical findings of rupture, laceration, or haematoma of solid organs with associated blood loss or perforation of hollow viscera. Some patients who have significant injuries may be difficult to diagnose, especially if the patient has multiple injuries or reduced level of consciousness making it difficult to get a good clinical picture. In addition to history and physical examination, haematological studies, urinalysis and urinary bladder catheterization, routine thoracic and abdominal radiography, especially with upright board lateral decubitus films CT, ultrasonography, or nuclear medicine procedures are used in the evaluation of these patients. Serial determinations of haematocrit and haemaglobin often give an indication of whether or not blood loss is present. It is also used to monitor the success of the transfusion replacement therapy. This is quite important as the current trend is to operate on the abdomen much less often (Howman–Giles *et al.*, 1978) and usually only when haemostasis cannot be maintained by transfusion.

The ability of the patient to void spontaneously is usually a good indication that there has not been trauma to the lower urinary tract. In a clean catheterized urine specimen the presence of erythrocytes, leucocytes or proteinuria suggest that there may be injury to either a kidney or the bladder. The presence of an air-filled viscus in the chest on an upright posterior or anterior radiograph indicates a traumatic diaphragmatic hernia. Fractured ribs when seen should raise the suspicion that there may be injury to either the liver or spleen. A lateral decubitus film of the abdomen is useful in detecting the presence of free air, which usually indicates that a hollow viscus has been ruptured. CT is now used routinely in the evaluation of patients with abdominal trauma. CT is almost always used to evaluate abdominal trauma in patients with either head or spinal injuries who are having neurological CT for the evaluation. CT is extremely sensitive in detecting solid organ injury as well as collections of fluid.

Ultrasonography is useful in detecting traumatic abnormalities to the spleen, liver, biliary tree, kidneys, pelvic organs, abdominal vasculature and the presence of haematoma.

Nuclear medicine can evaluate the presence of trauma to the kidneys, urinary tracts, bladder, liver, spleen and abdominal vasculature. The procedure is to inject a small quantity of ^{99m}Tc-labelled diethylenetriaminepentaacetic acid (DTPA) and evaluate the urinary tract for 15 min. Excellent results for detecting trauma to the urinary tract, especially the kidneys, have been

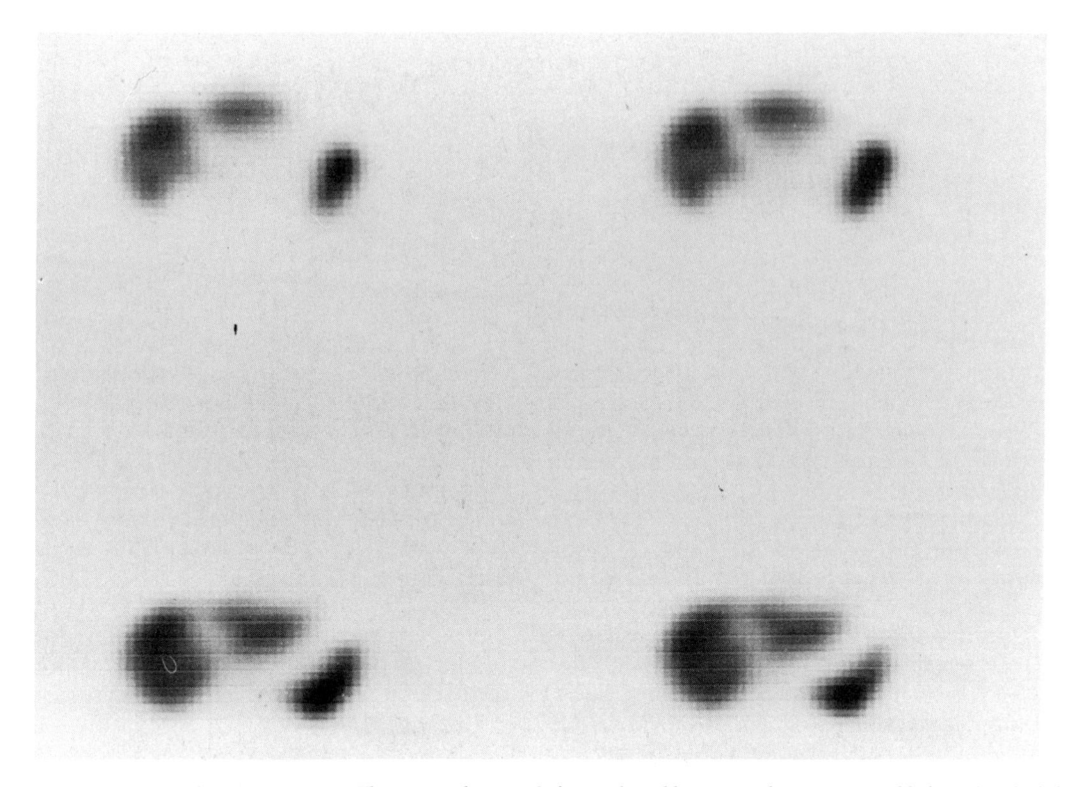

Figure 13.1 Hepatic shearing trauma. There is a photon-deficient band between the anatomical left and right lobes where the contusion is located.

obtained. In a study of 50 children at the Hospital for Sick Children comprised of intravenous urogram (IVU), ultrasound and dynamic renal imaging, four abnormalities were detected in the radionuclide study – two more than by either of the other techniques. Evaluation of the liver and spleen can be best performed by SPECT imaging. The major vessels are evaluated by radionuclide angiography after injecting ^{99m}Tc-labelled sulphur colloid. SPECT removes any problem of overlying renal activity. In addition, SPECT is significantly sensitive for detecting and characterizing traumatic abnormalities of the liver and spleen (Figure 13.1). At the Hospital for Sick Children a study of 50 patients with both planar and SPECT imaging showed three extra splenic abnormalities and two extra liver abnormalities not seen on planar imaging. This converted four patients to a diagnosis of injured liver or spleen.

13.1 EVALUATION OF RENAL ABNORMALITIES

The blood flow and blood pool image of the kidney are usually satisfactory to detect any cortical or medullary injury to the kidney. It is difficult to differentiate between laceration and haematoma. The usual abnormality is identified as a photon-deficient area. Occasionally if there is major injury to either the artery or vein no evidence of blood flow or functioning parenchyma will be seen. In such cases it is mandatory to have a secondary procedure to determine that in fact a kidney is present. This should be considered an emergency. Trauma to the drainage system of the kidney and bladder is usually evident by the presence of a leak. In such circumstances it is usual to image later to better define the leak prior to doing the SPECT liver and spleen scan.

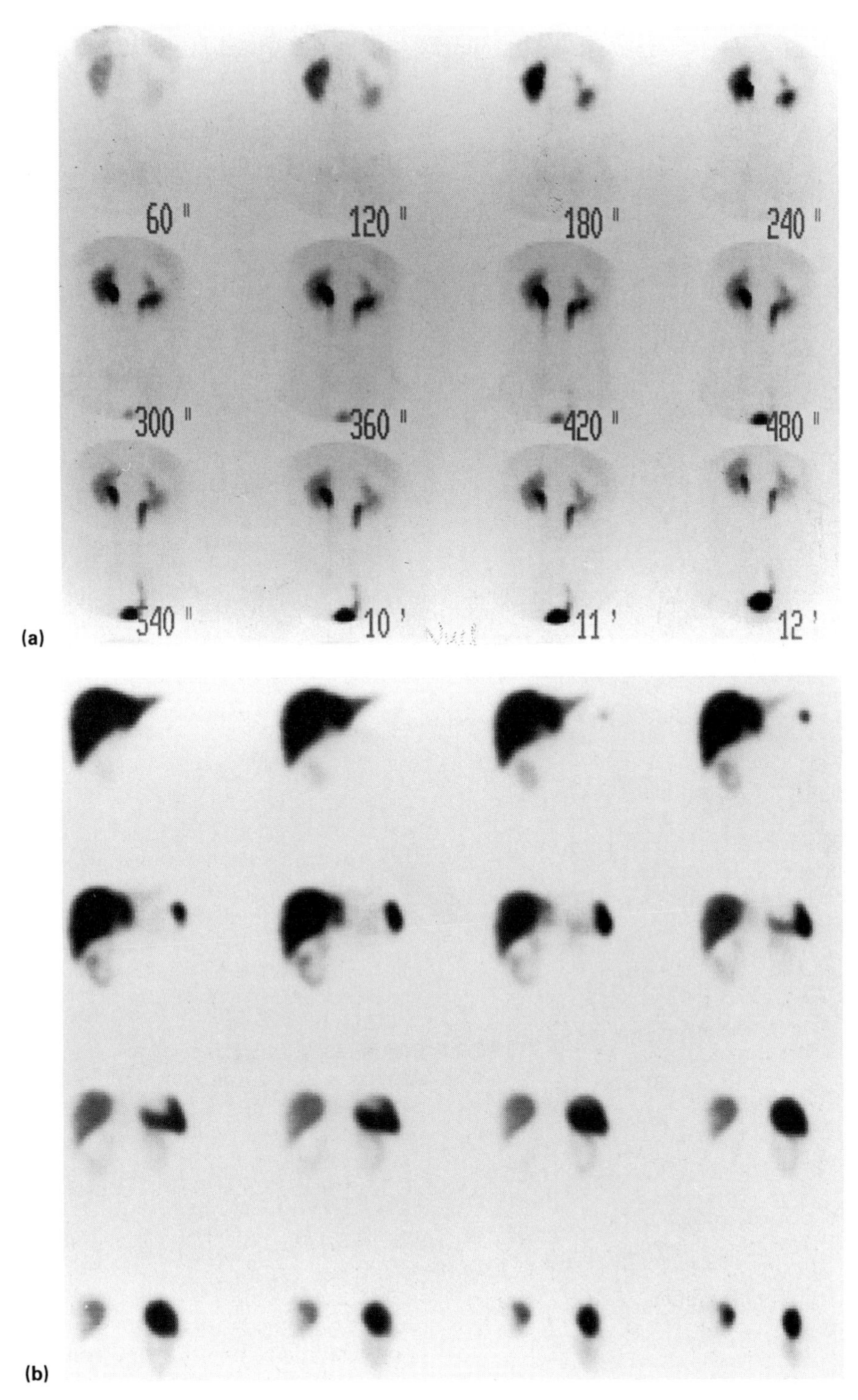

Figure 13.2 Renal contusion. The upper pole of the right kidney is seen to have absent function (a). The axial sections (b) and the coronal sections (c) demonstrate the separation of the liver and spleen from the kidneys. The contusion can be identified in the coronal images.

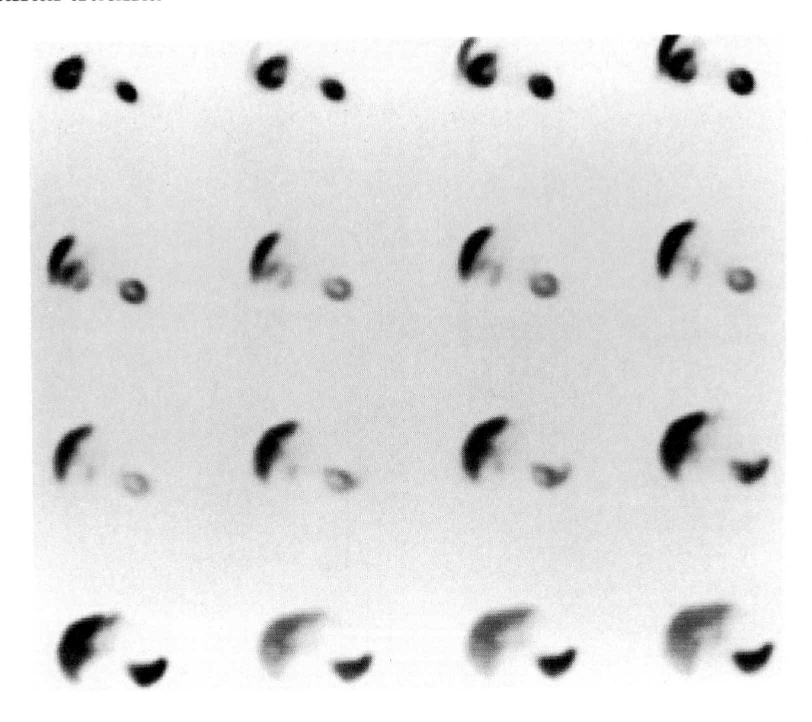

Figure 13.2 (cont'd)

13.2 LIVER AND SPLEEN EVALUATION

In evaluating either liver or spleen trauma the differentiation of laceration and haematoma is difficult. However, subcapsular haematoma is usually seen as a concave defect due to the lenticular shape that the haematoma develops as it is contained by the capsule of the liver. More commonly, laceration is seen as a linear band or wedge-shaped photon-deficient area in the tomographic slices. Frank rupture is identified when there is gross separation of components of the liver or spleen. A not uncommon type of injury to the liver secondary to blunt abdominal trauma is shearing along the line of the anatomic junction of the left and right lobes (Figure 13.2). This produces a band of decreased activity throughout the liver seen in many of the tomographic slices. One of the major assets of the tomographic technique is that it helps to characterize the abnormal findings far better than does planar imaging (Van Heertum, 1987). In addition, there is an increase in sensitivity (Brendel, 1984).

One of the main advantages of the radionuclide approach is that it is accurate and relatively inexpensive and can be performed quickly with only one technologist to do the study. Although it does not have the resolution of CT, and may not show all the abnormalities that procedure can, it has proved to be a very reliable technique for detecting abnormalities of the urinary tract, liver and spleen, and abdominal vasculature. As the current trend is to manage injury to the liver or spleen or a kidney conservatively, a reliable technique that is easily performed on an out-patient basis is necessary in the follow-up management of these patients. The SPECT study can provide such a service.

REFERENCES

Brendel A. J., Leccia, F., Drouillard, J. *et al.* (1984) Single photon emission computed tomography (SPECT), planar scintigraphy, and transverse computed tomography: a comparison of accuracy in diagnosing focal hepatic disease. *Radiology*, **153**, 527–32.

Freedman, G. S. (1973) Radionuclide imaging of the injured patient. *Radiol. Clin. N. Am.*, **11**, 461–77.

Froelich, J. W., Simeone, J. F. and McKusick, K. A. (1982) Radionuclide imaging and ultrasound in liver/spleen trauma: a prospective comparison. *Radiology*, **145**, 457–61.

Gilday, D. L. and Alderson, P. O. (1974) Scintigraphic evaluation of liver and spleen injury. *Semin. Nucl. Med.*, **4**, 357–70.

Howman-Giles, R., Gilday, D. L., Venugopal, S. *et al.* (1978) Splenic trauma: nonoperative management and long-term follow up by scintiscan. *J. Pediat. Surg.*, **13**, 121–6.

Van Heertum, R. L., Brunetti, J. C. and Yuetl, A. P. (1987) Abdominal SPECT imaging. *Semin. Nucl. Med.*, **17**, 230–46.

CHAPTER FOURTEEN

Hepatobiliary disease

D. M. Ackery

14.1 INTRODUCTION

A variety of investigations are now available to detect and classify hepatic disease. Ideally these should be used in a logical sequence to derive the maximum diagnostic information for the least inconvenience to the patient, at the lowest cost.

Tests for hepatic disorders vary in their ability to solve a particular problem because they measure different things. The appropriate investigation must be chosen to answer questions relevant to either structure or function. The slow acceptance of new tests into routine hospital practice makes the adoption of a rigid protocol difficult, and often patients are investigated in a random way. This may incur needless expense which is only justified if the waiting time for tests is so long that harm may result to the patient or alternative costs are incurred, such as those for bed occupancy. Alternatively a sequence of investigation should be planned, employing sensitive non-invasive tests first, followed if necessary by more complex ones, to lead to a specific diagnosis. Many hospitals have worked out such investigation pathways which suit local conditions and facilities. While not necessarily mandatory these are effective in providing a diagnosis in most patients.

14.2 RELEVANT PHYSIOLOGY AND ANATOMY

14.2.1 LIVER

(a) Physiology

The properties which determine adequate concentration of radioactive pharmaceuticals by the liver are vascular perfusion and cellular extraction. The product of these factors is termed the **effective hepatic blood flow**.

The liver has two afferent vascular supplies: the hepatic artery and the portal vein. The hepatic artery supplies approximately 25–30% of total blood flow, and 50% of available oxygen. The portal vein, draining from the splanchnic region and spleen, is responsible for the remaining blood perfusion but is relatively deficient in oxygen content. Both systems mix at the level of the hepatic lobule, and blood passes into hepatic veins and eventually into the inferior vena cava. Normal variations in detailed vascular anatomy are common, and those due to pathological causes may be relevant to the results of radiocolloid imaging. Hepatic fibrosis (cirrhosis) impedes the normal flow of blood through the liver, giving increased pressure in the portal system, with engorgement of the spleen and development of collateral venous return to the heart, and varices. Thrombosis of the portal vein gives few constitutional symptoms, and ligation or embolization of the hepatic artery, which is used as a therapeutic measure, does not usually give hepatic necrosis.

The liver macrophages (Kuppfer cells) comprise about 2% of the hepatic cellular volume. Their position as endothelial cells adjacent to the lumen of the vascular sinusoids permits effective removal of colloidal particles from the circulation. Extraction efficiency varies with colloid size, and is normally 80–90%. Radiocolloid uptake may be reduced by either impaired blood flow or extraction. In man 80–90% of the hepatic parenchymal volume is made up of hepatocytes. These are metabolically active, and are responsible for the excretion of dyes and other chemicals into bile. Their function becomes impaired by inflammation and obstructive jaundice.

(b) Anatomy

The liver is the largest solid organ of the human body. It occupies the right hypochondrium, the epigastrium and often extends into the left hypochondrium. Functionally it is a bilobed organ, the division between right and left lobes running from the fundus of the gall bladder to the vena cava. The radionuclide image can show a clear division at the attachment of the falciform ligament, but this should not be confused with the true anatomical division of the right and left lobes based upon blood supply and biliary drainage. The right lobe is contained by the rib cage and right hemidiaphragm, and variations in these will affect the morphological appearance. The lower costal edge can impress the liver so that a linear defect is shown in the right lateral image, and with hepatic enlargement the lower right lobe can often be seen to extend laterally where it is released from the constraint of the thoracic cage. The medial segment of the left lobe is thin, and shows in the left lateral view as a leaf of tissue which projects downwards and anteriorally (Figure 14.1). Abnormalities of the diaphragm affect the conformity of the superior surface of the right lobe.

Several anatomical variants can cause the hepatic images to show an apparent focal loss. The confluence of the portal vein, bile ducts and hepatic artery, the **porta hepatis**, may show prominently at the junction of the right and left lobes, particularly with extrahepatic biliary obstruction. The gall bladder, especially if enlarged, may indent the inferior surface of the right lobe. Enlargement of the right kidney may impress the posterior surface of the right lobe, causing anterior and caudal displacement, giving a characteristic appearance to the right lateral image. The confluence of the hepatic veins at the cephalic attachment of the falciform ligament can notch the upper hepatic border.

Morphological variations of the normal liver have been described as a result of follow up of a large series of hepatic images (McAfee *et al.*, 1965). In some cases these give rise to a palpable mass, e.g. Reidel's lobe (Figure 14.15). Others are related to distortion brought about by compression from adjacent organs. In order to minimize misinterpretation of hepatic pathology the possible normal variants need to be known.

14.2.2 SPLEEN

The spleen lies in the left hypochondrium between the fundus of the stomach and the diaphragm. It is closely related to the left kidney, the left colic flexure, and the tail of the pancreas. In the adult it is usually 12–13 cm in length and 7 cm in breadth. The splenic artery is supplied from the coeliac trunk, and the splenic vein joins the superior mesenteric vein to form the portal vein. Small encapsulated nodules of splenic tissue (accessory spleens or splenunculi) are frequently found in the neighbourhood of the spleen, and may enlarge after splenectomy. Splenic macrophages form an important part of the reticuloendothelial system, and are responsible for the uptake of radiocolloid and for erythrophagocytosis. The spleen is also responsible for erythrocyte storage, for cytopoiesis, and for functions connected with the immune response.

14.2.3 THE BILIARY TRACT

The biliary canals permit the passage of bile from the liver to the duodenum. The right and left hepatic ducts join at the porta hepatis to form the common hepatic duct, which in turn combines with the cystic duct to form the common bile duct. This is 10–15 cm long, and is joined at its distal end by the main pancreatic duct. They enter the wall of the duodenum at the ampulla of Vater. Anatomical variants in the junctions of the biliary ducts are common.

The gall bladder is attached to the inferior surface of the liver. It is usually about 10 cm in length and 3–5 cm in diameter. It serves as a reservoir of bile and renders it more concentrated. It connects with the biliary tree through the cystic duct. Acute inflammation of the gall bladder obstructs the cystic duct, thus preventing reflux of bile into it from the hepatic duct. Occasionally an intrahepatic gall bladder is responsible for producing a defect in radiocolloid image of the right hepatic lobe. A ^{99m}Tc-labelled iminodiacetic acid (IDA) image can readily show that this is due to the gall bladder (Figure 14.16).

14.3 METHODS OF INVESTIGATING THE LIVER

14.3.1 STRUCTURE

The simplest assessment of liver enlargement is by abdominal palpation. The lower edge may be felt on deep inspiration in non-obese patients. This does not necessarily indicate hepatomegaly because costal margin variants can expose the normal liver to palpation. Over-expansion of the lungs can cause downwards displacement.

A more exact guide to hepatic mass is given by either radionuclide, ultrasound or computed

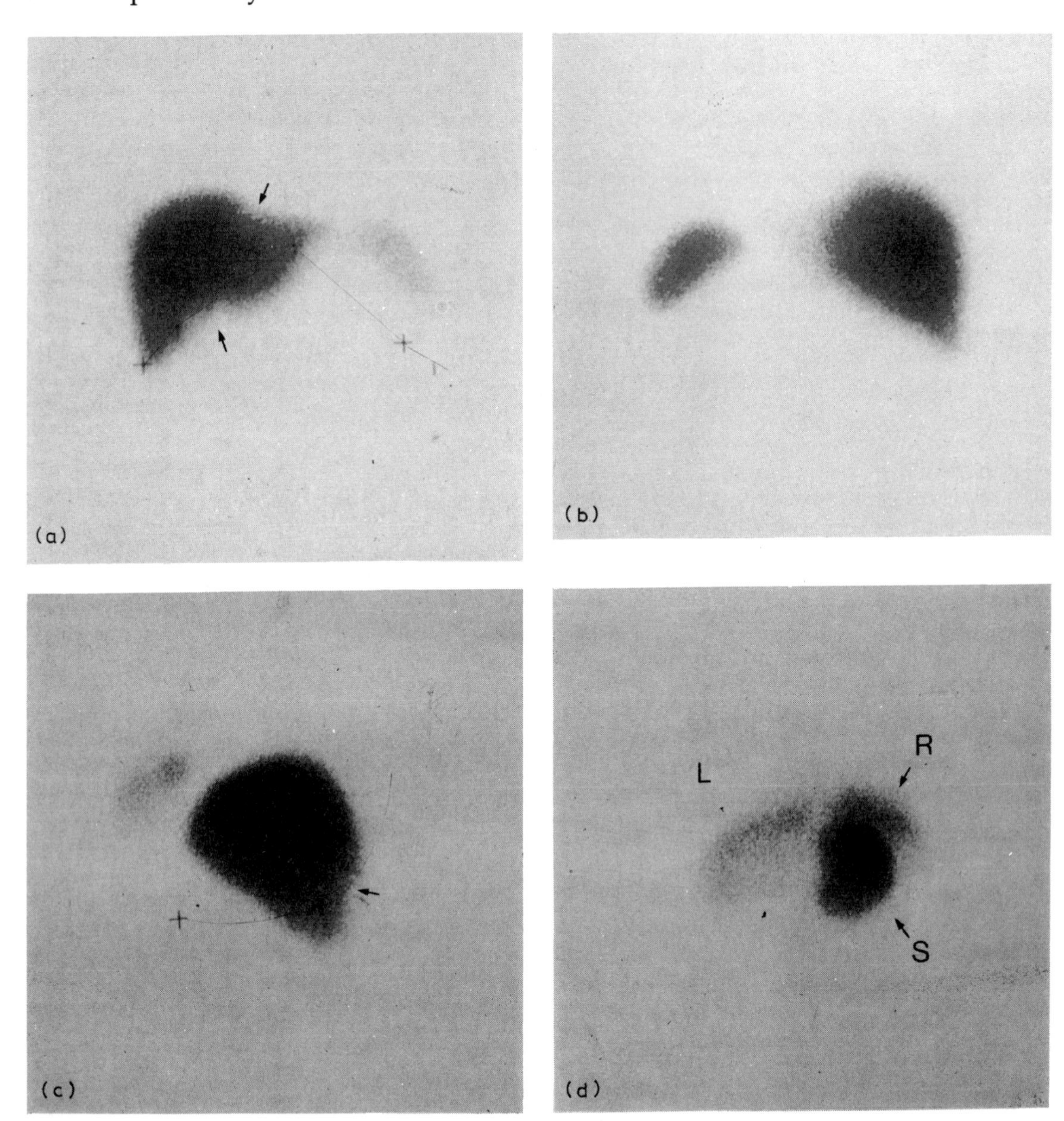

Figure 14.1 Normal liver. (a) Anterior: Hepatic image on left showing normal morphology; arrows show superior attachment of falciform ligament and inferior position of gall bladder. Splenic image on right is less well seen due to posterior site. (b) Posterior: Hepatic image on right. Splenic image on left. (c) Right lateral. (d) Left lateral: Left hepatic lobe (L), right hepatic lobe (R), spleen (S)

tomographic (CT) imaging. Of these, radionuclides give the best overall assessment of hepatic morphology. Anatomical detail is shown better by ultrasound and probably best by CT. These can demonstrate the caudate and quadrate lobes, specific hepatic segments, and other fine structure. All three techniques may demonstrate focal intrahepatic disease (Petasnick *et al.*, 1979; Ashare, 1980). For the demonstration of vascular detail hepatic angiography is necessary.

Hepatic microstructure is shown by histological examination of biopsy specimens. Direct percutaneous biopsy using the Menghini or Tru-cut needles and their derivatives is now a relatively

Table 14.1 Hepatic investigations

Investigation	*Indications*	*Limitations*	*Invasiveness*	*Sensitivity (SE) Specificity (SP)* Focal disease	Diffuse disease	*Complications*
Isotope colloid imaging	Focal disease Diffuse disease	Nil	No	SE 80% SP low	SE high SP low	Nil (low radiation dose)
Ultrasound imaging	Focal disease Extrahepatic disease Diffuse disease	Intestinal gas Obesity Scars, wounds, burns, etc. Operator experience	No	SE high SP high	SE low SP low	Nil
CT	Focal disease Extrahepatic disease Diffuse disease	Nil	No	SE high SP high	SE low SP low	Nil (moderate radiation dose)
Angiography	Pre-surgical Therapeutic embolization	Bleeding tendency Renal insufficiency	Yes	SE high SP moderate	SE low SP low	Rare
Percutaneous liver biopsy	Diffuse disease Focal disease	Bleeding tendency Biliary obstruction Hepatic congestion Haemangioma Hydatid cyst	Yes	SE low SP high	SE high SP high	Haemorrhage (0.2%) Mortality (0.1–0.01%)
Peritonoscopy (and biopsy)	Focal disease (surface) Lymphoma staging Portography	Gross bleeding tendency Surgical adhesions Obesity Tense ascites	Yes	SE } high for surface SP } lesions	SE high SP high	Complications (2%) Mortality (0.03%)

safe procedure and yields high-quality histological information (Hegarty and Williams, 1984; Lees *et al.*, 1985). This is of particular value in generalized hepatic disease when disturbances of architecture are identified and aetiological factors demonstrated by specialized staining techniques. It is less diagnostic for low-density focal disease unless guided by ultrasound or CT.

14.3.2 FUNCTION

Examination of the patient is the first step in the recognition of functional disturbance of the liver. Hepatomegaly is a common finding, and the presence of jaundice, spider naevi, liver palms, splenomegaly, ascites, varices and encephalopathy suggest increasing functional impairment and portal hypertension.

Measurement of liver function is common now that clinical chemistry laboratories are capable of analysing large numbers of samples by automated techniques. Although termed liver function tests these actually estimate the degree of hepatocellular functional impairment and bile duct patency. Diagnostic value is limited by the lack of specificity of most of the tests.

Radionuclide procedures also depend upon hepatic function, although the images are often of greater value in showing morphology. The factors which determine uptake of radioactivity are regional blood flow (both hepatic and portal), and the ability of the liver cells to extract the radiopharmaceutical. The output from the gamma camera can be quantified, and the time course of uptake and loss can be expressed as an index of total or regional hepatic function. Knowledge of normal physiology allows patterns of disturbed function to be interpreted. Table 14.1 summarizes investigations used for hepatic disorders.

14.4 METHODS OF INVESTIGATING THE HEPATOBILIARY SYSTEM

Conventional radiographic methods have been employed until recently to assess the functional integrity of hepatocytes and the patency of the biliary tract. During the last decade or so important advances with radiopharmaceuticals, ultrasound, CT and endoscopy have considerably altered the pattern of biliary investigation (Weissmann *et al.*, 1979a). Ultrasound and CT examine directly biliary structure, and can identify pathological lesions. Oral cholangiography and nuclear medical methods depend on adequate hepatocyte function to extract and excrete agents into the biliary tract. These indirect methods may fail when hepatocyte function is impaired by infection, cholestasis or toxins.

Table 14.2 gives a summary of procedures available for investigating the biliary tract. An appropriate investigation should be chosen to answer the particular diagnostic question that is asked. The choice will depend on the clinical status, and whether or not jaundice is present.

The technical ease and lack of complications associated with oral cholangiography make it the first choice for most gall bladder disorders, although accurate diagnosis of acute cholecystitis is now possible with nuclear medicine techniques. Ultrasound should be used initially when investigating the jaundiced patient, as bile duct dilatation is an early finding in extrahepatic biliary obstruction.

14.5 CLINICAL PROBLEMS

Requests for radionuclide investigation of the liver, spleen and biliary system are made when a disorder is suspected on clinical examination (e.g. palpable mass or jaundice) or as a result of abnormal liver function tests.

14.5.1 HEPATIC ENLARGEMENT

Manual palpation of the abdomen gives only an approximate assessment of hepatic size. The normal liver edge is often felt on deep inspiration, particularly if the lower costal margin is sharply angled. The left lobe is less easily palpated due to the rectus abdominis muscles, but usually lies well into the epigastrium. Displacement due to flattening of the hemidiaphragm by lung overinflation can give a misleading impression of liver enlargement, and it may be difficult to percuss the upper hepatic border (Halpern *et al.*, 1974; Sullivan *et al.* 1976). On the other hand a big liver may be masked by elevation of a paralysed hemidiaphragm.

Hepatic size is best demonstrated by the radionuclide colloid image. It is necessary to image in the anterior, posterior and right lateral projections to give the best assessment of liver bulk (Figure 14.1). The use of geometric modelling to quantify hepatic volume tends to be inaccurate and time consuming, and does not add to the

Table 14.2 Hepatobiliary investigations

Investigation	*Indications*	*Limitations*	*Invasiveness*	*Sensitivity (SE)* *Specifity (SP)*	*Complications*
Oral cholecystography	Cholecystitis Biliary calculi	Malabsorption Biliary obstruction (bilirubin 35 μmol l^{-1})	No	SE high for SP gall bladder function	Very rare
Intravenous cholangiography	Common duct lesions Non-opacified gall bladder (GB)	Macroglobulaemias Biliary obstruction (bilirubin 70 μmol l^{-1})	No	SE high SP limited	Occasional reaction
Ultrasound imaging	Dilated ducts GB distension Calculi Extrahepatic obstruction	Intestinal gas Obesity Scars, wounds, burns, etc. Operator expertise	No	SE high for biliary dilatation SP high for calculi	Nil
Isotope hepatobiliary imaging	Acute cholecystitis Partial biliary obstruction Biliary leaks	Biliary obstruction (bilirubin 85–170 μmol l^{-1})	No	SE high for cholecystitis SP and biliary patency	Nil (low radiation dose)
CT	Dilated ducts GB distension Calculi Extrahepatic obstruction	Nil	No	SE } similar to SP } ultrasound	Nil (moderate radiation dose)
Percutaneous transhepatic cholangiography	Duct obstruction Traumatic stricture Drainage	Pre-operative investigation only Bleeding tendency (unless corrected)	Yes	SE high SP high	Biliary leaks
Endoscopic retrograde cholangio-pancreatography (ERCP)	Jaundice	Severe cardiorespiratory insufficiency Acute pancreatitis	Yes	SE } high for cause and site SP } of obstruction	Sepsis Pancreatitis (1–3%)

qualitative assessment (Rollo and DeLand, 1968), but emission CT has been shown to give a more accurate prediction (Kan and Hopkins, 1979). The size of the patient should be known before hepatomegaly is intrepreted from the images, as liver mass will vary from one individual to another. The abdomen is palpated immediately following the imaging procedure so that anatomical landmarks and palpable masses are marked on the final image. Apparent hepatic enlargement can be due to a morphological variant of normal liver, and several of these have been described. True increase in hepatic mass is due usually to focal or diffuse disease, but at times the liver may show little increase in size when widely infiltrated.

14.5.2 FOCAL DISEASE

Radionuclide colloid imaging is particularly effective in identifying space-occupying lesions within the liver (McAfee *et al.*, 1965; McCready, 1972; Holder and Saenger, 1975; Oster *et al.*, 1975; Clarke *et al.*, 1986). It compares favourably with ultrasound for detecting focal masses, but is unable to distinguish solid from cystic lesions (Lerona *et al.*, 1974). CT is able to give solid–cystic discrimination, and is sensitive for detecting focal lesions (Alderson *et al.*, 1983), particularly now that fast scanning techniques with new contrast media are available (Robinson, 1985). Nuclear magnetic resonance imaging also has high sensitivity and specificity (Smith *et al.*, 1981).

(a) Metastatic disease

Radiocolloid imaging is undertaken frequently to determine the presence of hepatic metastases for both adults (Hatfield, 1975) and children (Miller and Greenspan, 1985). The liver is a common site for metastases from carcinoma of the stomach, intestines and oesophagus. It frequently shows malignant infiltration from carcinoma of the breast and lung, and less commonly from those arising from ovary, kidney and uterus. Melanoma and neuroblastoma may also metastasise to the liver.

The sensitivity of radiocolloid imaging for detecting metastases is reported to be between 0.75 and 0.85 (Lunia *et al.*, 1975; Rothschild and Rosenthal, 1976) when compared to histological evidence obtained by needle biopsy or at laparotomy. Recent advances in instrumentation and radiopharmaceuticals have not improved the diagnostic accuracy, although single-photon emission computed tomography (SPECT) can improve the results compared to planar imaging (Khan *et al.*, 1981; Carrasquillo *et al.*, 1983; Brendel *et al.*, 1984). A false-positive interpretation is particularly likely to occur with generalized hepatic dysfunction of obstructive jaundice or cirrhosis

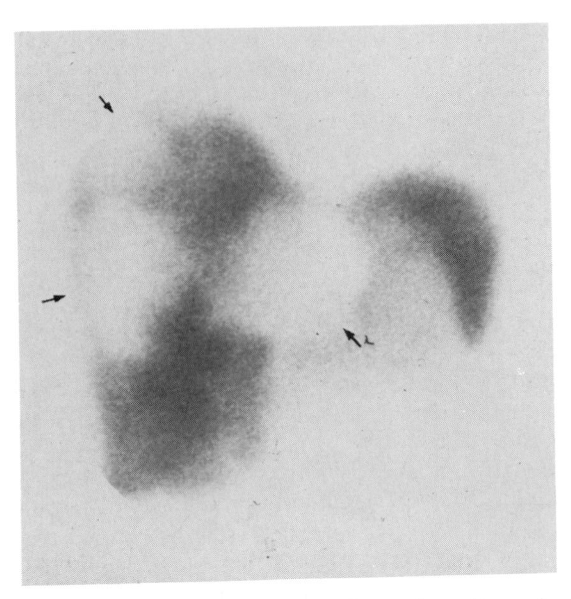

Figure 14.2 Colonic carcinoma. Large deposits can be seen in right and left hepatic lobes.

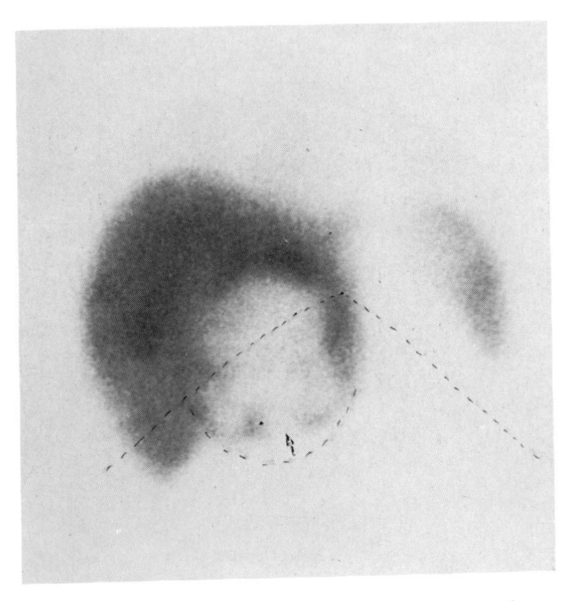

Figure 14.3 Carcinoid tumour. Anterior view showing large solitary deposit in left lobe.

(Rosenthal, 1976). On the other hand small focal lesions may not be resolved by the gamma camera, and can be missed if they lie deep in the liver. These two problems are minimized by using high-resolution SPECT imaging.

Metastases show widely varying image patterns. Single or a few large lesions arise typically from primary tumours of the gastrointestinal tract (Figures 14.2 and 14.3). Multiple small lesions are more common with poorly differentiated tumours and melanoma (Figure 14.4). Massive replacement of hepatic tissue can so impair Kupffer cell function that the pattern of diffuse liver uptake may be shown, with increase in the spleen/liver ratio of activity. Concentration of the bone radiopharmaceutical ^{99m}Tc-labelled hydroxymethylene diphosphonate in colonic metastases has been reported (Shih *et al.*, 1986).

The appearances are often diagnostic when multiple metastases are present, but in uncertain cases it is prudent to confirm the diagnosis by ultrasound or CT so as to exclude other causes of multiple focal disease (Taylor *et al.*, 1977), e.g. cysts.

(b) Primary hepatic tumours

Primary malignancy of the liver may present as hepatic enlargement at any age (Kido, 1975; Tonami *et al.*, 1975). It most often arises in a cirrhotic liver but can develop as a solitary lesion in an otherwise normal liver (Figure 14.5). Associated factors include the intake of carcinogens, regular administration of oral contraceptives, HBsAg-positive sera, and α_1-antitrypsin deficiency. High blood levels of α-fetoprotein are a common finding. No characteristic features are shown by the nuclide image to distinguish primary growths from other causes for focal disease. Active concentration of ^{67}Ga (James *et al.*, 1974; Pinsky and Henkin, 1976; Waxman *et al.*, 1980) and labelled selenomethionine (Kaplan and Domingo, 1972; Coakley and Wraight, 1980) by hepatocellular carcinoma has been reported. Uptake of hepatobiliary agents has also been shown (Utz *et al.*, 1980; Savitch *et al.*, 1983). None of these procedures is entirely diagnostic, and both money and time are saved by progressing direct to biopsy once a solid focal lesion has been confirmed by ultrasound.

(c) Hepatic abscesses

Pyogenic infection is largely responsible for hepatic abscesses in developed countries, although *Entamoeba histolytica* remains the commonest worldwide cause. The widespread use of antibiotics now means that pyogenic abscess is often a disease of the elderly, frequently with rather nonspecific symptoms. Solitary or confluent pyogenic abscesses which are restricted to a single hepatic lobe can be treated surgically. Amoebic or multiple

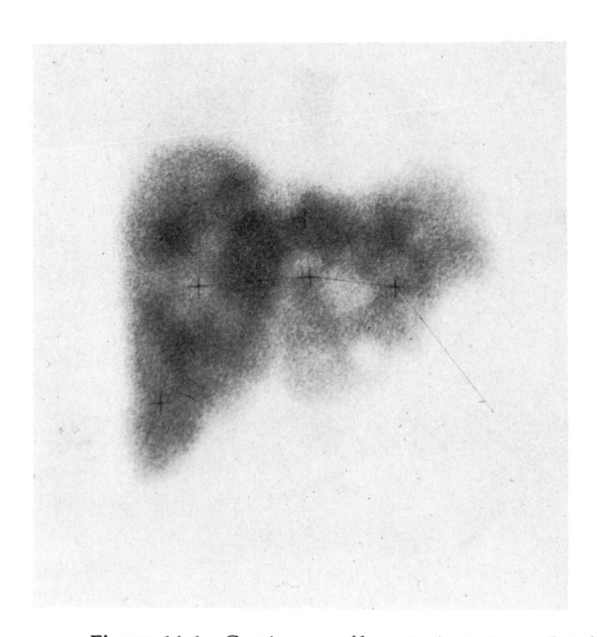

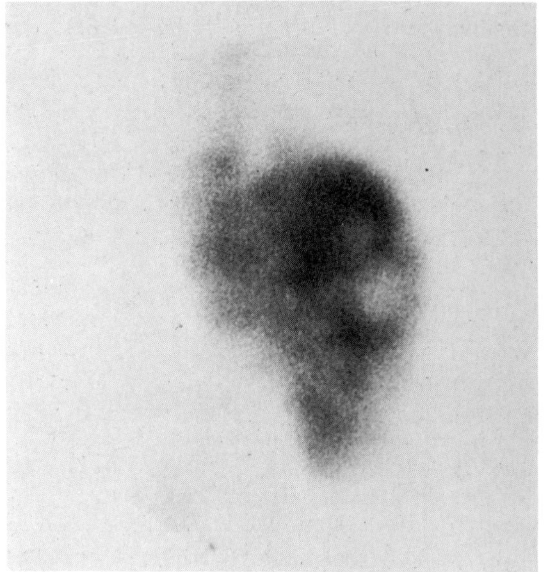

Figure 14.4 Carcinoma of breast. Anterior and right lateral views showing multiple hepatic deposits.

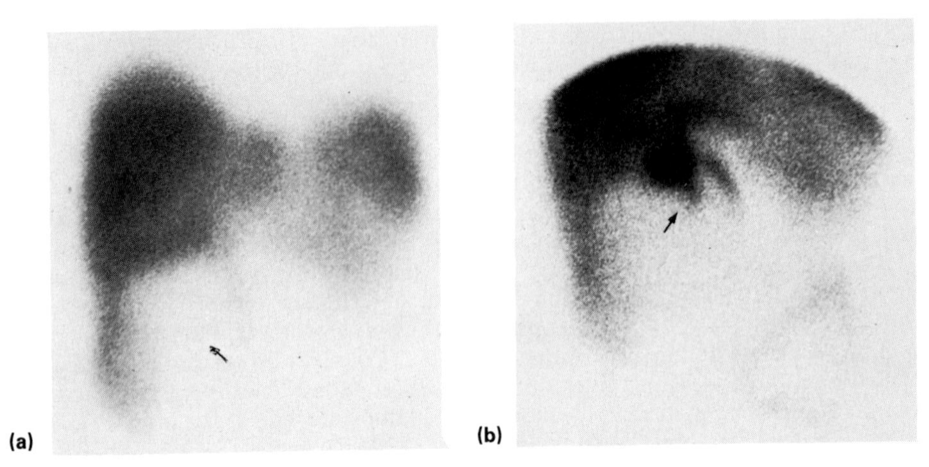

Figure 14.5 Hepatocellular carcinoma. (a) ^{99m}Tc-sulphur colloid. Arrow shows deficient colloid uptake at site of tumour. (b) ^{99m}Tc-imidodiacetic acid. Arrow shows displacement by tumour of gall bladder and common duct.

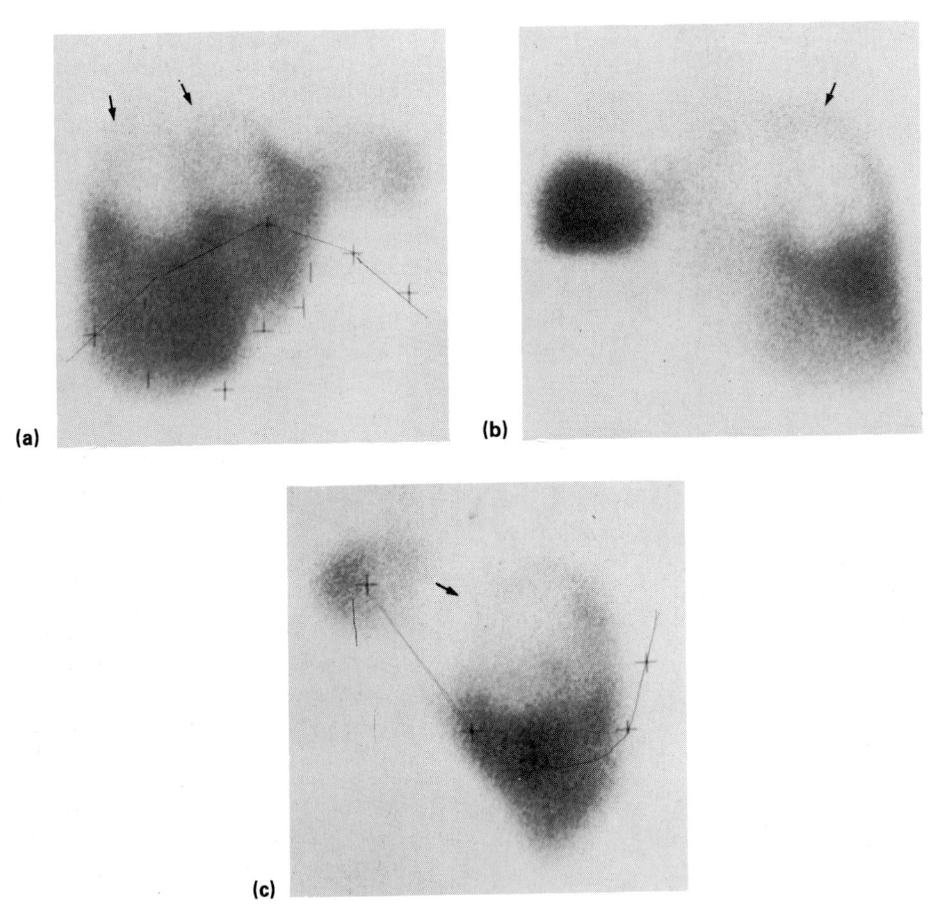

Figure 14.6 Pyogenic hepatic abscess. (a) Anterior; (b) posterior; (c) right lateral.

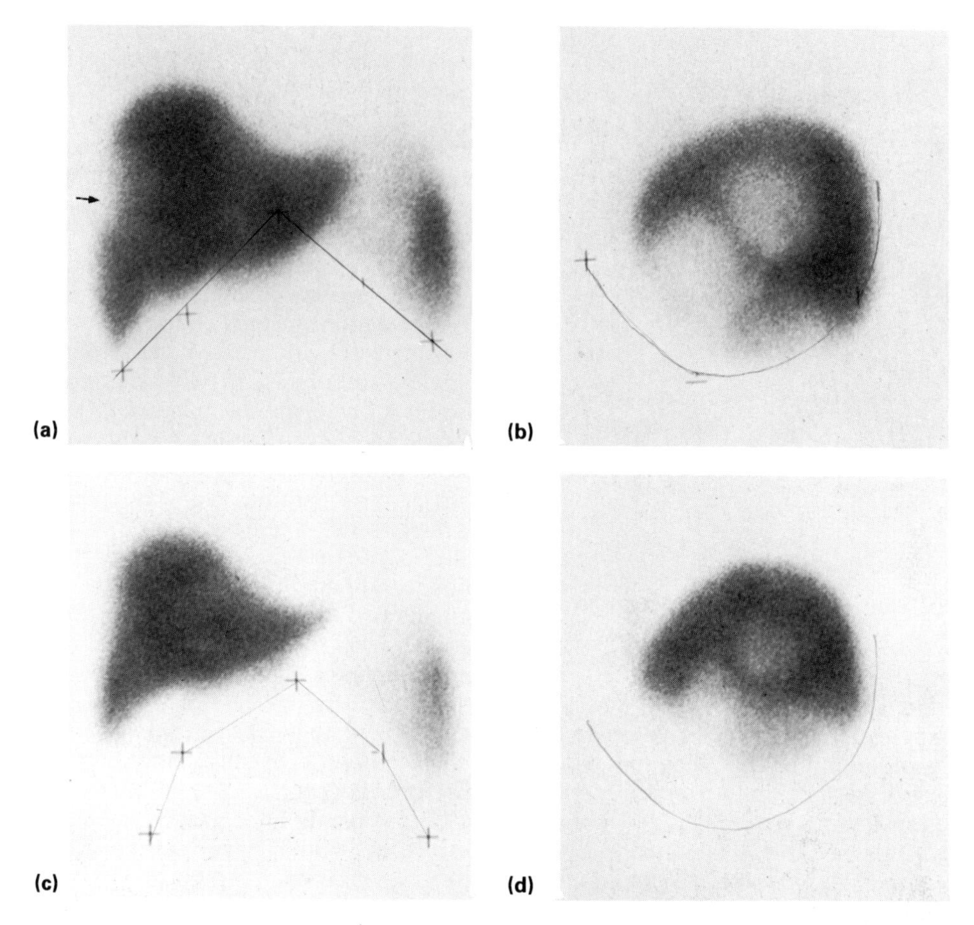

Figure 14.7 Amoebic abscess. (a), (b) Anterior and right lateral views showing confluent abscess cavities in right lobe with little hepatic enlargement, (c), (d) One week after metronidazole therapy. Liver and abscesses are smaller.

small pyogenic abscesses require medical treatment. Mortality from liver sepsis is high and early diagnosis is necessary to avoid complications. Both pyogenic (Figure 14.6) and amoebic abscesses (Figure 14.7) are readily localized by radionuclide imaging (Cuaron *et al.*, 1965; Schraibman, 1974; Ranson *et al.*, 1975). The position, size and extent of hepatic involvement can be ascertained from the image, and this gives guidance for drainage. When focal defects are shown in the clinical context of abdominal pain, pyrexia, nocturnal sweating, malaise and liver tenderness, the diagnosis is seldom in doubt. Rapidly growing hepatic metastases may rarely give a similar constitutional disturbance, and misdiagnosis is minimized by ultrasound imaging. Careful examination of all isotope views may be necessary to identify an abscess which lies deep in the right lobe.

(d) Hepatic cysts

Simple cysts of the liver, either solitary or few in number, are shown often at routine ultrasound scanning. These are usually small and not detected by radionuclide imaging. Larger cysts may enlarge the liver and show as non-specific focal lesions (Figure 14.8) which cannot be distinguished from solid masses. Ultrasound examination is necessary in doubtful cases to avoid a misdiagnosis of malignancy.

When hydatid disease is suspected (Joske, 1974) needle biopsy must be not be carried out because of the risk of dissemination. A positive diagnosis can be made by ultrasound identification of daughter foci within the main cyst. Skin testing and complement fixation tests give further confirmation.

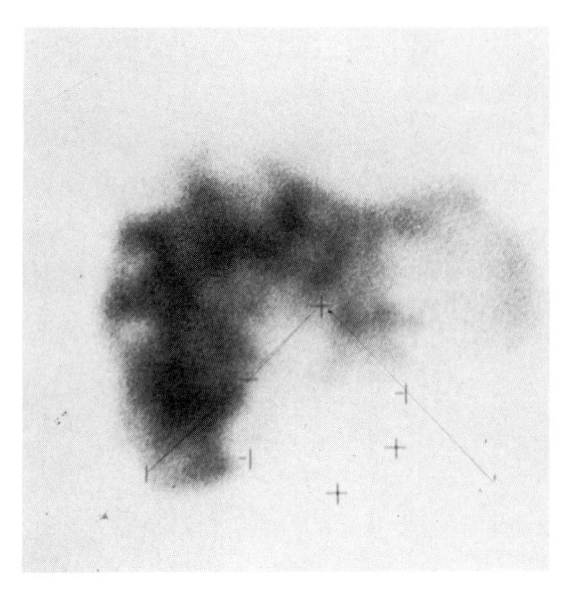

Figure 14.8 Multiple cysts with hepatic enlargement.

(e) Miscellaneous focal lesions

Certain other liver disorders can give rise to focal lesions in radiocolloid images. Commonly these occur in chronic liver disease as a result of regional functional impairment and fibrosis, and rarely are due to local tissue necrosis in fulminant hepatitis. Transient focal defects have been reported in children receiving chemotherapy (Abramson *et al.*, 1984). Benign hepatoadenoma can give a concave defect on the lateral border of the liver, and focal nodular hyperplasia can show focal losses (Biersack *et al.*, 1980), although hot-spots have also been reported in this condition (Uszler and Swanson 1975). Vascular disorders such as hepatic venous obstruction (Budd–Chiari syndrome) give patchy colloid uptake which can appear focal (Tavill *et al.*, 1975), and local vessel malformations also can show a focal loss. If haemangioma (Wiener and Parulekar, 1979) is suspected biopsy must not be undertaken. Blood labelling techniques can help to identify lesions of high vascularity (Intenzo *et al.*, 1988). Extrahepatic causes may also simulate the appearance of hepatic focal lesions (Figure 14.16).

14.5.3 DIFFUSE DISEASE

A wide variety of primary and secondary generalized liver disorders can give hepatic enlargement. The radiocolloid image shows irregular uptake of activity which is related to alterations in normal hepatic function and architecture. The mechanisms for these changes include impairment of normal macrophage function, alterations in blood flow, and replacement of liver parenchyma by fibrous tissue. The macrophages of spleen, bone marrow and lung comprise about 35% of the total reticuloendothelial system and when Kupffer cell function is impaired they become responsible for clearing a greater proportion of radiocolloid from the circulation. Images commonly show hepatic enlargement with patchy distribution of radioactivity, splenomegaly with high uptake, and increased activity in the marrow. Rarely activity is seen in the lungs. Of the many hepatic disorders responsible for these appearances, the commonest are chronic hepatitis, portal fibrosis, cirrhosis and extensive metastatic infiltration. Ultrasound can show a bright echo pattern in these conditions (Dewbury and Clark, 1979). Fulminant hepatic failure can show absent reticuloendothelial function, when hepatobiliary function is preserved (Gainey and Faerber, 1985).

With fatty infiltration alone, the liver is enlarged with little or no increase in splenic size or specific radioactivity. Increasing impairment of hepatic macrophage cell function (e.g. from excessive alcohol consumption) gives a characteristic pattern of hepatomegaly with patchy colloid distribution, and clear evidence of increased splenic and marrow uptake (Figure 14.9). These findings correlate reasonably well with the severity of the disease shown by histological examination (Geslien *et al.*, 1976), although the image alone gives no clue as to the cause of the functional impairment. Images are often interpreted as being typical of cirrhosis, but this may be misleading as this term decribes a histological appearance. It is likely that the poor hepatic concentration of colloid in these circumstances is related as much to such factors as macrophage blockade and intrahepatic vascular shunts, which are known to exist in conditions causing cirrhosis, as to the fibrosis itself. Patients with the characteristic histology of cirrhosis, but who no longer have evidence of hepatitis, may have a normal radiocolloid study. The relative uptake of activity between spleen and liver, often expressed as a quantitative ratio, has been used to monitor changes in function and response to therapy.

The non-specific appearance of the images in diffuse liver disease limits their diagnostic contribution. Patchy uptake may be due to infiltra-

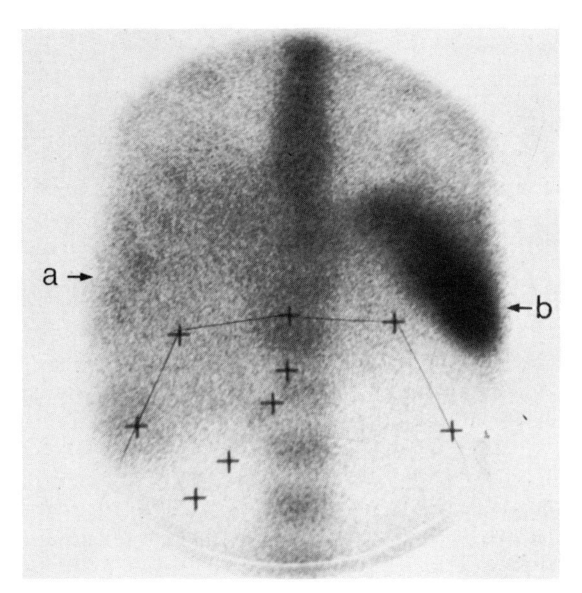

Figure 14.9 Alcoholic cirrhosis. Anterior view showing poor uptake in enlarged liver (a), high uptake in moderately enlarged spleen (b), and radiocolloid in marrow of spine and ribs.

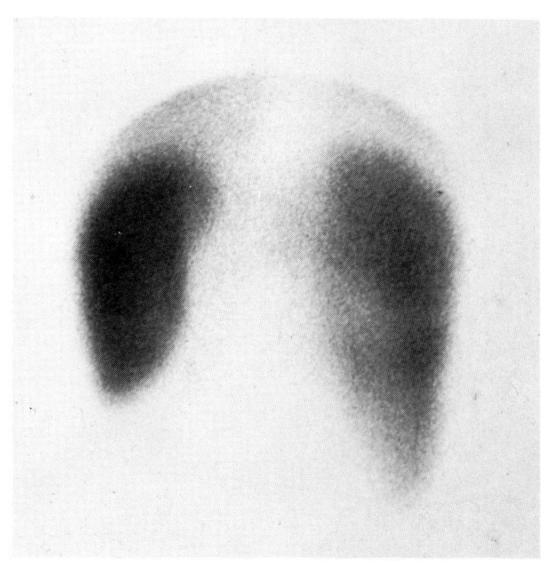

Figure 14.10 Non-Hodgkins lymphoma. Posterior view showing generalized increase in size of liver (Rt) and spleen (Lt).

tion, impaired blood flow or to biliary obstruction. Further investigation is usually necessary before a specific diagnosis can be made.

14.5.4 SPLENIC ENLARGEMENT

An enlarged spleen is usually felt by abdominal palpation, but may be missed in the obese patient or if the left hemidiaphragm is raised. Radiological screening may show the pressure deformity on the stomach of a large spleen. When splenic enlargement is suspected radiocolloid investigation should be undertaken. The posterior and left lateral projections will usually show the size and position of the spleen. Splenic mass varies with body size but a length of 13 cm on the posterior image is taken as a maximum for the normal adult value (McIntyre, 1972)).

(a) Splenomegaly not due to portal hypertension

The spleen size commonly increases in haematological disorders, and in viral, bacterial and parasitic infections. In these conditions enlargement is associated with little change in the spleen/liver ratio of activity. Uniform hepatosplenomegaly, in the absence of portal hypertension or haematological disturbance, suggests lymphoma (Figure 14.10). Generalized hepatosplenomegaly is shown in the acquired immunodeficiency syndrome (Smith, 1985).

Focal disease of the spleen is rare and may be due to tumour, e.g. lymphoma (Figure 14.11), cysts or abscesses. The clinical context with ultrasound scanning or CT usually gives a certain diagnosis.

(b) Portal hypertension

Splenomegaly is a common finding when pressure in the portal vein is raised due to increased intrahepatic vascular resistance. However, there is not a direct relationship between portal pressure and spleen size, and the spleen may not return to normal when the pressure is relieved. Other factors including impaired hepatic reticuloendothelial function also play a part. Collateral circulation and anastomoses develop, with the formation of varices. Apart from radiographic methods for showing the portal vein and its collaterals, a radionuclide estimate of the proportion of portal venous flow which is diverted from the liver through collateral vessels can be made by the direct injection of labelled particles into the spleen. Those particles which reach the liver are trapped in hepatic sinusoids, whereas the remainder drain into systemic veins and are eventually

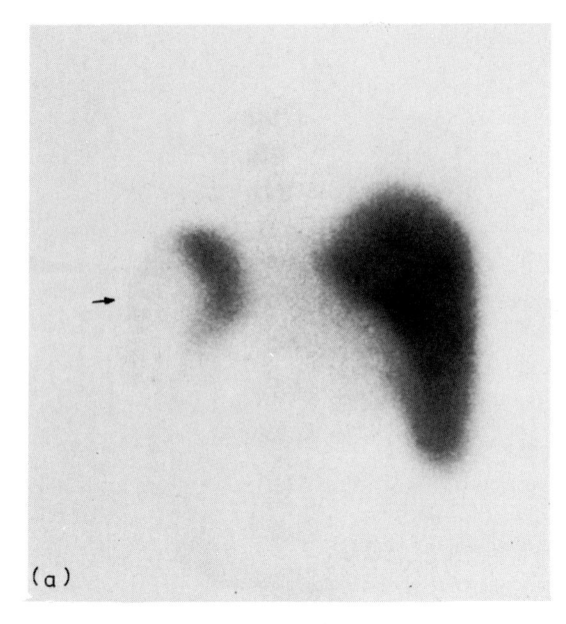

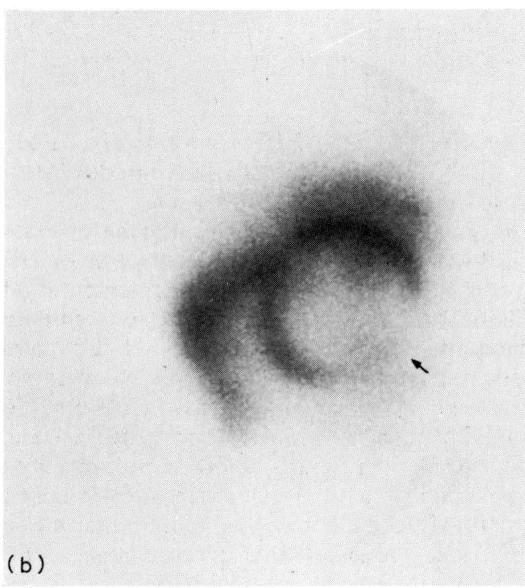

Figure 14.11 Non-Hodgkins lymphoma. (a) Posterior view showing splenic deposit; (b) left lateral view showing ring of splenic tissue surrounding lesion.

trapped in the pulmonary capillary bed. The activity at each site can be quantified to give the relative flows.

(c) Splenic displacement

The position of the spleen relative to the liver shown by the radiocolloid image is reasonably constant, and changes little with alterations in body posture (Chiles *et al.*, 1975). Significant displacement is readily recognized, and may be due to changes in the level of the left hemidiaphragm, gastric dilatation (Landgarten and Spencer, 1972), or to pathological masses in the abdomen, e.g. pancreatic pseudocyst (Grant and Ackery, 1976), which exert pressure on the spleen.

14.5.5 JAUNDICE

Cholestasis is an important component of many liver and biliary tract diseases. This stagnation of the bile may result in clinical evidence of jaundice and is characterized by a disturbance of the secretion by hepatocytes of whole bile into canuliculae. Cholestasis may be classified into extrahepatic biliary obstruction, which is caused by gallstones, tumours and cysts of the biliary ducts and adjacent organs, inflammation and pancreatic disease. Anatomical or physiological disorders of the biliary system, or parasitic infestation, may rarely cause biliary obstruction. Intrahepatic cholestasis is caused by those disorders which distort and narrow the intrahepatic bile ducts. This is shown in the terminal stages of metastatic disease, or with inflammation. Conjugated hyperbilirubinaemia and histological manifestations of cholestasis may also be associated with a number of conditions which affect the proper function of hepatocytes without causing demonstrable biliary obstruction. This may result from viral, alcoholic or drug-induced hepatitis, or from a variety of metabolic causes.

The principal diagnostic problems with the jaundiced patient are to distinguish between intra- and extrahepatic cholestasis, to identify the site of extrahepatic obstruction, to recognize unusual causes of hepatocellular or haemolytic jaundice which require special management or treatment, and to distinguish between acute and chronic hepatocellular disease.

Assessment of the jaundiced patient should rely initially on careful clinical examination and biochemical analysis of the serum and urine (O'Connor *et al.*, 1983). A diagnostic accuracy of 80% can be achieved by these means alone (Schenker *et al.*, 1962), and in most cases should permit haemolytic, familial or hepatic causes for the jaundice to be separated. When abnormalities of liver function tests persist for more than a week, and particularly if aminotransferases are not greatly raised, investigation must be undertaken to distinguish large bile duct obstruction from variants of intrahepatic cholestasis.

The best initial imaging investigations are ultrasound and CT (Gibson *et al.*, 1986), which are non-hazardous and easy to perform, and in experienced hands can rapidly and accurately identify dilation of the biliary ducts. They can distinguish between intrahepatic (medical) and extrahepatic (surgical) jaundice in over 90% of cases. Although a similar accuracy can be achieved with a computer diagnostic model, using clinical and biochemical data, the advantage of imaging is the low false-positive rate for diagnosing surgically correctable jaundice (Wheeler *et al.*, 1979). Ultrasound can establish the level of the obstruction in approximately 80% of patients (Dewbury *et al.*, 1979). It can also show calculi, tumours and other causes for obstruction, as well as providing detailed information about the gall bladder and liver. In over 40% of patients the cause of obstruction is identified. Failures can occur for technical reasons, and the investigation is of less value in partial obstruction when the biliary tree may not be dilated. Percutaneous transhepatic cholangiography is also useful in showing precise anatomical delineation and internal and external drainage patterns, either as a pre-operative procedure or as an alternative to surgery.

The radiocolloid image is of limited value in the investigation of patients with jaundice. Care must be taken when interpreting the images as the biliary ducts at the porta hepatis may be dilated and the gall bladder distended. Each can give the appearance of a circumscribed focal lesion which may be mistaken for a metastasic deposit (Agnew *et al.*, 1975). The distribution of radiocolloid in the liver may be patchy, with shift from the liver to the spleen and bone marrow, indicating secondary hepatic macrophage dysfunction.

The investigation of jaundice with radionuclides has for many years depended on the administration of ^{131}I-labelled Rose Bengal. This dye is concentrated by hepatocytes and excreted into bile, and the time-course of activity has been used to measure hepatic function and biliary patency (Gamlen *et al.*, 1975). The radiation dose of ^{131}I has permitted only low activities to be given to patients. This results in low counts and inferior images which cannot show detailed biliary anatomy or the level of extrahepatic biliary obstruction. These limitations of ^{131}I have been overcome by the introduction of hepatobiliary agents which can be labelled with ^{99m}Tc (Wistow *et al.*, 1977). ^{99m}Tc-labelled IDA, are rapidly concentrated by hepatocytes following intravenous administration and secreted promptly into the biliary tract. The high photon flux available with ^{99m}Tc ensures good images of the main biliary ducts and the gall bladder, and enables the flow of activity into the duodenum to be shown (Figure 14.12). These agents are also cleared to a small extent by the kidneys, and when hepatocyte function is impaired radioactivity in the urinary tract can sometimes give a misleading impression of intestinal transit. These IDA radiopharmaceuticals have a useful place in investigating jaundice and in measuring biliary flow (Pauwels *et al.*, 1980; Lieberman and Krishnamurthy, 1986; Krishnamurthy and Turner, 1990). They can show intermittent extrahepatic biliary obstruction when ultrasound gives no evidence of duct dilatation (Figure 14.13). They can also be used for assessing post-surgical biliary patency (Abu-Nema *et al.*, 1986; Siddiqui *et al.*, 1986), the patency of biliary stents, and for the assessment of biliary leakage after surgery (Scott-Smith *et al.*, 1983) or trauma.

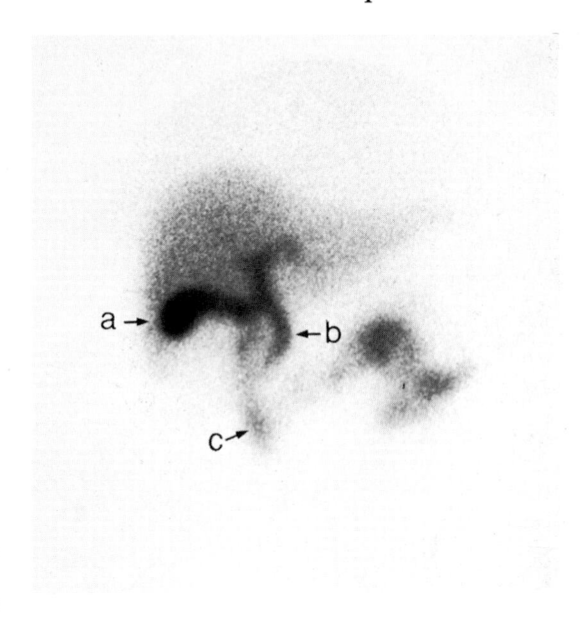

Figure 14.12 Normal hepatobiliary image at 30 min. (a) ^{99m}Tc-IDA has been concentrated in liver and excreted in gall bladder; (b) common duct; (c) duodenum.

Neonatal jaundice

^{131}I-labelled Rose Bengal has been used for several years to assess biliary patency in the jaundiced

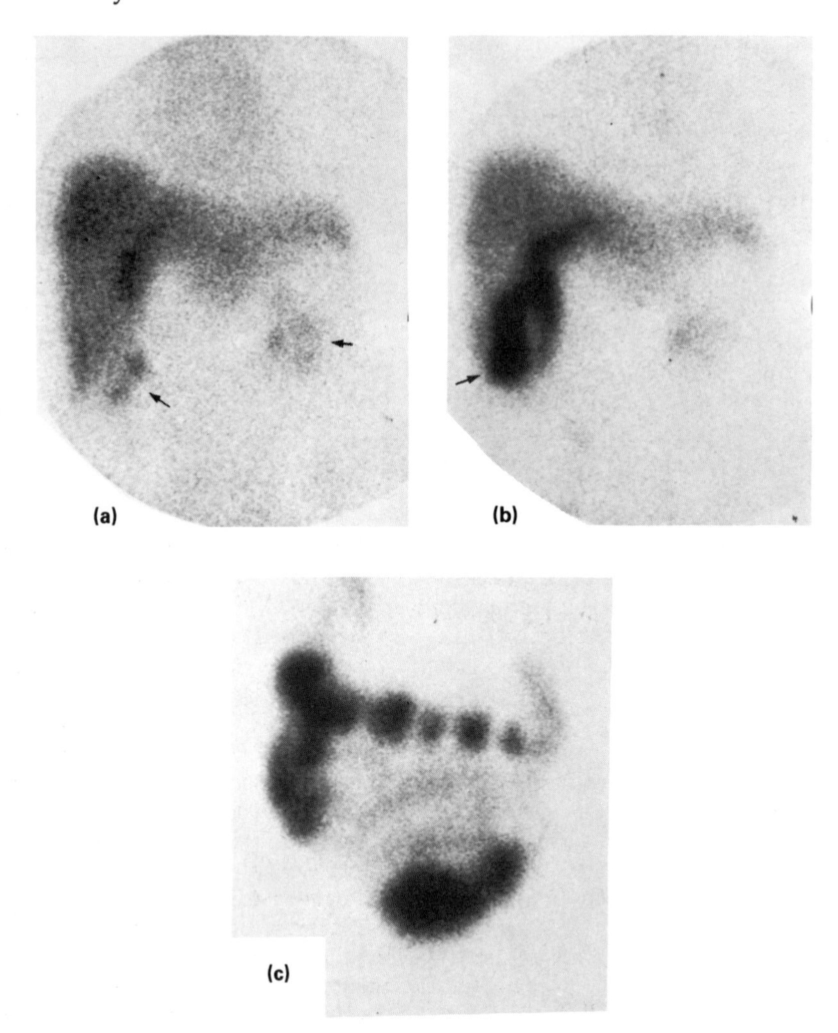

Figure 14.13 Partial obstruction of the common bile duct due to calculus. (a) Poor uptake of hepatobiliary agent by the liver, with activity showing in the renal pelvices (arrows). (b) Concentration in biliary ducts and gall bladder (arrow) at 1 h. (c) Activity in small and large intestine at 6 h.

infant. Measurements of stool activity are inaccurate due to contamination from activity excreted in the urine. Abdominal imaging overcomes this deficiency (Silverberg *et al.*, 1973) but suffers from statistical problems arising from the low activity which can be given. ^{99m}Tc-labelled IDA agents are reported to be good at distinguishing patients with biliary atresia from those with hepatitis and other causes for neonatal jaundice (Gerhold *et al.*, 1983), and it is recommended that phenobarbitone be given for at least three days before the test to enhance biliary excretion of the radiopharmaceutical (Majd *et al.*, 1981; Jaw *et al.*, 1984; Dick and Mowat, 1986). Imaging can be carried out up until 24 h, or the early ratio of activity in the heart compared to the liver may be used to give a 'hepatic index' (El Tumi *et al.*, 1987).

14.5.6 ABDOMINAL PAIN

(a) Acute cholecystitis

A confident diagnosis of acute cholecystitis can be made with a clinical picture of acute upper abdominal pain associated with fever, an acutely tender and usually palpable gall bladder, and transient jaundice. In more difficult cases investigation is required, and ^{99m}Tc-labelled hepatobiliary pharmaceuticals have been shown to have a place in the diagnosis (Weissman *et al.*, 1979b; Samuels *et al.*, 1983) as the gall bladder is unable to concentrate activity when the cystic duct is inflamed and obstructed. ^{99m}Tc-labelled IDA agents have been shown to be both sensitive and specific in this respect (Hall *et al.*, 1981), indicating that the demonstration of duct obstruction discriminates accurately between acute cholecystitis and other reasons for upper abdominal pain (Freitas *et al.*, 1980), particularly if investigation is carried out within 48 h of admission to hospital (O'Callaghan *et al.*, 1980). Interpretation can be more difficult if gall bladder filling is delayed. Hepatobiliary imaging is also of value in choledocholithiasis (Colletti *et al.*, 1986).

The results in chronic cholecystitis are less successful, with variable concentration of the radiopharmaceutical by the gall bladder. Further evaluation of these radiopharmaceuticals is required before their place in relation to other imaging procedures is established.

(b) Splenic infarction

Infarction of the spleen occurs principally in haematological disorders associated with splenic enlargement. Intense sharp pain is experienced in the left hypochondrium, and this may radiate to the left shoulder. A friction rub may be present. The splenic image usually shows a wedge-shaped defect at the site of the infarct.

14.5.7 POTENTIAL HEPATIC AND SPLENIC DISEASE

The liver and spleen may be infiltrated even when there is no clinical and biochemical evidence to suggest this, and in these circumstances it is often justified to carry out radiocolloid imaging to detect occult disease, particularly if ultrasound and CT are not available.

(a) Staging of malignancy

The limits imposed by spatial resolution on detecting small focal lesions question the efficacy of routine screening of the liver for the detection of early malignant spread (Fee Prokop *et al.*, 1974; Sears *et al.*, 1975; Operchal *et al.*, 1976). However, the predictive valve of a negative result remains high (McClees and Gedgaudas-McClees, 1984). In aggressive neoplastic conditions, such as small cell carcinoma of the lung and melanoma, it is common practice to screen patients by both radionuclide and ultrasound imaging before chemotherapeutic regimes are commenced. This provides a baseline for the evaluation of treatment. It is less effective in altering the management of a particular patient, as the detection rate in early disease is low (Evans *et al.*, 1980). Correct staging of Hodgkin's and non-Hodgkin's lymphoma helps in the subsequent management of these patients. Unfortunately radiocolloid imaging is of little value in providing definite evidence of hepatic and splenic involvement (Lipton *et al.*, 1972; Silverman *et al.*, 1972) because clear focal lesions appear only when the disease is at an advanced stage.

(b) Pyrexia of unknown origin

Although CT is the investigation of choice, radionuclide imaging continues to have a role in the difficult problem of a patient presenting with symptoms and signs of sepsis. Usually hepatic tenderness is present with intra- or perihepatic abscess, but this may not always be so, especially if the cavity is deep in the liver. An intrahepatic abscess usually gives a well-defined focal loss, and a right subphrenic collection often shows a concavity on the superior margin of the right lobe. This may be perceived more easily by undertaking a colloid image in combination with an isotope pulmonary image of either perfusion or ventilation to delineate the upper diaphragmatic border. The localization of a septic focus can be investigated further by using ^{111}In-labelled autologous leucocytes or ^{67}Ga-labelled citrate.

A diagnosis of amoebic abscess should be considered in those patients with unexplained fever who have travelled in regions where amoebiasis is endemic, even when hepatic enlargement and tenderness are absent. Liver imaging can give an early diagnosis in this condition.

(c) Abnormal liver function tests

Routine biochemical tests may identify liver dysfunction in the absence of clinical evidence. Single tests may be abnormal in non-hepatic conditions, and a small proportion of liver function tests will fall outside the usually quoted two standard deviation normal range for a laboratory. The likelihood of liver disease increases when several tests are abnormal.

The value of radionuclide imaging in the follow-up of patients with abnormal liver function tests is limited, particularly as biochemical tests do not show changes until significant generalized hepatic dysfunction exists. Radiocolloid uptake commonly confirms functional impairment without contributing further to a specific diagnosis. Patients with widespread metastases may sometime present with abnormal liver biochemistry and no hepatomegaly, and in these patients the radiocolloid image is helpful.

(d) Ascites

The most common hepatic causes for increased fluid in the peritoneal cavity are cirrhosis and malignancy, although other conditions such as the Budd–Chiari syndrome and subacute hepatic necrosis may rarely be responsible. Several factors contribute to the formation of ascitic fluid, including increased portal venous pressure, low serum albumin levels, increased hepatic lymph production and sodium retention. Hepatic and splenic size and morphology may be difficult to assess by palpation if the abdomen is tense with fluid, and then the radiocolloid study is required to provide this information.

In the Budd–Chiari syndrome the liver can show increased uptake of activity situated centrally in the anterior image, and posteriorly in the right lateral image (Tavill *et al.*, 1975). This is due to the caudate lobe being normal, as it is spared the effects of hepatic venous occlusion by independent venous drainage direct into the inferior vena cava. This appearance is not invariable, and in some cases only patchy liver distribution is shown which cannot be distinguished from other causes for impaired hepatic macrophage function. Further information may be gained by radionuclide venography (Huang *et al.*, 1986). Superior vena caval obstruction can show a similar irregular uptake when colloid is administered at the arm. This is due to collateral circulation which diverts the colloid via the umbilical vein into small segments of the liver (Holmquest and Burdine, 1973). Multiple thromboses of smaller hepatic veins also give a generalized uneven appearance which may be mistaken for metastatic infiltration.

(e) Screening of patients with familial disorders

A number of uncommon genetically linked conditions can affect hepatic function. Chemical liver function tests are the primary screening method for revealing asymptomatic liver involvement, but radiocolloid imaging of these patients and their relatives may also be justified. Conditions which lead eventually to cirrhosis are Wilson's disease, haemochromatosis, the glycogen storage diseases, α_1-antitrypsin deficiency and tyrosinosis. Polycystic disease may present with hepatomegaly, renal enlargement and renal failure. Ultrasound and radiocolloid imaging are used to confirm that hepatic cysts are present.

(f) Trauma

The liver and spleen are often affected by external injury or by penetrating wounds due to their fixed position in the abdomen. Small lacerations and subcapsular haematomas usually give few clinical manifestations. Larger lacerations or rupture can give considerable blood loss and the hepato-renal syndrome, with a high mortality, and early diagnosis is essential.

Radionuclide screening has been shown to be helpful in defining the extent of injury (Evans *et al.*, 1972; Gilday and Alderson, 1974), particularly in those patients with closed trauma, such as that resulting from road traffic accidents and falls. Radionuclide imaging can be carried out without difficulty as an emergency procedure, even in patients with multiple injuries, which enables assessment prior to angiography. Large focal lesions, concave defects on the liver surface, organ displacement, and minor patchy losses are reported. The limited resolution of radionuclide imaging may miss some smaller lesions, but the results of major injury are usually shown, and can guide surgical management. This problem is best evaluated by using a SPECT gamma camera as the patient only has to be moved once.

(g) Splenic hypofunction

This condition is suspected when Howell–Jolly bodies are detected in the peripheral erythrocytes. These can occur after splenectomy, or as a consequence of splenic atrophy following infarction, or with coeliac disease and ulcerative colitis (Figure 14.14). They are also often present with haemolytic and megaloblastic anaemias. Radiocolloid imaging shows the size and degree of hypofunction of the spleen, and the presence of splenunculi.

14.5.8 DISEASE PROGRESSION AND RESPONSE TO THERAPY

Serial radionuclide imaging is particularly well suited to show response to treatment or deterioration of function, during patient follow-up.

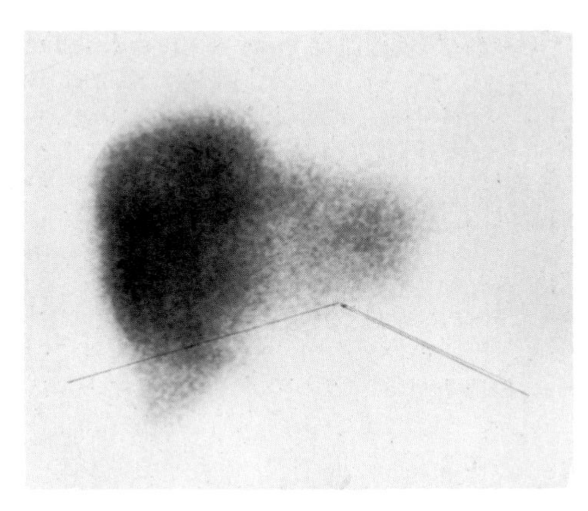

Figure 14.14 Coeliac disease. Anterior: Normal liver: absent splenic uptake.

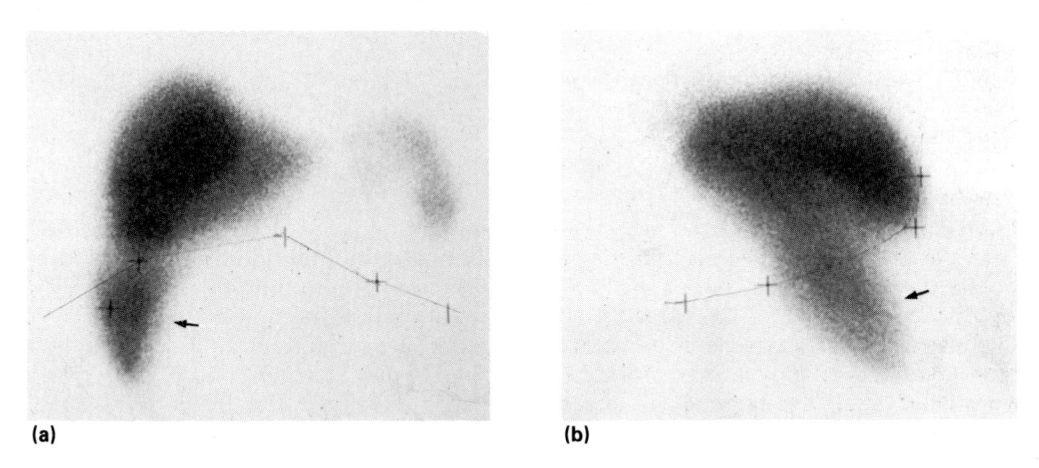

Figure 14.15 Normal liver with Riedels extension to right lobe (arrows). (a) Anterior; (b) right lateral.

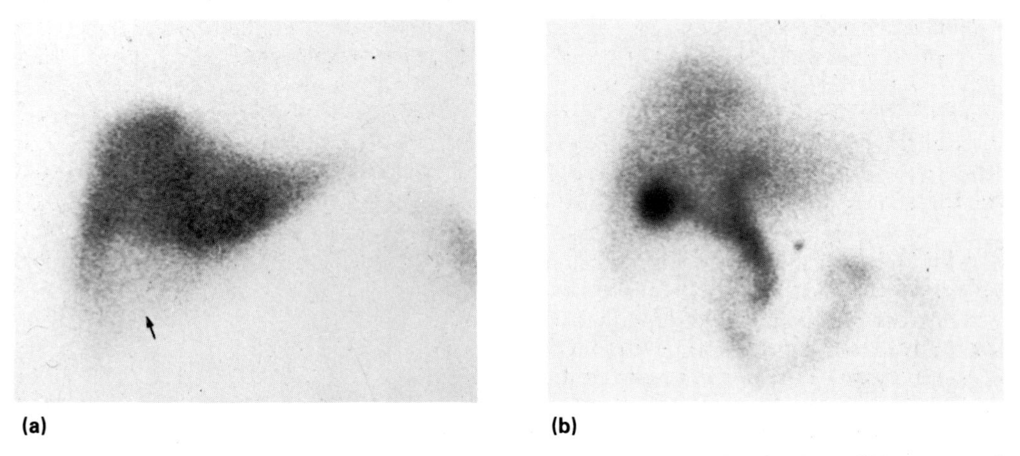

Figure 14.16 Normal liver. (a) Radiocolloid image shows defect in lower right lobe. (b) Hepatobiliary image shows intrahepatic gall bladder as cause.

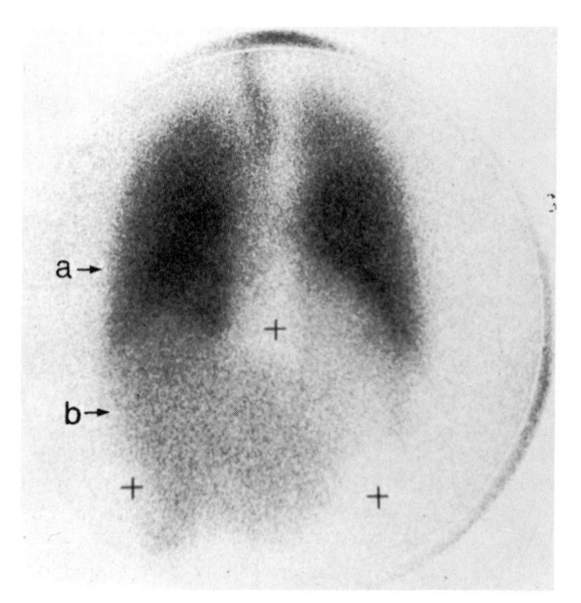

Figure 14.17 Eventration of the liver through foramen of Morgagni. (a) ^{81m}Kr activity in the lung; (b) liver radiocolloid image.

(a) Focal disease

Serial imaging, either by ultrasound, CT or radionuclides, can be used to detect the development of hepatic metastases in those patients with known primary malignancy. The growth or reduction in size of proven secondary deposits can also be monitored to assess the response to chemotherapy. Malignant change after radiotherapy is less successfully followed due to functional impairment induced in the liver by radiation damage (Herbst *et al.*, 1978). The effect of drainage procedures and medical therapy on the resolution of hepatic abscesses can be assessed both by radionuclide and ultrasound imaging.

(b) Diffuse disease

The radionuclide criteria for assessing alterations in diffuse liver disease are more difficult to define than for focal conditions. Progressive impairment of hepatic uptake of colloid gives an increasing value in the ratio of activity between spleen and liver. Serial quantitative measurements of the ratio can assess functional deterioration or improvement. Hepatoma should be suspected when a defined focal lesion develops in a cirrhotic liver.

(c) Response to surgery

The liver soon shows evidence of mitotic activity following partial resection. Regeneration of hepatic tissue takes place early, so that within a period of weeks to months the liver is restored to its pre-surgical volume. Radiocolloid imaging provides a simple method for measuring the rate of growth of the liver remnant (DeLand and Wagner, 1968; Karran *et al.* 1974) as well as providing data on the perfusion changes which precede regeneration.

^{99m}Tc-labelled IDA hepatobiliary agents have been used to assess cholecysto- and choledocho-intestinal anastomoses. They provide an easy method for showing post-operative biliary patency and the presence of bile leaks (Rosenthal, Fonseca, Arzoumanian, Hernandez and Greenberg, 1979). When used after hepatic transplantation ^{99m}Tc-IDA can help to distinguish between biliary tract obstruction and hepatocellular disease, although measurements of radioactivity retained in the blood have not been found to be a reliable index of transplant rejection because of variable renal excretion (Klingensmith, Fritzberg, Koep and Ronai, 1979). The radionuclide image may be wrongly interpreted if attention is not paid to possible technical problems (Johnson and Sweeney, 1967; Freeman *et al.*, 1969). It is not uncommon for structures overlying the liver to attenuate the photon emission and give rise to image non-uniformity. For instance the right breast, or a breast prosthesis, may overlie the upper surface of the right lobe (Figure 14.18). The rib cage may indent the liver, producing a linear defect, usually shown in the right lateral view. This can usually be identified by careful marking of the costal edge. Metal objects such as buckles, coins and jewellery must be removed before imaging to avoid attenuation artefacts. If the skin or

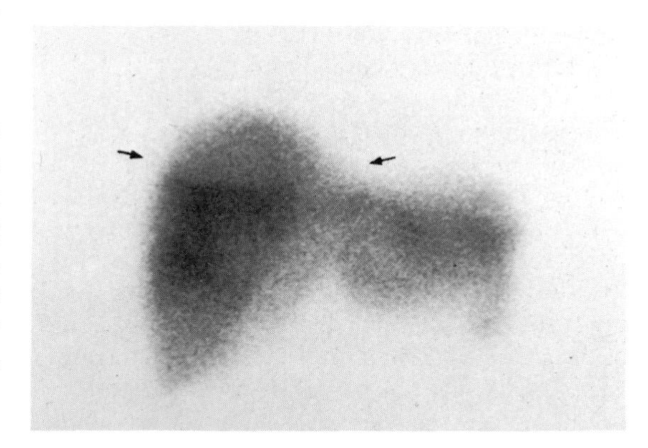

Figure 14.18 Normal liver. Arrows indicate line of reduced count rate in upper right hepatic lobe due to radiation attenuation by overlying breast.

clothing should become contaminated, either at the time of injection or from urinary activity, decontamination procedures must be carried out. Contamination can be recognized readily as small focal regions of high count rate.

14.6 TECHNIQUES

14.6.1 RETICULOENDOTHELIAL IMAGING

A number of different colloid preparations are commercially available as pharmaceutically approved products. The usual radioactive label is ^{99m}Tc. There are no clinical contraindications to the investigation. No special preparation of the patient is necessary.

Between 80 and 200 MBq are administered intravenously to the adult patient, and imaging is commenced after 15 min when the radiocolloid has been cleared maximally by the reticuloendothelial system. The patient may be imaged standing or lying, and views are taken from the anterior, posterior, and right and left projections, the liver having been centred in the field of the gamma camera for each view, using a storage oscilloscope display for positioning.

Anatomical landmarks pertinent to the particular projection are transferred to the final image display. These should include the lower costal margin in the anterior and right lateral projections with identification of the bisection of the midaxillary line, so that a reference coordinate is given for needle biopsy. If a radioactive marker source is used it is usually preferable to record these landmarks on a second film so that image detail is not obscured by the marker. The abdomen is palpated before the patient is moved so that the position of the hepatic border and abdominal masses are recorded on the final display. If a discrete focal mass is shown in the liver, the position of this is marked on the patient's skin as a guide for subsequent biopsy.

If deterioration of image resolution is encountered due to abnormal diaphragmatic movement the study may be acquired at breath hold, or if digital recording is available by respiratory gating of the acquired data using an electronic triggering circuit. Oblique views may assist in the identification of lesions not shown by conventional projections. SPECT studies will also improve the diagnostic accuracy of liver scanning (Fawcett and Sayle, 1989).

Quantitative studies

Digital acquisition of data is used with a bolus injection to provide an activity–time curve of the arrival of tracer in the liver, or when subtraction techniques are used for multiple isotope studies. Digital analysis is usually unnecessary for the interpretation of the routine colloid image although quantification of the uptake ratio between spleen and liver can be used to follow the degree of hepatic dysfunction in diffuse disease.

The effective perfusion rate of the liver can be determined using a mathematical model. This shows that the rate of uptake of radiocolloid is the same at all sites of accumulation (whether hepatic or extrahepatic), and that the relative effective perfusion rates can only be given by the equilibrium plateau values at individual sites (Karran *et al.*, 1979).

Rapid data acquisition following bolus injection can also be used to separate the hepatic and portal arrival of activity, and to determine the relative contribution of each to hepatic perfusion (Fleming *et al.*, 1981). Different techniques have been used to analyse these data (Fleming *et al.*, 1983; Leveson *et al.*, 1983). The mesenteric proportion of portal flow can be assessed in clinical situations (McLaren *et al.*, 1985). The hepatic/portal ratio of flow may be increased in gastrointestinal malignancy before metastases are evident in the liver (Leveson *et al.*, 1985). Radionuclides have also been used to assess the flow in percutaneous hepatic arterial catheters implanted for the direct perfusion of hepatic metastases with chemotherapeutic and other agents (Borzutzky and Turner, 1985). The perfusion pattern is shown by the injection of ^{99m}Tc-labelled microspheres or macroaggregated particles which can be imaged by planar or SPECT techniques (Ziessman *et al.*, 1985). Unlabelled microspheres can be used to obstruct temporarily the hepatic arterial flow and thus possibly enhance the therapeutic effect (Flowerdew *et al.*, 1987).

14.6.2 RADIOPHARMACEUTICALS WHICH GIVE POSITIVE UPTAKE IN HEPATIC FOCAL LESIONS

The lack of diagnostic specifity of the radiocolloid investigation has stimulated a search for alternative agents which might concentrate in hepatic focal lesions.

(a) ^{67}Ga-labelled citrate

This agent has shown its greatest promise in the identification of primary hepatocellular carcinoma. Reports suggest that over 90% of tumours show positive uptake, whereas less than 50% of metastases accumulate gallium. The precise mechanism of uptake is unknown. An adult intravenous dose of 150 MBq is followed by imaging at 48–72 h. Accumulation is shown in normal liver tissue and bone marrow, and frequently large intestinal uptake is also observed. Bowel cleansing with laxatives or enema is required for proper interpretation of ^{67}Ga images.

(b) Abscess localization

Inflammatory tissue may accumulate either ^{67}Ga-labelled citrate (Lavender *et al.*, 1971) or ^{111}In-oxine-labelled autologous leucocytes (Segal *et al.*, 1976; Fawcett *et al.*, 1980), and both techniques can show the site of intra- or extrahepatic sepsis. The gallium procedure is identical to that for tumour detection, but imaging at 24 h often successfully localizes the abscess. False-negative results may be obtained. ^{111}In-oxine-labelled autologous leucocytes separated from whole blood are re-injected and images taken between 24 and 48 h.

(c) Lesion vascularity

An assessment of the relative blood flow of a hepatic lesion compared to that of adjacent normal liver tissue can be made from the measurement of regional activity following a bolus intravenous injection (Waxman *et al.*, 1974). This technique is similar to contrast angiography, and can show an early 'blush' of activity in regions where blood flow is high. It can be carried out as part of the routine radiocolloid procedure by the administration of small volumes of high specific activity. Region of interest selection, using digitized images, permits construction of activity–time curves for different tissues. Alternatively regional vascularity can be demonstrated using an intravascular label which equilibrates in the vascular space and shows the regional vascular pool of blood (Lubin and Lewitus, 1972). The best agents for this are ^{99m}Tc-labelled human serum albumin or ^{99m}Tc-labelled red blood cells (Engel *et al.*, 1983). If ^{99m}Tc-labelled colloid is used for the routine liver image, it may be convenient to investigate the vascularity of a lesion immediately using an isotope of higher energy. Nuclides of indium, ^{111}In (170 keV) and ^{113m}In (390 keV), when injected intravenously, readily attach to circulating transferrin. Images are taken using the primary γ-emission of these isotopes with appropriate pulse-height analyser window settings to exclude the ^{99m}Tc activity. Vascular lesions can also be detected by the injection of labelled microspheres direct into the hepatic artery (Giotti, 1978).

14.6.3 DIAPHRAGMATIC LESIONS

Combined liver and lung imaging can assist in the diagnosis of lesions affecting the right hemidiaphragm (Gold and Johnson, 1975). Conventional colloid images of the liver taken simultaneously with images of either pulmonary perfusion (^{99m}Tc-labelled microspheres or macroaggregates), or ventilation (^{81m}Kr or ^{133}Xe gas) can demonstrate separation of adjacent surfaces of the liver and lung by space-occupying lesions, for instance subphrenic abscess, or apposition of the images in eventration (Soucek, 1975) and herniation of the liver into the chest (Figure 14.17).

14.6.4 HEPATOBILIARY FUNCTION

(a) ^{99m}Tc agents

Of the possible agents proposed for radionuclide imaging of the hepatobiliary system ^{99m}Tc-labelled IDA are best for routine clinical purposes (Lecklitner *et al.*, 1986). A variety of chemical derivatives have been proposed (Rosenthall, 1978; Klingensmith *et al.*, 1980; Shuman *et al.*, 1982; Lee *et al.*, 1986), the intention being to obtain good concentration in bile even when the serum bilirubin level is high (Schwarzrock *et al.*, 1986). Following fasting 160 MBq of the labelled IDA compound is given intravenously, with repeated anterior images taken over the first hour. Later images and right lateral views are taken as required (Krishnamurthy *et al.*, 1985). A milk drink can be given to stimulate biliary flow, and ingestion of a volume of water can help in discrimating between activity in the gall bladder and that in the duodenum (Wahl, 1984). Quantitative analysis of the results may be helpful (Krishnamurthy *et al.*, 1983; Brown *et al.*, 1986). The scintigraphic variations in healthy subjects, with response to intravenous cholecystokinin, have been described (Williams *et al.*, 1984). When assessment of biliary drainage is required over a period of several days the 6 h half-life of ^{99m}Tc may be a constraint. ^{97}Ru has been suggested as a longer-lived alternative (Schachner *et al.*, 1981).

(b) Rose Bengal

Most investigation of the biliary tract with the dye Rose Bengal has used an ^{131}I label. Rose Bengal is readily cleared from the circulation by the hepatocytes, and to a less extent by the kidneys. After overnight fasting an oral dose of 100–200 mg potassium iodide is given to reduce thyroidal uptake of free active iodide. The patient is rested supine for 15 min to stabilize hepatic blood flow, and then 4 MBq is administered intravenously with the gamma camera sited over the lower thorax and upper abdomen. Serial images are taken over a period of 30–40 min. If necessary biliary flow is encouraged by a milk drink towards the end of the imaging period. Time–activity curves are constructed for different regions from digital stored data. ^{123}I has also been used as a label for Rose Bengal; it has the advantage of a reduced radiation dose compared to ^{131}I, and therefore more activity can be administered, giving images of better quality.

14.6.5 SPLENIC FUNCTION

Radiocolloid is the nuclide investigation of choice to show splenic morphology and function. In some patients, however, more precise splenic imaging is required without interference by hepatic activity. For these circumstances autologous red cells labelled under aseptic conditions with ^{99m}Tc are used. These are damaged by heat, and then reinjected into the patient. The cells are rapidly sequestered by the spleen, and imaging can commence at 10 min. Posterior and left lateral views are taken. Quantitative serial imaging can be used to assess the functional capacity of the spleen.

14.6.6 NEEDLE BIOPSY

If histological confirmation of a focal lesion is required, the guidance provided for needle biopsy by radio nuclide, ultrasound or CT imaging greatly enhances the likelihood of a positive result. Blind biopsy has a large sampling error (Conn, 1972). Following a radionuclide image marking the position of the lesion on the skin can be useful if the biopsy is to be done away from the imaging department. Biopsy is usually avoided in those patients who have clotting abnormalities, or in biliary obstruction. When coagulation defects make conventional biopsy undesirable the internal jugular–hepatic vein approach can be used. Passive congestion of the liver increases the risk of biopsy, and suspicion of a hydatid cyst or haemangioma is an absolute contraindication.

REFERENCES

Abramson, S. J., Barash, F. S., Seldin, D. W. and Berdon, W. E. (1984) Transient focal liver scan defects in children receiving chemotherapy (pseudometastases). *Radiology*, **150**, 701–2.

Abu-Nema, T., Al-Suhaily, A. and Abdel-Dayem, H. M. (1986) Hepatobiliary imaging after Whipples' operation. *Clin. Nucl. Med.*, **11**, 572–3.

Agnew, J. E., James, O. and Bouchier, I. A. D. (1975) Liver and pancreas scanning in extrahepatic obstructive jaundice (with special reference to tumours of the bile and hepatic ducts). *Br. J. Radiol.*, **48**, 190–9.

Alderson, P. O., Adams, D. F., McNeil, B. J. *et al.* (1983) Computed tomography, ultrasound and scintigraphy of the liver in patients with colon or breast carcinoma: a prospective comparison. *Radiology*, **149**, 225–30.

Ashare, A. B. (1980) Radiocolloid liver scintigraphy: a choice and an echo. *Radiol. Clin. N. Am.*, **18**, 315–20.

Biersack, H. J., Thelen, M., Torres, J. F. *et al.* (1980) Focal nodular hyperplasia of the liver as established by ^{99m}Tc sulfur colloid and HIDA scintigraphy. *Radiology*, **137**, 187–90.

Borzutzky, C. A. and Turner, E. H. (1985) The predictive value of hepatic artery perfusion scintigraphy. *J. Nucl. Med.*, **26**, 1153–6.

Brendel, A. J., Leccia, F., Drouillard, J. *et al.* (1984) Single photon emission computed tomography (SPECT), planar scintgraphy, and transmission computed tomography: a comparison of accuracy in diagnosing focal hepatic disease. *Radiology*, **153**, 527–32.

Brown, P. H., Juni, J. E., Gray, L. L. and Krishnamurthy, G. T. (1986) Physiological manifestation of various liver diseases as measured by Tc-99m-IDA deconvolution analysis. *J. Nucl. Med.*, **27**, 937–8 (Abstract).

Carrasquillo, J. A., Rogers, J. V., Williams, D. L. *et al.* (1983) Single-photon emission computed tomography of the normal liver. *Am. J. Roentgenol.*, **141**, 937–41.

Chiles, J. T., Mintzer, R. A., Hoffer, P. B. and Gottschalk, A. (1975) Splenic mobility and its effect on estimates of splenic mass. *Radiology*, **114**, 407–10.

Clarke, D. P., Cosgrove, D. O. and McCready, V. R. (1986) Radionuclide imaging for liver malignancy and its relationship to other hepatic investigation. *Clin. Oncol.*, **5**, 159–81.

Coakley, A. J. and Wraight, E. P. (1980) Selenomethionine liver scanning in the diagnosis of hepatoma. *Br. J. Radiol.*, **53**, 538–43.

Colletti, P. M., Ralls, P. W., Lapin, S. A. *et al.* (1986) Hepatobiliary imaging in choledocholithiasis: a comparison with ultrasound. *Clin. Nucl. Med.*, **11**, 482–6.

Conn, H. O. (1972) Rational use of liver biopsy in the

diagnosis of hepatic cancer. *Gastroenterology*, **62**, 142–6.

Cuaron, A., Sepulveda, B. and Landa, L. (1965) Topographic distribution of amoebic abscesses studied by liver scanning. *Int. J. Appl. Radiat. Isot.*, **16**, 603–9.

Deland, F. H. and Wagner, H. N. (1968) Regeneration of the liver after hepatectomy. *J. Nucl. Med.*, **9**, 587–9.

Dewbury, K. C. and Clark, B. (1979) The accuracy of ultrasound in the detection of cirrhosis of the liver. *Br. J. Radiol.*, **52**, 945–8.

Dewbury, K. C., Joseph, A. E. A., Hayes, S. and Murray, C. (1979) Ultrasound in the evaluation and diagnosis of jaundice. *Br. J. Radiol.*, **52**, 276–80.

Dick, M. C. and Mowat, A. P. (1986) Biliary scintigraphy with DISIDA: a simpler way of showing bile duct patency in biliary atresia. *Arch. Dis. Child.*, **61**, 191–2.

El Tumi, M. A., Clarke, M. B., Barrett, J. J. and Mowat, A. P. (1987) Ten minute radiopharmaceutical test in biliary atresia. *Arch. Dis. Child.*, **62**, 180–4.

Engel, M. A., Marks, D. S., Sandler, M. A. and Puranchandar, S. (1983) Differentiation of focal intrahepatic lesions with ^{99m}Tc-red blood cell imaging. *Radiology*, **146**, 777–82.

Evans, G. W., Curtin, F. G., McCarthy, H. F. and Kiernan, J. H. (1972) Scintigraphy in traumatic lesions of liver and spleen. *JAMA*, **222**, 665–7.

Evans, R. A., Bland, K. I., McMurtrey, M. J. and Ballantyne, A. J. (1980) Radionuclide scans not indicated for clinical stage 1 melanoma. *Surg. Gynecol. Obstet.*, **150**, 532–4.

Fawcett, H. D., Lantieri, R. L., Frankel, A. and McDougall, I. R. (1980) Differentiating hepatic abscess from tumor: combined ^{111}In white blood cell and ^{99m}Tc liver scans. *Am. J. Roentgenol.*, **135**, 53–6.

Fawcett, H. D. and Sayle, B. A. (1989) SPECT versus planar liver scintigraphy: is SPECT worth it? *J. Nucl. Med.*, **30**, 57–9.

Fee, H. J., Prokop, E. K., Cameron, J. L. and Wagner, H. N. (1974) Liver scanning in patients with suspected abdominal tumor. *JAMA*, **230**, 1675–7.

Fleming, J. S., Humphries, N. L. M., Karran, S. J. *et al.* (1981) In vivo assessment of hepatic-arterial and portal-venous components of liver perfusion. *J. Nucl. Med.*, **22**, 18–21.

Fleming, J. S., Ackery, D. M., Walmsley, B. H. and Karran, S. J. (1983) Scintigraphic estimation of arterial and portal blood supplies to the liver. *J. Nucl. Med.*, **24**, 1108–13.

Flowerdew, A. D. S., Richards, H. K. and Taylor, I. (1987) Temporary blood flow stasis with degradable starch microspheres (DSM) for liver metastasis in a rat model. *Gut*, **28**, 1201–7.

Freeman, L. M., Meng, C. H., Johnson, P. M. *et al.* (1969) False positive liver scans caused by disease processes in adjacent organs and structures. *Br. J. Radiol.*, **42**, 651–6.

Freitas, J. E., Fink-Bennett, D. M., Thrall, J. H. *et al.* (1980) Efficacy of hepatobiliary imaging in acute abdominal pain. *J. Nucl. Med.*, **21**, 919–24.

Gainey, M. A. and Faerber, E. N. (1985) Disparate hepatic imaging with technetium-99m sulfur colloid and disofenin in Wilson's disease. *J. Nucl. Med.*, **26**, 368–72.

Gamlen, T. R., Triger, D. R., Ackery, D. M. *et al.* (1975) Quantitative liver imaging using ^{131}I Rose Bengal as an index of liver function and prognosis. *Gut*, **16**, 738–43.

Gerhold, J. P., Klingensmith, W. C., Kuni, C. C. *et al.* (1983) Diagnosis of biliary atresia with radionuclide hepatobiliary imaging. *Radiology*, **146**, 499–504.

Geslien, G. E., Pinksy, S. M., Poth, R. K. and Johnson, M. C. (1976) The sensitivity and specificity of 99m Tc-sulfur colloid liver imaging in diffuse hepatocellular disease. *Radiology*, **118**, 115–19.

Gibson, R. N., Yeung, E., Thompson, J. N. *et al.* (1986) Bile duct obstruction: radiologic evaluation of level, cause, and tumour resectability. *Radiology*, **160**, 43–47.

Gilday, D. L. and Alderson, P. O. (1974) Scintigraphic evaluation of liver and spleen injury. *Semin. Nucl. Med.*, **4**, 357–70.

Gold, R. P. and Johnson, P. M. (1975) Efficiency of combined liver–lung scintillation imaging. *Radiology*, **117**, 105–11.

Giotti, E. W. (1978) Microsphere angiography of the liver. *J. Nucl. Med.*, **19**, 433–4.

Grant, R. W. and Ackery, D. (1976) Displacement of the spleen in infected pancreatic pseudocyst: case report. *J. Nucl. Med.*, **17** 193–5.

Haaga, J. R. (1984) Magnetic resonance imaging of the liver. *Radiol. Clin. N. Am.*, **22**, 879–90.

Hall, A. W., Wisbey, M. L., Hutchinson, F. *et al.* (1981) The place of hepatobiliary isotope scanning in the diagnosis of gallbladder disease. *Br. J. Surg.*, **68**, 85–90.

Halpern, S., Coel, M., Ashburn, W. *et al.* (1974) Correlation of liver and spleen size. *Arch. Int. Med.*, **134**, 123–24.

Hatfield, P. M. (1975) Role of liver scanning in the diagnosis of hepatic metastases. *Med. Clin. N. Am.*, **59**, 247–76.

Hegarty, J. E. and Williams, R. (1984) Liver biopsy: techniques, clinical applications, and complications. *Br. Med. J.*, **288**, 1254–6.

Herbst, K. D., Corder, M. P. and Morita, E. T. (1978) Hepatic scan defects following radiotherapy for lymphoma. *Clin. Nucl. Med.*, **3**, 331–3.

Holder, L. E. and Saenger, E. L. (1975) The use of nuclear medicine in evaluating liver disease. *Semin. Roentgenol.*, **10** 215–22.

Holmquest, D. L. and Burdine, J. A. (1973) Caval-portal shunting as a cause of a focal increase in radiocolloid uptake in normal livers. *J. Nucl. Med.*, **14**, 348–51.

Huang, M.-J., Liaw, Y.-F. and Tzen, K.-Y. (1985) Radionuclide venography in Budd–Chiari syndrome with intrahepatic vena-caval obstruction. *J. Nucl. Med.*, **26**, 145–48.

Intenzo, C., Kim, S., Madsen, M., Desai, A. and Park, C. (1988) Planar and SPECT Tc-99m red blood cell imaging in hepatic cavernous hemangiomas and other hepatic lesions. *Clin. Nucl. Med.*, **13** (4), pp. 237–40.

James, O., Wood, E. J. and Sherlock, S. (1974) ^{67}Gallium scanning in the diagnosis of liver disease. *Gut*, **15**, 404–10.

Jaw, T.-S., Wu, C.-C., Ho, Y.-H. *et al.* (1984) Diagnosis of obstructive jaundice in infants: Tc-99m DISIDA in duodenal juice. *J. Nucl. Med.*, **25**, 360–3.

Johnson, P. M. and Sweeney, W. A. (1967) The false-positive hepatic scan. *J. Nucl. Med.*, **8**, 451–60.

Joske, R. A. (1974) The changing pattern of hydatid disease, with special references to hydatid of the liver. *Med. J. Aust.*, **1**, 129.

Kan, M. K. and Hopkins, G. B. (1979) Measurement of liver volume by emission computed tomography. *J. Nucl. Med.*, **20**, 514–20.

Kaplan, E. and Domingo, M. (1972) ^{75}Se-selenomethionine in hepatic focal lesions. *Semin. Nucl. Med.*, **2**, 139–49.

Karran, S. J., Leach, K. G. and Blumgart, L. H. (1974) Assessment of liver regeneration in the rat using the gamma camera. *J. Nucl. Med.*, **15**, 10–16.

Karran, S. J., Eagles, C. J., Fleming, J. S. and Ackery, D. M. (1979) *In vivo* measurement of liver perfusion in the normal and partially hepatectomized rat using Tc-99m sulfur colloid. *J. Nucl. Med.*, **20**, 26–31.

Khan, O., Ell, P. J., Jarritt, P. H. *et al.* (1981) Comparison between emission and transmission computed tomography of the liver. *Br. Med. J.*, **282**, 1212–14.

Kido, C. (1975) Primary liver cancer (angiography and scintigraphy). *Aust. Radiol.*, **19**, 129–39.

Klingensmith, W. C., Fritzberg, A. R., Spitzer, V. M. and Koep, L. J. (1980) Clinical comparison of ^{99m}Tc-diethyl-IDA and ^{99m}Tc-PIPIDA for evaluation of the hepatobiliary system. *Radiology*, **134**, 195–99.

Krishnamurthy, G. T., Bobba, V. R., McConnell, D. *et al* (1983) Quantitative biliary dynamics: introduction of a new noninvasive scintigraphic technique. *J. Nucl. Med.*, **24**, 217–23.

Krishnamurthy, G. T., Lieberman, D. A. and Brar, H. S. (1985) Detection, localization, and quantitation of degree of common bile duct obstruction by scintigraphy. *J. Nucl. Med.*, **26**, 726–35.

Krishnamurthy, G. T. and Turner, F. E. (1990) Pharmacokinetics and clinical application of technetium 99m-labelled hepatobiliary agents, *Semin. Nucl. Med.*, **20**, 130–49.

Landgarten, S. and Spencer, R. P. (1972) Splenic displacement due to gastric dilatation. *J. Nucl. Med.*, **13**, 223.

Lavender, J. P., Lowe, J., Barker, J. R. *et al.* (1971) Gallium 67 citrate scanning in neoplastic and inflammatory lesions. *Br. J. Radiol.*, **44**, 361–6.

Lecklitner, M. L., Austin, A. R., Benedetto, A. R. and Growcock, G. W. (1986) Positive predictive value of cholescintigraphy in common bile duct obstruction. *J. Nucl. Med.*, **27**, 1403–6.

Lee, A. W., Ram, M. D., Shih, W.-J. and Murphy, K. (1986) Technetium-99m BIDA biliary scintigraphy in the evaluation of the jaundiced patient. *J. Nucl. Med.*, **27**, 1407–12.

Lees, W. R., Hall-Craggs, M. A. and Manhire, A. (1985) Five years experience of fine-needle aspiration biopsy: 454 consecutive cases. *Clin. Radiol.*, **36**, 517–20.

Lerona, P. T., Go, R. T. and Cornell, S. H. (1974) Limitations of angiography and scanning in diagnosis of liver masses. *Radiology*, **112**, 139–45.

Leveson, S. H., Wiggins, P. A., Nasiru, T. A. *et al.* (1983) Improving the detection of hepatic metastases by the use of dynamic flow scintigraphy. *Br. J. Cancer*, **47**, 719–21.

Leveson, S. H., Wiggins, P. A., Giles, G. R. *et al.* (1985) Deranged liver blood flow patterns in the detection of liver metastases. *Br. J. Surg.*, **72**, 128–30.

Lieberman, D. A. and Krishnamurthy, G. T. (1986) Intrahepatic versus extrahepatic cholestasis: discrimination with biliary scintigraphy combined with ultrasound. *Gastroenterology*, **90**, 734–43.

Lipton, M. J., DeNardo, G. L., Silverman, S. and Glatstein, E. (1972) Evaluation of the liver and spleen in Hodgkin's disease I. The value of hepatic scintigraphy. *Am. J. Med.*, **52**, 356–61.

Loken, M. K., Ascher, N. L., Boudreau, R. J. and Natarian, J. S. (1986) Scintigraphic evaluation of liver transplant function. *J. Nucl. Med.*, **27**, 451–9.

Lubin, E. and Lewitus, Z. (1972) Blood. pool scanning in investigating hepatic mass lesions. *Semin. Nucl. Med.*, **2**, 128–32.

Lunia, S., Parthasarathy, K. L., Baksh, S. and Bender, M. A. (1975) An evaluation of ^{99m}Tc-sulfur colloid liver scintiscans and their usefulness in metastatic workup: a review of 1,424 studies. *J. Nucl. Med.*, **16**, 62–5.

Majd, M., Reba, R. C. and Altman, R. P. (1981) Hepatobiliary scintigraphy with ^{99m}Tc-PIPIDA in the evaluation of neonatal jaundice. *Pediatrics*, **67**, 140–5.

McAfee, J. G., Ause, R. G. and Wagner, H. N. (1965) Diagnostic value of scintillation scanning of the liver. *Arch. Int. Med.*, **116**, 95–110.

McClees, E. C. and Gedgaudas-McClees, R. K. (1984) Screening for diffuse and focal liver disease: the case for hepatic scintigraphy. *J. Clin. Ultrasound*, **12**, 75–81.

McCready, V. R. (1972) Scintigraphic studies of space-occupying liver disease. *Semin. Nucl. Med.*, **2**, 108–27.

McIntyre, P. A. (1972) Diagnostic significance of the spleen scan. *Semin. Nucl. Med.*, **2**, 278–87.

McLaren, M. I., Fleming, J. F., Walmsley, B. H. *et al.* (1985) Dynamic liver scanning in cirrhosis. *Br. J. Surg.*, **72**, 394–6.

Miller, J. H. and Greenspan, B. S. (1985) Integrated imaging of hepatic tumours in childhood. *Radiology*, **154**, 91–100.

O'Callaghan, J. D., Verow P. W., Hopton D. and Craven J. L. (1980) The diagnosis of acute gallbladder disease by technetium-99m-labelled HIDA hepatobiliary scanning. *Br. J. Surg.*, **67**, 805–8.

O'Connor, K. W., Snodgrass, P. J., Swonder, J. E. *et al.* (1983) A blinded prospective study comparing four current nonivasive approaches in the differential diagnosis of medical versus surgical jaundice. *Gastroenterology*, 84, 1498–504.

Operchal, J. A., Bowen, R. D. and Grove, R. B. (1976). Efficacy of radionuclide procedures in staging of bronchogenic carcinoma. *J. Nuclear. Med.*, **17**, 530 (Abstract).

Oster, Z. H., Larson, S. M., Strauss, H. W. and Wagner, H. N. (1975) Analysis of liver scanning in a general hospital. *J. Nucl. Med.*, **16**, 450–3.

Pauwels, S., Piret, L., Schoutens, A. *et al.* (1980) Tc-99m-diethyl-IDA imaging: clinical evaluation in jaundiced patients. *J. Nucl. Med*, **21**, 1022–8.

Petasnick, J. P., Ram, P., Turner, D. A. and Fordham, E. W. (1979) The relationship of computed tomography, gray-scale ultrasomography, and radionuclide imaging in the evaluation of hepatic masses. *Semin. Nucl. Med.*, **9**, 8–21.

Pinksy, S. M. and Henkin, R. E. (1976) Gallium-67 tumor scanning. *Semin. Nucl. Med.*, **6**, 397–409.

Ranson, J. H. C., Madayag, M. A., Localio, S. A. and Spencer, F. C. (1975) New diagnostic and therapeutic techniques in the management of pyogenic liver abscesses. *Ann. Surg.*, **181**, 508–18.
Robinson, P. J. (1985) Computed tomography of the liver. *Curr. Opinion Gastroenterol.*, **1**, 516–21.
Rollo, F. D. and DeLand, F. H. (1968) The determination of liver mass from radionuclide images. *Radiology*, **91**, 1191–4.
Rosenthal, S. N. (1976) Are hepatic scans overused? *Am. J. Dig. Dis.*, **21**, 659–63.
Rosenthall, L. (1978) Clinical experience with the newer hepatobiliary radiopharmaceuticals. *Can. J. Surg.*, **21**, 297–300.
Rosenthall, L., Fonseca, C., Arzoumanian, A. *et al.* (1979) 99m Tc-IDA hepatobiliary imaging following upper abdominal surgery. *Radiology*, **130**, 735–9.
Rothschild, M. A. and Rosenthal, S. (1976) Are hepatic scans overused? *Am. J. Dig. Dis.*, **21**, 655–9.
Samuels, B. I., Freitas, J. E., Bree, R. L. *et al.* (1983) A comparison of radionuclide hepatobiliary imaging and real-time ultrasound for the detection of acute cholecystitis. *Radiology*, **147**, 207–10.
Savitch, I., Kew, M. C., Paterson, A. *et al* (1983) Uptake of Tc-99m di-isopropylimino-diacetic acid by hepatocellular carcinoma. *J. Nucl. Med.*, **24**, 1119–22.
Schachner, E. R., Gil, M. C., Atkins, H. L. *et al.* (1981) Ruthenium-97 hepatobiliary agents for delayed studies of the biliary tract. 1: Ru-97. PIPIDA. *J. Nucl. Med.*, **22**, 352–7.
Schenker, S. Balint, J. and Schiff, L. (1962) Differential diagnosis of jaundice: report of a prospective study of 61 proved cases. *Am. J. Dig. Dis.*, **7**, 449–63.
Schraibman, I. G. (1974) Non-parasitic liver abscess. *Br. J. Surg.*, **61**, 709–12.
Schwarzrock, R., Kotzerke, J., Hundershagen, H. *et al.* (1986) ^{99m}Tc-diethyl-iodo-HIDA (JODIDA): a new hepatobiliary agent in clinical comparison with ^{99m}Tc-disopropyl-HIDA (DISIDA) in jaundiced patients. *Eur. J. Nucl. Med.*, **12**, 346–50.
Scott-Smith, W., Raftery, A. T., Wraight, E. P. and Calne, R. Y. (1983) Tc-99m labelled HIDA imaging in suspected biliary leaks after liver transplantation. *Clin. Nucl. Med.*, **8**, 478–79.
Sears, H. F., Gerber, F. H., Sturtz, D. L. and Fouty, W. J. (1975) Liver scan and carcinoma of the breast. *Surg. Gynecol. Obstet.*, **140**, 409–11.
Segal, A. W., Thakur, M. L., Arnot, R. N. and Lavender, J. P. (1976) Indium-III-labelled leukocytes for localisation of abscesses. *Lancet*, **ii**, 1056–8.
Shih, W.-J., Domstad, P. A., Lieber, A. *et al.* (1986) Localization of ^{99m}Tc-HMDP in hepatic metastases from colonic carcinoma. *Am. J. Roentgenol.*, **146**, 333–6.
Shuman, W. P., Gibbs, P., Rudd, T. G. and Mack, L. A. (1982) PIPIDA scintigraphy for cholecystitis: false positives in alcoholism and total parenteral nutrition. *Am. J. Roentgenol.*, **138**, 1–5.
Siddiqui, A. R., Ellis, J. H. and Madura, J. A. (1986) Different patterns for bile leakage following cholecystectomy demonstrated by hepatobiliary imaging. *Clin. Nucl. Med.*, **11**, 751–3.
Silverberg, M., Rosenthall, L. and Freeman, L. M. (1973) Rose Bengal excretion studies as an aid in the differential diagnosis of neonatal jaundice. *Semin. Nucl. Med.*, **3**, 69–80.
Silverman, S., DeNardo, G. L., Glatstein, E. and Lipton, M. J. (1972) Evaluation of the liver and spleen in Hodgkin's disease II. The value of splenic scintigraphy. *Am. J. Med.*, **52**, 362–6.
Smith, R. (1985) Liver–spleen scintigraphy in patients with acquired immunodeficiency syndrome. *Am. J. Roentgenol.*, **145**, 1201–4.
Soucek, C. D. (1975) Foramen of Morgagni hernia diagnosed by liver scan. *J. Nucl. Med.*, **16**, 261–3.
Sullivan, S., Krasner, N. and Williams, R. (1976) The clinical estimation of liver size: a comparison of techniques and analysis of the source of error. *Br. Med. J.*, **ii**, 1042–3.
Tavill, A. S., Wood, E. J., Kreel, L. *et al.* (1975) The Budd–Chiari syndrome: correlation between hepatic scintigraphy and the clinical, radiological and pathological findings in nineteen cases of hepatic venous outflow obstruction. *Gastroenterology*, **68**, 509–18.
Taylor, K. J. W., Sullivan, D., Rosenfield, A. T. and Gottschalk, A. (1977) Gray scale ultrasound and isotope scanning: complementary techniques for imaging the liver. *Am. J. Roentgenol.*, **128**, 277–81.
Tonami, N., Aburano, T. and Hisada, K. (1975) Comparison of alpha 1 fetoprotein radioimmunoassay method and liver scanning for detecting primary hepatic cell carcinoma. *Cancer*, **36**, 466–70.
Uszler, J. M. and Swanson, L. A. (1975) Focal nodular hyperplasia of the liver: case report. *J. Nucl. Med.*, **16**, 831–2.
Utz, J. A., Lull, R. J., Anderson, J. H. *et al.* (1980) Hepatoma visualization with Tc-99m pyridoxylidene glutamate. *J. Nucl. Med.*, **21**, 747–9.
Wahl, R. L. (1984) The 'water-ida': a simple means to separate duodenal from gallbladder activity on cholescintigraphic studies. *Eur. J. Nucl. Med.*, **9**, 335–6.
Waxman, A. D., Finck, E. J. and Siemsen, J. K. (1974) Combined contrast and radionuclide angiography of the liver. *Radiology*, **113**, 123–9.
Waxman, A. D., Richmond, R., Juttner, H. *et al.* (1980) Correlation of contrast angiography and histologic pattern with gallium uptake in primary liver-cell carcinoma: noncorrelation with alpha-feto protein. *J. Nucl. Med.*, **21**, 324–7.
Weissmann, H. S., Frank, M., Rosenblatt, R. *et al.* (1979a) Cholescintigraphy, ultrasonography and computerized tomography in the evaluation of biliary tract disorders. *Semin. Nucl. Med.*, **9**, 22–35.
Weissmann, H. S., Frank, M. S., Bernstein, L. H. and Freeman, L. M. (1979b) Rapid and accurate diagnosis of acute cholecystitis with 99mTc-HIDA cholescintigraphy. *Am. J. Roentgenol.*, **132**, 523–8.
Wheeler, P. G., Theodossi, A., Pickford, R. *et al.* (1979) Non-invasive techniques in the diagnosis of jaundice: ultrasound and computer. *Gut*, **20**, 196–9.
Wiener, S. N. and Parulekar, S. G. (1979) Scintigraphy and ultrasonography of hepatic hemangioma. *Radiology*, **132**, 149–53.
Williams, W., Krishnamurthy, G. T., Brar, H. S. and Bobba, V. R. (1984) Scintigraphic variations of normal biliary physiology. *J. Nucl. Med.*, **25**, 160–5.
Wistow, B. W., Subramanian, G., Van Heertum, R. L. *et*

al. (1977) An evaluation of ^{99m}Tc-labelled hepatobiliary agents. *J. Nucl. Med.*, **18**, 455–61.
Ziessman, H. A., Wahl, R. L., Juni, J. E. *et al.* (1985) The utility of SPECT for ^{99m}Tc-MAA hepatic arterial perfusion scintigraphy. *Am. J. Roentgenol.*, **145**, 747–51.

FURTHER READING

Krishnamurthy, S. and Krishnamurthy, G. T. (1988) Nuclear hepatology: where is it heading now? *J. Nucl. Med.*, **29**, 1144–9.
Seminars in Liver Disease (1989), 9th edition.

CHAPTER FIFTEEN

Haematology

A. M. Peters and S. M. Lewis

15.1 INTRODUCTION

Since the previous edition of this book the field of nuclear haematology has expanded considerably as a result of the introduction of new techniques for labelling blood cells, particularly platelets and leucocytes. These have led, for example, to improved methods for identifying and quantifying the causes of thrombocytopenia in the clinical setting and for understanding the normal kinetics of platelets and granulocytes in the context of clinical research.

15.2 BLOOD VOLUME

In normal subjects the relation between the packed cell volume (PCV; venous haematocrit) and the total red cell volume (RCV) is approximately linear. A peripheral blood count therefore provides a reasonably good indication of the circulating red cell mass. However, the plasma volume (PV) fluctuates in some circumstances so that the haemoglobin, red cell count and PCV do not always reflect the total RCV, and therefore may not provide an accurate assessment of anaemia or polycythaemia. By contrast, the RCV does not fluctuate to any great extent provided that erythropoiesis is in a steady state. Increased red cell production can result from abnormal proliferation of stem cells in primary proliferative polycythaemia (polycythaemia vera) or from increased erythropoietin production. The latter is an appropriate response to tissue hypoxia, e.g. in respiratory disease and in cyanotic congenital heart disease, but it may also arise inappropriately from erythropoietin-producing tumours (Table 15.1).

The control of PV is complex. Changes in PV are achieved by alterations in the distribution of water between the intravascular and extravascular fluid compartments across the capillary wall. PV is labile and influenced by bedrest, exercise, change in posture, food and ambient temperature. Short-term regulation of PV maintains the circulating blood volume at a constant level; as a rule, rapid adjustments take place immediately in shock or haemolysis or a few hours after blood transfusion or intravenous infusion. PV fluctuation may result in haemodilution or haemoconcentration, giving rise to pseudoanaemia or pseudopolycythaemia respectively. PV increases in pregnancy, especially in the first trimester, and in some cases may be a major factor in the anaemia of pregnancy.

Table 15.1 Causes of increased red cell volume

1. Primary proliferative polycythaemia
2. Idiopathic erythrocytosis
3. Autonomous high erythropoietin production
4. Secondary polycythaemia
   (a) *Hypoxic (with activation of normal erythropoietin mechanism)*
   High altitude
   Hypoxaemic lung disease (including intrinsic lung disease, hypoventilation, sleep apnoea)
   Cyanotic congenital heart disease
   High oxygen affinity haemoglobins
   Smoking
   Methaemoglobinaemia
   Red cell metabolic defect

   (b) *With 'inappropriate' secretion of erythropoietin*
   Renal tumour – hypernephroma, nephroblastoma
   Renal ischaemia (e.g. cysts, hydronephrosis, renal transplant)
   Hepatoma and liver disease
   Fibroids
   Cerebellar haemangioblastoma
   Bronchial carcinoma
   Phaeochromocytoma

   (c) *Miscellaneous*
   Androgen therapy
   Cushing's disease
   Hypertransfusion

Causes of a reduction in PV include fluid loss (e.g. in burns), diuretic therapy, alcohol, hypertension, smoking and prolonged confinement to bed. In some cases PV reduction is transient and in most of these conditions the cause is obvious. There are, however, patients in whom the reduction in PV is more prolonged, without apparent cause, and this gives rise to a syndrome which has been termed 'stress polycythaemia'; it occurs in subjects who are anxious or work under mental pressure; they are often hypertensive and obese.

15.2.1 CLINICAL INDICATIONS FOR MEASURING BLOOD VOLUME

The measurement of RCV and PV is necessary in the investigation of polycythaemia in order to establish an absolute increase in red cell mass as in true polycythaemia. These measurements are also useful in the exclusion of pseudoanaemia, i.e. an expanded PV with a normal RCV. Venous PCVs of greater than 0.56 in men or 0.52 in women are clearly above the upper limits of normal (0.50 and 0.47 respectively) and true polycythaemia is likely, whether primary proliferative or secondary. It is, however, important to exclude a lowered PV, i.e. pseudopolycythaemia. A smaller increase in PCV is not uncommon. When it is persistently above 0.50 in men or 0.45 in women but less than the abnormal limit, it is necessary to distinguish between a minor degree of true polycythaemia and pseudopolycythaemia; in addition there is a so-called 'physiological polycythaemia' in which both the RCV and PCV are within 2 standard deviations of the normal mean, but whereas RCV is on the high side, the PV is on the low side of the mean (Pearson *et al.*, 1984; Marsh *et al.*, 1987). It is not clear whether this is an early phase of pseudopolycythaemia or true polycythaemia or whether it is a transient phenomenon of no clinical significance. It is, however, important to identify and to document its occurrence, as an increasing PCV may be associated with the clinical effects of hyperviscosity and may thus require to be treated and controlled.

Blood volume should be measured when anaemia is accompanied by splenomegaly, since the latter is often associated with an expanded PV. Pseudoanaemia also occurs in cirrhosis (Maddney *et al.*, 1969) and in acute glomerulonephritis (Eisenberg, 1959).

The principle of measurement is that of dilution analysis. A small amount of a readily identifiable radionuclide is injected intravenously, either bound to the red cells or to a plasma protein, and its dilution is measured after complete mixing within the circulating red cell or plasma volumes, respectively.

Previously, ^{51}Cr was usually used to label red cells for measuring RCV; it is not ideal but is still used especially when this measurement is combined with a red cell survival study or measurement of gastrointestinal bleeding. Currently the most practical labels are ^{99m}Tc or indium (^{111}In or ^{113m}In). Plasma volume is measured with human serum albumin (HSA) labelled with ^{125}I or ^{131}I.

Whereas measurement of RCV should be accurate and reproducible, measurement of PV may only be approximate because of potential rapid fluctuation. There is a slow interchange of the labelled albumin between the plasma and extracellular fluids and some loss occurs by exchange with a small extravascular pool during the mixing period. For these reasons it is undesirable to calculate the RCV from PV using the observed haematocrit (see later). Total blood volume is obtained by adding together the separate direct measurements of the RCV and PV.

The subject of blood volume and its regulation in health and disease has a huge literature. Comprehensive reviews include those by Mollison (1979), Mayerson (1965) and Najean and Cacchione (1977). Practical information is provided in the recommendations on standardized techniques by the International Committee for Standardization in Haematology (ICSH) (1980b).

15.2.2 RED CELL VOLUME

(a) ***Sodium chromate (^{51}Cr)*** (ICSH, 1980b; Dacie and Lewis, 1984)

A dose of 0.1–0.2 μCi of $Na_2{}^{51}CrO_4$ per kilogram body weight in a volume of at least 0.2 ml is added to 5 ml of red cells. The ^{51}Cr becomes firmly bound to the red cells and elution *in vivo* is negligible during the time between administration and blood collection, even when the latter is delayed for an hour to allow for prolonged mixing. As the γ-photons from ^{51}Cr can easily be distinguished from those of ^{125}I, plasma volume can be measured simultaneously with this latter radionuclide. However, the major disadvantage of ^{51}Cr is its relatively long half-life (27.8 days), which is undesirable for frequent repeated measurements of RCV.

(b) ^{99m}Tc-pertechnetate

As this radionuclide has a short half-life, it can be used for repeated measurements. Unfortunately, 4–10% of the activity elutes from the cells in the first hour following injection (Ferrant *et al.*, 1974). In order to bind ^{99m}Tc, the red cells require to be 'tinned' by means of the prior addition of a stannous compound. This may be carried out either *in vitro* (Jones and Mollison, 1978) or *in vivo* (Pavel *et al.*, 1977), following which the cells are exposed to pertechnetate *in vitro*.

(c) Indium: ^{111}In or ^{113m}In

Both these isotopes of indium can be used for blood volume measurements but ^{113m}In is the more suitable for short-term investigations (Radia *et al.*, 1981). The labelling procedure is simpler than with ^{99m}Tc and since elution is less than with ^{99m}Tc during the first hour it is particularly suitable for delayed sampling. The indium may be complexed with oxine (Goodwin, 1978), tropolone (Danpure *et al.*, 1982) or acetylacetone (Sinn and Silvester, 1979); the latter two complexes are easy to prepare in aqueous solution (see Section 15.8.1).

(d) Measurement of RCV

At 10 and 20 min after the injection, 5 ml of blood are collected into ethylenediaminetetraacetic acid (EDTA). When intravascular mixing is likely to be prolonged, such as in splenomegaly (Toghill, 1964), another sample should be taken at 60 min.

Red cell volume (ml) =

$$\frac{\text{Radioactivity of standard (cpm ml}^{-1}) \times \text{dilution of standard} \times \text{volume injected (ml)}}{\text{Radioactivity of post-injection sample (cpm ml}^{-1})} \times \text{PCV}$$

Thus, although the measurement is of the RCV, it is more convenient to measure the radioactivity in a volume of whole blood and adjust by multiplying by 1/PCV to obtain radioactivity per millilitre of red cells. The PCV is that of the sample.

If delayed mixing is anticipated or there is a significant difference between the measurements at 10–20 and 60 min, the latter should be used for calculating RCV. In this event ^{51}Cr (or ^{113m}In) is to be preferred because of its lower rate of elution.

15.2.3 PLASMA VOLUME

The most commonly used tracer for plasma is ^{125}I-labelled HSA, but ^{131}I-labelled HSA is also commercially available. The albumin concentration should not be less than 20 g l^{-1} and must be from donors who are Australia-antigen and human immunodeficiency virus (HIV) antibody negative. ^{125}I has the advantage of being easily distinguished from ^{51}Cr, ^{99m}Tc and ^{113m}In and gives a lower radiation dose than ^{131}I. It can therefore be used in the simultaneous measurement of RCV and PV. Thyroid uptake of the radioiodine released following labelled HSA catabolism should be blocked with potassium iodide, 30 mg per day (Ellis *et al.*, 1977) given one to two days before injection and continued for two to four weeks.

Transferrin labelled with ^{113m}In has also been used as a plasma label (Wochner *et al.*, 1970). ^{113m}In has a short half-life (100 min) and is thus suitable for repeated measurements. Since its γ-photon energy is close to that of ^{51}Cr, ^{113m}In transferrin should be used in conjunction with ^{99m}Tc as the red cell label in the simultaneous measurement of PV and RCV. In practice, ^{113m}In transferrin as a plasma marker does not appear to confer any special advantage over ^{125}I-labelled HSA. ^{59}Fe and ^{52}Fe-labelled transferrin have also been used for PV measurements, but they are not routinely used unless ferrokinetic studies are undertaken at the same time.

When measuring PV, it is important to note that the dilution space varies with the labelled protein used and therefore does not necessarily represent the physiological volume of the plasma within the circulation. Thus, with ^{113m}In-labelled transferrin, the plasma volume is 1.05 that of albumin, whereas with an immunoglobulin tracer it is 0.95 (Valeri *et al.*, 1973; Wright *et al.*, 1975).

Measurement of PV

Details of the standard method recommended by ICSH have been published (1980b). ^{125}I-labelled HSA comes in vials containing 3–5 μCi ml^{-1} of albumin solution. One millilitre of labelled HSA is diluted with approximately 5 ml of saline. A measured volume (about 5 ml) is injected and the remainder kept as a standard. Blood samples of 5 ml are withdrawn at 10, 20 and 30 min. The zero time plasma activity is obtained by extrapolation from the clearance, which, initially, can be regarded as monoexponential.

Plasma volume (ml) =

$$\frac{\text{Radioactivity of standard (cpm ml}^{-1}) \times \text{dilution of standard} \times \text{volume injected (ml)}}{\text{Radioactivity of post-injection sample (cpm ml}^{-1}\text{ adjusted to zero time)}}$$

It has been suggested that if only a single 10 min blood sample is collected, the radioactivity at zero time can be approximated by multiplication by 1.015. This, however, is not reliable as disappearance rates vary from case to case. Accordingly, three samples are more reliable because a single 10 min estimation will be misleading when mixing is delayed.

15.2.4 EXPRESSION OF RESULTS OF BLOOD VOLUME ESTIMATIONS

Red cell and plasma volumes are usually expressed in terms of body weight and, for clinical interpretation, are compared with normal reference values. The mean ± 2 SD values for normal RCV are 30 ± 5 ml kg^{-1} for men and 25 ± 5 ml kg^{-1} for women (ICSH, 1980b). However, expression in terms of body weight may in some cases be unsatisfactory because the relation between blood volume and body weight varies according to body composition. For example, because fat is relatively avascular, low values are obtained in obese subjects. Blood volume is more closely correlated with lean body mass but the latter determination is not practical as a routine procedure. Alternatively an estimate of the so-called 'ideal weight' can be made from standard tables based on height, age, build and sex (Documenta Geigy, 1970), but this is somewhat arbitrary and tends to overcorrect for the avascularity of fat.

More complicated formulae, based on sex, height and weight of the subject, have been proposed for predicting the normal blood volume. They are slightly more reliable than body weight alone, especially in obesity. However, various criticisms can be made of them; for example, Hurley's tables (Hurley, 1975), although based on a large number of measurements, were derived from data available in the literature, but not always based on adequate methodology. In Nadler's series (Nadler *et al.*, 1962) the values for total blood volume were indirectly deduced from measurement of PV only and were dependent on the application of a body/venous haematocrit ratio of 0.91. The data on which these formulae were based came largely from selected groups of young people, e.g. volunteers, prisoners or soldiers. None of the prediction formulae have 95% confidence limits better than ± 10% and no one method can be recommended (ICSH, 1980b). Some of the formulae which appear to be fairly reliable are shown in Table 15.2. In practice, the diagnosis of absolute polycythaemia can be made from Hurley's tables if the RCV is greater than 125% of the predicted value for both men and women, and from Nadler's tables if the RCV is greater than 125% for men and greater than 130% for women (Lewis and Liu Yin, 1986).

In various series, estimates of PV in normal subjects have been more variable than those of RCV. This is because PV is labile and more dependent on such factors as activity and posture. Thus it is not possible to give well-based confidence limits for normal PV. The ICSH (1980b) has suggested 40–50 ml kg^{-1} for both men and women. Using Hurley's tables, PV is abnormally reduced if the estimated value is less than 80% of the predicted value for both men and women

Table 15.2 Blood volume reference values

Red cell volume

Men
- (a) $0.157H^3 + 0.014W + 0.258$*
- (b) $1486S^2 - 4106S + 4514$
- (c) $8.2H + 17.3W - 693$ or $1110S$
- (d) $8.6H + 18.6W - 830$ or $1550S - 890$

Women
- (a) $0.136H^3 + 0.013W + 0.070$*
- (b) $1167S - 479$
- (c) $16.4H + 5.7W - 1649$ or $840S$
- (d) $7.5H + 14.3W - 600$ or $1167S - 479$

Plasma volume

Men
- (a) $0.210H^3 + 0.018W + 0.346$*
- (b) $995 \exp(0.6085S)$
- (c) $1630S$
- (d) $(38.5H + 31.7W - 2830)(1 - 0.9\text{PCV})$ or $1580S - 520$

Women
- (a) $0.220H^3 + 0.020W + 0.113$*
- (b) $1278S^{1.289}$
- (c) $1410S$
- (d) $(16.5H + 38.4W - 1370)(1 - 0.9\text{ PCV})$

(a) Nadler *et al.* (1962).
(b) Hurley (1975).
(c) Retzlaff *et al.* (1969).
(d) Wennesland *et al.* (1959).

S = surface area, H = height, W = weight.
*Assumes normal PCV of 0.47 (men), 0.42 (women) and haematocrit ratio of 0.91.

(Lewis and Liu Yin, 1986). The normal range for total blood volume is 60–80 ml kg^{-1} (ICSH, 1980b).

Physical activity and changes in posture cause transient fluctuations in PV; hence the importance of resting the patient in a recumbent position for at least 15 min before carrying out blood volume measurements. Conversely, prolonged bedrest also causes a reduction in blood volume, and decreases up to 10% have been reported (Taylor *et al.*, 1945). Blood volume is higher in the summer than in winter; this is due to PV expansion, presumably related to changes in temperature and physical activity (Bazett *et al.*, 1940).

15.3 MEAN RED CELL LIFE SPAN (MRCLS)

There have been many studies of red cell survival in haemolytic anaemias (reviewed by Bentley and Miller, 1986). Nowadays, this procedure has a more limited use in clinical practice. Nonetheless, red cell survival studies continue to serve a useful function in cases of anaemia in which a haemolytic aetiology is suspected but not clearly diagnosed by other tests.

The majority of studies are carried out on autologous red cells. Donor red cell studies are sometimes useful to distinguish between an inherent red cell defect and an acquired abnormality leading to autologous red cell destruction. There are two methods using radionuclide markers, namely cohort and random labelling. In cohort labelling, a population, or cohort, of red cells is labelled during production in the bone marrow. Peripheral blood radioactivity is then monitored over a period of time to detect the release of these cells into the circulation and their subsequent removal, enabling measurement of MRCLS. Cohort labels are generally radiolabelled protein precursors (amino acids) such as glycine or lysine, or iron (^{59}Fe) (Cavill *et al.*, 1977a).

The major disadvantage of cohort labelling is that studies cannot be completed within a time period less than the MRCLS. Cohort labelling is thus of little value in clinical haematology. There are also other objections to these techniques. An 'ideal' cohort label would react with cells for only a very short period of time, would remain with the cell throughout its lifespan and would not be reutilized after red cell destruction. In practice, no cohort label meets these requirements. Furthermore, interpretation of cohort survival data is complex because the form of the curve depends on the rate of incorporation of the label into red cells and the extent of reutilization, in addition to the mode and rate of red cell destruction. In spite of these practical disadvantages, cohort labelling has one major advantage over random labelling: the use of precursor labels ensures that labelled cells are physiologically identical to normal cells.

With random labelling the age distribution of the labelled sample reflects the age distribution of the parent population. Red cell survival is then monitored from the disappearance of the labelled sample from the circulation. Ideally, a random red cell label must be equally distributed between cells of all ages (i.e. labelling must be truly random); it must be non-toxic to red cells; it must remain bound to the cell throughout its lifespan; and it should not be reutilized after red cell destruction. The opportunity for surface counting, to detect sites of red cell destruction, is an advantage.

Two compounds have been used for random labelling in red cell survival studies: sodium ^{51}Cr chromate (^{51}Cr) and diisopropyl fluorophosphonate (DFP), labelled with ^{32}P. ^{51}Cr is not ideal but has the advantage that, being a γ-emitter, is technically simple to use and may be measured at the body surface for detection of sites of red cell destruction. In clinical studies, a high level of accuracy is generally less important than technical simplicity and the potential for surface counting. Random labelling with ^{51}Cr is thus the method of choice in most clinical situations. However, it may be required to detect minor degrees of haemolysis or to monitor changes in MRCLS following disease progression or therapeutic intervention, in which cases DFP is preferred. Its major disadvantage is that surface counting is not possible as the label is exclusively a β-emitter. It is also less suitable for simultaneous measurement of the RCV.

15.3.1 THE RADIOACTIVE CHROMIUM METHOD

^{51}Cr which has a half-life of 27.8 days, is toxic to red cells, probably through oxidation; it inhibits glycolysis when present at a concentration of 10 $\mu g\ ml^{-1}$ of red cells and blocks glutathione reductase activity at a concentration exceeding 5 $\mu g\ ml^{-1}$. Blood should thus not be exposed to more than 2 μg of chromium per millilitre of packed red cells (Dacie and Lewis, 1984).

Lysis must be avoided when the red cells are washed. It may be necessary to use a slightly hypertonic solution, e.g. 12 g l^{-1} NaCl, specially if the blood contains spherocytes, or if an osmotic-fragility test has demonstrated lysis in 9 g l^{-1} NaCl. In patients whose plasma contains high-titre, high-thermal-amplitude cold agglutinins the blood must be collected in a warmed syringe and delivered into acid-citrate-dextrose (ACD) solution in a container previously warmed to 37 °C.

A procedure for labelling red cells and estimating MRCLS has been recommended by the ICSH (1971, 1980a). To ensure as little damage to red cells as possible, it is important to maintain the blood at optimal pH. This can be achieved by adding 10 volumes of blood to 1.5 volumes of the recommended (NIH-A) ACD solution or citrate-phosphate-dextrose (CPD) solution.

For a red cell survival study 0.5 μCi of $Na_2{}^{51}CrO_4$ per kilogram body weight is recommended. Ten minutes after injection (or 60 min in patients with cardiac failure or splenomegaly in whom mixing may be delayed), a sample of blood is collected into EDTA. The radioactivity in this sample provides a baseline for subsequent observations. By retaining some of the labelled cells to serve as a standard, the blood volume can be calculated if required.

Further 4–5 ml blood samples are taken from the patient 24 h later (day 1) and subsequently at a frequency depending on the rate of red cell destruction. It is recommended that three specimens be taken between days 2 and 7, and then two per week for the duration of the study. Sampling should be continued until at least half the radioactivity has disappeared from the circulation.

Hb or PCV should be measured in each sample. After lysis with saponin the radioactivity in each sample is measured and corrected for ^{51}Cr decay. Before the results can be analysed and interpreted, it is necessary to correct for the ^{51}Cr which elutes from intact red cells. The rate of elution is influenced by the anticoagulant solution into which the blood was collected prior to labelling. With ACD (NIH-A) and CPD, elution is about 1% per day. When MRCLS is markedly reduced elution is of minor importance and can be ignored. Otherwise it is essential to correct for elution, using the factors given in Table 15.3.

Sometimes, in addition to the elution which occurs continuously and at a constant rate, up to 10% of the ^{51}Cr may be lost within the first 24 h. The cause of this early loss is obscure and several components may be involved. If the early loss does not continue beyond the first two days, it is often looked upon as an artefact, in the sense that it does not denote an increased rate of lysis *in vivo*, and can usually be ignored. This is acceptable, at least for clinical studies, although it is possible that a small proportion of red cells are more prone to lysis and that the rate of elimination of the rest of the labelled cells is not representative of the entire cell population. It is common practice to calculate the T_{50}Cr, i.e. the time taken for the concentration of ^{51}Cr in the blood to fall to 50% of its initial value, after correcting the data for physical decay but not for elution. The chief objection to the use of T_{50}Cr is that it may be misleading and does not give the additional information on the pattern of the survival curve; moreover, the MRCLS cannot be calculated from it. With the technique described above, the mean value of T_{50} in normal subjects is about 30 days, with a range of 25–33 days.

Table 15.3 Normal range for ^{51}Cr survival curves with correction for elution

Day	*% ^{51}Cr (corrected for decay; not corrected for elution)*	*Elution correction factors*
1	93–98	1.03
2	89–97	1.05
3	86–95	1.06
4	83–93	1.07
5	80–92	1.08
6	78–90	1.10
7	77–88	1.11
8	76–86	1.12
9	74–84	1.13
10	72–83	1.14
11	70–81	1.16
12	68–79	1.17
13	67–78	1.18
14	65–77	1.19
15	64–75	1.20
16	62–74	1.22
17	59–73	1.23
18	58–71	1.25
19	57–69	1.26
20	56–67	1.27
21	55–66	1.29
22	53–65	1.31
23	52–63	1.32
24	51–60	1.34
25	50–59	1.36
30	44–52	1.47
35	39–47	1.53
40	34–42	1.60

(a) Blood volume changes

There is no need to correct the measurements of radioactivity per millilitre of whole blood for alterations in PCV provided that the total blood volume remains constant throughout the study. However, when it is suspected that the blood volume may be changing, e.g. in patients with renal disease or during red cell regeneration, serial determinations of blood volume should be carried out, and the observed radioactivity should then be multiplied by the observed blood volume and divided by the initial blood volume. In practice, if a patient receives a blood transfusion during a survival study, it can, as a general rule, be assumed that the blood volume will have returned to its pre-transfusion level within 24–48 h.

(b) Correction of survival data for blood loss

When there is a relatively constant loss of blood during a red cell survival study, the true MRCLS can be obtained from the following equation:

$$\text{True MRCLS} = T_a \times \frac{\text{RCV}}{\text{RCV} - (T_a \times L)}$$

where T_a = apparent MRCLS (days), RCV = red cell volume (ml), and L = mean rate of loss of red cells (ml per day), e.g. as measured in the stools in a case of gastrointestinal bleeding (see below).

(c) Analysis of survival data

Red cell survival data may be analysed in a variety of ways. With the widespread availability of small computers, much of the analysis may be automated. If the survival is fitted by a straight line on arithmetic paper, a linear survival function may be assumed and the MRCLS derived by extrapolation of the fitted line to zero activity. A plot that is linear on semi-logarithmic axes indicates an exponential survival, whereupon the MRCLS is the reciprocal of the rate constant of disappearance. If the plot is curvilinear on both arithmetic and semi-logarithmic axes, no conclusions can be drawn regarding the survival function. In this situation, extrapolation of the tangent to the curve at zero time to the time axis yields an estimate of the MRCLS.

If the day 0 results do not fit with the remainder of the points this may be due to 'early loss' because of elution of label from viable cells or because there has been rapid destruction of a proportion of labelled cells. In these circumstances it is acceptable to draw the best line through the later points, ignoring the day zero point.

A more complex mathematical treatment of the data may provide an improvement in the quality of the fit which may have value in physiological investigations but this is not likely to improve the overall accuracy of the results for clinical purposes. Computer programs for mathematical analysis have been described by ICSH (1980a); their applications have been reviewed by Bentley (1977).

15.3.2 PATTERNS OF SURVIVAL CURVES IN CLINICAL PRACTICE

The disappearance of labelled cells from the circulation is normally linear, with a MRCLS of 120 ± SD 15 days.

In congenital haemolytic anaemias the slope of the survival profile is also linear or slightly curvilinear. In the autoimmune haemolytic anaemias the red cell destruction is typically random and the curve of elimination therefore exponential.

In some cases of haemolytic anaemia the survival curve appears to consist of two components. This suggests the presence of cells of widely varying life-span. This type of 'double population' curve is seen in paroxysmal nocturnal haemoglobinuria, sickle-cell anaemia, some cases of hereditary enzyme-deficiency haemolytic anaemias, and when the labelled cells consist of a mixture of transfused normal cells and patient's cells. The MRCLS of the entire cell population can be deduced by extrapolation of the initial steep slope to the abscissa. The proportion of cells belonging to the longer-lived population can be estimated by extrapolating the second component to the ordinate.

An unusual curve may occur when transient (usually drug-induced) haemolysis occurs during the survival study. Another cause of an irregular rate of disappearance of the red cells is blood loss, e.g. from the gastrointestinal tract.

15.4 DETERMINATION OF THE SITES OF RED CELL DESTRUCTION

Supplementary information about the mechanism of haemolysis can be obtained from *in vivo* surface counting carried out in association with red cell survival studies. In clinical practice the main purpose of such studies has been to clarify the need for splenectomy. Thus, following injection of ^{51}Cr-labelled red cells, a progressive accumulation of activity in the spleen in haemolytic disease indicates active red cell destruction in that organ.

Most techniques are based on changes in radioactivity counts over the heart, spleen and liver. A standardized method has been described by the ICSH (1975). Using a shielded and collimated scintillation counter, or preferably a dual detector system, an initial measurement is taken about 30 min after injection and at varying intervals thereafter (usually two to three times weekly until time $T_{1/2}$). The surface sites chosen over the heart, spleen and liver are clearly marked with indelible ink. Small changes in positioning may introduce significant errors and it is very important to ensure that conditions are maintained as constant as possible throughout the investigation. The data are analysed by comparing the radioactivity over the heart with that over the spleen and liver.

Hepatic and splenic uptake can be expressed as the 'excess counts', which represents the difference between the counts actually observed over the organs and those expected from the contained RCV, calculated from the counts over the heart or in the blood. In addition the spleen : liver ratio is valuable in patients in whom there is accumulation of radioactivity in both the liver and spleen (ICSH, 1975; Najean *et al.*, 1975).

Four patterns of accumulation of ^{51}Cr have been noted in haemolytic anaemia: excess accumulation in the spleen alone; excess accumulation in the liver alone; no excess in either liver or spleen; excess accumulation in both liver and spleen. Splenectomy usually benefits patients with the first pattern, and to a more limited extent the last. The degree of improvement does not, however, correlate closely with the ^{51}Cr accumulation in the spleen and it must be emphasized that this is at best only a semi-quantitative measurement.

Even minor alterations in the conditions of counting and positioning of the patient may produce significant changes. Isolated readings may, therefore, be misleading. Amongst the variables which affect the count-rate are the volume of the organ counted in relation to its total volume, its depth and the elution rate of ^{51}Cr from the organ. Nevertheless, despite these difficulties, surface counting has proved to be of value in the management of patients with some types of haemolytic anaemia when used in conjunction with other clinical and laboratory investigations (Ahuja *et al.*, 1972; Ferrant *et al.*, 1982). ^{111}In-labelled red cells permit the use of quantitative gamma camera imaging (Heyns *et al.*, 1985). However, the higher rate of elution of ^{111}In from red cells and the shorter half-life of ^{111}In limit its use to severe haemolysis.

15.5 COMPATIBILITY TESTS

Short-term studies of donor cells in the circulation of a recipient can provide information on the likely outcome of a blood transfusion, especially when the patient has a high titre of low-avidity antibody which may react strongly with a wide variety of potential donor red cells in *in vitro* tests but which may not give rise to significant haemolysis *in vivo*, at least with some of the donor bloods. A study of behaviour of labelled donor cells is of particular value in the following circumstances:

1. when serological tests suggest that all normal donors are incompatible;
2. when in the presence of an allo-antibody no non-reacting donor can be found;
3. when the recipient has had an unexplained haemolytic reaction;
4. when the viability of the donor cells has been affected by adverse storage conditions.

There are, however, problems in interpreting results and the selection of the most reliable procedure is controversial (Mollison, 1984). The ICSH (1980a) has recommended measuring the disappearance of the labelled cells in the first 30–60 min after injection. Moroff *et al.* (1984) have proposed that the 24 h survival of stored red cells should be used and they have described two standardized methods based on the original ICSH recommendations.

The ICSH method is as follows. Blood (1–2 ml) is removed from the donor bag and 0.5 ml of the red cells are labelled with 20 μCi of ^{51}Cr in the standard way as described above. Alternatively, ^{113m}In or ^{99m}Tc can be used as the label. Blood is collected from the recipient at 3, 10 and 60 min after injection of the labelled cells and the radioactivities in whole blood and plasma expressed as percentages of the 3 min values.

With compatible blood the activity in the 60 min sample is, on average, 99% of that of the 3 min sample, but this may vary between 94% and 104%. If survival at 60 min is not less than 70% and the plasma activity is not more than 3%, the donor cells may be transfused with minimal hazard.

15.6 MEGALOBLASTIC ANAEMIAS

Megaloblastic anaemia may be suspected from macrocytosis in a peripheral blood film even in the absence of anaemia, and by an unusually high mean cell volume (MCV) in the peripheral blood. The commonest causes of megaloblastic anaemia are deficiencies of vitamin B_{12} and folate. The former is detected by estimation of the serum B_{12} and the latter by estimation of red cell and serum folate. There are microbiological assays for these but they are tedious and time consuming. Although still used, especially as reference methods, they have been largely replaced by radionuclide competitive protein binding assays. The assay for vitamin B_{12} is based on the principle that endogenous serum vitamin B_{12} will compete with radioactive vitamin B_{12} for binding to a limited amount of vitamin B_{12} binding protein. A similar system is used for folate assay.

The importance of distinguishing between B_{12} and folate deficiency cannot be emphasized sufficiently. Because of the close metabolic relationship between folic acid and vitamin B_{12} large doses of folic acid may relieve the anaemia of B_{12} deficiency but allow neurological damage to develop. Casual treatment of anaemia with multihaematinics which contain therapeutic amounts of folic acid can therefore be extremely deleterious in vitamin B_{12} deficiency. Obviously, when combined, both deficiencies should be given the appropriate therapy.

Elucidation of the causes of vitamin B_{12} or folate deficiency depends on both clinical and laboratory criteria. The latter include absorption studies, demonstration of serum antibodies to intrinsic factor or gastric parietal cells, and measurement of gastric secretion of intrinsic factor. Measurement of the absorption of vitamin B_{12} or folate helps in the differential diagnosis of the respective causes of their deficiencies, listed in Table 15.4. In this chapter only *in vivo* radionuclide absorption studies will be discussed.

Table 15.4 Causes of megaloblastic anaemia

1. Vitamin B_{12} deficiency
   - (a) Nutritional, especially vegans
   - (b) Malabsorption
     - Gastric pathology and gastrectomy (total or partial)
     - Addisonian pernicious anaemia
     - Intestinal causes
       - Stagnant loop syndrome (diverticulosis, strictures, etc.)
       - Ileal resection and Crohn's disease
       - Tropical sprue
       - Adult coeliac disease
       - Severe chronic pancreatitis
       - Transcobolamin II deficiency
       - Drugs (PAS, colchicine, anticonvulsants, alcohol)
2. Folate deficiency
   - (a) Poor diet
   - (b) Malabsorption
     - Gluten-sensitive enteropathy
     - Tropical sprue
     - Crohn's disease
     - Partial gastrectomy or jejunal resection
     - Drugs (anticonvulsants, cholestyramine, sulphasalazine)
   - (c) Excess requirements
     - Pregnancy
     - Prematurity and infancy
     - Malignancies (leukaemia, lymphoma)
     - Haemolytic anaemia, myelosclerosis
     - Inflammatory diseases (tuberculosis, malaria, rheumatoid arthritis)
   - (d) Liver disease
   - (e) Inborn errors of folate metabolism
3. Other causes
   - Congenital dyserythropoietic anaemia
   - Acquired dyserythropoiesis
   - Erythroleukaemia
   - Myelodysplastic syndromes
   - Drugs (antimetabolites, alcohol)

15.6.1 VITAMIN B_{12} ABSORPTION

There are two commonly used methods for quantifying the absorption of vitamin B_{12}. They require respectively measurement of urinary and faecal radioactivity. Plasma, hepatic or whole body radioactivities have been used (for review and bibliography, see Schilling, 1986). The method based on urinary excretion, originally described by Schilling (1953), is reliable and the most widely used. False positives are seen only in renal disease when the glomerular filtration rate is diminished below 20 ml min^{-1}, or when the urine is incompletely collected. In contrast, incomplete stool collection in the faecal test will lead to failure to detect an existing malabsorption. The ICSH (1981) has recommended whole body counting as a reference method and urinary excretion as the most reliable and convenient routine method.

Schilling (urinary excretion) test

A control urine must be collected within the 12 h preceding the test in order to exclude unexpected radioactivity from some other radionuclide investigation. For the test 1 μg of vitamin B_{12} (as cyanocobalamin) labelled with about 1 μCi of ^{57}Co and diluted in 100–200 ml of water is taken orally after an overnight fast. After 1–2 h 1 mg of non-radioactive cyanocobalamin is administered intramuscularly and urine is collected for 24 h after the start of the test. A standard is prepared from a similar dose of ^{57}Co diluted in about 100 ml of water.

The fraction of the dose excreted in the 24 h urine is measured. The normal urinary excretion is 10% or more. Less than 9% indicates defective absorption (provided that there is no abnormal urinary retention; when this is suspected it may be worthwhile continuing the urinary collection for a further 24 h, and measuring the fractional excretion in both 24 h specimens).

If absorption is abnormally low, a second study is performed giving the vitamin B_{12} together with a dose of intrinsic factor of known potency. This should preferably be human (gastric juice extract), but a preparation derived from hog stomach, e.g. Intrinsic Factor (IF) Concentrate (Amersham International plc), in a dose of 10 mg, is also usually satisfactory. The second test dose can be given 48 h after the first provided that an additional flushing-out injection of 1 mg of non-radioactive cyanacobalamin is given 24 h after the first oral dose and injection.

In pernicious anaemia, the addition of intrinsic factor to the dose of vitamin B_{12} will significantly increase absorption and subsequent excretion. In some cases, however, patients who have taken multivitamin preparations containing hog IF and have developed antibodies to this foreign protein will be unable to absorb the vitamin B_{12} bound to hog IF but will readily absorb the vitamin B_{12} bound to human gastric juice.

If the second test fails to improve the excretion, malabsorption must be considered. Causes include lesions in the small intestine, severe pancreatitis, blind loop syndrome and diverticulitis, tropical sprue, coeliac disease and Crohn's disease.

The terminal ileum is the major site of vitamin B_{12} absorption. In patients with small intestinal diverticulitis or blind loops, vitamin B_{12} malabsorption is due to competition with bacteria for host dietary vitamin B_{12}. The vitamin B_{12} malabsorption will not be corrected by IF but will be restored to normal following broad-spectrum antibiotics.

A test kit is available (e.g. Dicopac, Amersham) in which vitamin B_{12} is labelled with two different cobalt radionuclides, one as free B_{12} and the other as B_{12} bound to human gastric juice, so that the urinary excretion test can be performed in a single procedure. There have, however, been a number of discordant and confusing results with this method (Domstad *et al.*, 1981; England *et al.*, 1981; Fairbanks *et al.*, 1983).

15.6.2 FOLIC ACID ABSORPTION

Unlike vitamin B_{12} deficiency, the most common cause of folate deficiency is relative or absolute dietary deficiency. Defective absorption occurs in tropical sprue, idiopathic steatorrhoea and Crohn's disease. The use of radioactive folate has provided a relatively simple method to identify patients with poor folate absorption (Anderson *et al.*, 1960; Freedman *et al.*, 1973).

The test is analogous to the urinary excretion test for vitamin B_{12}. A flushing dose of 15–30 mg of non-radioactive folic acid is given by intramuscular injection followed by an oral dose of [^{3}H]folic acid. Various doses have been used (Chanarin, 1979). With one of 200 μg, about 80% is absorbed. Freedman *et al.* (1973) recommend a loading dose of 15 mg of folic acid intramuscularly 24 h before the initial test, and an oral test dose of 300 μg tritium-labelled folate in 100 ml water followed 30 min later by a second intramuscular injection of 15 mg of folic acid as a flushing dose. About 45% (SD 7%) is excreted in the urine in 24 hr in normal subjects, but significantly less in malabsorption.

15.7 IRON METABOLISM

There are three types of investigation which may provide useful clinical information:

1. iron absorption following an oral dose of ^{59}Fe;
2. distribution of radioactivity after an intravenous injection of ^{59}Fe;
3. imaging of radio-iron uptake.

15.7.1 IRON ABSORPTION

There is an enormous variation in the normal absorption which is affected by physiological differences in gastric secretion and gastrointestinal motility, and by differences between absorption of food iron and small amounts of soluble iron salt. This is further complicated by the role of ascorbic acid and chelating agents in the diet and the fact that iron may be absorbed but retained in the epithelial cells of the intestine and lost subsequently by the normal process of desquamation. Furthermore, iron absorption itself is a complex process so that interpretation of results must be treated cautiously (Bothwell *et al.*, 1979; Cook and Lipschitz, 1977).

The estimation of iron absorption requires a test dose of 15 mg of iron sulphate ($FeSO_4.7H_2O$) and 18 mg of ascorbic acid in 10 ml of 0.001 mol l^{-1}HCl, to which is added 2 μCi of ^{59}Fe-ferric chloride in 0.001 mol l^{-1} HCl. The solution is made up to 25 ml with water; 1 ml is retained as a standard and a measured volume of the remainder is administered by mouth following an overnight fast. The patient must not eat or drink for a further 3 h. The faeces are collected over the following five to seven days. Each specimen is counted in a large-volume counting system against a standard, diluted in about 100 ml of water, in a similar container.

An alternative method for measuring the radioactivity is by whole body counting, when it is necessary to take measurements only immediately after the dose is administered and again after seven days. In normal subjects absorption averages about 15–30% of the test dose; it increases to 50–80% in iron deficiency. There is likely to be malabsorption if less than 10% of the test dose is absorbed.

15.7.2 IRON DISTRIBUTION

Iron for incorporation into erythroblasts, which subsequently develop into mature red blood cells, is transported to the bone marrow or other sites of (extramedullary) erythropoiesis as transferrin-bound complex. At the surface of the erythroblasts the complex releases its iron which enters the cell to be incorporated into haem while the transferrin is recycled. Iron not bound to transferrin passes to the liver, and colloidal particles of iron (such as haemosiderin) are taken up by reticuloendothelial cells, mainly in the spleen.

Ferrokinetic studies providing information on erythropoiesis include the rate of clearance of injected ^{59}Fe from the plasma, plasma iron turnover, iron incorporation into red cells and surface counting to measure the uptake and turnover of iron by organs (Figure 15.1). These are relatively simple procedures but their interpretation depends on a model which is assumed to correspond to the biological mechanism. A number of models of varying complexity have been proposed (Ricketts *et al.*, 1975; Barosi *et al.*, 1976; Cavill, 1986) to take account of the interaction between the compartments which they define, as well as recirculation of iron which is released from destroyed red cells. Complex compartmental analysis with multiple sampling over an extended period is required (Cavill, 1986). Provided that the limitations of the simpler models are recognized, they provide clinically useful information. The more complex models provide data of marrow iron turnover, red cell iron turnover, ineffective iron turnover, non-erythroid iron turnover and tissue iron turnover. The mean red cell life-span can also be calculated. The reader is referred to Cavill (1986) for details of these methods.

15.7.3 PLASMA IRON CLEARANCE (PIC) AND PLASMA IRON TURNOVER (PIT)

In ferrokinetic studies it is necessary to have a sufficient amount of transferrin to ensure that all the radio-iron is transferrin bound. If the patient's plasma transferrin concentration is less than 0.6 g l^{-1} or if the unsaturated iron binding capacity is less than 20 μmol (1 mg) l^{-1}, normal, suitably screened, donor plasma should be used. About 5 μCi of ^{59}Fe-ferric citrate is added to 5–10 ml of plasma and incubated at 37 °C for 30 min. A measured volume is injected intravenously and 1 ml is retained as a standard. Commencing 10 min after injection, four to five blood samples are collected over a period of 1–2 h.

If the plasma iron concentration is known (measured in one or more of the collected specimens) PIT (mg l^{-1} per day) can be calculated from the rate constant (K) of the initial, mono-exponential, plasma ^{59}Fe clearance (i.e. as the product of K and plasma iron concentration).

15.7.4 IRON UTILIZATION (RCU)

Radioactivity is measured in blood samples collected at intervals (daily if possible) for about two weeks after administration of the ^{59}Fe. The RCU (%) is calculated from:

$$\frac{\text{red cell volume (ml)} \times \text{cpm ml}^{-1} \text{ red cells in daily specimens}}{\text{total radioactivity injected (cpm)}} \times 100\%$$

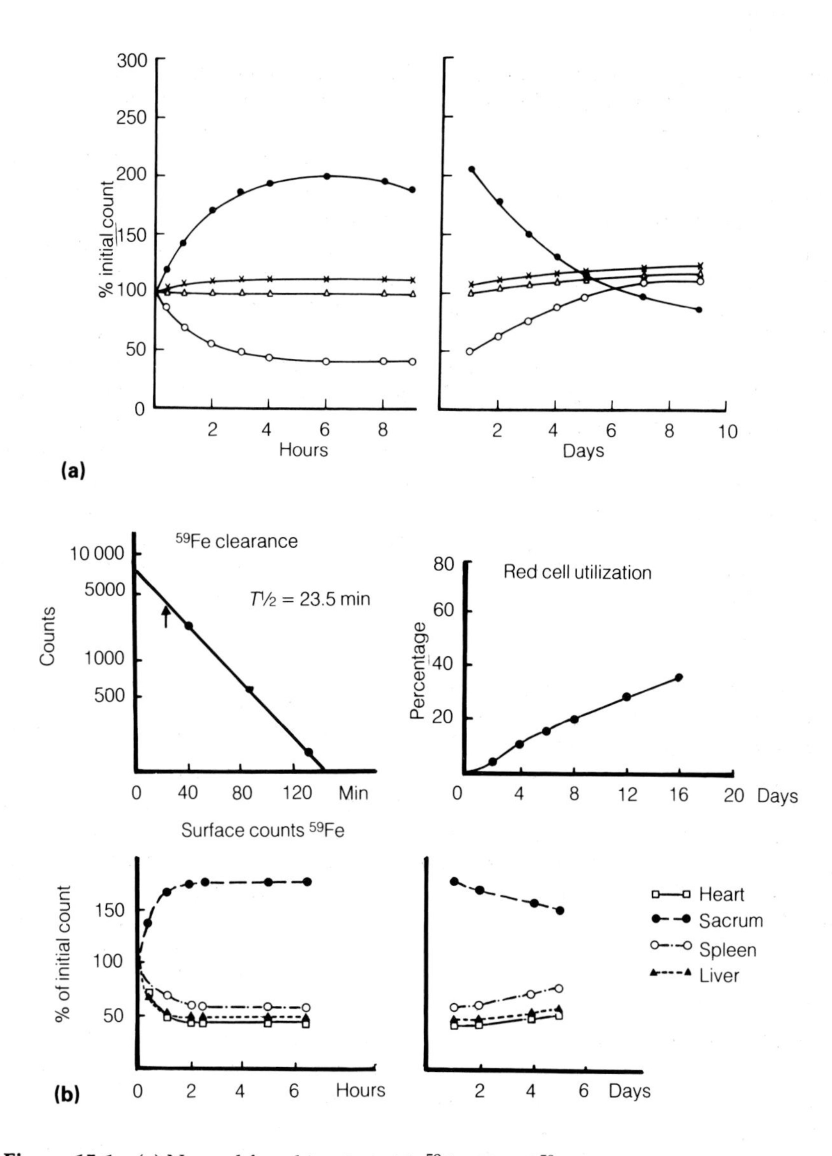

Figure 15.1 (a) Normal ferrokinetics with ^{59}Fe. Blood ^{59}Fe activity (○) initially falls as the iron is taken up into bone marrow (sacrum; ●), which consequently shows an early increase in activity. Over the ensuing days, however, blood activity rises as the ^{59}Fe reappears as haemoglobin ^{59}Fe in red cells, and bone marrow activity falls. Hepatic (×) and splenic (△) activities show little change throughout. (b) Ferrokinetics with ^{59}Fe in dyserythropoeisis. The plasma iron clearance is increased. There is rapid uptake of iron into sacral bone marrow, but the appearance of activity in blood over the ensuing days is less than expected.

Table 15.5 Ferrokinetic patterns in various diseases

	Plasma Clearance $T_{1/2}$	*Plasma iron turnover*	*Red cell utilization*
Normal	60–140 min	70–140 μmol l^{-1} d^{-1}	70–80%
Iron deficiency	↓	N	↑
Aplastic anaemia	↑	N	↓
Secondary anaemia	Slightly ↓	N	N
Dyserythropoiesis	Slightly ↓	↑	↓
Myelofibrosis	↓	↑	↓
Haemolytic anaemia	↓	↑	↑

↓ = short/decreased, ↑ = prolonged/increased.

The daily measured percentages are plotted against time on arithmetic graph paper. Maximum utilization is recorded.

15.7.5 INTERPRETATION (Table 15.5)

(a) Plasma iron clearance

The normal $T_{1/2}$ of PIC is 60–140 min. The clearance rate is influenced by the intensity of erythropoiesis and also by the activity of the macrophages of the reticuloendothelial system, especially in the liver, spleen and bone marrow, where the iron is retained as storage iron. Also, to a lesser extent, circulating reticulocytes may take up some of the iron. A rapid clearance indicates hyperactivity of one or more of these mechanisms, as for instance, in iron-deficiency anaemias, haemorrhagic anaemias, haemolytic anaemias (Figure 15.1) and polycythaemia vera. The clearance rate is decreased in aplastic anaemia (Figure 15.2). In leukaemia and in myelosclerosis the results are variable, depending upon the amount of erythropoietic marrow and the extent of extramedullary erythropoiesis; in myelosclerosis, however, rapid clearance is by far the more common finding. In dyserythropoiesis, the clearance may be normal or accelerated.

(b) Plasma iron turnover

The range of PIT in normal subjects is 4–8 mg l^{-1} per day (or 70–140 μmol l^{-1} per day). The PIT is increased in iron-deficiency anaemia, haemolytic anaemias, myelosclerosis and ineffective erythropoiesis, particularly in thalassaemia. In aplastic anaemia the PIT is normal or decreased, but when the plasma iron is raised the PIT may be above normal. The calculation of PIT assumes a constant rate of iron transport and, while it is an indicator of total erythropoiesis, it does not distinguish between effective and ineffective erythropoiesis.

(c) Red cell utilization

RCU gives a measure of effective erythropoiesis. In normal subjects it reaches a maximum of 70–80% on the 10th–14th day. A rapid plasma ^{59}Fe clearance is usually associated with early and relatively complete utilization; the converse also applies. The results are inconsistent in megaloblastic anaemias and in haemoglobinopathies in which there is ineffective erythropoiesis; and also in myelosclerosis and polycythaemia vera, depending on the extent of extramedullary erythropoiesis and whether the red cell life-span is reduced. If there is rapid haemolysis, the utilization curve will be distorted by destruction of some of the labelled red cells; this may be recognized if frequent (daily) samples are measured. In aplastic anaemia the utilization is usually 10–15%; in ineffective erythropoiesis it is as a rule 30–50%. The various ferrokinetic patterns in disease are illustrated in Table 15.5.

15.7.6 SITES OF ^{59}Fe DISTRIBUTION

Collimated surface scintillation counting over the liver, spleen, sacrum and heart (or measurement of blood radioactivity) at intervals after administration of ^{59}Fe demonstrates the ferrokinetic pattern. The first measurement should be made as soon as possible after the administration of the radionuclide, and again after 5, 20, 40 and 60 min, hourly for 6 h and then on alternate days for ten days. Results are corrected for physical decay of the isotope and normalized to the initial counts, which are expressed as 100% at each site. Results are plotted on arithmetical graph paper, as illustrated in Figures 15.2 and 15.3. This is a laborious

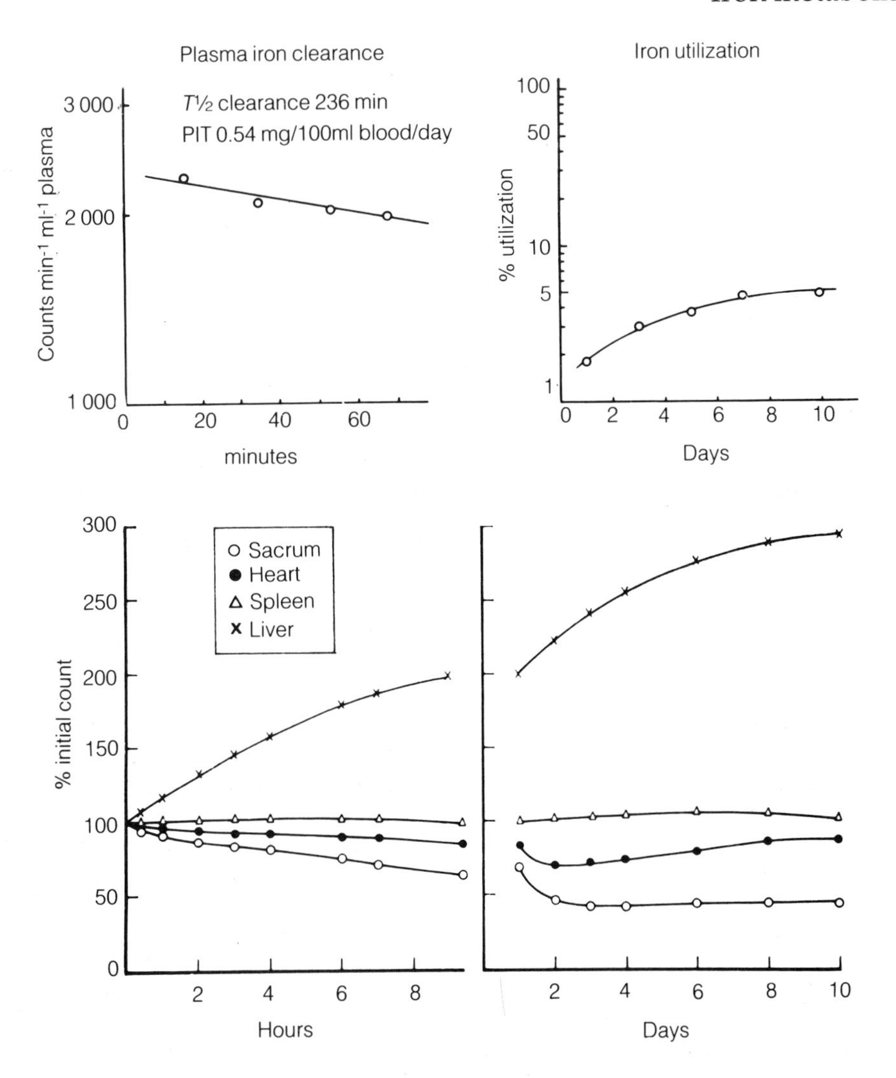

Figure 15.2 Ferrokinetics with ^{59}Fe in aplastic anaemia. Plasma iron clearance and red cell iron utilization are both markedly decreased with early appearance of iron in the liver. Hepatic iron uptake continues and there is no uptake by sacral bone marrow.

procedure which is only occasionally useful in the investigation of patients with myelosclerosis, aplastic anaemia, myelodysplasia or leukaemia, when it might be helpful to know the sites and extent of extramedullary erythropoiesis, especially if splenectomy is contemplated. Its main limitation is the assumption, often erroneous, that the sacrum is representative of the skeletal marrow.

(a) Imaging of iron uptake

When ^{52}Fe is available it can be used to visualize iron distribution and to identify the sites and extent of extramedullary erythropoiesis (Figure 15.4). The isotope is prepared and administered in the same way as ^{59}Fe for ferrokinetic studies. A dose of 100 μCi is usually suitable. In aplastic anaemia, radio-iron accumulates in the liver. ^{52}Fe (half-life 8 h) normally decays to ^{52m}Mn (half-life 21 min) which also accumulates in the liver (including the normal liver). Imaging is especially useful in myelofibrosis when there is extramedullary erythropoiesis, usually in the spleen, and a variable degree of bone marrow erythropoiesis (Pettit *et al.*, 1976, 1979; Ferrant *et al.*, 1986).

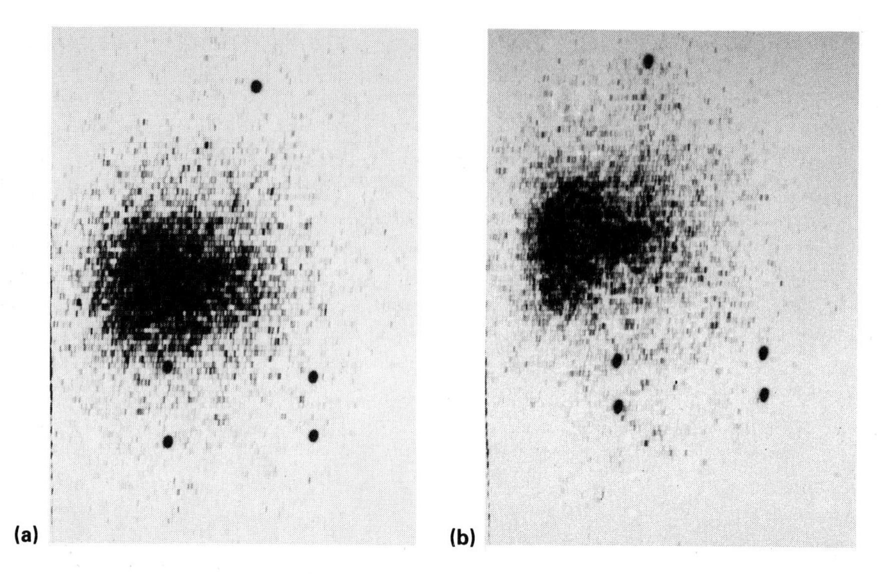

Figure 15.3 Images obtained in patients with aplastic anaemia following injection of (a) ^{59}Fe and (b) ^{52}Fe. Resolution is marginally superior with ^{52}Fe. Note marked hepatic activity and an absence of bone marrow and blood pool activities.

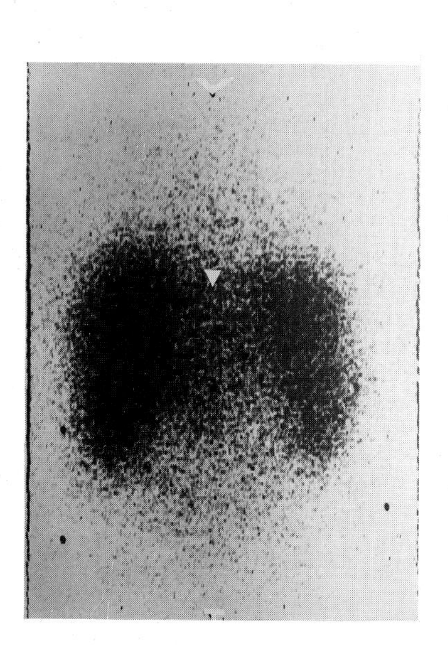

Figure 15.4 ^{52}Fe image in a patient with myelofibrosis, showing marked uptake into the liver and spleen, both of which are enlarged. The splenic activity indicates myeloid metaplasia and distinguishes the appearances from those of aplastic anaemia.

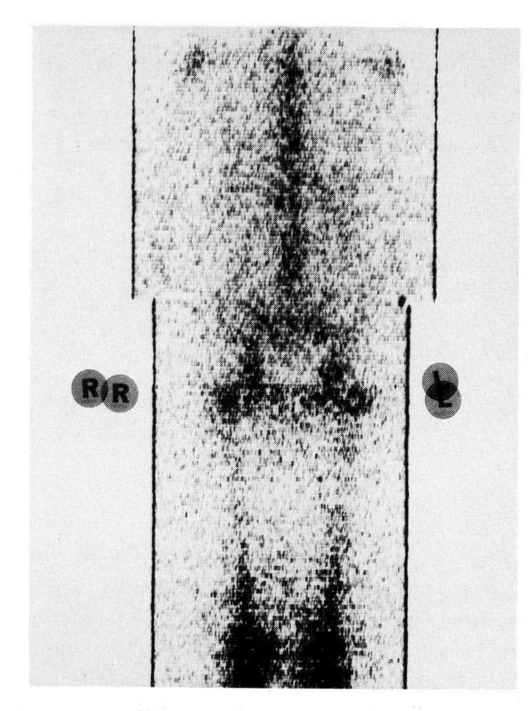

Figure 15.5 ^{52}Fe image in an adult with haemolytic anaemia, showing peripheral extension of active bone marrow (in particular, the erythron).

As ^{111}In-labelled chloride also binds to transferrin, it has been proposed as a convenient and more readily available substitute for ^{52}Fe (Arrago *et al.*, 1985; McNeil *et al.*, 1976). However, results with this isotope are inconsistent and do not always parallel that of iron (Ronai *et al.*, 1969; McIntyre *et al.*, 1974; Chipping *et al.*, 1980; Harnsberger *et al.*, 1982).

^{59}Fe can be imaged (Chaudhri *et al.*, 1974; Aubert *et al.*, 1983). Image quality is poor, however, because the long half-life limits the amount which can be administered and, in addition, the γ-ray energy of over 1 MeV is too high for most imaging devices. However, with suitable collimation and appropriate instrument settings reasonable images can be obtained (Figure 15.5).

15.8 RADIOLABELLED PLATELETS

Currently the best isotope with which to label platelets is ^{111}In and this has now almost replaced ^{51}Cr for this purpose (Peters *et al.*, 1986a). The indications within clinical haematology for radiolabelled platelets are measurement of mean platelet life-span (MPLS), quantification of splenic platelet pooling and identification of sites of platelet destruction. ^{111}In-labelled platelets are also used for imaging platelet deposition such as in deep vein thrombosis, arteriopathies and the rejecting renal transplant.

15.8.1 PLATELET LABELLING

(a) ^{51}*Cr*

^{51}Cr as chromate ion is actively incorporated into platelets, where it is reduced from the hexavalent to the trivalent state and is bound predominantly to adenyl nucleosides.

(b) ^{111}*In*

The mechanism by which the lipophilic ^{111}In complexes label platelets is not fully understood, but it is thought that the chelate transports the indium into the cell by passive diffusion. Inside the cell, the indium binds to a variety of intracellular components both in the cytoplasm and in the nucleus. The chelate is then thought to diffuse out of the cell. The role of the chelate, solely as a carrier for the ^{111}In, is difficult to prove because, in order to label cells, indium complex must be mixed with between 10^2 and 10^6 times more of the chelating agent than the amount required to complex the available ^{111}In.

All of the ^{111}In complexes formed with the chelates listed in Table 15.6 will label platelets in saline but only ^{111}In-labelled tropolonate (Danpure *et al.*, 1982) and ^{111}In-labelled mercaptopyridine oxide (merc) (Thakur and Sedar, 1987) will label cells satisfactorily in plasma. Cell labelling is simple and rapid and achieved either by adding the pre-formed ^{111}In complex to the cells or by mixing the chelate with the cells prior to adding the ^{111}In chloride. Although there are numerous techniques described in the literature for labelling platelets with ^{111}In they all share the same principles, which are as follows.

First, because ^{111}In labels blood cells indiscriminately, the platelets have to be separated from the other blood cells. This is achieved by differential centrifugation; since they are smaller than other blood cells platelets can be separated by centrifugation at a relatively low speed. After removal from the sedimented column of red cells and leucocytes, the supernatant containing the platelets (platelet-rich plasma, PRP) is centrifuged at a faster speed to sediment the platelets into a loosely packed pellet. Following removal of most of the platelet-poor plasma (PPP), the platelets are resuspended either in buffered saline or in a small volume of PPP (see below).

Second, platelets are very reactive and so must be inhibited during manipulation. The simplest way to achieve this is to reduce the pH of the PRP to about 6.5 with acid citrate dextrose (ACD). Alternatively, platelet-inhibitory prostaglandins can be added (Hawker *et al.*, 1980).

Third, the ^{111}In has to be complexed with a lipid-soluble chelating agent. ^{111}In-labelled oxine is the most widely used, largely because it is commercially available.

Fourth, depending on the chelates to be used, the platelets may require separation from plasma.

Table 15.6 Effect of labelling medium and chelating agent on the percentage of available ^{111}In incorporated by 2×10^7 granulocytes in 1 ml plasma (with 10% saline) or 1 ml HEPES–saline buffer at pH 7.6 using the optimum concentration of the chelating agent

^{111}*In complex*	*90% plasma (%)*	*HEPES saline (%)*
^{111}In-labelled tropolonate	54	80
^{111}In-labelled merc	36	87
^{111}In-labelled acetylacetonate	8	85
^{111}In-labelled oxine sulphate	9	67

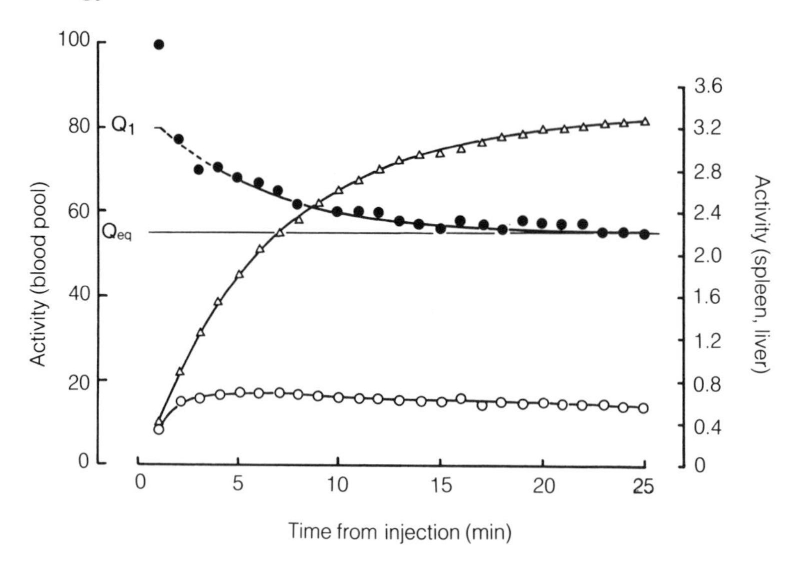

Figure 15.6 Time–activity curves recorded in regions of interest over the cardiac blood pool (●), liver (○) and spleen (△) in a normal subject following injection of ^{111}In-labelled platelets. Ordinate (left): percentage of maximum (blood pool); ordinate (right): counts per frame per pixel (liver and spleen). The subject was supine with the gamma camera below. The blood pool curve approaches an asymptote (Q_{eq}) which represents the recovery. Extrapolation of the blood pool curve to 1 min yields Q_1, which represents the total activity equilibrating between the blood and splenic pool, such that at equilibrium (reached at 20–25 min) splenic activity is represented by $Q_1 - Q_{eq}$ and blood activity by Q_{eq}. (Reprinted from *Thrombosis and Haemostasis*.)

^{111}In-labelled oxine and ^{111}In-labelled acetylacetonate bind avidly to plasma proteins and so the platelets have to be separated from plasma and resuspended in saline for labelling with these complexes. On the other hand, ^{111}In-labelled troplonate and ^{111}In-labelled merc can label platelets with adequate efficiency in plasma, providing the cell concentration is high.

A number of factors may affect the labelling efficiency, i.e. the percentage of available ^{111}In taken up by the platelets. The effect of plasma has already been mentioned and even at high cell concentration it is difficult to label platelets in plasma with ^{111}In-labelled oxine or ^{111}In-labelled acetylacetonate. Platelets are best maintained at a pH of 6.5. A pH of lower than this and particularly lower than 6 will lead to a fall in labelling efficiency. Labelling efficiency also critically depends on the concentration of the chelate and the optimal concentration varies from one chelate to another. Not surprisingly, labelling efficiency increases with increasing cell concentration, particularly in the presence of plasma. In effect, the cells and plasma compete with each other for the available ^{111}In. In plasma-free media, the cell concentration is less critical. Labelling efficiency usually reaches a maximum between 5 and 10 min at room temperature or earlier at 37 °C. Conversely the rate of labelling is greatly reduced at 4 °C.

(c) Problems encountered in thrombocytopaenia

Patients with thrombocytopaenia are frequently encountered when undertaking platelet kinetic studies, and, if the platelet count is less than about $20 \times 10^9\ l^{-1}$, homologous ABO/rhesus-matched platelets are likely to be necessary. When labelling autologous platelets from thrombocytopaenic patients more blood is required, usually in the range 100–150 ml. The addition of a red cell sedimenting agent, such as plasmasteril or hespan, to the whole blood (1 volume to 10 volumes of blood) prior to slow centrifugation improves the yield of PRP. When labelling with ^{111}In-labelled tropolonate it is usually necessary to reduce the proportion of plasma; a 25% concentration of plasma in saline markedly improves labelling efficiency whilst at the same time maintaining a physiological environment. Homologous platelets for use in patients with severe thrombocytopaenia may need to be HLA-matched, especially in patients with refractory thrombocytopaenia who have received multiple platelet transfusions (Peters *et al.*, 1985e).

(c) Evaluation of labelled platelet function

Platelet viability, following labelling, is usually assessed by nephelometric ADP platelet aggregometry. However, when ACD has been used to inhibit platelets, by reducing pH, the labelled platelets will remain relatively unresponsive to ADP unless they are first washed and resuspended at physiological pH. This is clearly not desirable and we would recommend *in vivo* methods to establish the functional status of the platelets. We perform dynamic gamma camera scintigraphy immediately following injection (Figure 15.6) when it can be shown that damaged or activated platelets undergo excessive irreversible or reversible liver uptake respectively (Figure 15.7).

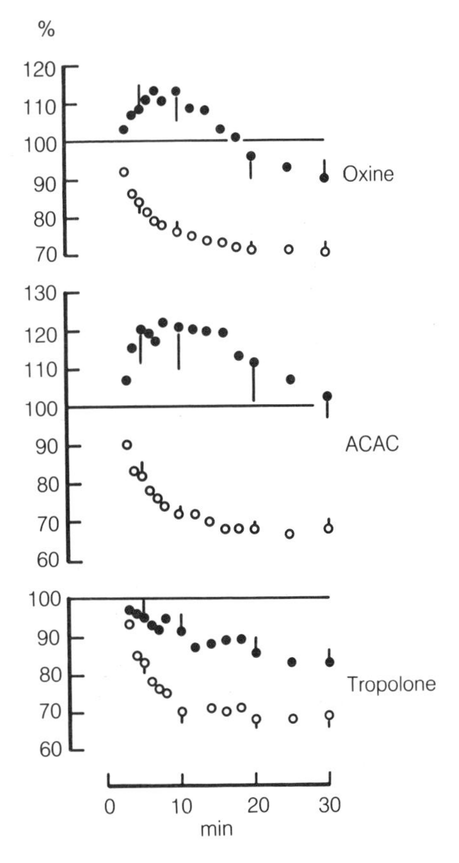

Figure 15.7 Composite time activity curves recorded in regions of interest over cardiac blood pool (○) and liver (●) in groups of patients following injection of platelets labelled in saline with ^{111}In-labelled oxine (upper panel, $n = 5$), in saline with ^{111}In-labelled acetylacetonate (middle panel, $n = 3$) and in plasma with ^{111}In-labelled tropolonate (lower panel, $n = 10$). Bars represent the SEM. Ordinate: percentage of initial value. Platelets labelled in saline, but not those labelled in plasma, show evidence of the 'collection injury'. (Reprinted from *Thrombosis and Haemostasis*.)

15.8.2 NORMAL PLATELET KINETICS

Platelet kinetics can be considered under three subheadings: platelet distribution, mean platelet life-span and sites of destruction.

(a) Platelet distribution

The total circulating platelet population is considerably greater than the product of the peripheral blood platelet count and the total blood volume. The difference, almost 50% of the total population, is represented by platelet pools throughout the body. Most of the total platelet pool resides within the spleen, where platelets are in continuous dynamic equilibrium with blood platelets (Heyns *et al.*, 1980; Peters *et al.*, 1980). Small platelet pools reside in the liver (Peters *et al.*, 1985b) and possibly also the lung (Biermann *et al.*, 1952; Martin *et al.*, 1981).

Any organ pool of blood cells can be defined and quantified in terms of the corresponding organ's plasma content. Thus a pool can be said to exist if the cell count, relative to plasma, is greater in the organ's vasculature than in reference blood such as peripheral venous or central blood. Alternatively, a cell pool can be quantified in terms of that cell's mean transit time through the organ expressed as a quotient of the organ's mean plasma transit time. The mean platelet transit time through a platelet pool has been expressed as a factor of the corresponding red cell transit time (Peters *et al.*, 1985b), although red cell transit time is not necessarily identical to plasma transit time, being longer in the spleen and shorter in the liver (Mollison, 1979). Thus red cells themselves pool in the spleen, as discussed elsewhere in this chapter.

The number of platelets residing in an organ is a function of the organ's blood flow (i.e. input rate) and the mean platelet residence time (i.e. output rate). Thus in the case of the spleen, which has a normal blood flow (SBF) of about 5% of the total blood volume per minute and a mean platelet

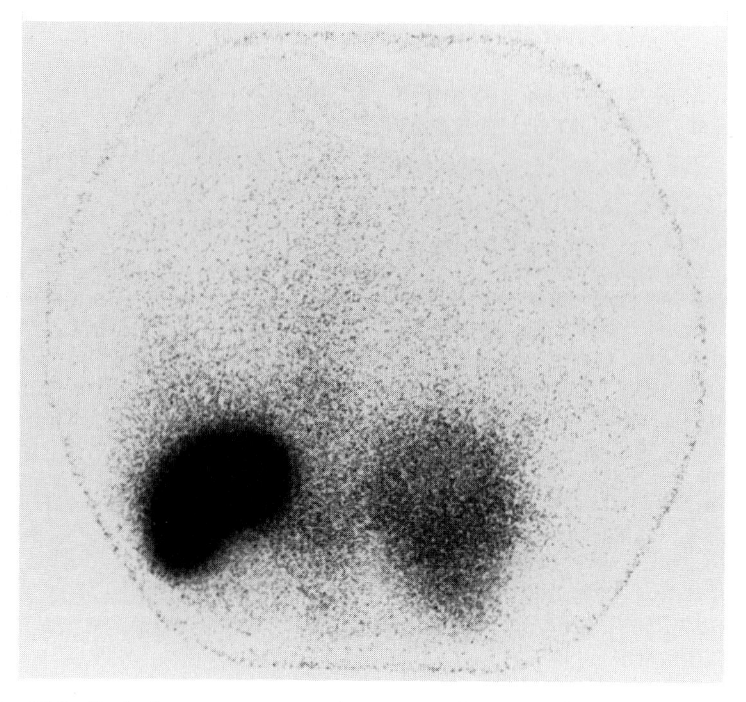

Figure 15.8 Posterior gamma camera image over the upper abdomen and chest five days following injection of ^{111}In-labelled platelets in a normal subject. There is intense splenic activity, moderate hepatic activity and minimal bone marrow activity.

residence time of 10 min (Peters *et al.*, 1980, 1985a), the platelet pool is about 40% of the total platelet population. The transit time relative to the red cell transit time is about 12 and to the plasma transit time about 36. The mean intrahepatic platelet transit time is only about 1.5 that of red cells and less than this relative to plasma transit time, since the intrahepatic haematocrit is less than the whole body haematocrit. In summary, therefore, the spleen is the location for essentially all of the platelet pooling in normal man.

(b) Mean platelet life-span (MPLS)

Following their release from bone marrow, normal platelets have a life-span in the normal circulation of about nine days. Given that about a third of the platelet population is at any time pooled in the spleen, a normal platelet spends a total of about three days in the spleen. Destruction of platelets, unlike that of polymorphonuclear leucocytes, but like that of red cells, is essentially non-random, although there may be a small superimposed component of random destruction. The disappearance of randomly labelled platelets from the circulation is therefore almost linear. The identification, interpretation and causes of reduced MPLS are discussed below.

(c) Sites of platelet destruction

Following their nine-day life-span in blood, platelets are destroyed in the reticuloendothelial system, principally the spleen and bone marrow (Figure 15.8). The quantitative role of the liver in platelet destruction is disputed, with estimates varying from greater than the spleen to less than the bone marrow (Table 15.7).

Table 15.7 Normal sites of senescent platelet disposal

	Liver (days)			*Spleen (days)*		
	0	3	7	0	3	7
Heyns *et al.* (1980)	16	24	34	26	28	32
Robertson *et al.* (1981)	9	18		42	50	
Klonizakis *et al.* (1980)	12		17	35		38
Scheffel *et al.* (1982)	13	14		38	45	

Values are percentages of injected radioactivity present in liver and spleen at different times after injection of ^{111}In-labelled platelets in normal subjects.

Following injection of radiolabelled platelets, the radioactivity in the spleen remains almost constant between equilibration of the platelets between splenic pool and blood, which is reached at about 30 min, and their complete removal from the circulation at about nine days (Figure 15.9) (Ries and Price, 1974; Peters *et al.*, 1984a). The explanation for this constancy is that as the activity signal from the platelets pooled in the spleen

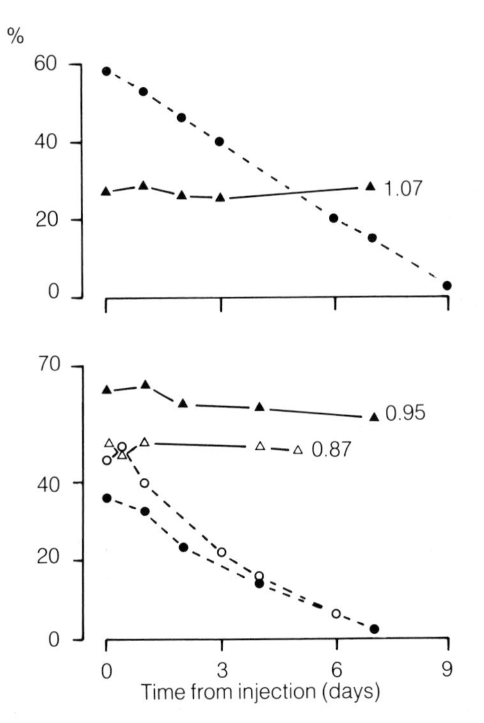

Figure 15.9 Time–activity curves based on peripheral venous blood samples (●) and a region of interest over the spleen (△) following injection of ^{111}In-labelled platelets in a normal subject (upper panel) and two patients with splenomegaly and reduced platelet survival (lower panel). Ordinate: percentage of injected dose. The figures are the D:P ratios, and indicate that in each case the spleen destroys almost the same fraction of the total platelet population as it pools. (Reprinted from *British Journal of Haematology*.)

declines with time the signal from radiolabel deposited in the spleen as a result of the intrasplenic platelet destruction increases at approximately the same rate. The total signal from the spleen therefore remains constant, indicating that the fraction of the whole body platelet population that is pooled in the spleen is equal to the fraction ultimately destroyed there.

15.8.3 DISORDERS OF PLATELET KINETICS

(a) Distribution

The only recognized abnormality of platelet distribution of clinical significance is the expanded splenic platelet pool of splenomegaly (Figure 15.10). When the spleen enlarges SBF increases, resulting in an increased rate of platelet input into the spleen (Peters *et al.*, 1984a). However, the mean transit time of platelets through the enlarged spleen remains essentially unchanged at 10 min. So, although platelets remain in dynamic equilibrium between blood and splenic pool, there is a net shift of platelets into the spleen,

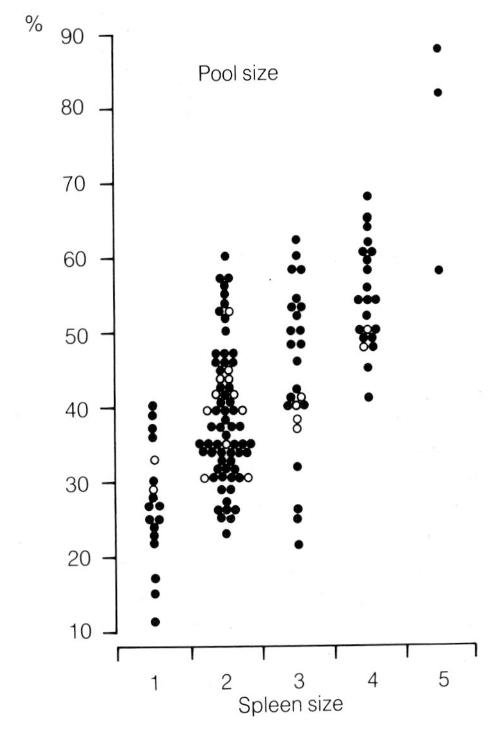

Figure 15.10 The relationship between the splenic platelet pool capacity and spleen size in patients with a variety of disorders. Ordinate: pool size as a percentage of the total platelet population. Spleen size (abscissa) has been graded according to the gamma camera posterior image, such that 1 and 2 correspond to the normal, 3 and 4 to increasing degrees of splenomegaly, and 5 to massive splenomegaly. In patients with secondary polycythaemia (○), splenic blood flow is inappropriately low for spleen size while intrasplenic platelet transit time is elevated above the normal. This results in a pool size which shows the same relationship to spleen size as in other patients. (Reprinted from *British Journal of Haematology*.)

resulting in peripheral thrombocytopenia. The thrombopoietic response of the bone marrow is dependent on the nature of the feedback mechanism, i.e. on whether platelet production is sensitive to the peripheral circulating platelet count, whole body platelet count or platelet biomass (product of platelet count and mean platelet volume) (Peters, 1986). Whichever of these is the most important, the severity of thrombocytopenia correlates closely with spleen size, although to produce clinically significant thrombocytopenia by this mechanism the spleen must be markedly enlarged.

The size of the splenic platelet pool, and therefore the effect of splenomegaly on the peripheral platelet count, can be quantified by measuring the recovery of ^{111}In-labelled platelets following intravenous injection (Harker and Finch, 1969). This is the percentage of the injected platelet-bound activity remaining in blood at the completion of equilibration between blood and splenic pool. This is reached at about 20–30 min in the normal spleen but earlier in splenomegaly (Figure 15.11). Normal recovery is about 65% but it may be as low as 10% in massive splenomegaly. The majority of unrecovered platelets, normally representing about 30% of the injected dose, enters the splenic pool, although minor pooling also occurs in the liver. The platelet recovery is also influenced by platelet damage and activation, sustained *in vitro* during isolation and labelling. Thus non-viable platelets are rapidly removed by the reticulo-endothelial system, while activated viable platelets are temporarily sequestered in the liver and occasionally also the lungs. Poor labelling technique will therefore result in a low recovery, perhaps 40% in the normal rising to about 50% a few hours after injection. When observed, this rise is therefore attributed to 'labelling' or 'collection' injury (Badenhorst *et al.*, 1982). Abnormal platelets may be more susceptible to the collection injury and it may therefore be difficult to quantify the volume of the splenic pool from recovery in such patients.

A more accurate picture of platelet distribution can be obtained from dynamic gamma camera imaging following intravenous injection of radiolabelled platelets. Because the blood and spleen behave as a closed two-compartmental system (Heyns *et al.*, 1980; Peters *et al.*, 1980, 1985a), the splenic time–activity curve increases monoexponentially to reach a plateau at 20–30 min after injection, while the blood activity, recorded from a region placed over the cardiac blood pool image, decreases with the same time constant to an asymptote which represents the recovery (Figure 15.6). In the absence of extensive platelet damage or activation, the hepatic time–activity curve peaks much earlier than the splenic (2–3 min normally but not later than 10 min) (Peters *et al.*,

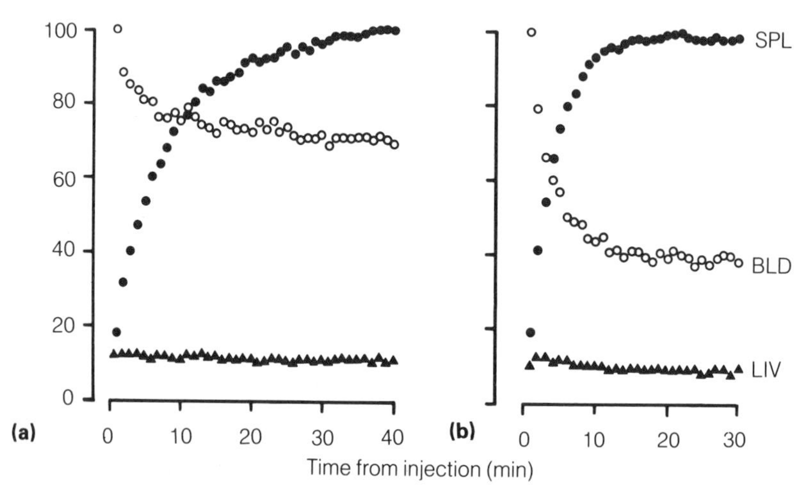

Figure 15.11 Time–activity curves recorded in regions of interest over the cardiac blood pool (○), liver (▲) and spleen (●) following injection of ^{111}In-labelled platelets in a normal subject (a) and a patient with splenomegaly (b). Ordinate (blood pool): percentage of initial value; ordinate (liver and spleen): percentage of maximal splenic activity (counts per pixel per frame). Note the lower recovery and earlier equilibration between blood and splenic platelet pool in splenomegaly.

1985b) and has a much smaller amplitude. After identification of the hepatic peak, the blood curve can be extrapolated back to zero time (Figure 15.6), enabling quantification of the partition of the platelets between blood and spleen; i.e. calculation of the splenic platelet pool volume. Further analysis of these kinetics yields SBF as a fraction of the total blood volume supplying the spleen in unit time and the mean intrasplenic platelet transit time (Peters *et al.*, 1980, 1985a).

(b) Disorders of platelet life-span

MPLS may be reduced as a result of intrinsic platelet disorders or abnormalities present within the circulation. When MPLS is only minimally reduced, the survival curve, instead of being almost linear, becomes distinctly curvilinear. When MPLS is markedly reduced, for example to a number of hours, the survival approaches an exponential function of time. Whereas there are many causes of minor to moderate reduction in MPLS, markedly shortened MPLS is usually due to idiopathic thrombocytopenic purpura (ITP).

Intravascular causes of reduced MPLS include severe arteriosclerosis, intracardiac prosthetic valves and prosthetic vascular grafts. In some cases, survival is reduced as a result of intravascular consumption, such as in thrombotic thrombocytopenic purpura (TTP). In others, such as patients with intracardiac valves, platelets age prematurely as a result of repeated mechanical insults and are removed into the normal sites of platelet destruction at an accelerated rate. The causes of reduced MPLS are summarized in Table 15.8.

Table 15.8 Causes and mechanisms of reduced mean platelet life-span

Causes	
Haematological	Idiopathic thrombocytopenia purpura (ITP) Thrombotic thrombocytopenia purpura (TTP) Leukaemia, lymphoma
Cardiovascular	Widespread arteriosclerosis Prosthetic materials (artificial valves, Dacron grafts) Deep vein thrombosis (DVT)
Pulmonary	Emphysema Eisenmenger's syndrome Adult respiratory distress syndrome Primary pulmonary hypertension
Renal	Allograft rejection Nephritis Nephrotic syndrome
Rheumatological	Systemic lupus erythematosus (SLE) Rheumatoid arthritis
Others	Cirrhosis Diabetes mellitus
Mechanisms	
Immune	Anti-platelet, e.g. ITP By-stander, e.g. SLE
Consumption	E.g. TTP, DVT
Accelerated ageing with premature removal	E.g. prosthetic cardiac valves, severe arteriosclerosis

Many analytical methods have been described for the calculation of MPLS from the platelet survival curve. A platelet survival which is perfectly linear indicates that platelet destruction is not random and that the frequency distribution of individual platelet life-spans is narrow. MPLS is then the time at which the survival curve cuts the time axis. In contrast, very short platelet survivals are essentially monoexponential and MPLS is the reciprocal of the rate constant of disappearance of labelled platelets. Abnormal survival curves between these two extremes, comprising the majority, require more complex analysis and a number of techniques have been proposed. Two of these, the multiple hit model and the Mills–Dornhorst technique, deserve mention because in addition to generating MPLS they give quantitative information about the mechanism of platelet destruction. For example, the multiple hit model proposes that a given platelet undergoes destruction after it has sustained a certain number of hits or insults. If destruction occurs after only a few insults then the survival curve is monoexponential. If a very large number of hits is required then survival is linear. In fact, MPLS = Na, where N is the number of hits required and a the average time interval between them. When survival is moderately shortened and curvilinear, useful information can be generated from estimations of a and N. The details of these procedures are available from the ICSH (1977).

(c) Identification of platelet destruction

The importance of identifying and quantifying the predominant sites of platelet destruction centres on the decision to undertake splenectomy in thrombyctopaenic patients shown to have a reduced MPLS. The physical characteristics of

^{111}In make this the best isotope with which to label platelets for the regional demonstration of excessive platelet destruction.

Various methods have been proposed for quantifying the role of the spleen in radiolabelled platelet destruction. When ^{51}Cr was routinely used for platelet labelling only surface counting with scintillation probes was possible. The relative contributions of the liver and spleen were expressed as their count rate ratio and as their respective count rates relative to the precordial count rate. With ^{111}In labelling, absolute quantification of liver and spleen activities as fractions of injected dose is possible (Table 15.7). Furthermore, since the initial splenic activity represents pooled platelet activity, the progressively increasing activity resulting from platelet destruction (analogous to 'excess' counts in red cell destruction) can be derived from total splenic activity by subtraction of the pooled activity, assuming the latter remains a constant fraction of the peripheral circulating activity (Klonizakis *et al.*, 1980). Since it has been demonstrated in a wide variety of disorders associated with splenomegaly and/or reduced MPLS that the splenic activity following injection of labelled platelets still remains essentially constant from beginning to end (Figure 15.9), i.e. that the spleen continues to destroy platelets in proportion to the numbers it pools, the finding of an increased rate of destruction of platelets in the spleen may well be appropriate for its size. The concept was formulated that the platelet itself determines the probability of its own life-span, which, however, can be modified by external intravascular factors (such as prosthetic valves), and that the probability of the platelet being in the spleen at its demise is a function of the size of the splenic platelet pool which itself is a function of spleen size (Peters *et al.*, 1984a). Support for this concept is the observation that splenomegaly *per se* is not necessarily associated with a reduced MPLS. A more appropriate parameter therefore with which to identify abnormal splenic platelet destruction is the percentage increase in splenic activity between the completion of mixing and the final removal of labelled platelets from the circulation: the destruction (*D*) to pooling (*P*) ratio (Figure 15.12). (Peters *et al.*, 1984a).

In immune thrombocytopaenia, the spleen undertakes an active role in that, through its macrophage Fc receptors, it may destroy platelets coated with IgG; under these circumstances total splenic activity progressively increases and the *DP* ratio is elevated. Platelets are, in other words, redirected to the spleen for destruction. Alternatively, antibody-coated platelets may be recognized by the liver and be destroyed there; because such platelets may continue to pool normally in the spleen, the *DP* ratio falls. Splenectomy would not therefore be expected to benefit the patient, unless the spleen is the source of antibodies. Abnormal liver destruction of platelets generally produces a very short MPLS, often less than 1 h, and severe thrombocytopaenia.

Abnormal liver destruction of platelets can usually be recognized from the initial dynamic scan as a progressively increasing hepatic signal. When both the liver and spleen destroy platelets in ITP, the *DP* ratio may paradoxically be normal yet the patient may benefit from splenectomy.

A reduced *DP* ratio may also be seen in abnormal peripheral platelet consumption such as in TTP. In such peripheral consumption, hepatic activity would not be expected to show any significant increase although data on this are not available. Destruction of platelets in bone marrow is a normal phenomenon. It is not known whether

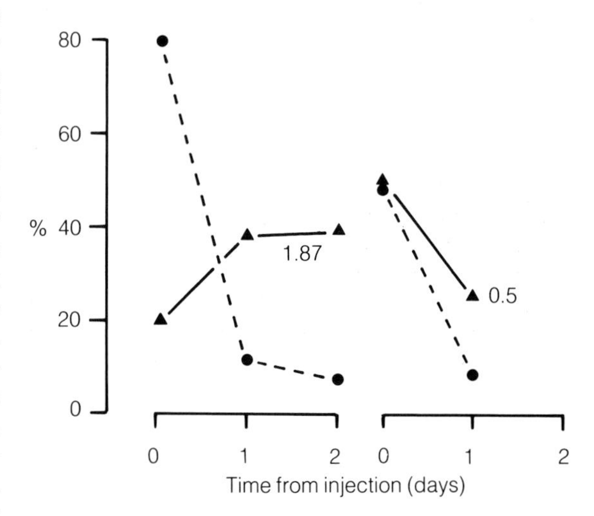

Figure 15.12 Platelet kinetics in severe ITP. The patient shown in the left panel has markedly reduced ^{111}In-labelled platelet survival (based on peripheral blood sampling, (●) and splenic activity (▲) which increases during the course of ^{111}In-labelled platelet removal from blood. The patient in the right-hand panel also has markedly reduced platelet survival, but in this case the splenic activity falls. Ordinate: percentage of injected dose. The figures are the destruction to pooling ratios.

the bone marrow ever exclusively causes thrombocytopenia by excessive platelet destruction.

15.8.4 INTERPRETATION OF THROMBOCYTOPAENIA

The main indication for performing labelled platelet kinetic studies is to define the cause of thrombocytopaenia. Thrombocytopaenia may be the result of (a) decreased platelet production, (b) increased splenic platelet pooling, or (c) decreased MPLS. The splenic platelet pool (SPP) as a fraction of the total circulating platelet population is slightly less than the difference between the recovery and 100% and is normally about one-third. Because of possible significant early hepatic uptake, the SPP is more reliably obtained by dynamic gamma camera imaging from which the hepatic uptake can then be corrected. The effective platelet production rate (PP) can then be calculated:

$$PP = \frac{\text{peripheral platelet count}}{(1 - \text{SPP}) \times \text{MPLS}}$$

Splenomegaly causes thrombocytopaenia by a dilutional effect. This tendency towards thrombocytopaenia can be quantified as an equivalent tendency caused by reduced MPLS. For example, the blood platelet volume is normally twice the splenic platelet volume. A fourfold increase in the latter would, in the absence of any thrombopoetic response, reverse this ratio, give an SPP of two-thirds of the total circulating platelet population, a recovery of approximately 30% and halve the peripheral platelet count. This would be the thrombocytopaenic equivalent of a reduction in MPLS to half normal. If thrombopoesis is sensitive to the total platelet population rather than the peripheral platelet count (P) then the latter can be predicted from the size of the SPP from

$$P = \frac{1 - (\text{SPP}) \times P(\text{norm})}{1 - \text{SPP}(\text{norm})}$$

P(norm) is the platelet count that would result from a reduced MPLS in the absence of splenomegaly. However, if platelet production is regulated by the peripheral platelet count then increased thrombopoesis would tend to reverse thrombocytopaenia due to splenomegaly. It is not, however, clear which of these regulatory mechanisms predominate.

It must be stressed, however, that platelet kinetic studies are often difficult to interpret, and although occasionally helpful the place of radionuclide studies in the management of patients with thrombocytopaenia is still not clear.

15.8.5 PLATELET IMAGING

Because ^{111}In is an efficient γ-emitter, ^{111}In-labelled platelets have been used to image a variety of thrombotic or microthrombotic disorders. The required doses of ^{111}In are somewhat higher (about 200–300 μCi) than those used in haematological studies.

(a) Deep vein thrombosis (DVT)

DVT can be located with ^{111}In-labelled platelets (Figure 15.13) and a limited number of clinical studies have demonstrated a reasonably high accuracy (Moser, 1985; Ezekowitz *et al.*, 1985). Sequential imaging is essential in order to avoid false positives resulting from high blood pool activity. Thus, as it falls, blood pool activity diverges from and can be distinguished from activity in thrombus. False negatives may be encountered if the patient has already been started on anticoagulant therapy because this inhibits further platelet deposition (Moser *et al.*, 1980). These two points limit the clinical useful-

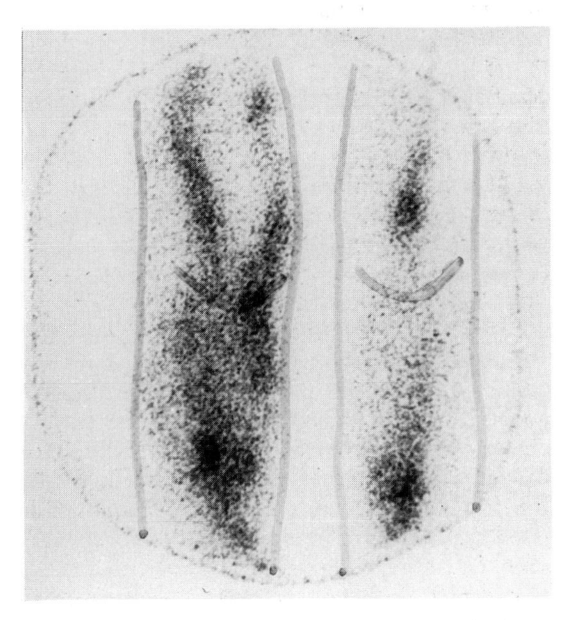

Figure 15.13 Gamma camera image over the lower limbs in a patient with bilateral deep vein thrombosis, 24 h after injection of ^{111}In-labelled platelets.

ness of platelet imaging in the diagnosis of DVT; thus clinicians are reluctant to withhold anti-coagulation while waiting for a diagnosis of DVT which may take 24 h from the time of referral to the nuclear medicine department.

(b) Renal allograft rejection

It is important to institute appropriate therapy for the rejecting renal transplant as early as possible. Because one of the earliest pathological features of acute rejection is platelet deposition in the micro-vasculature of the kidney, ^{111}In-labelled platelets have been useful for making an early diagnosis of rejection and distinguishing it from the other frequent complication of transplants, acute tubular necrosis (Fenech *et al.*, 1981). This distinction can also be made on ^{99m}Tc-labelled DTPA renography, although the use of maintenance immunopressive therapy, in particular cyclosporin A may confuse it. In spite of claims to the contrary, cyclosporin A does not itself appear to promote platelet deposition in the kidney or interfere with platelet imaging in the presence of rejection. ^{111}In-labelled platelets might therefore have a role in transplant management. However, in order to fully exploit this technique it is necessary for the radiolabelled platelets to be already circulating at the time of rejection; the patient in other words needs to be 'topped up' with labelled platelets at intervals of a few days and imaged at least daily. This regime clearly cannot be maintained for long periods but it may be practical over a limited period following transplantation, during which rejection is most likely. The interval would be dependent on the aggressiveness with which the recipient is immunosuppressed: thus in centres using low-dose maintenance immunosuppression rejection is likely to occur within the first few weeks.

(c) Left ventricular mural thrombus

^{111}In-labelled platelets have been used to diagnose left ventricular mural thrombus following myocardial infarction (Ezekowitz *et al.*, 1982). The main problem with this approach is to distinguish platelets that have become incorporated in clot from the much larger numbers that are circulating in the cardiac chambers. One solution is to subtract this large blood pool signal by labelling red cells with ^{99m}Tc. A fundamental problem common to any subtraction where background greatly exceeds target activity is that of excessive statistical noise following subtraction.

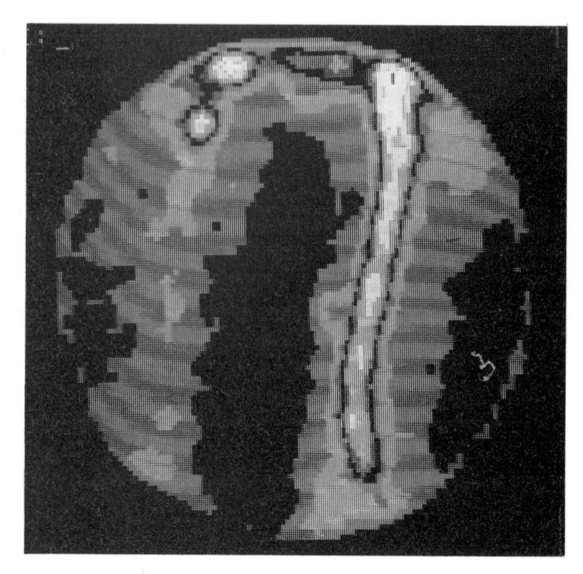

Figure 15.14 Gamma camera image over the thighs in a patient with a prosthetic femoro-popliteal Dacron graft. (Kindly supplied by Mr C. N. McCollum and reprinted from the *British Journal of Surgery*.)

(d) Arterial thrombus

There has been some interest in the use of ^{111}In-labelled platelets to image chronic focal arterial disease, mostly arteriosclerotic plaques in the carotid artery (Goldman *et al.*, 1983b). Also on the arterial side, ^{111}In-labelled platelets have been used to assess the thrombogenicity of prosthetic grafts such as Dacron aorto-bifemoral and femoro-popliteal grafts (Figure 15.14) (Goldman *et al.*, 1982; Stratton *et al.*, 1982). These have been used as quantitative models to evaluate anti-platelet therapy. Since the surface of these prosthetic materials appears to remain capable of accumulating radiolabelled platelets, i.e. to be thrombogenic, for many years, platelets are presumably in dynamic equilibrium between the artificial surface and blood. Apart from clinical research a role for radiolabelled platelets in the evaluation of such grafts is not clear, although Goldman *et al.* (1983a) have produced evidence to show that the extent of ^{111}In-labelled platelet uptake has prognostic significance for graft patency.

^{111}In-labelled platelets have not gained widespread clinical popularity for imaging thrombus largely because of the inconvenience and expense of the *in vitro* manipulation associated with labelling. There has been interest, therefore, in potential platelet-specific agents capable of labelling

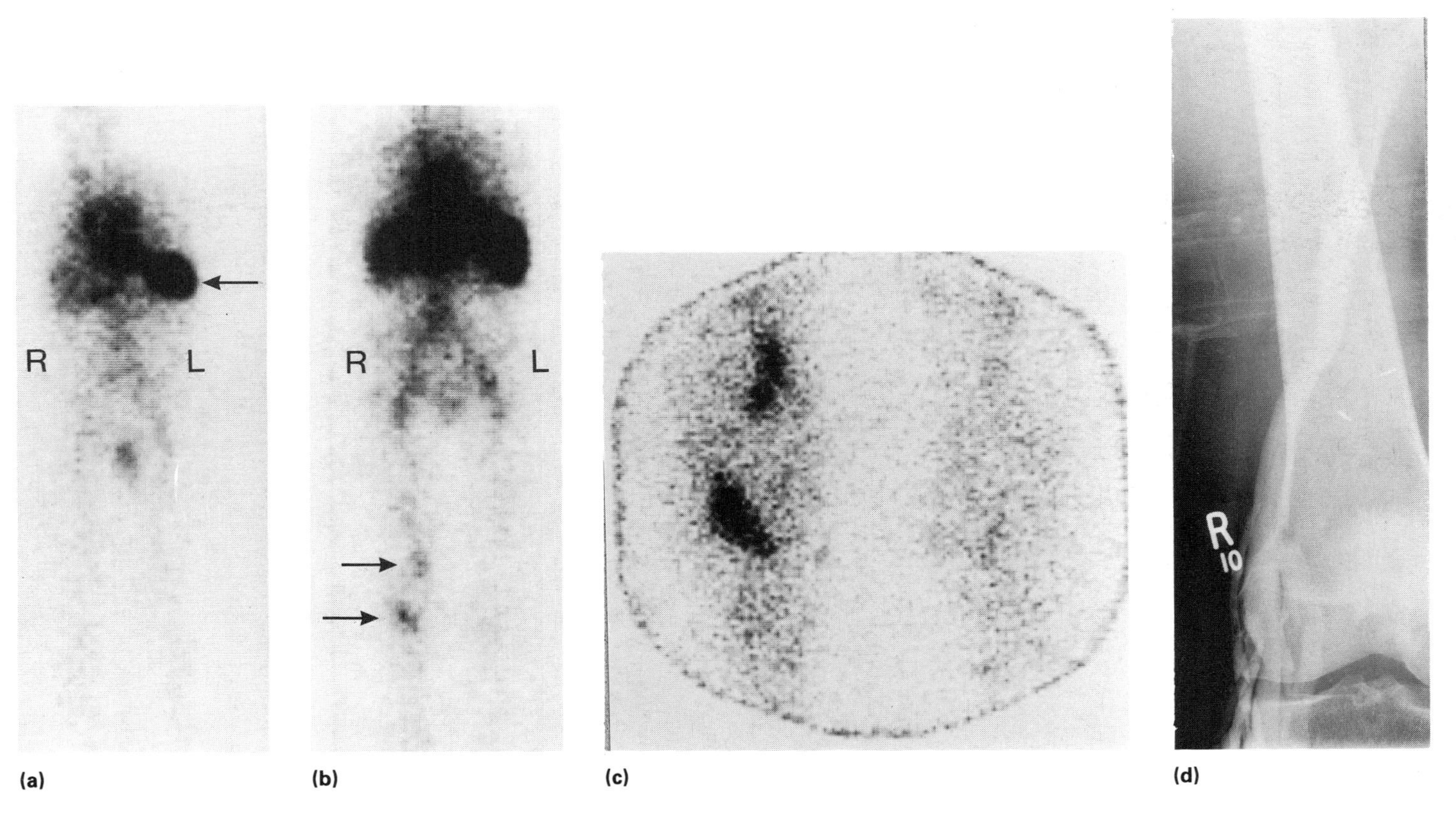

Figure 15.15 (a) Anterior whole body image in a patient without thrombosis obtained 24 h after injection of ^{111}In-labelled P256, a monoclonal antibody which recognizes the IIb/IIIa fibrinogen receptor of human platelets. The distribution of activity is very similar to the normal platelet distribution. The spleen is arrowed. (b) This patient has deep vein thrombosis involving the right lower extremity (arrowed). (c) Spot views, showing two separate foci of ^{111}In uptake. (d) Venogram confirming thrombus at the sites of ^{111}In uptake. (Reprinted from the *British Medical Journal*.)

platelets selectively in whole blood or even *in vivo*. One approach recently shown to be feasible is the use of radiolabelled monoclonal antibodies directed against platelet surface antigens. Thus an ^{111}In-labelled antibody which recognizes the IIb, IIIa fibrinogen receptor of primate platelets has been used successfully as an intravenous agent for localizing DVT (Figure 15.15) (Peters *et al.*, 1986b).

15.9 RADIOLABELLED GRANULOCYTES

15.9.1 GRANULOCYTE LABELLING

^{111}In-labelled leucocytes are widely used for imaging inflammation (Peters, 1989). Such cell populations are, in fact, heterogenous since, without separation techniques more elaborate than simple differential centrifugation, leucocytes cannot be separated from mononuclear leucocytes. However, provided the patient has a raised neutrophil count, such a mixed leucocyte preparation is adequate for imaging inflammation or abscess. Circumstances in which ^{111}In-labelled pure granulocytes may be clinically indicated are few. They include abscess imaging in patients with normal or low neutrophil counts, imaging focal granulocyte accumulation within the cardiovascular system (such as infected cardiac valve vegetations), and where quantitative studies are performed (such as quantification of faecal granulocyte excretion as an index of activity in inflammatory bowel disease); Saverymuttu *et al.*, 1983b).

The principles underlying leucocyte or granulocyte labelling are similar to those of platelet labelling: separation from other blood cells, inhibition during *in vitro* manipulation, separation from plasma and addition of a lipophilic ^{111}In-labelled chelate. Pure granulocytes can be separated by multiple density-gradient centrifugation. The sedimentation rate of cells suspended in fluids depends on the viscosity and density of the fluid, and the size and density of the cell. The principle of density-gradient centrifugation is that a cell will stop sedimenting when it meets a fluid with a density greater than its own. In an appropriate double density gradient, therefore, mononuclear leucocytes and platelets move no further than the interface between plasma and the first density, granulocytes sediment only as far as the interface between the two gradients and red cells move to the bottom of the tube. The granulocyte layer is removed, washed and resuspended for labelling.

Granulocytes appear to be more sensitive to removal from plasma than platelets and become activated, specially following separation in density-gradient columns made up with saline (Saverymuttu *et al.*, 1983a). However, the columns can be prepared with autologous plasma, although the densities, which must be exact, are less predictable and each laboratory must establish its own protocols. Activation is not detectable in most *in vitro* systems for measuring cell viability, since the tests themselves, by their very nature, induce activation and cannot therefore distinguish between quiescent cells and cells already activated by the separation procedure. Activated cells are of little use for abscess imaging because they become trapped in the lung on first pass following intravenous injection (Figure 15.16); following their release they are removed into the liver (Figure 15.17).

None of the currently used techniques for leucocyte or granulocyte separation utilize an inhibitory agent to prevent activation analogous to prostaglandins or acidification for platelet separation and labelling. However, use of heparin as anticoagulant appears to promote activation by causing micro-aggregation during leucocyte separation and we recommend ACD for anticoagulation in the same volume as used for platelet labelling. There is no need, however, to add further ACD prior to centrifugation as in platelet labelling.

^{111}In-labelled oxine or ^{111}In-labelled tropolonate should be used to label leucocytes, although we favour tropolone since it gives an acceptable labelling efficiency in plasma. ^{111}In-labelled acetylacetonate is not recommended because it has less selectivity for leucocytes than either ^{111}In-labelled oxine or ^{111}In-labelled tropolonate.

^{111}In-labelled granulocytes have no recognized role in the evaluation of granulocytopaenia, unlike ^{111}In-labelled platelets in thrombocytopaenia, yet the same general processes govern the peripheral granulocyte count: production, mean granulocyte life span and splenic pooling. Mean granulocyte life-span (MGLS) in blood is first order, rather than zero order, and is also very much shorter than MPLS. Granulocytes, however, display splenic pooling characteristics that are very similar to platelets with essentially the same intrasplenic transit time, about 10 min (Peters *et al.*, 1985c). Although reduced MGLS and increased splenic granulocyte pooling are recognized causes of a reduced peripheral granulocyte

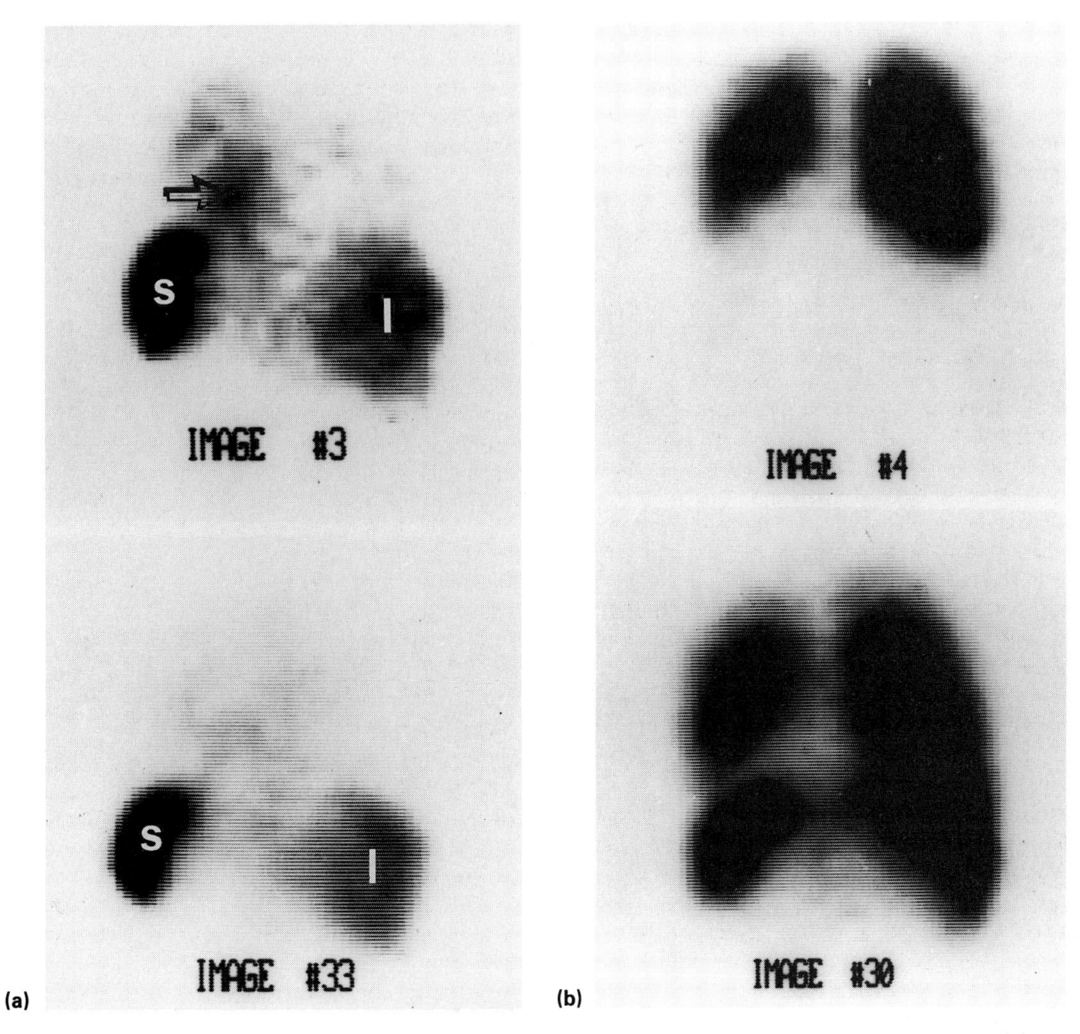

Figure 15.16 Posterior gamma camera images of the chest and upper abdomen in two patients following intravenous injection of ^{111}In-labelled 'pure' granulocytes. (a) The granulocytes were isolated on a density gradient enriched with autologous plasma, washed in plasma and labelled in plasma with ^{111}In-labelled tropolonate. (b) The granulocytes were isolated on a saline-based gradient, washed in saline and labelled in saline with ^{111}In-labelled acetylactonate. Image numbers are based on a frame rate of 1 per minute.

count, neither are regarded as accessible to diagnosis by radiolabelled granulocyte studies. ^{111}In-labelled granulocytes have not therefore become established in the work-up of patients with leucopaenia. Nonetheless an understanding of normal granulocyte kinetics is necessary for the interpretation of radiolabelled granulocyte imaging in inflammation.

A ^{99m}Tc agent, ^{99m}Tc-labelled haxamethylpropyleneamine oxime (HMPAO), has recently been described as a successful label for leucocytes and is becoming increasingly popular for white cell scanning (Peters *et al.*, 1986c). Although providing images of high count density and good resolution (Figure 15.18), this agent is less suitable than ^{111}In for granulocyte kinetic studies because of its short half-life and higher rate of elution. A comparison in inflammatory bowel disease has been made by Mountford *et al.* (1990).

15.9.2 GRANULOCYTE KINETICS

Granulocyte kinetics can be divided, like platelet kinetics, into distribution, MGLS and destruction.

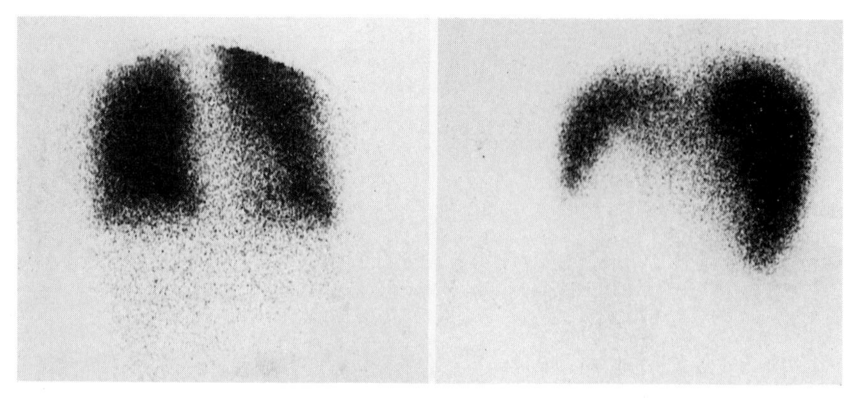

Figure 15.17 Initial lung sequestration of pure granulocytes manipulated and labelled with ^{111}In in saline with subsequent heavy uptake of activity by the liver, and to a lesser extent by the spleen. The recovery of labelled granulocytes (i.e. percentage of injected cells still circulating at 40 min) was less than 5%.

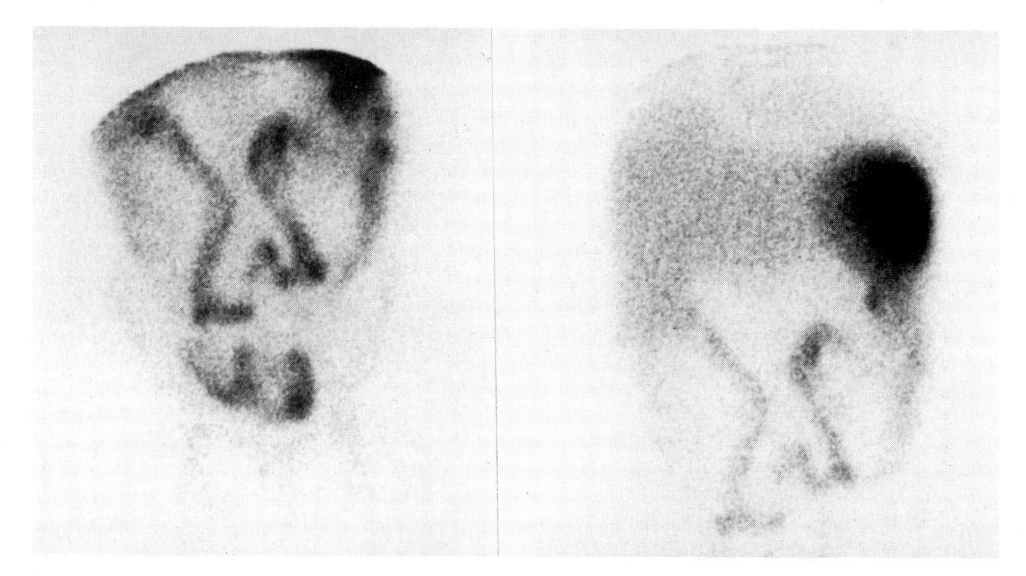

Figure 15.18 Inflamed small bowel, in a bone marrow recipient with graft-versus-host disease, imaged with ^{99m}Tc-HMPAO-labelled leucocytes. The scan was taken 23 min after injection.

(a) Distribution

Following release from bone marrow and prior to leaving the circulation, granulocytes are distributed and in dynamic equilibrium between two pools (Figure15.19): the marginating granulocyte pool and the circulating granulocyte pool. ^{111}In labelling has demonstrated that about one-third of the marginating granulocyte pool is located in the spleen (Figure 15.20). Most of the remainder is in the liver, lungs and probably bone marrow. The rest of the body accounts for substantially less than a quarter of the marginating granulocyte pool. The early studies from Wintrobe's group, based on ^{32}P-difluorophosphonate (DFP)-labelled granulocytes, demonstrated that following adrenaline or strenuous exercise granulocytes demarginate, resulting in an expansion of the circulating granulocyte pool (Athens *et al.*, 1961). The relevance of this is that the high activity seen in the spleen following ^{111}In-labelled leucocyte injection is physiological rather than an indicator of cell damage. Although a marginating granulocyte pool is almost certainly present in the liver,

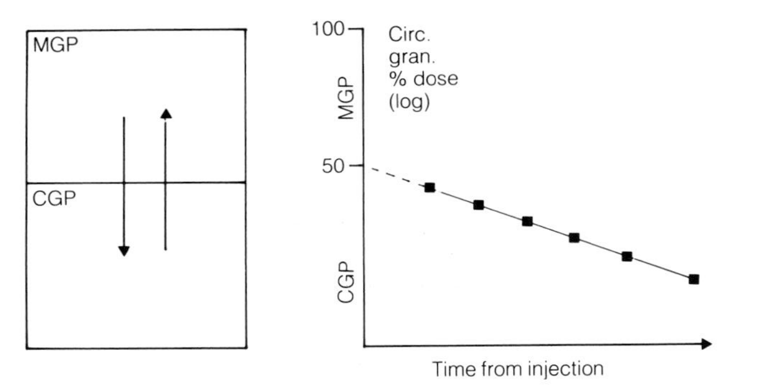

Figure 15.19 Diagrammatic representation of the distribution of blood granulocytes between the marginating granulocyte pool (MGP) and circulating granulocyte pool (CGP). Extrapolation of the monoexponential disappearance of radiolabelled granulocytes from blood to zero time leaves 50% of the injected cells unaccounted for. These cells have entered the MGP.

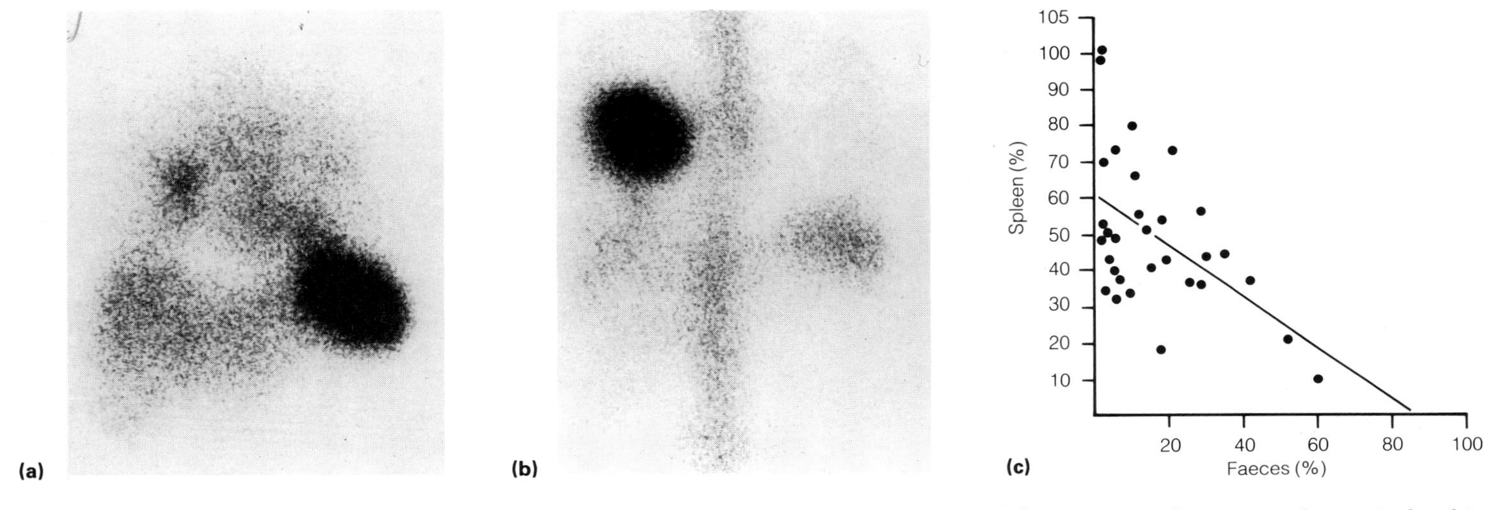

Figure 15.20 Splenic granulocyte pooling. (a) The anterior image over the chest, taken 40 min after injection of pure granulocytes isolated in plasma and labelled in plasma with ^{111}In-labelled tropolonate, shows the normal distribution of activity with, in addition, a small abnormal focus in the right mid-zone, corresponding to a suspected lung abscess. (b) The image at 24 h shows intense activity in the abscess but virtually no activity in liver or spleen. This is because of recruitment of previously pooled cells for migration into the abscess. (Reprinted from *Clinical Science*). (c) Relationship between the splenic activity at 3 hr after injection (expressed as a percentage of the activity 40 min after injection) and 4 day faecal ^{111}In excretion in 31 patients with inflammatory bowel disease (IBD) following injection of ^{111}In-labelled 'pure' granulocytes. Splenic activity at 40 min is represented almost entirely by pooled granulocytes which, depending on the severity of the IBD, are ultimately redirected for migration.

hepatic uptake of activity is sensitive to granulocyte damage and/or activation, with high uptake correlating with the degree of lung sequestration seen immediately following injection (Figure 15.17).

(b) MGLS

The $T_{1/2}$ of radiolabelled granulocyte clearance from blood is about 7 h. Maximum uptake in abscesses is not therefore seen until about 24 h after injection of labelled cells. However, positive scans should be detectable well before this time even though they are seen optimally at 24 h. If there is no evidence of abnormal activity on a white cell scan at 24 h further imaging in the hope that the scan will become positive is pointless. For reasons that are not clear the presence of inflammation does not shorten MGLS in blood (Saverymuttu *et al.*, 1985) and so, even in the presence of extensive sepsis, the maximum signal is still not achieved until about 24 h.

(c) Destruction

Other features of granulocyte kinetics that have been clarified by ^{111}In-labelled granulocytes are the normal disposal or destruction sites (Saverymuttu *et al.*, 1985). Contrary to the classical view that granulocytes continuously migrate to the tissues in the subclinical defence against infection, granulocytes do not normally migrate into the tissues but are destroyed in the reticuloendothelial system like platelets and red cells. The spleen and bone marrow are important in this respect and this explains why the spleen remains 'hot' and the bone marrow gets 'hotter' in the course of a labelled leucocyte study.

15.10 THE SPLEEN

Some functions of the spleen have already been referred to: its role in ferrokinetics, red cell pooling and destruction, platelet and granulocyte pooling and platelet and granulocyte destruction. In this section the central role of the spleen in blood cell kinetics and methods of evaluating splenic function and their indications will be reviewed.

15.10.1 SPLENIC IMAGING

Splenic imaging is routinely performed with ^{99m}Tc-labelled sulphur colloid or selectively with heat-damaged red cells (HDRBC). Splenic imaging may be useful for the evaluation of splenomegaly, detection of focal splenic disease, such as infarcts, or infiltration, such as lymphoma, and in the conservative management of splenic trauma. Occasionally it is necessary to selectively image the spleen during white cell scanning in which there is a question of sepsis in relation to the spleen or where, in the presence of a left-sided subphrenic abscess, there is doubt as to whether or not a patient is actually asplenic. Relapsing ITP may be associated with accessory splenic tissue which is best detected by selective imaging, either with HDRBC or, as part of a platelet kinetic study, with ^{111}In-labelled platelets.

The spleen has a central place in lymphocyte traffic and has immunological functions in relation to this, including the production of antibodies. Clinical nuclear medicine has little to offer in this field at present and it will not be discussed further. The other functions of the spleen are blood cell sequestration (pooling or trapping) and phagocytosis. Pooling can be distinguished from trapping by its reversibility. Trapping precedes phagocytosis. Thus it may be several hours before HDRBC, irreversibly sequestered (i.e. trapped) in the spleen, are actually phagocytosed (Klausner *et al.*, 1975).

Splenic congenital anomalies (asplenia, and right-sided spleen) have a high incidence of association (80–95%) with a peculiar complex type of serious cardiovascular malformation, consisting of one or more of the following (or variations of these):

1. atrial inversion or isomerism, and/or ventricular inversion;
2. single atrium or ventricle, or large ASD or VSD, or A–V communication;
3. transposition of the great arteries, truncus arteriosus, atresia of the aorta or pulmonary artery, or double outlet of either ventricle;
4. anomalous drainage of systemic or pulmonary veins or other major anomalies of central veins.

Therefore, selective splenic imaging may be helpful in the investigation of children suspected of having congenital heart disease, and conversely, the incidental discovery of asplenia, polysplenia or right-sided spleen, should immediately suggest the probability of coexistent complex cardiovascular malformation. In addition, there is a high incidence of coexistent anomalies of the liver, pancreas and lungs (heterotaxia syndrome).

15.10.2 SPLENIC RED CELL POOLING

The red cell volume of the normal spleen is about 5% of the total red cell volume (i.e. 100 ml in an adult). This corresponds to a mean intrasplenic red cell transit time of about 1 min. In splenomegaly, this red cell 'pool' is increased, by as much as five to ten times, e.g. in myelofibrosis, polycythaemia, hairy cell leukaemia and lymphoproliferative disorders (Pettit, 1977). An increase in the volume of the splenic red cell pool may, by itself, cause anaemia; measurement of the pool is therefore useful in the investigation of the anaemia associated with these conditions. It is also useful for determining the cause of erythrocytosis; thus, the increased pool in polycythaemia vera contrasts with secondary polycythaemia in which it is normal (Bateman *et al.*, 1978).

The splenic red cell volume is estimated from quantitative scanning, using the gamma camera or rectilinear scanner, after injection of red cells labelled with ^{99m}Tc or ^{113m}In. The red cell volume is measured in the usual way. The splenic area is scanned 20 min after the injection, and the fraction of the total radioactivity contained in the spleen is calculated. In order to delineate the splenic area more precisely, it is helpful first to give a small dose of labelled HDRBC.

In splenomegaly, equilibration of labelled red cells between blood and the splenic pool is delayed by up to 60 min because of the presence of a splenic pool with a slow red cell turnover (Toghill, 1964). For a given degree of splenomegaly, this pool size is greater for abnormal, as compared with normal, red cells.

15.10.3 SPLENIC POOLING OF OTHER BLOOD CELLS

Platelets, granulocytes and probably monocytes undergo splenic pooling to a much greater extent than red cells. The mean transit times of platelets and granulocytes are very similar. Pooling appears not to be coupled to intrasplenic cell destruction, at least for platelets, since transit time is unchanged in conditions such as ITP in which MPLS is markedly shortened as a result of excessive platelet destruction in the spleen (Peters *et al.*, 1985d). Almost nothing is known about the control mechanisms and purpose of splenic platelet and granulocyte pooling, which is remarkable for such a florid physiological phenomenon. Intrasplenic platelet transit time shows an inverse relationship with splenic perfusion (i.e. SBF/splenic volume) (Wadenvik and Kutti, 1987) but is otherwise rather invariable across a wide spectrum of disorders associated both with a reduced MPLS and splenomegaly (Peters and Lavender, 1982). The size of the splenic platelet pool is therefore a function only of SBF which itself correlates with spleen size. Adrenaline infusion shifts platelets from the spleen into blood by a reduction in SBF which is not compensated by the simultaneous increase in mean intrasplenic platelet transit time (Wadenvik and Kutti, 1987).

The spleen sequesters modified or effete blood cells. Red cells damaged by heating (HDRBC) at 49.5 °C for 20 min become rigid and are sequestered in the splenic pulp from where they either escape back into the circulation or are ultimately phagocytosed by splenic macrophages. On their return to the spleen, those that previously escaped are again subjected to the same probability of escape or erythrophagocytosis, and this results in a bi-exponential plasma disappearance curve (Figure 15.21). The mean transit time for the reversibly sequestered HDRBC is rather similar to that of normal platelets and granulocytes (Peters *et al.*, 1982).

HDRBC are useful for selective splenic imaging. Their rate of disappearance from plasma is also used as a quantitative index of splenic function,

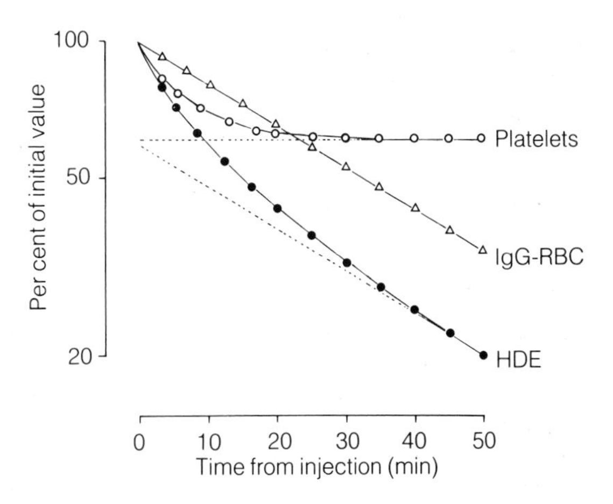

Figure 15.21 Blood clearance kinetics of radiolabelled platelets, antibody-coated red cells (IgG–RBC) and heat-damaged red cells (HDE). Platelets disappear from blood as a result of splenic pooling with negligible destruction over the observation period, while IgG–RBC are irreversibly removed into the spleen for destruction but show no pooling. Heat-damaged red cells undergo simultaneous pooling and irreversible removal, resulting in a bi-exponential blood clearance.

but this is only valid if conditions of heating are standardized and result in minimal extrasplenic uptake. Excessive damage for instance results in hepatic uptake. HDRBC clearance from plasma is commonly regarded as an index of splenic phagocytic function, but also reflects efficiency of trapping and SBF.

Coating red cells with anti-rhesus immunoglobulin is an alternative method of modifying them for splenic localization. Depending on the source of antibody, localization may be more specific for the spleen than HDRBC. IgG coating seems not to affect intrasplenic red cell transit time and their clearance from blood is essentially first order (Figure 15.21), with a time constant depending on SBF and splenic extraction efficiency (Peters *et al.*, 1984b). The latter is itself dependent on the number of IgG molecules present on the cell surface and the number of vacant Fc receptors on the splenic macrophages (Walport *et al.*, 1985).

The clearance of radiolabelled IgG-coated red cells from plasma has therefore been used to diagnose Fc receptor blockade in patients with disorders, such as systemic lupus erythematosis and essential cryoglobulinaemia, associated with elevated levels of immune complexes (Frank *et al.*, 1979). Since it may vary widely in these conditions, SBF should also be monitored so that the splenic extraction fraction can be calculated (Walport *et al.*, 1985).

Although clearly a function of splenic phagocytosis, the removal into the spleen of ^{99m}Tc-labelled colloids is not widely used as an index of splenic function. Indeed it is not certain what is the normal splenic extraction efficiency. Although widely assumed to be the same as the hepatic extraction efficiency, the splenic extraction efficiency for colloid is probably less and may be as low as 50% (Peters *et al.*, 1987).

15.11 BONE MARROW IMAGING

There are two separate cellular elements in bone marow which will concentrate radionuclides, thereby allowing bone marrow to be imaged: the reticuloendothelial system (RES) and the haematopoetic system. The latter is usually abbreviated to the 'erythron' although it also includes a myeloproliferative component. The two elements normally coexist throughout red (active) marrow, the distribution in the skeleton of which varies with age. Although the bone marrow normally can be imaged with agents selectively taken up by either component, in some pathological circumstances, such as aplastic anaemia, there is a divergence in the distribution of the elements, and the images obtained will depend on which group of agents is used.

15.11.1 INDICATIONS FOR BONE MARROW IMAGING

1. To define the distribution of active incorporation of iron into erythroid precursors (see above).
2. For the assessment of bone marrow replacement, e.g. by neoplastic tissue, which may be diffuse as in some haematological malignancies, or focal as in metastatic bone disease, or both, as in neuroblastoma.
3. Marrow infarction, e.g. in sickle cell disease. Other conditions which result in loss of functioning marrow include Paget's disease and radiation therapy (with loss of the erythron before the RES).
4. In conjunction with white cell scanning for the diagnosis of osteomyelitis in order to distinguish migrated neutrophils from those destroyed normally in the RES. This is especially useful in the infected prosthetic hip where variable amounts of bone marrow have been removed operatively.

15.11.2 AGENTS

(a) Colloids

Sulphur or tin colloids, as used in liver/spleen imaging, are useful for imaging the RES of bone marrow. Smaller particle size colloids, such as antimony sulphur colloid, have a relative selectivity for bone marrow, although uptake in the liver and spleen is still heavy. Information simultaneously acquired about spleen size is, however, often useful. Other radionuclides forming colloids include ^{198}Au and ^{113m}In.

(b) Iron

^{59}Fe and ^{52}Fe chloride will label the erythron, as described above. Although not usually regarded as 'imageable', reasonable images of ^{59}Fe can be obtained (Figure 15.5). ^{52}Fe is a positron emitter and can therefore be imaged either with a positron camera or with the rectilinear scanner collimated for the 511 keV annihilation photons.

(c) ^{111}In-labelled transferrin

^{111}In shows many of the properties of the iron isotopes and has therefore been used as a substitute for them. However, the biological behaviour of indium and iron is different in as many respects as they are similar, so the distribution of ^{111}In can only be extrapolated to the distribution of the erythron with great care, and this applies particularly to aplastic anaemia and myelofibrosis. Indeed, Chipping *et al.*, (1980) observed a distribution of ^{111}In and ^{52}Fe that was similar in only two of 15 patients with a variety of haematological conditions. However, in aplastic anaemia, McNeil *et al.* (1976) suggest that marrow ^{111}In uptake correlates with prognosis.

(d) Radiolabelled leucocytes

The agent which gives the best images of bone marrow is ^{99m}Tc HMPAO-labelled leucocytes. The intensity of the uptake seen within 40 min after injection raises the possibility that granulocytes normally pool in bone marrow sinusoids. However, because granulocytes, like platelets and red cells, are normally disposed of in bone marrow, the images presumably specifically represent the distribution of marrow RES. An alternative approach is to use ^{99m}Tc labelled antigranulocyte antibodies (Duncker *et al.*, 1990).

REFERENCES

Anderson, B., Belcher, E. H., Chanarin, I. and Mollison, P. L. (1960) The urinary and faecal excretion of radioactivity after oral doses of ^{3}H-folic acid. *Br. J. Haematol.*, **34**, 1191–2.

Ahuja, S., Lewis, S. M. and Szur, L. (1972) Value of surface counting in predicting response to splenectomy in haemolytic anaemia. *J. Clin. Pathol.*, **25**, 467–72.

Arrago, J. P., Rain, J. D., Vigneron, N. *et al.* (1985) Diagnostic value of bone marrow imaging with ^{111}Indium-transferrin and ^{99m}technetium-colloids in myelofibrosis. *Am. J. Hematol.*, **18**, 275–82.

Athens, J. W., Mauer, A. M., Ashenbrucker, H. *et al.* (1961) Leucocyte studies III. The distribution of granulocytes in the blood of normal subjects. *J. Clin. Invest.*, **40**, 159–64.

Aubert, B., Kahn, E., Parmentier, C. and Di Paola, R. (1983) Physical requirements of a ^{59}Fe bone marrow distribution digital scanning survey. *Eur. J. Nucl. Med.*, **8**, 162–6.

Badenhorst, P. N., Heyns, A. du P., Van Reenen, O. R. *et al.* (1982) The influence of the 'collection injury' on the survival and distribution of ^{111}In labelled canine platelets. *Br. J. Haematol.*, **52**, 233–40.

Barosi, G., Berzuini, C., Cazzola, M. *et al.* (1976) An approach by means of a mathematical model to the analysis of ferrokinetic data obtained by liquid scintillation counting of ^{59}Fe. *J. Nucl. Biol. Med.*, **20**, 8–22.

Bateman, S., Lewis, S. M., Nicholas, A. and Zaafran, A. (1978) Splenic red cell pooling: a diagnostic feature in polycythaemia. *Br. J. Haematol.*, **40**, 389–96.

Bazett, H. C., Sunderman, F. W. and Scott, J. C. (1940) Climatic effects on the volume and composition of blood in man. *Am. J. Physiol.*, **129**, 69–83.

Bentley, S. A. (1977) Red cell survival studies reinterpreted. *Clin. Haematol.*, **6**, 601–23.

Bentley, S. A. and Miller, D. T. (1986) Radionuclide blood cell survival studies. *Methods Hematol.*, **14**, 245–62.

Biermann, H. R., Kelly, K. H., Cordes, F. L. *et al.* (1952) The clearance of leukocytes and platelets from the pulmonary circulation by epinephrine. *Blood*, **7**, 683–92.

Bothwell, T. H., Charlton, R. W., Cook, J. D. and Finch, C. A. (1979) *Iron Metabolism in Man*, Ch. 12, Blackwell, Oxford.

Cavill, I. (1986) Plasma clearance studies. *Methods Hematol.*, **14** 214–44.

Cavill, I., Ricketts, C., Napier, J. A. F. and Jacobs, A. (1977a) Ferrokinetics and erythropoiesis in mean red cell production and destruction in normal and anaemic subjects. *Br. J. Haematol.*, **35**, 27–34.

Chanarin, I. (1979) *The Megaloblastic Anaemias*, 2nd edn, Blackwell, Oxford, p. 175.

Chaudhuri, T. K., Ehrhardt, J. C., De Gowin, R. L. and Christie, J. H. (1974). ^{59}Fe whole-body scanning. *J. Nucl. Med.*, **15**, 667–73.

Chipping, P., Klonizakis, I. and Lewis, S. M. (1980) Indium chloride scanning: a comparison with iron as a tracer for erythropoiesis. *Clin. Lab. Haematol.*, **2**, 255–63.

Cook, J. D. and Lipschitz, D. A. (1977) Clinical measurement of iron absorption. *Clin. Haematol.*, **6**, 567–81.

Dacie, J. V. and Lewis, S. M. (1984) *Practical Haemtology*, 6th edn, Churchill Livingstone, Edinburgh.

Danpure, H. J., Osman, S. and Brady, F. (1982) The labelling of blood cells in plasma with ^{111}In-tropolonate. *Br. J. Radiol.*, **55**, 247–9.

Documenta Geigy (1970) *Scientific Tables*, 7th edn, J. R. Geigy, Basel, p. 712.

Domstad, P. A., Choy, Y. C., Kim, E. E. and De Land, F. H. (1981) Reliability of the dual-isotope Schilling test for the diagnosis of penicious anaemia or malabsorption syndrome. *Am. J. Clin. Pathol.*, **75**, 723–6.

Duncker, C. M., Carrio, I., Berna, L. *et al* (1990) Radioimmunoimaging of bone marrow in patients with suspected bone metastases from primary breast cancer. *J. Nucl. Med.*, **31**, 1450–5.

Eisenberg, S. (1959) Blood volume in patients with acute glomerulonephritis as determined by radioactive chromium tagged red cells. *Am. J. Med.*, **27**, 241–5.

Ellis, R. E., Nordin, B. E. C., Tothill, P. and Veall, N. (1977) The use of thyroid blocking agents: a report of a working party of the MRC Isotope Advisory Panel. *Br. J. Radiol.*, **50**, 203–4.

England, J. M., Snashall, E. A. and de Silva, P. M. (1981) Comparison of the Dicopac with the conventional Schilling test. *J. Clin. Pathol.*, **34**, 1191–2.

Ezekowitz, M. D., Wilson, D. A., Smith, E. O. *et al.*

(1982) Comparison of ^{111}In platelet scintigraphy and two-dimensional echo-cardiography in the diagnosis of left ventricular thrombi. *N. Engl. J. Med.*, **306**, 1509–13.

Ezekowitz, M. D., Snyder, E. L., Pope, C. *et al.* (1985) in *Radiolabelled Cellular Blood Elements* (ed. M. L. Thakur), Plenum Press, New York, pp. 177–99.

Fairbanks, V. F., Wahner, H. W., Valley, T. B. and Schedit, R. M. (1983) Spurious results from dual isotope (Dicopac) vitamin B_{12} absorption test are due to rapid or variable rates of exchange of ^{58}Co-B_{12} for ^{57}Co-B_{12} bound to intrinsic factor. *Nucl. Med. Commun.*, **4**, 17–24.

Fenech, A., Nicholls, A. and Smith, F. W. (1981) Indium labelled platelets in the diagnosis of renal transplant rejection: preliminary findings. *Br. J. Radiol.*, **54**, 325–7.

Ferrant, A., Lewis, S. M. and Szur, L. (1974) The elution of ^{99}Tc^{m} from red cells and its effect on red cell volume measurement. *J. Clin. Pathol.*, **27**, 983–5.

Ferrant, A., Cauwe, F., Michaux, J. L. *et al.* (1982) Assessment of the sites of red cell destruction using quantitative measurement of splenic and hepatic red cell destruction. *Br. J. Haematol.*, **50**, 591–8.

Ferrant, A., Rodhain, J., Leners, N. *et al.* (1986) Quantitative assessment of erythropoiesis in bone marrow expansion areas using ^{52}Fe. *Br. J. Haematol.*, **62**, 247–55.

Frank, M. M., Hamburger, M. I., Lawley, T. J. *et al.* (1979) Defective reticuloendothelial system Fc receptor function in systemic lupus erythematosus. *N. Engl. J. Med.*, **300**, 518–23.

Freedman, D. S., Brown, J. P., Weir, D. G. and Scott, J. M. (1973) The reproducibility and use of the tritiated folic acid urinary excretion test as a measure of folate absorption in clinical practice: effect of methotrexate on absorption of folic acid. *J. Clin. Pathol.*, **26**, 261–7.

Goldman, M., Norcott, H. C., Hawker, R. J. *et al.* (1982) Femoro-popliteal by-pass grafts: an isotope technique allowing *in-vivo* comparison of thrombogenicity. *Br. J. Surg.*, **69**, 380–2.

Goldman, M., Hall, C., Dykes, J. *et al.* (1983a) Does ^{111}indium platelet deposition predict patency in prosthetic arterial grafts? *Br. J. Surg.*, **70**, 635–8.

Goldman, M., Leung, J. O., Aukland, A. *et al.* (1983b) ^{111}Indium platelet imaging, Doppler spectral analysis and angiography compared in patients with transient cerebral ischaemia. *Stroke*, **14**, 452–6.

Goodwin, D. A. (1978) Cell labelling with oxine chelates of radioactive metal ions: techniques and clinical implications. *J. Nucl. Med.*, **19**, 557–9.

Harker, L. A. and Finch, C. A. (1969) Thrombokinetics in man. *J. Clin. Invest.*, **48**, 963–74.

Harnsberger, H. R., Datz, F. L., Knochel, J. Q. and Taylor, A. T. (1982) Failure to detect extramedullary hematopoiesis during bone-marow imaging with indium-111 or technetium-99m sulfur colloid. *J. Nucl. Med.*, **23**, 589–91.

Hawker, R. J., Hawker L. M. and Wilkinson, A. R. (1980) Indium labelled human platelets: optimal method. *Clin. Sci.*, **58**, 243–8.

Heyns, A. du P., Lotter, M. G., Badenhorst, P. N. *et al.* (1980) Kinetics, distribution and sites of destruction of ^{111}In labelled human platelets. *Br. J. Haematol.*, **44**, 269–80.

Heyns, A. du P., Lotter, M. G., Kotze, H. F. *et al.* (1985) Kinetics, distribution and sites of destruction of ^{111}In-oxine labelled red cells in haemolytic anaemia. *J. Clin. Pathol.*, **38**, 128–32.

Hurley, P. J. (1975) Red cell and plasma volumes in normal adults. *J. Nucl. Med.*, **16**, 46–52.

International Committee for Standardization in Haematology (1971) Recommended methods for radioisotope red cell survival studies. *Br. J. Haematol.*, **21**, 241–50.

International Committee for Standardization in Haematology (1975) Recommended methods for surface counting to determine sites of red-cell destruction. *Br. J. Haematol.*, **30**, 249–54.

International Committee for Standardization in Haematology (1977) Recommended methods for radioisotope platelet survival studies. *Blood*, **50**, 1137–44.

International Committee for Standardization in Haematology (1980a) Recommended methods for the measurement of red-cell and plasma volume. *J. Nucl. Med.*, **21**, 793–800.

International Committee for Standardization in Haematology (1980b) Recommended methods for radioisotope red cell survival studies. *Br. J. Haematol.*, **45**, 659–66.

International Committee for Standardization in Haematology (1981) Recommended methods for the measurement of vitamin B_{12} absorption. *J. Nucl. Med.*, **22**, 1091–3.

Jones, J. and Mollison, P. L. (1978) Simple and efficient method of labelling red cells with ^{99m}Tc for determination of red cell volume. *Br. J. Haematol.*, **38**, 141–8.

Klausner, M. A., Hirsch, L. J., Leblond, P. F. *et al.* (1975) Contrasting splenic mechanisms in the blood clearance of red blood cells and colloidal particles. *Blood*, **46**, 965–76.

Klonizakis, I., Peters, A. M., Fitzpatrick, M. L. *et al.* (1980) Radionuclide distribution following injection of indium-111 labelled platelets. *Br. J. Haematol.*, **46**, 595–602.

Lewis, S. M. and Liu Yin, J. A. (1986) Blood volume studies. *Methods Hematol.*, **14**, 198–213.

Maddney, W. C., Boyer, J. L., Sen, N. N. *et al.* (1969) Plasma volume expansion in portal hypertension. *Johns Hopkins Med. J.*, **125**, 171–83.

Marsh, J. C. W., Liu Yin, J. A. and Lewis, S. M. (1987) Blood volume measurements in polycythaemia: when and why? *Clin. Lab. Haematol.*, **9**, 452–6.

Martin, B. A., Dahlby, R., Nicholls, I. and Hogg, J. C. (1981) Platelet sequestration in the lung with hemorrhagic shock and reinfusion in dogs. *J. Appl. Physiol.*, **50**, 1306–12.

Mayerson, H. S. (1965) Blood volume and its regulation. *Ann. Rev. Physiol.*, **27**, 307–22.

McIntyre, P. A., Larson, S., Eikman, E. A. *et al.* (1974) Comparison of the metabolism of iron labelled transferrin and indium labelled transferrin by the erythropoietic marrow. *J. Nucl. Med.*, **15**, 856–62.

McNeil, B. J., Rappeport, J. M. and Nathan, D. G. (1976) Indium chloride scintigraphy: an index of severity in patients with aplastic anaemia. *Br. J. Haematol.*, **34**, 599–604.

Mollison, P. L. (1979) *Blood Transfusion in Clinical Medicine*, 6th edn, Ch. 3, Blackwell, Oxford.

Mollison, P. L. (1984) Methods of determining the post

transfusion survival of stored red cells. *Transfusion*, **24**, 93–6.

Moroff, G., Sohmer, P. R. and Button, L. N. (1984) Proposed standardization of methods for determining the 24-hour survival of stored red cells. *Transfusion*, **24**, 109–14.

Moser, K. M. (1985) in *Radiolabelled Cellular Blood Elements* (ed. M. L. Thakur), Plenum Press, New York, pp. 155–76.

Moser, K. M., Spragg, R. G., Bender, F. *et al.* (1980) Study of factors that may condition scintigraphic detection of venous thrombi and pulmonary emboli with indium-111 labelled platelets. *J. Nucl. Med.*, **21**, 1051–8.

Mountford, P. J., Kettle, A. G., O'Doherty, M. J. *et al.* (1990) Comparison of Technetium ^{99m} leukocytes with Indium^{111} oxine leukocytes for localising intrabdominal sepsis. *J. Nucl. Med.*, **31**, 311–15.

Nadler, S. B., Hidalgo, J. U. and Bloch, T. (1962) Prediction of blood volume in normal human adults. *Surgery*, **51**, 224–32.

Najean, Y. and Cacchione, R. (1977) Blood volume in health and disease. *Clin. Haematol.*, **6**, 543–66.

Najean, Y., Cacchione, R., Dresch, C. and Rain, J. D. (1975) Methods of evaluating the sequestration site of red cells labelled with ^{51}Cr: a review of 96 cases. *Br. J. Haematol.*, **29**, 495–510.

Pavel, D. G., Zimmer, A. M. and Patterson, V. N. (1977) *In vivo* labelling of red blood cells with ^{99m}Tc: a new approach to blood pool visualization. *J. Nucl. Med.*, **18**, 305–8.

Pearson, T. C., Botterill, C. A., Glass, U. H. and Wetherley-Mein, G. (1984) Interpretation of measured red cell mass and plasma volume in males with elevated venous PCV values. *Scand. J. Haematol.*, **33**, 68–74.

Peters, A. M. (1986) in *Platelet Kinetics and Imaging* (eds A. du P. Heynes, P. N. Badenhorst and M. G. Lotter), CRC Press, Florida, pp. 71–96.

Peters, A. M. (1989) Imaging with white cells. *Clin. Radiol.*, **40**, 453–4.

Peters, A. M. and Lavender J. P. (1982) Factors controlling the intrasplenic transit of platelets. *Eur. J. Clin. Invest.*, **12**, 191–5.

Peters, A. M., Klonizakis, I., Lavender, J. P. and Lewis, S. M. (1980) Use of ^{111}Indium labelled platelets to measure spleen function. *Br. J. Haematol.*, **46**, 587–93.

Peters, A. M., Ryan, P. F. J., Klonizakis, I. *et al* (1982) Kinetics of heat damaged autologous red blood cells. *Scand. J. Haematol.*, **28**, 5–14.

Peters, A. M., Saverymuttu, S. H., Wonke, B. *et al.* (1984a) The interpretation of platelet kinetic studies for the identification of sites of abnormal platelet destruction. *Br. J. Haematol.*, **57**, 637–49.

Peters, A. M., Walport, M. J., Elkon, K. B. *et al.* (1984b) The comparative blood clearance kinetics of modified radiolabelled erythrocytes. *Clin. Sci.*, **66**, 55–62.

Peters, A. M., Lane, I. F., Sinclair, M. *et al.* (1985a) The effects of thromboxane antagonism on the transit time of platelets through the spleen. *Thromb. Haemost.*, **54**, 495–7.

Peters, A. M., Saverymuttu, S. H., Malik, F. *et al.* (1985b) Intrahepatic kinetics of indium-111-labelled platelets. *Thromb. Haemost.*, **54**, 595–8.

Peters, A. M., Saverymuttu, S. H., Keshavarzian, A. *et al.* (1985c) Splenic pooling of granulocytes. *Clin. Sci.*, **68**, 283–9.

Peters, A. M., Saverymuttu, S. H., Bell, R. N. and Lavender, J. P. (1985d) The kinetics of short-lived indium-111 radiolabelled platelets. *Scand. J. Haematol.*, **34**, 137–45.

Peters, A. M., Porter, J. B., Saverymuttu, S. H. (1985e) The kinetics of unmatched and HLA-matched 111-In-labelled homologous platelets in recipients with chronic marrow hypoplasia and anti-platelet immunity. *Br. J. Haematol.*, **60**, 117–27.

Peters, A. M., Saverymuttu, S. H., Danpure, H. J. and Osman, S. (1986a). Cell labelling. *Methods Haematol.*, **14**, 79–109.

Peters, A. M., Lavender, J. P., Needham, S. G. *et al.* (1986b) Imaging thrombus with a radiolabelled monoclonal antibody to platelets. *Br. Med. J.*, **293**, 1525–7.

Peters, A. M., Danpure, H. J., Osman, S. *et al.* (1986c) Preliminary clinical experience with Tc-99m HM-PAO for labelling leucocytes and imaging inflammation. *Lancet*, **ii**, 946–9.

Peters, A. M., Gunasekera, R. D., Henderson, B. L. *et al.* (1987) Non-invasive measurement of blood flow and extraction fraction. *Nucl. Med. Comm.* **8**, 823–37.

Pettit, J. (1977) Splenic function. *Clin. Haematol.*, **6**, 639–56.

Pettit, J. E., Lewis, S. M., Williams, E. D. *et al.* (1976) Quantitative studies of splenic erythropoiesis in polycythaemia vera and myelofibrosis. *Br. J. Haematol.*, **34**, 465–75.

Pettit, J. E., Lewis, S. M. and Nicholas, A. W. (1979) Transitional myeloproliferative disorder. *Br. J. Haematol.*, **43**, 167–84.

Radia, R., Peters, A. M., Deenmamode, M. *et al.* (1981) Measurement of red cell volume and splenic red cell pool using ^{113m}indium. *Br. J. Haematol.*, **49**, 587–91.

Retzlaff, J. A., Tauxe, W. N., Kieley, J. M. and Stroebel, C. F. (1969) Erythrocyte volume, plasma volume and lean body mass in adult men and women. *Blood*, **33**, 649–67.

Ricketts, C., Jacobs, A. and Cavill, I. (1975) Ferrokinetics and erythropoiesis in man: the measurement of effective erythropoiesis, ineffective erythropoiesis and red cell lifespan using ^{59}Fe. *Br. J. Haematol.*, **31**, 65–75.

Ries, C. A. and Price, D. C. (1974) ^{51}Cr platelet kinetics in thrombocytopenia: correlation between splenic sequestration of platelets and response to splenectomy. *Ann. Intern. Med.*, **80**, 702–7.

Robertson, J. S., Dewanjee, M. K., Brown, M. L., Fuster, V. and Chesebro, J. H. (1981) Distribution and dosimetry of ^{111}In-labelled platelets. *Radiology*, **140**, 169–76.

Ronai, P., Winchell, H. S., Anger, H. O. and Lawrence, J. H. (1969) Whole-body scanning of ^{59}Fe for evaluating body distribution of erythropoietic marrow, splenic sequestration of red cells and hepatic deposition of iron. *J. Nucl. Med.*, **10**, 469–74.

Saverymuttu, S. H., Peters, A. M., Danpure, H. J. *et al.* (1983a) Lung transit of 111-indium labelled granulocytes: relationships to labelling techniques. *Scand. J. Haematol.*, **30**, 151–60.

Saverymuttu, S. H., Peters, A. M., Pepys, M. B. *et al.* (1983b) Quantitative fecal indium-111 labelled leukocyte excretion with assessment of disease activity in Crohn's disease. *Gastroenterology*, **85**, 1333–9.

Saverymuttu, S. H., Peters, A. M., Keshavarzian, A. *et al.* (1985) The kinetics of 111-indium distribution following injection of 111-indium labelled autologous granulocytes. *Br. J. Haematol.*, **61**, 675–85.

Scheffel, U., Tsan, M. F., Mitchell, T. G. *et al.* (1982) Human platelets labelled with In-111-8-hydroxyquinoline: kinetics, distribution and estimates of radiation dose. *J. Nucl. Med.*, **23**, 149–56.

Schilling, R. F. (1953) Intrinsic factor studies. II. The effect of gastric juice on the urinary excretion of radioactivity after the oral administration of radioactive vitamin B_{12}. *J. Lab. Clin. Med.*, **42**, 860–6.

Schilling, R. F. (1986) Absorption and excretion studies. *Methods Hematol.*, **14**, 185–97.

Sinn, H. and Silvester, D. J. (1979) Simplified cell labelling with indium-111-acetylacetone. *Br. J. Radiol.*, **52**, 758–9.

Stratton, J. R., Thiele, B. L. and Ritchie, J. L. (1982) Platelet deposition on dacron aortic bifurcation grafts in man: quantitation with indium-111 platelet imaging. *Circulation*, **66**, 1287–93.

Taylor, H., Erickson, L., Henschel, A. and Keys, A. (1945) The effect of bed rest on the blood volume of normal young men. *Am. J. Physiol.*, **144**, 227–32.

Thakur, M. L. and Sedar, A. W. (1987) Ultrastructure of human platelets following indium-111 labelling in plasma. *Nucl. Med. Commun.*, **8**, 69–78.

Toghill, P. (1964) Red cell pooling in enlarged spleens. *Br. J. Haematol.*, **10**, 347–57.

Valeri, C. R., Cooper, A. G. and Pivacek, L. D. (1973) Limitation of measuring blood volume with iodinated I-125 serum albumin. *Arch. Int. Med.*, **132**, 534–8.

Wadenvik, H. and Kutti, J. (1987) The effect of an adrenaline infusion on the splenic blood flow and intrasplenic platelet kinetics. *Br. J. Haematol.*, **67**, 187–92.

Walport, M. J., Peters, A. M., Elkon, K. B. *et al.* (1985) The splenic extraction ratio of antibody coated erythrocytes and its response to plasma exchange and pulse methylprednisolone. *Clin. Exp. Immunol.*, **65**, 465–73.

Wennesland, R., Brown, E., Hopper, J. Jr *et al.* (1959) Red cell, plasma and blood volume in healthy men measured by radiochromium (^{51}Cr) cell tagging and hematocrit: influence of age, somatotype and habits of physical activity on the variance after regression of volumes to height and weight combined. *J. Clin. Invest.*, **38**, 1065–77.

Wochner, R. D., Adatepe, M., van Amburg, A. and Potchen, E. J. (1970) New method for estimation of plasma volume with the use of the distribution space of transferrin- ^{113m}indium. *J. Lab. Clin. Med.*, **75**, 711–21.

Wright, R. R., Tono, M. and Pollycove, M. (1975) Blood volume. *Semin. Nucl. Med.*, **5**, 63–78.

CHAPTER SIXTEEN

Body composition

R. F. Jewkes

16.1 INTRODUCTION

Radionuclide studies have made a major contribution to our understanding of the changes that the body undergoes in health and disease. Moore *et al.* (1963) used them to develop their concept of the body being made up of a number of distinguishable physiological compartments. First, the body cell mass, the 'engine', which comprises all the cells of the body, characteristically oxygen consuming and energy exchanging. Second, the extracellular tissues, the 'chassis', with a predominantly supporting role and characteristically very low metabolic activity. Third, the body fat, neutral triglyceride. Much of the extracellular compartment is fluid and includes the blood plasma, the interstitial fluid, cerebrospinal fluid, localized effusions and digestive juices.

Investigations with administered radionuclides depend on the dilution principle (Table 16.1). If an administered radioactive marker spreads itself evenly throughout a part of the body, then the mass or space through which it spreads can be calculated from its eventual dilution.

The starting point for a comprehensive measurement of body composition is total body water measured with tritiated water. The total body water normally comprises about 73% of the weight of hydrated body tissue, that is excluding the non-aqueous constituents such as bone mineral and the triglyceride stores.

Total body water (TBW) is normally approximately equally divided between the extracellular (ECW) and the intracellular (ICW) compartments. There are many markers which spread predominantly in the ECW, of which radiobromine (^{82}Br or ^{77}Br) is probably the most popular. Unfortunately there is no unique marker for ICW. It must be calculated by subtraction of the measured ECW from TBW. The plasma volume can be measured separately by the dilution of radioiodinated human serum albumin.

Another view of the cellular and extracellular compartments comes from the measurement of the two major cations in the body. Body potassium is almost entirely intracellular and radiopotassium appears to mix fairly freely with 98% of it. Body sodium is predominantly located in the extracellular compartment with only a small intracellular contribution. Radiosodium mixes with about 70% of total body sodium within 24 h. The other 30% is mostly within bone mineral and metabolically less accessible.

Table 16.1 Radionuclide investigation of body composition

Aspects of body composition	*Relevant measurement*	*Radionuclide or radiopharmaceutical*
1. Total body mass	Body weight	
2. Aqueous compartment	Total body water	THO
3. Body cell mass	Total exchangeable potassium	^{42}K, ^{43}K
	Intracellular water (calculated)	
4. Extracellular compartment	Total exchangeable sodium	^{24}Na, ^{22}Na
	Extracellular water	^{82}Br, ^{77}Br
	Plasma volume	^{125}I-labelled human serum albumin
5. Body fat	Calculated from body weight and total body water	

It is of limited value to make any of these measurements in isolation. Much more information can be gained by using the radionuclides simultaneously or in close sequence to obtain a comprehensive view of body composition. Such studies can usually be completed in 24–48 h and there are many descriptions of such combined studies in the literature (Moore *et al.*, 1963; Veall and Vetter, 1958; Skrabal *et al.*, 1970; Smith and Edmonds, 1987). Making certain assumptions it is possible to calculate from these measurements the total body fat, body solids other than fat, and dry skeletal weight. The measurements can be compared to predicted values (Skrabal *et al.*, (1973) or using the system of Moore *et al.* (1963) to a comprehensive prediction of body composition derived from the patient's age, sex and weight. In most cases this latter is more satisfactory as the 'normal range' for each measurement tends to be too wide to be helpful (Fig. 16.1).

Table 16.2 Body composition measurements; mean values in normal subjects related to body weight

Percentage of total body weight	*Men*	*Women*
Total body water	*59–51	*51–47
Extracellular water	24	22
Intracellular water	*31–26	24
mmol kg^{-1} body weight		
Total exchangeable sodium	40	37
Total exchangeable potassium	*48–37	*38–30
TENa/TEK ratio	†0.8–1.0	1.0

*Decreasing with advancing age.
†Increasing with advancing age.
After Moore *et al.*, 1963.

16.2 SOME COMMON PATTERNS OF BODY COMPOSITION

16.2.1 SEX, AGE AND RACE

There are considerable differences in body composition between men and women, summed up by saying that men, at least before middle age, tend to be much more muscular and so have relatively high indices of body cell mass. Women have less skeletal muscle and proportionately more fat. The relative cell dominance of the two sexes is indicated by the ratio of the total exchangeable sodium (TENa) to total exchangeable potassium (TEK). This is typically 0.8 for young men and 1.0 for women. Some comparative figures for body composition measurements for men and women are given in Table 16.2. Advancing age has relatively little effect on the body composition of women except that obesity becomes more common. Men change more fundamentally as skeletal muscle mass shrinks after middle age with the result that the differences in body composition between the sexes diminish.

There is very little known about differences in body composition between races though there are hints that these may be significant (Kojo Addae *et al.*, 1978). Body composition of West African and West Indian negroes shows an exaggeration of the predominance of skeletal muscle in young men, and a relative diminution in body fat. There is some evidence that this is also found, though to a lesser degree, in West African women. Caution is therefore desirable in applying published 'normal values' to such subjects, especially in the young.

16.2.2 OBESITY

The body's neutral triglyceride store varies from 10% of body weight in a particularly fit muscular male to 50% of body weight in an extremely obese individual. Excess fat, however, hides the state of the rest of the body. The absolute quantities of body water and body electrolytes will appear low relative to body weight, but in the fit obese subject these quantities will appropriate to each other, and match some lower body weight which may be regarded as the subject's 'normal'.

However, some subjects, particularly the elderly, show a body composition which is less satisfactory. Although the extracellular tissue is preserved, the large fat deposits hide a shrinkage in the body cell mass, as shown by changes of the indicators of the cellular compartments. ICW falls as a proportion of TBW and the TENa/TEK ratio rises. Such subjects usually show a decline in physical performance and frequently manifest intercurrent diseases such as hypertension and diabetes.

16.2.3 BODY WASTING

Wasting is probably the commonest response of body composition to disease. There is obvious loss of body fat and cell mass, mainly skeletal muscle.

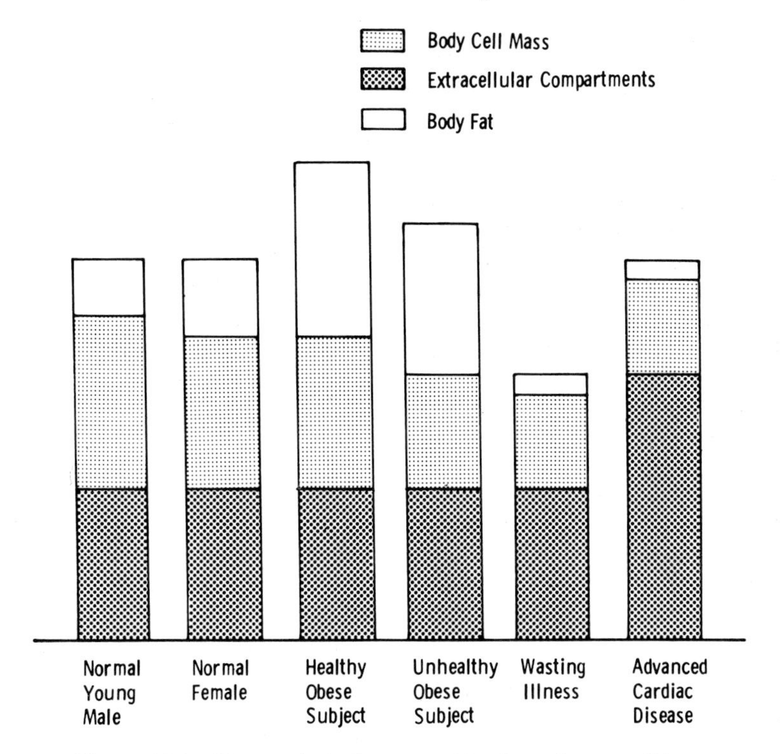

Figure 16.1 Changes in body composition in various conditions.

The extracellular tissue is, however, maintained at a level appropriate to the weight of the patient before illness. The loss of fat is shown by a rise in total body water relative to body weight. TEK and ICW, the indices of body cell mass, shrink, while TENa and ECW, the indices of extracellular tissue, are relatively increased. The TENa/TEK ratio rises from a normal of 1.0, and in severe illness may reach 2.0 or even higher.

The plasma volume rises relative to body weight as a result of two processes. First, it is maintained as part of the maintenance of extracellular tissue as a whole. Secondly, it may rise to compensate for a fall in red cell mass, as most severe disease processes are associated with anaemia. The basic pattern of wasting may be modified by the underlying disease. Surgical conditions of the gastrointestinal tract may predispose to potassium loss in excess of the loss of body cell mass as shown by the intracellular water. Disorders of the heart, lungs, liver and kidneys may cause retention of salt and water with consequent expansion of the extracellular compartment (Figure 16.1).

16.2.4 RESPONSE TO INJURY OR EXTENSIVE INFLAMMATORY DISEASE

The immediate effect of injury may be external blood loss, but of equal importance may be the formation of sequestrated extracellular fluid volume in the form of inflammatory exudate, traumatic oedema or haematoma. In some cases of peritonitis, multiple fractures or extensive burns, 10, 20 or even 50% of total extracellular fluid volume may be so sequestered. The total extracellular fluid volume does not alter but the 'effective' extracellular fluid is considerably reduced, best shown by a fall in plasma volume.

The immediate response, aided by effective treatment, is restoration of the 'effective' extracellular fluid volume by expanding the ECW by the amount equivalent to that 'lost'. ECW, TENa and TBW measured at this stage will be high. There then follows a period of post-traumatic catabolism, frequently aggravated by relative starvation. The body cell mass is eroded with an absolute fall in TEK and ICW and body fat. The TENa/TEK ratio rises progressively throughout.

The first obvious healing process is the reabsorption of sequestered extracellular fluid and excretion via the kidneys. The TENa and ECW return towards pre-illness values. The rebuilding of body cell mass occurs later. Full restoration of TEK and ICW may take months as muscular tissue is resynthesized and body fat stores laid down.

16.2.5 DISTURBANCE OF BODY TONICITY

The body is a homogeneous osmotic system with electrolytes by far the most important determinants of body fluid osmotic pressure. Sodium and potassium together represent 92% of soluble cations and so body fluid osmotic pressure closely follows the concentrations of these two elements.

Anions are of course present in equivalent amounts but are more diverse and their relative quantities more variable. Chloride is the predominant anion in the extracellular water but there are substantial quantities of carbonate and proteins. The non-electrolyte crystalloids in body fluid, such as glucose, urea, creatinine and amino acids, contribute little to the osmolality of body fluids in normal subjects. However, in advanced liver disease and renal failure, these and other unidentified crystalloids may be present in such quantities that the concentration of plasma sodium falls to a very low level as a compensatory mechanism.

16.2.6 HYPOTONICITY

The quantity of water in the body is nicely gauged to balance the quantity of osmotically active substances. This is shown by the ratio (TENa + TEK)/TBW, which is remarkably constant in health. However, in many serious disease states hypotonicity may develop, as shown by a fall in plasma sodium. In a vast majority of cases this is an expression of inappropriate retention of water, as renal excretion is impaired for reasons that are often poorly understood. It is usual for the TENa to be increased though the ECW is proportionately even more expanded.

Rarely, the condition is aggravated by loss of sodium or potassium, most commonly via the gastrointestinal tract. When potassium loss occurs disproportionate to any decrease in body cell mass, the intracellular hypotonicity usually initi-

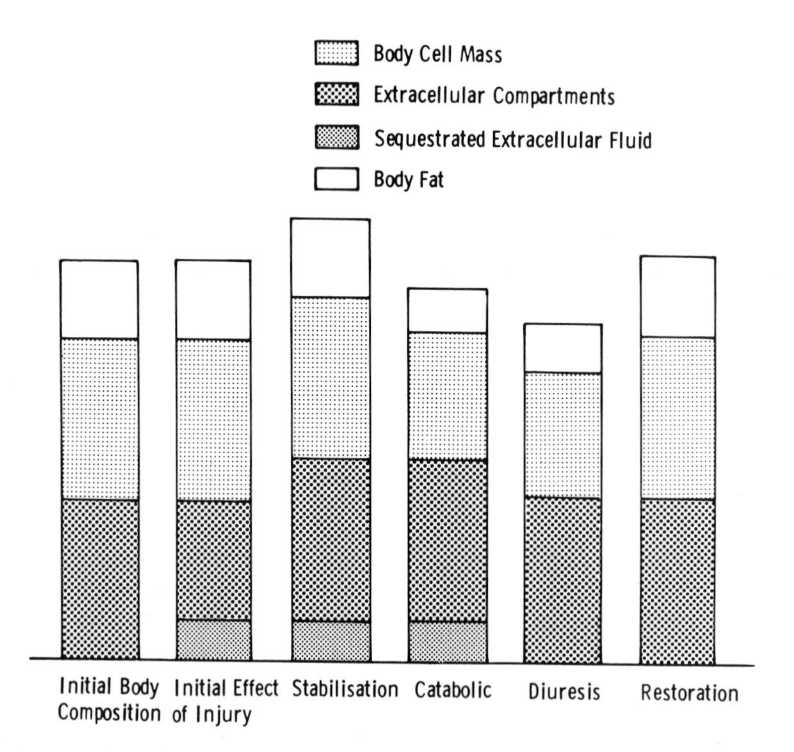

Figure 16.2 Changes in response to severe injury and subsequent recovery.

ates a corresponding extracellular hypotonicity, with a fall in plasma sodium. Significant movement of sodium into the cells to replace the lost potassium is probably a very rare event.

16.2.7 HYPERTONICITY

Hypertonicity is infrequent and almost always the result of relative water loss. The most common cause is probably a solute-induced diuresis as occurs with the hyperglycaemia of uncontrolled diabetes, but which may also occur following overenthusiastic tube feeding regimes providing high protein loads or from excessive catabolism following extensive trauma, burns or gastrointestinal bleeding. Sometimes hypertonicity is a result of excessive water loss from lungs or skin, perhaps associated with water deprivation in an unconscious subject. Very rarely is it due to excessive salt administration or failure of antidiuretic hormone.

16.3 THE PLACE OF BODY COMPOSITION STUDIES

Body composition studies using radionuclides have delineated the changes produced by a great range of disease processes. However, in spite of the fact that they have been available for over 20 years, they have not really moved out of the research environment into everyday clinical practice. The reasons are partly technical but also largely physiological.

What is wanted in clinical practice is a single test which can be rapidly carried out on a patient and which will:

1. measure body fluid and accurately quantify intra- and extracellular water, and allow an accurate estimate of the appropriateness of these volumes;
2. identify and quantify the degree of tissue wasting and indicate if recent or longstanding;
3. indicate any unusual abnormalities of concentration of body composition or elements, particularly intracellular potassium.

Unfortunately, no such test exists. Multiple radionuclide studies can answer most of these questions but are cumbersome and relatively prolonged, requiring a patient to be in a stable state for measurement. There is usually delay before the results are available.

After completion of the test there is the task of interpretation of the results, which may not be straightforward. First, there is the problem of establishing the 'normal' for comparison. The 'normal range' for each measurement is frequently too large to be useful. However, it is usually possible to work out a coherent body composition prediction for any individual (Moore *et al.*, 1963). Though these predictions are based on a fairly large study of 'normals' from many centres, the combined results may not be appropriate to particular populations, especially non-European races.

The first requirement is knowledge of the subject's body weight. Current weight, however, may be only a very approximate guide to the patient's healthy weight and normal body build, and may need to be interpreted with care. Total body water is the starting point from which to determine the amount of body fat on the assumption that the non-adipose body structure will be approximately 73% water, normally a very constant figure. But this may not be so in severely waterlogged patients. There is therefore the possibility of serious error for such patients and in repeated measurements in those who may be markedly improving or deteriorating.

A further problem is the absence of a direct measurement of intracellular water. Though TBW measurements are reasonably precise, doubts can sometimes remain over the methods for ECW. Many radioactive and non-radioactive tracers have been advocated for this: radiosulphate, inulin, thiosulphate, manitol, sucrose, ^{51}Cr-labelled ethylenediaminetetraacetic acid (EDTA), thiocyanate, radiochloride and radioactive and non-radioactive bromide. These distribute in spaces ranging from 15 to 30% cent of body weight (Swales, 1975). Clearly the ease with which these molecules penetrate the extremities of the extracellular fluid varies. Furthermore these substances may extend beyond the ECW. There is often some cellular penetration and it is usual to compensate for this in the case of bromine by multiplying the measured distribution space by 0.95. This, however, cannot be more than an approximation and intracellular penetration may increase markedly in very sick patients. In addition, gastrointestinal fluid accumulation could cause loss of radioactivity from the ECW into fluid volumes that are actually 'outside' the body.

Sodium, the indicator of extracellular tissue, is occasionally in doubt. Only 80–90% of the 24 h exchangeable sodium is in ECW. The location of the other 10–20% is uncertain and may not always be the same in all patients. Most of it is in the bone mineral in normal subjects but there is sodium associated with other extracellular structures such as proteins and mucopolysaccharides. There is a small amount of sodium which appears to be intracellular and this varies between different tissues, being higher in smooth muscle than skeletal muscle. Again this is of small importance in normal subjects but may assume importance in disease (Carroll *et al.*, 1965).

Finally, the reliability of total exchangeable potassium in some situations has been questioned (Telfer *et al.*, 1975) because of discrepancies between TEK and total-body potassium as measured in a whole-body counter (see below). It appears that the mixing time for radiopotassium in the total-body potassium may be occasionally prolonged and TEK may be underestimated if samples for measurement are taken too early.

This catalogue of doubts certainly overestimates the difficulties encountered in studies confined to homogeneous populations whose body composition has not been grossly distorted. Also the studies will have increased validity when repeated on individuals. But clearly reliable results are only obtained as a result of constant watchfulness.

When it comes to the applications of these studies we find that a wide variety of clinical conditions produce a relatively limited range of changes in body composition. Illness of almost any kind tends to be associated with loss of body fat and body cell mass, with maintenance or frequently expansion of the extracellular compartment. Though measurements have demonstrated, and more particularly quantified, the changes, it is clear that a knowledge of the expected trends is often sufficient for effective management, without the need for specific measurements. Should a more rapid or reliable test appear this complacent clinical view may change markedly, but at present the tests are too laborious to be routinely applied.

16.4 TOTAL-BODY POTASSIUM BY MEASUREMENT OF ENDOGENOUS RADIOPOTASSIUM (^{40}K)

Natural potassium is faintly radioactive from its content of the nuclide ^{40}K (0.12%) but this very low level of radioactivity in the human body can be measured. It requires a very sensitive whole-body counter which unfortunately is rarely to be found in nuclear medicine departments, but is available in a number of larger medical physics or health physics institutions. The very low level of radioactivity limits the accuracy of the measurements to the order of ±4% but this is comparable to that of measurement of exchangeable potassium (Boddy *et al.*, 1971). The advantages of this are the convenience of measurements without the need to administer radioactivity, and the ability to complete the measurement in under an hour.

16.5 ASPECTS OF BODY COMPOSITION DETERMINED WITH THE AID OF WHOLE-BODY NEUTRON ACTIVATION

A further development of the availability of sensitive whole-body counters has been the study of body composition after induction of radioactivity by whole-body neutron activation, using neutrons from a reactor, cyclotron or neutron generator. The great problem is the large number of different radionuclides produced, some of those of potential use being very short-lived. However, the technique has successfully measured body content of sodium, chloride, nitrogen, calcium and phosphorus (Cohn and Dombrowski, 1971; Boddy *et al.*, 1973). The extensive facilities required will make it unlikely that this attractive technique will be widely available in the foreseeable future.

REFERENCES

Boddy, K., King, P. C., Tothill, P. *et al.* (1971) Measurement of total body potassium with a shadow shield whole-body counter: calibration and errors. *Phys. Med. Biol.*, **16**, 275–82.

Boddy, K., Holloway, I. and Elliott, A. (1973) A simple facility for total body *in vivo* activation analysis. *Int. J. Appl. Radiat. Isot.*, **24**, 428–30.

Carroll, H. J., Gotterer, R. and Altshuler, B. (1965) Exchangeable sodium, body potassium, and body water in previously edematous cardiac patients: evidence for osmotic activation of cation. *Circulation*, **32**, 185–92.

Kojo Addae, S., Dakubu, S., Larmie, E. T. *et al.* (1978) Total body water, total exchangeable sodium and related variables in the Ghanaian. *Clin. Sci. Mol. Med.*, **54**, 477–9.

Moore, F. D., Oleson, K. H., McMurrey, J. D. *et al.* (1963) *The Body Cell Mass and Its Supporting Environment*. Saunders, Philadelphia.

Skrabal, K., Arnot, R. N., Helus, F. *et al.* (1970) A

method for simultaneous electrolyte investigations in man using 77Br, 43K and 24Na. *Int. J. Appl. Radiat. Isot.*, **21**, 183–91.

Skrabal, K., Arnot, R. N. and Joplin, G. F. (1973) Equations for the prediction of normal values for exchangeable sodium, exchangeable potassium, extracellular water and total body water. *Br. Med. J.*, **2**, 37–8.

Smith, T. and Edmonds, C. J. (1987) Measurement of exchangeable sodium: 22Na or 24Na? *Nucl. Med. Commun.*, **8**, 655–9.

Swales, J. D. (1975) *Sodium Metabolism in Disease*. Lloyd Luke Medical Books, London, p. 12.

Telfer, N., Weiner, J. M. and Merrill, Q. (1975), Distribution of sodium and potassium in chronic obstructive pulmonary disease. *Am. Rev. Resp. Dis.*, **111**, 166.

Veall, N. and Vetter, H. (1958) *Radioisotope Techniques in Clinical Research and Diagnosis*. Butterworth, London.

CHAPTER SEVENTEEN

Special clinical problems in paediatrics

D. L. Gilday

17.1 INTRODUCTION

Paediatric nuclear medicine has quite a different mix of studies than does the average adult practice (Table 17.1).

Performing effective nuclear medicine procedures in the paediatric population requires certain modifications of techniques used when studying adult patients. The modifications can be categorized under the following headings:

1. child interaction
2. sedation
3. injection techniques
4. radiopharmaceutical dosage
5. image recording.

17.1.1 CHILD INTERACTION

The reaction and response of a child to a nuclear medicine procedure is largely dependent on the approach of the staff towards that individual, the technique used in performing the study and the general environment of the department. All staff members dealing with patients should have a calm, relaxed manner with a kind, confident and sympathetic approach.

All patients old enough to comprehend should have their procedure explained to them in words appropriate to their level of understanding. Positive aspects of the study should be emphasized, negative aspects minimized. It is crucial never to mislead the child about what is about to happen. A child's trust in the staff may be difficult to obtain; once obtained it is easily jeopardized.

Table 17.1 Distribution of studies by system

Renal	51%
Skeleton	18%
GI	7%
CSF	5%
Lung	3%
Brain	3%
Miscellaneous	13%

Maintaining close physical contact with the patient and talking to them while the study is being performed distracts their attention from the procedure itself and often gains greater cooperation. Consoling the child is frequently helpful. Encouraging the child to watch their picture on the television monitor, providing them with toys, soothers and used saline syringes goes a long way towards achieving a successful result. We have found that providing an FM stereo Walkman for older children having a single-photon emission computed tomography (SPECT) study does wonders for gaining cooperation and lack of motion.

Parents are usually present in the department unless the procedure requires a sterile field. It has been our experience that with well-trained staff parental involvement is rarely required but the child is usually much happier with a parent(s) present. Some children who are a disciplinary problem are more uncooperative when a parent is present. In these circumstances we ask the parent to stay in the waiting room.

Careful restraint is frequently necessary in the younger patient but should be used in moderation. Babies can be restrained by the use of sandbags alongside the body and across the knees and arms. Wrapping the baby in a 'papoose'-like manner with blankets is often the best approach. This provides adequate restraint without causing discomfort. Older uncooperative children are best immobilized with restrainers strapped around the stretcher top using Velcro straps.

17.1.2 SEDATION

If moderate restraint is not successful then sedation is required for a technically satisfactory study.

This is especially true for SPECT studies as the sandbags cause attenuation and the procedure is lengthy. Sedation is recommended in overly anxious patients who refuse to cooperate, very young or hyperactive patients who are unable to remain still and retarded patients who lack the mental capacity to follow simple instructions.

Sedation may take several forms. Intramuscular Nembutal (pentobarbital sodium 6 mg kg^{-1} in patients weighing less than 15 kg, 5 mg kg^{-1} in larger children up to 100 mg, after which the dose should be increased more gradually) administered 30 min prior to imaging works best in the majority of patients. It has the desired 'knockout' effect which is much preferred to the 'calming' effect of milder sedatives, without causing major cardiorespiratory depression. Children usually awake within 2 h. With all sedatives, the child's cardiac and respiratory status must be closely monitored. We currently use an automated cardiorespiratory monitor.

Nembutal is contraindicated in neonates less than 2 months of age. This group lacks adequate levels of the liver enzymes which are required to metabolize Nembutal before it acts *in vivo*. In place of Nembutal we use an elixir of Phenergan (promethazine) and chloral hydrate, 30–45 min before scanning. The effect is less pronounced than with Nembutal but it is usually adequate and the patient arouses readily.

Valium and Nembutal suppositories have all been found to be inadequate. None produces the deep sleep required to perform nuclear medicine procedures on the patient. When all else fails, intravenous Nembutal or Valium (diazepam) is usually the best of the very strong sedatives, as it can be titrated to the child's sedation level.

17.1.3 INJECTION TECHNIQUES

Injection of radiopharmaceuticals in small children presents several minor problems, all of which are easily surmounted by modifying techniques used in adults. Very small children will be completely covered by the head of a large field of view camera. This increases the child's anxiety and makes injection difficult. This can often be solved by placing the child supine on the stretcher top and having the camera underneath. Lucite stretcher tops prevent excessive attenuation of photons. In smaller children or head, feet or hand imaging the camera collimator can act as an extension of the stretcher.

Finding a suitable vein for intravenous injections is rarely a problem providing several points are remembered. Although the anticubital fossa frequently has the largest vein, the elbow is less easily immobilized than the hand or foot and the latter are often preferable injection sites. Scalp veins are also easily accessible but are used as a last resort as a small area of hair must be shaved to find them. Jugular injections are mandatory for left-to-right shunt evaluations and are also useful in procedures where repeated blood samplings are required (e.g. glomerular filtration rate (GFR) determination), when the child's other veins have been used for repeated venipunctures in the past.

Our injection apparatus is a 12 cm^3 syringe of saline connected with extension tubing to a three-way stop-cock to which is also connected the syringe of radiopharmaceutical and a butterfly (23 or 25 gauge) needle. This allows the dose syringe to be completely isolated from the saline while the needle is inserted into the vein. Once the needle is properly positioned (confirmed by injecting some saline into the patient) the injection is carried out by pushing the bolus into the extension set and then forcing it through the needle by injecting the contents of the saline syringe.

17.1.4 RADIOPHARMACEUTICAL DOSAGE

The amount of radioactivity can be readily calculated by referring to Figure 17.1. The patient's dose is determined by weight and the percentage of the standard adult dose is determined according to the patient's body surface area. This dose calculation permits distribution of tracer per unit area of organ rather than per kilogram of body weight.

It is very important to establish a minimum dose for each radiopharmaceutical. To get an adequate study, especially a dynamic one, there have to be enough photons detected per unit time to adequately assess the patient's problem. It is better to ensure a slightly higher delivered radiation dose than to have an uninterpretable study. The risk of the higher radiation dose is negligible, especially if we have helped the patient.

17.2 IMAGE RECORDING

If a computer is available there are major advantages in recording all image data into the computer. First, no repeat imaging is required if there are film processing problems as the images may be

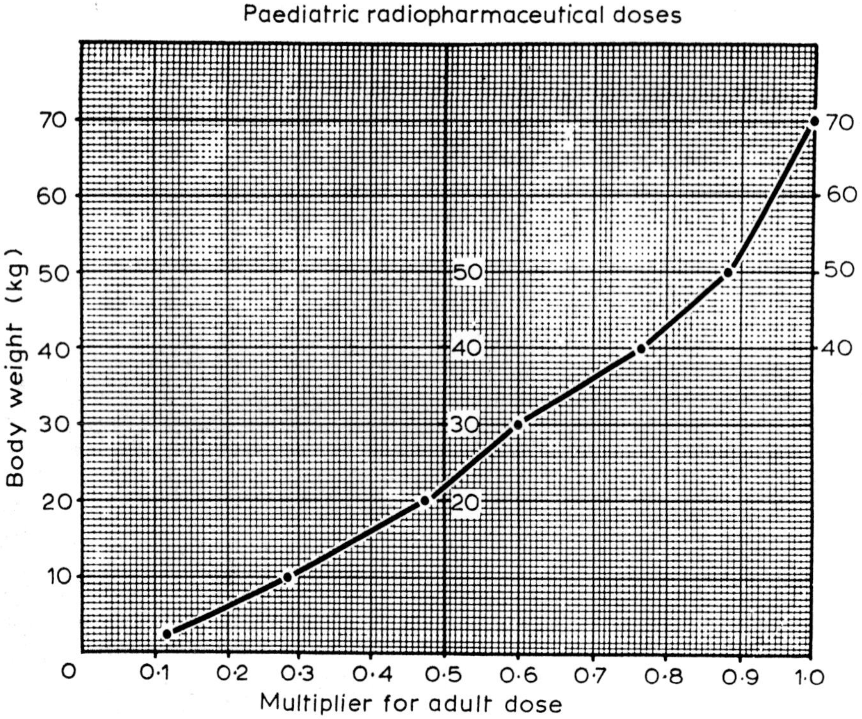

Figure 17.1 Radiopharmaceutical dosage schedule based on a body surface area using weight to determine the percentage of adult dose to administer.

re-recorded on the film imager. Second, the same data (image) may be displayed (filmed) using different windows, eliminating the need for repeat views in bone imaging of the ends of long bones (growth zones).

17.3 LOCOMOTOR PROBLEMS

The major indication for imaging the osseous system other than in malignancies is to determine the cause of bone pain. This is very often done after all the traditional investigations have failed to detect any significant abnormality. Today we recommend and follow a policy at the Hospital for Sick Children that if the plain films are normal then the bone scan is the next procedure. In spinal problems this is always done by high-resolution SPECT imaging. Our technique is fairly standard except that we always perform a three-phase study consisting of blood flow, blood pool and delayed images. The highest resolution system is used to obtain the best images.

17.3.1 AVASCULAR NECROSIS OF THE FEMORAL HEAD

Avascular necrosis of the femoral head, as in Legg–Perthes disease, is usually detected radiologically. However, in some cases the radiographs are normal when there is a very definite absence of blood flow to the femoral head (D'Anigelis *et al.*, 1975). We have found that the children who present with the clinical symptoms of transient synovitis fit into one of two categories. The first is that of a typical transient synovitis with mild hyperaemia involving the whole of the hip joint (acetabulum and femoral head). The second and much less frequent scan finding is that of partial or total absence of radiotracer in the femoral head. These children who present as if they have transient synovitis in fact have Legg–Perthes disease. Radiographs subsequently become abnormal sometime between 6 and 15 months. In a 24-month period a total of 105 scans were done for suspected synovitis or Legg–Perthes; seven showed decreased radioactivity in the femoral head (five had normal and two had equivocal

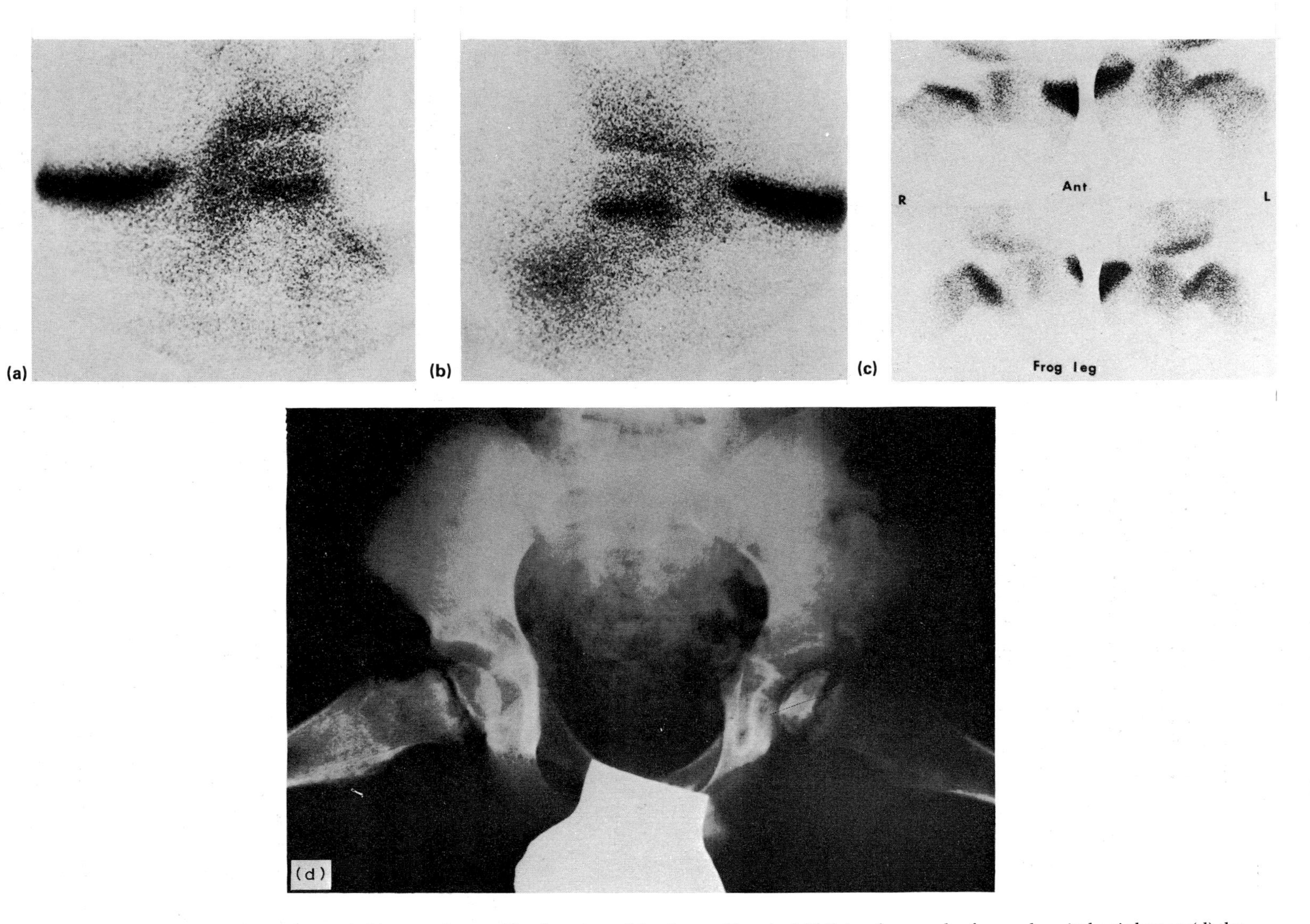

Figure 17.2 Legg–Perthes disease: (a, b) normal magnification view of the femoral heads; (c) bilateral avascular femoral capital epiphyses; (d) the radiograph demonstrated a typical Legg–Perthes involvement on the left and probably a normal right one.

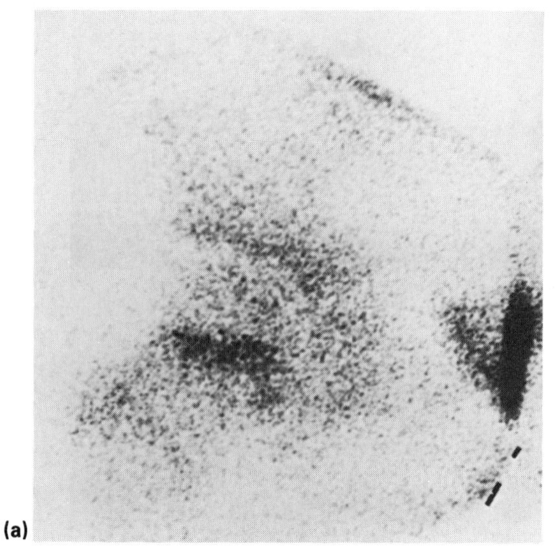
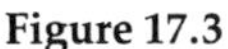

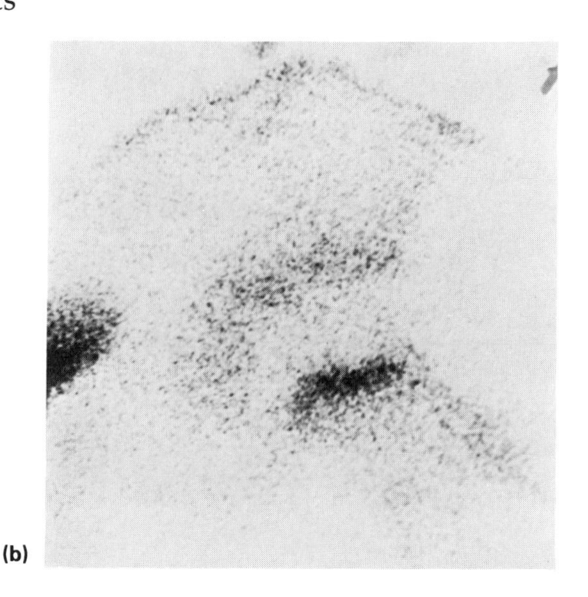

(a) (b)

Figure 17.3

radiographs). Thirty-six patients with Legg–Perthes were studied to stage the disease. Patients with synovitis showed either normal uptake or slight diffuse increase of the affected hip (Figure 17.2); none with these appearances later developed Legg–Perthes disease. Those with Legg–Perthes showed either partial or total absence of radiotracer in the femoral head initially (Figure 17.2). When revascularization occurs, a band of increased activity is seen laterally in the head. Since the bone-scan abnormalities antedate the radiographic changes by several months, we feel that the scan in the initial stages is a very good differentiator of whether or not the child will develop the classical radiological changes of Legg–Perthes disease.

17.4 INFECTION

Septic arthritis of the hip can frequently cause symptoms very similar to Legg–Perthes disease or transient synovitis. The important feature of this entity is that it may cause compression of the arterial supply to the proximal femoral capital epiphysis (Figure 17.3). When this occurs, there will be decreased blood flow and thus decreased tracer accumulation within the femoral head. This appearance in the scan is seen as a reduction in femoral capital epiphyseal activity in the pinhole magnification images which we still find better than SPECT imaging. This is a surgical emergency and requires the decompression of the hip joint by a drainage of the pus. Subsequently, the hip will become hyperaemic, which is the normal response to inflammation and infection.

In children, the diagnosis of osteomyelitis is frequently difficult. The child may present with bone pain, joint tenderness, soft tissue swelling and erythema, fever and bacteraemia, but the differentiation from pure cellulitis may be difficult. Unfortunately, the radiological examination may yield a wide range of findings: normal, soft tissue swelling and, in some, the frank bone changes of osteomyeltis. The therapeutic management of osteomyelitis usually involves a minimum of 21 days on intravenous antibiotics whereas cellulitis usually requires only 10 days of therapy. Therefore, it is imperative to make the correct diagnosis as soon as possible.

Using combined 'blood pool' and bone imaging, it is possible to differentiate osteomyelitis from cellulitis and to do so very early in the course of the patient's illness (Gilday *et al.*, 1975). The typical bone scan appearance of osteomyelitis (Figure 17.4) is a well-defined focus of increased radioactivity within bone, associated with an identical area of hyperaemia in the 'blood pool' images. Occasionally, the focal increase is superimposed on a more diffuse increase secondary to generalized hyperaemia. This appears to be quite specific for osteomyelitis and is readily differentiated from the patterns of cellulitis and septic arthritis. The 'blood pool' images are less valuable in the spine due to the underlying abdominal and thoracic organs. The bone images easily demonstrate the abnormal vertebral bodies involved in

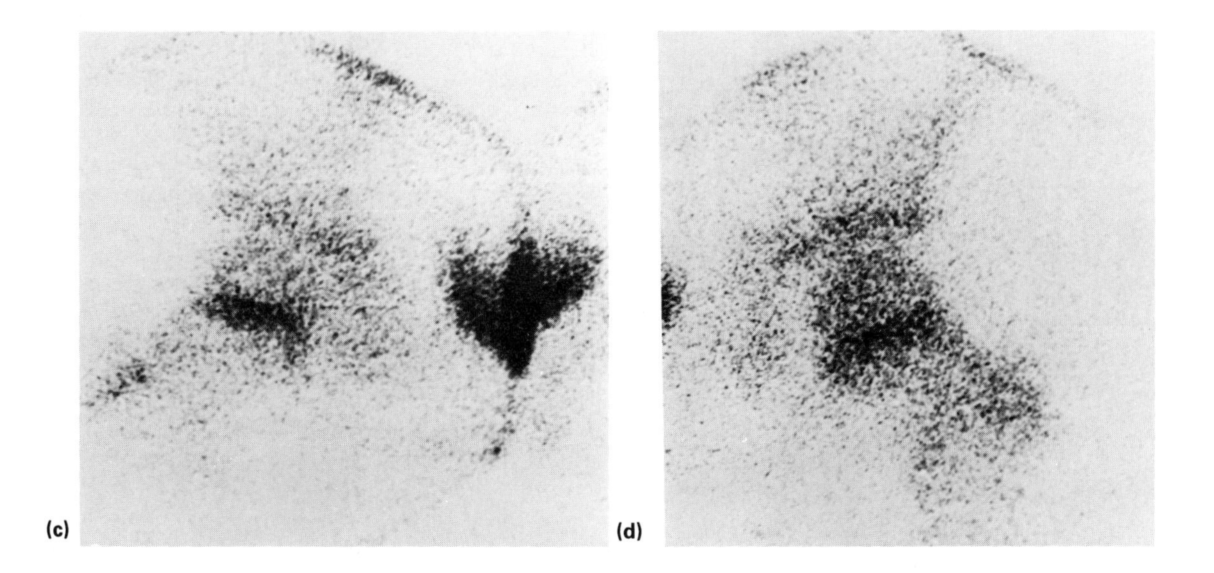

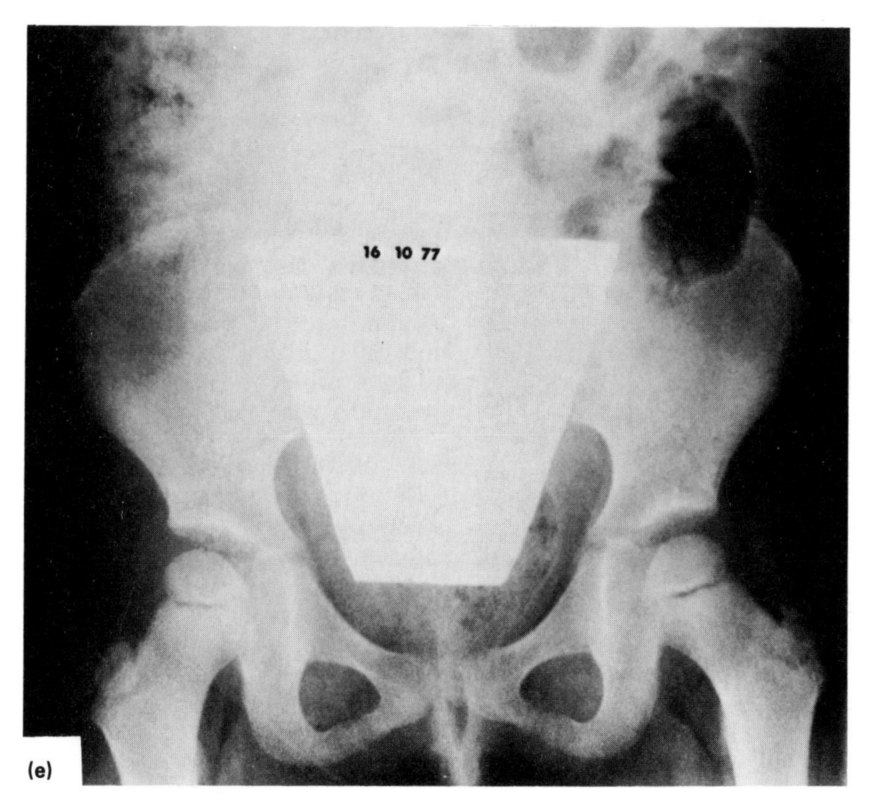

Figure 17.3 Septic arthritis. Initially the left femoral capital epiphysis showed reduced tracer accumulation (b) and after surgical relief of the increased intracapsular pressure there was increased tracer metabolism in the femoral head (d) indicating a return of blood flow.

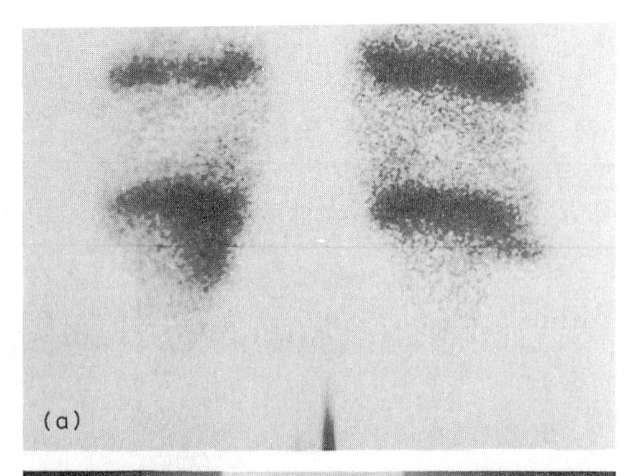

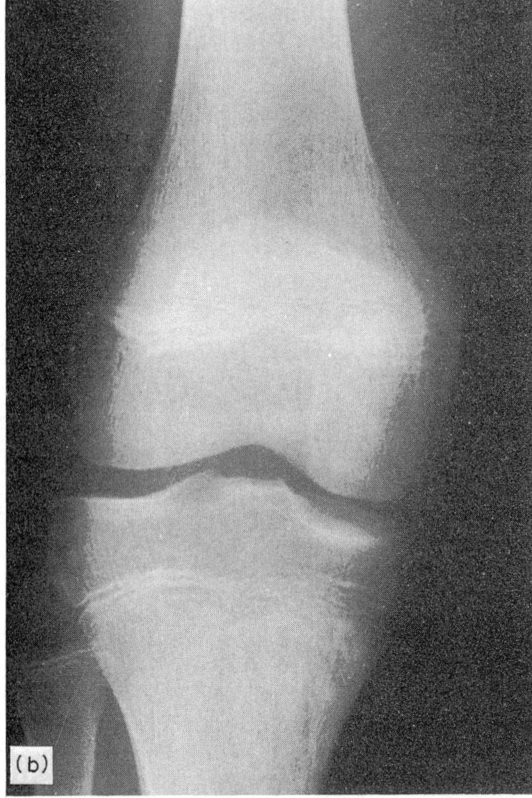

Figure 17.4 Acute osteomyelitis. There is focal increased tracer metabolism medially in the proximal metaphysis of the right tibia (a). This is typical in location and appearance of acute osteomyelitis. Radiographic changes became evident seven days after the bone scan (b).

the diskitis–osteomyelitis, usually confirming the radiological diagnosis of diskitis (Figure 17.5).

The appearance of cellulitis was that of a diffuse increase in radioactivity involving both the soft tissues and bone. This was readily apparent in both the 'blood pool' and bone images as being due to diffuse soft tissue hyperaemia. Septic arthritis has a very similar appearance due to the hyperaemia involving the joint. The subchondral bones on either side of the affected joint have increased tracer metabolism.

The bone image was found to be positive as early as 24 h after the onset of symptoms and always by three days, which was well before any bony changes were evident in the radiographs. Occasionally, however, soft tissue swelling or indistinct fat lines permit the presumptive radiological diagnosis of osteomyelitis.

The bone image has its greatest value in assessing areas difficult to evaluate by standard radiological means, such as the pelvis and spine. These areas do not have the easily seen fat planes of the long bones and, therefore, the early diagnosis of osteomyelitis is usually made by bone imaging.

We are now confident that if a child has clinical symptoms suggesting osteomyelitis then the examination which can most readily give the correct answer is bone imaging. This is especially true early in the illness or if the axial skeleton is involved. However, in some unusual cases (less than 5%) the scan may be normal in spite of very definite clinical signs; then gallium citrate imaging has proven very useful in detecting occult osteomyelitis. We do not use gallium as the primary test due to its higher radiation dose and 24 h delay in getting good images.

The infant who is less than 6 weeks of age at the time of onset of osteomyelitis frequently has a very aggressive destructive type of osteomyelitis. The radiograph usually becomes abnormal by the time the disease is suspected clinically. The gross destruction of the bone is evident radiologically and, unfortunately, at the same time the bone scan appears to be normal in a high number cases. This is in spite of very careful technique and optimum bone imaging with magnification collimators (Ash and Gilday, 1980). Our original experience using older cameras is still valid but a number of these osteomyelidities appear as 'cold' defects with newer higher-resolution cameras.

It would appear that this type of destructive lesion does not allow a bony reaction in the destructive phase. This destruction is what we see as a photopenic area. It is interesting to note that an osteomyelitis which starts after the age of 6 weeks, even though the patient is at the same physical

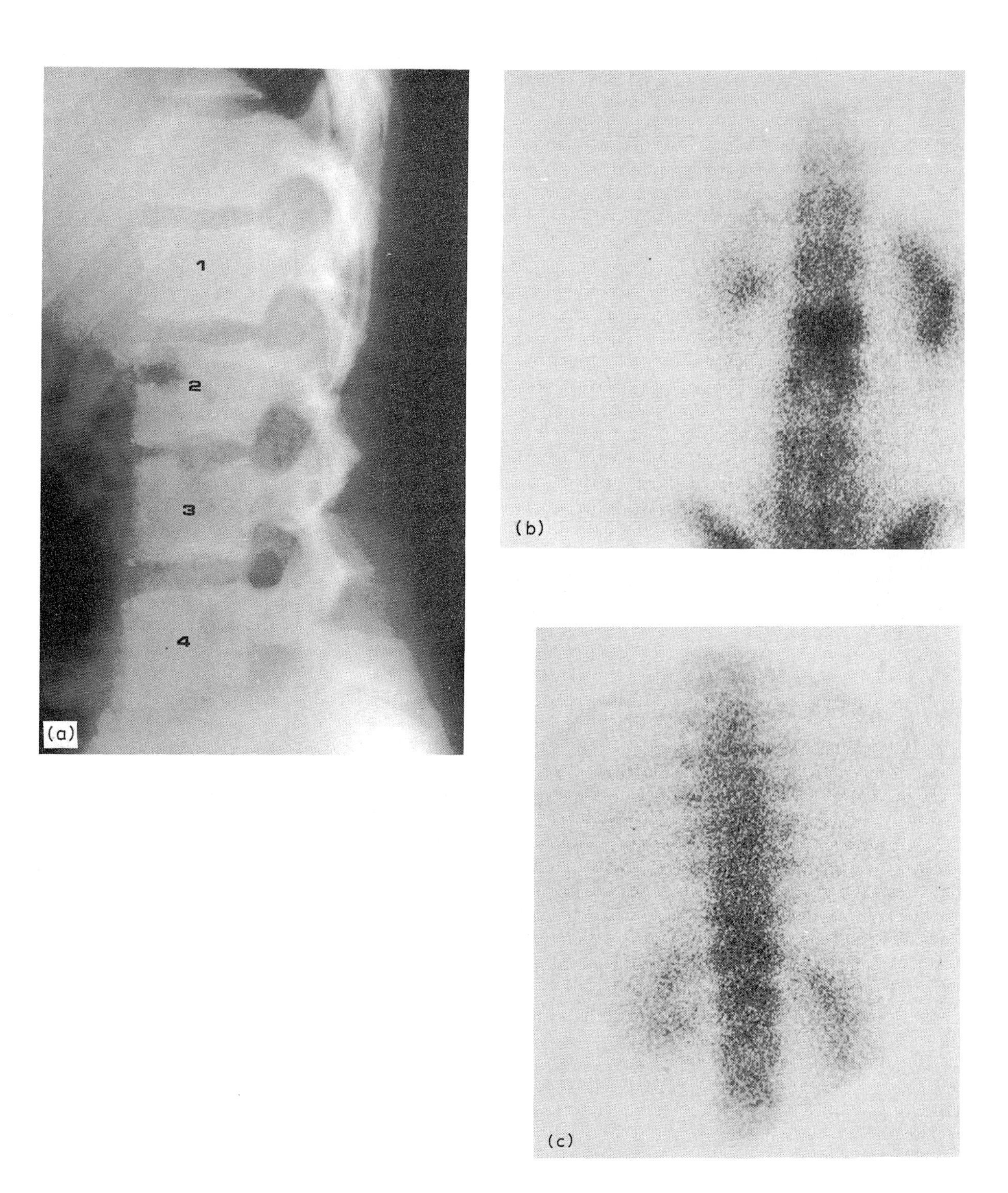

Figure 17.5 Diskitis–osteomyelitis. The second–third lumbar disk space is narrowed (a). The second lumbar vertebra has increased tracer metabolism indicating osteomyelitis (b). Follow-up study three weeks later shows the response to antibiotic therapy (c).

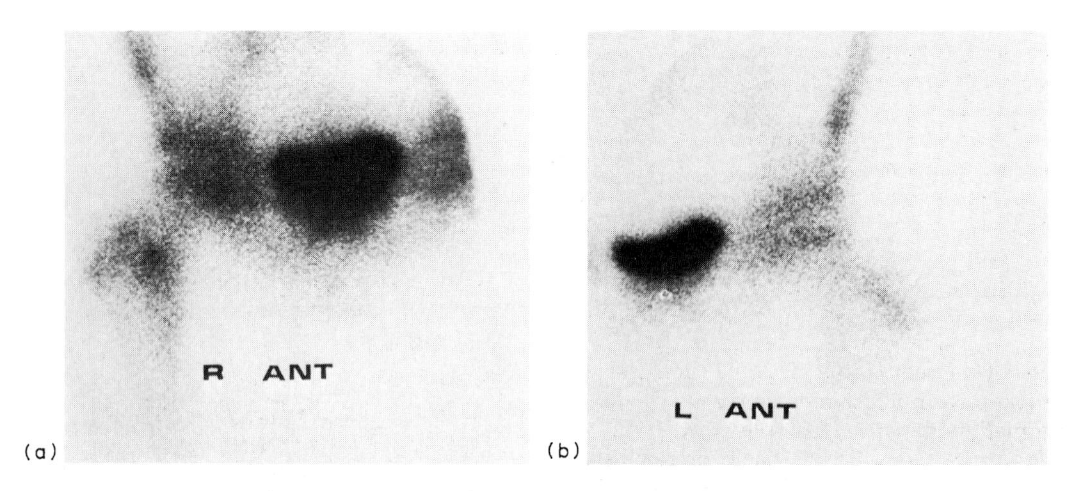

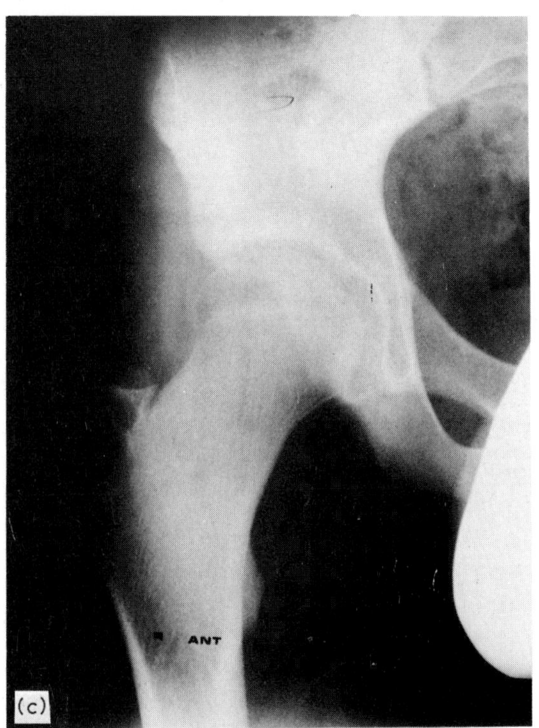

Figure 17.6 Osteoid osteoma. Focal increase adjacent to the right lesser trochanter (a); normal (b). Radiographs performed with sedation, and, thus, proper anatomical positioning demonstrates a subtle lucent nidus (c).

age when imaged, will have an abnormal scan whereas the patient with the earlier onset of osteomyelitis will have a normal scan.

17.4.1 OSTEOID OSTEOMA

This is the largest group of benign bone neoplasms that we have encountered. In a 15-year review we have diagnosed 78 osteoid osteomas, 70 of which have been confirmed surgically and eight are being followed clinically (Smith and Gilday, 1980). The most common indication for studying this group was to determine the cause of bone pain. We perform about 140 bone scans a year in children with undiagnosed bone pain. The commonest pathological cause was osteoid osteomas. Almost invariably the history was atypical and the diagnosis was in question radiologically. When there was a suspicious radiological change, confirmation of the presence of an osteoid osteoma was possible by the bone scan. In the talus and spine the scan was most helpful as one and four, respectively, had normal radiographs.

Radiologically, it is difficult to evaluate osteoid osteomas in certain areas of the body, namely the spine, the femoral neck region and the small bones of the feet (Table 17.2). In such instances, the complete nuclear medicine study with high information density, multiple-view bone scans and pinhole magnification has been necessary in the diagnosis of an osteoid osteoma. Subsequent radiological tomography, in the appropriate projection, often confirmed the presence of the osteoid osteoma. In several of our cases, CT or radiographic tomography was not positive and the bone scan had to be used to locate the lesion immediately prior to surgery. Some institutions use probes to locate the lesion intra-operatively.

We have found that it is almost always necessary to perform pinhole imaging of the hip region to delineate the exact location of femoral neck or intertrochanteric region osteoid osteomas (Figure 17.6). Quite frequently, the child's severe pain precludes proper positioning for the standard radiographs of the femur. However, once a lesion has been demonstrated by bone scan, it is imperative to obtain appropriate radiographic views of the area, using sedation and analgesics if necessary.

It is usually necessary to use the bone scan in evaluating long bones, as the radiological diagnosis is usually definitive. The converse is true in the spine. Not only is it difficult to detect osteoid osteomas in this area radiologically, but frequently the children are treated for other causes of back pain and the investigation for osteoid osteoma is not performed. We helped several children, each with a long and complicated history. The symptoms were present for more than two years and each child had significant orthopaedic and, in one case, neurosurgical intervention for back pain. In all the cases it was obvious from the nuclear medicine study that there was an osteoid osteoma present in the spine (Figure 17.7). In one case, the additional radiographs subsequently demonstrated a very abnormal superior articular facet of the vertebral body. This was removed with immediate resolution of the patient's symptoms. In the others, tomograms were normal and one boy had to have a preoperative localization of the osteoid osteoma by bone scanning. This was successful and enabled the surgeons to find the osteoid osteoma, which was confirmed pathologically.

Table 17.2 Location of osteoid osteomas in children

Femur	34
Tibia	12
Talus	6
Acetabulum	5
Spine	17
Humerus	2
Ulna	1
Skull	1

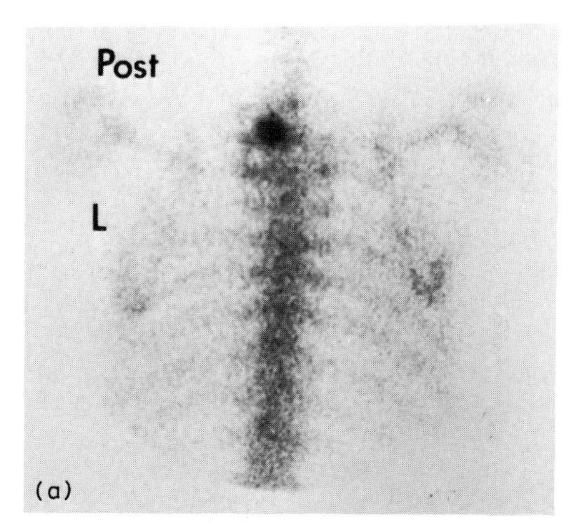

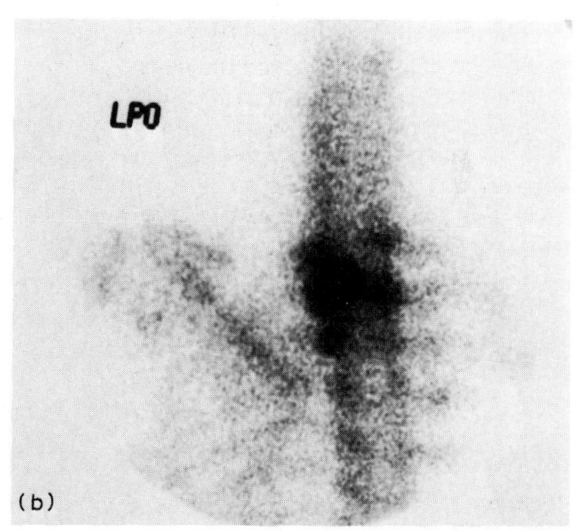

Figure 17.7 Osteoid osteoma of C5. The posterior (a) and magnified oblique view (b) demonstrate the occult osteoid osteoma to be in the left lateral vertebral mass.

Ivory osteomas in the skull are also highly vascular and have the same highly intense concentration of the bone radiopharmaceutical as the osteoid osteoma.

17.5 SPONDYLOLYSIS

In many cases of spondylolysis the pars interarticularis defect may not be 'easily' identified on the spinal radiographs. SPECT bone imaging has the ready advantage of being able to detect not only the reparative attempts of the defect but also to see the increase bone stress at the articular facets. By doing SPECT the location of the increased bone metabolism can help decide whether it is a bilateral defect or bone stress. The defect abnormalities will be more posterior (Figure 17.8).

17.6 CHILD ABUSE

Our socio-legal system has developed an enlightened sensitivity to child abuse. In most paediatric hospitals the total-body scan has become the first test to determine if the child has had any bony damage. If one or more areas is found to be abnormal then high detail radiography is performed to confirm the abnormality and to help date it as well. With greater recognition of this problem more studies are being performed. In highly suspicious cases we recommend that skull radiography be performed even if the bone scan is normal as it has a lower sensitivity for detecting trauma to the calvarium.

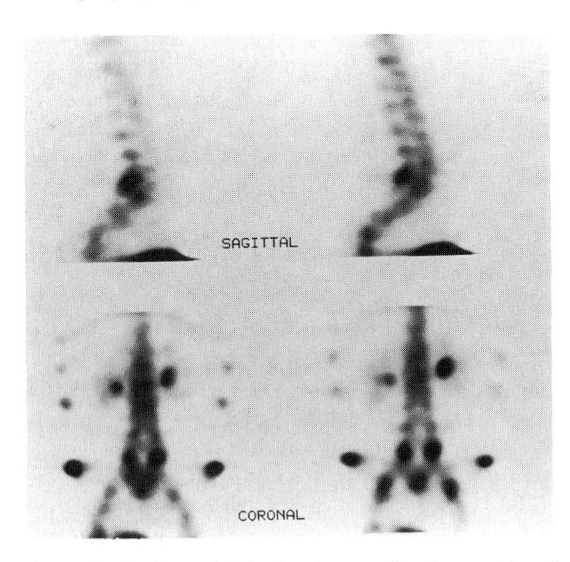

Figure 17.8 Spondylolysis. An excellent example of attempted repair of the pars articularis defects bilaterally seen on the SPECT bone scan.

17.7 MEDIASTINAL GALLIUM IMAGING

Gallium imaging plays a major role in the evaluation of children with lymphomas. The mediastinum is often a difficult area to evaluate due to the presence of the thymus. The thymus may enlarge in viral and other illnesses, which can cause confusion (Figure 17.9). The best way to differentiate lymphomatous involvement (Figure 17.9a) from the normal (Figure 17.9b) is to compare the chest radiograph with the scan. The normal thymus appears as a 'sail'-shaped structure.

17.8 GASTROINTESTINAL PROBLEMS

17.8.1 LIVER DISEASE

The liver/spleen scan is probably the easiest, cheapest and most readily available means of detecting metastases to the liver and spleen. The addition of ultrasound in obscure or questionable presence of metastases makes the detection almost 100%. The usual scan findings are those of focal lesions within the liver. Primary hepatic lesions such as hepatoblastoma are usually single, although the occasionally multilobular or multicentric variety can occur.

More common is the evaluation of benign disease of the liver or spleen. One of the main indications for liver and spleen scanning is abdominal trauma. With the current trend by paediatric surgeons to manage splenic and hepatic trauma conservatively, the role of the spleen and liver scan has become paramount in their clinical investigation and management. Usually the findings are those of well-localized areas of absent activity within the spleen or in some cases of rupture of the spleen – actual separation of pieces of splenic tissue which still accumulate the tracer within them. Sequential studies demonstrate a gradual resolution of the defect and/or drawing together of the shattered components of the spleen (Figure 17.10). Usually liver trauma results in a solitary haematoma which appears as a large, focal defect. These are occasionally treated surgically with partial resection of the liver. The scan is then used to follow the liver regeneration.

Subphrenic abscesses are readily detected by the liver/spleen scan. These usually cause a concave defect in the contour of the liver. In those

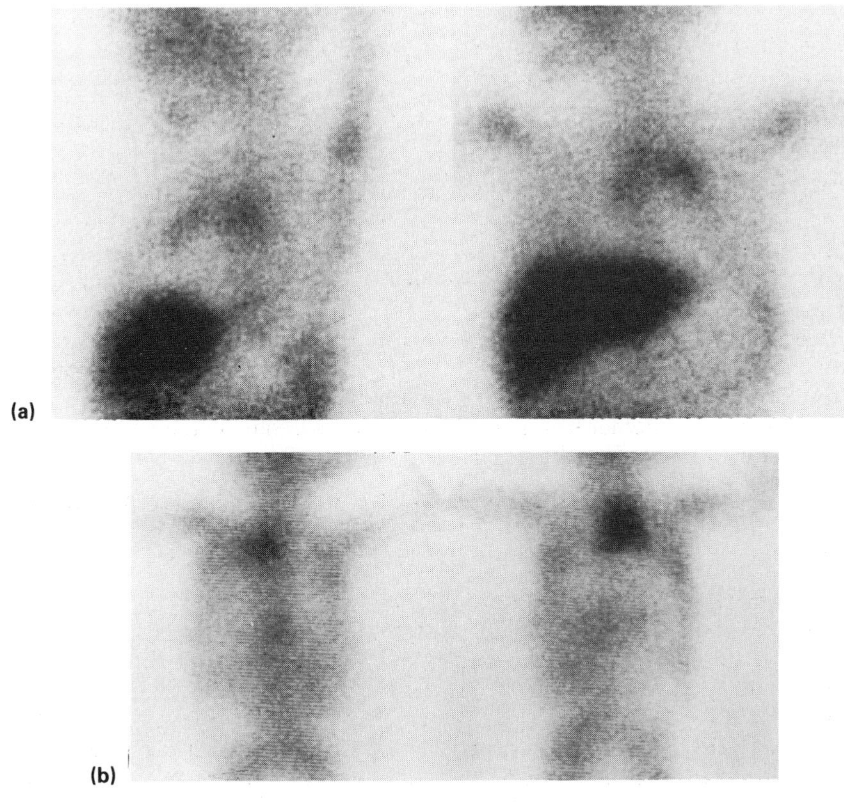

Figure 17.9 Mediastinal lymphoma. Typical 72 h Ga scan shows irregular increased tracer in a Hodgkin's lymphoma of the mediastinum (a). Normal thymic tracer activity is seen in a 'sail' shape (b).

abscesses which are not adjacent to the liver, a gallium scan offers a very good means of detecting the intra-abdominal abscess. Subtraction of the liver image from the gallium image provides a greater degree of confidence in the diagnosis (Figure 17.11). Its accuracy rate is greater than 95% in the detection of active abscesses.

17.8.2 BILIARY DISEASE

One of the more difficult and therefore interesting areas of investigation in paediatrics is the evaluation of biliary disease. The problem of differentiating neonatal hepatitis from biliary atresia is extremely difficult to achieve with 100% reliability (Majd *et al.*, 1981b). The main criteria for separation of these two entities is that after injection of ^{99m}Tc-labelled DISIDA or equivalent radiopharmaceutical the tracer is never seen to be excreted into the bowel throughout 24 h in babies with biliary atresia (Figure 17.12). In the baby with neonatal hepatitis, the radiopharmaceutical would appear in the bowel within 24 h. A most important feature of this type of study is to premedicate the patient for five days with phenobarbitol (2.5 mg kg^{-1} twice a day for five days) before injecting the ^{99m}Tc-labelled DISIDA (Majd *et al.*, 1981a).

Another important role for biliary imaging in paediatrics is the evaluation of a choledocal cyst. A choledocal cyst is usually detected as a cystic structure on ultrasound. The radionuclide evaluation is to determine the physiological nature of this cyst. It is important that the cyst be seen to communicate with the hepatic duct system and to fill. In the post-operative period the study demonstrates the easy flow of the radiopharmaceutical through the biliary tract.

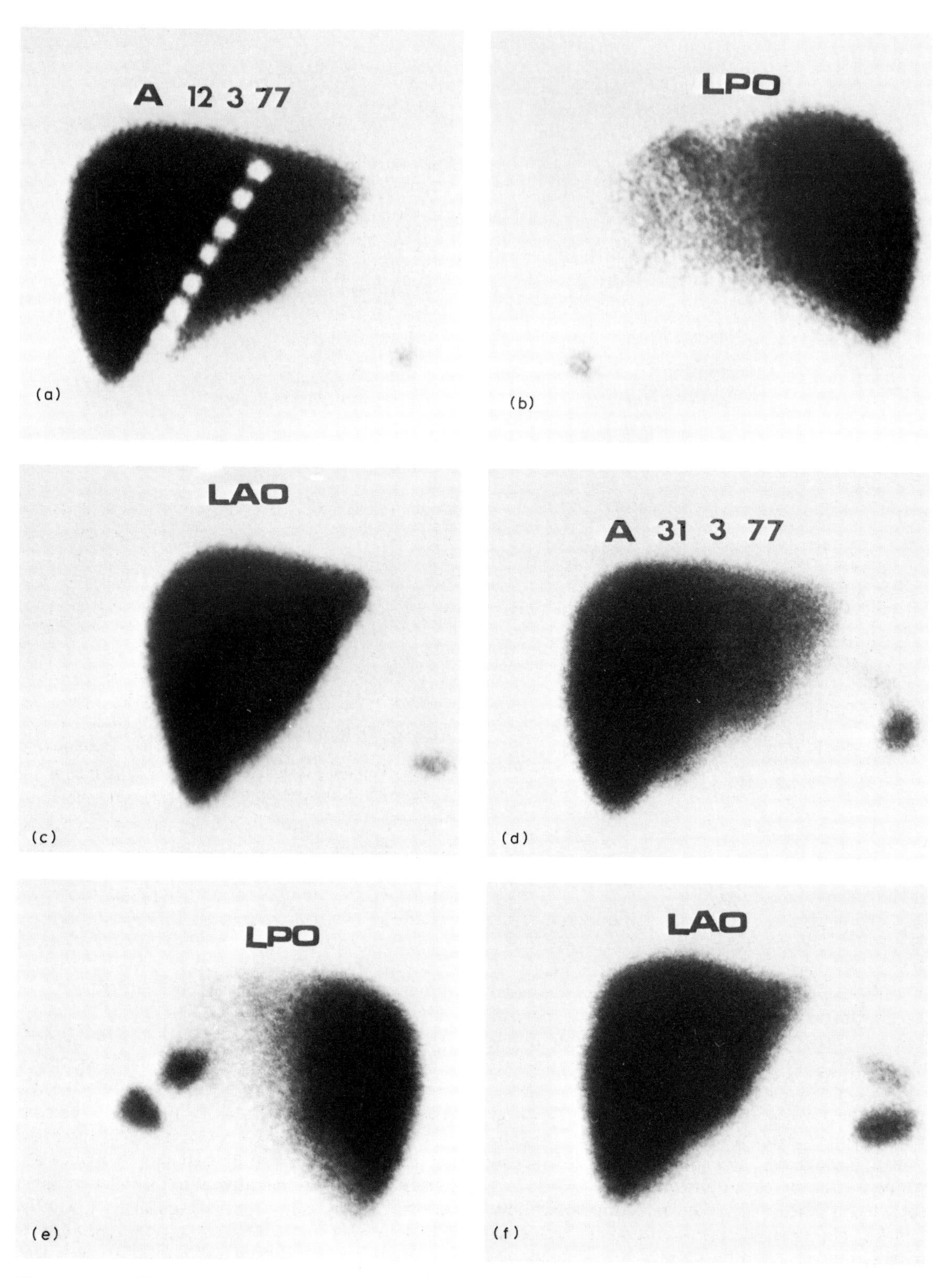

Figure 17.10 Shattered spleen. The spleen is shattered and only two fragments accumulated sulphur colloid (a–c). Follow-up study 19 days later shows the resolution of the space-occupying haematoma (d–f). The follow-up at two months shows that the two components are contiguous (g–i).

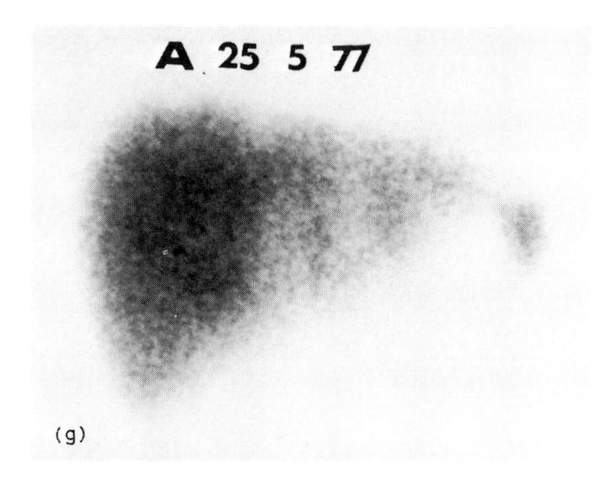

(g)

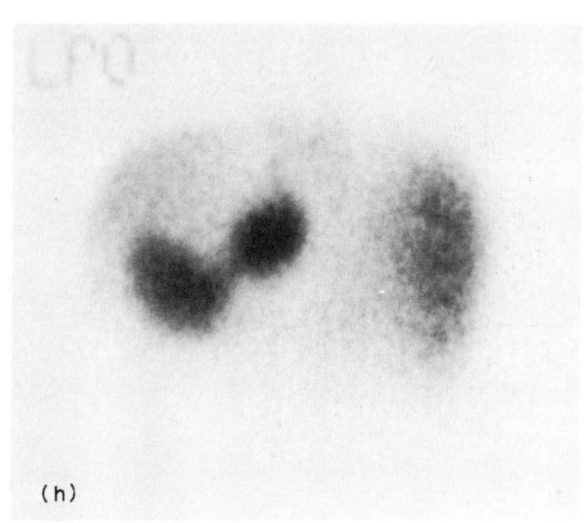

(h)

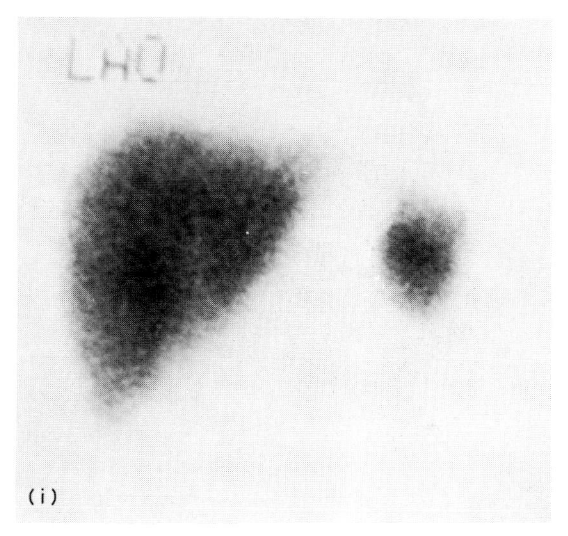

(i)

17.8.3 GASTRO-OESOPHAGEAL REFLUX

The role of gastro-oesophageal reflux in the cause of both symptoms and more specifically lung disease is well defined. However, what is not well defined is how to determine whether or not reflux which is taking place is the cause of the repeated pulmonary infections. There have been strong advocates of using ^{99m}Tc-labelled milk to monitor reflux and aspiration in children who are suspected of having this combination. Unfortunately, we as many others have not found this study to be that sensitive in detecting aspiration. This is due to the fact that aspiration secondary to reflux is a very intermittent occurrence and we are only able to monitor the situation for a short period of time. What has become apparent though is that the milk scan is very valuable in detecting reflux in children. The main advantage is that one can monitor the gastro-oesophageal junction to determine in which position the reflux occurs. This allows for better determination of what circumstances will produce reflux and thus permit the paediatrician to better treat the patient by correct postural positioning.

The rate of gastric emptying, which is very important in many gastroenteric problems, can be readily assessed as part of the reflux procedure by measuring the emptying of the stomach contents. We usually use the percentage retention at 60 min (Di Lorenzo *et al.*, 1987). The amount retained should be less than 65% at 3 months of age and this gradually decreases to 44% by 6 years. Oesophageal motility problems can be evaluated using computerized dynamic imaging of the tracer moving down the oesophagus.

17.8.4 PERTECHNETATE ABDOMINAL IMAGING

The aetiology of rectal bleeding in infants and children is often obscure (Shandling, 1965). In a 10-year period from 1952 to 1962, 801 patients were admitted to the Hospital for Sick Children with a history of rectal bleeding, i.e. approximately 80 per year. Of 61 patients in whom all examinations were negative who underwent laparotomy, 31 had negative findings and a Meckel's diverticulum was present in 24, 20 with gastric mucosa. Meckel's diverticulum is a common congenital anomaly (0.3–3% in mature individuals) (Valdes *et al.*, 1970); however, a relatively small percentage (average 20%) of these patients

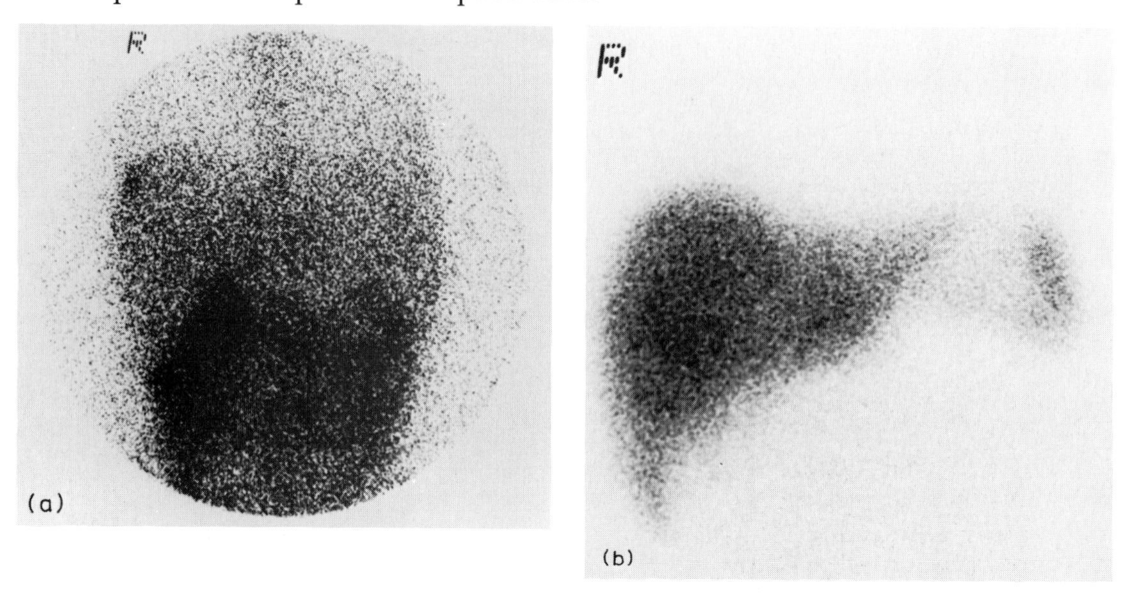

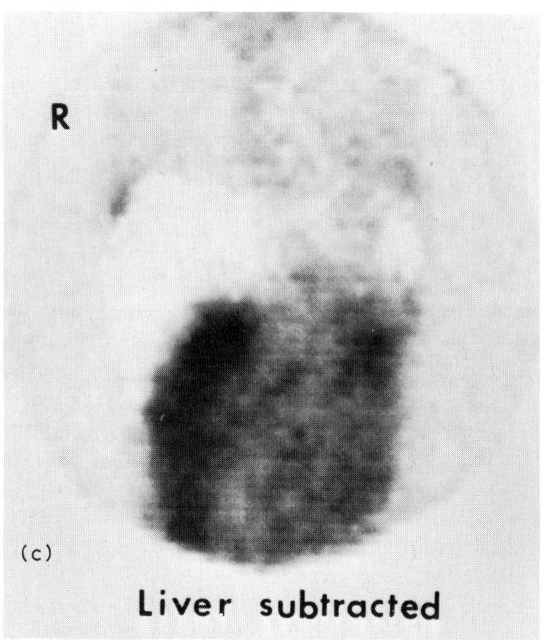

Figure 17.11 Small subphrenic abscess. Ga scan (48 h) shows increased tracer in the gut and a suggestion of a focal increase superficially on the right side of the liver (a). Liver scan was normal (b). Computer subtraction image provides the diagnostic information that a small subphrenic abscess is present (c) (surgically confirmed).

have ectopic gastric mucosa within their Meckel's diverticulum.

The initial descriptions by Duszinski *et al.*, (1970a) describe successful detection of Meckel's diverticulum with a rectilinear scanner. However, the test was not specific in their hands (as intussusceptions and polyps were also positive) and it took 2 h from the time of injection to complete the study. Rosenthall, who performed this study using a gamma camera, had an accuracy rate of 5/8 but still did not have a specific study (Rosenthall *et al.*, 1972). He carried out his studies using a gam-

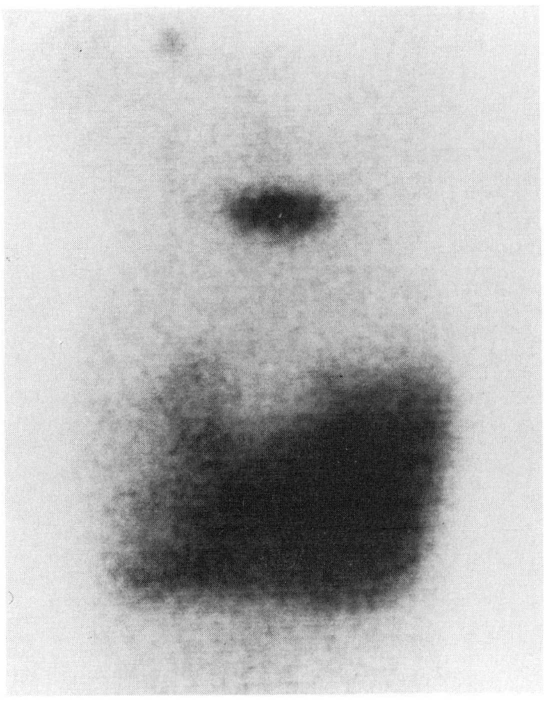

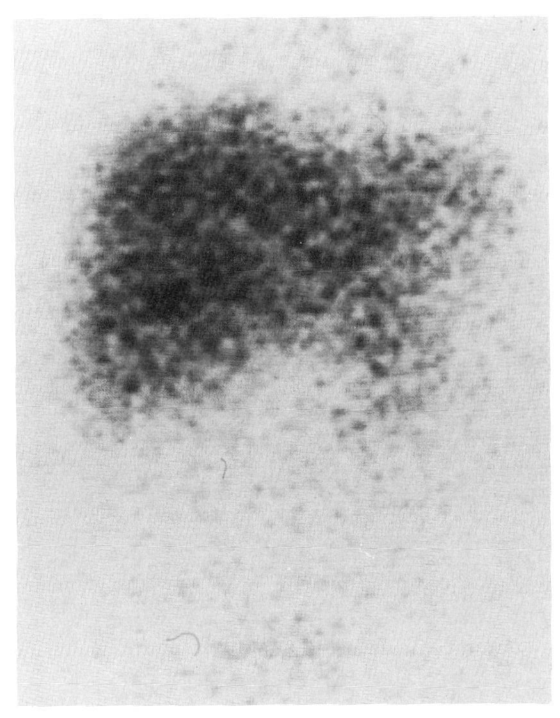

(a) (b)

Figure 17.12 Biliary atresia. At 4 h (a) and 24 h (b) after the injection of ^{99m}Tc-labelled DISIDA no radiotracer is seen in the bowel.

ma camera and imaging at 15, 30, 45 and 60 min after injection. In a multi-institutional paper presented by Conway, the results had greater than 80% accuracy in children who had a laparotomy (Conway, 1976a).

There is a rapid increase in radioactivity in the stomach as the pertechnetate is secreted by the gastric mucosa. Renal and bladder activity are present as 20% of the injected pertechnetate is excreted by the kidneys. The early sequential views permit monitoring of the rate of accumulation of pertechnetate in the stomach during the first 15 min. The posterior views at 15 and 30 min demonstrate the location of the renal pelves. Other than these normal structures there should not be any focus of activity throughout the abdomen in the area of the small bowel, although ureters and the iliac vessels are sometimes seen.

In the child with a Meckel's diverticulum the time sequence of radioactive concentration within the ectopic gastric mucosa parallels that in the normal gastric mucosa of the stomach (Figure 17.13). This important feature helps differentiate ectopic gastric mucosa from inflammatory causes which tend to accumulate the radioactivity at a slower rate; it also can help to differentiate an extrarenal pelvis from a Meckel's diverticulum.

Problems occur in interpreting this study. The early appearance of the radiopharmaceutical in the ureters may simulate a focal lesion posteriorly at the pelvis brim due to a slight hold-up at this location while the child is supine. This fades with time and usually disappears during the prone and lateral views, and in the subsequent anterior views there should not be much activity within the ureter. Occasionally a Meckel's diverticulum may overlie an existing structure which contains radioactivity such as the ureter. Then the diagnosis of Meckel's diverticulum is difficult unless the bowel moves during the study. If not, a repeat study may show the focal accumulation to have moved. In some patients there is rapid movement of the tracer into the duodenum, which causes confusion; however, the lateral and posterior views help to demonstrate the location of such increased activity. To minimize the excretion of the pertechnetate into the lumen of the stomach or out the ectopic gastric mucosa we suggest pre-

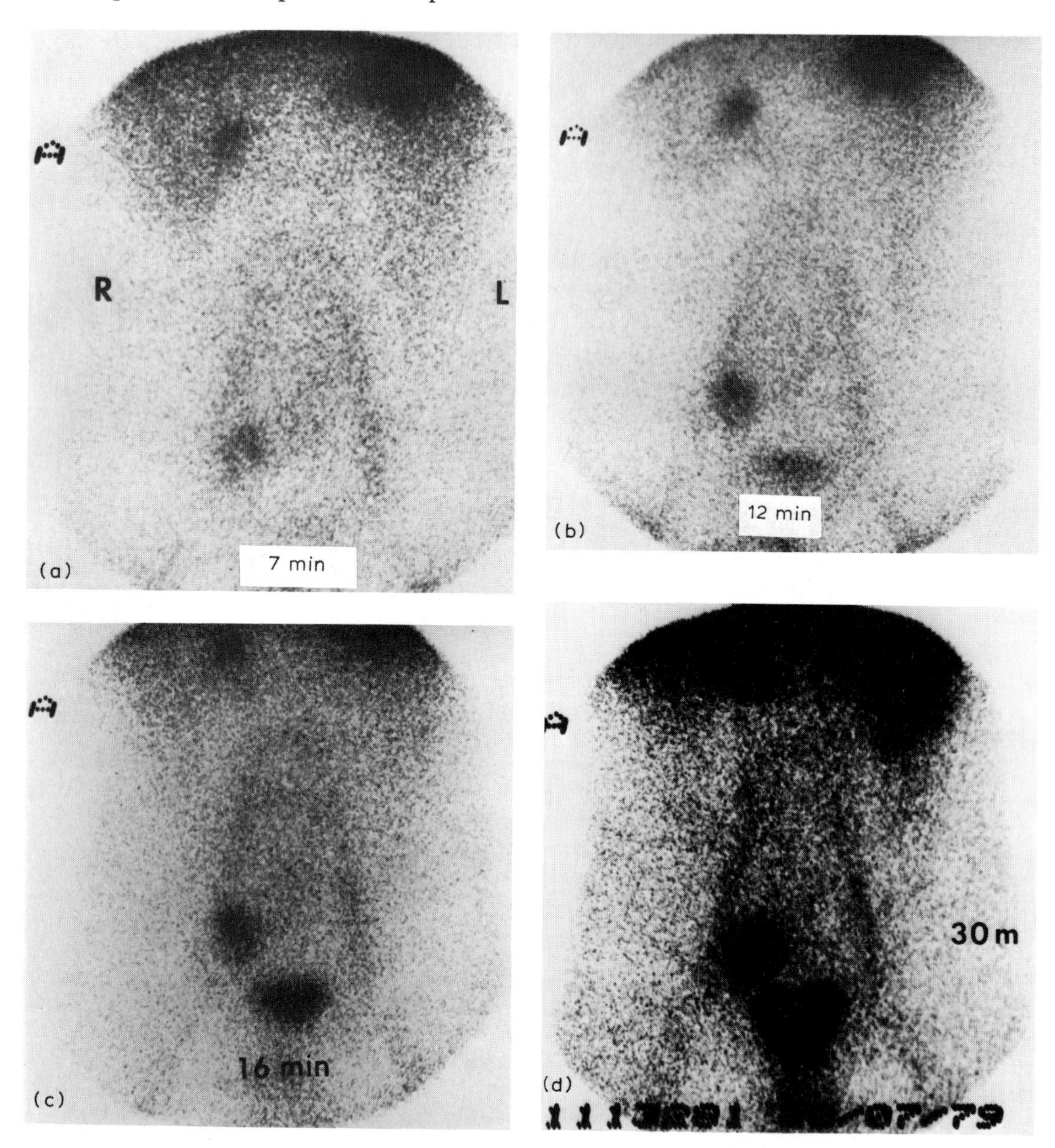

Figure 17.13 Meckel's diverticulum containing ectopic gastric mucosa. The images from 7 to 30 min (a–d) show pertechnetate accumulation in the ectopic gastric mucosa paralleling that of the stomach.

medication with 5 mg kg^{-1} of cimetidine to a maximum of 300 mg infused in 20 ml of saline over 20 minutes. Any other lesion which contains ectopic gastric mucosa can produce the correct time sequence but may assume a different shape, such as duplication of the small bowel. Inflammatory bowel disease such as gastroenteritis or regional enteritis produces abnormal scans but the distribution of activity is diffuse or the time sequence is different.

Our results would suggest that the pertechnetate abdominal scan can detect ectopic gastric mucosa with an accuracy of at least 95%. This is a significant improvement over previously published reports which is due to the sequential early imaging and the multiple views at 15 and 30 min., and the use of cimetidine.

17.9 GENITOURINARY PROBLEMS

From infancy to puberty the radionuclide renal study is widely used to evaluate renal function. In conjunction with ultrasound it has almost replaced the intravenous urogram. In the newborn, the renal study also permits visualization of renal morphology during the period when the intravenous urogram may not adequately delineate the kidneys (especially in patients with ectopic or poorly functioning kidneys). In neonates with compromised renal function the study is the most accurate method for determining the function of each or both kidneys (Martin *et al.*, 1975).

In children under 2 years of age the injection is via a pedal vein so that we may evaluate the possibility of inferior vena cava (IVC) obstruction. The child must not Valsalva during the injection

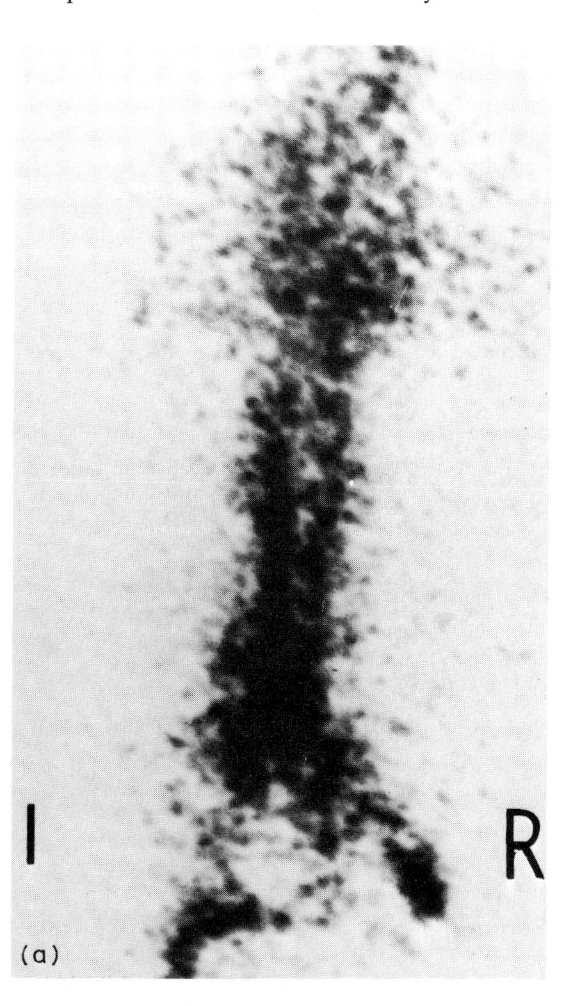

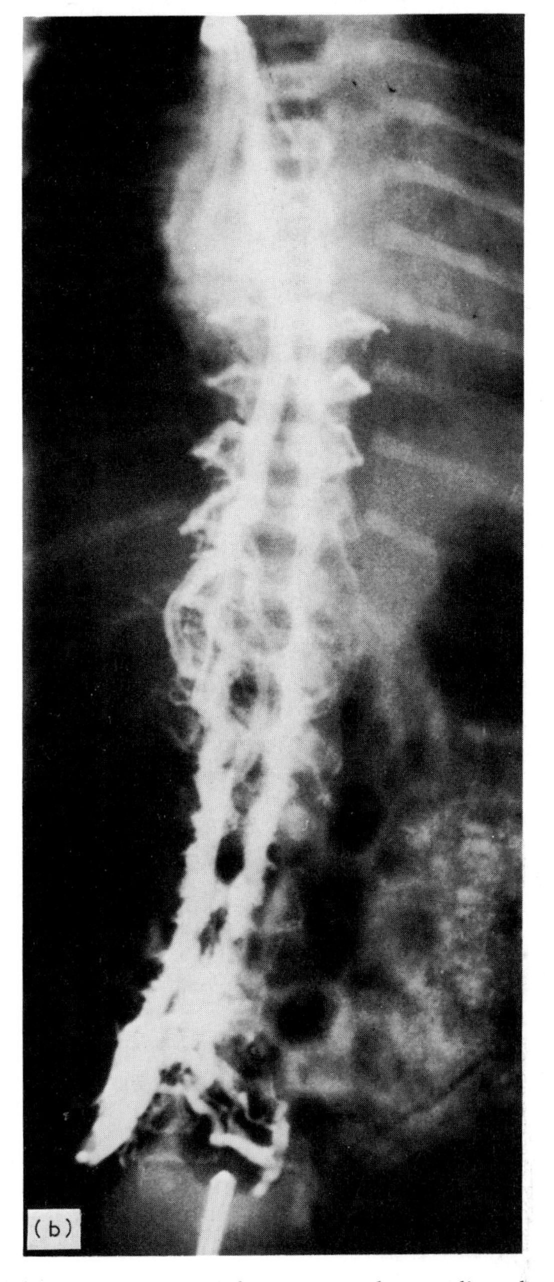

Figure 17.14 Inferior vena cava occlusion. The radionuclide vena cavagram (a) demonstrates the vessel's occlusion by the interruption of flow through it and the tracer passing up Batson's plexus. This was confirmed by contrast angiography (b).

or the IVC will occlude due to increased physiological intra-abdominal pressure (Figure 17.14; McDonald *et al.*, 1974).

Serial assessment of renal function forms an important aspect of paediatric urology, particularly in children with hydronephrosis, vesicoureteral reflux and chronic pyelonephritis who may require repeated evaluation both pre- and post-operative. The decision of whether to do a nephrectomy or a reconstructive procedure may be a difficult one, especially in the child whose contralateral kidney is already jeopardized. One of the factors influencing this decision is the degree of function of the affected kidney. In the past, this has been difficult to assess as the intravenous urogram does not measure renal function and 24 h urinary creatinine clearances can be difficult to collect in children and have a varying degree of accuracy. In addition, split creatinine clearances for individual function require ureteral catheterization unless the patient has undergone nephrostomy or ureterostomy. In our centre we have found that renal scanning with technetium-labelled diethylenetriamine pentaacetic acid (^{99m}Tc-labelled DTPA), which has greater than 95% excretion by glomerular filtration, provides a simple and relatively non-invasive method for assessing the relative function on each side and for measuring the glomerular filtration rate. A separate filtration rate for each kidney may be calculated from these two measurements and used to assess the patient pre-operatively and to follow post-operative changes.

We record the radionuclide angiogram of the kidneys during the intravenous bolus injection of ^{99m}Tc-labelled DTPA (8.5 mCi m^{-2} body surface area). Beginning 1 min after the injection, sequential images of the kidneys are taken every minute for 15 min with a further one at 30 min and thereafter as necessary. In this way, a visual renogram or renal scan is obtained. All of the data is recorded by a computer which is then used to measure differential renal function during the first 2 min. Regions of interest are placed over each kidney and the appropriate background flagged (Figure 17.15). The background activity is subtracted from each renal curve to produce curves which represent the radioactivity in the kidneys,

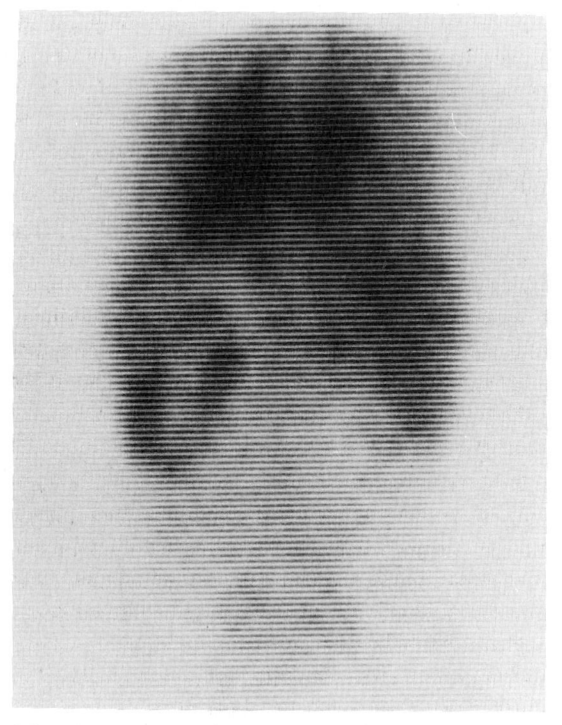
(a)

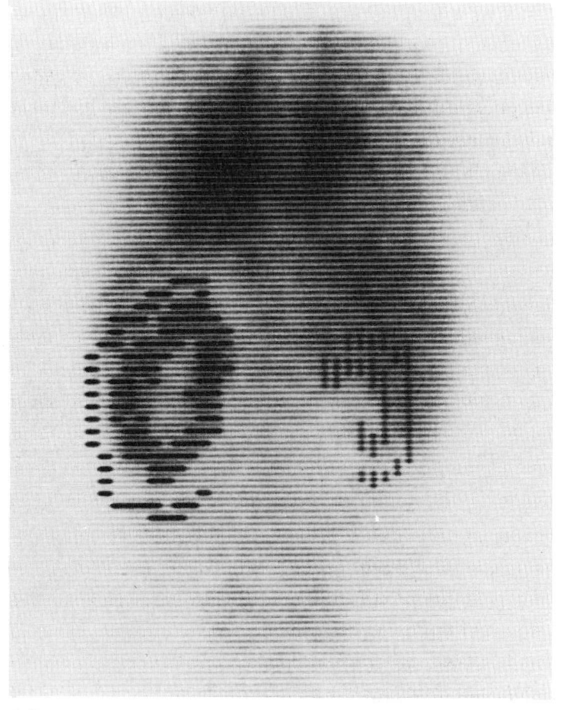
(b)

Figure 17.15 Differential renal scan evaluation. The composite 0–120 s image (a) and the superimposed regions of interest on the right (b). Each kidney has its own background.

between 0 and 2 min. The activity under each curve is readily calculated and the total radioactivity in the two kidneys obtained by summing the two. The amount of activity in each kidney is then expressed as a percentage of the total. This provides a measure of the functioning renal mass on one side relative to the other. Although DTPA is essentially a glomerular filtration agent and theoretically may not reflect tubular function, we have found that in almost all cases this provides a simple and useful index and does not differ significantly from the percentages obtained using ^{99m}Tc-labelled glucoheptonate (of which 80% is filtered and 20% is tubular bound) or DMSA (80% bound, 20% filtered). Furthermore, there were no differences between the glucoheptonate percentages calculated at 1–3 min reflecting the amount filtered by each kidney and at 24 h reflecting the tubular binding by each kidney. Correction factors for kidney depth have been used in other centres (Maneval *et al.*, 1990), but we have not found these to be necessary. In a series of 13 cases in which the differential renal function measured by radionuclide techniques was compared with split creatinine clearances, the correlation coefficient was 0.96 (Pieretti *et al.*, 1974).

One advantage of using ^{99m}Tc-labelled DTPA is that the glomerular filtration rate (GFR) may be measured at the same time by taking two plasma samples at 90 min and at least 30 min later and then plotting the plasma disappearance. The results show a good correlation coefficient of 0.91 when compared with 24 h urinary creatinine clearances. This method is reproducible in that the GFRs repeated on the same patients who were clinically stable did not differ significantly from each other. By multiplying the percentage obtained from the differential renal functional analysis by the GFR, individual filtration rates for each kidney may be determined (Ash and Gilday, 1980). A variety of gamma camera techniques such as that by Gates and Piepz have been used to evaluate GFR without taking a blood sample. These are referred to as uptake GFR measurements. In paediatrics these techniques have not correlated with the two-sample method as well as in adults.

If one kidney has markedly decreased or delayed function and is not well visualized between 1 and 3 min, the differential renal analysis cannot be performed between the two kidneys. It is also difficult to assess kidneys which are extremely hydronephrotic with thinned parenchyma containing less radioactivity than background due to large amounts of non-radioactive urine in the calyces and renal pelvis. In these cases, we feel that the differential renal analysis has less validity as it is difficult to define accurately the functioning parenchyma and avoid the areas not containing radioactivity. If the information is vital we will repeat the study with DMSA and measure the relative renal mass at 4 h. The differential renal function analysis is a relative measure only and an apparent decrease on one side may be due to improvement on the other side. Although the images obtained from the renal scan usually indicate which is the side that has changed, accurate diagnosis may be difficult unless a GFR is performed at the same time.

This method is helpful in assessing renal function in patients with vesicoureteral reflux, ureteropelvic junction obstruction, ureterovesical junction obstruction, posterior urethral valves and prune belly syndrome. It is particularly useful in the neonate and young infant in whom a drastic improvement in renal function may be seen following surgery and as much as a 20 percentile increment (for example from 10 to 30%) in the renal differential obtained. In many of these children, the affected kidney(s) may be poorly visualized on IVP and the function erroneously underestimated from this. As a result, radionuclide measurement has become an integral part of the urological assessment in paediatrics.

The child with either reflux problem or obstructive hydronephrosis is usually evaluated pre- and post-operatively for the degree of relative renal function, absolute renal function and rate of egress of the radioactive urine from the kidneys. In cases where an obstructive component to urine flow is suspected a Lasix stress test is begun between 10 and 30 min after the injection of ^{99m}Tc-labelled DTPA. Intravenous Lasix (furosemide) (0.1 mg kg^{-1} maximum 2.0 mg) is given and images recorded for 30 min, into the computer. The clearance rate is calculated using the computer. This permits a quantitative method of determining the effect of surgery and/or post-operative complications on the renal drainage system. Normal *T*/2 values are less than 8–10 min. This value may be higher (up to 20 min) in grossly dilated pelves or after surgery. The Lasix washout study appears to reflect the state of urinary flow better than the Whitaker test in the post-operative period (Figure 17.16; Krueger *et al.*, 1980).

In large hydronephrotic kidneys or after repair

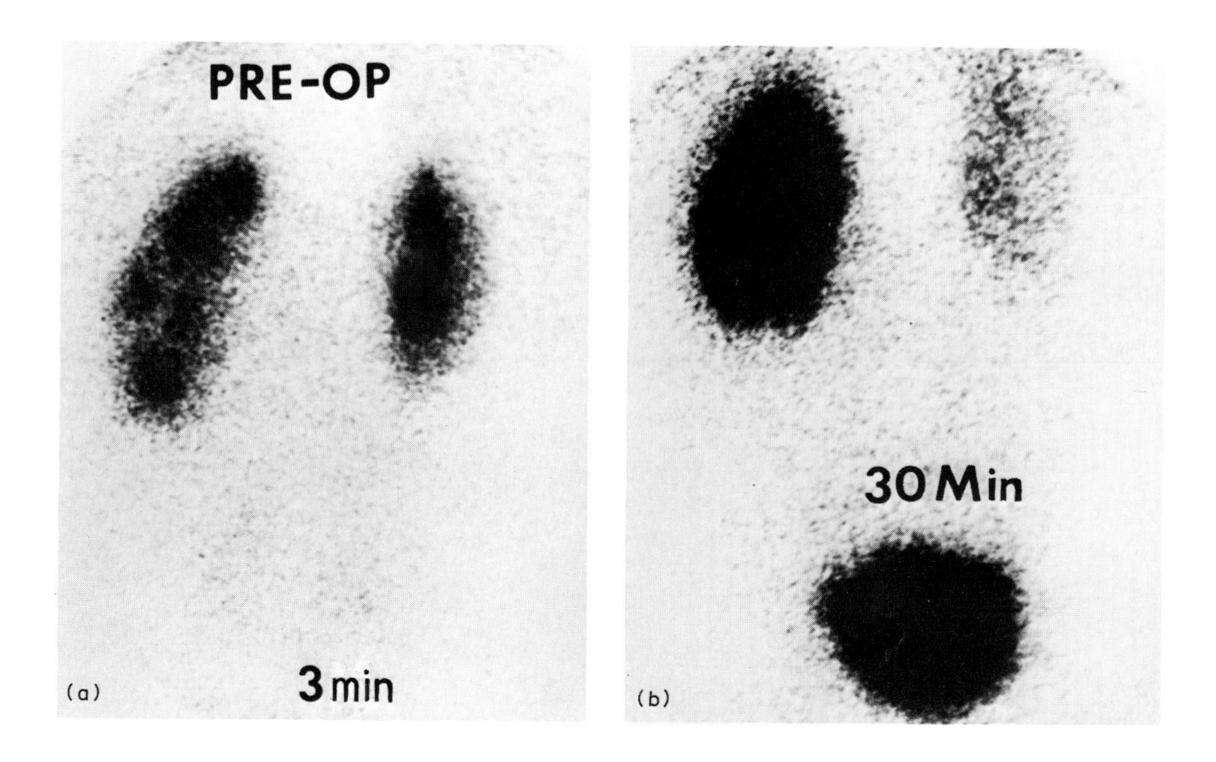

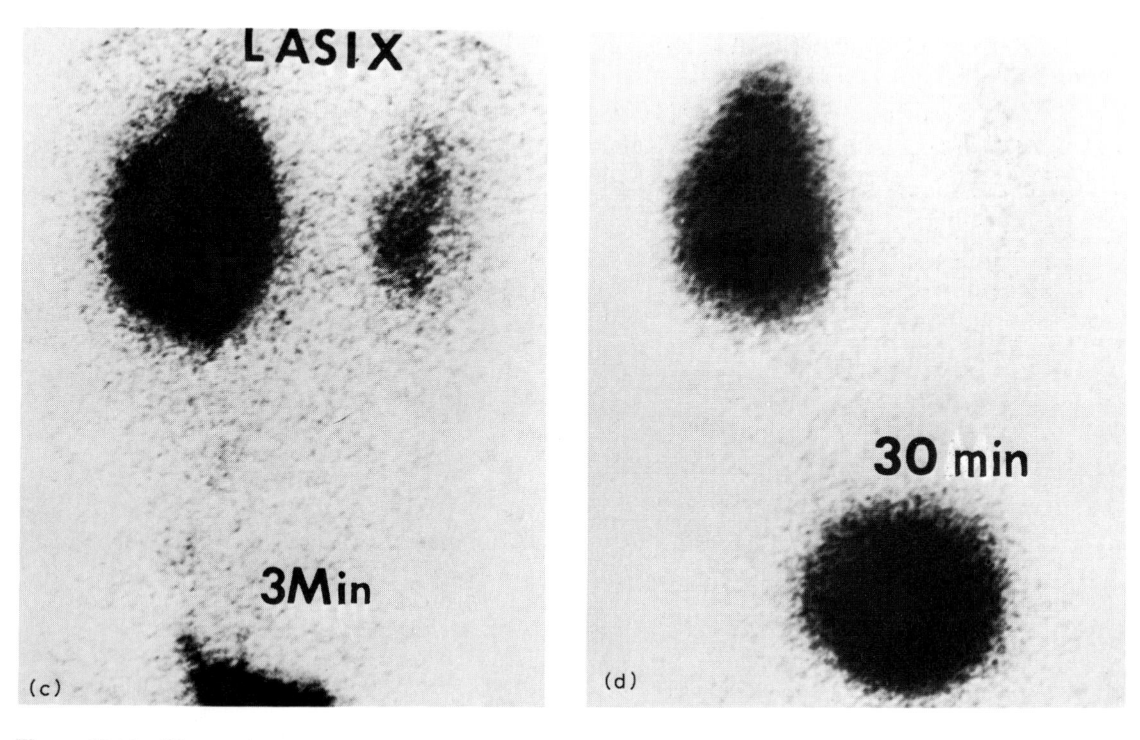

Figure 17.16 Obstructive uropathy. The pre-operation study shows almost complete left pelvi-ureteric function obstruction (a, b), even with Lasix stimulation (c, d).

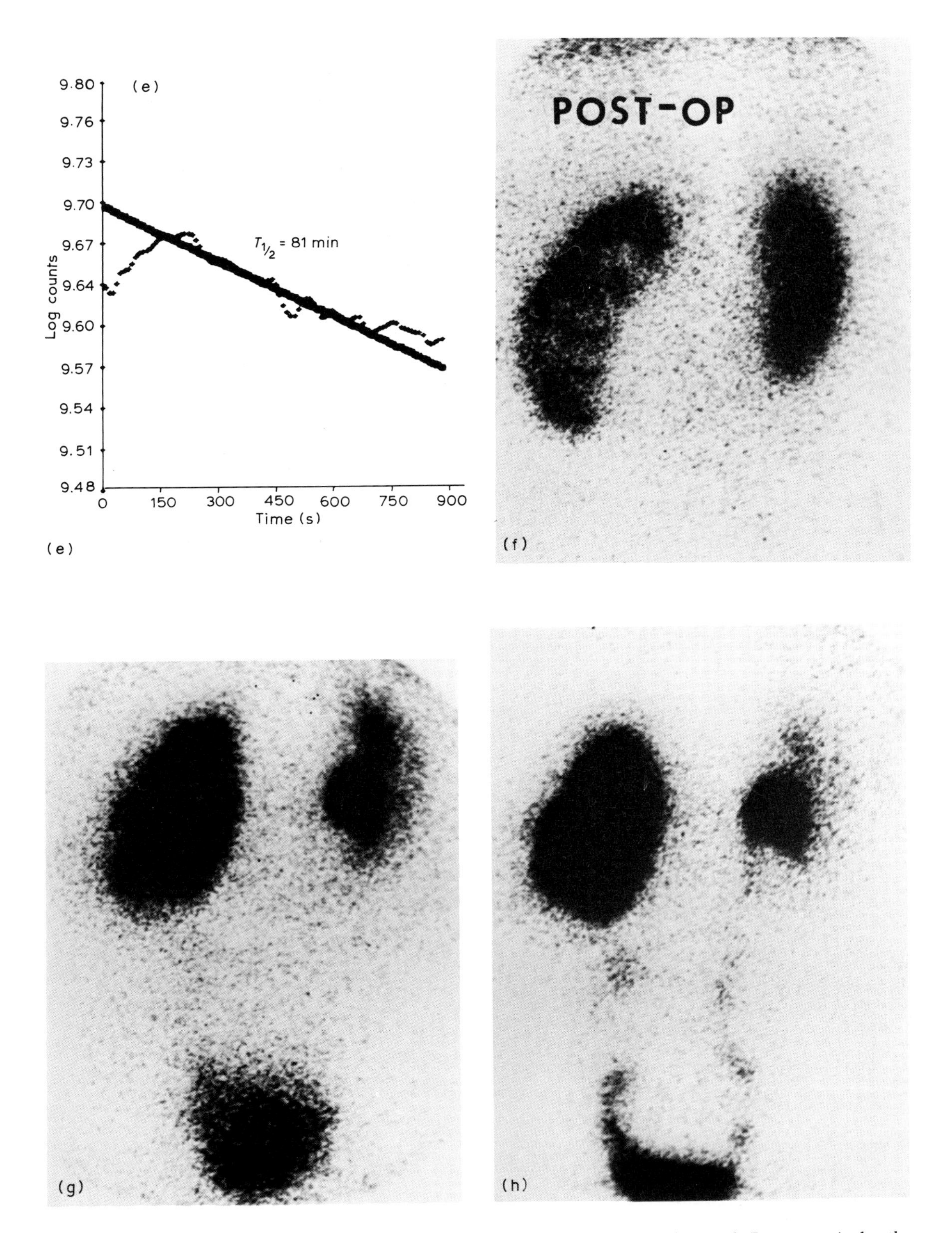

Figure 17.16 (cont'd) The clearance curve (e) has a $T/2$ of 81 min, which is abnormal. Post-operatively, the appearance is very similar (f–i) but the clearance curve (j) has a $T/2$ of 10 min, which is at the upper limit of normal.

Figure 17.16 continued overleaf

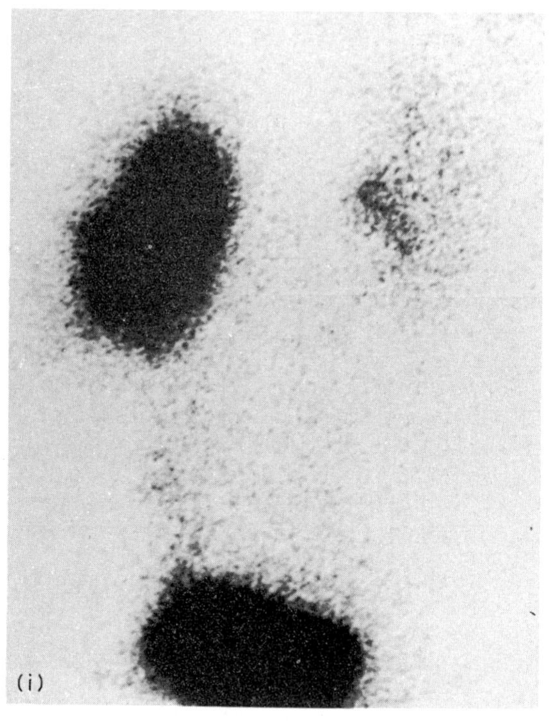

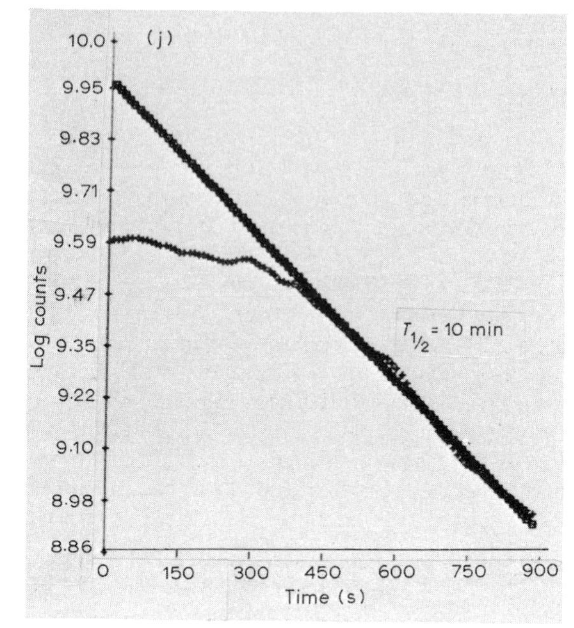

Figure 17.16 (cont'd).

of an obstruction a delay in the drainage of radioactive urine is present immediately after reimplantation of ureters (anti-reflux surgery) and will slowly improve over about six months. After that they usually drain normally. Care must be used in assessing Lasix washout curves performed on normal kidneys that have already emptied their pelves as the *T*/2 is invalid. The same applies to very poorly functioning kidneys.

In patients with decreased renal function such as haemolytic uraemic syndrome, in which case the kidneys do not appear on the intravenous pyelogram, the renal scan may show some sign of renal function and thus is very useful in such patients. The GFR determines the residual degree of renal function.

In kidney transplant patients, the renal scan is used sequentially during the first two weeks after transplantation for the evaluation of the viability of the transplant and, subsequently, for an estimate of its function using two main parameters in addition to the images (Ash *et al.*, 1990). One is the percentage of cardiac output to the kidney using the method of Peters *et al.* (1987) and the other is the measurement of the GFR of the kidney. These have become invaluable adjunctive indicators to the images in the assessment of whether or not the kidney is being rejected. The blood flow estimator is extremely sensitive in the first two weeks after transplantation, whereas the GFR is generally a better indicator of function later and quite useful to detect early chronic rejection.

Radionuclide cystography is a well-tried technique which has proven to be very successful (Conway and Kruglik, 1976). Recently, computer-analysed antegrade voiding cystograms have been tried and appear to be as accurate as the retrograde version. This could be preferred as it is more physiological. However, due to reflux and other problems the generally preferred method is still the catheter voiding cystogram. The detection rate of reflux is at least as good or better than that of the X-ray. In the voiding cystourethrogram, however, the radiation dose is considered to be approximately one hundredth to one thousandth of that of the radiological study (Pollet *et al.*, 1979). In addition, the monitoring of the bladder and ureters is constant throughout both filling and emptying phases – something not feasible using fluoroscopy.

17.10 NEUROLOGICAL PROBLEMS

17.10.1 CEREBROSPINAL FLUID DISORDERS

The cerebrospinal fluid (CSF) is produced primarily in the choroid plexi of the ventricles, but is also produced throughout the subarachnoid space. The predominant flow is normally directed from the ventricles out into the foramina in the fourth ventricle, and from there out into the subarachnoid cisterns, and around the brain stem, then up through the tentorial hiatus between and over the hemispheres. Although water and ions are secreted and absorbed throughout the system, albumin and chelates do not readily diffuse across the subarachnoid membrane. The CSF protein is mainly reabsorbed parasagittally at the arachnoid villae projecting into the venous sinuses and by the epidural veins in the vertebral column.

The major indications for the use of CSF imaging in children are:

1. diagnosis and classification of hydrocephalus;
2. detecting CSF leaks;
3. localizing subarachnoid blocks and abnormal flow;
4. demonstrating subarachnoid and porencephalic cysts;
5. demonstrating patency of lumboperitoneal, ventriculoatrial and ventriculoperitoneal shunts;
6. demonstrating function of third ventriculostomies;
7. evaluation of obstructive hydrocephalus.

The technique for performing cisternographic studies in children is as follows. Injection is carried out under sterile conditions using ^{99m}Tc-labelled DTPA (or ^{111}In-labelled DTPA). Two hours after a lumbar injection, radioactivity is seen in the basal cisterns, suprasellar cisterns and some in the sylvian cisterns and cerebellopontine angle. By 4 h radioactivity is through the tentorium, around the frontal lobes anteriorly with more in the sylvian cisterns and basal cisterns. At 24 h radioactivity is over the hemispheres and concentrated parasagittally.

When evaluating CSF leaks, well counting should be done of the nasal packs which were placed adjacent to the sphenoid, posterior and anterior ethmoids, and images taken at 1, 6 and 24 h.

The following is the clinical technique for imaging the ventricular flow patterns in children. Imaging should be carried out immediately after the injection of the tracer into the ventricle. Radioactivity should flow into the opposite ventricle immediately and into the cisterna magna and basal cisterns within minutes and should be over the hemispheres and into the parasagittal region by 24 h.

In shunt-function studies the tracer is injected either into the reservoir of the shunt if it is a ventriculoatrial or ventriculoperitoneal type, or directly into the spinal subarachnoid space in the lumboperitoneal type. The amount of tracer used is of the order of 1 mCi of ^{99m}Tc-labelled DTPA in 0.1 ml volume. In ventriculoperitoneal shunts the radioactivity should move through the tube in 15–30 min and clear the reservoir in 30–45 min. The flow through the lumboperitoneal shunt tubing is rapid but clearing of the lumbosubarachnoid space may take up to 2–3 h.

17.10.2 HYDROCEPHALUS

(a) *Non-communicating hydrocephalus*

The flow pattern appears normal since there is no ventricular filling. There may possibly be obstruction at the basal cisterns because of pressure phenomena.

(b) *Communicating hydrocephalus – ex vacuo*

Dilated ventricles may be seen with radioactivity refluxing into them but they clear within 24 h. There may be normal or slightly delayed flow over the hemispheres with large subarachnoid spaces.

Communicating hydrocephalus – extraventricular obstructive, Radioactive CSF rapidly refluxes into dilated ventricles, where it remains with or without flow over the hemispheres and no concentration parasagittally. The ventricles appear as a broad 'C' of radioactivity on the lateral views, and as heart-shaped on the anterior, whereas on the posterior they are rounded rectangular areas of radioactivity seen superiorly and sagittally. The vertex view is the most valuable in assessing ventricular stasis, as one can see the ventricles very clearly with few confusing structures (Figure 17.17). This study is used after the detection of dilated ventricles to determine the functional nature of the CSF flow. When the tracer remains in the ventricles at 24 h then the child invariably benefits from a CSF diversionary shunt.

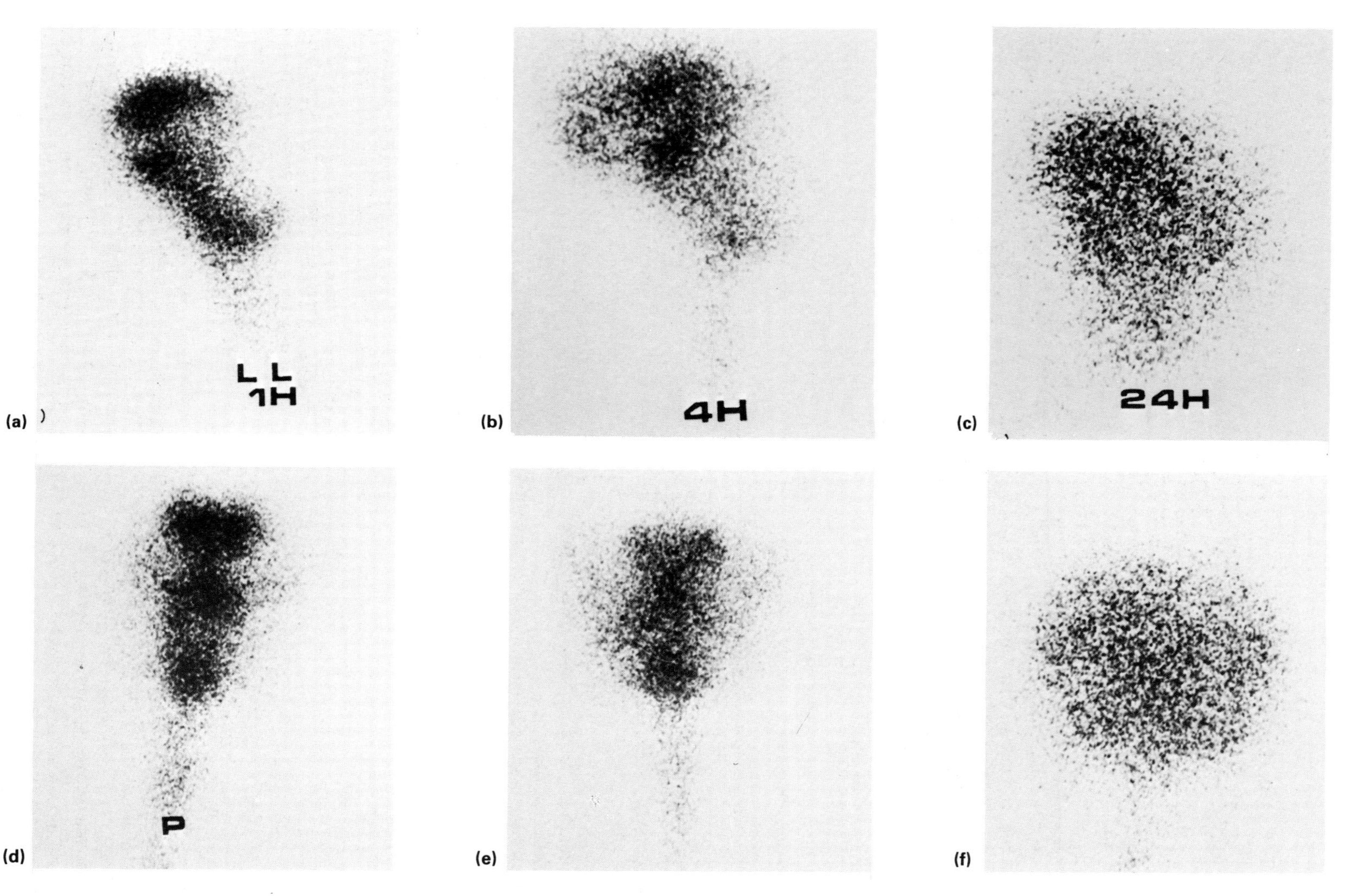

Figure 17.17 Extraventricular obstructive hydrocephalus. There is ventricular reflux at 1 h (a, d) with stasis through 24 h (b, c, e, f), which is fairly uniform over the surface of the brain.

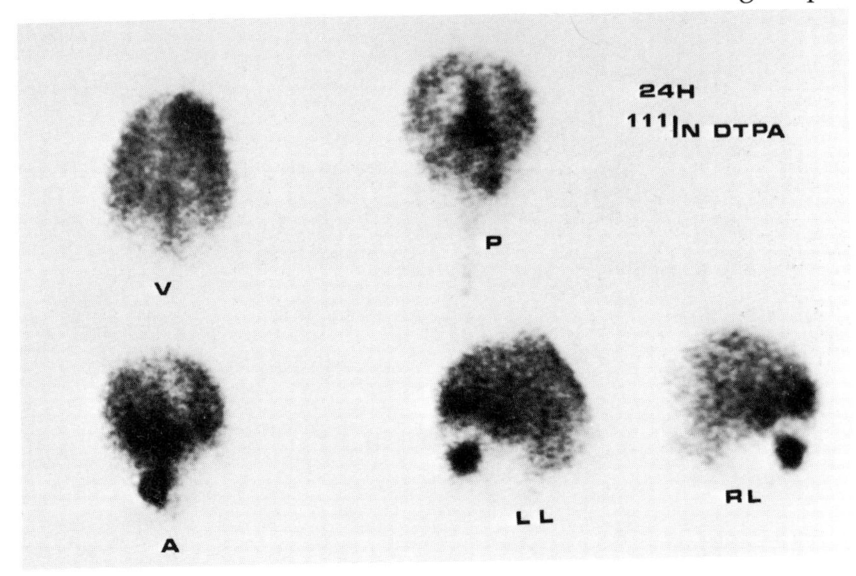

Figure 17.18 Rhinorrhoea. The 24 h images demonstrate the tracer leaking into the left nasopharynx via a fracture in the cribiform plate. There is increased tracer pooling there.

17.10.3 CSF LEAKS

In children with rhinorrhoea, radioactivity can be found in the nose, nasopharynx or sinuses. Its more precise localization may be determined by counting the nasal packs which were placed in the anterior, middle and posterior nasopharynx (Figure 17.18).

In those with otorhinorrhoea, radioactivity may be found in the nasal pharynx when it has passed through the Eustachian tube. If the eardrum is ruptured, it can be detected on a cotton ball in the ear.

17.10.4 EVALUATION OF CSF DIVERSIONARY SHUNTS

The clinical evaluation of CSF diversionary shunt function is often difficult. Usually, the problem of whether or not the overall shunt function is adequate is apparent from a change in symptomatology. However, shunt function is usually evaluated clinically by observing the compression of the reservoir and its subsequent refilling. If the reservoir is difficult to compress the obstruction is usually considered to be distal, whereas if the reservoir compresses easily but fills slowly it is suspected of being proximal.

Once the needle is introduced into the reservoir then 0.1 ml of ^{99m}Tc-pertechnetate in saline is introduced into the reservoir and an image taken in two modes. Initially, these are identical, i.e. an image is taken for information density of 1000 counts per square centimetre over the reservoir. Subsequently, images are repeated for the same count density and also for the same time as the initial image. The latter series of images permits an 'eyeball' assessment of the clearance of the tracer from the reservoir. The former is used to give anatomical detail. A second series of images is carried out monitoring the distal end of the tracer as it flows down the tube.

The images are compared to determine the clearance of the tracer from the reservoir during the supine phase of the study and the effect of hydrostatic pressure on the system is evaluated after the upright images. At this point, the patient is allowed to sit or walk so that the increased hydrostatic pressure in the ventricles will drive the CSF through the system to its destination. Usually this will occur in all patients with a functioning shunt. If there is no flow of the tracer through the shunt apparatus at this point, then the reservoir is compressed five to ten times in patients with ventriculoperitoneal shunt, and the head and torso images repeated to confirm the lack of flow. One additional manoeuvre is carried out in the situation where the tracer readily enters the abdomen but does not disperse throughout the peritoneal cavity. The patient is rotated and

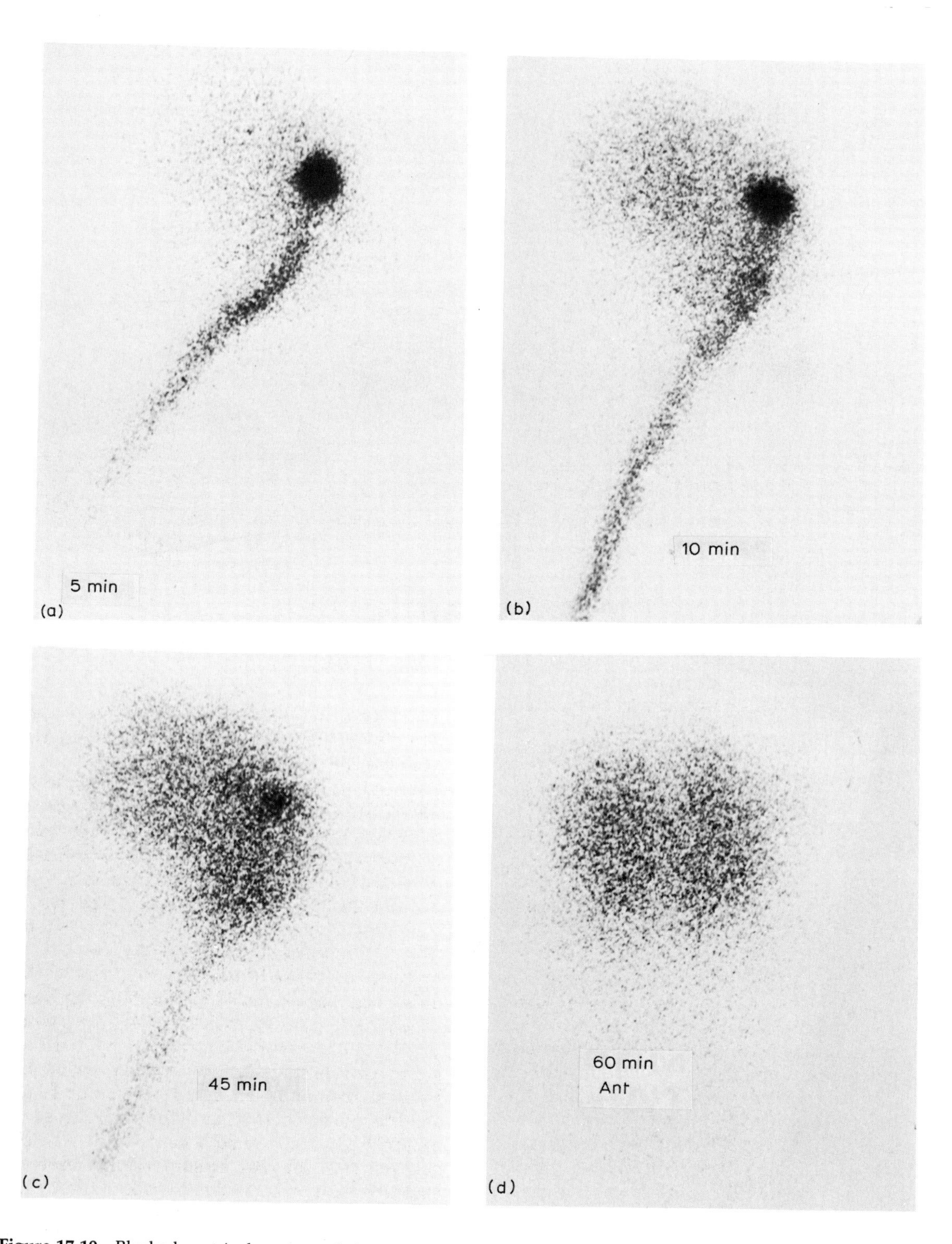

Figure 17.19 Blocked ventriculoperitoneal shunt. Images taken at 5 min (a), 10 min (b), 45 min (c) and 60 min (d) after injection of the reservoir show rapid egress of the tracer down the tube and refluxing back into the ventricle (e). The abdominal end of the catheter (f, g) shows that the tracer never leaves the tube. The catheter tip was embedded in the peritoneum.

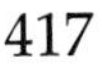

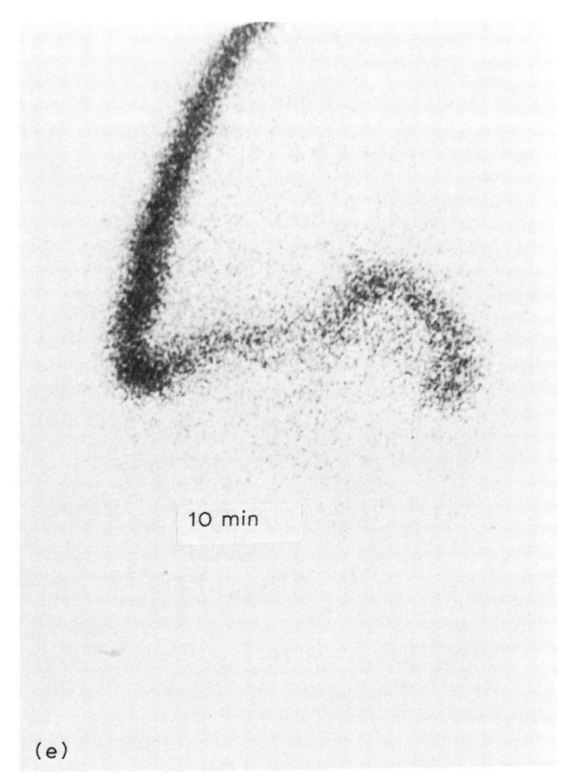

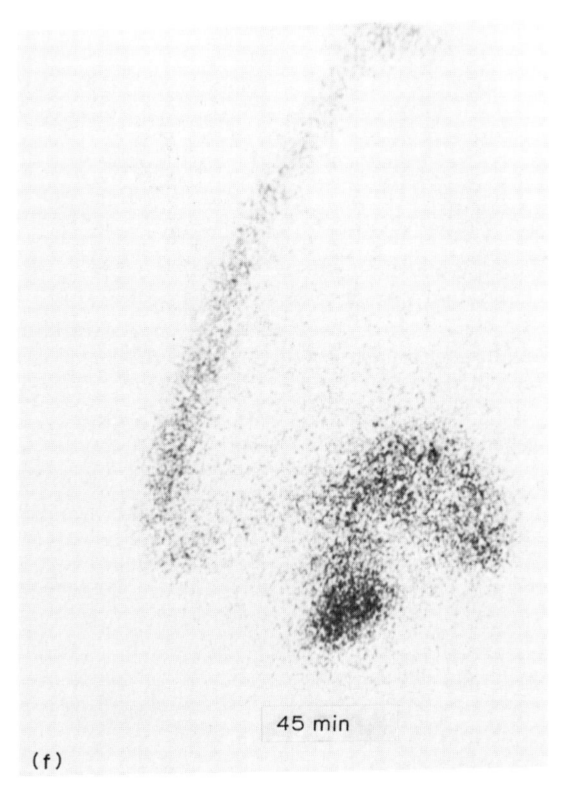

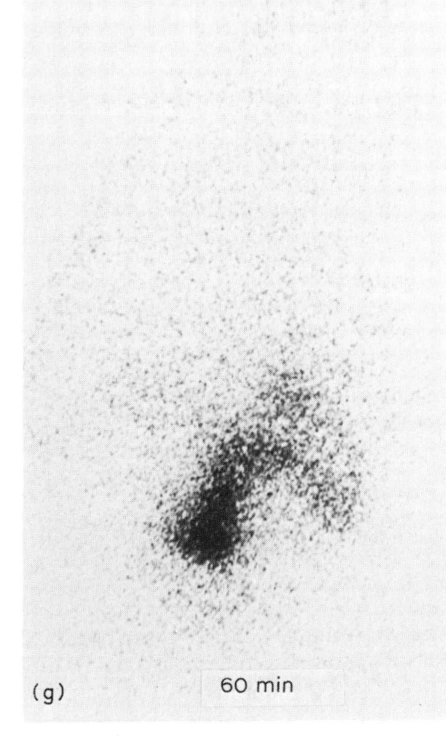

moved about so as to try and disperse the tracer to differentiate between a loculation and normal pooling.

In our review we studied 67 ventriculoatrial and 164 ventriculoperitoneal shunts. Of these 105 normal studies occurred and none had subsequent documentation of shunt malfunction. Of the 103 blocked shunts, 98 had the site correctly predicted. A variety of clinical and surgical results were found for the 23 poorly functioning shunts (Figure 17.19).

These results indicate that in general the radionuclide assessment of shunt function is quite satisfactory. However, in some of the cases when there was a discrepancy between the radionuclide results and the clinical or surgical findings, it must be remembered that the shunt study only evaluates the function at the time of the study. This was exemplified in one child whose shunt was obstructed by scan, but at surgery the reservoir externalized and there was no sign of malfunction. However, when the surgeon had reconnected the reservoir to the distal tube, it suddenly appeared to be blocked, and indeed was. This type of intermittent obstruction can occur when the distal catheter imbeds itself into the peritoneum or the bowel. Our overall evaluation of the distal tubing is very much better than that of the ventricular tube assessment as the latter requires an indirect means for determining its state of function.

17.11 SEIZURES

Since the advent of ^{99m}Tc-labelled HMPAO the evaluation of seizures has altered significantly. At the Hospital for Sick Children we now routinely evaluate all children with seizures that are refractory to normal treatment and who may be considered for surgical removal of the focus. We now perform interictal and where possible ictal SPECT perfusion scans. The typical finding in the interictal phase is decrease in perfusion at the seizure focus site (Figure 17.20). In most ictal scans the focus is seen as an increase in perfusion (Figure 17.21). This simple technique has greatly assisted our neurologists and neurosurgeons in selecting the appropriate surgical approach. Cerebral perfusion techniques are being extended to other cerebrovascular disorders (Shahar *et al.*, 1990) and cerebral palsy (Denays *et al.*, 1990).

17.12 PAEDIATRIC CARDIOLOGY

Nuclear cardiology procedures are important in the diagnosis and management of many cardiac abnormalities in infants and children as they are in adults. Both functional and structural information which was previously obtained by cardiac catheterization and contrast angiography can now be derived non-invasively. In paediatrics, particularly in neonatal patients, where catheterization has significant mortality and morbidity, physiological functional information is essential and should be obtained non-invasively.

Information which could only previously be obtained primarily by cardiac catheterization and contrast angiography can now be derived non-invasively. Echocardiography is used to detect morphological abnormalities and nuclear cardiology is used to gain further functional information. Neonates present special problems in diagnosis. The important differential diagnosis of the cyanotic newborn include the respiratory distress syndrome and other pulmonary disorders, and cyanotic heart disease due to right-to-left shunting through a patent ductus arteriosus or foramen ovale. In transposition of the great vessels or other causes of a large right-to-left shunt with pulmonary stenosis, the tracer is visualized in the aorta before the appearance in the lungs. This abnormality of flow will not be seen in neonates whose cyanosis has a pulmonary cause. Confirmation of abnormal flow may be obtained by placing a computer-generated region of interest over the carotid vessels to generate time–activity curves and show the premature arrival of tracer in the systemic circulation.

The presence of a raised pulmonary vascular resistance may affect the amount of shunting through a septal defect, and sequential studies may be necessary in the estimation of pulmonary/systemic flow ratio and to determine when surgery should be considered.

17.12.1 RADIONUCLIDE ANGIOCARDIOGRAM

For diagnosis, the radionuclide angiocardiogram allows separation of the cardiac chambers in time as well as in space so that individual chambers, particularly when in an unusual location, can be identified and the direction of blood flow through the chamber determined. However, the small size of the cardiac chambers and the more rapid transit of activity through the central circulation in children limits the anatomical resolution that is possible. The indications in congenital heart disease, are as follows:

1. in patients at high risk from a cardiac catheterization to indicate the presence or site of disease, particularly the newborn and premature;
2. the asymptomatic patient with a murmur suggestive of congenital heart disease such as a ventricular septal defect;
3. repetitive evaluation when a diagnosis has already been established to define changes;
4. documentation of ventricular reserve during exercise as a guide to the timing of surgery, or the effectiveness of surgery;
5. determination of patency of temporary surgical shunts.

The first-pass technique involves the injection of tracer as an intravenous bolus, preferably via a jugular vein. The sequential passage of the bolus is followed through the heart with a scintillation detector. A Bender–Blau autofluoroscope has advantages in sensitivity at the expense of resolution but the newer high count rate versions of the

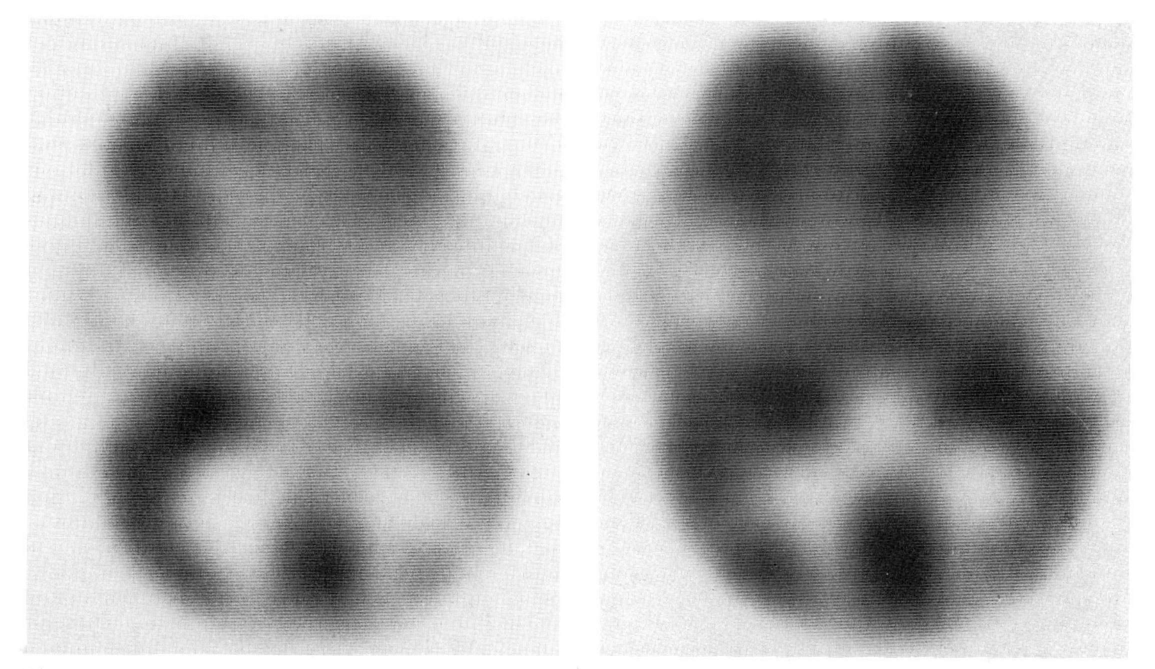

Figure 17.20 Interictal seizure focus. The left temporal lobe demonstrates decreased perfusion on two adjacent 1 cm SPECT (^{99m}Tc-labelled HMPAO) slices.

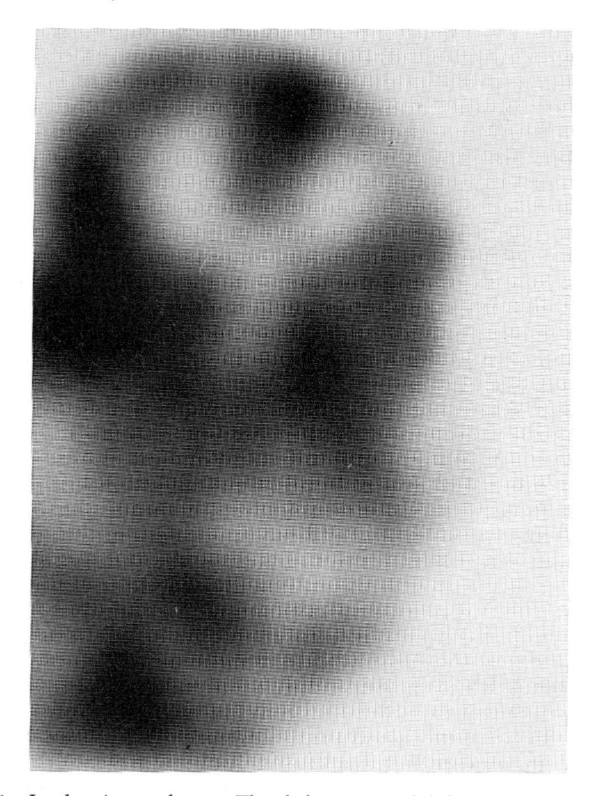

Figure 17.21 Ictal seizure focus. The left temporal lobe demonstrates increased perfusion in the SPECT (^{99m}Tc-labelled HMPAO) slice.

Anger camera will give excellent results, with improved resolution.

^{99m}Tc-pertechnetate is the most frequently used tracer and when combined with *in vivo* labelling of red blood cells gated equilibrium studies can be performed following the angiogram.

The nuclear angiogram is performed by injecting a small bolus, less than 0.5 ml of ^{99m}Tc-pertechnetate (15 mCi m^{-2} body surface area), into an external jugular vein via a 19 or 21 gauge scalp vein needle. The needle is attached to a three-way stopcock and extension tube. The radioactivity is injected into the extension tube by the stopcock once the needle is properly placed in the vein. The dose is then flushed with 10 ml of saline into the vein. A short, sharp bolus results. If prolongation or fragmentation of the bolus occurs erroneous results are usually produced. The bolus may also be delayed when there is obstruction to the venous return to the heart, elevated pulmonary venous pressures or obstructive valvular disease. Computer-processed images are used for interpretation. Currently, we record the transit of the bolus at 10 frames per second. The computer system permits magnification of the image so that we can zoom in on the pertinent portion of the camera field of view. This is of particular value in the very small child, especially the neonate.

The analysis of the radionuclide angiocardiogram is divided into several components. First is the qualitative analysis or visual inspection and assessment of the images using the computer in both static and dynamic modes. This is a very important aspect of the study, as often a peculiarity of anatomy may be demonstrated by an abnormal flow pattern.

17.12.2 SHUNT QUANTIFICATION

(a) Left-to-right shunts

Left-to-right shunt estimation is the commonest indication for the radionuclide angiocardiogram. Computer quantification was first described by Maltz and Treves in 1973. A time–activity histogram is generated from the passage of the radioactive bolus through the lungs. By applying a least-squares fit to a gamma variate function of this pulmonic flow, one can accurately estimate the pulmonary flow. By subtracting the fitted curve from the raw data a pulmonary recirculation curve is obtained. The ratio of the area under the first transit curve to the area under the recirculation curve is the pulmonary/systemic flow ratio (*QP*/*QS*; Figure 17.22).

This analysis is comparable to the dye dilution technique and is more readily performed. We obtained good correlation (r=0.82, $p < 0.001$) in a group of 86 patients. The main difficulty with this technique is to determine whether or not the gamma variate fit to the raw data is satisfactory. Using a computerized curve-fit-analysis routine, the ease of obtaining a fit of good quality is improved. Experience is most valuable in obtaining correct and consistent results. Our computer program minimizes this difficulty by automatically obtaining the points which are most adequate and selecting the best-fitting curve from various attempts. When necessary, the operator is able to override the program. Poor bolus injection, superior vena cava (SVC) obstruction, a large heart in a small chest causing difficulty in placing a region of interest over the lung alone, single ventricle or large VSD chamber mixing are all difficulties in left-to-right shunt quantification.

(b) Right-to-left shunts

^{99m}Tc-labelled microspheres embolize in the pulmonary circulation and normally do not appear in the systemic circulation following an intravenous injection. If there is a right-to-left shunt, the microspheres appear in the systemic circulation and may be detected with a computerized whole-body imaging system. The shunt can be measured by whole-body imaging using the following:

$$\%\ \text{right-to-left shunt} = \left(\frac{\text{total body count} - \text{total lung count}}{\text{total body count}}\right) \times 100$$

Imaging of the body should not be delayed after injection of microspheres as rapid loss of ^{99m}Tc occurs from the particles, possibly due to fragmentation, and a consequent overestimate of shunt size will occur. Since there is distribution of particulates to the systemic circulation, the number of microspheres should be restricted to about 50 000.

17.12.3 EQUILIBRIUM BLOOD POOL IMAGING

Equilibrium blood pool imaging is frequently used after radionuclide cineangiography to obtain high-count-rate, high-resolution images for determination of ejection fraction, and to allow mul-

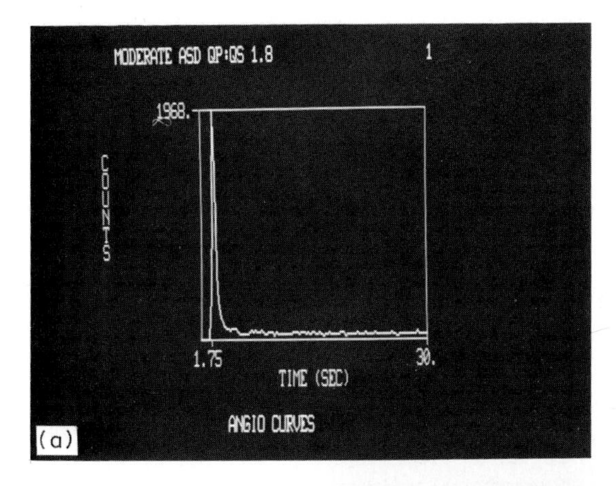

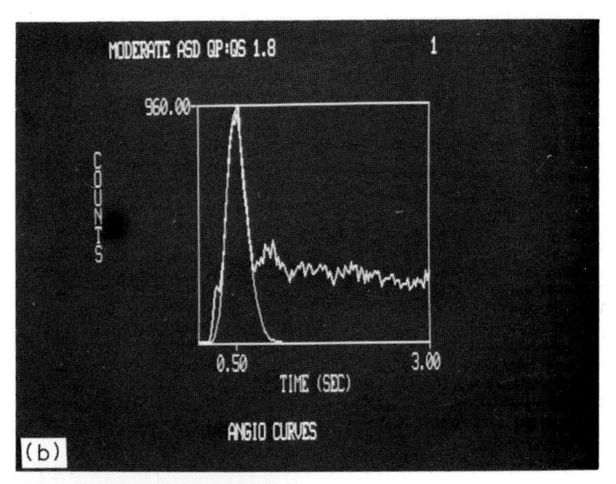

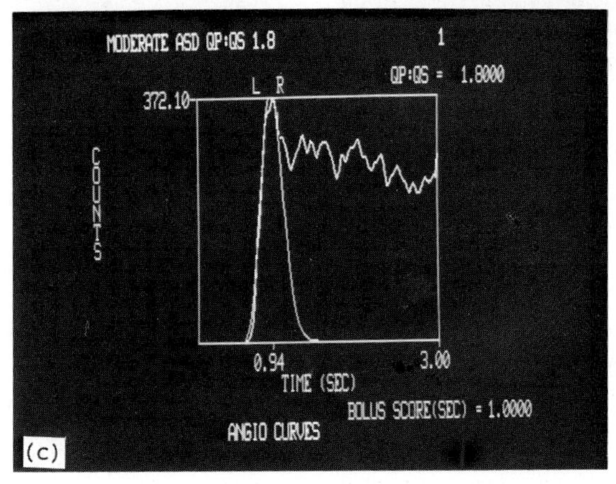

Figure 17.22 Moderate atrial septal defect shunt. The bolus was very compact as demonstrated by the superior vena cava curve (a). The computer gamma variate fits the pulmonary curve (b) well, showing a smaller recirculation. The computer fit to the recirculation curve (c) yields a *QP/QS* of 1.8, which is moderate.

tiple projections of the heart to be obtained. This may be helpful when the cardiac anatomy was not clear from the first-pass study.

Once the tracer has equilibrated in the blood, the heart cavity can be studied by using standard ventricular function analysis (MUGA) (Strauss *et al.*, 1977). We now only use *in vitro* labelled RBC as we have found that the *in vivo* technique gives poor labelling in too many cases.

The acquisition length varies from 2 min in stress studies to 20 min in resting studies. The data are viewed in movie mode and the wall motion of the heart chambers observed. The resting gated study is usually performed in two views. The left anterior oblique (LAO) view is angled along the septum usually with a 15° caudal tilt, giving the best delineation of the ventricles. The other view is usually anterior. The positioning must be modified if the child has congenital heart disease.

From the gated images ventricular wall motion is studied and dyskinetic or akinetic segments determined. This is of particular value in conditions of poor ventricular contraction, such as ischaemia and cardiomyopathies (Figure 17.23). Segmental wall motion abnormalities may be noted in areas of ischaemia such as anomalous left coronary artery disease.

Besides wall motion, quantification of ventricular function, i.e. ejection fraction (EF), stroke volume, systolic and diastolic volumes, and atrial kick contribution to the EF can be readily obtained. These are important parameters in determining the extent or severity of the disease and are a rapid, non-invasive method of following the patient's clinical course. Differentiation of time–

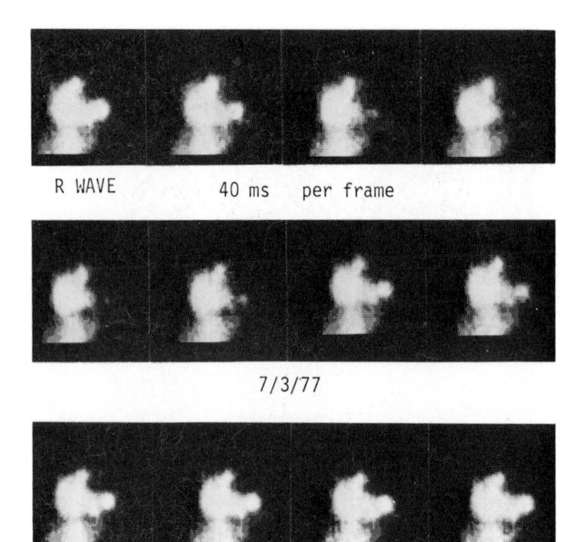

Figure 17.23 Atrophic cardiomyopathy. This child with viral myocardiopathy has good contraction of the left ventricle but poor contraction of the right. This is due to the ischaemic changes secondary to the viral illness affecting solely the right ventricle.

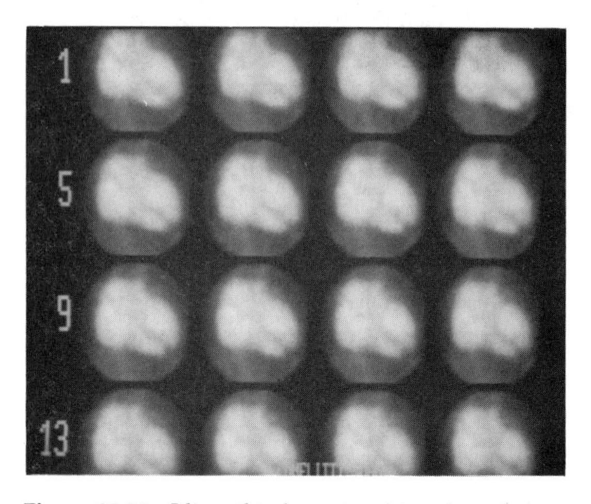

Figure 17.24 Idiopathic hypertrophic subaortic stenosis. The typical appearance of the small, very hypercontractile left ventricle is present. The superior portion of the septal space between the ventricles is increased.

activity curves also allows the maximum rate of construction and expansion to be determined.

An interesting example of the use of gated blood pool studies is the diagnosis of idiopathic hypertrophic subaortic stenosis. (Figure 17.24; Pohost *et al.*, 1977). In these patients, the gated images show a small left ventricular cavity usually displaced towards the apex. Asymmetrical thickening of the left ventricular myocardium may be seen, especially in the upper septum, with distortion of the right ventricular blood pool. The ejection fraction is high due to the hypercontractile left ventricle.

17.12.4 MYOCARDIAL PERFUSION IMAGING

Thallium myocardial scanning is well established in the adult patient; however, there has not been the same demand for its use in paediatrics. The dose of ^{201}Tl is 1.15 mCi m^{-2}. Imaging is carried out as soon as possible after the injection. The highest-resolution tomographic system should be used with a 20% window around the 69–83 keV mercury X-ray photopeak. We use a 180° rotation and collect 64 128 × 128 pixel array images.

In childhood, myocardial ischaemia usually occurs secondary to a severe hypoxic episode during birth, which can be precipitated by severe aortic stenosis or coarctation of the aorta. An anomalous left coronary artery, the effect of surgery such as the total anomalous great vessels switch procedure and atrophic cardiomyopathies may also cause ischaemia. Evaluation of the extent and progression of ischaemia can accurately be determined by ^{201}Tl scanning.

Although the presence of an anomalous left coronary artery is uncommon, it is important to make this diagnosis in the child presenting with cardiac symptoms. Similarly, after coronary artery surgery the vessel flow may be compromised and all such patients should be evaluated six months after surgery. The extent of myocardial ischaemia and infarction can readily be obtained from careful interpretation of the ^{201}Tl tomogram. Additionally, some prognostic information can be derived by observing the amount of left ventricular myocardium rendered ischaemic by the anomalous origin of the left coronary artery. In some patients with extensive collateralization between the right and left coronary systems, the degree of ischaemia may be small. Repeat studies can follow the progression of ischaemia and help determine timing of surgical intervention. Pre- and post-operative ^{201}Tl studies help evaluate the results of surgical correction. In children over 6 years of age, exercise ^{201}Tl scans can be performed to assess ischaemia under stress.

A fascinating area for ^{201}Tl scanning is its use in the neonate who was thought to have compromised blood flow at birth to assess the status of

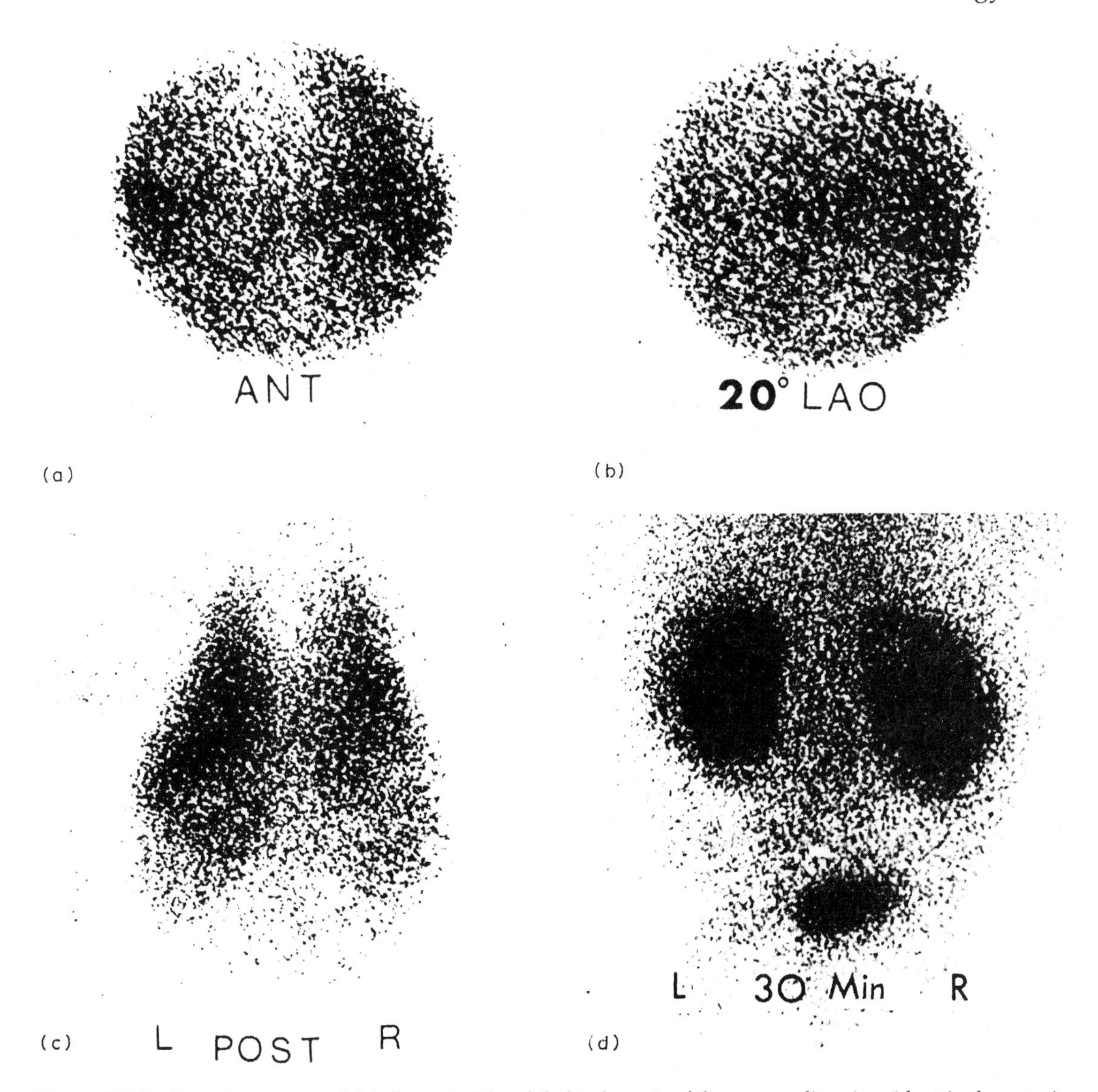

Figure 17.25 Transient myocardial ischaemia. The global ischaemia of the myocardium is evident in the anterior (a), 20° lateral (b) and posterior (c) views as the heart is not identifiable. The post-myocardial images of the kidneys demonstrated multicystic disease (d), a totally unrelated coincidental disease.

myocardial perfusion. In such children we use gated 45% LAO, anterior and lateral projections as the heart is too small for SPECT imaging. It has been well shown that the tracer distribution depends on blood flow (Wesselhoeft *et al.*, 1972) and removing the tracer from the blood (Na^+-K^+ ATPase pump) (Treves and Collins-Nakai, 1976). Weich *et al.* (1977) have shown that ^{201}Tl extraction is decreased by hypoxia and acidosis. Non-structural myocardial dysfunction of the newborn is often due to transient myocardial ischaemia (TMI) (Finley *et al.*, 1979). In a group of neonates at birth, ^{201}Tl scans in the first week showed no discernible tracer accumulation in the ventricular myocardium, but there was retention of tracer in the lungs. At about 4–5 weeks, there was improvement of ^{201}Tl uptake (Figure 17.25). This, however, appeared to lag behind the clinical and ECG improvement by about five to seven days. Several other neonates had similar uptake of tracer into the myocardium as seen in normal adults. In those babies with TMI, relative myocardial/pulmonary activity ratios initially are low, i.e. 1.3:1, and later show improvement to greater than 2:1. The other neonates without TMI had values greater than 2:1. The important clinical application of ^{201}Tl scanning in the newborn is that non-structural myocardial dysfunction of ischaemic origin can be diagnosed and often differentiated from other structural abnormalities, and appropriate therapy instituted. With echocardiography and/or radionuclide angiograms demonstrating poor function and normal structural anatomy, the diagnosis of myocardial ischaemia can be confirmed by ^{201}Tl myocardial scans (Finley *et al.*, 1979).

Several neonates with critical aortic stenosis and coarctation had large concentrically hypertrophied left ventricles with areas of decreased tracer distribution in their apical inferior regions. This was suggestive of local ischaemia and corresponded to the ischaemic changes seen on their ECGs. Other neonatal conditions such as hypertrophic cardiomyopathies, myocarditis and ventricular hypertrophy as a result of left-to-right shunts have scan findings similar to those described for the older patient. Transposition of the great arteries has fairly symmetrical uptake in both ventricles. ^{201}Tl scanning has also been used in the diagnosis of single ventricle where there is no visualization of the interventricular septum. These non-invasive tests may decrease the number of cardiac catheterizations in these sick neonates.

REFERENCES

Ash, J., De Souza, M., Peters, M., Wilmot, D., Hausen, D. and Gilday, D. (1990) Quantitative assessment of blood flow in pediatric recipients of renal transplants. *J. Nucl. Med.*, **31**, 580–5.

Ash, J. M. and Gilday D. L. (1980) Renal nuclear imaging and analysis in pediatrics. *Urol. Clin. N. Am.*, **7**, 201.

Conway, J. J. (1976a) The sensitivity, specificity and accuracy of radionuclide imaging of Meckel's diverticulum. *J. Nucl. Med.*, **17**, 553.

Conway, J. J. (1976b) Effectiveness of direct and indirect radionuclide cystography in detecting vesicoureteral reflux. *J. Nucl. Med.*, **17**, 81.

D'Angilelis, J. A., Fisher, R. L., Ozonoff, M. B. and Sziklas, J. J. (1975) 99m Tc-pertechnetate bone imaging in Legg–Perthes disease. *Radiology*, **115**, 407.

Denays, R., Tondeur, M., Toppet, V. *et al.* (1990) Cerebral palsy: initial experience with Tc-99m HmPAO SPECT of the brain. *Radiology*, **175**, 111–16.

Di Lorenzo, C., Piepsz, A., Ham, H and Cadranel, S. (1987) Gastric emptying with gastro-oesophageal reflux. *Arch. Dis. Child.*, **62**, 449–53.

Duszynski, D. O., Jewett, T. C. and Allen, J. E. (1970a) The visualization of Meckel's diverticulum with 99m Tc-pertechnetate. *Surgery*, **68**, 567–70.

Finley, J. P., Howman-Giles, R. B., Gilday, D. L. and Rowe, R. D. (1979) Transient myocardial ischaemia of the newborn infant demonstrated by thallium myocardial imaging. *J. Pediat.*, **94**, 263–70.

Gilday, D. L. (1976) in *Neuroradiology in Infants and Children* (eds D. C. F. Harwood-Nash and C. R. Fitz), Mosby, St Louis, pp. 572–608.

Gilday, D. L., Paula, D. J. and Patterson, J. (1975) Diagnosis of osteomyelitis in children by combined blood pool and bone imaging. *Radiology*, **117**, 331.

Krueger, R., Ash, J. M., Silver M. *et al.* (1980) Primary hydronephrosis: assessment of the diuretic renogram, pelvic perfusion pressure, post operative findings and renal and ureteral histology. *Urol. Clin. N. Am.*, **7**, 231.

Maltz, D. L. and Treves, S. (1973) Quantitative radionuclide angiography: determination of QP:QS in children. *Circulation*, **47**, 1049–56.

Majd, M., Reba R. C. and Altman R. P. (1981a) Effect of phenobarbital on 99Tc-IDA scintigraphy in the evaluation of neonatal jaundice. *Semin. Nucl. Med.*, **11**.

Majd, M., Reba R. C. and Altman, R. P. (1981b) Hepatobiliary scintigraphy with 99mTc-PIPIDA in the evaluation of neonatal jaundice. *Pediatrics*, **67**, 140–5.

Maneval, D. C., Magill, H. L., Cypress, A. M. and Rodman, J. H. (1990) Measurement of skin-to-kidney resistance in children: implications for quantitative renography. *J. Nucl. Med.*, **31**, 287–91.

Martin, D. J., Gilday, D. L. and Reilly B. J. (1975) Evaluation of the urinary tract in the neonatal period. *Radiol. Clin. N. Am.*, **13**, 359.

McDonald, P., Tarar, R., Gilday, D. L. *et al.* (1974) Some radiologic observations in renal vein thrombosis. *Am. J. Roentgenol.*, **120**, 368.

Peters, A. M., Gunasekera, R. D., Henderson, B. L. *et al.* (1987) Noninvasive measurement of blood flow and extraction fraction. *Nucl. Med. Commun.*, **8**, 823–37.

Pieretti, R., Gilday, D. and Jeffs, R. (1974) Differential kidney scan in pediatric urology. *Urology*, **4**, 665.

Pohost, G. M., Vignola, P. A., McKusick, K. E. *et al.* (1977) Hypertrophic cardiomyopathy: evaluation of gated cardiac blood pool scanning. *Circulation*, **85**, 92–9.

Pollet, J. E., Sharp, F. and Smith, F. W. (1979) Radionuclide imaging for vesicorenal reflux using intravenous 99mTc-DTPA. *Pediat. Radiol.*, **8**, 165–7.

Rosenthall, L., Henry, J. N., Murphy, D. A. and Freeman, L. M. (1972) Radiopertechnetate imaging of the Meckel's diverticulum. *Radiology*, **105**, 371–3.

Shahar, E., Gilday, D., Hwang, P., Cohen, E. and Lambert, R. (1990) Diatric cerebrovascular disease. Alterations of regional cerebral blood flow directed by Tc 99m-HmPAO SPECT. *Arch. Neurol.*, **47**, 578–84.

Shandling, B. (1965) Laparotomy for rectal bleeding. *Pediatrics*, **35**, 787.

Smith, F. W. and Gilday, D. L. (1980) Scintigraphic appearances of osteoid osteoma. *Radiology*, **137**, 191–5.

Strauss, H. W., Singleton, R., Burow, R. *et al.* (1977)

Multiple gated acquisition (MUGA): an improved non-invasive technique for evaluation of regional wall motion (MWM) and left ventricular function (LVF). *Am. J. Cardiol.*, **39**, 284.

Treves, S. and Collins-Nakai, R. L. (1976) Radioactive tracers in congenital heart disease. *Am. J. Cardiol.*, **38**, 711–21.

Valdes, Papena and Stein (1970) *Morphologic Pathology of the Alimentary Canal*, Saunders, Philadelphia, p. 482.

Weich, H. F., Strauss, H. W. and Pitt, B. (1977) The extraction of thallium-201 by the myocardium. *Circulation*, **56**, 188–91.

Wells, R. G., Sty J. R. and Starshak, R. J. (1987) Hepatobiliary imaging in neonatal jaundice. *Appl. Radiol.*

Wesselhoeft, H., Hurley, P. T., Wagner, H. M., Jr and Rowe, R. D. (1972) Nuclear angiocardiography in the diagnosis of congenital heart disease in infants. *Circulation*, **45**, 77–91.

CHAPTER EIGHTEEN

Tumour imaging

S. E. M. Clarke

18.1 INTRODUCTION

The adequate management of any malignancy depends on several factors. The first is an accurate diagnosis. For the diagnosis to be accurate, not only must the site of the tumour be identified, but the exact tissue in which the tumour is arising must be determined. Although the histogenic type of the tumour may be readily apparent on light microscopy, more detailed investigations including histochemical techniques of resected tumour are often necessary to correctly characterize the malignancy in terms of tissue origin and degree of differentiation of the tumour. A further factor in contributing to decisions on management is the stage of the malignancy at the time of presentation or at the time of investigation.

Current theories of tumour formation include the 'single cell theory', which postulates that a neoplasm derives from a single cell which undergoes neoplastic change. Monoclonal gammopathies, for example, appear to arise from a single clone of plasma cells which become malignant and which by local proliferation and metastatic spread replace the normal clones of immunoglobulin-forming cells. It is possible that lymphomas and tumours of the haemopoietic tissues develop similarly.

The second commonly held theory is the 'field of growth' theory. This is based on the tendency for multiple tumours to arise in a restricted area of tissue and for apparently recurrent tumours to develop near the site of removal of a primary tumour. Examples of multiple primary tumours arising in a particular field include transitional cell tumours of the urinary tract, uterine leiomyomas, breast cancer which is bilateral in about 9% of cases, and polyposis coli. The factors that may produce a 'field of growth' have been recognized as:

1. extrinsic physical and chemical agents;
2. hereditary predisposition;
3. chronic disease, generally inflammatory;
4. hormones;
5. viruses.

The extrinsic agents include ionizing and ultraviolet radiations. The first case of carcinoma of the skin arising after the local application of ionizing radiation was reported in 1902. Since then animal experiments using ionizing radiation on normal and inflamed tissues have resulted in skin cancers, subcutaneous sarcomas, osteosarcomas, frequently after a latent interval of many months. In man, squamous carcinoma of the skin was a well-recognized hazard for early radium workers and irradiated lupus vulgaris frequently underwent malignant change. In bone, osteosarcoma may develop several years following local irradiation of a benign tumour or an inflammatory lesion. There is also a well-proven association between thymic irradiation in childhood and the subsequent development of thyroid cancers up to 18 years later. The sequelae of the Nagasaki and Hiroshima atomic bomb attacks are still being investigated but the increased incidence of leukaemia in the survivors confirms the long-term effect of ionizing radiations on the bone marrow.

The association of long-standing exposure to ultraviolet radiation and multiple squamous carcinomas in exposed areas of the body is well recognized and basal cell cancers are also frequently encountered in this group.

Chemical agents that are associated with the development of tumours subdivide into those occurring naturally and synthesized chemicals. Natural chemicals such as aflatoxin produced by the mould *Aspergillus flaveus* contaminate foodstuffs such as ground nutmeal. Aflatoxin is a powerful liver carcinogen and has been implicated as the causative agent in areas of Africa where hepatic cancer is prevalent. Synthetic chemical carcinogens have been implicated in many occupational cancers. The polycyclic hydrocarbons were demonstrated in the 1920s to produce skin cancers by Japanese workers when rabbit's ears were painted with tar. 3,4-Benzypyrene has been subsequently shown to be the most important carcinogenic constituent of coal tar. The tumours occur at the site of application of the carcinogen, with squamous carcinomas following application to the skin, and sarcomas forming after subcutaneous injection.

Workers in the aniline dye industry, exposed to the aromatic amines, α-naphthylamine, β-naphthylamine and benzidine have been observed to have a higher incidence of bladder carcinomas than the rest of the population.

Whilst there is little significant hereditary predisposition to most of the common types of cancer, cancer of the breast has recently been recognized as occurring more commonly in relatives of affected women than in the general population. There are a number of uncommon neoplastic diseases which are inherited. Important examples of these disease are polyposis coli, retinoblastomas and the multiple endocrine neoplasias. The recent discovery of the 'oncogene' has opened up a new area of research in the factors causing cancer.

Virchow believed that cancer was the result of prolonged stimulation of the tissues through 'chronic irritation'. Although this theory is now discounted as the explanation for most tumours, certain chronic inflammatory conditions of surface epithelia are now recognized as giving rise to cancers. Chronic varicose ulcers, sinuses of chronic osteomyelitis and old burn scars occasionally give rise to squamous cell carcinomas. Ulcerative colitis is also an important precancerous condition. About 4% of all cases undergo neoplastic change, and at least one third of all cases lasting 12 years develop cancer, usually multifocal.

Chronic metabolic and deficiency diseases are associated with cancer. About 90% of primary liver cell cancer in man is superimposed on previous cirrhosis and in Paget's disease bone osteosarcoma is an occasional complication, occurring in about 1% of cases.

The relationship between hormones and neoplasia has been clarified over the years. In 1932 Lacassagne successfully produced mammary cancers in mice of both sexes by administering large doses of oestrogen. The contraceptive pill has now been implicated in the occurrence of breast cancer in women who have taken the pill over a long period. There is also a significant incidence of breast cancer in individuals undergoing sex-change surgery, augmented by high-dose oestrogens.

Although hormones appear to play a relatively small role in the aetiology of human cancer, they are of great importance in maintaining the growth of some tumours. These hormone-dependent tumours require specific hormones for their continued growth and undergo regression when the hormone is withdrawn. Many of these hormone-dependent tumours undergo evential transition to complete hormone independence. Prostatic carcinoma was the first neoplasm in man to be successfully repressed by hormonal therapy. It is usually androgen dependent and following castration there is dramatic relief with regression of tumour and its metastases.

Doses of stilboestrol are also given either as an adjunct to orchidectomy or alone.

Breast cancers manifest hormone dependence in less than half the affected women. In premenopausal women oophorectomy often produces remission but this is usually of short duration. In post-menopausal women, oestrogen receptor-positive tumours have been found to regress with tamoxifen, which competes with the oestradiol for receptor sites. The exact mechanism of action of tamoxifen remains unclear. Papillary and follicular cancers of the thyroid are commonly TSH dependent and doses of thyroxine are used to suppress the TSH level.

Tumour-producing oncogenic viruses are of great importance as some human tumours are associated with, if not actually caused by, viruses. Several human tumours have a proven association with viruses. Burkitt's lymphoma is associated with the Epstein–Barr virus. Virus has been cultured from the neoplastic lymphocytes and all patients have high antibody titres to the virus. Infected origins of the tumour also explain the geographical distribution of the tumour as it is found when there is high instance of endemic malaria. Carcinoma of the cervix is a tumour in which there is a significant association between the tumour and the herpes simplex virus type 2. Epidemiological studies support the theory that the herpes simplex virus is a contributory factor in the development of cervical cancer.

18.1.1 STAGING

The stage of a malignancy is defined in terms of local and distant spread of the primary tumour. The 'TNM' system of staging is a system that has been developed as applicable to all sites, irrespective of treatment and which may be supplemented by information which subsequently becomes available from histopathology and from surgery. The system is based on the assessment of the primary tumour (T), the regional lymph nodes (N) and on the presence or absence of distant metastases (M). Numbers are then added to these three components to indicate the extent of disease, e.g. $T_2 N_1 M_0$. Accurate staging not only affects management but also assists in the evaluation of treatment results and facilitates the exchange of information between treatment centres without ambiguity. As well as affecting management decisions, the stage of the tumour at presentation has significant prognostic implications. This is exemplified in rectal cancers in which the staging classification devised by Dukes (1942) aids in the assessment of prognosis (Dukes, 1958). Stage A tumour, i.e. rectal tumour confined to the muscular wall, has an 80–90% survival rate at five years, whereas patients with stage C disease, i.e. tumour invading pararectal tissue and involving lymph nodes, have a less than 25% five-year survival rate.

18.1.2 SPREAD

The mode of spread of tumour cells remains a poorly understood process. Local infiltration follows natural clefts or tissue planes and dense fascial sheets may confine malignant cells for some time. In osteosarcoma of bone, the tumour enlarges but is confined within the periosteum and cartilage is also resistant to tumour infiltration. Infiltration can also occur into individual cells, as occurs in malignant melanoma when epidermal invasion is seen.

Invasion into the lymphatics occurs with carcinoma at an early stage in the spread of the tumour. Sarcoma, however, only rarely involve the local lymphatics. Venous invasion is seen commonly in lung cancers and hypernephromas. The invading tumour becomes covered with thrombus and may eventually totally block the vessel, resulting in venous stasis distal to the invading tumour.

Metastatic spread occurs in the lymphatics when a group of tumour cells in an invaded lymphatic becomes detatched and lodges in the subcapsular sinus of the regional lymph node. As the cells divide the node becomes replaced by tumour and further spread occurs to the next group of glands by way of the efferent channel. This commonly occurs in carcinoma and melanoma but is rarely seen in sarcoma. The extent of lymphatic involvement is important in assessing prognosis and is one of the factors taken into consideration when staging tumours.

Blood spread, following invasion of small vessels or veins by tumour and subsequent detachment of tumour emboli, occurs early in the development of sarcomas. These emboli impact in capillary beds of the lungs and liver, which explains why these organs are a common site of secondary spread. What is less easily explained is why systemic metastases may develop in the absence of apparent lung deposits. It is possible that microscopic lung metastases are present which may be missed on post-mortem examination or that some tumour emboli may be small enough to pass through the lung capillary network. Tumour cells have been demonstrated in the circulation (Nedalkott *et al.*, 1962) but it is probable that most die as a result of cytoxic reaction mediated by the T_H and T_c cells of the immune system.

18.1.3 SITES OF METASTATIC SPREAD

The commonest organ in which blood-borne metastases occur is the liver. Gastrointestinal, genitourinary, lung and breast cancers, melanomata and sarcomata regularly metastasize to the liver.

The lungs are the second most common site for metastatic spread and are frequently involved in sarcoma, carcinoma of the thyroid, breast and kidney. Testicular tumours and choriocarcinoma also favour the lungs.

After the liver and lungs the skeleton is the next most frequent site of secondary deposits. The primary tumour is usually a carcinoma of the lung, breast, prostate, kidney or thyroid. Of the lung cancers, it is the oat cell carcinoma that is particularly liable to metastasize to the skeleton in contrast to the squamous cell carcinoma, adenocarcinoma and undifferentiated carcinoma. With thyroid tumour, follicular carcinomas commonly metastasize to bone, unlike papillary carcinomas which rarely spread to the skeleton. These distinctive patterns of metastases indicate the biological individuality of different cancers arising from a single organ.

Bone metastases may be osteosclerotic or osteolytic. In the former there is the deposition of new bone and the resultant secondaries are hard and, on X-ray, radiopaque. The osteogenesis is reflected in the raised level of serum alkaline phosphatase whilst the serum calcium and phosphatate levels remain normal. Most osteosclerotic secondaries are due to prostatic carcinoma.

Other secondary tumours, carcinoma of the breast and colon and neuroblastomas may also occasionally be sclerotic, but more commonly they and other tumours that metastasize to bone are osteolytic. This is seen on X-ray as an area of lucency and may lead to spontaneous fracture. If much of the marrow is replaced by tumour, a leucoerythroblastic anaemia may result.

The brain is also a site for secondary spread, the commonest primary source being the lung. Carcinoma of the breast and melanoma may also spread to the brain. It has been postulated that there is direct communication between the bronchial veins and the vertebral plexus but this is not proven.

Of the endocrine glands the adrenal gland is the one that most commonly contains metastases. Usually the medulla is involved, but discrete cortical deposits are not uncommon. Oat cell carcinoma of the lung frequently metastasizes to this site and it has been estimated that one-third of fatal lung cancers show adrenal deposits. Cancer of the breast also often spreads to the adrenals and may metastasize to the ovaries.

The skin is the site of metastases that tend to occur as discrete nodules, the primary source being usually the lung or breast. Multiple cutaneous deposits are also a common feature of the malignant melanoma.

Secondary tumours are usually multiple although the solitary cannon-ball lung metastases sometimes seen in hypernephroma and seminomas are obvious exceptions.

18.2 CENTRAL NERVOUS SYSTEM

Tumours of the central nervous system (CNS) account for 9% of all primary tumours and the variety and behaviour of these tumours reflect the complexities of both the nervous system and of the tumour processes involved.

The clinical presentation of an intracranial tumour depends principally upon the combination of three factors: raised intracranial pressure, epilepsy and focal neurological defects. The nature of the tumour and its site contribute to its characteristic presentation.

Raised intracranial pressure may be caused by any expanding lesion within the skull. Initially cerebro spinal fluid (CSF) is displaced from the ventricular and subarachnoid space, followed by displacement of cerebral tissue. Slowly growing tumours may cause gross displacement with remarkably little neurological disturbance, but more rapidly expanding lesions may produce early neurological signs. Posterior fossa lesions cause displacement of the cerebellar tonsils through the foramen magnum, which may cause fatal medullary compression. In addition to the growth of the tumour itself, cerebral oedema and the development of hydrocephalus may contribute to the raised pressure. The symptoms of headache, vomiting and visual disturbance as papilloedema develops are seen with most tumours but are usually most marked in posterior fossa tumours.

An epileptic attack may occur at any stage during the growth of a tumour and may be the presenting symptom. Usually the lesion is supratentorial and the seizures are generally grand mal in type, although focal seizures may occur and assist in clinical localization.

Pressure, infiltration and oedema of cerebral tissue may result in loss of function. In addition, there may be non-localizing signs such as bilateral sixth nerve palsies caused by raised intracranial pressure. The degree of neurological disturbance depends on the nature of the tumour, its rate of growth and the destruction of infiltrated tissue. Some tumours, such as astrocytomas in the brain stem, may be very extensive and yet produce very little evidence of neurological dysfunction. Other, more rapidly growing tumours undergo necrosis, form cysts or cause haemorrhage with much surrounding tissue oedema which may produce dramatic and sudden impairment of neurological function.

18.2.1 GLIOMAS

Gliomas represent 45% of all primary brain tumours and the astrocytoma is the commonest glioma. The classification of gliomas is based on the degree of differentiation of the tumour and correlation with embryonic development. The differentiated tumours are composed of cells resembling astrocytes with abundant glial processes.

Radionuclide brain imaging using ^{99m}Tc-pertechnetate, diethylenetriamine pentaacetic acid (DTPA) or glucoheptonate provide a method of investigating patients with signs of an intracranial lesion with a sensitivity of 80–90% (O'Mara and Mozley, 1971) but a low specificity. Glioblastoma multiforme or astrocytoma grade IV is a highly vascular tumour and hypervascularity is observed in dynamic radionuclide brain imaging in 50–80% of cases (Quinn, 1971). The often cystic nature of the rapidly growing malignant astrocytoma may be identified on planar radionuclide imaging but SPECT imaging will increase the ability to define the non-homogeneous nature of these tumours (Cowan and Watson, 1980).

Computed tomography (CT) has replaced planar radionuclide imaging for the detection of primary and secondary intracerebral tumours in most centres. In district general hospitals in which there is no ready access to CT, there remains a role for radionuclide imaging in the initial evaluation of a patient with symptoms and signs suggestive of an intracerebral lesion. The clinical usefulness of radionuclide brain imaging lies in its low false-negative rate, estimated as 4% by Boucher and Sear (1980) and 2% by Carril *et al.* (1979) and it therefore provides a cheap, cost-effective method of assessing neurological symptoms particularly in the elderly. The addition of single-photon emission CT (SPECT) increases the predictive accuracy of radionuclide brain imaging to that achieved with CT (Carril *et al.*, 1979; Ell *et al.*, 1980).

SPECT imaging with ^{99m}Tc-labelled hexamethyl propylene amine oxine (HMPAO) demonstrates the alteration in blood flow associated with cerebral tumours. High-grade gliomas show an increased uptake of HMPAO (Flower *et al.*, 1986) but in most gliomas the tracer uptake is reduced (Lindegaard *et al.*, 1986).

Positron-emitting tomographic imaging has been used by Di Chiro *et al.* (1982) to evaluate the glucose utilization of cerebral gliomas and this has been shown to be increased when compared with utilization in normal tissue and can be used for staging.

18.2.2 MENINGIOMAS

Meningiomas account for 15% of all primary intracranial tumours, and arise from meningeal cell elements, particularly those around the arachnoid villi in the walls of the dural veins and sinuses. They arise most frequently in the parasagittal region, but are also found in the sphenoid region, the olfactory groove and the basi cranium. Malignant meningiomas are rare and malignant change is most commonly seen in the angioblastic type of meningioma. CT will demonstrate that these tumours are highly vascular. The addition of early first-pass imaging using ^{99m}Tc-pertechnetate, glucoheptonate or DTPA will demonstrate the increased perfusion and increased blood pool of a meningioma corresponding to the blush on contrast angiography. Its classical position close to but not crossing the mid-line on an anterior vertex view will also aid in the primary diagnosis of a meningioma. CT is now, however, the most commonly used imaging technique in the investigation of a meningioma and again the demonstration of contrast enhancement will confirm the highly vascular nature of these tumours.

18.2.3 POSTERIOR FOSSA TUMOURS

Tumours of the posterior fossa present with certain characteristic features, including symptoms and signs of raised intracranial pressure as the cerebellar tonsils are displaced through the foramen magnum causing medullary compression. CT of posterior fossa tumours has a lower sensitivity than with supratentorial tumours owing to the artefact from sphenoid ridges. Unlike supratentorial gliomas where there is close correlation between the malignancy of the tumour and the degree of enhancement, posterior fossa gliomas commonly enhance even when low grade. Radionuclide brain imaging in multiple projections will usually successfully demonstrate the posterior fossa, and tumours such as acoustic neuromas may be accurately located.

18.2.4 INTRACRANIAL METASTASES

Some 15–20% of all intracranial tumours are metastatic in origin. Of these, 65% are bronchogenic in origin and about 30% arise from the breast. Other important sites include kidney, colon, pancreas and testes, with malignant melanoma accounting for 15% in some series. Whilst intracranial metastases usually present during the clinical course of established malignant disease, these may be the cause of presentation and pre-

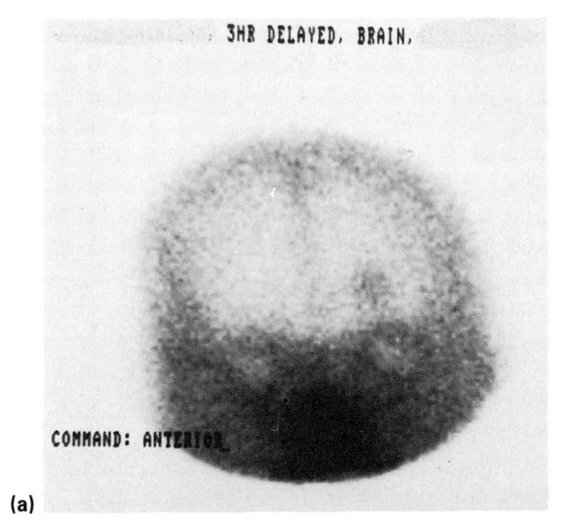

(a)

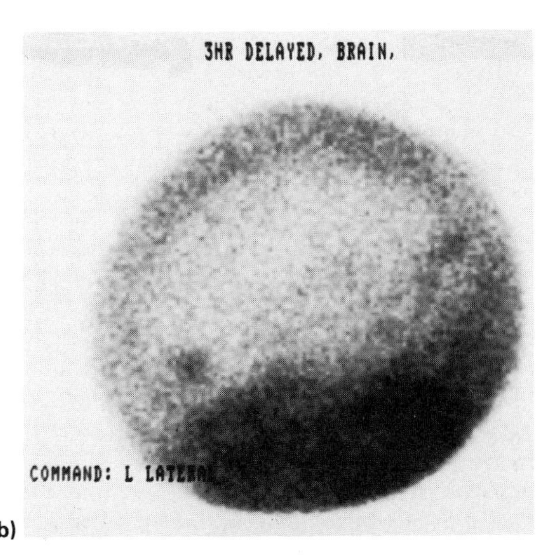

(b)

Figure 18.1 75-year-old female with a history of increasing confusion. ^{99m}Tc-labelled glucoheptonate brain scan demonstrates focal uptake in the left frontal region (a) with a further area of abnormality in the left temporoparietal region (b). Metastases were diagnosed and subsequently a small carcinoma of the bronchus was discovered.

cede the discovery of the primary. Blood-borne metastases are rarely solitary although one lesion may dominate the clinical picture at presentation. Uncommonly a solitary metastases may occur long after successful treatment of a primary tumour, such as with hypernephroma and in these cases surgical excision followed by radiotherapy is justified. In most cases, however, the treatment of intracranial metastases is palliative. Radionuclide brain imaging provides a simple, well-tolerated technique for the detection of cerebral metastases that may be suspected at the time of initial presentation or which develop during the follow-up of a patient with known malignancy (Figure 18.1).

18.3 TUMOURS OF THE HEAD AND NECK

The commonest malignant tumour of the head and neck is a squamous carcinoma, usually poorly differentiated with little or no keratinization. The second commonest is the malignant lymphoma.

18.3.1 SQUAMOUS CARCINOMA

Symptoms of squamous carcinomas at presentation depend on the site of the primary tumour, with pain referred to the ear being a significant feature. Dysphagia is another common symptom of pharyngeal tumours, whilst laryngeal tumours frequently present with symptoms of hoarseness. Tumours of the head and neck are often visible on direct or indirect inspection and involved lymph nodes are commonly palpable at presentation.

Treatment is undertaken using a combination of surgery and radiotherapy with five-year survival rates ranging from 90% for glottic carcinomas, 40% for carcinomas of the maxillary antram and tongue, down to 15% for carcinoma of the piriform fossa.

The primary tumour is usually visible either on direct examination or on indirect mirror examination. Examination under general anaesthetic may be necessary to adequately visualize the tumour and clinical evaluation has proved the most sensitive means of assessing the involvement of local lymph nodes. A chest X-ray and lateral view of the neck should be performed in all cases to assess mediastinal node involvement and pulmonary metastases, and a barium swallow should be performed where dysphagia is a prominent symptom. X-rays of the skull and sinuses should be performed when carcinoma of the ear, nasopharynx, nasal fossa or paranasal sinuses are suspected and CT is now essential in delineating lesions in and around the base of the skull. Assessment of nodal involvement has proved disappointing with CT in view of the common inflammatory lymph node enlargement that is present coincidentally.

Radionuclide imaging with ^{67}Ga has been used to evaluate patients with squamous carcinomas of the head and neck. Unfortunately, the normal distribution of ^{67}Ga in the salivary glands and nasal mucosa lowers the sensitivity of this technique in tumours of the sinuses or nasopharynx. Pinsky and Henkin (1976), however, reported a 65% correlation with pathological findings in patients with squamous carcinomas of the head and neck, but only 33% of metastatic nodes showed definitely a positive gallium uptake, Silberstein *et al.* (1974). Kashima *et al.* (1974), however, reported positive scans in 86% of patients having primary tumours of the head and neck with all lesions detected of 2 cm or greater (Figure 18.2). ^{67}Ga imaging has been used by Higashi *et al.* (1977) to distinguish chronic maxillary sinusitis from maxillary malignancy, and has been shown to be useful as a prognostic indicator in patients who have received pre-operative irradiation. Patients whose scans demonstrated uptake of ^{67}Ga all died within six months of scanning, whereas those patients without ^{67}Ga uptake in residual tumour were all alive 8–14 months after treatment.

The most crucial clinical question prognostically, however, remains that of involvement of lymph nodes at the time of presentation and ^{67}Ga has not proved to be clinically useful in satisfactorily answering this problem, although with the increasing use of SPECT and high doses of ^{67}Ga further evaluation is warranted.

Recently a new tumour imaging agent, ^{99m}Tc-labelled pentavalent dimercaptosuccinic acid (V DMSA), has been reported to be taken up in squamous carcinomas of the head and neck. Initial reports (Ohta *et al.*, 1984) appeared promising, Watkinson *et al.* (1989) have shown that although ^{99m}Tc V DMSA is taken up to a variable extent by squamous carcinomas, the sensitivity of detection does not exceed that of clinical examination, and is much lower than clinical examination for the detection of involved lymph nodes. In addition pre- or post-operative radiotherapy causes significant false-positive uptake which may last for up to a

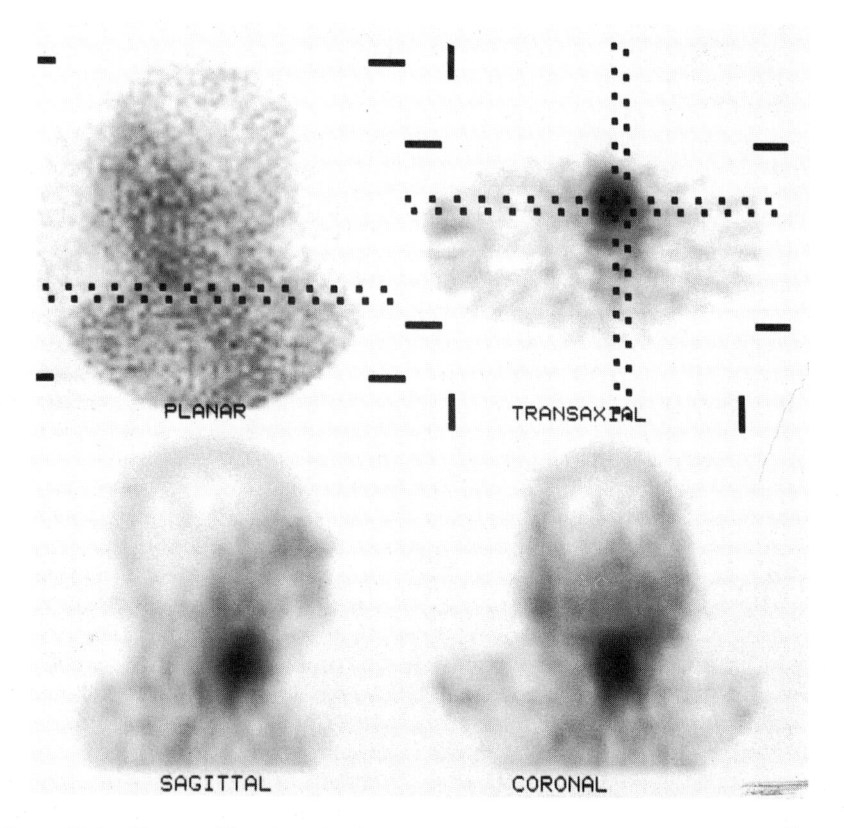

Figure 18.2 82-year-old male with a known squamous carcinoma of the larynx. ^{67}Ga imaging with SPECT shows significant uptake at site of known tumour.

year after treatment. The role of radionuclides in imaging head and neck cancer has been reviewed by Watkinson and Maisey (1988).

18.3.2 LYMPHOMAS

The second commonest tumour of the oropharynx is the malignant lymphoma which is usually of the non-Hodgkin type. These tumours frequently present as a mass, with pain being an unusual and late feature. Lymph nodes in the neck are frequently involved and systemic spread occurs in 50% of cases. Treatment is by wide-field radiotherapy.

CT has been used to assess the extent of lymph node involvement and also to determine the presence of systemic spread. ^{67}Ga, although not specific, has a reported sensitivity of almost 90% in untreated patients with malignant lymphoma (Kashima *et al.*, 1974; Pinsky and Henkin, 1976; Silberstein *et al.*, 1974; Gould *et al.*, 1978). It has proved a useful means of staging lymphomas by detecting remote sites of involvement. In order to accurately determine the presence of liver or spleen involvement a ^{67}Ga scan should be combined with a ^{99m}Tc liver colloid scan. Subtraction imaging using these two techniques increases the sensitivity of detection of the hepatic and splenic lesions and upper abdominal para-aortic nodes.

18.3.3 GLOMUS JUGULARE TUMOURS

The glomus jugulare tumour is benign or of low-grade malignancy. It arises from paraganglionic chemoreceptor tissue situated in or close to the middle ear. It occurs mainly over the age of 40 and is commoner in females than males. Histologically the tumours are chemodactomas. Patients present with a long history of oral symptoms, with deafness being the commonest presenting symptom. The tumour is visible on examination of the tympanic membrane if the tympanic membrane is involved and a bruit may be audible. X-rays, including CT to assess involvement of the temporal bone should be performed. A ^{99m}Tc-labelled MDP bone scan and SPECT may also provide information about local bone involvement. Arteriography shows the tumour as a characteristic blush.

Radionuclide studies using ^{131}I or ^{123}I-meta-iodobenzylguanidine (MIBG) have recently been reported (Khafagi *et al.*, 1987; Bomani *et al.*, 1987). MIBG is a guanethidine analogue that is taken up by some neuroectodermally derived tumours, including phaeochromocytomas and neuroblastomas. Encouraging results in imaging and therapy have been reported using MIBG to image patients with paragangliomas.

18.4 ENDOCRINE TUMOURS

18.4.1 THYROID

Malignant tumours of the thyroid are classified according to histological type. Thyroid cancer is uncommon, accounting in most countries for less than 0.5% of all cancer deaths. Females are affected more commonly than men, and there is a steady increase in incidence with age in men but a substantial incidence in young adult women (25–35 years). There has been a significant decrease in the incidence in children since about 1955 and this relates to the virtual cessation of irradiation of the neck in children for benign disease. Follicular carcinoma appears to be more common in low-iodine endemic goitre areas. Papillary carcinoma occurs more commonly in iodine-rich areas. Anaplastic cancer is mainly a disease of the elderly and thyroid lymphoma occurs when thyroiditis and thyroid antibodies are prevalent.

(a) Papillary carcinoma

These tumours are characterized histologically by recognizable small papillae and small, spherical, calcified psammoma bodies. The pure papillary tumour is relatively uncommon and the pattern is more commonly mixed with follicular elements present. Papillary tumours spread to local lymph nodes (30–55%) but distant metastases are very uncommon 4–6% (Freitas *et al.*, 1985).

Papillary tumours present as nodules in the thyroid which are usually circumscribed. The patient may also complain of pain in the nodule and dysphagia if the nodule is enlarged or compressing the oesophagus. Rarely, hoarseness will be present due to recurrent laryngeal nerve involvement. An involved lymph node may be palpable at presentation. The patient is usually clinically and biochemically euthyroid except in the uncommon circumstance with papillary tumour arising in a toxic multinodular goitre.

Thyroid imaging is undertaken to evaluate the palpable nodule anatomically and functionally. Imaging using ^{99m}Tc pertechnetate will demonstrate a non-functioning area of the thyroid in the region of the palpated nodule and on ultrasound the nodule will be observed to be solid. Thoracic inlet views may be performed if the patient complains of symptoms suggestive of oesophageal or tracheal compression and a chest X-ray should be performed to exclude lung metastases, although these are uncommon. Fine-needle aspiration of the thyroid nodule may be undertaken to confirm the diagnosis.

Following thyroid surgery and confirmation of the histological diagnosis, a ^{131}I scan of the neck should be undertaken to assess the presence of remnant thyroid tissue. If the scan demonstrates thyroid tissue, thyroid ablation is undertaken using 50–80 mCi (1850–3000 MBq) of ^{131}I. Whole-body iodine imaging may then be used to follow the patient whose primary tumour has follicular elements to assess recurrent local or distant disease. Thyroxine therapy must be stopped for one month before ^{131}I imaging.

(b) Follicular carcinoma

Follicular cancer of the thyroid represents 10–20% of all thyroid cancers. Follicular tumours are usually unifocal, tend to occur at an older age and are usually larger in size. Follicular carcinomas closely resemble mature normal thyroid tissue and a well-differentiated tumour may be difficult to distinguish on fine-needle aspiration from a benign adenoma. Hurtle or clear cells may be present and may, as a clear cell variety of follicular carcinoma, resemble a renal carcinoma. 28% of follicular cancers spread to local lymph nodes and 14% metastasize to bone or lung. Although patients with follicular thyroid tumours are usually clinically and biochemically euthyroid, patients with large primary tumours or widespread distant metastases may occasionally have biochemical evidence of hyperthyroidism. As with papillary tumours, patients present with an asymptomatic lump in the thyroid, or less commonly complain of pain, hoarseness or symptoms of compression. Following surgery the management is identical to that of papillary cancer with follicular elements, using ^{131}I whole-body iodine to detect recurrence (Figure 18.3).

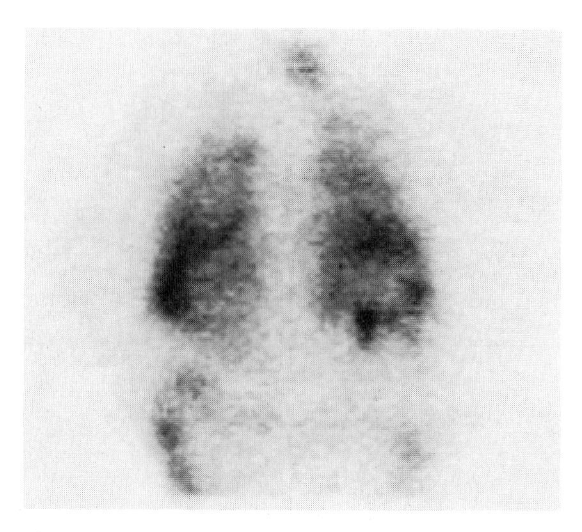

Figure 18.3 78-year-old male, one year after total thyroidectomy and ^{131}I ablation for follicular carcinoma of the thyroid. ^{131}I whole-body scan shows uptake in the neck and lung fields with non-specific activity in the gut. Chest X-ray confirmed metastases.

(c) Medullary carcinoma of the thyroid (MTC)

MTC is an uncommon tumour, accounting for less than 10% of thyroid malignancies; 90% of these tumours are sporadic but 10% occur as part of the multiple endocrine neoplasia syndrome, types 2a and 2b being inherited as an autosomal dominant trait. The tumours arise in the parafollicular or C cells of the thyroid that arise from neuro-ectoderm and secrete calcitonin. C cell hyperplasia is believed to be a pre-malignant condition in patients with the inherited form of the disease and the tumours are usually multifocal, involving both lobes of the thyroid. Sporadic forms of the disease are unifocal.

Patients may present with the symptoms of a nodule or nodules in the thyroid gland. They may also present with symptoms caused by vasoactive peptide secretion that occurs commonly with these tumours, i.e. flushing and diarrhoea. ^{99m}Tc pertechnetate imaging of the thyroid will demonstrate an area of reduced uptake corresponding to the site of the nodule that is solid on ultrasound. In familial forms of the disease the scan may show the classical 'owl eye' appearance of cold nodules in both lobes of the thyroid (Anderson *et al.*, 1978). Recently, a newly developed radiopharmaceutical, ^{99m}Tc-labelled V DMSA has been shown to be selectively taken up into sites of primary and recurrent MTC with a sensitivity variably reported as 65% (Patel *et al.*, 1988) to 88% (Clarke *et al.*, 1988; Figure 18.4). This ^{99m}Tc-labelled tumour imaging agent is remarkable for its low, non-specific uptake in organs such as the liver and bone marrow, which facilitates the identification of liver and bone metastases. This imaging agent is now contributing significantly to patient management with its ability to define both local soft tissue

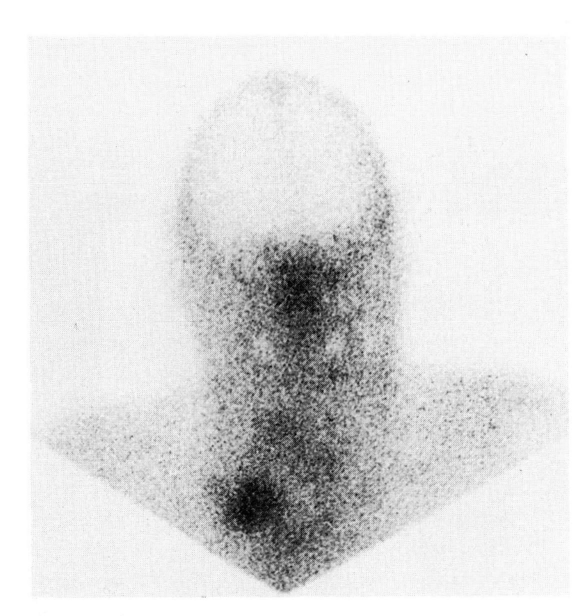

Figure 18.4 65-year-old male with a five-year history of medullary thyroid cancer, and elevated calcitonin levels following removal of primary tumour. ^{99m}Tc-labelled V DMSA imaging identifies focal area of uptake in region of right sternoclavicular joint which was confirmed at surgery to be at the site of recurrent tumour.

recurrence and distant metastases. Its use to identify the presence and site of residual tissue post-surgery and to locate the site of recurrence in patients whose calcitonin levels become elevated again have been described by Clarke *et al.* (1988).

^{131}I-MIBG has also been used to image patients with MTC (Endo *et al.*, 1984a; Connel *et al.*, 1984; Baulieu *et al.*, 1986). Its low sensitivity in these patients means that it has no role in the identification of primary or recurrent disease. Its use in therapy, however, has been reported (Clarke *et al.*, 1987a) but experience is too limited at present to determine whether it is a significant therapeutic option in those patients whose tumours do take up ^{131}I-MIBG.

^{201}Tl-thallous chloride has been shown to be taken up into all types of thyroid cancer, including MTC (Tonami *et al.*, 1978). Its poor imaging characteristics are a disadvantage in the detection of distant metastases but neck recurrence in patients with all types of thyroid cancer has been reported. One particular use of ^{201}Tl-thallous chloride is the assessment of recurrence in patients with follicular or mixed tumours whose thyroglobulin levels rise whilst on suppressive doses of thyroxine and in whom neck evaluation is needed without the time delay of stopping thyroxine or the risk of TSH-stimulated tumour growth.

(d) *Anaplastic thyroid cancer*

Anaplastic thyroid cancer constitutes only 4–6% of thyroid cancers. It is locally invasive, grows and metastasizes rapidly, and death commonly occurs within months of the initial diagnosis. ^{99m}Tc-pertechnetate imaging demonstrates the non-functioning nature of the nodule. ^{131}I is not taken up into the metastases and surgery with external beam radiotherapy remains the only therapeutic option at present. ^{201}Tl-thallous chloride uptake has been reported in anaplastic thyroid cancer (Hoefnagel *et al.*, 1986a).

18.4.2 PARATHYROID TUMOURS

Carcinoma of the parathyroid gland occurs in 2–3% of primary tumours and up to 7% in recurrent disease. The tumours are either chief or a mixed cell variety and the majority are left inferior tumours. Although the majority are well differentiated, one-third have spread to the cervical lymph nodes, lungs, liver or bones at the time of primary diagnosis (Esselstyn, 1977). The three classical forms of clinical presentation are bone disease without evidence of renal stones, renal stones without evidence of bone disease and asymptomatic patients with hypercalcaemia. Parathyroid carcinoma has been described with multiple endocrine neoplasia syndromes types 1 and 2, peptic ulceration and pancreatitis. Imaging of the neck with ultrasound will identify enlargement of the involved parathyroid gland. ^{99m}Tc-pertechnetate and ^{201}Tl-thallous chloride subtraction imaging may also be used, although as the majority of these carcinomas are palpable radionuclide imaging is usually not necessary (Ferlin *et al.*, 1983).

18.4.3 ADRENAL TUMOURS

Tumours arising from the adrenal gland may be subdivided into those arising from the adrenal cortex and those from the adrenal medulla.

(a) *Adrenocortical tumours*

Adrenocortical carcinomas occur rarely and may be functional or non-functioning. Functioning carcinomas produce a variety of syndromes dependent upon their hormone secretion. Large or cortical tumours tend to be malignant and arbitrarily 100 g defines benign from malignant. Well-differentiated cortical carcinomas can be difficult to distinguish from adenomas unless there is vascular invasion and metastases. Histology usually defines the poorly differentiated variety. Metastases to regional lymph nodes occur in 25% of cases, liver in 30–70% of cases, lungs in 50% and bones in 20–40% (Grenberg and Marks, 1978). Imaging of the adrenocortical tumours may be undertaken using ultrasound and CT; 25% of adrenal carcinomas show patchy calcification and this may be identified using both these imaging techniques. Other investigations include venography with selective adrenal venous sampling and arteriography, which will demonstrate the vascularity of the primary tumour and may also show liver secondaries. Radionuclide imaging with ^{75}Se-seleno-cholesterol has a limited role but may be used early in the investigative pathway in symptomatic patients to differentiate Cushing's disease, when both adrenals will be visualized from Cushing's syndrome, when only the involved adrenal will be visualized due to suppression of the contralateral gland. ^{75}Se-seleno-cholesterol imaging fails to distinguish benign adrenal cortical tumours from well-differentiated carcinomas, but poorly differentiated carcinomas will generally take up the tracer poorly. Rarely the metastases may take up the tracer (Thrall *et al.*, 1978).

(b) Adrenal medullary tumours

Phaeochromocytomas, arise from the primitive ganglion cells of the adrenal medulla and 10% are malignant. About 75% of tumours secrete catecholamines or their precursors.

Phaeochromocytomas arise in the adrenal medulla in 80% of patients; the remainder arise in any of the sympathetic ganglia from neck to pelvis, the majority (98%) being intra-abdominal. In adults the tumours are bilateral and multiple in 5–10% higher in children (25%) and greatest in the hereditary syndromes (50–70%). Most adrenal medullary tumours secrete adrenaline whereas the extra-adrenal tumours secrete noradrenaline. The reported incidence of malignant adrenal phaeochromocytoma varies owing to a lack of accepted diagnostic criteria. The incidence ranges from 7% to 15% but if diagnosed by the presence of metastases is only 1–2.5% (Goodall and Symington, 1983). Histologically benign and malignant tumours have similar appearances regarding mitotic figures, nuclear pleomorphism and even capsular and intravascular invasion (Symington, 1969). The only absolute criteria for malignancy is the presence of metastases in sites where chromaffin tissue is not normally found, such as lung, liver, lymph nodes and bone. Malignant phaeochromocytomas may also arise in extra-adrenal sites. Sizes vary from small to very large (1000 g). The large tumours are metabolically less active and are often missed.

Patients present with a variety of different symptoms, ranging from paraoxysmal headaches, sweating and palpitations to persistent fatigue, tachycardia and abdominal pain. Occasionally patients present with complications of a malignant phaeochromocytoma such as a cerebrovascular accident.

Investigations are predominantly biochemical and include the measurement of catecholamines and catecholamine metabolites in the urine. Because a significant number of malignant phaeochromocytomas occur outside the adrenal medulla, imaging to locate the tumour should be undertaken. CT is now the imaging modality of choice in most centres, but the development of ^{131}I-MIBG by Wieland *et al.* (1980) has provided a radionuclide technique for imaging these tumours. Studies have been published using ^{131}I and ^{123}I-MIBG showed a high sensitivity and specificity (Ackery *et al.*, 1984; Lynn *et al.*, 1984) of tumour detection (Figure 18.5). SPECT imaging further increased sensitivity of ^{131}I-MIBG imaging (Hoefnagel *et al.*, 1987a).

18.5 LUNG

The incidence of carcinoma of the lung has been steadily rising. Its incidence varies around the world, with industrial areas having a higher incidence than rural areas. Although predominantly a disease of men earlier in the century, the incidence in women is steadily increasing.

The epidemiology of lung cancer reflects the pattern of smoking and it is now universally accepted that this disease is causally related to tobacco smoking, with cigarette smokers being at a higher risk than pipe smokers. Discontinuation of the habit reduces the risk of lung cancer. The carcinogen is believed to reside in the tar and the relative danger of tobacco depends on its tar yield. Tobacco smoking is associated mainly with squamous carcinoma and to a lesser extent oat cell carcinoma of the lung. Lung cancer has also been

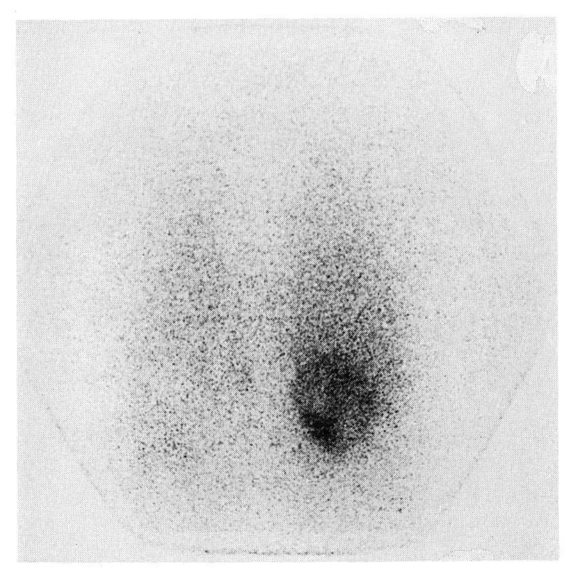

(a)

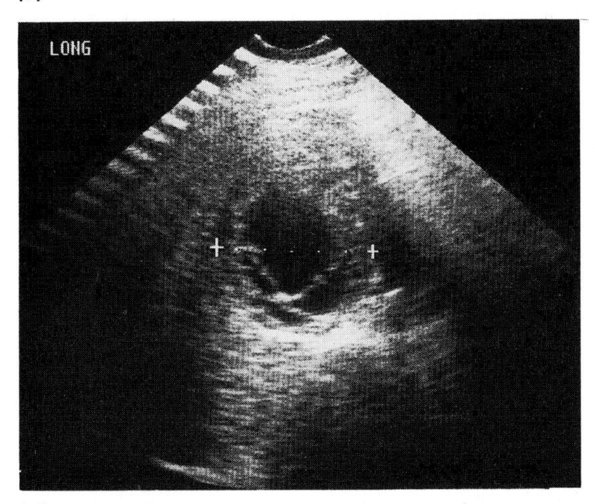

(b)

Figure 18.5 35-year-old female with a history of hypertensive episodes and elevated VMA levels. ^{123}I-MIBG imaging of posterior chest and abdomen identifies area of uptake in the region of right adrenal gland (a) and ultrasound confirmed a large mass with cystic and solid components (b). A malignant phaeochromocytoma was removed at surgery.

associated with certain industries such as gas and coke, chrome and nickel ore industries and the asbestos industry.

Malignant change can occur in any tissue which constitute the human airway, from the trachea to the alveoli.

18.5.1 SQUAMOUS CARCINOMA

These lesions are the most common carcinomas of the bronchus, comprising 40% of all lung cancers. They have a high correlation with smoking. A degree of differentiation is related directly to prognosis, with well-differentiated tumours having a better prognosis. Although lymph node metastases are common, blood-borne metastases occur late in the course of the disease.

18.5.2 ADENOCARCINOMA

These lesions comprise 20% of all lung cancers and are the most frequent types among non-smokers. They are usually situated peripherally in the lungs and metastasize early to lymph nodes. Blood-borne metastases occur early in the disease.

18.5.3 ANAPLASTIC SMALL CELL CARCINOMA

These tumours comprise approximately 35% of all tumours. The majority arise from the large central bronchi and are highly malignant. The histological appearance is characteristic, with small oat-shaped or spindle-shaped cells. The primary lesion may be a small undetected lesion in a patient who is found to have widespread blood-borne metastases. Lymph node metastases also occur early and 50–70% of patients have malignant cells in their bone marrow, compared with 10% of patients with other lung neoplasms. Oat cell carcinoma is related to the bronchial carcinoids and both are thought to arise from the Kulchitzy cells. These tumours are frequently responsible for ectopic hormone production.

18.5.4 ANAPLASTIC LARGE CELL CARCINOMA

This group of tumours includes the very poorly differentiated or anaplastic lesions of squamous or adenocarcinomatous origin. The tumours spread early to the lymph nodes and blood-borne metastases are common.

18.5.5 CLINICAL PRESENTATION AND MANAGEMENT

Sixty per cent of patients present with chest symptoms of cough, dyspnoea, haemoptysis or chest pain. Superior vena caval obstruction is also strongly suggestive of carcinoma of the bronchus. In addition patients complain of general symptoms of weight loss, lassitude and anorexia. An apically situated tumour or pancoast tumour may give local pain due to infiltration of the brachial plexus.

The chest X-ray will show an abnormality in the majority of patients studied: either a hilar mass or a discrete peripheral lesion. Persistent segmental lobar atelectasis caused by a small central obstructing lesion is a common finding. Pleural effusions are also a common feature on the X-ray of a patient with carcinoma of the lung and in those with severe lymphatic involvement; reticular shadowing due to lymphangitis carcinomatosa may be observed. CT is used when assessing the centrally placed lesions and the involvement of mediastinal lymph nodes.

The diagnosis is confirmed on sputum cytology, bronchial brushings or node biopsy. Peripheral lesions may be biopsied percutaneously and mediastinoscopy can be used to biopsy central lesions.

Radionuclide imaging may contribute to management in patients with proven lung carcinoma. Detection of the primary tumour using ventilation–perfusion imaging has proved difficult because of the frequency of coexisting pulmonary disease (Vatz *et al.*, 1979). Pulmonary scintigraphy may be used for the pre-operative assessment of lung function to assess the function of the 'normal' lung (Olsen *et al.*, 1974). ^{67}Ga has been widely used to assess the extent and location of lung tumours (Siemsen *et al.*, 1978) and uptake has been shown by Higashi *et al.* (1980) to vary with histological type, although his work has since been challenged (DeLand *et al.*, 1974). Sensitivity of imaging in lung cancer is variously reported, ranging from 85% to 95% (Larson *et al.*, 1975; Demeester *et al.*, 1979). De Meester *et al.* (1979) have reported that the predictive value of a positive ^{67}Ga scan for primary carcinoma of the lung is 91%, with a predictive value of a negative scan being 76%. ^{67}Ga scintigraphy has been found by Muhe (1971) to be more accurate than sputum cytology and bronchoscopy. The most common cause for a false-negative study is tumour size of less than 1.5 cm (DeLand *et al.*, 1974), hepatic activity that obscures the lower right lobe (Hjelms and Dyrbye, 1975), tumour degeneration and necrosis (Becherman *et al.*, 1976), associated lung pathology (Cellerino *et al.*, 1973) and the recent administration of cytostatic drugs (Alazraki *et al.*, 1978).

The role of ^{67}Ga imaging in detecting hilar mediastinal tumour extension remains unclear. The reported sensitivity of detection of mediastinal node involvement ranges from 100% (Alazraki *et al.*, 1978) to 56% (Demeester *et al.*, 1979; Richardson *et al.*, 1980), whilst specificity ranges from 97% (Richardson *et al.*, 1980) to 71% Alazraki *et al.* (1978). Waxman *et al.* (1984) have used two distinct sets of criteria to determine the sensitivity and specificity of ^{67}Ga imaging in patients with mediastinal spread, comparing the results of imaging with the findings at surgery. They concluded that high specificity is associated with selective evaluation of the mediastinum and unilateral hilar uptake. High sensitivity is achieved only if the hilar and mediastinum are considered together.

The use of ^{67}Ga in the assessment of tumour resectability has been assessed (Richardson *et al.*, 1980). The high sensitivity of tumour detection means that if the hilar is included as a determinant of central tumour involvement, patients with negative hilum and negative mediastinum may be considered as candidates for surgery provided no other sites of abnormality are present. However, with the non-specificity of hilar uptake of ^{67}Ga, uptake in the hilar region is an indication for mediastinoscopy.

SPECT techniques have been applied to ^{67}Ga imaging in an attempt to overcome the problem of non-specific bone uptake in the sternum and ribs (O'Donnell *et al.*, 1983). Quantification has also been used by Higashi *et al.* (1980) to increase the predictive value of imaging in primary lung cancer.

^{201}Tl-thallium chloride was first described as a tumour-seeking radiopharmaceutical by Cox *et al.* (1976), who observed uptake of ^{201}Tl in a left lung mass whilst performing a myocardial scan. Subsequently, Salvatore *et al.* (1976) investigated 71 patients with a variety of different lung pathologies, including 43 patients with lung cancer. Hilar uptake was seen in 20 of the 23 patients with known hilar metastases, and focal peripheral uptake was seen in 18 of the 20 patients with peripheral lesions. Uptake was also seen in lung metastases and patients with hilar involvement in Hodgkin's lymphoma. Sehweil *et al.* (1988) have studied 97 patients with proven malignancy, including 56 patients with lung carcinoma. They demonstrated abnormal uptake in 48 of the 56 patients with lung cancer and also concluded that the optimum time for imaging based on calculations of tumour:background ratios was 18 min. Adenocarcinoma of the lung has been reported as taking up ^{201}Tl-thallium chloride more avidly than ^{67}Ga (Togawa *et al.*, 1985, 1989), but many reports of imaging in lung cancer fail to specify the histological types of tumour being studied.

The use of ^{201}Tl imaging to differentiate benign from malignant lesions visualized on chest X-ray has been studied by Tonami *et al.* (1989) using SPECT and high doses of ^{201}Tl-thallium chloride. The technique is highly sensitive, identifying all the malignant tumours imaged, and specific with uptake in only two of the seven patients studied with benign disease. Delayed imaging also showed a slower clearance from malignant than benign lesions. ^{201}Tl clearance in squamous cell carcinoma was faster than those in that of adenocarcinoma and small cell carcinoma.

Monoclonal antibodies have been used with some success to image lung tumours (Zimmer *et al.*, 1985; Okabe *et al.*, 1985), including small cell tumours with high target:background ratios reported (Okabe *et al.*, 1985). Positron-emitting radiopharmaceuticals are now being used to study protein synthesis, glucose metabolism and blood flow in lung tumours (Kubota *et al.*, 1985).

18.6 SKIN

The skin is most commonly affected by malignant changes. In the majority of patients who develop skin cancer, an aetiological factor can be identified. Since the nineteenth century the importance of carcinogens in the development of skin tumours has been recognized. These include coal tar, creosote, mineral oils, paraffin and arsenicals. Radiation has also been identified as a cause of skin tumours and the past use of X-rays to treat ringworm has resulted in the development of basal cell carcinomas up to 60 years after the original treatment. Racial factors have also been identified, with skin cancers developing in those of Celtic extraction rather than in Anglo-Saxons. This is believed to be due to the relative lack of pigmentation in those racial groups. Long-term sun exposure is also a potential risk factor, with an increased incidence of skin tumours in fair-skinned individuals with outdoor occupations. Serious efforts to educate populations at risk are now being made. The classifications of skin tumours is essentially histological.

18.6.1 DIAGNOSIS

Most skin lesions are diagnosed by their appearance and histological characteristics. Many skin tumours are locally invasive only at the time of diagnosis. Malignant melanomas, however, have frequently metastasized to local lymph nodes by the time of presentation and diagnostic techniques for assessing regional lymph nodes are therefore needed. Lymphangiography and CT have been the main techniques used recently; however, work with anti-melanoma antibodies has been reported, initially using a ^{131}I label (Larsen *et al.*, 1983a, 1985) but subsequently using a ^{111}In-DTPA chelated label (Halpern *et al.*, 1985; Murray *et al.*, 1985; Taylor *et al.*, 1988). Taylor *et al.* (1988) have also used SPECT to increase the sensitivity of detection of small lesions <1 cm in diameter in the chest and axilla. Lesions in the liver are missed if they accumulate monoclonal antibody to the same extent as the rest of the liver. The largest study is that of Siccardi *et al.* (1986).

Carrasquillo *et al.* (1987) have also used both ^{131}I and ^{111}In-DTPA-labelled monoclonal antibody T101 to image tumour and nodal sites in patients with cutaneous T-cell lymphoma. The ^{111}In-DTPA-labelled antibody gave significantly better results than ^{131}I owing to loss of ^{131}I from the antibody leading to markedly different biodistribution.

18.7 LIVER

Primary liver tumours are uncommon tumours in Europe and North America, accounting for less than 2% of all new cancer cases (Fisher, 1976). Hepatoma is the commonest primary liver tumour (75–80% in most series), with the cholangiocarcinomas accounting for 15–20%. Other rarer tumours include haemangioendothelioma, haemangiosarcoma and Kupffer cell sarcoma. Hepatoma is one of the most rapidly growing solid organ tumours, with untreated patients dying within six months of diagnosis. In Europe and North America hepatomas usually occur in patients with pre-existing cirrhosis.

18.7.1 PRIMARY LIVER TUMOURS

Ultrasound examination of the liver, together with ^{99m}Tc-labelled sulphur or tin colloid imaging, provide first-line screening methods of imaging patients with suspected primary liver tumours. In 73% of patients with hepatoma, a single discrete defect is seen on the scan (Patton, 1982) which differentiates the scan appearance from that of uncomplicated cirrhosis or liver metastases. Hepatomas also demonstrate a high avidity for ^{67}Ga-gallium citrate in more than 90% of cases (Lomas *et al.*, 1972; Waxman *et al.*, 1980) and in patients with a single defect on the ^{99m}Tc-labelled sulphur colloid scan, with the remainder of the liver showing poor uptake suggestive of cirrhosis. A ^{67}Ga avid lesion has a high probability of being due to a hepatoma. ^{75}Se-seleno-methionine has also been used in the past to image hepatomas (Coakley and Wraight, 1980) but poor imaging characteristics, high cost and high radiation dose to the patient mean that it has no clinical use at the present time.

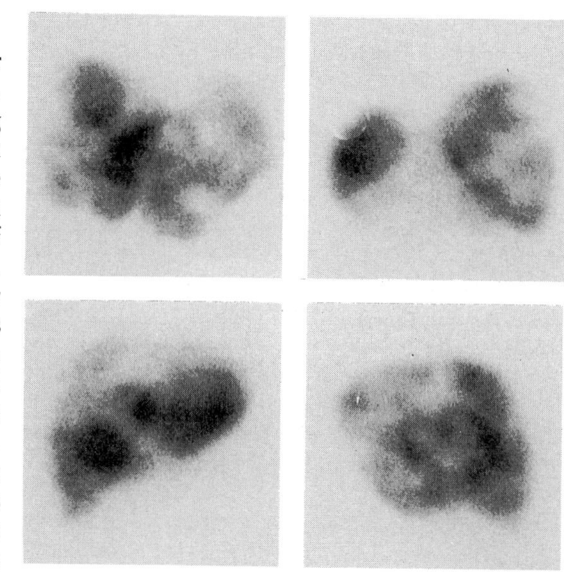

Figure 18.6 42-year-old female with carcinoma of the breast. ^{99m}Tc-labelled colloid imaging performed to assess known liver metastases prior to chemotherapy.

18.7.2 LIVER METASTASES

Approximately 30–50% of all cancer patients will develop metastases disease at some stage in their disease and the demonstration of liver metastases at the time of initial diagnosis and staging will significantly affect management with many types of tumour. Ultrasound imaging is an extremely cost-effective imaging modality, readily differentiating between cystic and solid lesions. It is, however, an operator-dependent technique. ^{99m}Tc-labelled colloid imaging is a more expensive imaging technique which does not rely on operator expertise; however, its main use is in following patients with liver metastases to assess progression of disease and response to therapy because a series of planar images enables both the number and size of lesions to be compared more easily (Figure 18.6).

The sensitivity of ^{99m}Tc-labelled colloid imaging for the detection of secondaries is reported as between 75% and 85% (Lumia *et al.*, 1957; Rothschild and Rosenthal, 1976). The addition of SPECT increased the sensitivity by about 10% (Ell and Khan, 1981). Scan features vary from single or a few large lesions seen typically with gastrointestinal secondaries to multiple small lesions seen with breast and melanoma metastases. Large solitary deposits may also be observed in patients with clinical features of hepatic spread from a primary carcinoid tumour.

Patients with diffuse metastatic disease are occasionally treated with intra-arterial infusions of cytotoxic agents, and ^{99m}Tc-labelled albumin macroaggregates have been used to assess the position of the catheter tip before giving chemotherapy (Mansfield and Park, 1985).

18.8 BREAST

Breast cancer is the commonest cancer in women in the UK over the age of 40. The prevalence of the disease is low in developing countries and uncommon in China and Japan. Aetiology is thought to be multifactorial. Race is one factor since deaths in the Western world from breast cancer are common whereas in Japan, deaths are relatively unknown. Breast cancer is also more common in higher socio-economic groups. Endocrine factors play a significant role. Nulliparous women are at greater risk of developing breast cancer and women with more than four children are at lower risk (MacMahan *et al.*, 1990). Breast feeding is also believed to play a protective role. There is much debate at the present time as to the role of the contraceptive pill in the development of breast cancer. Familial factors are also significant since daughters of women with breast cancer have a 15 times greater probability of developing breast cancer than the general population.

18.8.1 PATHOLOGY

Breast tumours are classically divided between the non-invasive and invasive breast cancers. They may also be subdivided into those that express oestrogen receptors and those that do not. Oestrogen receptors are less commonly found in pre-menopausal women (30%) compared with post-menopausal women (60%).

Patients are staged by evaluation of the primary tumour mass, regional lymph nodes and assessing the presence of distant metastases.

18.8.2 CLINICAL

Patients present with a painless lump in the breast, or may be discovered to have an unsuspected lump during examination or screening. Up to 75% of patients have involved nodes at time of presentation (Fisher, 1976). Haematogenous spread is common, often occurring early in the disease. The most commonly involved distant sites are the skeleton, lungs and liver. Although bone metastases are classically osteolytic, 5–10% are sclerotic. Metastases in the lungs are usually discrete and focal, but retrograde infiltration of the peribronchial lymphatics may result in lymphangitis carcinomata.

18.8.3 INVESTIGATIONS

Following physical examination, mammography is performed to differentiate diffuse fibroadenosis and breast cysts from suspicious focal lesions. Biopsies of suspicious lesions may be performed using Trucut or excision biopsy techniques to determine the histology. Clinical assessment of the axillary nodes is highly unreliable since 40% of patients in whom there is no clinical evidence of nodal involvement would be discovered to have nodal metastases at surgery. By comparison, 20% of patients with palpable nodes would be found at histology to have no evidence of tumour involvement.

18.8.4 MANAGEMENT

Surgical treatment of breast cancer remains a subject of considerable debate, with many surgeons now opting for smaller, less disfiguring operations such as simple mastectomy or even lumpectomy as opposed to the classical radical mastectomy that was held to be the optimum operation since 1894. Adjunctive treatment with radiotherapy has been shown to improve the long-term survival in patients undergoing conservative surgery. The results of adjuvant chemotherapy are at present unclear. The most significant therapeutic development in recent years has been the use of hormonal therapy in the form of the anti-oestrogen tamoxifen.

18.8.5 RADIONUCLIDE IMAGING IN BREAST CANCER

Radionuclide imaging in breast cancer plays no role in diagnosis of the primary tumour. Various attempts have been made to use radionuclide studies to assist in staging the patients with known breast malignancies but limited success has been reported. McClean and Ege (1986) have used axillary lymphoscintigraphy and internal mammary lymphoscintigraphy in a large series of patients with breast cancer. Results show an association between asymmetrical uptake of tracer and histologically demonstrated metastases (Murray *et al.*, 1985). Radiolabelled antibodies have been used by a number of workers (Clarke *et al.*, 1989; Tjandra *et al.*, 1989) but attempts to image involved lymph nodes using this technique have been disappointing.

The main role for radionuclide imaging has been in the detection and follow-up of bone metastases. The incidence of abnormal scans in patients with stage 1 disease is less than 5% and less than 10% in patients with stage 2 disease (Kinkler *et al.*, 1985). With stage 3 disease, a significant number of patients have abnormal bone scans at the time of presentation and scans should therefore be performed routinely in this group at presentation as a positive scan may modify the initial surgery (Wilson *et al.*, 1980). Bone scanning provides a highly sensitive means of detecting bone metastases and the scan is frequently positive before any abnormality can be detected on X-ray (Coleman *et al.*, 1986). Its lack of specificity, however, makes the use of X-rays important when assessing whether the observed lesion is metastatic or benign. Bone metastases in breast cancer may rarely be solitary and the sternum may be the only site of abnormality (Boxer *et al.*, 1989).

^{99m}Tc-labelled colloid liver spleen imaging may be used in conjunction with ultrasound to confirm the presence of clinically suspected liver metastases. The radionuclide scan has a significant role in the follow-up of patients with known liver metastases, enabling the clinician to clearly visualize the number and size of metastases following treatment.

18.9 BONE

Whilst the skeleton is one of the most common sites for metastatic disease, primary bone tumours are rare and account for approximately 1–1.5% of all deaths from malignant disease. The aetiology of primary bone tumours is poorly understood and although certain oncogenic animal viruses have been implicated, no causal relationship has been proved. There are a number of well recognized predisposing causes, namely fibrous dysplasia, Paget's disease, osteochondroma and irradiation.

The classification of malignant primary bone tumours is based on the tissue from which the tumour originates. There are three important aspects of the diagnosis of a primary bone tumour: histological type, local extent and distant spread. Bone scintigraphy has been evaluated by Goodgold *et al.* in an attempt to differentiate benign from malignant bone tumours (1983). Using a combination of shape and size of the lesion and the pattern of tracer uptake they correctly identify the majority of lesions studied. In general, lesions that have been identified on X-rays that do not show abnormal accumulation on bone scan are unlikely to be malignant. Those lesions that take up tracer avidly with significant blood pool activity are more likely to be malignant. Gandsman *et al.* (1983) have studied three-phase bone scanning in benign and malignant disease and have shown that in osteomyelitis blood flow was increased over a significantly larger area than the bone lesion itself. In bone tumours the increase in blood flow is restricted to the area of the tumour. In early Paget's disease there was mild local increase in blood flow, but in advanced Paget's the blood flow pattern resembled that of tumours. The most useful investigations to delineate the local extent of the tumour are arteriography, CT scanning, X-ray tomography and skeletal scintigraphy. The importance of defining the local extent of the tumour relates to management as the excision of the tumour, usually by amputation, must include all local disease. Arteriography and CT scanning are particularly useful in determining the extent of soft tissue involvement. Skeletal scintigraphy using ^{99m}Tc-labelled diphosphonate is useful in identifying 'skip' lesions which may determine the level of amputation. Determination of local extent also has prognostic significance since smaller tumours have a better prognosis than larger ones.

18.9.1 OSTEOGENIC SARCOMA

Although rare, this tumour is the commonest primary malignant tumour of bone. It can develop at any age but is particularly common during childhood and the adolescent growth spurt or as a complication of Paget's disease. The tumour arises from the metaphysis, the commonest site being the lower end of the femur (26%), the upper end of the tibia (18%) and the upper end of the humerus (9%). It may be multiple. Patients present with symptoms of pain followed by a palpable bone mass. Current treatment consists of amputation and adjuvant to chemotherapy.

Classical bone scan appearances are those of patchy intense tracer uptake and distortion of the normal bone contour. Three-phase bone studies confirm the vascular nature of the tumour. The ability of the bone scan to define accurately the extent of the disease has been debated. Papanicolaou *et al.* (1982) concluded that the bone scan was a highly accurate method of determining the local extent of the tumour. Chew and Hudson (1982), however, found that the scan accurately identified the extent of the tumour in less than half of the patients studied. This finding may be explained by the observation of Golderman *et al.* (1975) of generalized increased tracer uptake in the whole of the affected limb which is attributed to marrow hyperaemia, medullary reactive bone or periosteal new bone.

The major role of the bone scan in patients with osteogenic sarcoma is its role in determining the presence of distant metastases. Amputation is reserved for those patients in whom no evidence of metastases can be found. Increased tracer uptake is commonly seen at the site of metastases, although occasionally absent tracer uptake may be observed (Goris *et al.*, 1980; Siddiqui and Ellis, 1982).

Although the lungs are the most common sites of metastatic spread, evidence is now appearing that suggests that adjuvant chemotherapy is altering the natural history of the disease and that distant bone metastases are occurring earlier in the disease, and before the appearance of lung metastases (McKillop *et al.*, 1981; Giulano *et al.*, 1984). Bone scanning should therefore be performed routinely in patients undergoing adjuvant chemotherapy. ^{18}F scintigraphy has been used by McNeil *et al.* (1973) to study the effects of radiotherapy in patients with osteosarcoma. Decreased ^{18}F uptake was seen in those patients who responded to radiotherapy, whereas persistently increased uptake was seen in patients with recurrence or local infection.

Osteosarcoma lung metastases have been shown in numerous studies to take up bone-seeking radiopharmaceuticals to a variable extent (Ghaed *et al.*, 1974; McClean and Murray, 1984). The majority of lung metastases studied, however, do not take up tracer (Giulano *et al.*, 1984).

18.9.2 CHONDROSARCOMA

These tumours generally occur in the 30–60-year-old age group, although they may occur in younger individuals. Whilst generally occurring as a primary tumour in the young age group, in older patients condrosarcomas are usually secondary to malignant change in the osteochondroma. Patients present with an alteration of size or symptoms within existing known osteochondroma.

The bone scan in patients with chondrosarcoma reveals moderately increased tracer uptake in the lesion, with minimal distortion of the bone contour (Pearlman and Steiner, 1978). Intensity of uptake and tracer distribution cannot be used to distinguish benign from malignant but the bone scan is useful in detecting lesions in the spinal column (Smith *et al.*, 1982).

18.9.3 EWING SARCOMA

This usually occurs in the 5–20-year age group and affects males more commonly than females. It arises in the diaphysis of long bones, particularly the tibia, followed by the fibula, humerus and femur. The lesions may be multiple. Patients present with complaints of pain and the development of a slow-growing lesion. Systemic symptoms of fever may also be experienced.

^{99m}Tc-labelled diphosphonate bone scanning reveals intense uniform tracer uptake with distortion of the bone contours and an ill-defined margin (McClean and Murray, 1984).

^{67}Ga-gallium citrate has been compared with bone scanning by Frankel *et al.* (1974) and has been shown to be an equally sensitive method of detecting the primary tumour. Radiotherapy to the primary tumour results in markedly reduced ^{67}Ga accumulation in the primary tumour. Bone metastases may be demonstrated in patients when investigated with bone scintigraphy (Goldstein *et al.*, 1986; McNair, 1985), with an incidence ranging from 11% to 47%. Bone metastases are associated with the poor prognosis and bone scanning shows an increased sensitivity in detecting metastases when compared with conventional X-rays (McNair, 1985).

Lumbroso *et al.* (1989) have assessed the uptake of ^{123}I-MIBG into sites of Ewing sarcoma because of the proposed neuroectodermal origin of these tumours. No significant uptake was seen at the site of primary tumour or metastases in the 15 children studied.

18.9.4 MULTIPLE MYELOMA

Although not strictly a primary bone tumour skeletal involvement is a major component of multiple myeloma. This malignant disease of the plasma cells accounts for 1% of all malignancies. Patients present with back or rib pain, precipitated by movement, sudden onset and severe in nature. Persistent localized pain may indicate a pathological fracture at the site of a bone lesion. In addition to bone symptoms, patients are anaemic and may develop renal failure, hypercalcaemia and neurological complications.

Comparative studies between X-rays and bone scanning have shown that although the bone scan is often abnormal in patients with multiple myeloma the number of lesions detected is far fewer than may be identified with conventional X-rays (Wahner *et al.*, 1980; Woolfenden *et al.*, 1980; Waxman *et al.*, 1981). In particular, large lytic lesions clearly visible on X-ray may not be detected by bone scanning. Anscombe and Walkenden (1983) have reported a 'super scan' appearance in some patients. ^{67}Ga accumulation in myelomatous deposits occurs in less than half of patients studied and uptake is associated with a particularly poor prognosis (Waxman *et al.*, 1981).

18.9.5 SKELETAL METASTASES

The skeleton is one of the commonest sites of metastatic disease, and metastases account for more than half of the cases of malignant bone tumours. The tumours that commonly metastasize to bone are prostate, breast, thyroid, renal and bronchogenic. The skeleton may be involved as a result of direct spread from the primary tumour or via the bloodstream. These occur more commonly in the axial skeleton.

Bone scanning is a sensitive and cost-effective method of screening the patient at the time of primary diagnosis, for investigating the patient with known malignancy and symptoms of bone pain and assessing the effects of therapy on known metastases. Sensitivity of bone scanning exceeds that of X-rays for the detection of metastases (Charkes *et al.*, 1968). The incidence of a false-negative scan result in bone metastases is less than 3% (Pistenma *et al.*, 1975; Citrin and McKillop, 1978). Metastases from most tumours are associated with increased osteoblastic activity and increased diphosphonate accumulation which is usually multiple and asymmetrical (Figure 18.7). In patients with widespread bone metastases the scan may show diffusely increased tracer uptake throughout the skeleton with low soft tissue background. Renal images are only faintly visualized. The appearance of the super-scan may be difficult to distinguish from the metabolic super-scan but on close inspection irregularities of uptake may be identified in the ribs and long bones (Fogelman *et al.*, 1977). Unusually, tracer uptake at the site of the metastases may be reduced or absent resulting in a 'cold' area which may be surrounded by a 'hot' rim (Stadalnik, 1979). This finding occurs commonly with multiple myeloma (Weingrad *et al.*, 1984) and in renal carcinoma (Kim *et al.*, 1983; Figure 18.8). Around 2% of metastases are associated with reduced tracer uptake. The explanation for the cold area is thought to be due to metastases that fail to excite an osteoblastic response or rapidly growing metastases.

Although ^{99m}Tc-labelled diphosphonate bone scanning provides a highly sensitive method of detecting and evaluating bone metastases, its specificity is low, with focal increased tracer uptake being also associated with trauma, infection, inflammation and benign bone tumours.

Solitary areas of increased uptake may prove particularly difficult to evaluate on the bone scan as, although not conforming to the standard accepted pattern of metastatic disease, they may be due to a solitary metastasis. McNeil (1984) demonstrated that up to 17% of solitary rib lesions are metastatic, and around 80% of vertebral lesions. Boxer *et al.* (1989) have recently reviewed scans from patients with breast cancer and shown that 21% had solitary metastasis, the commonest site being the spine in 52% of cases. Polyostotic Paget's disease of bone may also prove difficult to distinguish from metastatic disease although the uniform involvement of the whole vertebra rather than the pedicle or uniform skull and maxillary uptake may give an indication of the underlying pathology. X-rays of the affected area should be performed to confirm the diagnosis.

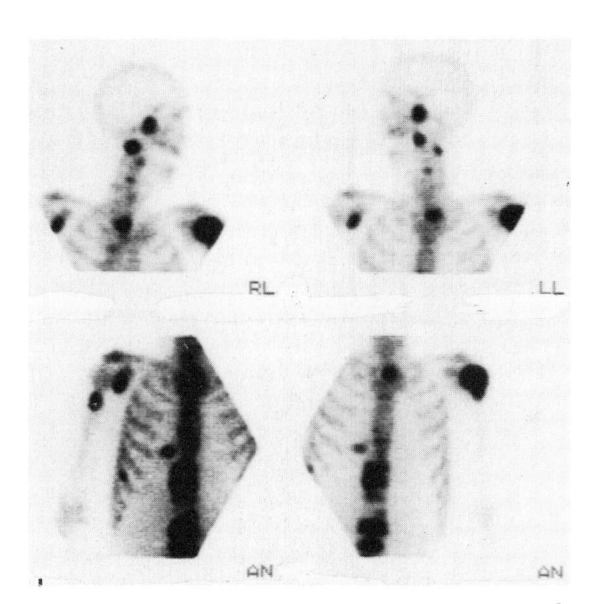

Figure 18.7 65-year-old male with known cancer of the prostate and widespread bone pain. ^{99}Tc-labelled MDP bone imaging confirms multiple metastases throughout the skeleton.

Modern high-resolution gamma cameras allow anatomical resolution of the spine so that lesions can be correctly sited in the transverse process, pedicle or body of the vertebra. The addition of SPECT further facilitates the correct anatomical localization of abnormal uptake and may differentiate uptake due to degenerative change from that due to metastatic disease. Again local X-rays should be performed to fully evaluate the affected vertebra. The bone scan provides an excellent method of assessing the response of metastases to therapy, whether chemotherapy or radiotherapy (Figure 18.9). In successfully treated patients the uptake of tracer would decrease gradually until the bone scan returns to normal. In

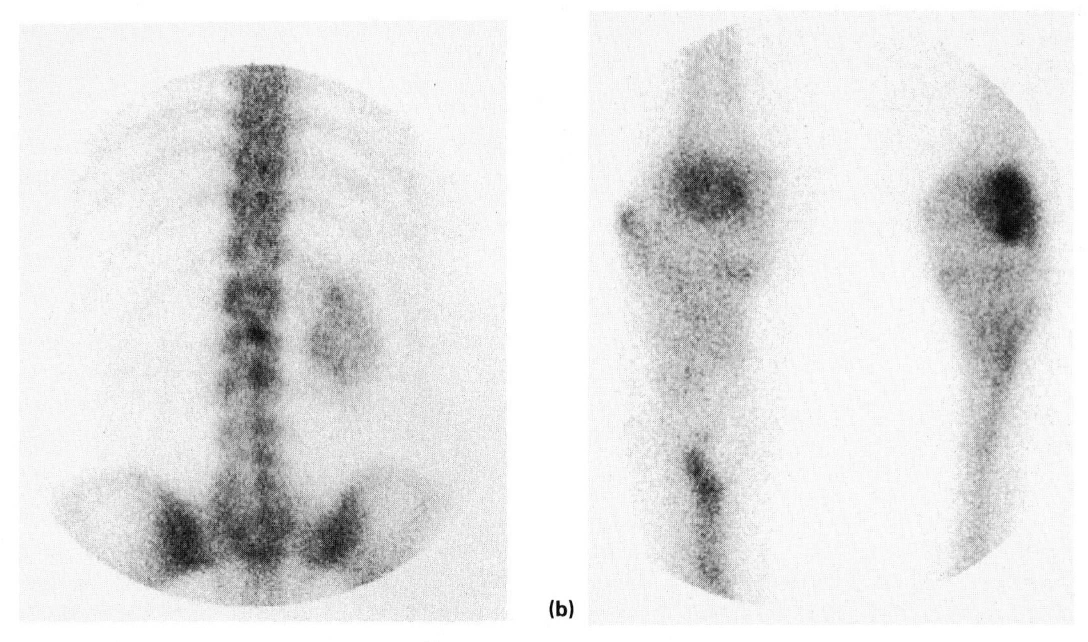

Figure 18.8 56-year-old female imaged with ^{99m}Tc-labelled MDP two years after left nephrectomy for a hypernephroma (a). Tibial views identify an area of reduced uptake in the right upper tibia with increased uptake in the mid-tibia at the site of a large metastases (b).

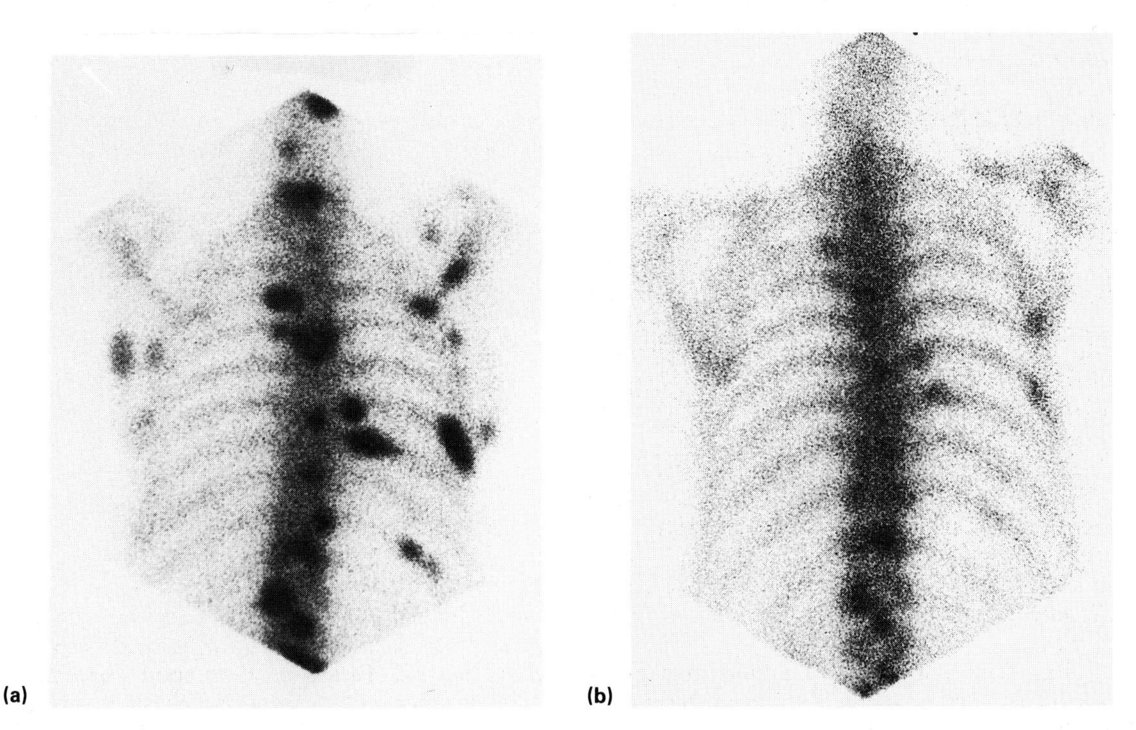

Figure 18.9 67-year-old female with known cancer of breast. ^{99m}Tc-labelled MDP bone scan (a) shows multiple metastases in the spine and ribs. Bone scan (b) one year later shows marked improvement in metastases following treatment with tamoxifen and prednisone.

addition, reduced tracer uptake may be observed in the surrounding bone lying within the radiotherapy field. If bone scans are performed within a few months of successful treatment, an increase in tracer uptake or 'flare' phenomenon may be observed corresponding to the healing osteoblastic response (Gillespie *et al.*, 1975; Alexander *et al.*, 1976). New sites of uptake may also be observed in specific tumours (Rossleigh *et al.*, 1982).

New radiopharmaceuticals are being developed to image soft tissue and bone metastases simultaneously. ^{99m}Tc-labelled V DMSA has been used to image patients with a variety of tumours, including medullary carcinoma of the thyroid and squamous carcinoma of the head and neck. Studies in a series of patients with MTC give a sensitivity of about 80% and a specificity of 70% in detecting both soft tissue and bone metastases (Clarke *et al.*, 1987b; Watkinson *et al.*, 1987). ^{123}I, and ^{131}I-MIBG have been used in patients with a number of different neuroendocrine tumours, particularly phaeochromocytoma and neuroblastomas, and uptake in soft tissue recurrence and bone metastases has been demonstrated.

18.10 TECHNIQUES

18.10.1 ^{67}GA, GALLIUM CITRATE

Edward and Hayes (1969) first described the use of ^{67}Ga for scanning neoplastic lesions in 1969. Since then much has been discovered about the mechanism of gallium accumulation in tumours and the types of tumour into which it accumulates.

^{67}Ga has three major photopeaks, 91, 185 and 300 keV, and a half-life of 78.1 h. Its normal biodistribution includes the salivary glands, liver, spleen and skeleton with excretion into the gut. In addition to tumour accumulation, ^{67}Ga also is taken up by inflammatory tissue and into metabolically active bone.

^{67}Ga is almost 100% protein bound in normal plasma (Hayes *et al.*, 1981) and has been shown to be bound to transferrin. Lactoferrin and ferritin have also been shown to bind ^{67}Ga (Hoffer *et al.*, 1977; Weiner *et al.*, 1983) and under certain circumstances transfer of ^{67}Ga from the transferrin–^{67}Ga complex to ferritin may be demonstrated (Weiner *et al.*, 1983). Changes in ^{67}Ga biodistribution and excretion patterns, due to alterations in the unsaturated iron binding capacity, have been reported (Hayes *et al.*, 1981). Tsan and Scheffel (1986) have postulated the factors that affect the accumulation of ^{67}Ga in tumours and have identified increased capillary permeability, specific tumour cell accumulation, inflammatory cells, ^{67}Ga binding proteins and pH. Hoffer *et al.* (1977) suggests that this specific tumour cell accumulation is due to binding ^{67}Ga by lactoferrin present in some tumours. The mechanism by which ^{67}Ga crosses the cell membrane is still not understood, however, although Larson *et al.* (1979) have postulated the presence of transferring receptors in tumour cell surfaces which are responsible for the internalization of the transferrin–^{67}Ga complex.

^{67}Ga is taken up by a variety of neoplasms, including lymphomas (both Hodgkin and non-Hodgkin) where the sensitivity ranges from 50% to 70% (Johnston *et al.*, 1974) and where its clinical role in staging has been established. Although the standard dose is 100 MBq and recently reviewed McLaughlin *et al.* (1990), recent studies using 370 MBq have reported increased sensitivity of detection (Southee *et al.*, 1989). The sensitivity in detecting hepatic or splenic involvement is only 38% due to the non-specific accumulation of gallium by these organs (Beckerman *et al.*, 1985). In those patients with ^{67}Ga-avid tumours, repeat ^{67}Ga

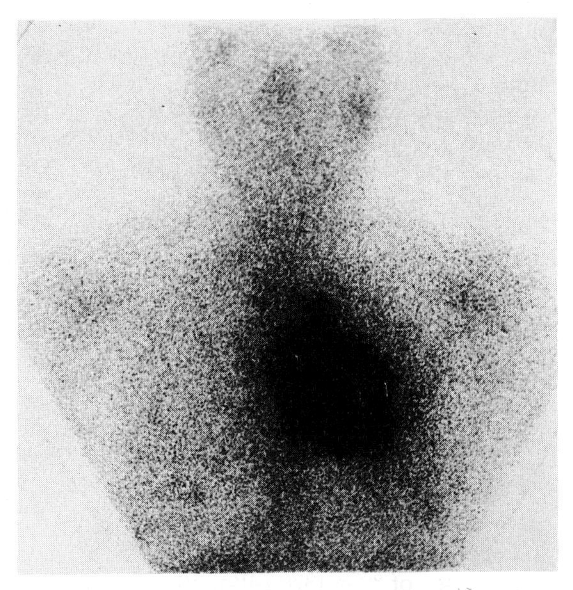

Figure 18.10 49-year-old female with nodular sclerosing Hodgkin's disease. ^{67}Ga-Gallium citrate scan shows marked uptake in mediastinum. CT imaging confirmed tumour in the anterior mediastinum extending to the left pulmonary artery.

imaging permits the follow-up of the tumour following surgery, radiotherapy or chemotherapy (Figure 18.10).

^{67}Ga has also been used to stage carcinomas of the lung, particularly to determine the involvement of the mediastinum. Alazraki *et al.* (1978) studied the value of ^{67}Ga imaging in detecting mediastinal disease in a group of patients with potentially resectable lesions and recommend that if the primary tumour concentrates gallium and the mediastinum does not, the patient may be saved a staging mediastinoscopy and referred directly for thoracotomy. Demeester *et al.* (1979) have shown that a ^{67}Ga positive scan signifies the presence of mediastinal disease with a 90% probability. Uptake of ^{67}Ga by lung carcinomas correlates with the incidence of metastases and survival.

The role of ^{67}Ga in imaging hepatoma is now well established. Less than 10% of cirrhotic pseudo-tumours accumulate ^{67}Ga in contrast to 90% of hepatomas (Suzuki *et al.*, 1971).

The main role of ^{67}Ga in the management of patients with malignant myeloma is the identification of bone metastases. ^{67}Ga has been shown to accumulate avidly in some bone lesions that appear only marginally abnormal on a diphosphonate bone scan (Waxman *et al.*, 1981). In some patients ^{67}Ga also accumulates in soft tissue lesions and plasmacytomas (Wolfenden *et al.*, 1980).

In vitro studies have shown that melanomas have a strong avidity for ^{67}Ga. The mechanism of tumour binding is unclear, but it has been demonstrated that melanin binding of gallium is not the mechanism, since uptake is seen in both melanotic and amelanotic tumours (Lavender *et al.*, 1971). Milder *et al.* (1973) have reported a sensitivity of 54% for the detection of involved sites with a high specificity of 98%. Factors affecting sensitivity included tumour size and metastatic site. Tumours that were greater than 2 cm in diameter were detected by gallium scanning in 75% of cases, whereas those less than 2 cm were only detected in 11% of cases. All bone metastases were detected but lesions in the gastrointestinal tract, kidneys and adrenals were visualized in only 45% of cases.

Recently studies have been performed using high doses of ^{67}Ga (370 MBq, 10 mCi) and tomographic imaging and the sensitivity of lesion detection increased to 82% (Kirkwood *et al.*, 1982).

Although less clinically useful than in the tumours already mentioned, ^{67}Ga is also taken up by a number of other tumours, including some brain tumours, cancers of the head and neck, breast cancer, testicular malignancies and primary bone tumours. Studies, however, have failed to demonstrate any advantage of ^{67}Ga in these tumours over CT or clinical examination. Although occasionally clinically valuable ^{67}Ga imaging does not have a place in the routine management of these tumours.

18.10.2 METAIODOBENZYLGUANIDINE (MIBG)

Since 1979 when Wieland *et al.* first successfully imaged dog adrenal medulla using the *para* isomer of an arakylguandine, much work has been done to develop, evaluate and confirm the clinical usefulness of the guanethidine noradrenaline analogue MIBG (Troncone *et al.*, 1990). Iodination with ^{131}I and ^{123}I has enabled this agent to be successfully used to image many neuroectodermally derived tumours including phaeochromocytomas, neuroblastomas, carcinoids and medullary carcinomas of the thyroid. The mechanism of uptake of MIBG in these tumours remains unclear but it has been demonstrated that MIBG localizes within the intracellular storage granules. This is not the only explanation for the retention of MIBG within neuroectodermally derived tumours, however, since MIBG is also taken up and retained in non-secretory tumours.

Uptake of ^{131}I-MIBG in benign phaeochromocytoma occurs in over 80% of tumours studied, with a specificity greater than 90% (Shapiro *et al.*, 1986). Studies were initially performed with ^{131}I-MIBG and although image quality is not ideal small tumours have been visualized. Recently ^{123}I-MIBG has been used by Lynn *et al.* (1984) with no loss of sensitivity and a significant improvement in image quality.

Uptake in malignant phaeochromocytoma, which accounts for 10% of all phaeochromocytoma, has also been demonstrated and MIBG imaging has proved a valuable clinical tool for assessing patients with benign or malignant phaeochromocytomas pre-operatively to ensure that the patient is not one of the 10% with bilateral disease or one of the 15% with tumour outside the adrenals. Post-operatively MIBG has been used to assess recurrent disease and to screen for metastases. In those patients with significant MIBG uptake at recurrent or metastatic sites, therapy with high-activity doses of MIBG may be performed, with reports of limited success (Marchandise *et al.*, 1987).

Uptake of ^{131}I- and ^{123}I-MIBG by neuroblastomas has been extensively investigated and successfully demonstrated (Geatti *et al.*, 1985; Hoefnagel *et al.*, 1985). Although ^{99m}Tc-labelled MDP successfully demonstrates the extent of skeletal involvement by neuroblastomas, MIBG provides an imaging method for assessing the extent of both soft tissue and bone disease. Like phaeochromocytomas, high sensitivity of tumour detection greater than 90% is reported in patients with neuroblastoma. Since there is good uptake and prolonged retention of ^{131}I-MIBG in neuroblastomas, ^{131}I-MIBG has been used in therapy in a significant number of children. Although most children treated have been clinically stage IV with no response or relapse following chemotherapy, complete remissions have been achieved in a few cases and nearly half the reported cases have experienced partial remission (Hoefnagel *et al.*, 1987b).

In 1984 Fischer *et al.* (1984) described uptake of ^{131}I-MIBG in a patient with a mid-gut carcinoid tumour. Since then reports in the literature have indicated that more than 50% of carcinoids are able to concentrate ^{131}I-MIBG. There appears no relation between the urinary excretion of 5-hydroxyindoleacetic acid (5-HIAA) and the degree of ^{131}I-MIBG uptake. In order to identify liver metastases, imaging up to seven days should be performed which precludes the use of ^{123}I-MIBG (Figure 18.11). As in other neuroectodermally derived tumours, therapy has been undertaken with limited success, palliative responses only being achieved in patients with large tumour volumes (McEwan *et al.*, 1987).

Endo *et al.* in 1984 published a first case report of ^{131}I-MIBG uptake in a primary medullary carcinoma of the thyroid. Further case reports appeared in the literature but it was not until the publication of the first series of patients studied with ^{131}I-MIBG that its relatively low sensitivity in the detection of primary and recurrent disease was established (Poston *et al.*, 1985). The combined sensitivity of tumour detection on review of current literature is only 40%, which confirms that ^{131}I-MIBG has no role in screening for MCT. Therapy in patients whose tumours accumulate ^{131}I-MIBG has been attempted by several groups with palliative responses only reported (Clarke *et al.*, 1987).

Following the success of ^{131}I-MIBG and ^{123}I-MIBG in imaging patients with phaeochromocytomas and neuroblastomas, numerous studies have been performed to assess the uptake of MIBG in other neuroectodermally derived tumours.

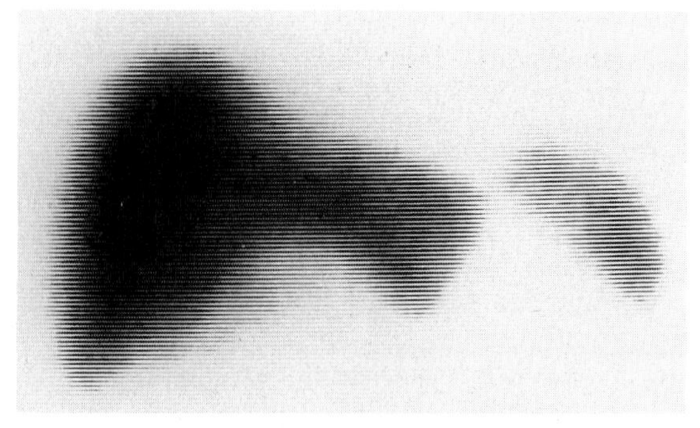

(a)

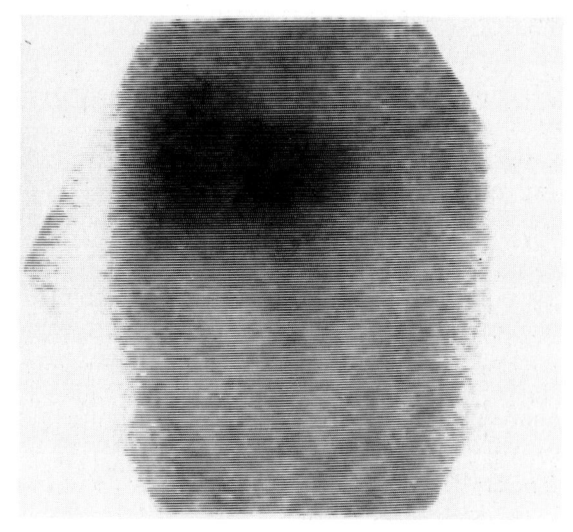

(b)

Figure 18.11 63-year-old female with a history of carcinoid and abnormal liver function tests. ^{99m}Tc-labelled colloid scan demonstrates an area of reduced uptake in the left lobe of the liver (a). ^{131}I-MIBG scan of the abdomen shows uptake of MIBG in the cold area on the colloid scan, confirming a carcinoid deposit (b).

Moderate results have been obtained in paragangliomas (Baulieu *et al.*, 1988; Van Gils *et al.*, 1989), chemodectomas (Van Gils *et al.*, 1989), ganglioneuromas (Hoefnagel *et al.*, 1986b), schwannomas and islet cell tumours. Consistently negative results have been obtained in neurofibromas, melanomas and oat cell carcinomas (Hoefnagel *et al.*, 1987c). Therapy has been attempted in patients with paragangliomas, achieving pain relief but no significant or long-term evidence of tumour regression.

18.10.3 THALLOUS CHLORIDE (^{201}Tl)

Although established as a myocardial imaging agent, ^{201}Tl-thallous chloride has also been used with varying successes as a tumour imaging agent. First described as a lung tumour imaging agent by Cox *et al.* (1976) it has been used to successfully image thyroid, bronchial and breast carcinomas, lymphomas, osteosarcomas, Ewing's sarcomas, soft tissue sarcomas, hepatomas and oesophageal cancers (Hisada *et al.*, 1978; Salvatore *et al.*, 1976; Marks and Caroll, 1978; Temi *et al.*, 1984). Its use in imaging thyroid cancer has been most widely reported and uptake has been demonstrated in all forms of thyroid cancer, including medullary carcinoma of the thyroid. Hoefnagel *et al.* (1986a) shows 100% sensitivity when imaging patients with MCT. The normal biodistribution of ^{201}Tl-thallous chloride in the liver, heart and lungs may obscure metastases at any of these sites. The poor imaging characteristics compared with its relatively high radiation dose when compared with ^{99m}Tc-labelled V DMSA limits its usefulness in this disease. The main role at present in thyroid cancer is the ability to image recurrent tumours while the patient is on suppressive doses of thyroxine, unlike ^{131}I.

18.10.4 PENTAVALENT DMSA

In 1984, Endo *et al.* reported uptake of a new tumour imaging agent in a wide variety of benign and malignant tumours. ^{99m}Tc-labelled V DMSA is prepared using a standard renal DMSA kit with a pH adjusted to alkaline, and 370 MBq of ^{99m}Tc are added. Its normal pattern of distribution includes the nasal mucosa, salivary glands, breasts and testes and faint uptake is also seen in bone. Although uptake in squamous carcinoma of the head and neck has been demonstrated (Watkinson *et al.*, 1989), ^{99m}Tc-labelled V DMSA has been shown not to be superior to clinical evaluation and therefore has no role in the management in this tumour. In medullary carcinoma of the thyroid, however, intense uptake is seen and sensitivities of 86% have been reported (Clarke *et al.*, 1987c; Patel *et al.*, 1988; Guerra *et al.*, 1989) with both soft tissue and bone uptake seen. Its role in management is under investigation but at present it is recommended as the imaging agent of choice in patients with suspected recurrence of MCT (Clarke *et al.*, 1988). Although sensitivity is high, specificity is lower due to false-positive uptake in bone at sites of surgery or trauma, and diffuse uptake following radiotherapy (Watkinson *et al.*, 1989).

18.10.5 MONOCLONAL ANTIBODIES

In recent years significant advances have been made in the isolation of tumour-specific antigens with the development of antibodies to these antigens. Although initially work was done with polyclonal antibodies, results were disappointing. In 1975 a breakthrough came with the introduction by Kohler and Milstein of a technique for the production of monoclonal antibodies using the hybridoma technique.

IgG-type antibodies are the main class used in immunoscintigraphy and they consist of two long chains (heavy or H chains) and two short chains (light or L chains) which are linked together by disulphide bridges.

(a) Labelling with radionuclides

Many factors must be considered when selecting the radionuclide with which a monoclonal antibody for immunoscintigraphy should be labelled. A fundamental factor is that immunoreactivity must be preserved during the labelling procedure. Other factors to be considered are the radiation dose to the patient, the emitted radiation from the radionuclide, the half-life of the radionuclide, the accumulation kinetics of the monoclonal antibody and finally the cost and availability of the radionuclide. Currently four radionuclides are in use in immunoscintigraphy and these are ^{131}I, ^{123}I, ^{111}In and ^{99m}Tc.

(a) ^{131}I

Since the iodination of complex molecules is a technique that is widely used, the use of ^{131}I in immunoscintigraphy was used initially. The advantages of ^{131}I in immunoscintigraphy are its cheapness and its availability. The half-life of eight days is long enough to permit studies to be carried out over a relatively prolonged period. Disadvantages of ^{131}I include β-radiation and high-energy γ-emissions which increase the radiation dose to the patient and also result in poor-quality images. The β-emission may ultimately prove advantageous, however, if localization is adequate since therapy with high doses of ^{131}I-labelled monoclonal antibodies may then be undertaken.

(b) ^{123}I

Again, the ease with which immunoglobulins may be iodinated gives this radionuclide an advantage for immunoscintigraphy. Its single γ-emission of 159 keV is well suited to the gamma camera. Its main disadvantages include its expense, restricted availability and its short half-life since maximum tumour background ratios occur in some tumours, especially liver metastases, up to 96 h after injection. This may prove less of a problem with Fab fragments which are cleared more rapidly from the circulation and therefore have earlier optimal imaging times. One further disadvantage of both ^{131}I and ^{123}I is the *in vivo* loss of label from the antibody, resulting in free iodine.

(c) ^{111}In

Because of its favourable physical characteristics of a half-life of 2.8 days and single γ-emissions of 172 and 274 keV, ^{111}In is well suited for immunoscintigraphy. The direct labelling of antibodies by ^{111}In is not possible, however, and a chelating agent must be used to bind the metal ion to protein. The most commonly used chelating agent at present is DTPA. Care must be taken when conjugating the antibody or fragment with the chelate to avoid cross-reaction of the DTPA chelate with the amino groups on the specific immunoreactive area with a loss of immunoreactivity. Once prepared the ^{111}In DTPA-labelled antibody shows good *in vivo* stability with no dissociation of ^{111}In from the complex. A further disadvantage of ^{111}In-labelled DTPA monoclonal antibodies is the accumulation of these labelled antibodies in the liver and bone marrow, which reduces the sensitivity of tumour detection in these areas.

(d) ^{99m}Tc

Although ^{99m}Tc has an established place as the radionuclide of choice for radiopharmaceutical labelling, with its ideal γ-energy, low cost and availability, its use in labelling monoclonal antibodies has been limited by two factors. The first is the difficulties that have been experienced in successfully labelling monoclonal antibodies with ^{99m}Tc, with poor preservation of immunoreactivity of the labelled compound. Recently success in labelling has been reported by several groups

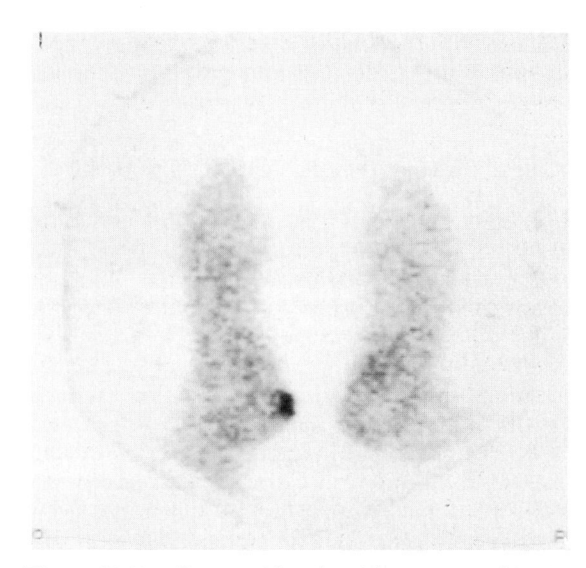

Figure 18.12 42-year-old male with a one-year history of a melanotic lesion on the right heel. ^{111}In-labelled DTPA anti-melanoma antibody localizes at site of lesion.

(Mather *et al.*, 1989) and work with ^{99m}Tc-labelled PRIA3 in colorectal cancer appears extremely promising (Granowska *et al.*, 1989). The main and only other disadvantage of ^{99m}Tc for labelling monoclonal antibodies is its short half-life of 6.4 h, which may restrict its use in tumours that accumulate antibodies slowly either because of low avidity or poor blood supply.

(e) Clinical use of radiolabelled monoclonal antibodies

The role of imaging in the management of patients with cancer varies with tumour type and this is proving true as immunoscintigraphy develops and becomes more widely used. Its role in primary diagnosis remains at present limited for most tumour types due to the relatively low sensitivity and specificity at present reported.

(f) The future

Non-specific uptake of antibody reduces the sensitivity and specificity of the technique and also increases the radiation burden to the patient. Various manoeuvres are at present being explored attempting to reduce non-specific uptake of antibody. New chelating agents are being tried (Brechbiel *et al.*, 1986; Paik *et al.*, 1987).

'Cocktails' of antibodies have been used in an attempt to increase sensitivity (Klapdor *et al.*,

1985) and more recently bispecific antibodies have been produced with different specificities associated with the two arms of the 'Y' (Scheidhauer *et al.*, 1986).

The route of administration has also been varied and peritoneal and subcutaneous routes have been used with some success (Nelp *et al.*, 1987; Colcher *et al.*, 1987).

Finally, the production of human antibodies as opposed to mouse antibodies has been attempted both to reduce the human anti-mouse antibody response (HAMA) and also in an attempt to increase specificity.

During the past few years recombinant DNA technology has been used to address the problem of antigenicity of mouse antibodies. Recently an advanced molecular biological approach has been successful that reduces the mouse portion of the monoclonal antibody to the minimum essential part, the rest of the molecule being human.

18.11 POSITRON EMISSION TOMOGRAPHY (PET)

Although few centres have the facility to perform PET, the technique is making significant contributions to the understanding of tumour pathophysiology and metabolism. With the development of small cyclotrons it is hoped that PET imaging will increase and be incorporated into the routine management of patients with tumours. The aspects of tumour pathophysiology that may be studied using PET with the appropriate radiopharmaceuticals are listed in Table 18.1. In addition to studying tumour pathophysiology, PET

Table 18.1

Aspects of tumour pathophysiology	*PET radiopharmaceutical*
Oxygen utilization	$^{15}O_2$
Regional blood flow	$C^{15}O_2$ $H_2{}^{15}O$
Tissue pH	$^{11}CO_2$
Amino acid metabolism	^{11}C-Methionine
	^{18}F-Fluorotyrosine
	^{11}C-Leucine
	^{11}C-Tyrosine
	^{11}C-Glycine
Glucose metabolism	^{18}F-Fluorodeoxyglucose
	^{11}C-Glucose
Permeability	^{68}Ga-labelled EDTA
	^{82}Rb
Proliferation	^{11}C-Thymidine
	^{77}Br-labelled deoxyuridine
	^{18}F-Fluorouracil

may be used to study drug uptake in tumours and identify the presence of tumour receptors.

^{15}O-Oxygen is used to determine oxygen utilization and is often combined with the measurement of blood flow. After inhalation of $^{15}O_2$ a steady state in the tissue is obtained and imaging is performed (Jones *et al.*, 1976). For quantitative determination of oxygen metabolism, pO_2, pCO_2, haemoglobin, haematocrit and the pH values of blood must be obtained (Kyrento *et al.*, 1983).

The tissue pH may be assessed using $^{11}CO_2$. The pH within the tumour is usually elevated. Tumour cells are also frequently hypoxic and ^{18}F-fluoromisonidazole has been used to image the hypoxic cells within tumours.

Amino acid metabolism may be determined to assess tumour growth, metabolic activity and the protein synthesis that occurs in response to therapy. Various positron-emitting radiopharmaceuticals may be used, including ^{11}C-methionine, ^{11}C-leucine, ^{11}C-tyrosine, ^{11}C-glycine, ^{18}F-fluorotyrosine. Fujiwara *et al.* (1989) have shown that ^{11}C-methionine uptake varies with histological type in lung cancer tumours.

Glucose metabolism reflects tumour proliferation rates and is generally assessed using ^{18}F-fluorodeoxyglucose (^{18}FDG). ^{18}FDG enters the metabolic cycle like glucose, but is trapped in tissue in the form of ^{18}FDG phosphate. Sokoloff *et al.* (1977) have developed a model for calculating regional glucose metabolic rate on the basis of *in vitro* measurements of glucose metabolism using ^{14}C-deoxyglucose. Wolleman and Lajta (1972) have shown that glucose metabolism is positively correlated with the histological grade of malignancy in human and animal tumours.

Tumour proliferation may also be studied using positron-emitting nucleotides and nucleosides, such as ^{11}C-thymidine, ^{18}F-labelled uridine and ^{18}F-labelled uracil to assess DNA synthesis. The uptake of nucleotides and nucleosides in tumours is dependent on blood flow, endogenous synthesis, local reutilization and the rate of removal of degradation products.

The effect of tumours in the brain is to disrupt the blood–brain barrier. ^{68}Ga-labelled EDTA and ^{82}Rb have both been used to assist the permeability of the blood–brain barrier during chemotherapy treatments of patients with primary cerebral lymphoma (Iannotti *et al.*, 1987).

Recently positron-emitting radionuclides have been used to successfully label both drugs and receptors such as ^{18}F-fluoroestradiol (Mintun *et al.*, 1988).

With the advancement of PET and the development of new radiopharmaceuticals, it appears hopeful that in the near future PET imaging will play a key role in the management of cancer (Table 18.2). At the time of primary diagnosis PET imaging can assist with both the detection and the grading of tumours and in the determination of the prognosis. In the treated patient the use of PET to assess tumour response to therapy is now established.

Table 18.2 The application of PET in the management of cancer

Tumour detection and differentiation
Tumour grading
Prognosis
Tumour therapy response
Imaging hypoxic cells
Drug uptake
In vivo receptor assay

Table 18.3 Characteristics of an ideal therapeutic radiopharmaceutical

1. Easily prepared or readily available
2. Stable *in vivo* binding of radionuclide to pharmaceutical
3. Minimal non-specific uptake
4. High tumour accumulation
5. Long tumour residence time
6. Cheap

18.12 THERAPY

One of the areas of development in nuclear medicine over the past ten years has been in the field of therapy. Although ^{131}I has been used successfully to treat patients with recurrent or metastatic folicular or mixed thyroid cancer for over 40 years, most of the nuclear medicine research has concentrated on diagnostic techniques rather than therapy.

Recently new radiopharmaceuticals have been developed that are incorporated into metabolic pathways, thereby facilitating the uptake of the agent by the target organ. The incorporation of a β-emitting radionuclide into the radiopharmaceutical then provides the clinician with a potential new therapy tool. Factors to be taken into account when assessing a radiopharmaceutical for therapy are listed in Table 18.3.

18.12.1 ^{131}I-MIBG

MIBG is a guanethidine analogue developed for imaging the adrenal medulla. Since the first publication of Wieland *et al.* in 1980 many reports have appeared confirming uptake of MIBG in other neuroectodermally derived tumours, including neuroblastomas, paragangliomas, carcinoids and medullary carcinomas of the thyroid. Following the publication of a report by Sisson *et al.* in 1984 of uptake by MIBG in a malignant phaeochromocytoma a number of reports have appeared in the literature describing experience in therapy with MIBG (McEwan *et al.*, 1988; Marchandise *et al.*, 1987). Most authors use 3.7–7.4 GBq doses infused slowly at three- to six-month intervals. Cumulative results from the limited experience show partial response in one-third of patients treated for malignant phaeochromocytoma and palliation in over 50%. No complete remissions have been recorded. Treatment is well tolerated and reported side effects are minimal. Cumulative experience of ^{131}I-MIBG uptake in patients with neuroblastoma yields a sensitivity of over 90%. MIBG has now been used to treat many children with neuroblastomas in whom other forms of therapy have failed (Fisher *et al.*, 1987; Bestagno *et al.*, 1987; Voute *et al.*, 1987). All patients treated had extensive disease. When the data are reviewed 5% of patients treated have undergone complete remission, 40% have experienced partial remission, 25% remain unchanged and in 10% the disease progresses. Doses used are up to 7.5 GBq and the treatment interval is about 8–12 weeks. Side effects are common due to the frequent involvement of the bone marrow. Inevitable radiation dose to the marrow with therapy results in anaemia, reduction in platelets and white count and occasionally complete marrow suppression. Marrow harvesting is now performed as a precautionary manoeuvre in patients with extensive disease prior to treatment.

Case reports and small series of therapy with MIBG in other neural crest tumours have been reported, with limited success. These include medullary carcinoma of the thyroid (Clarke *et al.*, 1987), carcinoid (McEwan *et al.*, 1987) and paraganglioma (Baulieu *et al.*, 1988).

18.12.2 STRONTIUM (^{89}Sr)

^{89}Sr has a half-life of 50.5 days and a β-particle energy of 1.49 kV. It is a bone-seeking radiopharmaceutical that is taken up, like ^{99m}Tc-technetium diphosphonate, into sites of increased osteoblastic activity. It has been used successfully by Lewington (1989) to palliate pain in patients with severe bone metastases from prostatic cancer. The palliative effect has been proved to be greater than just a placebo effect through a double-blind cross-over trial comparing stable strontium with ^{89}Sr.

18.12.3 YTTRIUM (^{90}Y)

^{90}Y has a short half-life (2.7 days) and a high β-particle energy, E_{max} = 2.3 MeV with no γ-emissions. Although its use in treating synovial disease is established, preliminary studies have been carried out to assess its use in tumour therapy. When complexed with the bone-seeking tetraphosphonate EDTMP, significant bone uptake occurs and initial studies suggest ^{80}Y-labelled EDTMP may be successful in the therapy of primary bone tumours (Keeling *et al.*, 1989). ^{90}Y antibodies have been used intraperitoneally in an attempt to treat ovarian cancer, with little success (Stewart *et al.*, 1989). ^{90}Y glass microspheres have been administered via the hepatic artery in patients with hepatic metastases, with partial response in 55% of patients treated (Shapiro *et al.*, 1989).

18.12.4 SAMARIUM (^{153}Sm)

^{153}Sm has a half-life of 46.3 h and a β-energy of 0.81 kMeV. It also emits 103 keV γ-photons which may be used for imaging. When labelled to EDTMP it has been used to treat patients with widespread bone metastases, with palliation of bone pain in 75% and evidence of stabilization or regression of disease in 62% of patients studied (Harvey Turner *et al.*, 1989).

18.12.5 ANTIBODIES

Although imaging results with radiolabelled monoclonal antibodies have proved generally disappointing, good results with high tumour uptake have been observed with a few tumours. Malignant melanoma has successfully been imaged using a number of different monoclonal antibodies and a few reports of partial response to therapeutic doses of ^{131}I-labelled melanoma antibody have been reported (Larson *et al.*, 1983b). Evaluation of tumour response is difficult as most patients survive only a short time after treatment. Studies suggest single doses up to 170 GBq can be tolerated with resultant high tumour radiation doses (Larson *et al.*, 1983). A general limitation to the use of multiple courses of treatment is the development of HAMA, which significantly alter the biodistribution of the labelled antibody, reducing tumour uptake and increasing liver accumulation.

Regional application of radiolabelled monoclonal antibodies has been used by some workers in an attempt to improve the local delivery of antibody and reduce non-specific uptake. Stewart *et al.* (1987) have used intraperitoneal administration of ^{131}I-labelled HMFG1 and HMFG2 in patients with ovarian cancer in doses up to 8.5 GBq of ^{131}I on 30 mg of antibody. Best responses were seen in patients with microscopic disease, where some complete remissions were obtained. Patients with nodules more than 2 cm in diameter showed no response to therapy. Stewart *et al.* have also used ^{90}Y-labelled monoclonal antibodies intraperitoneally in patients with ovarian cancer. The maximum dose administered was 0.9 GBq and tumour response was observed in only one patient.

Lashford *et al.* (1988) have used a variety of ^{131}I-labelled monoclonal antibodies administered intrathecally to treat patients with malignant

Table 18.4 Radiopharmaceuticals in therapy

Radiopharmaceutical	*Tumour*
^{131}I	Follicular Thyroid carcinoma Mixed thyroid Carcinoma
^{131}I-labelled monoclonal antibody	Ovarian Melanoma
^{32}P	Polycythaemia rubra
^{90}Y-labelled microspheres	Bone
^{90}Y-labelled EDTMP	Bone
^{90}Y-labelled MoAb	Ovarian
^{131}I-MIBG	Phaeochromocytoma Neuroblastomas Paragangliomas Medullary thyroid carcinoids
^{89}Sr	Disseminated prostatic cancer
^{153}Sm-labelled EDTMP	Skeletal metastases

meningitis (Table 18.4). The tumours treated were medulloblastomas, pineoblastomas, lymphomas, teratomas, gliomas and metastatic carcinomas. Doses up to 2.7 GBq were used. Six of the ten patients treated showed marginal complete response to treatment. Two patients experienced status epilepticus following administration of labelled antibody.

REFERENCES

Ackery, D. M., Tillett, P. A., Condon, B. R. *et al.* (1984) New approach to the localization of phaeochromocytoma imaging with ^{131}MIBG. *Br. Med. J.*, **288**, 1587–91.

Alazraki, M. P., Ramsdell, J. W., Taylor A. *et al.* (1978) The reliability of gallium scan, chest radiography compared with mediastinoscopy for evaluating mediastinal spread in lung cancer. *Am. Rev. Resp. Dis.*, **117**, 415–20.

Alexander, J. L., Gillespie, P. J. and Edelstyn, G. A. (1976) Serial bone scanning using ^{99m}technetium diphosphonate in patients undergoing cyclical combination chemotherapy for advanced breast cancer. *Clin. Nucl. Med.*, **1**, 13–17.

Anderson, R. J., Sizemore, G. W. and Wahner, H. W. (1978) Thyroid scintigraphy in familial medullary Ca of the thyroid gland. *Clin. Nucl. Med.*, **3**, 147.

Anscombe, A. and Walkenden, S. B. (1983) An interesting bone scan in multiple myeloma: ?myeloma super scan. *Br. J. Radiol.*, **56**, 489–92.

Baulieu, J. C., Guilloteau, D., Calmettes, C. *et al.* (1986) MIBG uptake in MTC: a feature of multiple endocrine neoplasia. *J. Nucl. Med.*, **27**, 1009.

Baulieu, J. L., Guilloteau, D., Baulieu, F. *et al.* (1988) Therapeutic effectiveness of iodine-131 MIBG metastases of a non-secreting paraganglioma. *J. Nucl. Med.*, **29**, 2008–13.

Becherman, C., De Meester, T. R. and Skinner D. R. (1976) in *Medical Radionuclide Imaging* (Vol. II), IAEA, Vienna, p. 351.

Beckerman, C., Hoffer, P. B. and Bitran, J. D. (1985) The role of gallium 67 in the clinical evaluation of cancer. *Semin. Nucl. Med.*, **15**, 72–103.

Bestagno, M., Guerra, P., Puricelli, G. P. *et al.* (1987) Treatment of neuroblastoma with ^{131}I MIBG: the experience of an Italian study group. *Med. Paediatr. Oncol.*, **15**, 203–5.

Bomani, J., Levison, D. A., Flatman, W. D. *et al.* (1987) Uptake of iodine-123 MIBG by phaeochromocytomas, paragangliomas and neuroblastomas: a histopathological comparison. *J. Nucl. Med.*, **28**, 973–8.

Boucher, B. J. and Sear, R. (1980) A summary of the results of radioisotope brain scans on a large series of patients. *Br. J. Radiol.*, **53**, 1174–6.

Boxer, D., Todd, C., Coleman, R. and Fogelman, I. (1989) Bone secondaries in breast cancer: the solitary metastases. *J. Nucl. Med.*, **30**, 1318–20.

Brechbiel, M. W., Gansow, O. A., Atcher, R. W. *et al.* (1986) Synthesis of 1-(*p*-isothiocyanotobenzyl) derivatives of DTPA and EDTA: antibody labelling and tumour imaging studies. *Chemistry*, **25**, 2772–81.

Carrasquillo, J. A., Foon, K. A. Mulshine, J. M. *et al.* (1987) Radioimmunoscintigraphy of chronic lymphocytic leukaemia with monoclonal antibodies. *J. Nucl. Med.*, **28**, 602.

Carril, J. M., Macdonald, A. F., Dendy, P. P., *et al.* (1979) Cranial scintigraphy: value of added emission computed tomographic sections to conventional pertechnetate images. *J. Nucl. Med.*, **20**, 117–23.

Cellerino, A., Filippi, P. G. and Chian Taretto, A. (1973) Operative and pathologic survey of 50 cases of peripheral lung tumours scanned with gallium 67. *Chest*, **64**, 700.

Charkes, N. D., Young, I. and Sklaroff, D. M. (1968) The pathological basis of the strontium bone scan. *JAMA*, **206**, 2482–88.

Chew, F. S. and Hudson, T. M. (1982) Radionuclide bone scanning of osteosarcoma: falsely extended uptake patterns. *Am. J. Roentgenol.*, **139**, 49–54.

Citrin, D. L. and McKillop, J. H. (1978) *Atlas of Technetium Bone Scans.* Saunders, Philadelphia.

Clarke, S. E. M., Lazarus, C. R., Edwards, S. *et al.* (1987a) Scintigraphy and treatment of MCT with ^{131}I MIBG. *J. Nucl. Med.*, **28**, 1820.

Clarke, S. E. M., Lazarus, C. R., Watkinson, J. *et al.* (1987b) ^{99m}Tc(v) DMSA: experience in imaging. *Nucl. Med. Commun.*, **8**, 265.

Clarke, S. E. M., Lazarus, C., Mistry, R. and Maisey, M. N. (1987c) The role of ^{99m}Tc (v) DMSA in the management of patients with MCT. *Br. J. Radiol.*, **60**, 1089–92.

Clarke, S. E. M., Lazarus, C., Wraight, P. *et al.* (1988) Pentavalent ^{99m}Tc DMSA, ^{131}MIBG and ^{99m}Tc MDP: an evaluation of three imaging techniques in patients with MCT. *J. Nucl. Med.*, **29**, 33–8.

Clarke, S., Allen, S. J., Twelves, C. *et al.* (1989) Immunoscintigraphy in breast cancer with 131 and 125 iodine labelled SM3. *Eur. J. Nucl. Med.*, **15**, 548.

Coakley, A. J. and Wraight, E. P. (1980) Selenomethine liver scanning in the diagnosis of hepatoma. *Br. J. Radiol.*, **53**, 538–43.

Colcher, D., Esteban, J., Carrasquillo, J. A. *et al.* (1987) Complementation of intra cavitary and intravenous administration of a monoclonal antibody B72.3 in patients with carcinoma. *Cancer Res.*, **47**, 4218–24.

Coleman, R. E., Habibollahi, F., Rubens, R. D. and Fogelman, I. (1986) Bone scintigraphy in early breast cancer: the relevance of tumour characteristics in identifying patients with serial scanning. *Nucl. Med. Commun.*, **7**, 292.

Connel, J. C., Hilditch, T., Elliott, A. and Sample, P. (1984) ^{131}I MIBG and medullary thyroid cancer. *Lancet*, **ii**, 1273–4.

Cowan, R. J. and Watson, N. E. (1980) Special characteristics and potential of single photon emission computed tomography in the brain. *Semin. Nucl. Med.*, **10**, 335–44.

Cox, P. H., Belfer, A. J. and Van Der Pompe, W. B. (1976) Thallium 201 chloride uptake in tumours, a possible complication in heart scintigraphy. *Br. J. Radiol.*, **49**, 767–8.

DeChiro, G., Delapaz, R. L. and Brooks, R. M. (1982) Glucose utilization of cerebral gliomas measured by (18F)fluoro-deoxy-glucose and positron emission tomography. *Neurology*, **32**, 1323–9.

DeLand, F. M., Sauerbrunn, B. J. Z. and Boyd, C. (1974) 67 Gallium citrate in untreated primary lung cancer:

preliminary report of a co-operative group. *J. Nucl. Med.*, **15**, 408.

Demeester, T. R., Golomb, H. M. and Kirchner, P. (1979) The role of gallium-67 scanning in the clinical staging and preoperative evaluation of patients with carcinoma of the lung. *Ann. Thorac. Surg.*, **28**, 451.

Dukes, C. E. (1942) *J. Pathol. Bacteriol.*, **50**, 527.

Dukes, C. E. (1958) in *Cancer*, (ed. R. W. Karen), Butterworths, London, p. 136.

Edward, C. L. and Hayes, R. L. (1969) Tumour scanning with 67 gallium citrate. *J. Nucl. Med.*, **10**, 103–105.

Ell, P. J., and Khan, O. (1981) Emission computerized tomography clinical application. *Semin. Nucl. Med.*, **11**, 50–60.

Ell, P. J., Deacon, J. M. and Jarritt, P. H. (1980) *Atlas of Computerised Emission Tomography*, Churchill Livingstone, Edinburgh.

Endo, K., Shiomi, K., Kasagi, K., *et al.* (1984a) Imaging of MTC with ^{131}I MIBG. *Lancet*, **ii**, 233.

Endo, K., Ohta, M. and Sakahara, M. (1984b) in *Radiopharmaceuticals and Labelled Compounds*, IAEA, Vienna, p. 201.

Esselstyn, C. B. (1977) Parathyroid pathology: its relation to choice of operation for hyperparathyroidism. *World J. Surg.*, **1**, 701–8.

Ferlin, G., Borsato, N. and Camerani, N. (1983) New perspectives in localizing enlarged parathyroid by technetium–thallium substraction scan. *J. Nucl. Med.*, **24**, 438–41.

Fischer, M., Kamanabroo, D. and Sandercaup, H. (1984) Scintigraphic imaging of carcinoid tumours with ^{131}I MIBG. *Lancet*, **ii**, 165.

Fisher, B. (1976) Pathological findings from the national surgical adjuvant breast project (protocol no 4): significance of regional node histology other than sinus histiocytes in invasive mammary cancer. *Am. J. Clin. Pathol.*, **65**, 21–30.

Fisher, M., Wehinger, H., Kraus, C. *et al.* (1987) Treatment of neuroblastoma with ^{131}I MIBG: experience of the Munster Kassel Group. *Med. Paediatr. Oncol.*, **15**, 196–9.

Flower, M. A., Babich, J. W. and Keeling, F. (1986) Clinical evaluation of new radioactive tracer (^{99m}Tc-ceretex) for imaging regional cerebral blood flow in patients with brain tumours, *Proceedings of the 26th Annual Scientific Conference of Biological Engineering Society*, 'Blood flow in the brain'. Strachclyde University, September 1986.

Fogelman, I., McKillop, J. H., Grieg, W. R. and Boyle, I. T. (1977) Absent kidney sign associated with symmetrical and uniformly increased uptake of tracer by the skeleton. *Eur. J. Nucl. Med.*, **2**, 257–60.

Frankel, R. S., Jones, A. E., Cohen, J. A. *et al.* (1974) Clinical correlations of ^{67}gallium radionuclide studies with radiography in Ewing's sarcoma. *Radiology*, **110**, 597–603.

Freitas, J. E., Gross, M. D., Ripley, S. and Shapiro, B. (1985) Radionuclide diagnosis and therapy of thyroid cancer: current status report. *Semin. Nucl. Med.*, **15**, 106–31.

Fujiwara, T., Matsuzawa, T., Kubota, K. *et al.* (1989) Relationship between histologic type of primary lung cancer and ^{11}C methionine uptake with PET. *J. Nucl. Med.*, **30**, 33.

Gandsman, E. J., Deutsch, S. D. and Tyson, I. B. (1983) Use of dynamic bone scanning in the differential diagnosis of osteomyelitis, Paget's disease and primary bone tumours. *J. Nucl. Med.*, **24**, 83.

Geatti, O., Shapiro, B. and Sissan, J. C. (1985) ^{131}I MIBG for the locating of neuroblastoma: preliminary experience in 10 cases. *J. Nucl. Med.*, **26**, 736–42.

Ghaed, N., Thrall, J. H., Pinsky, S. M. and Johnson, M. C. (1974) Detection of extra osseous metastases from osteosarcoma with ^{99m}technetium pyrophosphate bone scanning. *Radiology*, **112**, 373–5.

Gillespie, P. J., Alexander, J. L. and Edelstyn, G. A. (1975) Changes in ^{87m}strontium concentrations in skeletal metastases in patients responding to cyclical combination chemotherapy for advanced breast cancer. *J. Nucl. Med.*, **16**, 191–3.

Giulano, A. E., Feig, S. and Eilber, F. R. (1984) Changing metastatic patterns of osteosarcoma. *Cancer*, **54**, 2160–4.

Goldman, A. B., Becker, M. H., Braumstein, P. *et al.* (1975) Bone scanning: osteogenic sarcoma correlation with surgical pathology. *Radiology*, **124**, 83–90.

Goldstein, H., McNeil, B. J., Zinfall, E. and Treves, S. (1986) Is there still a place for bone scanning in Ewing's sarcoma? *J. Nucl. Med.*, **21**, 10–12.

Goodall, A. L. and Symington, T. (1983) Studies in phaeochromocytoma: clinical aspects: diagnosis by adrenergic blocking drugs and treatment. *Glasgow Med. J.*, **34**, 95–7.

Goodgold, H. M., Chen, D. C., Majd, M. and Nolan, N. G. (1983) Scintigraphy of primary bone neoplasia. *J. Nucl. Med.*, **24**, 57.

Goris, M. C., Basso, L. V. and Etcubanas, E. (1980) Photopaenic lesions in bone scintigraphy. *Clin. Nucl. Med.*, **5**, 299–301.

Gould, A. A., Hubner, K. F. and Greenlaw, R. H. (1978) Gallium 67 citrate imaging in malignant lymphoma: final report of a co-operative group. *J. Nucl. Med.*, **19**, 1013–19.

Granowska, M., Mather, S. J., Britton, K. E. *et al.* (1989) Colorectal cancer immunoscintigraphy, RIS with a ^{99m}Tc-labelled monoclonal antibody, PR1A3. *Nucl. Med. Commun.*, **10**, 221.

Greenberg, P. H. and Marks, C. (1978) Adrenal cortical carcinoma: a presentation of 22 cases and a review of the literature. *Ann. Surg.*, **44**, 81–5.

Guerra, U. P., Pizzocaro, C., Terzi, A. *et al.* (1989) New tracers for the imaging of the medullary thyroid carcinoma. *Nucl. Med. Commun.*, **10**, 285–95.

Halpern, S. E., Dillman, R. O. and Witzun, K. F. (1985) Radioimmuno detection of melanoma using indium-111 96.5 monoclonal antibody: a preliminary report. *Radiology*, **155**, 493–9.

Harvey Turner, J., Martindale, A., Sorby, P. *et al.* (1989) SM-153 EDTMP therapy of disseminated skeletal metastases. *Eur. J. Nucl. Med.*, **15**, 400.

Hayes, R. L., Rafter, J. J. and Byrd, B. L. (1981) Studies of the *in vivo* entry of gallium 67 into normal and malignant tissue. *J. Nucl. Med.*, **22**, 325–32.

Higashi, T., Auyuma, W. and Mori, Y. (1977) Gallium 67 scanning in the differentiation of maxillary sinus carcinoma from chronic maxillary sinusitis. *Radiology*, **123**, 117.

Higashi, T., Wakao, H. and Nakamura, K. (1980) Quantitative gallium 67 scanning for predictive value in primary lung cancer. *J. Nucl. Med.*, **21**, 628.

Hisada, K., Tonami, N., Miyamae, T. *et al.* (1978) Clinical evaluation of tumour imaging with ^{201}thallium chloride. *Radiology*, **129**, 497–500.

Hjelms, E. and Dyrbye, M. (1975) Uptake of ^{67}gallium in malignant lesions of the lung and lymphatic tissue. *Scand. J. Resp. Dis.*, **56**, 251.

Hoefnagel, C. A., Voute, P. A. and DeKraker, J. (1985) Total body scintigraphy for detection of neuroblastoma. *Diagn. Imag. Clin. Med.*, **54**, 21–7.

Hoefnagel, C. A., Delprat, C. C., Marcuse, H. R. and DeVijlder, J. J. M. (1986a) Thallium-201 total body scintigraphy in follow up of thyroid cancer. *J. Nucl. Med.*, **27**, 1854–7.

Hoefnagel, C. A., DeKraker, J., Marcuse, H. R. and Voute, P. A. (1986b) in *Nuklearmedizin: Nuclear Medicine in Research and Practice* (eds H. A. E. Schmidt, P. J. Ell and K. E. Britton, Schattauer-Verlag, Stuttgart, pp. 473–6.

Hoefnagel, C. A., Klumper, A. and Voute, P. A. (1987a) Single photon emission tomography using ^{131}MIBG in malignant phaeochromocytoma and neuroblastoma case reports. *J. Med. Imag.*, **1**, 57–60.

Hoefnagel, C. A., Voute, P. A., DeKraker, J. and Marcuse, H. R. (1987b) Radionuclide diagnosis and therapy of neural crest tumours using iodine-131 MIBG. *J. Nucl. Med.*, **28**, 308–14.

Hoefnagel, C. A., Marcuse, H. R., DeKraker, J. and Voute, P. A. (1987c) Methodik und problematik der ^{131}I MIBG mit SPECT. *Nuclearmediziner*, **4**, 317–23.

Hoffer, P. B., Huberty, J. and Khayam-Bashi, J. (1977) The associated of gallium 67 and lactoferrin. *J. Nucl. Med.*, **18**, 713–17.

Iannotti, F., Fieschi, C. and Alphano, B. (1987) *J. Comput. Assist. Tomogr.*, **11**, 390–7.

Johnston, G., Benna, R. S. and Teates, C. D. (1974) 67 Gallium citrate imaging in untreated Hodgkin's disease: preliminary report of a co-operative group. *J. Nucl. Med.*, **15**, 399.

Jones, T., Chesler, D. A. and Ter-Pogossian, M. (1976) Continuous inhalation of ^{15}oxygen for assessing regional oxygen extraction in the brain of man. *Br. J. Radiol.*, **49**, 339–43.

Kashima, H. K., McKusik, K. A. and Malmud, L. S. (1974) Gallium 67 scanning in patients with head and neck cancer. *Laryngoscopy*, **84**, 1078.

Keeling, A. A., Vaughan, A. T. M. and Beaney, R. P. (1989) Yttrium-90-EDTMP bone seeking radiotherapeutic agent. *Nucl. Med. Commun.*, **10**, 224.

Khafagi, F., Egerton-Vernon, J., Van Doorn, T. *et al.* (1987) Localization and treatment of familial malignant non-functional paraganglioma with ^{131}iodine MIBG: report of two cases. *J. Nucl. Med.*, **28**, 528–32.

Kim, E. E., Bledin, A. G., Gutierre, Z. C. and Hayne, T. P. (1983) Comparison of radionuclide images and radiographs for skeletal metastases from renal cell carcinoma. *Oncology*, **40**, 284–6.

Kinkler, I. H., Merrich, M. V. and Rodger, A. (1985) Bone scintigraphy in breast cancer: a nine year follow up. *Clin. Radiol.*, **36**, 279–82.

Kirkwood, J. M., Myers, J. E. and Vlock, D. R. (1982) Tomographic gallium 67 citrate scanning: useful new surveillance for malignant melanoma. *Ann. Intern. Med.*, **66**, 694.

Klapdor, R., Montz, R., Lauder, H. *et al.* (1985) Untersuchungen zur intratumeralen: Radio immunotherapie transplantierte pankreas karzinoma mit 131J-anti CA19-9/CEA. *Nucl. Compact*, **16**, 424–7.

Kohler, G. and Millstein, C. (1975) Continuous cultures of few cells secreting antibody of predefined specificity. *Nature*, **256**, 495–7.

Kubota, K., Matsuzawa, J., Ito, M. *et al.* (1985) Lung tumour imaging by positron emission tomography using C-11 L-methionine. *J. Nucl. Med.* **26**, 37–42.

Kyrento, A. L., Brownell, G. L., Schleiderburg, G. and Elmullay, D. R. (1983) Regional blood flow measurement in rabbit soft tissue tumour with positron imaging using the $C^{15}O_2$ study state and labelled microspheres. *J. Nucl. Med.*, **24**, 1135–42.

Larson, S. M., Rasey, J. S. and Allen, D. R. (1979) A transferrin mediated uptake of gallium 67 by EMT-6 sarcoma: studies in tissue culture. *J. Nucl. Med.*, **20**, 837–42.

Larson, S. M., Brown, J. P. and Wright, P. W. (1983a) Imaging of melanoma with 131I labelled monoclonal antibodies. *J. Nucl. Med.*, **24**, 123–9.

Larson, S. M., Carrasquillo, J. A., Krohn, K. A. *et al.* (1983b) Localization of ^{131}I labelled p. 97 specific Fab fragments in human melanoma as a basis for radiotherapy. *J. Clin. Invest.*, **72**, 2101–14.

Larson, S. M., Carrasquillo, J. A. and McGuffin, R. W. (1985) Use of 131I labelled muirine Fab against a high molecular weight antigen of human melanoma: preliminary experience. *Radiology*, **155**, 487–92.

Larson, S. M., Milders, M. S. and Johnston, G. J. (1975) in *Radiopharmaceuticals* (eds G. Subramanian, B. A. Rhodes and J F. Cooper), Society of Nuclear Medicine, New York, p. 413.

Lashford, L. S., Mosely, R., Richardson, R. *et al.* (1988) Intrathecal administration of radiolabelled antibodies for therapy of malignant meningitis. *Nucl. Med. Commun.* **9**, 181.

Lavender, J. O., Lowe, J. and Barker, J. R. (1971) Gallium 67 citrate scanning in neoplastic and inflammatory lesions. *Br. J. Radiol.*, **44**, 361.

Lewington, V. J. (1989) Strontium-89 therapy in disseminated prostatic carcinoma. *Nucl. Med. Commun.*, **10**, 224.

Lindegaard, M. W., Skretting, A. and Hager, B. (1986) Cerebral and cerebellar uptake of ^{99m}Tc-(*d,l*)hexamethyl-propyleneamine oxime (HM-PAO) in patients with brain tumours studied by single photon emission computerised tomography. *Eur. J. Nucl. Med.*, **12**, 417–20.

Littenberg, R. L., Alazraki, N. P. and Taketa, R. M. (1973) A clinical evaluation of gallium 67 citrate scanning. *Surg. Gynaecol. Obstet.*, **137**, 424.

Lomas, F., Dibso, P. E. and Wagner, H. M. (1972) Increased specificity of lung scanning with the use of gallium 67 citrate. *N. Engl. J. Med.*, **286**, 1323–9.

Lumbroso, J., Oberlin, O., Terrier, P. H. *et al.* (1989) May 123-I MIBG contribute to imaging Ewing's sarcoma of bone. *Eur. J. Nucl. Med.*, **15**, 451.

Lumia, S., Parthasarathy, K. L., Baksh, S. and Bender, M. A. (1957) An evaluation of ^{99m}Tc-sulfur colloid liver scintiscans and their usefulness in metastatic workup: a review of 1424 studies. *J. of Nucl. Med.*, **16**, 62–5.

Lynn, M. D., Shapiro, B., Sisson, J. C. *et al.* (1984) Portrayal of phaeochromocytoma and normal neural human adrenal medulla, by *m*-123 I-MIBG. *J. Nucl. Med.*, **25**, 436–40.

MacMahan, B., List, N. and Eisenberg, H. (1990) in *Prognostic Factors in Breast Cancer*, Livingstone, p. 56.

Mansfield, C. M. and Park, C. H. (1985) Radionuclide imaging in radiation oncology. *Semin. Nucl. Med.*, **15**, 28–45.

Marchandise, X., Brendel, A. J., Laudry, M. *et al.* (1987) Treatment of malignant phaeochromocytoma with ^{131}I MIBG: results of a French multi center study. *Nucl. Med.*, **26**, 51–2.

Marks, D. S. and Caroll, K. L. (1978) ^{201}Thallous chloride uptake by non-Hodgkin's lymphoma: Radiographic exhibit. *Henry Ford Hosp. Med. J.*, **201**, 56–7.

Mather, S. J., Ellison, D., Bentley, S. *et al.* (1989) Antibody labelling with ^{99m}technetium. *Nucl. Med. Commun.*, **10**, 245.

McClean, R. and Ege, G. (1986) Prognostic value of axillary lymphoscintigraphy in breast carcinoma patients. *J. Nucl. Med.*, **27**, 1116–24.

McClean, R. J. and Murray, P. C. (1984) Scintigraphic patterns in certain primary malignant tumours. *Clin. Radiol.*, **35**, 379–383.

McEwan, A. J., Catz, Z., Fields, A. L. *et al.* (1987) ^{131}I MIBG in the diagnosis and treatment of carcinoid syndrome. *J. Nucl. Med.*, **28**, 658.

McEwan, A. J., Blake, G., Hall, V. L. and Ackery, D. M. (1988) Therapy of malignant phaeochromocytoma with ^{131}I MIBG. *Eur. J. Nucl. Med.*, **11**, A17.

McKillop, J. H., Etcubanas, E. and Goris, M. L. (1981) The indications for and limitations of bone scintigraphy in osteogenic sarcoma: a review of 55 patients. *Cancer*, **48**, 1133–8.

McLaughlin, A. F., Magee, M. A., Greenough, R. *et al.* (1990) Current role of gallium screening in the management of lymphoma. *Eur. J. Nucl. Med.*, **16**, 755–71.

McNair, N. (1985) Bone scanning in Ewing's sarcoma. *J. Nucl. Med.*, **26**, 349–52.

McNeil, B. J. (1984) Value of bone scanning and malignant disease. *Semin. Nucl. Med.*, **14**, 277–86.

McNeil, B. J., Cassady, J. R., Geiser, C. F. *et al.* (1973) Fluorine 18 bone scintigraphy in children with osteosarcoma or Ewing's sarcoma. *Radiology*, **109**, 627–31.

Milder, M. S., Frankel, R. S. and Bulklox, G. B. (1973) Gallium 67 scintigraphy in malignant melanoma. *Cancer*, **32**, 1350.

Mintun, M. A., Welch, M. J. and Seege, B. A. (1988) Radiology, **169**, 45.

Muhe, E. Von (1971) Scintigraphic demonstration of bronchial carcinoma using gallium-67 citrate. *Thorax Chir.*, **10**, 440.

Murray, J. L., Rosenblum, M. G. and Sobel, R. E. (1985) Radioimmuno imaging in malignant melanoma with indium-111 labelled monoclonal antibody 96.5. *Cancer Res.*, **45**, 2376–81.

Nedalkott, B., Christopherson, W. M. and Harter, J. S. (1962) *Acta Cytol.*, **6**, 319.

Nelp, W. B., Eary, J. F., Jones, R. F. *et al.* (1987) Preliminary studies of monoclonal antibodies lymphoscintigraphy in malignant melanoma. J. Nucl. Med., **28**, 34–41.

O'Donnell, J. K., Go, R. T., Macintyre, W. J. *et al.* (1983) Gallium 67 emission tomography in the detection of suspected pulmonary lesions. *J. Nucl. Med.*, **24**, 114.

Ohta, H., Endo, K., Fujita, T. *et al.* (1984) Imaging of soft tissue tumours with ^{99m}Tc(v) DMSA: a new tumour seeking agent. *Clin. Nucl. Med.*, **9**, 568–73.

Okabe, T., Kaizu, T. and Fujisawa, M. (1985) Clinical application of monoclonal antibodies to small cell lung cancer. *Jpn. J. Nucl. Med.*, **24**, 250–65.

Olsen, G. N., Block, A. J. and Tobias, J. A. (1974) Prediction of post pneumonectomy pulmonary function using quantitative macroaggregate lung scanning. *Chest*, **66**, 13–16.

O'Mara, R. E. and Mozley, J. M. (1971) Current status of brain scanning. *Semin. Nucl. Med.*, **1**, 7–30.

Paik, C. H., Quadri, S. M. and Reba, R. C. (1987) In vivo comparison of antibody DTPA conjugates with different linkages. *J. Nucl. Med.*, **28**, 572.

Papanicolaou, N., Kozakewich, H., Treves, S. *et al.* (1982) Comparison of the extent of osteosarcoma between surgical pathology and skeletal scintigraphy. *J. Nucl. Med.*, **23**, 7.

Patel, M. C., Patel, R. B., Ramanathan, P. *et al* (1988) Clinical evaluation of ^{99m}Tc(v)-dimercaptosuccinic acid (DMSA) for imaging MCT and its metastases. *Eur. J. Nucl. Med.*, **13**, 507–10.

Patton, D. D. (1982) (eds L. M. Freeman and H. S. Weissman), in *Nuclear Medicine Annual* Raven Press, New York, pp. 35–79.

Pearlman, R. J. and Steiner, C. E. (1978) Chondrosarcoma: correlative study of nuclear imaging and histology. *Bull. Hosp. Joint Dis. Orthop. Inst.*, **39**, 153–64.

Pinsky, S. M. and Henkin, R. (1976) Gallium-67 tumour scanning. *Semin. Nucl. Med.*, **6**, 397–410.

Pistenma, D. A., McDougall, I. R. and Kriss, J. P. (1975) Screening for bone metastases: are only scans necessary? *JAMA*, **231**, 46–50.

Poston, G. J., Thomas, H., Macdonald, D. W. *et al.* (1985) ^{131}I MIBG uptake by medullary carcinoma of the thyroid. *Lancet*, **ii**, 560.

Quinn, J. L., III (1971) Serial brain scans in glioblastoma multiforme. *Radiology*, **101**, 367–70.

Richardson, J. V., Zenke, B. A. and Rossi, N. P. (1980) Preoperative non-invasive mediastinal staging in bronchogenic carcinoma. *Surgery*, **88**, 382–385.

Rossleigh, M. A., Lovegrove, T. A., Reynolds, P. M. and Byrne, M. J. (1982) Serial bone scans in the assessment of response to therapy of advanced breast cancer. Clin. Nucl. Med., **7**, 397–402.

Rothschild, M. A. and Rosenthal, S. (1976) Are hepatic scans ever used? *Am. J. Digest, Dis.*, **2**, 655–9.

Salvatore, M., Carratu, L. and Porta, E. (1976) Thallium 201 as a positive indicator for lung neoplasms preliminary experiments. *Radiology*, **121**, 487–8.

Scheidhauer, K., Stefani, F., Markl, A. *et al.* (1986) Radioimmunoscintigraphy with ^{99m}Tc labelled monoclonal antibodies in primary occular melanomas. *Nucl. Med.*, **25**, A45.

Sehweil, A., McKillop, J. H., Ziada, G. *et al.* (1988) The optimum time for tumour imaging with thallium 201. *Eur. J. Nucl. Med.*, **13**, 527–9.

Shapiro, B., Sissan, J. C., Geatti, O. *et al.* (1986) in

Nuclear Medicine in Clinical Oncology (ed. C. Winckler), Springer-Verlag, Berlin, pp. 129–37.

Shapiro, B., Andrews, J., Fig, L. *et al.* (1989) Therapeutic intraarterial administration of yttrium-90 glass microspheres for hepatic tumours. *Eur. J. Nucl. Med.*, **15**, 401.

Siccardi, A. G., Buraggi, G. L., Callegaro, L. *et al.* (1986) Multicentre study of immunoscintigraphy with radiolabelled monoclonal antibodies in patients with melanoma. *Cancer Res.*, **46**, 4817–22.

Siddiqui, A. R. and Ellis, J. H. (1982) Cold spots on bone scan at the site of osteosarcoma. *Eur. J. Nucl. Med.*, **7**, 480–1.

Siemsen, O. K., Grebe, S. F. and Waxman, A. D. (1978) The use of gallium-67 in pulmonary disorders. *Semin. Nucl. Med.*, **13**, 235.

Silberstein, E. B., Kornblut, A. and Shumrich, D. A. (1974) Gallium 67 as a diagnostic agent for detection of head and neck tumours and lymphoma. *Radiology*, **110**, 605–8.

Silverberg, E. (1981) Cancer statistics. *Cancer*, **31**, 20.

Sisson, J. L., Shapiro, B. and Beier Walters, W. H. Radiopharmaceutical treatment of malignant phaeochromocytoma. *J. Nucl. Med.*, **25**, 197–206.

Smith, T. W., Nandi, S. C. and Mills, K. (1982) Spinal chondrosarcoma demonstrated by ^{99m}technetium MDP bone scan. *Clin. Nucl. Med.*, **7**, 111–12.

Sokoloff, L., Rivitch, M. and Kennedy, C. (1977) The ^{14}C deoxyglucose method for the measurement of local cerebral glucose utilization: theory procedure and normal values on the conscious and anaesthetised rat. *J. Neurochem.*, **28**, 897–916.

Southee, A. E., McLaughlin, A. F., Joshua, D. E. *et al.* (1989) Gallium scanning as a predictor of outcome in mediastinal Hodgkin's disease. *Eur. J. Nucl. Med.*, **15**, 547.

Stadalnik, R. C. (1979) 'Cold spot': bone imaging. *Semin. Nucl. Med.*, **9**, 2–3.

Stewart, J. S. W., Griffiths, M., Munro, A. J. *et al.* (1987) Intraperitoneal radioimmunotherapy for ovarian cancer in immunotherapy and scintigraphy of tumours with monoclonal antibodies. *Satellite Symposium 3rd International Conference in Hormones and Cancer*, pp. 65–73.

Stewart, J. S. W., Hird, V., Snook, D. *et al.* (1989) Intraperitoneal yttrium-90 labelled monoclonal antibody in ovarian cancer. *Nucl. Med. Commun.*, **10**, 226–89.

Suzuki, T., Honjo, I. and Hamamoto, K. (1971) Positive scintophotography of cancer of the liver with 67 gallium citrate. *Am. J. Roentgenol. Rad. Therapy Nucl. Med.*, **113**, 92.

Symington, T. (1969) in *Functional Pathology of the Human Adrenal Gland*, Livingstone, London, pp. 219–324.

Taylor, A., Milton, W., Eyre, H. *et al.* (1988) Radioimmuno detection of human melanoma with indium-111 labelled monoclonal antibody. *J. Nucl. Med.*, **29**, 329–37.

Temi, S., Oyamada, H., Nishikawa, K. *et al.* (1984) Thallium-201 chloride scintigraphy for bone tumours and soft part sarcomas. *J. Nucl. Med.*, **25**, 114.

Thrall, J., Freitas, J. E. and Beierwaltes, W. (1978) Adrenal scintigraphy. *Semin. Nucl. Med.*, **8**, 23–41.

Tjandra, T. J., Sacks, N. P., Thompson, C. A. *et al.* (1989) The detection of axillary lymph node metastases from breast cancer by radiolabelled monoclonal antibodies: a prospective study. *Br. J. Cancer*, **59**, 296–302.

Togawa, T., Suziki, A. and Kato, K. (1985) Relation between thallium-201 to gallium-67 uptake ratio and histological type in primary lung cancer. *Eur. J. Cancer Clin. Oncol.*, **21**, 925.

Togawa, T., Yui, N., Koakubu, M. and Kinoshita, R. T. (1989) Two cases of adenocarcinoma of the lung in which thallium-201 gave a better delineation of metastatic lesions than gallium-67. *Clin. Nucl. Med.*, **14**, 197–200.

Tonami, N., Bunko, H., Mishi Gishi, T. *et al.* (1978) Clinical application of ^{201}thallium scintigraphy in patients with cold thyroid nodules. *Clin. Nucl. Med.*, **3**, 217–21.

Tonami, N., Skuka, N., Yokoyama, K. *et al.* (1989) Thallium 201 single photon emission computed tomography in the evaluation of suspected lung cancer. *J. Nucl. Med.*, **30**, 997–1004.

Troncone, L., Rufini, V., Montemaggi, P., Danza, F. M., Lasorella, A. and Mastrangelo, R. (1990) The diagnostic and therapeutic utility of radioiodinated metaiodobenzylguanidine (MIBG) *Eur. J. Nucl. Med.*, **16**, 325–35.

Tsan, M. and Scheffel, U. (1986) Mechanism of gallium 67 accumulation in tumours. *J. Nucl. Med.*, **27**, 1215–19.

Tsan, M. F., Scheffel, E. U. and Tzen, K. Y. (1980) Factors affecting the binding of gallium 67 in serum. *Int. J. Nucl. Med. Biol.*, **7**, 270–3.

Vallabhajosula, S. R., Harwig, J. F. and Siemsen, J. K. (1980) Radiogallium localization in tumours: blood binding and transport and the role of transferrin. *J. Nucl. Med.*, **21**, 650–6.

Van Gils, A. P. G., Van der Mey, A. G. L., Hoogma, R. P. J. M. *et al.* (1989) Iodium-123 MIBG scintigrafie bij chemodactomen een oprallend resultaat. *Nucl. Geneeskd. Bull.*, **II**, 61.

Vatz, R. D., Alderson, P. O. and Tochman, M. S. (1979) Ventilation perfusion imaging in the early detection of lung cancer. *J. Nucl. Med.*, **20**, 612.

Voute, P. A., Hoefnagel, C. A., De Kraker, J. *et al.* (1987). Radionuclide therapy of neural crest tumours. *Med. Paediatr. Oncol.*, **15**, 192–5.

Wahner, H. W., Kyle, R. A. and Beabont, J. W. (1980) Scintigraphic evaluation of the skeleton in multiple myeloma. *Mayo Clin. Proc.*, **55**, 739–46.

Walleman, N. and Lajta, T. H. A. (eds) (1972) *Handbook of Neurochemistry*, Plenum Press, New York, p. 583.

Watkinson, J. C., Clarke, S. E. M. and Shaheen, O. H. (1987) An evaluation of the uptake of Tc^{99m} (v) DMSA in patients with squamous carcinoma of the head and neck. *Clin. Otolaryngol.*, **12**, 405–11.

Watkinson, J. C. and Maisey, M. N. (1988) Imaging head and neck cancer using radioisotopes: a review. *J. R. Soc. Med.*, **81**, 653–7.

Watkinson, J. C., Todd, C., Allen, S. *et al.* (1989) ^{99m}Tc(v) DMSA imaging: does it have a role in the management of patients with head and neck SCC? *Nucl. Med. Commun.*, **10**, 239.

Waxman, A. D., Richmond, R., Duffner, H. *et al.* (1980) Correlation of contract angiography and histologic pattern with gallium uptake in primary liver-cell carcinoma: non-correlation with alpha-feta protein. *J. Nucl. Med.*, **21**, 324–7.

Waxman, A. D., Siemsen, J. K. and Levine, A. M. (1981) Radiographic and radionuclide imaging in multiple myeloma: the role of gallium scintigraphy. *J. Nucl. Med.*, **22**, 232–6.

Waxman, A. D., Julian, P. J., Brackman, M. B. *et al.* (1984) Gallium scintigraphy and bronchogenic carcinoma: the effect of tumour location on sensitivity and specificity. *Chest*, **86**, 178–83.

Weiner, R. E., Schrieber, G. J. and Hoffer, P. B. (1983) In-vitro transfer of gallium-67 from transferrin to ferretin. *J. Nucl. Med.*, **24**, 608–14.

Weingrad, T., Heyman, S. and Alari, A. (1984) Cold lesions on bone scan in paediatric neoplasms. *Clin. Nucl. Med.*, **9**, 125–30.

Wieland, D. M., Wu, J. L., Brown, L. E., Mangner, T. J. *et al.* (1980) Radiolabelled adrenergic neuroblocking agents: adreno-medullary imaging with ^{131}iodobenzylguanidine. *J. Nucl. Med.*, **21**, 349–53.

Wilson, G. S., Rich, M. A. and Brennan, M. J. (1980) Evaluation of bone scan in the preoperative clinical staging of breast cancer. *Arch. Surg.*, **115**, 415–19.

Woolfenden, J. M., Pitt, M., Durle, B. G. M. and Moon, T. E. (1980) Comparison of bone scintigraphy in radiology and multiple myeloma. *Radiology*, **134**, 723–8.

Zimmer, A. M., Rosen, S. T. and Spies, S. M. (1985) Radioimmuno imaging of human cell lung carcinoma with I131 tumour specific monoclonal antibody. *Hybridoma*, **4**, 1–14.

CHAPTER NINETEEN

Clinical otolaryngology

N. D. Greyson and A. M. Noyek

19.1 INTRODUCTION

Otolaryngology is primarily involved with diagnosis and treatment of diseases involving the mucosal structures of upper air and food passages, adnexal organs such as salivary glands, deep visceral cervical structures such as lymph nodes and the thyroid gland, as well as the cartilaginous and bony structures of the skull and larynx which support the soft tissue organs and enclose the mucosal-surfaced air spaces.

Most of these structures lend themselves to traditional methods of diagnosis by history, physical examination and conventional radiographs. The air-containing bony structures of the temporal bone and paranasal sinuses, and the orbits and mandible permit radiographic recognition of organic disease when significant osteolysis, osteoblastosis or opacification is present. However, radiological signs require significant changes in bone mineralization for visualization, and replacement of the air cavities by water density has an obscuring effect on the underlining bone.

The recent advances in imaging techniques, computed tomography (CT), ultrasound and magnetic resonance imaging enhance diagnosis, especially in the evaluation of deeply placed clinically inaccessible areas such as the temporal bones, paranasal sinuses and orbits. Magnetic resonance imaging (MRI) has superior soft tissue delineation, compared with CT, although it does not demonstrate bone directly. It is thus less influenced by overlying osseous or dental structures, and is being used increasingly in diseases of the head and neck (Mandelblatt *et al.*, 1987; Teresi *et al.*, 1987; Harris and Wilk, 1987; Mancuso and Hanafee, 1985).

Nuclear medicine adds a physiological dimension to diagnostic imaging with a variety of radiopharmaceuticals, whose localization in specific tissues or within organs rely on metabolic functions which may be affected by pathological processes.

Table 19.1 outlines some of the most common applications of diagnostic nuclear medicine in otolaryngology.

19.2 THREE-PHASE BONE SCANNING

Radiography of the skull and facial bones remains the primary diagnostic imaging modality and generally provides fine detailed anatomical images of these structures. However, problems are often encountered due to overlying soft tissue densities and the inability to position the patient, particularly following trauma. Difficulties in interpretation may arise due to the complexity of the anatomical structures, especially differentiation between suture lines, vascular markings and fracture lines. Subtle bone changes due to local inflammatory or neoplastic infiltration may not be resolved on the radiographs, as 30–50% alteration in calcium content may be required to produce visible density changes.

Bone scanning provides functional images of altered bone physiology. Any lesion producing osteoblastic reaction, increased or decreased blood flow or increased calcium turnover will result in altered deposition of the bone scanning agent. Although anatomical resolution is generally poor, compared with radiographs, physiological changes are sensitively detected, sufficient to confirm or exclude pathological osseous involvement (Alexander, 1976; Gates and Goris, 1976; Noyek *et al.*, 1977; Greyson and Noyek, 1978; Noyek, 1979; Matteson *et al.*, 1980; Bergstedt and Lind, 1981; O'Mara, 1985).

In assessing the head and neck, we have found the addition of the radionuclide angiogram and blood pool images to be of significant value (Figure 19.1). The patient is positioned under the

Table 19.1 Common applications of nuclear medicine in ear, nose and throat diagnosis

Clinical indication	*Technique*	*Findings*
Neoplasm	Three-phase bone scan (±SPECT) Whole-body bone scan	Soft tissue v. bone invasion Remote secondary
	^{67}Ga-Gallium citrate whole-body	Lymphoma staging
Inflammation	Three-phase bone scan ^{67}Ga-Gallium citrate	Soft tissue v. bone sepsis Acute v. chronic osteomyelitis
Trauma	Three-phase bone scan (±SPECT)	Detect fractures, age fractures and healing
Trismus	Bone scan TM joint (SPECT)	Local bony lesion v. non-bony or referred pain
Laryngeal lesions	Bone scan	Trauma, arthritis, inflammation
Bone sclerosis or lysis	Three-phase bone scan and whole body survey	Paget's, fibrous dysplasia, eosinophilic granuloma, myeloma – local or systemic
	Brain scan	Meningioma
Bone graft	Three-phase bone scan (±SPECT)	Assess viability
Salivary lesions	^{99m}Tc-Pertechnetate	Overall function (Sjogren's) Obstruction Function of masses
	^{67}Ga-Gallium citrate	Inflammatory lesions, neoplasms
Excess tearing	^{99m}Tc-Pertechnetate tear duct scan	Functional tearing v. obstruction
Thyroid	^{99m}Tc-Pertechnetate or ^{123}I scan	Neck mass, ectopic thyroid, post-irradiation
Tinnitus or hearing problem	^{99m}Tc-labelled DTPA or glucoheptonate brain scan and flow	Acoustic neuroma, AV malformation 1° or 2° tumour, abscess
	Bone scan – skull	Paget's disease of temporal bone

gamma camera in the appropriate projection (neutral anterior, extended anterior 'Water's' (for face and mandible), or flexed anterior 'Towne's' (for frontal regions)). Following intravenous injection of 15–20 mCi (550–740 MBq) ^{99m}Tc-labelled methylene diphosphonate or other bone-seeking radiopharmaceutical, rapid sequential images are taken at 3 s intervals. These images of the first transit of the radiopharmaceutical through the major vascular channels are similar to a low-resolution angiogram and the activity seen on the scan is related to the local blood flow.

Within the first few minutes following injection, when the radiopharmaceutical is in equilibration in the vascular compartment, but has not yet localized in bone, a 'blood pool' image is obtained. The intensity of radioactivity indicates the size of the vascular compartment (arterial, venous and capillary).

In the case of both blood pool and delayed images, multiple views are obtained. These should include anterior, posterior, and both lateral and oblique projections. In many cases, standard radiographic views (Water's, Towne's and oblique temporal bone views) are of value (Gates and Goris, 1976). Improved resolution may be obtained using converging or pin-hole collimators when small structures are encountered.

The delayed image two or more hours after injection, shows bone reaction to a lesion, but the addition of the blood flow and blood pool images add specificity to the diagnoses. Demonstrating increased vascularity in an inflammatory process indicates activity, as opposed to a chronic, more indolent inflammation where hyperaemia is minimal. Neovascularity of a tumour is seen in the blood pool image, whether soft tissue or bone, while the delayed scan indicates bony involvement. The hyperaemia of repair seen on the blood pool is a feature of a recent or healing fracture, as opposed to an older traumatic lesion (Greyson and Noyek, 1978; Noyek, 1979). Table 19.2 summarizes three-phase bone scan findings.

In interpreting bone scans of the skull and face,

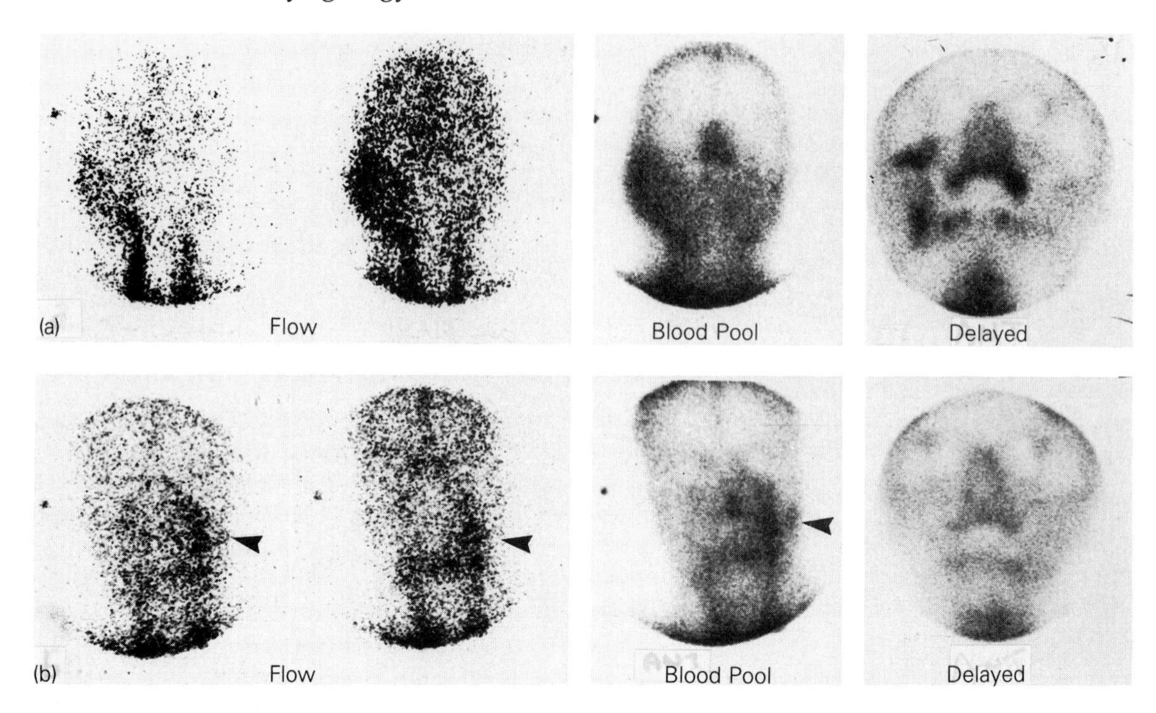

Figure 19.1 Three-phase bone scanning in malignant neoplasm of the head and neck. (a) Adenocarcinoma of the right parotid gland. The neoplasm is highly vascular and shows increased flow and hyperaemia on the blood pool image. The delayed scan shows uptake in the ascending ramus of the mandible which was not apparent on the radiograph, but confirmed at surgery. (b) Vascular carcinoma of the buccal mucosa demonstrated on the flow and blood pool images (arrows), but the normal appearance on the delayed image shows that the lesion is confined to the soft tissues.

Table 19.2 Three-phase bone scanning of face

Lesion	*Flow and pool*	*Delayed scan*
Neoplasm		
Soft tissue	+	−
Bony infiltration	+	+
Inflammation		
Acute sinusitis/cellulitis	+	− or mild +
Acute osteomyelitis	+	++
Chronic osteomyelitis	−	+
Trauma		
Recent fracture	+	+
Delayed union	+	+
Non-union	−	− or mild +
Bone graft		
Free (non-vascularized)	−	− early post-op. → + late
Vascularized	+	+ initial post-op.

care should be taken to avoid misinterpretation of activity in the mandible and maxillary alveolar ridges, which are common sites of uptake due to dental infection, extractions, or malfitting dentures (Tow *et al.*, 1978). Accurate interpretation depends on familiarity with the normal features of the bone scan of cervical area, face and skull (Jones and Patton, 1976; Noyek, 1979).

Single photon emission computed tomography (SPECT) permits the demonstration of anatomy and pathology in three dimensions. Lesion to background contrast is enhanced, and overlying structures which might obscure the lesion can be separated. This augmentation to the routine bone scan is useful in evaluating facial and skull fractures, localizing tumours and sepsis, assessment of viability of grafts, and detecting temporomandibular joint disease (Brown *et al.*, 1977; Collier *et al.*, 1983; O'Mara, 1985; Cawthorn *et al.*, 1986; Nobuharu, 1986).

19.2.1 MALIGNANT NEOPLASMS

Although primary bone tumours may arise within the facial structures, most primary neoplasms which involve the oropharyngeal cavity, sinuses, salivary glands or auditory canal are soft-tissue tumours which may invade local bony structures or may have distant metastases. Radiographs and physical examination are often insufficient to detect subtle bony infiltration.

Blood flow and blood pool phases of the three-phase bone scan may demonstrate the hypervascularity of the soft-tissue component of the tumour, and when compared with the delayed image give an indication of whether the lesion is confined to soft tissue or has extended into bone. Because the radiopharmaceutical is distributed throughout all bony structures, a whole-body metastatic survey may be performed with the same radiopharmaceutical injection, without increased radiation dose to detect the presence of distant bony metastases.

Figure 19.1(a) shows a hypervascular adenocarcinoma of the parotid gland demonstrated in the blood flow and pool phases. The conventional radiographs of the mandible failed to demonstrate bony involvement whereas the delayed bone scan clearly shows extensive tumour infiltration, which was confirmed surgically.

Figure 19.1(b) demonstrates a vascular squamous carcinoma of the left buccal mucosa which was demonstrated in the blood flow and blood pool phases. The delayed bone scan shows no bony involvement, indicating that the tumour was confined to the soft tissues.

The pre-operative bone scan may be of greater value to the surgeon than clinical assessment or conventional radiographs to determine whether conservative or radical excision is indicated.

Metastases to the facial bones and the calvarium are not unusual, particularly in carcinoma of the lung, urinary tract and breast. When bone scanning for metastases from primary neoplasms remote from the head and neck, at least three views, anterior and both laterals, are recommended to exclude lesions here.

A special category of primary neoplasms of the head and neck are the lymphomas, which may have local or systemic manifestations. These may be imaged using 3–6 mCi (111–222 MBq) of ^{67}Ga-gallium citrate, which localizes in a variety of neoplastic and inflammatory lesions. Although it is not useful in specific diagnosis of lymphomas, it localizes in almost 90% of untreated patients with malignant lymphoma. (Kashima *et al.*, 1974; Pinsky and Henkin, 1976; Silberstein *et al.*, 1974; Smith *et al.*, 1975; Gould *et al.*, 1978). It is thus useful as a means of staging lymphoma by detecting remote sites of involvement.

Figure 19.2 shows a ^{67}Ga scan of a patient presenting with a right cervical swelling which was lymphoma infiltration in the right parotid gland. This avidly accumulates gallium and moderate uptake is noted in a right axillary node which was barely palpable, but was confirmed to be an additional site of lymphoma.

^{67}Ga scanning has been used in a variety of head and neck malignancies and in post-therapy evaluation (Higashi *et al.*, 1977a). Uptake of ^{67}Ga by other neoplasms has been less reliable than

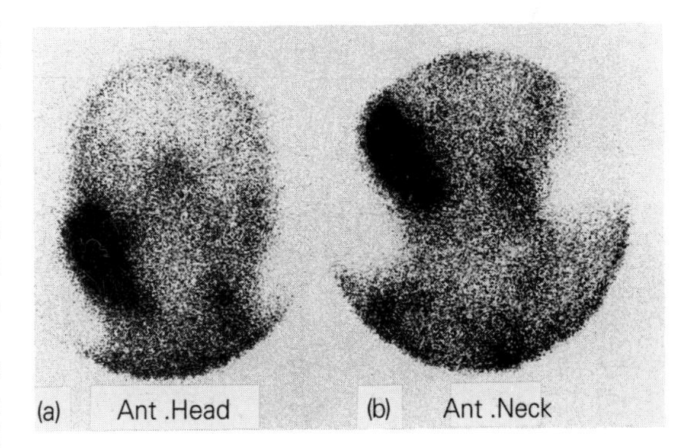

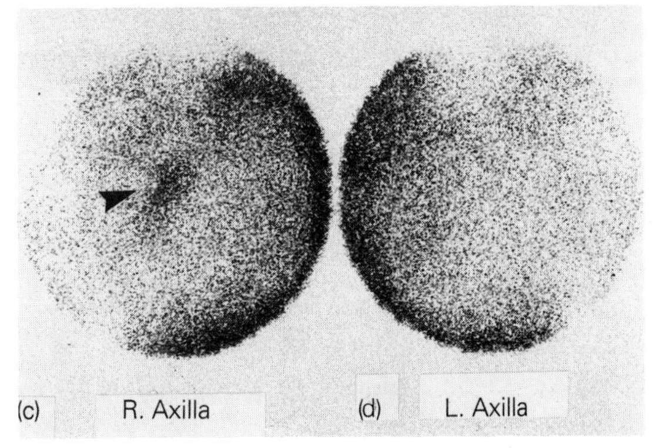

Figure 19.2 ^{67}Ga scanning in lymphoma. The right parotid mass shows intense concentration of gallium due to lymphomatous infiltration. A small right axillary node was considered clinically insignificant prior to the gallium scan which shows radiopharmaceutical accumulation (arrow). This was confirmed to be an additional site of lymphoma. (a) Anterior head; (b) neck; (c) right axilla; (d) left axilla.

lymphoma. Only about 60% of laryngeal primary neoplasms are visualized, as opposed to over 85% of lung and bronchial malignancies. Uptake is capricious, occasionally demonstrating the primary while missing the cervical node metastases, or vice versa. It is thus of limited value in these situations.

19.2.2 INFLAMMATORY LESIONS

Paranasal sinuses are a common site of acute and chronic inflammation. Opacification or local mucosal thickening on the radiographs indicates local pathology, but the extent of bony involvement and biological activity may be less definite (Noyek *et al.*, 1983; Noyek *et al.*, 1984). In the

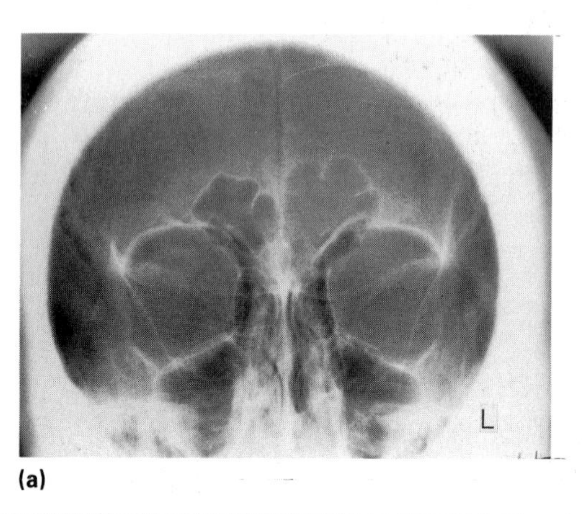

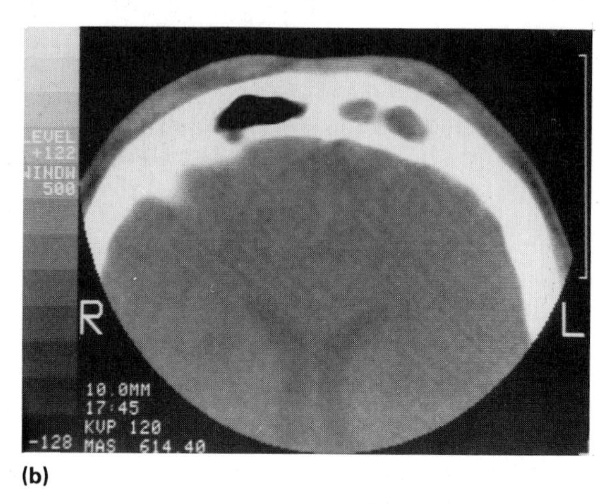

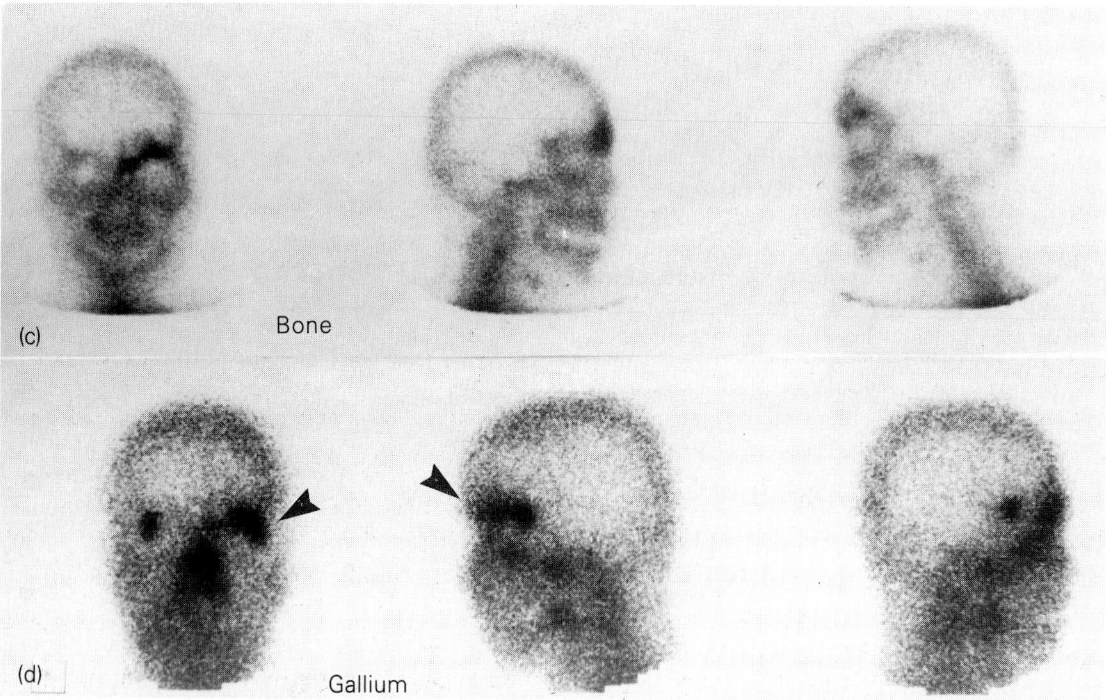

Figure 19.3 Acute frontal sinusitis with osteomyelitis. (a) Plain radiographs of frontal sinuses showing no significant abnormality. (b) CT of frontal sinuses. Left frontal sinus is partly opacified. (c) ^{99m}Tc-labelled MDP bone scan showing intense increased uptake in left frontal sinus area. (d) ^{67}Ga scan shows marked increased uptake in left frontal sinus area (arrow), in addition to the normal lacrimal gland uptake, as seen on right side.

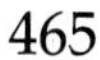

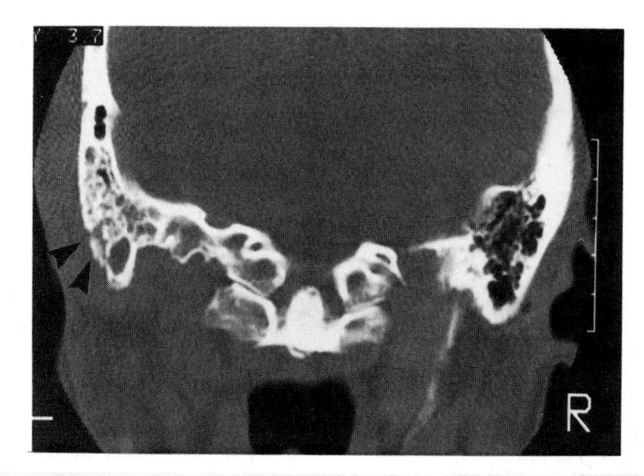

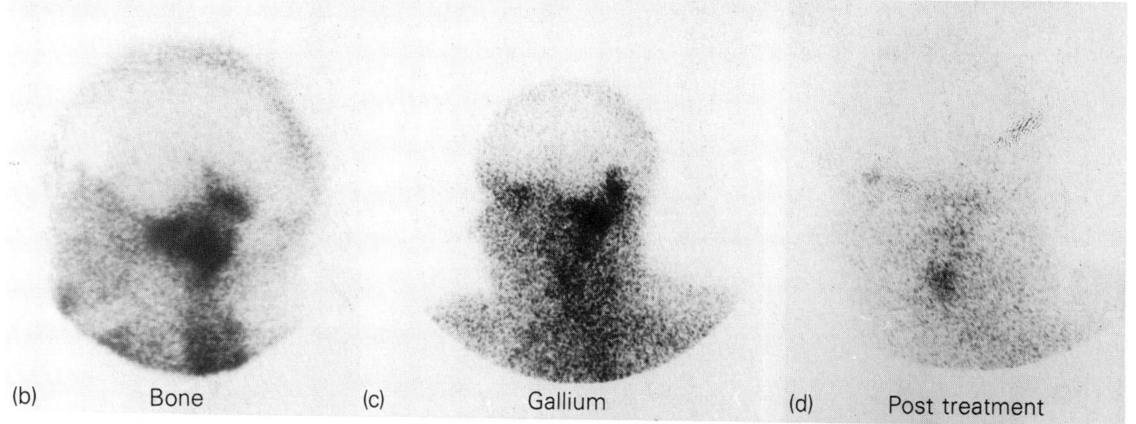

Figure 19.4 Resolving malignant external otitis (*Pseudomonas* infection in diabetic male). (a) CT of mastoid region. Left mastoid is opacified with cortical destruction (arrows) due to active sepsis. (b) ^{99m}Tc-labelled MDP left lateral bone scan showing extensive involvement of left temporal bone. (c) ^{67}Ga scan during active phase shows marked gallium activity in left temporal area. (d) ^{67}Ga scan following six weeks of antibiotic therapy demonstrates resolution of the active sepsis. Both bone scan and CT will remain abnormal for a prolonged period during repair after treatment, and thus cannot be used to evaluate activity of the lesion.

presence of acute osteomyelitis, radiographic changes may not be apparent for 10–14 days.

In acute sinusitis without osteomyelitis, soft-tissue hyperaemia is seen on the flow and blood pool images, while the delayed bone scan may show only slight increased uptake due to increased local blood flow. In chronic sinusitis, less hyperaemia is present, but there may be more uptake on delayed scans due to chronic osteitis with increased osteoblastic activity. A disparity exists in both cases between the soft-tissue hyperaemia and bony involvement, evident when blood pool and delayed scans are compared (Table 19.2).

In the presence of osteomyelitis complicating sinusitis, hyperaemia is evident on the blood flow and blood pool images and the delayed bone scan shows intense uptake. Figure 19.3 shows a patient with left frontal sinusitis and local osteomyelitis, while the radiograph was considered negative and the CT scan showed mild opacification.

^{67}Ga localizes in acute inflammatory processes but the ability to concentrate diminishes as the infection subsides (Figure 19.4). It does not accumulate in chronic osteomyelitis (Lisbona and Rosenthall, 1977) (Figure 19.5). It does, however, outline an active focus within chronic osteomyelitis.

Radiographically, it may be difficult to differentiate between chronic sinusitis and carcinoma because of the increased soft-tissue densities and bone reaction in both of these diseases. ^{67}Ga provides a means of distinguishing these processes by accumulating in the malignant process but not

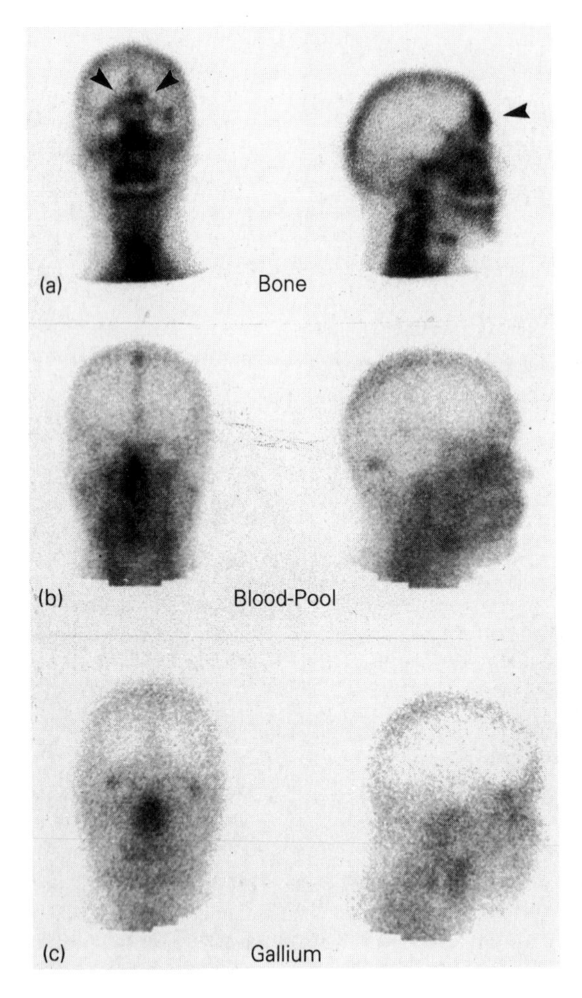

Figure 19.5 Chronic frontal sinusitis without osteomyelitis. (a) Delayed ^{99m}Tc-labelled MDP bone scan of skull shows moderate increased uptake in the frontal sinus area (arrows). (b) Blood pool image shows normal appearance. (c) ^{67}Ga scan shows no abnormal uptake. The chronic inflammatory reaction has produced mild osteoblastic response (osteitis), but absence of hyperaemia and negative gallium scan indicate that this is a quiescent lesion.

in the chronic sinusitis (Higashi *et al.*, 1977; Shafer *et al.*, 1981).

19.2.3 TRAUMA

Following severe facial trauma, some fractures may be obvious radiographically, but more subtle fractures, such as blow-out fractures of the orbit (especially when there is pre-existing sinus disease), medial maxillary antral fractures, fractures of the base of the skull and pterygoid areas may be difficult to demonstrate on a radiograph. Demonstration of a fracture on a radiograph requires that the X-ray beam passes parallel to the fracture line. This is not always possible to accomplish due to difficulties in manoeuvring the traumatized patient, and fractures may be obscured by overlying soft tissue oedema or haemorrhage.

The uptake of the radiopharmaceutical in a fracture occurs early, as the mechanisms of increased blood flow, hyperaemia of repair and osteoblastic activity in the callus of a healing fracture are all factors which encourage intense local uptake. Uptake in the fracture is demonstrated on the scan, regardless of the plane of projection relative to the fracture line, and a positive scan is sufficient evidence of the fracture even when the radiographs are normal (Hisada *et al.*, 1976; Greyson and Noyek, 1978; Noyek, 1979; Noyek *et al.*, 1977, 1983; Roub *et al.*, 1979). Absence of uptake 24–48 h after an injury substantially excludes a fracture, although this has been identified in a patient with very marked osteoporosis whose fracture eventually went on to heal (Noyek, 1979).

Figure 19.6 shows a patient who sustained multiple facial and mandibular fractures. The hyperaemia on the blood pool images shows that the fractures are recent and healing. The delayed scan shows the sites of bone injury including mandibular, zygomaticofrontal and other facial fractures, many of which were not apparent on the initial radiographs.

The delayed bone scan remains positive for a prolonged period throughout healing as well as during the remodelling phase. However, the blood pool image, reflecting hyperaemia of repair, is positive only during the active healing phase and is not apparent during the relatively quiescent remodelling. In delayed union, hyperaemia persists as long as the reparative process is active (Table 19.2). Absence of hyperaemia of repair despite radiographic evidence of the separated fracture line in bones such as the mandible or extremities is a prognosticator of poor healing, usually representing non-union.

Bones of membrane origin, such as the skull, heal very slowly and a fracture line on a radiograph cannot be accurately aged. Recent fractures are hot, but lose their osteoblastic activity when old. The ability to determine the age of a fracture using bone scan may have medico-legal implications.

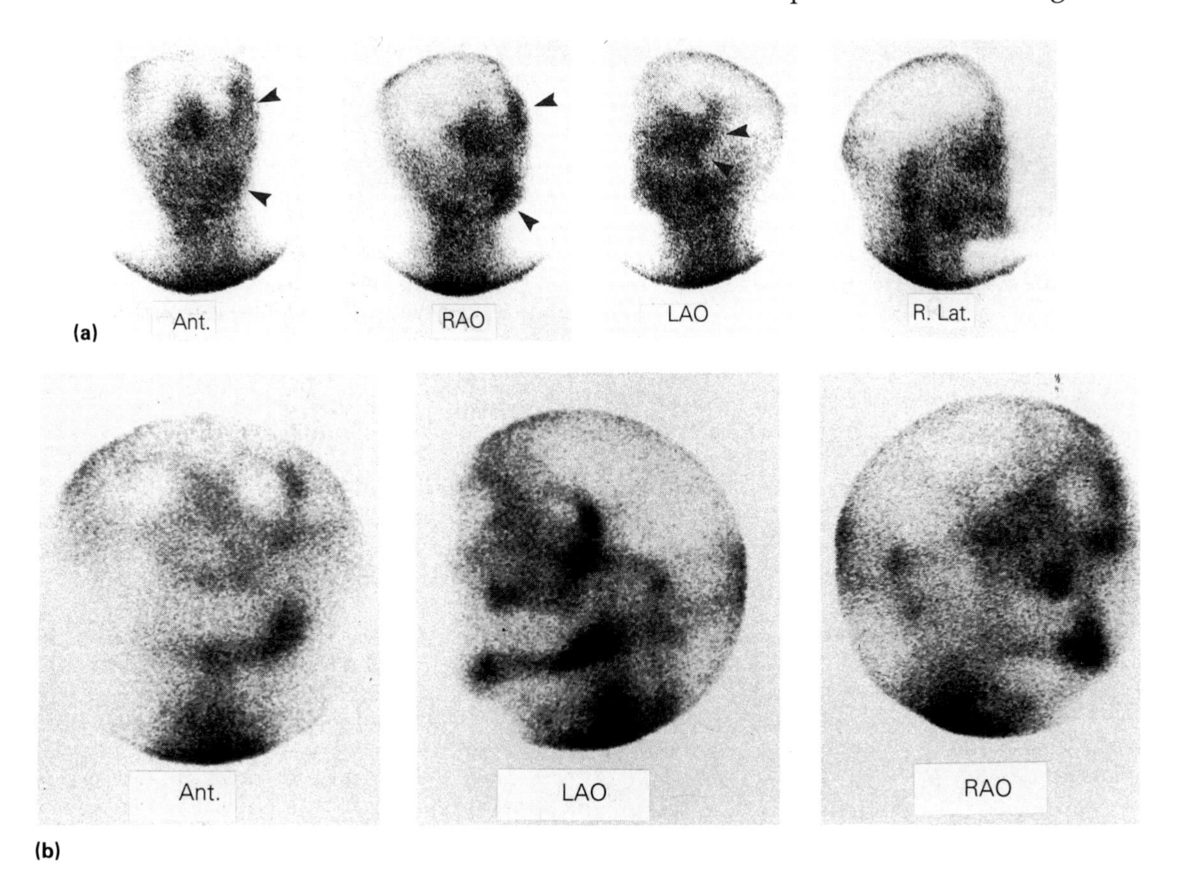

Figure 19.6 Bone scanning in multiple facial fractures. (a) Blood pool images show marked hyperaemia in the area of the zygoma and mandible indicating recent fractures. (b) Delayed bone scan showing uptake in multiple facial fractures indicating a tripod fracture of the zygoma, and fracture of the left mandible. Several of these fractures were not visible on radiographs because of overlying soft tissue swelling, and difficulty in positioning the patient.

19.2.4 TEMPOROMANDIBULAR PAIN

Trismus may be due to local bony factors such as temporomandibular (TM) joint arthritis, fractures, loose bodies or infection, or may be due to non-osseous causes such as muscle spasm, fibrous adhesions or referred pain. Radiographic assessment of TM joints demonstrates bony anatomy and spatial alteration of the joint. Arthrography is invasive, requiring an often painful injection of iodinated contrast. MRI produces high-resolution images which show alterations in the disc itself (Harms and Wilk, 1987), although symptoms may occur with an intact or non-displaced disc. Radionuclide images demonstrate subtle physiological changes occurring in adjacent bones due to local pathology or altered stress on the articular surface, prior to gross morphological changes.

In the normal lateral bone scan of the skull there is some uptake in the floor of the middle cranial fossa and temporal bones, but no focal uptake in the TM joint. The ascending ramus of the mandible is also not usually visualized on a bone scan. Local uptake on the delayed scan indicates bony TM joint disease and is a sensitive indicator of inflammatory or degenerative arthritis. We have been able to detect early degenerative changes due to dental extractions or new dentures, post-facial trauma, and wear and tear changes in the TM joints in patients with bruxism and in gum-chewers. The altered dynamics produce peri-articular bone deposition visible on bone scans in reaction to this stress. This focal uptake is not present in non-articular causes of trismus and directs the clinician away from surgical intervention of the structure of the joint. The sensitivity of detection of internal derangement of TM joints increased from 76% with planar imaging to 94% with SPECT. This is comparable to arthrography (96%), but non-invasive. Conventional radiography show only 4% of surgically proved lesions (Collier *et al.*, 1983).

Figure 19.7 shows uptake in the TM joint of a renal transplant patient complaining of TM pain. This was proved to be avascular necrosis of the head of the mandible, secondary to steroids.

19.2.5 LARYNGEAL LESIONS

Although the larynx is primarily cartilaginous in structure, with age there is progressive calcification and ossification, with occasional marrow production. Ossified laryngeal structures behave like bone and localize bone scanning agents. The mature larynx is commonly seen on a bone scan as a diffuse area of slightly increased uptake in the anterior cervical region.

Focal lesions involving the larynx may show hyperaemia on blood pool images and intense uptake of the bone-seeking radiopharmaceutical on delayed scan. Laryngeal fractures, carcinoma of the larynx and chondritis producing reactive changes may be detected. The hyoid bone, faintly seen normally, shows marked osteoblastic response when fractured or invaded by tumour.

The cricoarytenoid joints are subject to arthritic changes, which like the peripheral arthritides may be demonstrated on scans, although changes are invisible on conventional radiographs. Thus, patients with systemic arthritis such as rheumatoid arthritis or gout, presenting with dysphagia or neck pain, may have focal uptake in the larynx suggestive of arthritic changes in these small laryngeal joints (Greyson and Noyek, 1978; Noyek, 1979).

Lateral views of the larynx are necessary to separate laryngeal structures from the cervical spine, which commonly has increased uptake due to degenerative arthrosis or bony lesions (Oppenheim and Cantez, 1977).

19.2.6 MISCELLANEOUS BONY LESIONS

The facial and skull bones may be involved in a wide variety of non-neoplastic, non-inflammatory lesions which may present difficult differential diagnosis when initially detected on radiograph.

Sclerotic changes such as Paget's disease, fibrous dysplasia and sclerotic reaction due to underlying meningioma may be further assessed by bone scanning. A whole-body survey may reveal areas of unsuspected involvement such as an isolated vertebra, rib or extremity, which may have a more characteristic appearance or be accessible to biopsy.

The addition of a brain scan or CT of the head may be necessary to demonstrate a meningioma as the underlying cause of an osteoblastic lesion in the base of the skull or orbits. Osteomas of sinuses

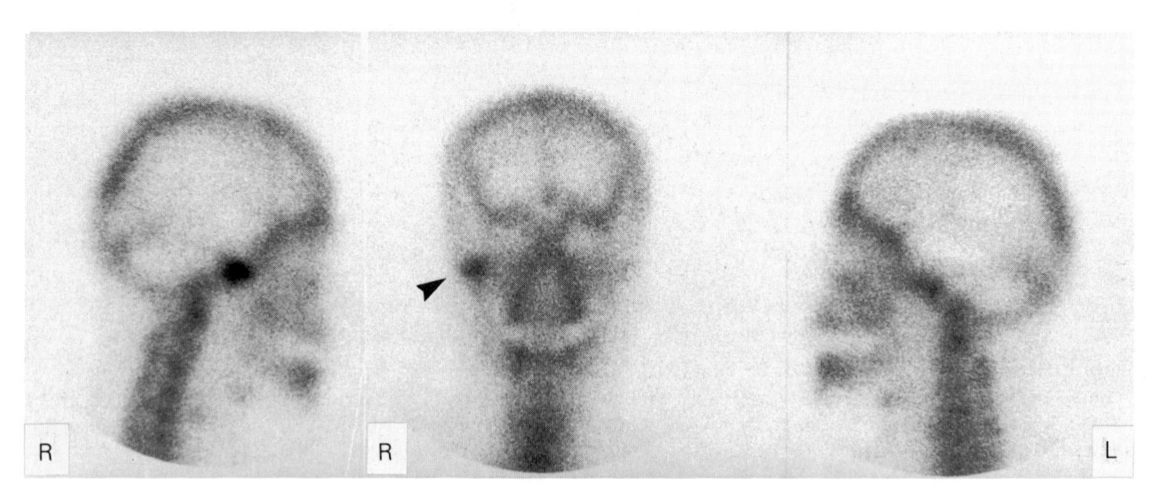

Figure 19.7 TM joint disease. Bone scan in renal transplant patient complaining of acute onset of pain in the right TM joint which persisted, while radiographs were normal. Bone scan shows focal increased uptake in the right TM joint, compared with normal appearing left side. Radiographic changes occurred later. Resected TM head showed avascular necrosis, secondary to steroid therapy.

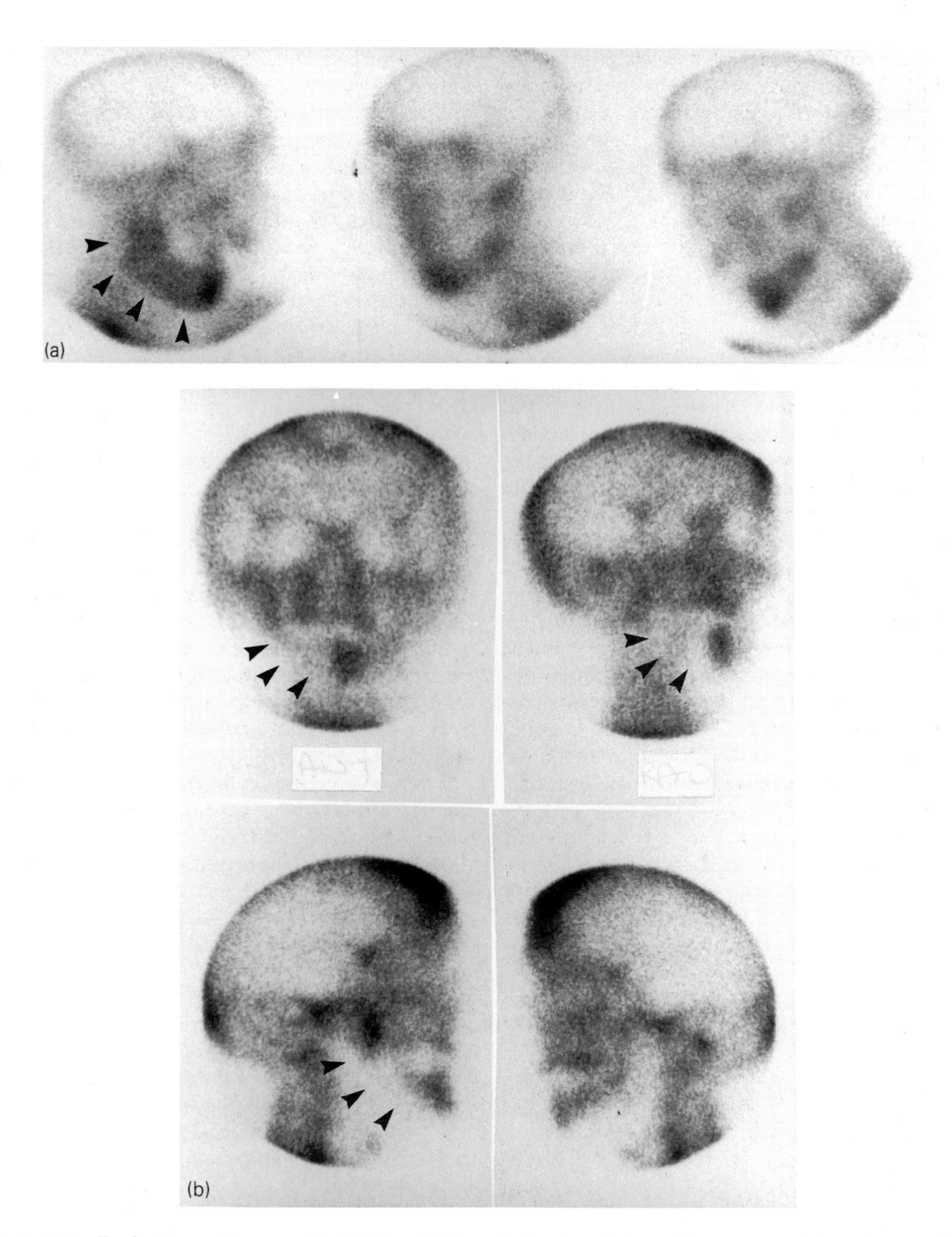

Figure 19.8 Evaluation of bone graft viability. (a) Vascularized graft from iliac crest used in reconstruction of extensive resection of the mandible (arrows) in a patient undergoing a Commando procedure for carcinoma of the mouth. Vascularized grafts show uptake of MDP immediately after surgery. (b) Non-vascularized mandibular graft shows defect on bone scan until it is invaded by neovascularity and osteoblasts.

are generally quiescent, but occasionally they become active and involve adjacent bony structures, a feature easily recognized on bone scans. Lytic lesions may be due to eosinophilic granuloma or multiple myeloma which may have systemic manifestations, necessitating a whole-body survey to establish the extent of involvement. Post-operative assessment following osteotomies, dental extractions, etc. may show complications of non-union or osteomyelitis.

Of particular recent interest is the ability of the bone scan to detect the viability of bone grafts. Non-vascularized ('free') grafts are initially cold on bone scan but eventually become incorporated into the body by 'creeping substitution' of neovascularity and osteoblasts. In this later stage, the graft becomes hot on a bone scan, and is an indication of a successful graft.

Vascularized grafts which are transplanted along with soft tissue and vessels anastomosed by microvascular surgical techniques should continue to function as viable bone showing normal or slightly increased uptake, particularly at the osteotomy ends, in the early post-operative period (Noyek, 1979). This technique is of particular value in assessing successful bone grafts in patients undergoing radical excision of the mandible (Commando procedure) (Figure 19.8).

19.3 SALIVARY GLAND DISEASE

The conventional imaging method of salivary glands is by contrast sialography, which requires cannulation of one or more of the salivary ducts and injection of radioiodinated contrast material into the duct system with retrograde filling of the canaliculi and demonstration of the acinar pattern within the glands.

Contrast sialography is not without difficulty, often requiring dilatation or incision of the duct orifice. This may be uncomfortable for the patient during and after the procedure. There is a frequent post-procedure inflammatory response secondary to the contrast material. CT, ultrasound and MRI demonstrate the soft tissue structure of the salivary glands. These give an anatomical, but not a functional assessment of the gland.

Salivary gland scanning using ^{99m}Tc-pertechnetate provides physiological images of the salivary gland, providing assessment of function and drainage (Schall and DiChiro, 1972; Greyson and Noyek, 1978; Greyson and Noyek, 1982; Lunia *et al.*, 1978; Ohrt and Shafer, 1982; Blue and Jackson, 1985).

Metabolism of pertechnetate is analogous to iodide. It is trapped but not organified in the thyroid gland, and is secreted in saliva, breast milk, gastric epithelium and excreted by the kidneys. Iodide is secreted by the ductal epithelium of the salivary glands and this is also the secretory site of pertechnetate.

The patient is placed in the Water's position under the gamma camera and following an intravenous injection of 15 mCi (555 MBq) of ^{99m}Tc-pertechnetate rapid sequential images are obtained to show the blood flow to the salivary glands. Serial images every 3 min show progressive concentration of activity within the gland and accumulation in the mouth. The thyroid gland is included in the field of view and the intensity of activity of the salivary and thyroid glands are normally approximately equal. After 20 min the patient is given some lemon or sour candy. This causes prompt salivation with drainage of the glands when the salivary ducts are patent. This provocative test is useful in demonstrating obstruction of ducts, when intermittent pain or gland swelling occurs, whether radiographs show opaque calculi or not.

Relative blood flow as well as excretory function of each salivary gland can be easily assessed either visually or with a computer. A mass lesion may be characterized as being either vascular or non-vascular, and functioning or non-functioning. Functioning salivary gland tumours tend to be those with large numbers of oncocytes, such as Warthin's tumour, oncocytomas and oxyphilic adenomas. These are consistently benign.

Depending on the proportions of cell types, mixed tumours are commonly cool or cold on the scan. Malignant neoplasms are generally vascular but non-functioning on the salivary gland scan, as are lymphomas and abscesses. Simple cysts are non-vascular and non-functioning on the scan.

Overall salivary gland function is useful in assessing xerostomia, particularly due to Sjogren's syndrome as a complication of rheumatoid arthritis. Figure 19.9 and Table 19.3 summarize a variety of salivary gland scan findings.

^{67}Ga localizes faintly in normal salivary glands, probably because of their lactoferrin content. Focal increased accumulation could represent a primary or secondary malignant neoplasm or septic focus. Diffuse increased uptake occurs in asep-

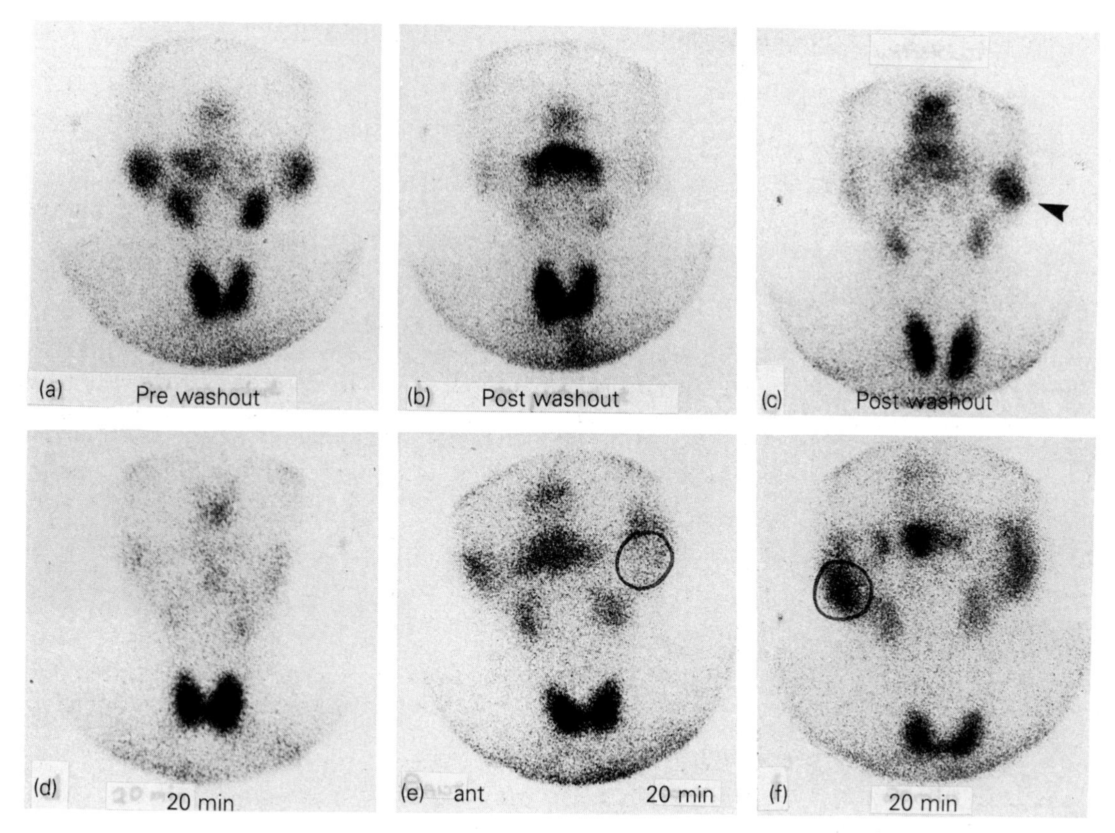

Figure 19.9 Patterns of salivary gland imaging. (a) Normal (20 min pre-washout). Note approximately uniform uptake in parotid, submandibular and thyroid glands. Some activity in the mouth. (b) Washout images (20 min post-washout) following lemon. Salivary glands have drained uniformly and activity is now in the oral cavity. (c) Washout image in patient with intermittent left parotid swelling. No stone demonstrated. Obstruction due to stricture of the duct. (d) Sjogren's syndrome (20 min). Very poor concentration seen in all salivary glands. (e) Benign mixed tumour of the left parotid gland (anterior view, 20 min). A mass (outlined) does not accumulate pertechnetate. (f) Warthin's tumour (20 min). The right parotid mass (outlined) concentrates pertechnetate. This is characteristic of Warthin's tumour and the rare oncocytomas.

tic inflammatory diseases, such as sarcoidosis or Mickulicz's syndrome (Greyson and Noyek, 1982; Singer *et al.*, 1984). Salivary symptoms in sarcoidosis may be mild and overlooked with the systemic or pulmonary manifestations. We routinely perform serial whole-body gallium imaging in sarcoidosis to evaluate the effect of therapy, or progression of disease (Lubat and Kramer, 1985) (Figure 19.10).

19.4 LACRIMAL DRAINAGE SCANNING

Tumours, trauma and inflammatory conditions of the paranasal sinuses may produce obstruction to tear duct drainage with clinical symptoms of excessive tearing.

The conventional imaging modality, contrast dacrocystography, involves intubation of the canaliculi and manual injection of contrast to fill the tear ducts. Where there is gross distortion of anatomy or infection, manipulation may be difficult or contraindicated. Similarly, the pressure injection is not physiological and may not reflect a true functional state of the 'tear pump mechanism'.

Following the instillation of a tiny drop of ^{99m}Tc-pertechnetate on to the inferior recess, the material spreads over the globe of the eye by capillary action, labelling the tears and outlining the drainage pathways. Sequential images using a gamma camera fitted with a pin-hole collimator (preferably 1 mm aperture) produces high-

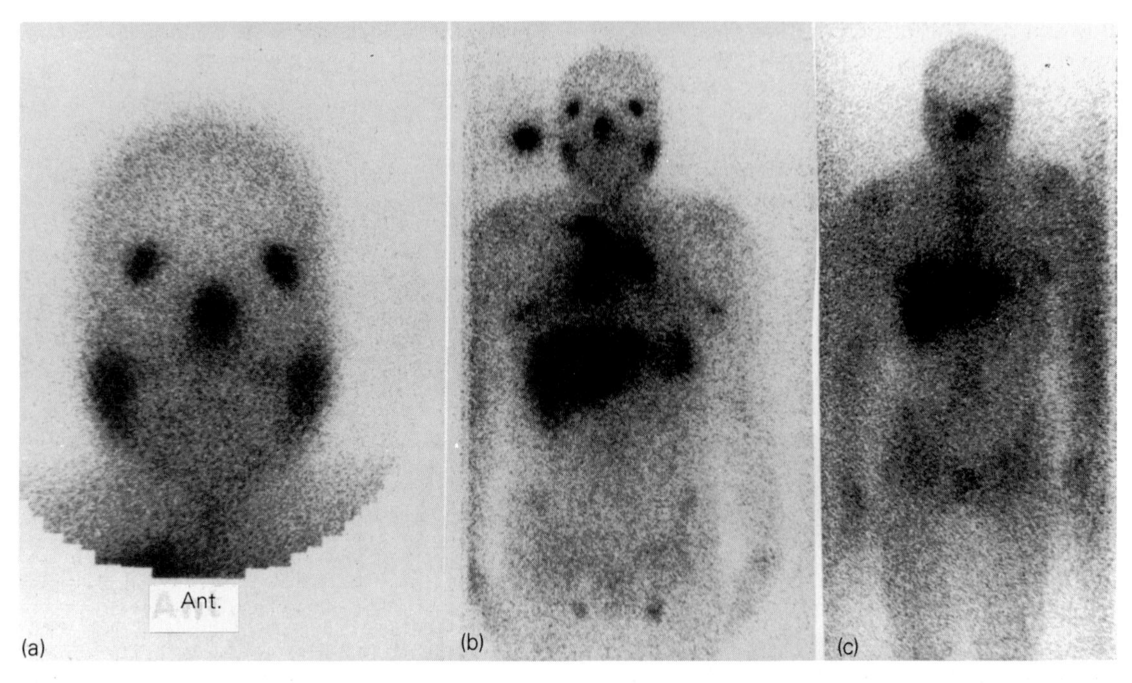

Figure 19.10 Gallium scanning in sarcoidosis. (a) Intense increased uptake in lacrimal and salivary glands indicating uveoparotitis commonly seen in sarcoidosis. (b) The whole-body image of the same patient also demonstrates marked bilateral perihilar, peritracheal, supraclavicular and inguinal adenopathy, with breast and spleen uptake indicating multifocal inflammatory reaction. (c) Same patient four months later, following spontaneous remission of the disease, now shows normal gallium distribution throughout the body.

Table 19.3 Salivary scan findings

	Flow	*Function*	*Washout*
Sjogren's syndrome	↓	↓	↓
Obstruction	↓	± ↓	↑
Warthin's tumour	↑	↑	↑
Benign mixed tumour	± ↑	↓	↓
Malignant tumour	↑	↓	↓
Cyst	↓	↓	↓
Acute inflammation	↑	↓	↑

Arrow direction depicts activity compared with normal.

resolution images of the canaliculi, nasolacrimal sac and duct. Normally, drainage into the nose is seen within the first minute. Delayed drainage is easily recognized with stasis often persisting for longer than 20 min, and the level of obstruction may be characterized as being proximal or distal to the nasolacrimal sac (Carlton *et al.*, 1973; Greyson and Noyek, 1978; Denffer, *et al.*, 1984). As this procedure is atraumatic and rapid, pre- and post-operative assessment may be readily obtained.

19.5 HEARING DISORDERS

Acoustic neuromas (8th nerve neuroma) may be detected on a radionuclide brain scan, particularly when specific attention is paid to the posterior fossa and converging collimator posterior and oblique views are obtained. More than 75% of lesions may be detected; however, these are often very small when symptomatic, and when less than 2 cm in diameter, lying close to the base of the skull, they may be difficult to detect on a planar brain scan.

Tomographic brain imaging (SPECT) improves detection of lesions in this area, but (CT) or MRI are superior techniques for posterior fossa lesions.

Meningiomas at the base of the skull, in the region of the temporal bone, may produce auditory symptoms. Sphenoid wing meningiomas may produce sclerotic reaction in the orbit and combined brain and bone scans are useful to detect the intracranial component.

Arteriovenous malformations in the temporal bone may be a cause of pulsatile tinnitus. Arteriovenous malformations are easily detected on the flow study phase of the brain scan by the early arterial blush, fading on the delayed scan. These may be contrasted with temporal lobe primary and secondary tumours, and cerebral infarction involving the auditory pathways, which are commonly best seen on the delayed brain scan.

Paget's disease of the temporal bone, easily detected on a bone scan, may produce auditory symptoms because of nerve compression. Pulsatile tinnitus may be noted if there is a high blood flow in this region.

REFERENCES

Alexander, J. M. (1976) Radionuclide bone scanning in diagnosis of lesions of the maxillofacial region. *J. Oral Surg.*, **34**, 249–56.

Bergstedt, H. F. and Lind, M. G. (1981) Facial bone scintigraphy: VIII. Diagnosis of malignant lesions in maxillary, ethmoidal and palatal bones. *Acta Radiol. (Diag.)*, **22**, 609–18.

Blue, P. W. and Jackson, L. (1985) Stimulated salivary clearance of technetium-99m pertechnetate. *J. Nucl. Med.*, **26**, 308–11.

Brown, M. L., Keyes, J. W., Leonard, P. F. *et al.* (1977) Facial bone scanning by emission tomography. *J. Nucl. Med.*, **18**, 1184–8.

Carlton, W. H., Trueblood, J. H. and Rossomondo, R. M. (1973) Clinical evaluation of microscintigraphy of the lacrimal drainage apparatus. *J. Nucl. Med.*, **14**, 89–92.

Cawthorn, M. A., Hartshorne, M. F. and Bauman, J. M. (1986) SPECT confidence building: subtle skull bone lesions made conspicuous. *Clin. Nucl. Med.*, **11**, 805–6.

Collier, B. D., Carrera, G. F., Messer, E. J. *et al.* (1983) Internal derangement of the temporomandibular joint: detection by single-photon emission computed tomography. *Radiology*, **149**, 557–61.

Denffer, H. V., Dressler, J. and Pabst, H. W. (1984) Lacrimal dacryoscintigraphy. *Semin. Nucl. Med.*, **14**, 8–15.

Gates, G. F. and Goris, M. L. (1976) Maxillary-facial abnormalities assessed by bone imaging. *Radiology*, **121**, 677–82.

Gould, A. A., Hubner, K. F. and Greenlaw, R. H. (1978) Ga-67 citrate imaging in malignant lymphoma: final report of cooperative group. *J. Nucl. Med.*, **19**, 1013–19.

Greyson, N. D. and Noyek, A. M. (1978) Nuclear medicine in otolaryngological diagnosis. *Otolaryngol. Clin. North Am.*, **11**, 541–60.

Greyson, N. D. and Noyek, A. M. (1982) Radionuclide salivary scanning. *J. Otolaryngol.*, **11** (Suppl. 10), 1–47.

Higashi, T., Aoyama, W., Mori, Y. *et al.* (1977a) Gallium-67 scanning in the differentiation of maxillary sinus carcinoma from chronic maxillary sinusitis. *Radiology*, **123**, 117–22.

Higashi, T., Kashima, D., Shimura, K. *et al.* (1977b) Gallium-67 scanning in evaluation of therapy of malignant tumours of the head and neck. *J. Nucl. Med.*, **18**, 243–9.

Hisada, K., Suzuki, Y. and Iimori, M. (1976) Technetium-99m pyrophosphate bone imaging in the evaluation of trauma. *Clin. Nucl. Med.*, **1**, 18–24.

Harris, S. E. and Wilk, R. M. (1987) Magnetic resonance imaging of the temporomandibular joint. *Radiographics*, **7**, 521–41.

Jones, B. E. and Patton, D. D. (1976) Bone scans of facial bones: normal anatomy. *Am. J. Surg.*, **132**, 341–5.

Kashima, H. K., McKusick, K. A., Malmuk, L. S. *et al.* (1974) Gallium-67 citrate scanning in patients with head and neck cancer. *Laryngoscope*, **84**, 1078–89.

Lisbona, R. and Rosenthall, L. (1972) Observations on the sequential use of ^{99m}Tc-phosphate complex and ^{67}Ga imaging in osteomyelitis, cellulitis and septic arthritis. *Radiology*, **123**, 123–8.

Lubat, E. and Kramer, E. C. (1985) Gallium-67 citrate accumulation in parotid and submandibular glands in sarcoidosis. *Clin. Nucl. Med.*, **10**, 593.

Lunia, S., Chodos, R. B., Lynia, C. *et al.* (1978) Oxyphilic adenoma of the parotid gland. *Radiology*, **128**, 690.

Mancuso, A. A. and Hanafee, W. N. (1985) *Computed Tomography and Magnetic Resonance Imaging of the Head and Neck.* Wiliams and Wilkins, Baltimore.

Mandelblatt, S. M., Braun, I. F., Davis, P. C. *et al.* (1987) Parotid masses: MR imaging. *Radiology*, **163**, 441–4.

Matteson, S. R., Staab, E. V. and Fine, J. T. (1980) Bone scan appearance of benign oral pathologic conditions. *J. Oral Surg.*, **38**, 759–63.

Nobuharu, Y. (1986) Single photon emission computed tomography in the diagnosis of skull base invasion of nasopharyngeal carcinoma. *J. Nucl. Med.*, **23**, 367–73.

Noyek, A. M. (1979) Bone scanning in otolaryngology. *Laryngoscope*, **89**, (Suppl. 18), 1–87.

Noyek, A. M., Dolan, D., Zizmor, J. *et al.* (1983) The thick walled usually opacified maxillary sinus: conventional CT radionuclide ultrasound correlative studies. *Rev. Laryngol.*, **104**, 255–261.

Noyek, A. M., Holgat, R. C., Wortzman, G. *et al.* (1977), Sophisticated radiology in otolaryngology. *J. Otolaryngol.*, **6** (Suppl. 3), 73–117.

Noyek, A. M., Kassel, E. E., Wortzman, G. *et al.* (1983) Contemporary radiologic evaluation in maxillary facial trauma. *Otolaryngol. Clin North A.*, **16**, 473–508.

Noyek, A. M., Kirsh, J. C., Greyson, N. D. *et al.* (1984) The clinical significance of radionuclide bone and gallium scanning in osteomyelitis of the head and neck. *Laryngoscope*, **94** (Suppl. 34), 1–21.

O'Mara, R. E. (1985) Role of bone scanning in dental and maxillofacial disorders. *Nucl. Med. Ann.*, **1985**, 265–84.

Oppenheim, B. E. and Cantez, S. (1977) What causes lower neck uptake in bone scans? *Radiology*, **124**, 749–52.

Ohrt, H. J. and Shafer, R. B. (1982) An atlas of salivary gland disorders. *Clin. Nucl. Med.*, **8**, 370–6.

Pinsky, S. M. and Henkin, R. E. (1976) Gallium-67 tumour scanning. *Semin. Nucl. Med.*, **6**, 397–409.

Roub, L. W., Gumerman, L. W., Hanley, E. N. *et al.* (1979) Bone stress: a radionuclide imaging perspective. *Radiology*, **132**, 431–8.

Schall, G. L. and DiChiro, G. (1972) Clinical usefulness

of salivary gland scanning. *Semin. Nucl. Med.*, **2**, 270–7.

Shafer, R. B., Marlette, J. M., Browne, G. A. *et al.* (1981) The role of ^{99m}Tc-phosphate complexes and ^{67}Ga in the diagnosis and management of maxillofacial disease. *J. Nucl. Med.*, **22**, 8–11.

Silberstein, E. B., Kornblut, A., Shumrick, D. A. *et al.* (1974) Gallium-67 as a diagnostic agent for detection of head and neck tumours. *Radiology*, **110**, 605–8.

Singer, I., McLaughlin, A. and Morris, J. (1984) Appearance of Ga-67 citrate scanning in a patient with Mikulicz's syndrome associated with non-Hodgkin's lymphoma: a case report. *Clin. Nucl. Med.*, **9**, 283–5.

Smith, N. J., Teates, C. D., El-Mahdi, A. M. *et al.* (1975) The value of gallium-67 scanning in the evaluation of head and neck malignancies. *Laryngoscope*, **85**, 778.

Teresi, L. M., Lufkin, R. B., Worthham, D. G. *et al.* (1987) Parotid masses: MR imaging. *Radiology*, **163**, 405–9.

Tow, D. E., Garcia, D. A. and Jansons, D. *et al.* (1978) Bone scan in dental diseases. *J. Nucl. Med.*, **19**, 845–7.

CHAPTER TWENTY

Radioimmunoscintigraphy

K. E. Britton, M. Granowska and P. S. Shepherd

20.1 INTRODUCTION

Nuclear medicine techniques are known for their sensitivity to changes of function induced by disease but not for their specificity in determining the nature of the disease process. To address this problem, nuclear medicine has developed new procedures for tissue characterization additional to functional measurements, through the use of receptor binding techniques and antigen–antibody interactions. The technique of using radiolabelled antibodies to image and characterize the nature of disease process *in vivo* is called radioimmunoscintigraphy (RIS). It is applicable, in principle, to any type of pathology: benign, as in the identification of myocardial infarction by radiolabelled antimyosin, or malignant.

Cancerous tissue differs from normal tissue in a number of subtle ways which enables it to invade surrounding tissues. This ability appears to be determined mainly by the surface properties of the cancer cell and differences have been found in the biochemistry, the receptor characteristics and the antigenic determinants of the cancer cell surface in comparison with the equivalent population of normal cells. Thus the modern approach to the detection of cancer attempts to exploit these features and to demonstrate the presence of a cancer not by relying on its physical attributes, size, shape, position, space occupation, density, water content or reflectivity, etc., as for conventional radiology, X-ray computed tomography (CT), nuclear magnetic resonance (NMR) or ultrasound (US), but through the essential and specific cancerousness of a cancer. The special biochemistry is being demonstrated through the enhanced uptake of glucose as ^{18}F-labelled desoxyglucose, amino acids such as ^{11}C-methionine and such compounds as ^{57}Co-labelled bleomycin, ^{201}Tl and ^{99m}Tc-labelled hexamethylpropyleneamineoxime (HMPAO). The use of a *meta*-iodobenzylguanidine to detect and treat neuroblastoma takes advantage of the altered receptor characteristics of the tissue. This chapter is concerned with techniques designed to take advantage of the different antigenic determinants of cancerous from normal tissue in order to demonstrate the tumour, its recurrence and its metastases.

Previous nuclear medicine approaches to imaging cancer have relied on non-specific alterations in function or metabolism of surrounding tissue such as the osteoblastic response of bone, the loss of liver Kupffer cells or the alteration of the blood–brain barrier; or else upon non-specific uptake by cancer tissue as well as other inflammatory conditions as occurs with ^{67}Ga-gallium citrate. RIS is still a long way from achieving the goal of specific cancer detection but the signposts along the way are becoming more clearly discerned.

Four factors are required for RIS: an antibody capable of detecting the cancer; a radiolabel to give the best signal; a radiolabelling method with appropriate quality control to give a reagent suitable for human use while maintaining the full immunoreactivity of the antibody; and an imaging system appropriate to the radionuclide and the region under study.

The selective localization of cancer tissue by radiolabelled antibodies carries with it the hope of selective therapy, and explains much of the motivation behind the development of radioimmunoscintigraphy. However, there are two additional requirements for radioimmunotherapy (RIT): the ratio of uptake of radiolabel by the target cancer compared to that in the most critical non-target organ should be a value of at least 10 : 1; and estimates of the absorbed radiation dose delivered to the tumour, to the critical non-target organ, to the bone marrow, and to the whole body for which a reasonable maximum would be 2 Gy (200 rad), poses severe limitations on current techniques.

20.2 THE ANTIGEN

The key to RIS is the discovery of an antigen that is specific to the disease process under study. Three decades of saturation analysis techniques using antigen–antibody binding characteristics to measure hormones and other biological substances *in vitro* have shown the feasibility and specificity of this approach when the appropriate antigen, or ligand, is identified and purified, and an avid and specific antibody is raised against it. The part of an antigen with which an antibody reacts is called an epitope or antigenic determinant.

It is the lack of the specificity of the antigen to the disease process that is the first problem for RIS. Thus myosin is released by the destruction of cardiac tissue from any cause, e.g. myocarditis, cardiac transplant rejection, and so RIS with antimyosin can never be specific for myocardial infarction. However, an antibody, for example, against parathormone, or against hormone receptor sites, might be more selective in identifying parathyroid tissue or the appropriate endocrine receptor sites on the end organ tissues.

The development of the oncogene–antioncogene theory of cancer has raised hopes for the demonstration of cancer-specific oncoproteins. The discovery that specific genes are involved in the regulation of growth led to the concept that the uncontrolled growth of cancer cells is due to aberrant expression of these genes – oncogenes – and that these may be the final common pathway for genetic damage, virus and carcinogenic induction of cancer. Such transforming genes have been demonstrated. Since genes are made up of specific DNA sequences, then RNA sequences equivalent to them and thence amino acid sequences equivalent to these can be produced, thus cancer-related oncoproteins are derived and give the hope that cancer-specific antigens will be discovered, leading in turn to cancer-specific antibodies. Work in this direction has been undertaken in lung cancer (Chan and Sikora 1987), where a monoclonal antibody against the oncoprotein equivalent to the c-myc oncogene has been raised and used for RIS.

The expression of antigen by the cell is a dynamic process. Clearly it needs to be on the surface accessible to antibody, and the higher its density the greater the amount of antibody likely to be bound. The possibility of binding is given by the binding constant of the reaction between antigen and antibody. Current antibodies have values of K_B 10^{-9} to 10^{-10} l mol^{-1}. Density of antigen can be increased by certain circumstances, e.g. exposure to γ-interferon. Nuclear antigens would require the internalization of the antibody by endocytosis, a less probable interaction. Modulation of antigen means that the degree of antigen expression changes with time and antigen can be reduced after exposure to a specific antibody. Such an event can lead to internalization and metabolism of the labelled antibody with either loss of the label or its fixation in the cell. Important for detection, and crucial to radioimmunotherapy, is the requirement that the antigen expression is not heterogeneous. Ideally, all the cancer cells should express the antigen. In practice this is rare, and more usually clumps of cells are antigen positive and others antigen negative. Some cancers do not express a particular antigen at all. Thus antibodies against placental alkaline phosphate (PLAP) are excellent for RIS of ovarian cancer, but only 70% of ovarian adenocarcinoma express this antigen.

Current tumour-associated antigens are chosen in different ways. The de-differentiation antigens are widely used, such as carcinoembryonic antigen (CEA), human choriogonadotrophin (HCG) and α-fetoprotein (AFP). These are expressed in greater numbers in malignant cells than in normal tissues. They are secreted from such cells and are easily detectable in blood and body fluids. Surprisingly, injected antibody is not inactivated by, for example, circulating CEA and immune complex formation does not appear to be a problem. However, these cancer antigens are not specific, e.g. CEA occurs in lung and gastric cancer as well as colorectal. They can be increased in non-malignant disease, e.g. Crohn's disease, and are present in the related normal tissues – colonic mucosa. Virus-related antigens may be used, e.g. anti-hepatitis antibody for liver cancer. Idiotypic antigen may be used for the leukaemias and lymphomas. An alternative approach is to use normal epithelial tissue antigens lining ducts which by their situation are not normally exposed to blood. Human milk fat globule (HMFG) is a glycoprotein found in the lining epithelium of the lactiferous ducts of the breast, the internal lining of an ovarian follicle and in the crypts of the colon. The architectural disruption by the malignant process exposes these antigens in increased density directly to the bloodstream and antibodies against these, such as HMFG1 and HMFG2, are used for RIS. The preferred antigen is membrane fixed and specific to the cancer. The nearest conventional antigen to this ideal is the high-molecular-weight melanoma antigen against which an antibody called 225.28S is widely used in Europe for RIS both for cutaneous and for ocular melanoma. P-97 and 96.5 monoclonal antibodies are also relatively specific for cutaneous melanoma. A membrane-stable antigen called TAG72 against which an antibody B72.3 has been made is proving useful for RIS in colorectal, ovarian and breast cancer. The list is growing rapidly and over 20 different malignancies are under intensive study using RIS.

20.3 THE ANTIBODY

Antibodies are bifunctional molecules. One part of the molecule is highly variable in terms of its structure (variable region) and is associated with binding to antigen, while the second part varies little between different classes of antibodies (constant region). Biological functions of antibodies such as complement activation and binding to cell surface receptors are controlled by their C regions. The basic structure of an IgG antibody molecule contains four polypeptide chains – two heavy and two light chains – held together by a variable number of disulphide bonds (see Figure 20.1). It can be cleaved into smaller fragments that retain their ability to bind antigen by the two enzymes pepsin and papain. These fragments have markedly different imaging properties when radiolabelled and compared to the whole antibody molecule because they are smaller and have lost their biological Fc regions.

The specificity and accuracy of RIS depends on the production, in a form acceptable to human use, of a pure antibody against the selected anti-

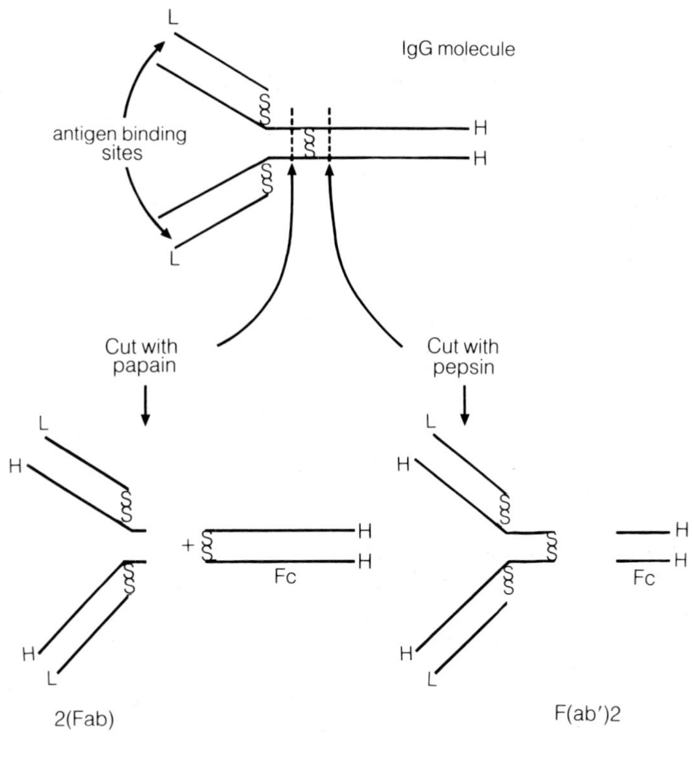

Figure 20.1 Structure of the IgG molecule.

gen. This has been made possible through the development of monoclonal antibody technology.

20.3.1 WHAT IS A MONOCLONAL ANTIBODY?

A monoclonal antibody is a secreted product of a single B-lymphocyte clone. Since each B-lymphocyte and its descendants are genetically destined to make a single antigen combining site (idiotype), all the antibody molecules produced by a B-cell clone are homogeneous in terms of their structure and antigen-binding specificity. In pathological terms a malignant transformation of a single B-lymphocyte may give rise to a plasma cell tumour known as a myeloma or plasmacytoma that produces a homogeneous antibody product or myeloma protein. Tumours of this type produce monoclonal gammopathies that can be diagnosed serologically by detecting them as sharp narrow bands on serum electrophoretic scans. In the past these monoclonal antibodies have been invaluable in elucidating the structure of antibodies (Figure 20.1) but of little use practically. However, in 1975, Kohler and Milstein in Cambridge devised a way of making monoclonal antibodies in the laboratory by the technique of somatic cell hybridization (Kohler and Milstein, 1975). This involved the fusion of B-lymphocytes with a myeloma cell line adapted for growth *in vitro* to make hybrid cells known as hybridomas. Essentially these hybridomas retain the two important functions of their parental cells, namely the ability to produce specific antibodies and to grow indefinitely in tissue culture. To make a hybridoma secrete a single antibody specificity, a non-antibody-secreting myeloma mutant is used as one of the fusion partners. This avoids the possibility of two different antibody specificities being secreted, which would occur if both parents synthesized antibody, as well as mixed hybrid antibody molecules made up of heavy and light chains from each of the parents.

20.3.2 HOW DOES A MONOCLONAL DIFFER FROM A POLYCLONAL ANTIBODY?

In a normal antibody response to a foreign antigen a large number of B-lymphocytes are activated to secrete specific antibodies that bind to antigenic determinants (small chemical groupings, or haptens) expressed on the surface of the antigen. Added together these antibodies constitute a polyclonal antibody response to a given antigen and they will have a range of antibody affinities. The term antibody affinity refers to the summation of the attractive and repulsive forces existing between a single antibody combining site and its antigenic determinant. Each time a polyclonal antiserum is made to a given antigen it will contain a different mix of antibody affinities which collectively give a mean value or avidity for their binding to the antigen. This means polyclonal antisera are difficult to standardize from one batch to another. Also these antisera will contain only a small proportion (±1%) of their total IgG antibody as antigen-specific antibody, and so further purification steps are required to remove the 99% non-specific IgG before they can be radiolabelled and used as imaging agents. This can be done if a supply of purified antigen is available, and this is not often the case, by coupling it to an insoluble support matrix and using this to absorb out the specific antibodies from the antisera. These specific antibodies are then eluted off the antigen with low-pH and high-salt buffers, a procedure that can be very damaging to them. Most of these problems can be avoided by using monoclonal antibodies. Unlike polyclonal antibodies, monoclonal antibodies bind to antigen with one specificity and one affinity and can be produced in large amounts in the laboratory under standard conditions. All these factors make them ideal standard reagents for a wide range of biological and clinical applications. A list of advantages and disadvantages of monoclonal antibodies over polyclonal antisera is presented in Table 20.1.

20.3.3 HOW ARE MONOCLONAL ANTIBODIES MADE?

The preparation of hybridoma cell lines secreting specific monoclonal antibodies is now approaching a routine laboratory procedure. An outline of the technique is given in Figure 20.2.

20.4 PREPARATION OF MONOCLONAL ANTIBODIES

There are three essential requirements for the production of monoclonal antibodies: (1) a source of antigen-stimulated B-lymphoblasts from an appropriately immunized animal, usually a spleen cell preparation; (2) a non-immunoglobulin-secreting myeloma cell line; and (3) a way of isolating hybridomas from unfused

Table 20.1 Advantages and disadvantages of monoclonal antibodies compared with polyclonal antibodies

	Type of antibody	
	Monoclonal	*Polyclonal*
Advantages		
Specificity and affinity	Constant	Variable
Standardization as a reagent	Good	Difficult
Amount of specific antibody produced	Unlimited	Variable
Preparation of internally labelled antibody	Yes	No
Stability of IgG fragments e.g. Fab, F(ab′)$_2$	Depends on Ig subclass	Variable
Potential for biotechnological alteration, e.g. changes to constant-region genes	Good	None
Disadvantages		
Removal of non-specific cross-reactions by absorption	No	Possible
Antigen binding affinity/avidity	Usually low (10^5–10^8 l m^{-1})	High (10^8–10^{12} l m^{-1})
Risk of reduced binding to antigen when labelled at high specific activity	High	Low
Cost of production	High	Low

myeloma cells in a fusion mixture (Figure 20.2). The latter is achieved by using a myeloma mutant that lacks the enzyme hypoxanthine guanine-phosphoribosyl transferase (HGPRT), which is essential for DNA synthesis via the alternate biosynthetic pathway that utilizes exogenous sources of purines and pyrimidines. These calls must synthesize DNA via their *de novo* pathways, which means they can be killed in culture by blocking this pathway with an anti-folate drug such as aminopterin. The choice of which myeloma cell line to use in making hybridomas depends on whether mouse (Galfre and Milstein, 1981), or human (James and Bell, 1987) monoclonal antibodies are being raised.

To produce mouse hybridomas the animals are immunized twice with the antigen, in as pure a form as possible, in the presence of an adjuvant, e.g. Freund's complete adjuvant. Three days before the fusion the mice are boosted with an intravenous dose of antigen and then on fusion day their spleens are removed and made into a single-cell suspension. Meanwhile the mouse myeloma cells are grown in spinner culture vessels in the laboratory. The fusion procedure involves mixing these two parental cells types together (at a ratio of 2:1 B-cells:myeloma cells) and then spinning them down and removing the supernatant. Next a 50% solution of polyethyleneglycol (PEG, mol. wt 1500) is added to the pelleted cells for 1–2 min with mixing to ensure cell membrane fusion. The cell mixture, containing fused and unfused cells, is resuspended in tissue culture medium and plated out into culture trays for incubation at 37 °C in a 5% CO_2 atmosphere. The culture medium in which the hybrids are grown contains all the necessary nutrients for growth plus hypoxanthine, aminopterin and thymidine (HAT). This medium containing HAT selects for hybrid growth only because unfused myeloma cells (HGPRT negative) die in the presence of aminopterin, which blocks their only route for DNA synthesis. Hybrids, on the other hand, use their HGPRT enzyme acquired from the antibody-secreting B-cell parent to take up hypoxanthine and thymidine (HT) from the medium for their survival. Normal unfused B-cells die in culture after a week because they are not adapted for continuous growth under these conditions.

20.4.1 HOW IS A HYBRIDOMA SELECTED?

The selection and cloning of hybrids secreting antibodies of a desired specificity begins at three to four weeks after fusion, when the growing hybrids have secreted enough antibodies into the culture medium for them to be detected in an immunoassay system. Depending on the type and availability of the antigen/s to which monoclonal antibodies are being raised, there follows a primary screening to select those wells containing hybrids secreting specific antibody. Tissue culture supernatant taken from wells containing actively growing hybrids is incubated in the presence of the antigen (either attached to microtitre plate

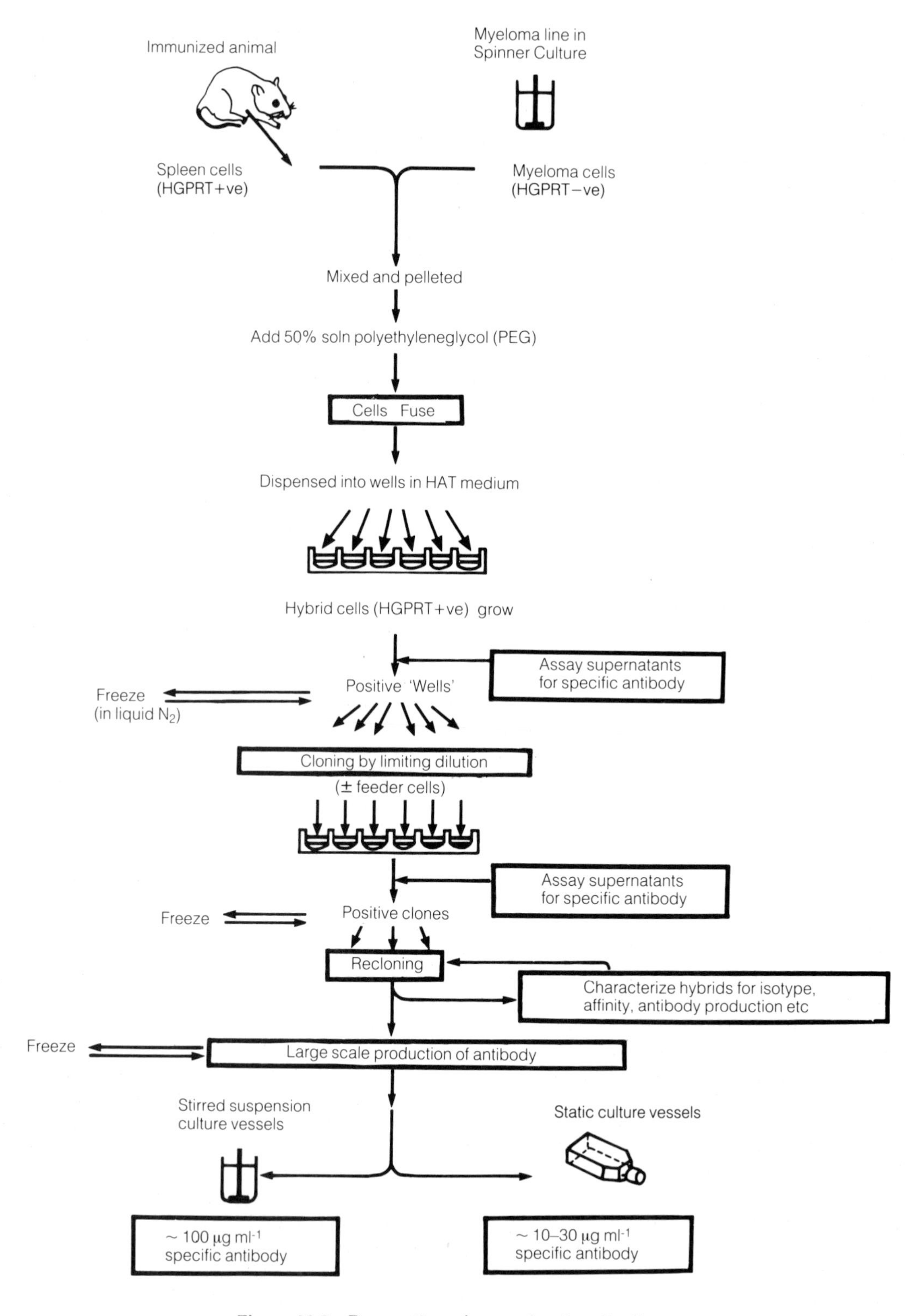

Figure 20.2 Preparation of monoclonal antibodies.

wells or expressed on cell membranes, etc.) and then removed. After washing away unbound antibody, the specific antibody bound to antigen is detected using a second anti-mouse antibody which can be either radiolabelled for radioimmunoassay type screens, or enzyme labelled for enzyme-linked immunosorbent assays (ELISA), or have a fluorescent compound attached to it so that localization of antibodies on tissue sections can be visualized under fluorescent microscopy. Positive wells on this initial screen are then cloned by limiting dilution techniques in the presence of feeder cells (usually mouse macrophages or spleen cells) to supply additional growth factors. When these have grown up they are rescreened against antigen and the positive wells recloned for a second time. Regular testing and recloning of hybrids grown in continuous culture is essential to ensure stability of antibody production.

20.4.2 HOW ARE MONOCLONAL ANTIBODIES PURIFIED?

The isolation and purification of monoclonal antibodies for clinical purpose comes from tissue culture medium harvested from bulk cultures of cloned hybridomas. The methods used to isolate antibodies from tissue culture media containing 5–10% serum (usually fetal calf) and other products (mainly salts and antibiotics), depends on their antibody classes (isotypes). A number of mouse antibodies (IgG2a, IgG2b, IgG3, and some IgGl isotypes) bind to a staphylococcal protein A product via their Fc ends (see Figure 20.1) and this property is made use of in their purification. The culture medium containing antibody is passed down a column of protein A covalently linked to gel beads, and the antibody binds to it. After washing the column with an alkaline buffer to remove extraneous proteins, etc., the antibody is eluted by lowering the pH and raising the salt concentration of the buffer to give highly purified material. Unfortunately many antibodies do not bind to protein A and have to be purified by first making a 50% ammonium sulphate precipitation of the culture medium and then additional purification on ion-exchange chromatography or gel filtration (Weir, 1978). However, the development of high-performance liquid chromatography (HPLC) systems capable of purifying high-molecular-weight proteins, such as antibodies, has made the task simpler, more reproducible and quicker than using traditional low-pressure systems. The purified antibody must then be assessed for purity on 10% sodium dodecyl sulphate (SDS) polyacrylamide gels, and for biological activity in an antigen-specific assay. The preparation of antibody for use in patient studies should comply with the National Institute for Biological Standards and Control (NIBSAC) guidelines covering their preparation and testing for viral and pyrogen contamination (see Section 20.5).

20.4.3 MONOCLONAL ANTIBODY CHARACTERIZATION

The first investigation carried out on a newly acquired antibody is to determine its isotype (class of antibody). This is done by simple immunodiffusion in agar using class-specific antisera. The antigen specificity of the antibody will have been defined by the screening procedure employed during its isolation. However, the antibody specificity has to be evaluated against normal tissues before it can be used as an *in vivo* imaging agent (Mason *et al.*, 1985). Some antibodies can bind to several antigens that are very similar in structure with different binding affinities. These cross-reactions between structurally similar antigens and antibodies may reduce their imaging specificity, but this depends to some extent on the biodistribution of the antigens. Another problem that confronts the use of antibodies in RIS is the expression of a given antigen on different cell types. In this situation a reduction in imaging specificity will result because all the tissues and organs expressing a common antigen will be identified by the radiolabelled antibody. Although tissue and organ binding studies *in vitro* may help to identify useful antibodies for RIS, they cannot fully predict the results that will be obtained when tested in patients.

Also included in a full characterization of a monoclonal antibody is a measure of its binding affinity (K) to its specific antigen (Steward and Steensgaard, 1983). The affinity of an antibody is a constant value derived from the summation of forces (ionic, hydrophobic, hydrogen bonding, steric, and van der Waals') involved in the association and dissociation between a single antigenic determinant and its antibody combining site. Put simply it is a value of how tightly an antibody will bind to its antigen and how useful it will be as an imaging agent *in vivo*. Methods of measuring antibody affinity depend on the availability and physicochemical composition of the antigen. Normally the antigen is radiolabelled, and then a range of antigen concentrations reacted with a constant amount of antibody. When this reaction reaches equilibrium the amount of bound and free antigen is measured and the results expressed as a Scatchard plot (bound/free versus bound) to give the K value (and the antibody valence if you require it). Most values for K are approximations because almost all antigens used as targets for imaging purposes are not true haptens and so their reaction kinetics do not fit the hapten model system. However, they are a guide in choosing between the antibodies for radiolabelling techniques in relation to the antigen-combining site of an antibody.

20.4.4 BIOLOGICAL FACTORS AFFECTING UPTAKE

At present, only antibodies against tumour-associated antigens have been used for RIS. Apart from specificity the antibody must have access to the antigen, so that local factors are very important. The arrival of the antibody in the vicinity of the antigenic binding sites on the cells depends on physical factors: the flow to the tumour, the capillary permeability and the effects of the cellular environment on the diffusion and convection of the antibody. The higher the avidity of the antibody for the antigen, the greater the probability of an interaction and binding on the cell membrane. The blood supply to the tumour is a major determinant of the kinetics of uptake of an antibody. The higher the flow, the more rapid the uptake, the earlier the imaging and the more short-lived the radionuclide label may be. Tumour blood supply is not under autonomic control, so attempts are being made to enhance tumour uptake by pharmacological intervention, reducing blood flow to the rest of the body. Tumour capillaries are more leaky than normal, so allowing proteins to pass from the circulation to the tumour. This enabled early workers to use radiolabelled albumin or fibrinogen to image tumour and accounts for the uptake of non-specific antibody by tumours. Extracellular fluid to cell ratio of tumours is greater than normal tissues and the charge and composition of this fluid may affect the rate of uptake of antibody onto tumour cell antigens. Locally secreted antigen, such as CEA, from colorectal cancer may enhance the uptake in the environment of the tumour. Tumour growth leads to deprivation of central blood supply, with necrosis and cyst formation – areas without specific antigen. In general, the larger the tumour the smaller the fraction of cancer cells to tumour mass and the greater the degree of non-specific uptake. Thus, the specific uptake of labelled antibody is designed best for demonstrating small tumours.

Other factors are also important in determining the uptake of antibody by cancer cell antigens. If the amount of antibody administered per study is increased, the amount taken up by both the tumour and its environment is greater, so the tumour to mucosa ratio does not change, but this may not be true for doses over 20 mg. The relationship between tumour weight and uptake is not linear, for the reasons given above – the larger the tumour the proportionally greater the stroma and cystic and necrotic changes. The degree of differentiation of the tumour is important, poorly differentiated tumours taking up much less antibody per gram than well-differentiated tumours – a fourfold difference in a study of colorectal cancer (Granowska *et al.*, 1988b). Staging of cancer *in vivo* is not possible if normal lymph nodes draining the site of cancer take up a secreted antigen more avidly than the involved nodes, as occurs with CEA. Coexisting disease may compete for the antibody and benign tumours may also take up antibody as well as malignant tumours. Another considerable influence on detection of small tumours is the degree and distribution of uptake in the tissue background, in normal bowel, liver, in the urinary tract and/or in bone marrow depending on the nature of the antibody and the radiolabel.

Kinetic factors play an important part in the differentiation of specific antibody uptake from non-specific uptake and in the choice of radiolabel. Whereas after an initial distribution period non-specific uptake decreases with time due to a falling blood and tissue fluid concentration and due to local metabolism by reticulo-endothelial cells (Figure 20.3), specific uptake of antibody continues to increase with time over the first day (Figure 20.4) although at a progressively slower rate as its concentration in the supplying blood falls. Kinetic analysis is helpful in the demonstration of tumours under 2 cm in diameter.

One of the problems of RIS is the development of human anti-mouse antibodies (HAMA; Van Kroonenburgh and Pauwels, 1988). This occurs in response to most injections of whole mouse

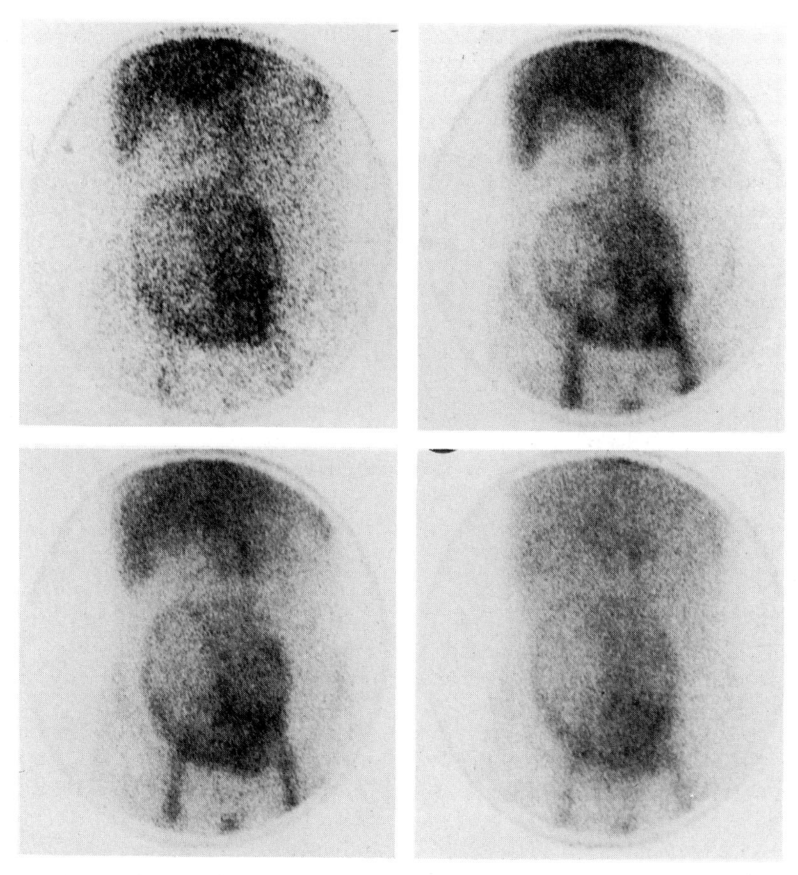

Figure 20.3 RIS with ^{123}I-labelled HMFG2 in a patient with large fibroids in the uterus, anterior abdominal views at top left, 1 min; top right, 10 min; bottom left, 4 h; and bottom right, 22 h. Note the high early activity fading with time and typical of non-specific uptake and compare with **Figure 20.4**.

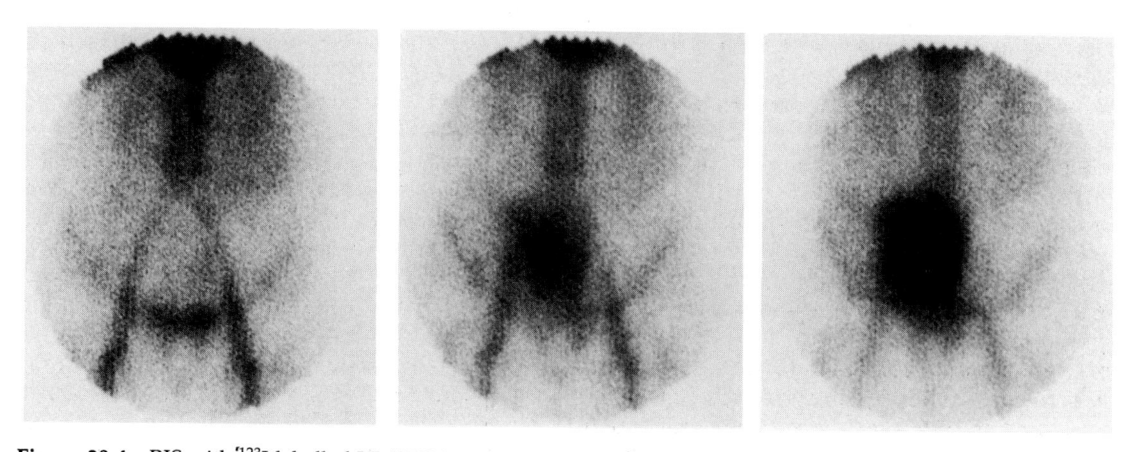

Figure 20.4 RIS with ^{123}I-labelled HMFG2 in a patient with a large ovarian adenocarcinoma, anterior abdominal views: left, 10 min; centre, 4 h; right, 22 h. Note the increasing uptake with time typical of specific uptake and compare with **Figure 20.3**.

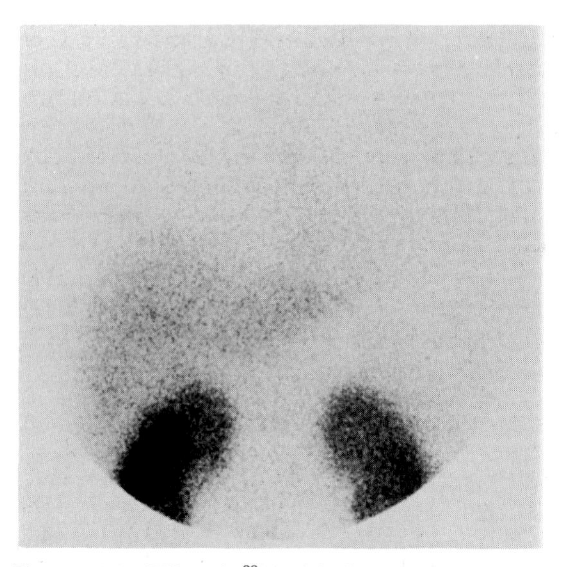

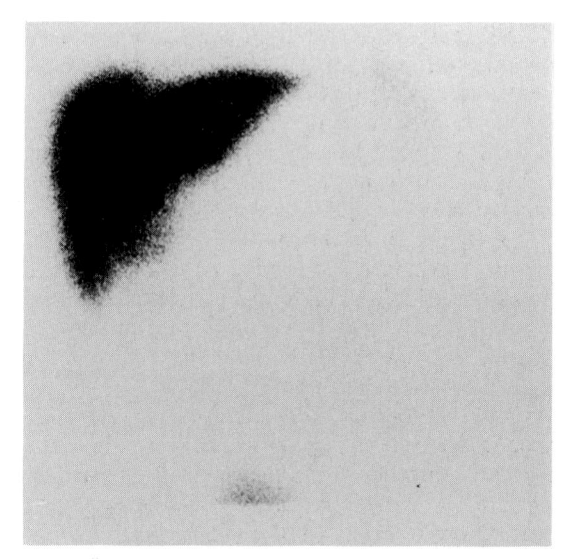

Figure 20.5 RIS with ^{99m}Tc-labelled F(ab′)$_2$ fragment of 225.28S monoclonal antibody against high-molecular-weight melanoma antigen. Both images are at 20 min. Left: normal distribution with high renal uptake due to filtration, reabsorption, metabolism and deposition of ^{99m}Tc in the proximal tubules. Right: abnormal distribution due to allergic reaction (skin test negative, no previous exposure to antibody). There is very high liver uptake and low renal excretion due to immune complex formation which is too large to be filtered.

monoclonal IgG γ-globulin, particularly when intradermal skin testing is combined with intravenous injection. This is the main reason why skin testing is being abandoned. There is usually no HAMA response to the first injection of F(ab′)$_2$ fragments and a response is 50% to a second injection. The biodistribution may be much altered in the second injection of whole antibody for RIS in the presence of a strong HAMA response, with a more rapid blood clearance of the labelled antibody to liver and other reticuloendothelial systems. Occasionally a systemic reaction occurs (frequency about one per 1000 studies) and the liver uptake may be rapid. This is illustrated in Figure 20.5. On the left is the normal renal uptake of ^{99m}Tc-labelled F(ab′)$_2$ 225.28S antimelanoma monoclonal antibody with low liver uptake at 20 min. On the right is the 20 min image in a patient having an episode of nausea and faintness shortly after injection of the same antibody. Although the skin test was negative, the liver uptake is high and rapid.

20.5 QUALITY CONTROL

Since monoclonal antibodies are a biological product derived from cell culture stringent quality-control procedures are necessary to prevent undesirable products, particularly genetically active material and virus, from being present in the final product. A reasonable set of guidelines has been set out by a working party on the clinical use of antibodies (Begent, 1986), but some legislators are demanding tests for numbers of unlikely viruses at all stages of the production which, apart from the expense, are unnecessary – given proper procedures. The essential requirements are knowledge of: the name, source and characteristics of the parent myeloma line; the source of the immune parental spleen cell; the source of its immunogen and the immunization procedure; a description of the fusion and cloning processes and the method of cell culture; the class and subclass of the monoclonal antibody secreted and the precautions taken to avoid contamination of the cell seed suspension and subcultures; the use and nature of antibiotics in the culture and any preservatives in the purification of the antibody; the capacity of the purification procedure to remove DNA and RNA viruses; the pharmaceutical quality of the final antibody product; and its characterization against normal and pathological tissues in terms of its specificity and avidity by immunocytochemistry. The rationale for its use in RIS should include its demonstrated specificity for the chosen tumour and absence of reactivity with clinically relevant other tissues or tumours. Human tumour xenograft uptake in an experimental animal such as the nude mouse is not required and may give misleadingly optimistic results since the human tumour antigens have no competition in the mouse, the ratio of tumour mass to mouse is inappropriately large and the tumour stroma is made up by mouse connective tissue, or be misleadingly pessimistic if antigenic modulation or cytochemical modification has occurred.

20.6 THE RADIOLABEL

What are the properties of an ideal radiolabel for radioimmunoscintigraphy and how do the available radionuclides match up? The key requirement for static imaging of a tumour through the distribution of a radiotracer is a high count rate delivered from the tissue of interest to the imaging system. The major determinant of the suitability of radionuclide for antibody labelling is its half-life of decay. The shorter the half-life, the greater the activity that may be administered and the higher the count rate obtained, given an upper limit of the absorbed dose of radiation that is permitted for diagnostic nuclear medicine. Ideally the half-life should be matched with kinetic information on the rate of antibody uptake by the target. If the uptake of antibody follows Michaelis–Menton kinetics, as would be expected at a first approximation, then the uptake rate is initially greatest, the fractional uptake of the amount administered decreasing with time as the concentration in the blood supplying the target decreases with time. The temporal requirement concerns the rate of clearance of the injected antibody from the blood and tissues providing the environment for the target, in relation to its residence time on the target tissue. A typical biological half-life of clearance of whole antibody from blood is 43 h, with a range of 24–64 h, and an antibody fragment is cleared at approximately twice this rate, a biological half-life of 21.5 h with a range of 15–30 h. For a typical whole antibody and a typical compact reasonably vascular tumour about 75% of the total uptake of labelled antibody occurs in the first 12 h, favouring the use of a radionuclide with about a 12-h physical half-life, such as ^{123}I (13.2 h). For some antibodies uptake will be more rapid, as Buraggi *et al.* (1985) have shown for anti-melanoma antibody, giving an optimal time between 6 and 12 h, favouring a radiolabel with a physical half-life of 6 h such as ^{99m}Tc (Buraggi, 1986). Other malignancies, such as colorectal cancer and particularly relatively avascular tumours such as scirrhous carcinoma of the breast, may show slower uptake requiring a longer-lived radionuclide such as ^{111}In (67.4 h physical half-life; Table 20.2).

An appreciation of the need for higher sensitivity in order to detect small tumours requires an understanding of the sources of signal degradation. Noise is a term used generally for anything that degrades the signal and has many sources, but the most important is the signal itself. Since one of the aims of radioimmunoscintigraphy is to visualize recurrences or spread of cancer not detectable by conventional radiology, X-ray com-

Table 20.2 Radiolabels for radioimmunoscintigraphy

	^{123}I	^{111}In	^{99m}Tc	^{131}I
Availability	Twice weekly	Twice weekly	Twice daily	Daily
γ-ray energy (keV)	159	171 250	140	360
β-particles	Absent	Absent	Absent	Present
Half-life	13 h	67 h	6 h	8 d
Suitability for gamma camera crystal	Excellent	Good	Excellent	Poor
Collimator (keV)	200	300	160	400
Dose administered (mCi)	3–4	3–4	15	1
(MBq)	120–160	120–160	550	40
Expected counts per pixel per injection taking ^{131}I as unity	25×	10×	80×	1
Reduction of absorbed dose per injection, taking ^{131}I as unity	10×	2×	20×	1
Thyroid blocking required	Yes	No	No	Yes
Appropriateness to the kinetics of antibody uptake	Very good	Excellent	Very good	Inappropriate

puted tomography, nuclear magnetic resonance or ultrasound through the properties of a specifically targeted antibody, then the optimization of a significant signal from a small target is essential. Most of the noise that prevents this objective is due to the weakness of the signal itself, for the radioactive decay of a radionuclide with the emission of γ-rays is a random process governed by Poisson statistics. Poisson noise depends on the square root of the count rate, so that the lower the count rate the disproportionally high is the noise. Thus at 10 000 counts per minute (cpm) the noise is 100 cpm; i.e. 1% of the counts recorded, whereas at the count rate of 100 cpm the noise is 10 cpm, i.e. 10% of the counts recorded. This primary type of degradation of the signal severely reduces tumour detectability. Low count rates give 'noisy' images where the tumour is less separable from background and the high variability of the background itself may give 'noise blobs' which may be falsely interpreted as tumour signals. This may be illustrated by consideration of RIS in a child with neuroblastoma using 40 MBq ^{131}I-labelled UJ13A (an antibody reacting with neuroblastoma) on one occasion (Figure 20.6a) and 40 MBq ^{123}I-labelled UJ13A three weeks later (Figure 20.6b). For the same tumour in the same child, the same administered activity, and the same antibody with ^{131}I as the radiolabel, the tumour is lost in the noisy background of liver, heart and spleen at 21 h and can just be visualized at 70 h, whereas with ^{123}I as the radiolabel the spleen and liver are clearly outlined at 10 min, and by 4 h the space seen superior to the spleen had been replaced by a focal area of high uptake in the tumour, and at 21 h. With ^{131}I the signal to noise ratio at 70 h was 25:1 but the signal was poor, whereas with ^{123}I at 21 h the signal to noise ratio was 1.5:1 yet the tumour is evident. The tumour is also evident at 4 h on a colour-coded image (Plate 9) when the tumour to background ratio was only 1.23:1. This pair of studies demonstrates the greater importance of the signal itself over the calculated signal to background ratio. For ^{123}I the count content per pixel was 25 times that from ^{131}I for the same administered activity. A good signal enables detection, however high the non-specific background activity (Britton and Granowska, 1987).

Thus, in principle a radioactively labelled tumour the size of a pinhead will be visualized if it gives a good enough signal, just as a high note on the trumpet can be heard above the noise of the battle. Whilst the avidity, affinity and selectivity of the antibody are crucial to that signal, the choice of a radiolabel itself is very important. Thus the number of radiolabels allowable per antibody while retaining its immunoreactivity, the efficiency and abundance with which the γ-rays are emitted from the radiolabel, their γ-ray energy, their interaction with the crystal of the gamma camera, the total number of radioactive molecules that may be injected into the patient and the availability of the radiolabel, all contribute to the choice of ideal radionuclide. The emitted γ-ray must be sufficiently energetic so that tissue absorption does not reduce sensitivity too much but not so energetic that it passes through the thin crystal of the gamma camera. The ideal energy of a γ-ray to interact efficiently with the crystal of the gamma camera is between 100 and 200 keV, and the nearer to the top of this scale the less the tissue absorption. Thus, ^{99m}Tc and ^{123}I are to be preferred to ^{111}In and ^{131}I on these grounds. The choice of collimator is important. The more energetic the γ-ray, the thicker the lead septa of the collimator will have to be, so that in this circumstance less crystal can be exposed than for a lower-energy γ-ray, so the sensitivity for detection is reduced. Too thin septa for too energetic a γ-ray allows septal penetration and thus degrades resolution. Thus, due to their γ-ray energies, collimators with septa designed for up to 400 keV for ^{131}I, for up to 300 keV for ^{111}In, for up to 200 keV for ^{123}I, and for up to 160 keV for ^{99m}Tc, have to be used. The lower the energy specification of the collimator the greater is the crystal exposure and thus its contribution to sensitivity.

A further reason for using radionuclides with a short half-life is so that a large amount of activity may be administered to the patient and yet give a low radiation exposure, since the absorbed dose depends on the activity received integrated over time. To reduce the radiation exposure to the patient it is also important that the radionuclide is free from β-particle radiation. Even ignoring its excessive γ-ray energy, for these two factors ^{131}I, with its eight-day half-life and β-emission which gives 80% of the radiation due to this radionuclide *in vivo*, should no longer be used for modern radioimmunoscintigraphy but limited to radioimmunotherapy. A comparison of approximate absorbed doses is given in Table 20.3. These matters are discussed further by Britton and Granowska (1987).

The immunoreactivity of the antibody must be preserved during the radiolabelling. This usually

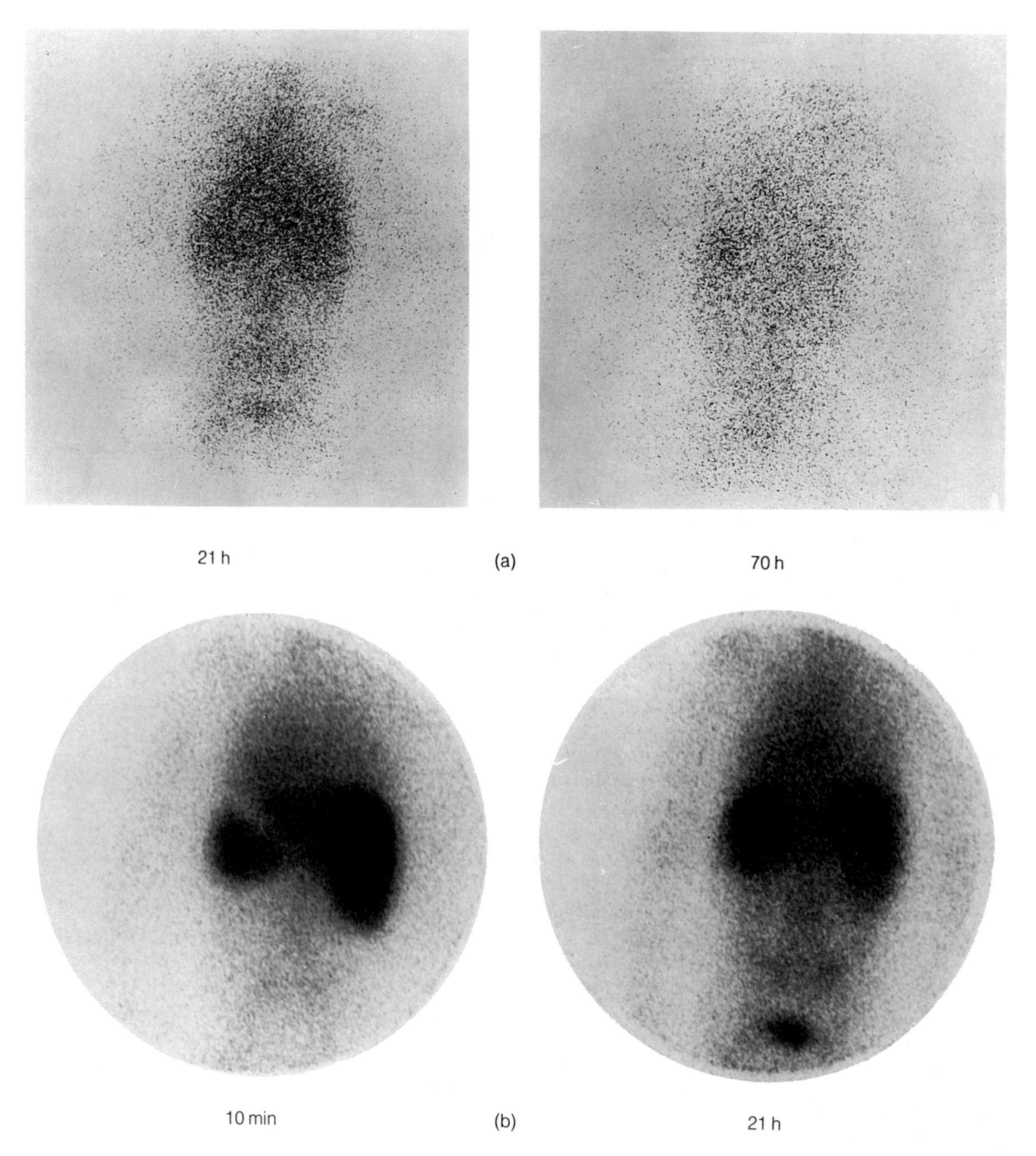

Figure 20.6 RIS of neuroblastoma using radioiodinated UJ13A in a 4-year-old child. (a) Posterior abdominal images 21 and 70 h after injection of 40 MBq ^{131}I-labelled UJ13A. General uptake is seen in the liver, spleen and blood pool at 21 h. Focal low contrast uptake is seen at 70 hrs in the tumour (**arrowed**). (b) Posterior abdominal images at 10 min and 21 h, after injection of 40 MBq ^{123}I-labelled UJ13A in the same child. At 10 min the spleen and liver are identified with an area of reduced uptake superior to the spleen. At 21 h, a focal area of increased uptake is evident in the tumour superior to the spleen.

Table 20.3 Absorbed radiation doses (cGy) for radioimmunoscintigraphy: an approximate comparison taking ^{131}I-labelled IgG as 100%

Agent	*Activity (MBq)*	*Liver*	*Kidney*	*Gonad*	*Marrow*	*Spleen*	*Whole body*
^{131}I-labelled IgG	40	2.0	7.8	0.02	0.77	25	1.6
^{131}I-labelled F(ab')$_2$	60	70%	22%	15%	42%	40%	25%
^{111}In-labelled IgG	120	470%	12%	20%	70%	20%	46%
^{111}In-labelled F(ab')$_2$	120	58%	112%	10%	35%	10%	23%
^{123}I-labelled IgG	120	75%	0.6%	20%	32%	4%	3%
^{123}I-labelled F(ab')$_2$	120	43%	0.4%	10%	18%	0.3%	2%
^{99m}Tc-labelled IgG	400	0.5%	1.0%	5%	0.3%	0.1%	0.02%

requires that the radiolabel to antibody molar ratio is 1:1 or 2:1 since labelling of the antigen-combining site of the antibody must be avoided. Site-specific labelling of the constant-region parts of the antibody molecule away from the antigen-combining site is being developed to overcome this problem. Methods for labelling must therefore be 'gentle' so as not to denature the molecule by altering its three-dimensional conformation. Genetically engineered mouse antibodies can be 'humanized' to make them less immunogenic, have a specific labelling site introduced, and improvements made to their antigen specificity as well as being produced by a continuous fermentation-like process. All these technological improvements will eventually overcome many of the present problems relating to quality control (Britton and Granowska, 1988).

20.6.1 LABELLING WITH RADIOIODINE

Experience with labelling antibodies with ^{125}I for *in vitro* saturation analysis hormone assays led to the use of ^{131}I and then ^{123}I as the radiolabel for RIS. The chloramine T or iodogen techniques are preferred, labelling the protein through a tyrosine radical. Because of its low solubility in water, iodogen is dissolved in an organic solvent, dichloromethane, and dispensed into sterile polypropylene plastic tubes. The solvent is evaporated to dryness at 20 °C, leaving the iodogen fixed to the tubes, which are stable on refrigeration for several months. For labelling, the antibody is added to the tube, and then 10 mCi (400 MBq) ^{123}I, 0.1–0.2 ml 0.1 M citrate buffer pH 6 400 μg antibody (2 mg ml^{-1} in 0.1 M citrate/Tris buffer pH 7.4) and 10 μl potassium iodide (6 × 10^{-5} M in water) are added and mixed together by gentle shaking for 10 min. Extra carrier iodine is added since the ^{123}I is almost carrier free, having a specific activity of about 8 × 10^{-4} mg mCi^{-1} iodine with a chemical concentration of 8 × 10^{-3} μg ml^{-1}. To remove free ^{123}I the mixture is decanted onto a Sephadex G50 filtration column in a 20 ml syringe which has been pre-washed with 1% serum albumin in phosphate-buffered saline. After a 5 ml void volume, the eluate is collected and the activity assayed. Chromatographic quality control is undertaken and the reagent used if there has been over 70% labelling efficiency. Immunoreactivity is tested by radioimmunoassay or ELISA.

20.6.2 INDIUM LABELLING OF ANTIBODIES

Radiolabelling monoclonal antibodies with ^{111}In has some advantages over other isotopes such as iodine (^{123}I and ^{131}I). Although ^{111}In has similar imaging properties to ^{123}I and ^{99m}Tc it is superior to ^{131}I and is not taken up by the thyroid gland. It is also currently more available than ^{123}I, and with a longer physical half-life (67 h) it is better suited for *in vivo* biodistribution studies than ^{123}I; Table 20.3).

The method most commonly used to label antibodies with ^{111}In is that described by Hnatowich *et al.* (1983), in which the bicyclic anhydride of diethylenetriaminepentaacetic acid (DTPA) is first coupled to the antibody and then ^{111}In is chelated to this conjugate in a second step. An outline of the method is given below.

1. DTPA anhydride is dissolved in dry dimethylsulphoxide (DMSO) at 10 mg ml^{-1} and the antibody concentration should be 10 mg ml^{-1} in 0.05 M bicarbonate or Hepes buffer pH 8.0.
2. The desired amount of DTPA (approximately 50 μg for a 2:1 molar ratio of DTPA:antibody) is added to the antibody and mixed rapidly before being left to stand for 15 min.
3. Separation of free DTPA from that bound to antibody is done on a gel filtration column

pre-run with a 0.1 M acetate buffer pH 5.5, and then the antibody conjugate can be aliquoted and stored frozen at −20 °C until required.

4. Radiolabelling of DTPA–antibody conjugates with ^{111}In is done by adding 40 µl of 5 M sodium acetate to pharmaceutical-grade [^{111}In]indium chloride (74 MBq in 200 µl of 0.04 M HCl, Amersham, UK) to form the acetate derivative. This is then added to the DTPA–antibody conjugate, mixed and left at room temperature for 30 min. Separation of the free ^{111}In from that bound to the conjugate is achieved on a gel filtration column pre-run in phosphate-buffered saline (PBS) pH 7.4 containing 1% human serum albumin. The sample is then filter sterilized through a 0.22 µm disposable filter and is ready for use.

Although the preparation of conjugates is technically simple to perform, some care is required to ensure that the molar ratios between antibody and DTPA are optimal and that contamination with heavy metals is avoided. The use of plastic or polypropylene equipment and the best grades of chemicals and distilled water should reduce the risks of heavy metals binding to conjugates. To achieve good ^{111}In labelling a balance has to be struck between the amount of DTPA attached to the antibody and the effects of this DTPA coupling on the physicochemical and biological properties of the antibody. An illustration of how the latter can be assessed is shown using a mouse monoclonal antibody (IgG2a) to human thyroglobulin. Conjugates were made at 0:1 (hydrolysed DTPA:ab), 1:1, 2:1, 5:1 and 50:1 (DPTA:ab), and at antibody concentrations of 5, 10, 15 and 20 mg ml^{-1}. The structural changes resulting from these different amounts of DPTA coupled to this antibody are shown in Figure 20.7. Essentially there is a gradual increase in the molecular weights of both light and heavy chains as the ratio of DTPA:ab is raised. These increases are due to DTPA binding directly to the polypeptide chains themselves mainly via lysine residues and through interchain cross-linking to give heavy–light and heavy–heavy chain dimers as shown on 10% SDS polyacrylamide gels. These structural alterations produced a 10% loss of binding activity to thyroglobulin at molar ratios of 5:1 and 50:1 (Figure 20.8) when the conjugates were labelled with ^{111}In. The optimum DTPA:ab conjugation ratio for this antibody (1D4) was 2:1, giving comparable labelling efficiency to those achieved at higher molar ratios (Figure 20.9) and the least detectable damage to its structure (Figure 20.7) and antigen-binding capacity (Figure 20.8).

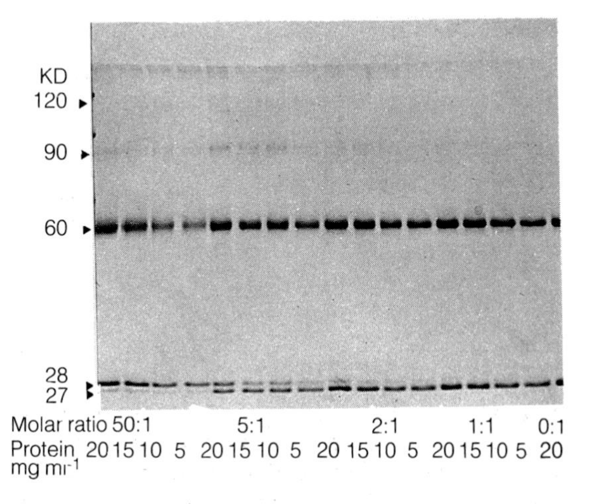

Figure 20.7 Effect of molar ratio and protein concentration on DTPA conjugates. Structural changes seen when run on 10% polyacrylamide gels under reducing conditions.

A general finding with all ^{111}In-labelled antibodies given intravenously to patients is the high uptake of ^{111}In in the liver. This probably occurs for a number of reasons: the transchelation of ^{111}In onto transferrin in plasma (6–10% per day), its binding to liver cells, and the localization of antibodies in liver by virtue of its large blood supply, and antibody uptake by Kupffer cells of the reticuloendothelium system. Certainly new types of metal chelates and different methods of linking them to antibodies will help reduce this problem in the future.

20.6.3 TECHNETIUM LABELLING OF ANTIBODIES

In vivo stability of ^{99m}Tc-labelled monoclonal antibodies was a problem until the method of Schwarz and Steinstraesser (1987). This approach has been modified by Mather and Ellison (1990).

The S–S bonds holding the heavy chains together in the hinge region of the gamma globulin are opened using 2-mercaptoethanol (2-ME). The antibody is concentrated by ultrafiltration to approximately 10 mg/ml. To a stirred solution of antibody, sufficient 2-mercaptoethanol is added to provide a molar ratio of 1000:1 2-ME: antibody. The mixture is incubated at room temperature for 30 minutes with continuous rotation. The reduced

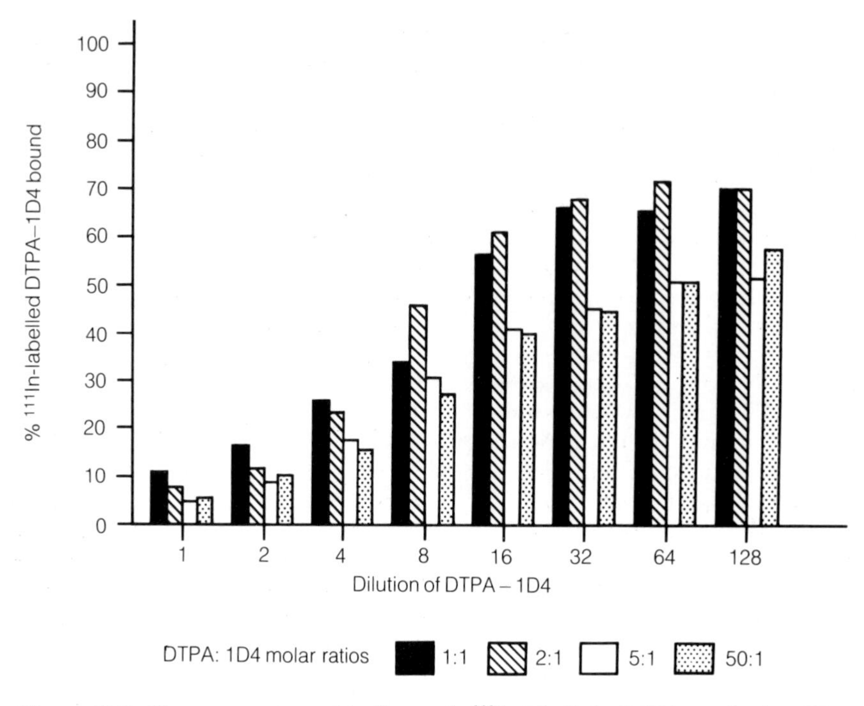

Figure 20.8 The percentage binding of ^{111}In-labelled DTPA–antibody (ID4) conjugates, at four different molar ratios, to thyroglobulin in a solid-phase radio-immunoassay.

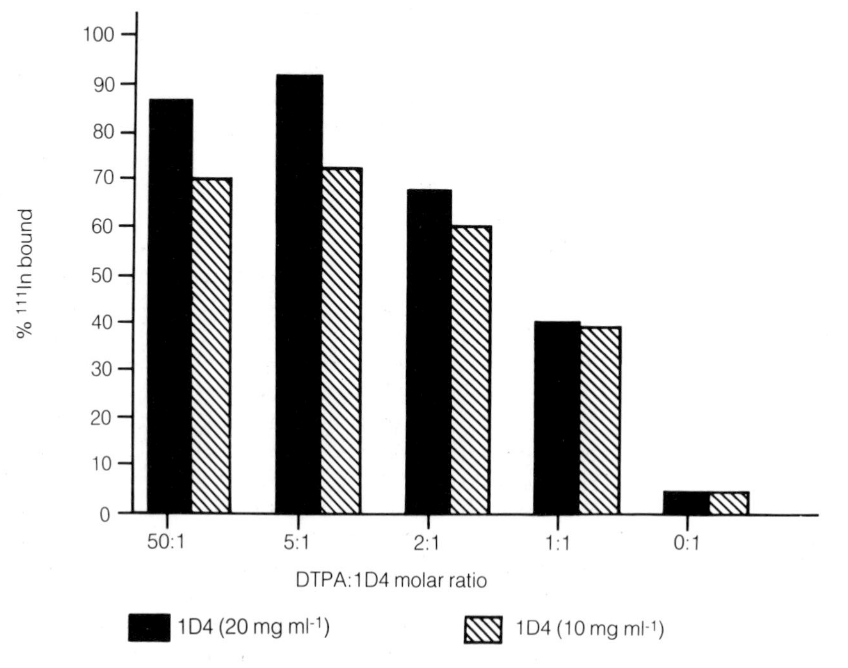

Figure 20.9 Radiolabelling efficiency of different molar ratios of DTPA–antibody (ID4) conjugates with ^{111}In.

antibody is purified by gel filtration on Sephadex –G50 using phosphate buffered saline as mobile phase. The antibody fractions are collated and divided into 0.5 mg aliquots. These are frozen immediately at $-20°$ C and stored ready for use.

When imaging is required the antibody aliquot is thawed and reconstituted using an Amerscan methylene disphosphonate, MDP, kit with 5ml 0.9% sterile saline. Thirty-five microlitres of MDP solution are added to antibody aliquot and mixed well. Then the required amount of ^{99m}Tc-pertechnetate (700 MBq approx.) is added to antibody/MDP mixture, which is gently shaken for 10 minutes. The labelling efficiency is assessed by thin layer chromatography (ITLC) developed in 0.9% saline and should be over 95%. If below this, the labelled antibody can be further purified by gel-filtration of Sephadex–G50 prior to injection The labelled antibody is stable for some hours *in vitro* after preparation. The ^{99m}Tc-labelled antibody is stable *in vivo*. There is no thyroid uptake of ^{99m}Tc even after 24 hours in patients who have received no thyroid blocking medication. This technique has been successfully used for four different antibodies in clinical use in this department to date.

20.7 CLINICAL PROTOCOLS AND DATA ANALYSIS

Before injection of a labelled monoclonal antibody, the patient must be asked about allergies. A history of severe allergic reactions or sensitivity to foreign protein is a contraindication to RIS. Skin testing by intradermal injection of 0.1 ml of the antibody against a saline control 30 min befor the study is often performed. A greater than 1 cm wheal within 30 min would indicate hypersensitivity. However, there are two disadvantages. First, a non-reaction does not exclude anaphylactic reaction to the subsequent intravenous injection, because skin hypersensitivity is not the correct sensitivity test, and secondly intradermal injection of antibody may sensitize the patient against further injections. Skin testing is therefore being abandoned.

A typical protocol is as follows: the nature of the test is explained to the patient and informed consent is obtained. Potassium iodide, 60 mg twice daily, is given the day before, during and for three days after the test for ^{123}I and for two weeks for ^{131}I. In addition, for these labels and when ^{99m}Tc is used, potassium perchlorate 400 mg is given just before the injection. No such preparation is required when ^{111}In is a label. The patient is then positioned supine on the scanning couch under the gamma camera fitted with an appropriate collimator and set up for the particular radionuclide. The labelled antibody in the appropriate dose is injected intravenously and, for example, in the context of ovarian or colorectal cancer images are obtained of the upper abdomen anteriorly and posteriorly, and similarly for the lower abdomen at 10 min, 6 h and 22 h for ^{123}I and ^{99m}Tc, and at 10 min, 22 h and 48 h or 72 h for ^{111}In.

20.7.1 TRANSPARENT FILM DISPLAY

The detection of a lesion is dependent on the darkening in the level of greyness of the 'grey scale' caused by the greater count density recorded from the lesion. The considerable distortion and degradation of image data that occurs when it is presented in a transparent film should be appreciated. The dynamic range of film is deliberately non-linear, being related to a log scale with respect to count rate, to encompass both high- and low-activity areas. Detection depends not only on the absolute magnitude of the signal but also on its statistical significance with respect to background, which itself shows considerable statistical fluctuations as well as biological variation. The image also superimposes counts arising from different depths with different attenuations. The eye's ability to perceive lesions depends on the contrast in the image and on the training and familiarity of the observer with the particular display, the types of abnormalities found in the primary or recurrent cancer under study and the features and normal variations to be expected in such images. It is therefore necessary to stress that the gamma camera should be tuned to perfection and the focus and intensity setting of the display film checked and optimized before undertaking the study.

The series of transparent films are evaluated for the distribution of uptake in normal structures: vascular activity, bone marrow, liver, spleen, kidneys, gastrointestinal and urinary activity; for sites of abnormal uptake and how the distribution of uptake varies with time. Thus the activity in vascular structures, tissue background and at sites of non-specific uptake after an initial increase tends to decrease with time (Figure 20.3) whereas areas of specific uptake show increasing uptake with time during the first 24 h (Figure 20.4).

However, gastrointestinal, liver and marrow activity for ^{111}In, and stomach and urinary activity for ^{123}I, may increase with time. Focal tumour uptake may be best seen at 6 h for ^{99m}Tc-labelled $F(ab')_2$ RIS in ocular melanoma (Siccardi *et al.*, 1986), and at 24 h for ovarian cancer (Granowska *et al.*, 1990a) and colorectal cancer (Granowska *et al.*, 1990b), and for ovarian cancer with ^{123}I-labelled HMFG2 (Granowska *et al.*, 1984). For example, in a blinded prospective study in recurrent ovarian cancer, accurate localization of the site or sites of the recurrences were made correctly using transparent film displays in 18 out of 20 patients and confirmed by maps made at laparotomy (Granowska *et al.*, 1986a). In colorectal cancer 24 or 48 h may give the best contrast using ^{111}In-labelled anti-CEA (Plates 10 and 11). The key to identifying the tumour site is the changes occurring in the series of transparent films between the 10 min, 4 h and later images.

20.7.2 IMAGE ENHANCEMENT

The following additional techniques are used to improve the contrast between the target and its background: the use of $F(ab')_2$ fragments (Wahl *et al.*, 1983); SPECT (Berche *et al.*, 1982); background subtraction using a second radiopharmaceutical (Goldenberg *et al.*, 1980), subtracting an early image from a later image (Granowska *et al.*, 1983), kinetic analysis with probability mapping (Granowska *et al.*, 1986), and the use of a second antibody to speed the clearance of the radiopharmaceutical from the blood (Begent *et al.*, 1983).

Fab is a monovalent fragment and $F(ab')_2$ a bivalent fragment obtained by enzyme digestion of the whole antibody so as to remove the Fc portion, leaving the active antigen-binding site intact.

The advantages of using an $F(ab')_2$ fragment include: the absence of the Fc protein which binds particularly to the reticuloendothelial cells, tending to increase liver, marrow, lymph node and splenic uptake; a more rapid clearance from blood by a factor of about twofold; and a more rapid diffusion into tumour tissue. The disadvantages include: usually a lower avidity than the whole antibody; loss by glomerular filtration into the kidney followed by absorption and metabolism in the proximal tubules, depositing the metal ^{111}In and ^{99m}Tc there (but not ^{123}I, which is released by deiodinases); greater diffusibility into a wider volume of distribution than the whole antibody, contributing to tissue background; and a further preparative step. However, matched to a short-lived radionuclide such as ^{99m}Tc or ^{123}I the advantages probably outweigh the disadvantages. For ^{111}In a reduced liver uptake is balanced by greater renal uptake and the benefits are less evident.

The main requirement for SPECT is a high count rate from the target, so that the rotation can be completed in a time that is reasonable to expect a patient to remain still. This favours the use of the shorter-lived radionuclides for labelling the antibody. It is the registration of sites of suspected abnormality in relation to anatomical landmarks that is the main problem for interpretation. Major vessel activity and incidental bone marrow uptake help but the presence of activity in the bowel makes for difficulties. Superimposition of the image on that of X-ray CT has been performed (Liehn *et al.*, 1987). The advantage of SPECT is the increased contrast of the target in the plane of the section and particularly the ability to separate objects from in front of and behind the target, e.g. the bladder from a pelvic tumour, which may overlap on a conventional view. Another potential advantage is the ability to quantify the amount of activity in a region of the transverse section, for example, for dosimetry; however, this is much more difficult than expected. Errors occur due to less than perfect rotation and linearity of response of the camera, Poisson statistical noise, algorithm noise, artefacts due to overlapping tissue activities – the partial volume effect, patient and organ movement and difficulties in correcting for tissue attenuation. Accuracy is thereby considerably reduced and the anatomical relationships of tissues and target may be difficult to visualize and to interpret. SPECT sections, once created, cannot be repositioned. The technique is a potentially useful adjunct to, but not a substitute for, planar imaging.

Background subtraction techniques have a long history. The earliest approach to improve the signal by reducing tissue background was to subtract the distribution of one radiopharmaceutical from another. Classically an image of the pancreas is obtained by subtracting a liver image from a liver plus pancreatic image (Kaplan *et al.*, 1966). This approach was applied by Goldenberg *et al.* (1980) to RIS.

A distribution of ^{131}I-labelled antibody, representing blood and tissue activity plus tumour uptake, has a blood and tissue activity distribution of ^{99m}Tc-labelled albumin subtracted from it to enhance the tumour contrast. Unfortunately this approach is fraught with difficulties because of the different energies of the γ-rays of ^{131}I and ^{99m}Tc. Thus the tissue attenuation and γ-ray scattering is quite different for the two radionuclides. As a result edge artefacts and variable noise make image interpretation difficult. In principle it is very difficult to correct for this effect (Ott *et al.*, 1983). The technique of Green *et al.* (1984) overcomes this to some extent by taking a region of interest (ROI) in the subtracted picture and then calculating the ratio of ROI signal to background in the albumin picture and comparing this with the ratio of the ROI signal to background in the ^{131}I-labelled antibody image. If the ratio of these signal to background ratios is greater than four, then that represents, in their hands, a statement of detectability of a significant abnormality, although there is a degree of overlap of the normal with the abnormal. An improved method for radionuclides of similar energies is described by Liehn *et al.* (1987).

In any tumour, part of the uptake is due to non-specific features: the blood flow, the tumour blood volume and vascular transit time, the leakiness of the tumour capillaries, which is greater than for normal tissues, the extracellular fluid content, and the lack of lymphatic drainage. Such non-specific uptake improves sensitivity but reduces the specificity of any imaging agent. Thus, if the specificity of a monoclonal antibody against a tumour-associated antigen is to determine the uptake, the tumour or metastasis should be small so that non-specific uptake plays a minimal role.

It is clearly important to distinguish specific tumour uptake from non-specific uptake, and to reduce the effects to tissue and blood background. The concept was introduced of subtracting an image taken early after injection before significant tumour uptake, which shows the distribution of blood and tissue activity, from an image taken after the specific uptake of the radiolabelled antibody has taken place (Granowska *et al.*, 1983). This approach overcomes the problem of subtracting the distribution of two radionuclides with differing energies, and allows considerable enhancement of tumour uptake. However, it requires the repositioning and normalization of the two images. The repositioning must be reasonably accurate between the first and second visits of the patient, and then the computer images must be completely superimposed. For each image of the patient, marker images are also obtained. For the latter the patient's bony landmarks, xiphisternum, costal margins, anterior superior iliac spines and symphysis pubis are marked with indelible ink and point-source radioactive markers are positioned over these. Transparent films of the marker positions on the persistence scope are made at the early visit. At each subsequent visit, the markers are replaced on the patient and the patient is repositioned until the image of the marker on the persistence scope fits that on the previously recorded films placed over the scope. The computer is also programmed so that the recorded images can be moved and fixed one pixel at a time, vertically, horizontally or by rotation so that an exact superimposition of the later image over the earlier image may be made in order that detailed analysis of the images may be performed by proportional subtraction of the early image from the later image (Granowska *et al.*, 1987).

A more sophisticated approach makes use of the kinetic information as well as the count rate distribution. As noted above, specific tumour uptake increases with time after injection of the radiolabelled antibody, whereas blood and tissue non-specific activity decreases with time after the initial distribution phase is over. By analysing pairs of images separated in time, for example, the 10 min image with the 22 h image or the 4 h image with the 22 h image, in terms of the temporal changes in the count rate distribution that have occurred between the pairs of images, then sites of specific uptake will be identified as positive derivations from a line of correspondence calculated from the count rate frequency distribution of the two images for the areas where there has been no change between the two images. This technique of kinetic analysis with probability mapping satisfies the basic requirements of detectability of low contrast differences and insensitivity to statistical noise over the range encountered in a typical RIS study. Biopsy-proven deposits of 0.5 cm diameter have been correctly identified using this approach (Granowska *et al.*, 1986, 1988). The use of second anti-mouse immunoglobulin antibody to clear the circulation of the residual radiolabelled mouse monoclonal antibody was pioneered by Begent *et al.* (1983), who first encapsulated the second antibody in liposomes and more recently has used the second antibody directly. Experimental work in rats showed a dramatic reduction in the circulating level of the radiolabelled monoclonal antibody by injecting the second antibody 24 h after the first. This reduction is associated with a sharp increase in the liver content of the radiolabel, which then declines due to the uptake of the immune complex. One problem is that the second antibody reduces the tumour uptake of the first antibody and this may be due to using a second antibody of too high an avidity for the first. This approach is probably not required for imaging but should have benefits in reducing the absorbed radiation dose to normal tissue of radioimmunotherapy.

20.8 CLINICAL STUDIES

The crucial requirement when introducing any new technique of imaging is to define the clinical circumstances under which it should be able to contribute to clinical management if successful; for relevant diagnostic tests are those whose results alter clinical management. However, many diagnostic tests are undertaken in relation to a particular clinical problem and this strict criterion of a successful test is only recently being met by RIS for the technique is still in its early stages. When the results of prospective studies already underway are available with existing antibodies, the present clinical indications will be better defined. Nevertheless, a number of generalizations about the technique in the management of malignant disease may be made.

RIS has no role as a screening test for well people for the presence of cancer since it involves the injection of a foreign protein, a radioactive source, and an antibody that is not cancer specific.

RIS is gaining a role in the evaluation of patients picked up as a result of a preliminary investigation. The demonstration of a cyst in the pelvis may be supplemented using RIS to determine whether it contains ovarian cancer. The demonstration of an eye tumour ophthalmoscopically leads to ultrasound, which is not specific as the cause, and then RIS, which is 92% specific for ocular melanoma (Bomanji *et al.*, 1987a). RIS is expected to be applied to the differential diagnosis of the shadow in the chest X-ray and the lesion on mammography.

RIS is a natural counterpart to the increasing search for tumour markers in serum. However, the ideal antigen for detection in serum has to be released easily from the tumour as is CEA or AFP, and most markers do not show a rise in serum until some tumour necrosis has occurred; whereas for RIS an antigen well fixed to tumour gives more specific results. In colorectal cancer, positive identification of primary or recurrent tumour is successful even when the serum CEA is still normal. A raised serum marker is increasingly leading to RIS with the appropriate radiolabelled antibody (Green *et al.*, 1984; Chatal *et al.*, 1984). However, circulating tumour markers are also not cancer specific.

RIS may have a role in the primary staging of a known cancer. However, for secreted antigens such as CEA the uptake by normal local lymph nodes is greater than that by involved lymph nodes in colorectal cancer (Beatty *et al.*, 1986; Granowska and Britton, 1987). The reverse should be true for fixed membrane antigens such as PRIA3 (Granowska *et al.* 1990b). Colloid lymphoscintigraphy showing 'missing' nodes in a chain could be supplemented with positive identification of such nodes using the appropriate labelled antibody. A limitation of RIS in demonstrating liver metastases is evident due to the high uptake of the labelled antibody by the liver, and in the case of ^{111}In there is transchelation and deposition of this metal in the liver. This may be circumvented in future by the introduction of a metabolizable 'spacer' between the metal and the antibody.

RIS has a prime role in the re-evaluation of the patient after the management of the primary cancer by surgery, radiotherapy or chemotherapy or combinations of these. It is of no clinical benefit to image by RIS the large metastases already evident on ultrasound or X-ray computed tomography. It is of particular benefit to demonstrate that a mass in the pelvis is not due to post-surgical fibrosis but is a tumour recurrence; that an enlarged lymph node does not contain metastases; and that a clinically or radiologically normal abdomen does in fact contain tumour. This role in demonstrating previously unsuspected metastases has been confirmed in cutaneous melanoma (Siccardi *et al.*, 1986), in peritoneal plaques and pelvic recurrence of ovarian cancer (Granowska *et al.*, 1986a) where X-ray computed tomography (Blaquiere and Husband, 1983) and ultrasound (Khan *et al.*, 1983) are unreliable, in colorectal cancer recurrences (Chatal *et al.*, 1984), and in bone marrow metastases from breast cancer (Rainsbury *et al.*, 1983).

RIS is an essential precursor to radioimmunotherapy to demonstrate *in vivo* the uptake of the chosen antibody. Immunohistochemistry showing evidence of specific binding to the patient's tumour cells by the antibody is important but not sufficient evidence to justify radioimmunotherapy.

20.8.1 OVARIAN CANCER

Ovarian cancer is the third most frequent lethal cancer in women and it presents late. Case finding in well women using ultrasound is being attempted, in which case a specific antibody to distinguish malignant from benign disease would be helpful. Antibodies against PLAP (H17E2, Epenetos *et al.*, 1986b; and H317, Critchley *et al.*, 1986) are more specific than HMFG 1 and 2 (Granowska *et al.*, 1986a) but only react with about 75% of ovarian cancers, unlike HMFG1 and 2, which react with over 95% of ovarian adenocarcinoma. Antibody B72.3 against the TAG72 surface antigen does not cross-react with mesothelial cells and is taken up by the majority of ovarian cancers. Serum markers for ovarian cancer are not sufficiently specific to be useful in screening. However, a positive serum marker such as PLAP or OC125 should lead to a request for RIS with an antibody against the most positive antigen.

The management of ovarian cancer is primary surgery followed by appropriate chemotherapy. RIS can help in staging the disease by demonstrating deposits in the pelvis, lateral abdomen, omentum and subdiaphragmatically, particularly peritoneal plaques which are not susceptible to ultrasound (Khan *et al.*, 1983) or X-ray computed tomography (Calkins *et al.*, 1987). Laparoscopy with peritoneal washings is successful in only 50% of patients when compared to staging laparotomy. RIS is rarely helpful, however, in demonstrating liver metastases.

At primary surgery the tissue should be screened against a series of monoclonal antibodies to find the most avidly bound in the particular patient. After completion of the chemotherapy, the patient should then undergo RIS with the appropriate antibody labelled with ^{123}I (Granowska *et al.*, 1984) or ^{99m}Tc (Granowska *et al.*, 1990a) to detect residual disease if it is not apparent clinically or radiologically. Conversely a mass demonstrable by X-ray computed tomography can be shown to be viable tumour rather than post-treatment fibrosis by RIS. In the first case, RIS may prevent the need for second-look laparotomy since evidence of small subclinical or subradiological deposits of viable tumour is an indication for further chemotherapy (Granowska *et al.*, 1986a). Alternatively radioimmunotherapy may be considered, particularly if there is malignant ascites, with minimal residual disease. Demonstration of large viable tumour mass should lead to further salvage laparotomy to debulk the tumour where appropriate.

The detection of subclinical and subradiological disease is a severe test of RIS and a prospective study using kinetic analysis probability mapping has been shown to be reasonably successful (Granowska *et al.*, 1988b), whereas traditional transparent film imaging is less accurate. A prospective study in 23 patients presenting with pelvic masses confirmed its sensitivity for detecting ovarian cancer (100% correct), its 75% accuracy in localizing subclinical disease and its 75% specificity in demonstrating absence of residual disease in patients who underwent multiple biopsies at subsequent second-look surgery.

The goal is to reduce the need for second-look laparotomy by the non-invasive demonstration of disease. In some centres the policy of always performing second-look laparotomy to evaluate chemotherapy is being modified as a result of RIS.

20.8.2 COLORECTAL CANCER

The release of CEA by colorectal cancer led to the early application of RIS in its management (Mach *et al.*, 1980, 1983; Chatal *et al.*, 1984). While RIS is effective in primary diagnosis (Plate 10) conventional radiology and endoscopy is the established and reliable method of diagnosis, with biopsy to confirm the malignant change. The staging of colorectal cancer cannot be performed using anti-CEA since CEA is trapped by normal nodes more effectively than by involved nodes (Plate 10). This is because once the carcinoma has broken through the basement membrane the shed antigen travels in the local lymphatics and is held by the sinusoidal lining cells of the lymph nodes (Granowska and Britton, 1987). This is one of the disadvantages of using an antigen that is shed. An epithelial surface membrane antigen such as B72.3 (Colcher *et al.*, 1986), AUAI (Arklie, 1981) or PRIA3 (Granowska *et al.*, 1990b) does not appear to have this problem.

RIS is also poor at detecting liver metastases since the normal antibody is cleared by the reticuloendothelial system. The liver retention is increased when immune complex formation occurs, due to antibody reaction with circulating antigen, and is severe when ^{111}In is used as a label. This metal is fixed in the liver by transchelation when it is taken up, whereas radioiodine-labelled antibodies have the radioiodine split off by the liver iodinases so that the free iodine is excreted in the urine. Conventional liver ultrasound and liver colloid scanning remain good methods for looking for liver metastases, particularly in combination. Subtraction of a colloid scan from the RIS image of the liver and the use of SPECT are being evaluated. The determination of the hepatic artery to total liver blood flow hepatic artery/liver ratio using the ^{99m}Tc-labelled colloid liver scan has aided the detection of early metastases (Levenson *et al.*, 1983) ^{99m}Tc anti CEA has recently shown to be successful (Baum *et al.*, 1989).

Recurrence of colorectal cancer, however, can be well demonstrated by RIS, both before circulating tumour markers rise and also as a consequence of demonstrating a rise of such markers. Again these markers have only moderate specificity and sensitivity, but an increasing or sustained rise is usually diagnostic of recurrence. The particular marker may be used in the selection of the most appropriate antibody for RIS. X-ray, CT and ultrasound are less reliable in the demonstration of small tumour recurrences since the bowel wall is difficult to distinguish from tumours for the former, and bowel gas may interfere with the latter. A mass that is detected by X-ray, CT or ultrasound may be due to post-surgical fibrosis and one of the important uses of RIS is to show that such a mass is due to viable tumour recurrences. RIS may also demonstrate tumour recurrence not detectable radiologically. Demonstration of such recurrences is leading to further salvage surgery or local radiotherapy.

There is a possible role for RIS in prognosis through imaging and examination of the specimen after injectiing the radiolabelled antibody before surgery. It is possible that lymph nodes that are image positive and tumour cell negative indicate a good prognosis; and those that are image negative and tumour cell positive indicate a poor prognosis if such findings are taken to represent degrees of host response to a cancer-related antigen (Granowska and Britton, 1987).

20.8.3 MELANOMA

The most clinical experience of RIS is in the context of melanoma, where a multicentre trial of the Ferrone monoclonal antibody (Buraggi *et al.*, 1985) against the high-molecular-weight melanoma antigen 225.28S has been sucessfully completed (Siccardi *et al.*, 1986). This trial concerned the use of ^{99m}Tc and ^{111}In-labelled F(ab')$_2$ fragments of this antibody in 254 melanoma patients. 250 of 412 known lesions were visualized in 159 out of 191 patients known by other criteria to have metastases, and 95 new lessions not previously demonstrated were seen in 61 patients of this group. Usually it was the small lesions less than 2 cm that were not detected but the percentage of lesions visualized with ^{99m}Tc F(ab)$_2$ was 74%, significantly better than with ^{111}In (59%), supporting the argument set out earlier in this text. Higher false-negative rates were found in stage IV disease (21%) than the stage III disease, partly due to lack of expression of the antigen. Skin nodules were the most frequent lesions that were not visualized. But many lesions not evident clinically or radiologically were correctly identified. Reanalysing these data by the authors showed that taking stage I to stage III disease and considering only the use of the ^{99m}Tc labelled antibody, 78 of 84 patients (93%) were correctly shown to have metastases by RIS and in those 146 out of 199 lesions (79%) were correctly identified. Other antibodies used for melonama are p-97 (Larson *et al.*, 1983) and 96.5 (Halpern *et al.*, 1985).

Ocular melanoma, although somewhat different from skin melanoma, also cross-reacts with the 225.28S (Bomanji *et al.*, 1987a) and may be used to help, in conjunction with conventional investigations, in the differential diagnosis of a non-pigmented melanoma from other metastases or benign choroidal haemangioma (Bomanji *et al.*, 1987b; Plate 4).

20.8.4 OTHER MALIGNANCIES

At least 20 malignancies have been studied with RIS. The use of monoclonal antibodies in neuroblastoma (Goldman *et al.*, 1984) has largely been replaced by radioiodinated MIBG (*meta*-iodobenzyl guanidine) and similar antibodies are applicable to brain glioma (Richardson *et al.*, 1986). Carcinoma of the breast has been studied but, because of the scirrhous nature and poor expression of antigen *in vivo*, RIS has been less successful than in ovarian and colonic cancer (Rainsbury *et al.*, 1983). Carcinoma of the lung has not yet had a specific antigen identified but remarkably successful RIS has been undertaken using an anti-CEA monoclonal antibody (Riva *et al.*, 1986). Carcinoma of the thyroid has been investigated with anti-thyroglobulin (Fairweather *et al.*, 1983; Shepherd *et al.*, 1985). Carcinoma of the cervix shows some uptake of HMFG antibodies (Pateisky *et al.*, 1985). Seminoma shows marked expression of placental alkaline phosphatases which can contribute to the management of the patient (Epenetos *et al.*, 1986b). Hepatoma is detectable through its common expression of hepatitis viral antigens and this is being used to develop RIS (Bergmann *et al.*, 1987). Chorion carcinoma is demonstrable by the uptake of anti-HCG (Begent *et al.*, 1987).

Prostatic cancer is an obvious candidate for RIS and antibodies against, for example, prostatic specific antigen are likely to be better than those presently available (Vihko *et al.*, 1984). Osteosarcoma has also been visualized using RIS (Perkins *et al.*, 1984), and renal carcinoma (Belitsky *et al.*, 1978).

The many monoclonal antibodies available against lymphocyte antigens has led to their direct use in therapy, their application in RIS in lymphoma (Carrasquillo *et al.*, 1986) and in radioimmunotherapy (De Nardo *et al.*, 1986).

20.9 RADIOIMMUNOTHERAPY

The reasoned approach to the demonstration of cancerous tissue by the intravenous injection of radiolabelled antibodies is tending to be submerged in an emotionally over-optimistic demand for a cure for cancer by targetting treatment in the same way – radioimmunotherapy (RIT). In addition to all the requirements for RIS, RIT requires an absolute amount of antibody, whether carrying a radionuclide, a toxin or a chemotherapeutic agent, to be taken up and to remain attached to the tumour cell. For RIS it does not matter if only some fraction of the cells of a tumour mass take up the antibody, but for RIT heterogeneity of uptake is a major problem. For RIS the strength of the signal for detection can be improved and the background manipulated, but for RIT the ratio of tumour uptake to that by normal tissue is paramount. This therapeutic ratio depends on the uptake by the target to that by the most critical target organ. Whereas for RIS the imaging may be completed in 24 h, for RIT the residence time of the antibody on the tumour should be as long as possible, as the absorbed dose by the tumour depends on the area under the activity/residence time curve. Indeed, increasing the difference between the tumour residence time and that in normal tissue may be the key to the problem.

The radiosensitivity of the tumour is important. Well oxygenated tumour is more radiosensitive than hypoxic tissue, so therapy is more effective in small, well-perfused tumours. The killing rate is inversely proportional to tumour volume (10^4 cells = 0.3 mm, 10^6 cells = 2 mm, and 10^9 cells = 1 cm diameter). The radiation dose to kill cells is about tenfold more than that to stop cells dividing so repeated treatment may be necessary, and cure almost certainly requires the help of a host immune response against the tumour.

For non-tumour tissue the bone marrow and gastrointestinal tract are sensitive to 100–500 rads (1–5 Gy). If the bone marrow has already been irradiated or damaged by chemotherapy it will be even more critically radiosensitive. Vascular damage – nephritis, hepatitis and pneumonitis – occurs at 1000–2000 rads (10–20 Gy). It is therefore necessary to estimate the total absorbed doses delivered to the tumour, to the critical non-target organ, to the bone marrow and to the whole body. The absorbed dose depends on the amount of activity taken up, the volume of the tumour or tissue and the time course of activity. Dose assessment has to be made by a combination of practical measurements and theoretical modelling with an array of assumptions. Quantification of uptake whether by combined planar imaging (geometric mean of anterior and posterior, combination of views at right angles) or by SPECT is not straightforward. Specification of the volume is inaccurate by radionuclide imaging, depending on a decision as to the cut-off boundary chosen for the count distribution. Volume is more accurate by X-ray computed tomography, but much tumour tissue may not be evident, particularly peritoneal plaques, or have clearly defined edges in the absence of body fat. The time course of change in activity properly requires repeated measurements of the uptake phase and the biological half-life in the tumour and non-tumour tissues. The microdosimetry, particularly the effective energy and range of the radiation and the compactness of the tumour, are important. Electron capture and Auger electrons have very high effective energy deposition but a nanometre range, so much radiolabelled antibody would need to be internalized to affect the nucleus. α-Particles have high effective energy deposition and micrometre range, so that every cancer cell would need to bind the α-labelled antibody. Such incorporation of α-particle emitters, e.g. ^{211}At (half-life 7.2 h, 5.87 MeV, decaying to ^{211}Po, 0.52 s, 7.45 MeV) would have a great therapeutic effect but only if uptake were homogeneous (Bloomer *et al.*, 1984). With β-emitting radionuclides, the choice for therapy depends on the β-ray energy, the abundance of the β-emission and the physical half-life. β-Radiation has low energy deposition and up to 400 traverses of a cell by a β-particle are needed to destroy it. However, they have a millimetre range which increases with the β-energy: for ^{131}I up to 2 mm, so that heterogeneous uptake of antibody by tumour could allow the radiation of adjacent cells; and for ^{90}Y up to 10 mm, allowing action over some spacial separation of clumps of cells provided a sufficient activity can be taken up by the tumour (Humm, 1986; Humm and Cobb, 1990).

The currently available antibodies are against tumour-associated and not tumour-specific antigens, so the uptake by normal tissues for a therapeutic approach is a major drawback. After intravenous injection the percentage uptake of the administered dose by the tumour is very small, usually less than 1%, depending on tumour size and between 0.01 and 0.0001% per gram, so that over 99% of the activity is irradiating normal tissues.

Thus, the therapeutic ratios for intravenously administered ^{131}I-labelled monoclonal antibody are generally low and cannot yet be used to justify the intravenous route for RIT of solid tumours (Vaughan *et al.*, 1986). Some lymphomata (De Nardo *et al.*, 1987) and childhood neuroblastomas are exceptions. Uptakes of up to 7% of intravenously administered ^{131}I-labelled UJ13A anti-neural crest antibody have been demonstrated in neuroblastoma (Goldman *et al.*, 1984). If the upper limit of whole-body dose that is acceptable is taken as 2 Gy, then the absorbed dose to a typical solid tumour will be subtherapeutic. For this reason the intracavity or regional approach is preferred.

Intraperitoneal therapy with ^{131}I-labelled HMFG2 or HI7E2 for ovarian cancer presenting as peritoneal seedlings with ascites after full conventional chemotherapy has been applied and is being evaluated (Hammersmith Oncology Group, 1984). Initial enthusiasm is being tempered with findings that uptake of non-specific antibody may sometimes be similar, but ratios of specific to non-specific antibody uptake of 2:1 to 10:1 are more usual. However, high uptake of specific antibody has been confirmed in malignant cells in the ascitic fluid and in superficial peritoneal malignant cells (Ward *et al.*, 1986; Colcher *et al.*, 1987b) but kinetic studies comparing intravenous and intraperitoneal simultaneous administration of the same antibody labelled with different radionuclides shows, on analysis of surgical specimens, that subserosal tumours receive at least 50% of their antibody uptake via the blood supply after the antibody has been absorbed into the circulation from the peritoneal fluid (Ward *et al.*, 1987).

The critical test of making a comparison with the earlier non-specific agents such as ^{199}Au has not yet been performed. Similar approaches have been made to malignant pleural or pericardial effusions. In colon cancer the treatment of liver metastases by intra-arterial infusion of ^{131}I anti-CEA is under study (Delaloye *et al.*, 1985) as well as intraperitoneal administration of ^{131}I-labelled AUAI, anti-colon membrane antibody, for peritoneal spread with ascites. ^{131}I-labelled antiferritin is being assessed for therapy in hepatoma (Order, 1982). For glioma, introduction of ^{131}I-labelled UJ13A via the cerebrospinal fluid has been described (Coakham *et al.*, 1986) and ^{131}I-labelled H17E2 given by intra-arterial infusion is being undertaken (Hooker *et al.*, 1985). Work is in progress on alternative β-emitters: ^{90}Y (Hnatowich *et al.*, 1985; Despande *et al.*, 1990), and ^{109}Pd (Fawwaz *et al.*, 1984) for antibody labelling. The lymphatic route is also being considered for cancer therapy. All these approaches attempt to improve the therapeutic ratio of specific to non-specific uptake and increase the amount of specific uptake, so an adequate irradiation dose is achieved. Since the smaller the tumour, the greater the proportion of specific to non-specific uptake of monoclonal antibody, the aim should be to sterilize the small tumour deposits (less than 2 cm diameter) and not attempt to tackle the clinically and radiologically evident larger masses. The problem of determining accurate dosimetry remains considerable, however.

20.9.1 TECHNIQUE OF INTRAPERITONEAL THERAPY

The preparation of radiolabelled antibody for therapy demands a high degree of skill to meet the requirements of both the sterility and radiation safety. The labelled antibody must be used within 2 h because of progressive radiolysis and loss of immunoreactivity due to the radionuclide's β-emission. The recoil of α-emitters makes the stable labelling of antibodies very difficult.

For ^{131}I labelling the rapid, highly efficient technique using *N*-bromosuccinic acid avoids the need to separate free iodine using a column (Mather and Ward, 1987). For ^{90}Y a similar technique to that for ^{111}In uses a bifunctional chelate (Hnatowich *et al.*, 1985).

For iodine therapy, potassium iodide 60 mg b.d. is given for two days before and for four weeks during the treatment. After a full explanation to the patient and signed consent has been obtained, the patient is transferred to the designated therapy side ward. Under local anaesthesia using an aseptic technique, a Hickman intravenous cannula is introduced into the peritoneal cavity and secured with a suture. In the absence of ascites, 1 l of sterile peritoneal dialysis fluid is suspended above the patient on a stand and is instilled by gravity feed and the system is tested for leaks. Wearing appropriate protective clothing, the radiolabelled antibody in a shielded vial has a needle inserted, below the fluid level, connecting it to the peritoneal catheter and another inserted above the fluid level connecting it to a suspended 1 l bag of dialysis fluid. By gravity feed, the radiolabelled antibody is forced out of the vial and into the peritoneum. If ascites is present, this is first drained off as far as possible and the same procedure adopted. The appropriate instructions for handling a patient containing a radioactive therapy dose are issued to the nursing staff and visitors as for radioiodine therapy of thyroid cancer. The patient is monitored daily. Whole-body counting and abdominal imaging are undertaken on the third or fourth and seventh days after administration.

Results

The effects of intraperitoneal therapy in ovarian cancers are not yet satisfactory. Malignant ascites can be treated and recurrence of ascites prevented or delayed. After second-look operation reduction of residual tumour to under 2 cm diameter masses followed by intraperitoneal RIT appears to cause resolution in perhaps 10%, partial remission in about 15% and no benefit in 75%. Tumour masses over 2 cm in diameter are not successfully treated by RIT (Epenetos, 1987).

Selection of patients is difficult and depends therefore on the demonstration of minimal residual disease by second-look laparotomy, laparoscopy or by RIS with kinetic analysis. The isolation of the patient has to be discussed and the side effects are not negligible, particularly if tumour involves the gastrointestinal tract. Oesophagitis, small intestinal radiation damage and recto-vaginal fistulae have occurred in our experience. Nevertheless in a few selected cases RIT has a place to play at present. The use of more avid and selective antibodies, more effective labelling and labelling methods, and a better understanding of the biological and immunological factors involved should lead to greater success in the future. Perhaps the key to success is in damaging the tumour cell sufficiently to alter its immunological nature, while sparing the immune system, which is usually damaged by chemotherapy, so that an adequate host response may be mounted against the cancer.

The new approach under evaluation reduces the irradiation of normal tissues through a three-stage process using biotin antibody/avidin/biotin radionuclide (Paganelli *et al.*, 1990), or a two-stage process with a bifunctional, bispecific antibody; one hypervariable region reacting with the tumour and the other with the radiotherapy ligand. The bispecific antibody labelled with ^{99m}Tc or ^{111}In to prove uptake is injected first and binds to the tumour. Unbound antibody clears to the reticuloendothelial system and is metabolized. A few days later the radiotherapy ligand is injected and binds to the tumour. Unbound ligand is excreted through the kidneys. By using a long-lived radionuclide such as ^{32}P ($T_{1/2}$ 14 days β 1.71 MeV) the tumour is irradiated. With metabolism and release of ^{32}P locally, it is taken up by cytoplasm and DNA of the dividing cells increasing its radiotherapeutic effect. Systemic effects are reduced by giving effervescent phosphate (Sandoz) orally. The advantage of a long-lived radionuclide such as ^{32}P is greater irradiation of the tumour to compensate for the difficulties in increasing the amount of antibody bound to the tumour (Britton, 1991).

REFERENCES

Arklie, J. (1981) Studies of the human epithelial cell surface using monoclonal antibodies, D. Phil. thesis, University of Oxford.

Baum, R. P., Hertel, A., Lorenz, M. *et al.* (1989) ^{99m}Tc-labelled anti-CEA monoclonal antibody for tumour immunoscintigraphy: first clinical results. *Nucl. Med. Commun.*, **10**, 345–50.

Beatty, J. D., Duda, R. B., Williams, L. E. *et al.* (1986) Preoperative imaging of colorectal carcinoma with 111-In-labelled anticarcino-embryonic antigen monoclonal antibody. *Cancer Res.*, **46**, 6494–502.

Begent, R. H. J. (1986) Working party on clinical use of antibodies. *Br. J. Cancer*, **54**, 557–68.

Begent, R. H. J., Keep, P. A., Green, A. J. *et al.* (1983) Liposomally entrapped second antibody improves

tumour imaging with radiolabelled (first) anti-tumour antibody. *Lancet*, **ii**, 739–41.
Begent, R. H. J., Bagshawe, K. D., Green, A. J. and Searle, F. (1987) The clinical value of imaging with antibody to human chorio gonadotrophin in the detection of residual chorio carcinoma. *Br. J. Cancer*, **55**, 657–60.
Belitsky, P., Ghose, T., Aquino, J. *et al.* (1978) Radionuclide imaging of metastases from renal cell carcinoma by 131-I labelled anti-tumour antibody. *Radiology*, **126**, 515–17.
Berche, C., Mach, J.-P., Lumbroso, J. D. *et al.* (1982) Tomoscintigraphy for detecting gastrointestinal and medullary thyroid cancers: first clinical results using radiolabelled monoclonal antibodies against carcinoembryonic antigen. *Br. Med. J.*, **285**, 1447–51.
Bergmann, J. F., Lumbroso, J. D., Manil, L. *et al.* (1987) Radiolabelled monoclonal antibodies against alphafeto protein for *in vivo* localization of human hepato cellular carcinoma by immunotomoscintigraphy. *Eur. J. Nucl. Med.*, **13**, 385–90.
Blaquiere, R. M. and Husband, J. F. (1983) Conventional radiology and computed tomography in ovarian cancer. *J. R. Soc. Med.*, **76**, 574–9.
Bloomer, W. D., McLaughlin, W. H., Lambrecht, R. M. *et al.* (1984) 211-At radiolabelled therapy: further observations with radiocolloids of 32-P 165-Dy and 90-Y. *Int. J. Radiat. Oncol. Biol. Phys.*, **10**, 341–8.
Bomanji, J., Garner, A., Prasad, J. *et al.* (1987a) Characterization of ocular melanoma with cutaneous melanoma antibodies. *Br. J. Ophthalmol.*, **71**, 647–50.
Bomanji, J., Hungerford, J. L., Granowska, M. and Britton, K. E. (1987b) Radioimmunoscintigraphy of ocular melanoma with 99-Tc-m labelled cutaneous melanoma antibody fragments. *Br. J. Ophthalmol.*, **71**, 651–8.
Britton, K. E. (1991) Overview of radioimmunotherapy. *Ant. Immunoconj. Radiopharm.*, (in press).
Britton, K. E. and Granowska, M. (1987a) Radioimmunoscintigraphy in tumour identification. *Cancer Surveys*, **6**, 247–67.
Britton, K. E. and Granowska, M. (1987b) in *Radiolabelled Monoclonal Antibodies for Imaging and Therapy: Potential, Problems and Prospects* (ed. S. R. Srivastava), NATO Advanced Science Institute, Barga, 1986, Plenum Press, New York.
Britton, K. E. and Granowska, M. (1988) Radioimmunoscintigraphy: a way ahead. *Nucl. Med. Commun.*, **9** (in press).
Britton, K. E., Granowska, M., Mather, S. and Nimmon, C. C. (1985) in *Immunoscintigraphy* (*Monographs in Nuclear Medicine*, Vol. I) (eds L. Donato and K. E. Britton) Gordon and Breach, London, pp. 51–66.
Buraggi, G. L. (1986) in *Multicentre Study of Immunoscintigraphy of Melanoma* (Coordinator A. G. Siccardi), National Tumour Institute, Milan, p. 50.
Buraggi, G. L., Turrin, A., Cascinelli, N. *et al.* (1985) in *Immunoscintigraphy* (eds L. Donato and K. E. Britton), Gordon and Breach, London, pp. 215–53.
Calkins, A. R., Stehman, F. B., Wass, J. L. *et al.* (1987) Pitfalls in interpretation of computed tomography prior to second look laparotomy in patients with ovarian cancer. *Br. J. Radiol.*, **60**, 975–9.
Carrasquillo, J. A., Bunn, P. A., Keenan, A. M. *et al.* (1986) Radioimmunodetection of cutaneous T-cell lymphoma with 111-In-labelled T101 monoclonal antibody. *New Engl. J. Med.*, **315**, 673–80.
Chan, S. and Sikora, K. (1987) The potential of oncogene products as tumour markers. *Cancer Surveys*, **6**, 185–207.
Chatal, J. F., Saccavini, J. C., Furnoleau, P. *et al.* (1984) Immunoscintigraphy of colon carcinoma. *J. Nucl. Med.*, **25**, 307–14.
Coakham, H. B., Richardson, R. B., Davies, A. G. *et al.* (1986) Antibody guided radiation therapy via the CSF for malignant meningitis. *Lancet*, **ii**, 860–1.
Colcher, D., Esteban, J. M. Carrasquillo, J. A. *et al.* (1987a) Quantitative analyses of selective radiolabelled monoclonal antibody localisation in metastastic lesions of colorectal cancer patients. *Cancer Res.*, **47**, 1185–9.
Colcher, D., Esteban, J., Carrasquillo, J. A. *et al.* (1987b) Complementation of intracavity and intravenous administration of a monoclonal antibody (B72.3) in patients with carcinoma. *Cancer Res.*, **67**, 4218–24.
Critchley, M., Brownless, S., Pattern, M. *et al.* (1986) Radionuclide imaging of epithelial ovarian tumours with ^{123}I-labelled monoclonal antibody (H317) specific for placental-type alkaline phosphatase. *Clin. Radiol.*, **37**, 107–12.
Delaloye, B., Bischof-Delaloye, A., Volant, J. C. *et al.* (1985) First approach to therapy of liver metastases in colorectal carcinoma by intrahepatically infused 131-I labelled monoclonal anti-CEA antibodies. *Eur. J. Nucl. Med.*, **11**, All.
De Nardo, S. J., De Nardo, G. L., O'Grady, L. F. *et al.* (1987) Treatment of a patient with B cell lymphoma by I-131 LYM-1 monoclonal antibodies. *Int. J. Biol. Mark.*, **2**, 49–53.
Despande, S. V., De Nardo, S. J., Kukis, D. L. *et al.* (1990) Yttrium-labelled monoclonal antibody for therapy: labelling by a new macrocycle bifunctional chelating agent. *J. Nucl. Med.*, **31**, 473–9.
Epenetos, A. A. (1987) Antibody guided diagnosis and therapy. *Br. J. Cancer*, **86**, 517.
Epenetos, A. A., Mather, S., Granowska, M. *et al.* (1981) Targetting of iodine-123-labelled tumour-associated monoclonal antibodies to ovarian, breast and gastrointestinal tumours. *Lancet*, **ii**, 999–1004.
Epenetos, A. A., Snook, D., Rawlinson, F. and Hooker, G. (1986a) Prospects for antibody targeted radiotherapy of cancer. *Lancet*, **ii**, 579–80.
Epenetos, A. A., Carr, D., Johnson, P. M. *et al.* (1986b) Antibody guided radiolocalisation of tumours in patients with testicular or ovarian cancer using two radioiodinated monoclonal antibodies to placental alkaline phosphatase. *Br. J. Radiol.*, **59**, 117–25.
Fairweather, D. S., Bradwell, A. R., Watson-James, S. F. *et al.* (1983) Detection of thyroid tumours using radiolabelled antithyroglobulin. *Clin. Endocrinol.*, **18**, 563–70.
Fawwaz, R. A., Wang, T. S. T., Srivastava, S. C. *et al.* (1984) Potential of palladium-109 labelled antimelanoma monoclonal antibody for tumour therapy *J. Nucl. Med.*, **25**, 796–9.
Galfre, G. and Milstein, C. (1981) Preparation of monoclonal antibodies: strategies and procedures. *Methods Enzymol.*, **73B**, 1–46.
Goldenberg, D. M., Kim, E. E., Deland, F. H. *et al.*

(1980) Radio-immunodetection of cancer with radioactive antibodies to carcinoembryonic antigen. *Cancer Res.*, **40**, 2984–92.

Goldman, A., Vivian, G., Gordon, I. *et al.* (1984) Immunolocalisation of neuroblastoma using radiolabelled monoclonal antibody UJ13A. *J. Paediatr.*, **105**, 252–6.

Granowska, M. and Britton, K. E. (1987) in *Radioaktiv Isotope in Klinik and Forschung*, Vol. 17 (*Gasteiner International Symposium 1986*, Vol. 17) (ed. R. Hofer and H. Bergmann), Ergman-Verlag, Vienna, pp. 377–81.

Granowska, M., Britton, K. E. and Shepherd, J. (1983) The detection of ovarian cancer using 123-I monoclonal antibody. *Radiobiol. Radiother. (Berlin)*, **25**, 153–160.

Granowska, M., Shepherd, J., Britton, K. E. *et al.* (1984) Ovarian cancer: diagnosis using 123-I monoclonal antibody in comparison with surgical findings. *Nucl. Med. Commun.*, **5**, 485–99.

Granowska, M., Britton, K. E., Shepherd, J. H. (1986a) A prospective study of 123-I-labelled monoclonal antibody imaging in ovarian cancer. *J. Clin. Oncol.*, **4**, 730–6.

Granowska, M., Britton, K. E., Crowther, M. *et al.* (1987) in *Radiolabelled Monoclonal Antibodies for Imaging and Therapy: Potential, Problems and Prospects* (ed. S. R. Srivastava), NATO Advanced Science Institute, Barga, 1986, Plenum Press, New York.

Granowska, M., Jass, J. R., Britton, K. E. *et al.* (1988a) A prospective study of the use of In-111 labelled anti-carcinoembryonic antigen, CEA, in colorectal cancer and of some biological factors affecting its uptake. *Int. J. Colorect. Dis.*, **4**, 97–108.

Granowska, M., Mather, S. J., Jobling, T. *et al.* (1990a) Radiolabelled stripped mucin, SM3, monoclonal antibody for immunoscintigraphy of ovarian tumours. *Int. J. Biol. Mark.*, **5**, 89–96.

Granowska, M., Mather, S. J., Britton, K. E. *et al.* (1990b) ^{99m}Tc radioimmunoscintigraphy of colorectal cancer. *Br. J. Cancer*, **62**, Suppl. X, 30–3.

Granowska, M., Nimmon, C. C., Britton, K. E. *et al.* (1988b) Kinetic analysis and probability mapping applied to the detection of ovarian cancer by Radioimmunoscintigraphy. *J. Nucl. Med.*, **29**, 599–607.

Green, A. J., Begent, R. H. J., Keep, P. A. and Bagshawe, K. D. (1984) Analysis of radioimmunodetection of tumours by the subtraction technique. *J. Nucl. Med.*, **25**, 96–100.

Halpern, S. E., Dillman, R. O. and Witztium, K. F. (1985) Radioimmunodetection of melanoma utilizing ^{111}In-96.5 monoclonal antibody. *Radiology*, **155**, 493–9.

Hammersmith Oncology Group (1984) Antibody guided irradiation of malignant lesions: three cases illustrating a new method of treatment. *Lancet*, **i**, 1441–3.

Hnatowich, D. J., Childs, R. L., Lanteigne, D. and Najafi, A. (1983) The preparation of DTPA-coupled antibodies radiolabelled with metallic radionuclides: an improved method. *J. Immunol. Methods*, **65**, 147–57.

Hnatowich, D. J., Virzi, F. and Doherty, P. W. (1985) DTPA coupled antibodies labelled with yttrium-90. *J. Nucl. Med.*, **26**, 503–9.

Hooker, G., Snook, D., Pickering, D. *et al.* (1985) Antibody guided irradiation of brain gliomas. *Eur. J. Nucl. Med.*, **11**, All.

Humm, J. L. (1986) Dosimetric aspects of radiolabelled antibodies for tumour therapy. *J. Nucl. Med.*, **27**, 1490–7.

Humm, J. L. and Cobb, L. M. (1990) Non uniformity of tumour dose in radioimmunotherapy. *J. Nucl. Med.*, **31**, 75–83.

James, K. and Bell, G. T. (1987) Human monoclonal antibody production: current status and future prospects. *J. Immunol. Methods*, **100**, 5–40.

Kaplan, E., Ben-Porath, M., Fink, S. *et al.* (1966) Elimination of liver interference from the selenomethionine pancreas scan. *J. Nucl. Med.*, **7**, 807–9.

Khan, O., Cosgrove, D. O., Wiltshaw, E. *et al.* (1983) Role of ultrasound in the management of ovarian carcinoma. *J. R. Soc. Med.*, **76**, 821–7.

Kohler, G. and Milstein, C. (1975) Continuous cultures of fused cells secreting antibody of proven defined specificity. *Nature*, **256**, 495–7.

Larson, S. M., Brown, J. P., Wright, P. W. *et al.* (1983) Imaging of melanoma with I-131-labelled monoclonal antibodies. *J. Nucl. Med.*, **24**, 123–9.

Levenson, S. H., Wiggins, P. A., Nasim, T. A. *et al.* (1983) Improved detection of hepatic metastases by the use of dynamic flow scintigraphy. *Br. J. Cancer*, **47**, 719–21.

Liehn, J.-C. (1987) in *Radiolabelled Monoclonal Antibodies for Imaging and Therapy: Potential, Problems and Prospects* (ed. S. R. Srivastava), NATO Advanced Science Institute, Barga, 1986, Plenum Press, New York.

Liehn, J. C., Hannequin, P., Nasea, S. *et al.* (1987) A new approach to image subtraction in immunoscintigraphy: preliminary results. *Eur. J. Nucl. Med.*, **13**, 391–6.

Mach, J. P., Carrel, S., Forni, M. *et al.* (1980) Tumour localisation of radiolabelled antibodies against carcinoembryonic antigen in patients with carcinoma. *New Engl. J. Med.*, **303**, 5–10.

Mach, J. P., Chatal, J. F., Lumbruso, J. D. *et al.* (1983) Tumour localisation in patients by radiolabelled monoclonal antibodies against colon cancer. *Cancer Res..*, **43**, 5593–600.

Mason, D. Y., Naiem, M. Abdulaziz, Z. *et al.* (1985) in *Monoclonal Antibodies in Clinical Medicine* (eds A. J. McMichael and J. W. Fabre) Academic Press, London, pp. 585–635.

Mather, S. J. and Ellison, D. (1990) Reduction mediated Technetium 99m-labelling of monoclonal antibodies. *J. Nucl. Med.*, **31**, 692–7.

Mather, S. J. and Ward, B. (1987) High efficiency iodination of monoclonal antibodies for radiotherapy. *J. Nucl. Med.*, **28**, 1034–7.

Order, S. E. (1982) Monoclonal antibodies: potential role in radiation therapy and oncology. *Int. J. Radiat. Oncol. Biol. Phys.*, **8**, 1193–201.

Ott, R. J., Grey, L. J., Zivanovic, M. A. *et al.* (1983) Limitations of dual radionuclide subtraction technique for detection of tumours by radioiodine labelled antibodies. *Br. J. Radiol.*, **58**, 101–8.

Paganelli, G., Malcovati, M., Fazio, F. (1990) Monoclonal antibody pretargeting techniques for tumour localization: the avidin-biotin system. *Nucl. Med. Commun.* (in press).

Pateisky, N., Philipp, K., Skodler, W. D. *et al.* (1985) Radioimmunodetection in patients with suspected ovarian cancer. *J. Nucl. Med.*, **26**, 1369–76.

Perkins, A. C., Armitage, N. C., Hardy, J. G. *et al.* (1984) Immunoscintigraphy of bone tumours using an 131-I-labelled antiosteosarcoma monoclonal antibody. *Nucl. Med. Commun.*, **5**, 539 (abstr.).

Rainsbury, R. M., Ott, R. J., Westwood, J. H. *et al.* (1983) Location of metastatic breast carcinoma by a monoclonal antibody chelate labelled with Indium-111. *Lancet*, **ii**, 934–48.

Riva, P., Paganelli, G., Riceputi, G. *et al.* (1986) Radioimmunodetection of lung cancer by means of an anti-CEA monoclonal antibody. *J. Nucl. Med.*, **27**, 881 (abstr.).

Schwarz, A., Steinstraesser, A. (1987) A novel approach to ^{99m}Tc-labelled monoclonal antibodies. *J. Nucl. Med.*, **28**, 721.

Shepherd, P. S., Lazarus, C. R., Mistry, R. D. and Maisey, M. N. (1985) Detection of thyroid tumour using a monoclonal ^{123}I anti-human thyroglobulin antibody. *Eur. J. Nucl. Med.*, **10**, 291–5.

Siccardi, A. G., Buraggi, G. L., Callegaro, L. *et al.* (1986) Multicentre study of immunoscintigraphy with radiolabelled monoclonal antibodies in patients with melanoma. *Cancer Res.*, **46**, 4817–22.

Steward, M. W. and Steensgaard, J. (1983) *Antibody Affinity: Thermodynamic Aspects and Biological Significance*, CRC Press, Boca Raton.

Van Kroonenburgh, M. J. P. G. and Pauwels, E. K. J. (1988) Human immunological response to mouse monoclonal antibodies in the treatment and diagnosis of malignant disease. *Nucl. Med. Commun.*, **9** (in press).

Vaughan, A. T. M., Bradwell, A. R., Dykes, P. W. and Anderson, P. (1986) Illusions of tumour killing using radiolabelled antibodies. *Lancet*, **i**, 1492–3.

Vihko, P., Heikkila, J., Kontturi, M. (1984) Radioimaging of the prostate and metastases of prostatic carcinoma with 99-Tc-m labelled prostatic acid phosphatase specific antibodies and their Fab fragments. *Ann. Clin. Res.*, **16**, 51–2.

Wahl, R. L., Parker, C. W. and Philpott, G. (1983) Improved radioimaging and tumour localisation with monoclonal (Fabl) 2. *J. Nucl. Med.*, **24**, 316–25.

Ward, B. G., Mather, S. J., Shepherd, J. H. *et al.* (1986) Prospects for antibody targeted radiotherapy of cancer. *Lancet*, **ii**, 580–1.

Ward, B. G., Mather, S. J., Hawkins, L. *et al.* (1987) Localisation of radioiodine conjugated to the monoclonal antibody HMFG2 in human ovarian cancer: assessment of intravenous and intraperitoneal routes of administration. *Cancer Res.*, **47**, 4719–23.

Weir, D. M. (ed.) (1978) *Handbook of Experimental Immunology*, 3rd edn, Blackwell Scientific Publications, Oxford.

CHAPTER TWENTY-ONE

Lymph node scanning

R. F. Jewkes

21.1 INTRODUCTION

The lymphatic system is not easily investigated. Until 1955 when Kinmonth *et al.* (1955) introduced radiographic lymphangiography, its anatomy could only be demonstrated by biopsy and its physiology could not be demonstrated at all. In the 1960s a more aggressive therapeutic attack on primary and secondary malignancies led to widespread use of lymphangiography and its results were impressive. It demonstrates an otherwise inaccessible system of the body with very high resolution so that nodes can be seen in considerable detail. Its obvious advantages hide its less obvious disadvantages, which are sufficiently great to justify pursuing radionuclide lymph node scanning as a possible alternative. The disadvantages of radiographic lymphangiography might be listed as follows:

1. It is invasive and requires considerable patient cooperation or at least tolerance. The test is not readily repeated.
2. It requires technical expertise and a considerable investment of time.
3. In spite of the detail it reveals, any series still contains a substantial number of false-positive, false-negative and inconclusive results (Brown *et al.*, 1979).
4. The process is non-physiological.
5. Degenerative changes have been reported in lymph nodes following radio-contrast administration (Kazem *et al.*, 1971; McIvor, 1980).
6. There are a number of adverse reactions and complications, though these may be rendered infrequent with care.

Radionuclide lymph scans (lymphoscintigraphy) have probably been undervalued. This was initially because much of the original published work was carried out using ^{198}Au, which was not a very satisfactory radiopharmaceutical. With modern agents there has been marked improvement in the quality of the images but they continue to be underused owing to the prominence of radiographic lymphangiography.

There is also a great dependence on ultrasound and computed tomography (CT) scanning to evaluate the lymphatic system. These require recognizable node enlargement to identify abnormality. It is well known that nodes may be replaced with tumour without being enlarged. Also elongation of nodes is difficult to recognize on transverse sections. These techniques also fail to provide evidence as to the functional integrity of the system. In the relatively uncomplicated situation of the parasternal nodes, CT scanning has been unfavourably compared to internal mammary lymphoscintigraphy (Collier *et al.*, 1983). Unfortunately no systematic comparison of techniques seems to have been carried out for other regions.

The extreme simplicity of the radionuclide scan is a great merit and it is probably adequate for the investigation of many cases with much saving in time and effort. The technique depends on normal lymphatic drainage. If a radioactive colloid is injected interstitially in the drainage area of a group of nodes, it will enter the lymphatic channels and be concentrated in the lymph nodes. This concentration has been shown to depend on phagocytosis and not merely passive physical filtration (Cox, 1974). It is important that the colloidal particles should be of optimum size, as large particles stay at the site of injection and small particles are not retained in lymph nodes. The first colloid used for this investigation was ^{198}Au (Glassburn *et al.*, 1972). This was an excellent colloid but a very poor radionuclide, as its energy was too great for sensitive delineation of individual lymph nodes, while its powerful β-emission caused an unacceptable radiation dose at the site of the injection. ^{99m}Tc-labelled antimony sulphide colloid (Fairbanks *et al.*, 1972) is the most commonly accepted substitute, injections of 100–500 μCi giving satisfactory images of regional lymph nodes within 1–4 h.

Many other agents have been tried and have their advocates but have failed to gain widespread acceptance. These include ^{99m}Tc-labelled stannous phytate (Ege and Warbrick, 1979), [^{197}Hg]mercuric sulphide colloid (Cox, 1971, 1974), ^{99m}Tc-labelled rhenium sulphide colloid (Stewart *et al.*, 1985), ^{99m}Tc-labelled dextran (Juma *et al.*, 1985), ^{99m}Tc-labelled autologous red cells (Kaplan *et al.*, 1981) and ^{99m}Tc-labelled hydroxyethyl starch (Sadek *et al.*, 1987).

21.2 INVESTIGATION OF LYMPH NODES BELOW THE DIAPHRAGM AND LYMPH DRAINAGE OF THE LOWER LIMBS

A radionuclide lymph node scan of the lower part of the body is shown in Figure 21.1. This was produced in the most common way by bilateral injections of radiocolloid subcutaneously between the first and second toes. Compared with radiographic study definition is poor but an approximately symmetrical distribution of radioactivity is clearly identified in the inguinal, external iliac and para-aortic nodes. There is a faint haze of radioactivity identified in the liver and this is important as it indicates patency of the lymphatic channels. This study was of a patient with a metastasizing fibrosarcoma and shows asymmetry of the inguinal nodes with increased uptake on the right and filling defects on the left.

Figure 21.2 was a case of Hodgkin's disease with abnormal inguinal and external iliac nodes but no abnormality detected higher up in the abdomen. Figure 21.3 was a case of reticulosarcoma with more pronounced changes than in

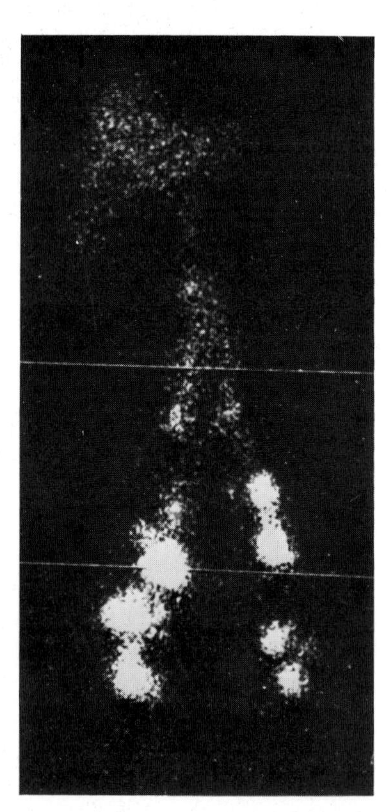

Figure 21.1 Inguinal and abdominal lymphoscintigraphy. Inguinal metastases from fibrosarcoma.

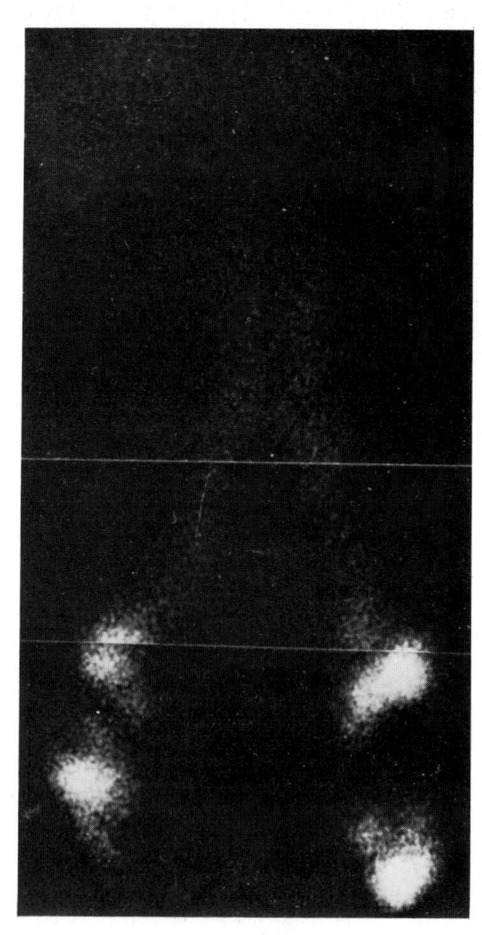

Figure 21.2 Inguinal and abdominal lymphoscintigraphy. Hodgkin's disease with inguinal node involvement.

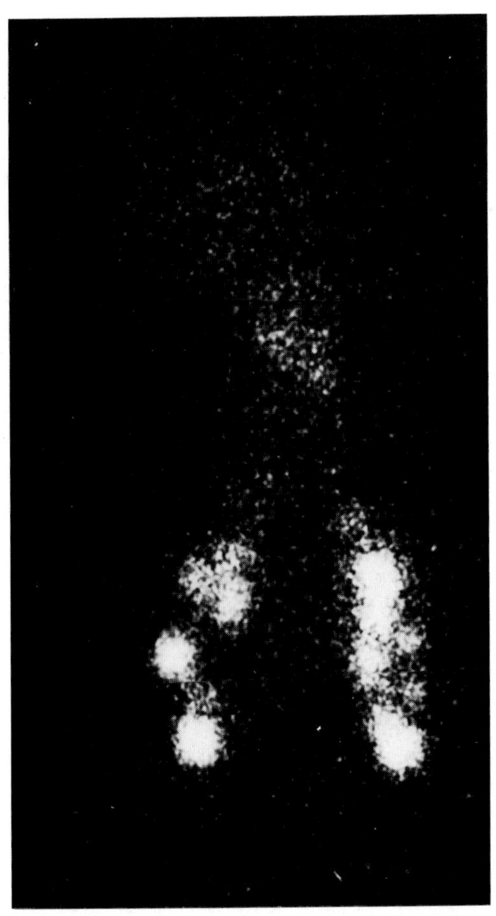

Figure 21.3 Inguinal and abdominal lymphoscintigraphy. Reticulosarcoma with inguinal and abdominal node involvement.

Figure 21.2 and also with abnormal mid-abdominal accumulation of radiocolloid. Figure 21.4 was a case of vaginal carcinoma. The normal anatomy has become almost unrecognizable and the radioactive colloid is widely distributed within abdominal masses.

From this it is possible to discern some criteria of abnormality:

1. A marked asymmetry of distribution of radioactivity due to increased or decreased uptake by lymph nodes;
2. Failure to visualize an expected group of nodes;
3. Breaks in the lymph node chains;
4. Ballooning of lymph node groups;
5. Mottled texture;
6. Absent liver activity.

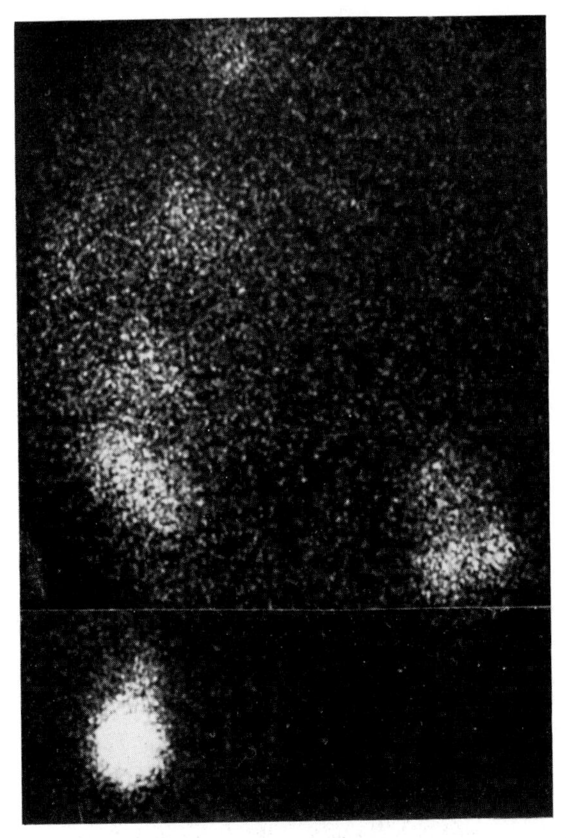

Figure 21.4 Inguinal and abdominal lymphoscintigraphy. Vaginal carcinoma with massive abdominal node involvement.

There remain considerable difficulties, which may also be listed.

1. Normal anatomical variation. The lack of detail makes it possible to be misled by lymph node groups which may be occasionally absent or sparse for no pathological reason.
2. Both 'hot' spots and 'cold' spots can be abnormal. This reflects the fact that filtration by the lymph nodes is an active process and that phagocytes may be both stimulated or depressed or replaced.
3. Any series will have a relatively high percentage of inconclusive studies, perhaps 30%. In such cases it is necessary to resort to other investigations (though there is no guarantee that they will provide a better answer!).
4. Interpretation may be made more difficult by the effect of local infection or X-irradiation.

The advantages which justify continuing interest

in radionuclide lymph scans are, however, very substantial.

1. The test is virtually non-invasive and requires minimal cooperation from the patient. It can easily be done on outpatients.
2. The process is fundamentally physiological. It shows the direction of normal lymph flow rather than the way in which lymph can be made to flow.
3. It is applicable to regions other than the lower half of the body, a most important advantage.
4. It can be repeated frequently if necessary.
5. It requires minimal technical expertise and machine time.

Though lymphoscintigraphy does not provide exactly the same type of information as radiographic lymphangiography, a number of studies have compared the two (Glassburn *et al.*, 1972; Fairbanks *et al.*, 1972; Breit *et al.*, 1969) and, in the majority of patients, perhaps 80%, the final conclusion is the same whichever technique is used. This type of comparison is, however, not definitive as radiographic lymphangiography is not an entirely statisfactory standard. A more correct study would require comparison of lymph node scanning with widespread lymph node biopsy. No such study has been carried out to date.

Both X-ray lymphography and bipedal lymphoscintigraphy fail to show the internal iliac lymph nodes or to give information about the immediate lymphatic drainage from the lower urinary tract or reproductive organs. Some information can be obtained by lymphoscintigraphy using an appropriate site for injection of the radiocolloid. Many sites have been tried in the pelvis but the most satisfactory and the easiest is into the two ischiorectal fossae.

Useful information can be obtained in a high percentage of cases but the technique has not been routinely used. It has been reviewed quite comprehensively (Kaplan, 1983).

21.3 INTERNAL MAMMARY LYMPH NODES

Internal mammary lymph nodes have considerable importance as sites of metastatic malignant disease and there is no other practical method of investigating them. Handley (1975) found in his biopsy series that 20% of all operable breast cancers already had metastases in these nodes, and this percentage rose to 32% for medial and central lesions. The internal mammary chain, particularly on the right, is also responsible for drainage of the peritoneal cavity and the liver and may obtain malignant metastases from these sites.

The technique has been extensively studied by Ege (1977; Ege and Clark, 1985). The test is simple, requiring an injection of radiocolloid into the posterior rectus sheath beside the xiphisternum, with images of the front of the chest being made 2 h later. It is usual to study one side first and then the other, as this sequence identifies drainage patterns which may involve crossover between chains at various possible levels.

The criteria for abnormal nodes are similar to those for nodes seen in the lower part of the body and interpretation may at times be similarly difficult. Recognition of the variability in the numbers of nodes and their position is of importance if radiation is planned, as conventional radiation fields may irradiate non-existent lymph nodes and totally miss those which do exist. The presence of cross-drainage and sometimes the total absence of one or other internal mammary chain may also change the therapeutic approach markedly (Collier *et al.*, 1983).

The results of the test have been shown to have prognostic significance and have been recommended as an element to be taken into consideration in the staging of breast carcinoma (Ege and Clark, 1985).

21.4 AXILLARY NODE SCANNING

Axillary lymph nodes are important sites of metastatic spread and have been investigated by several workers (MacLean and Ege, 1986; Black *et al.*, 1980).

Imaging can be carried out after subcutaneous injection into the breast, but similar results can be obtained by injections into the interdigital regions of the backs of the hands. Unlike the internal mammary system, the axillary lymphatics are a meshwork and the axillary lymph nodes do not lie in a simple chain. Individual nodes cannot be reliably distinguished and abnormal nodes may be proximal to normal nodes. The value of such studies in predicting outcome has been extensively studied (MacLean and Ege, 1986) and shown to be comparable to lymph node histology. There are deficiencies but what is perhaps poorly recognized are the deficiencies of lymph node histology in predicting outcome.

Development of the technique has possibly

been hindered by the surgical accessibility of the axillary lymph nodes. The literature has shown considerable variation in the purpose of different investigators as well as in criteria of interpretation. Until recently routine removal of nodes has seemed to make prior assessment unnecessary. It is possible that more recent surgical conservatism will renew interest in this investigation.

21.5 LYMPHOSCINTIGRAPHY OF CUTANEOUS MALIGNANT MELANOMA

The treatment of malignant melanoma usually requires extensive resection of the lesion followed by excision of draining lymph nodes. There must therefore be correct identification of the routes of drainage. In some situations, for instance the lower limbs, the route is obvious as all lymphatic channels pass to the inguinal nodes. However, in many other sites the route is less constant and this is particularly so in the case of lesions which lie at the boundaries of the conventionally accepted lymphatic drainage territories. In these situations, lymphoscintigraphy has been employed in numerous centres in an effort to display the drainage patterns. Work from four centres has been summarized by Bennett and Lago (1983). Other series have been published by Wanebo *et al.* (1985).

Technique is a simple of variation of what has already been described. The lesion is ringed by small subcutaneous injections of radiocolloid and images of possible drainage areas made up to 3 h later. Lymphatic drainage as so displayed has been shown to correlate well with the location of nodal metastases and to be much superior to assumptions made on the basis of conventional anatomical diagrams. The appearance of the nodes, however, gives no guidance as to the presence or absence of metastases. It is important to study patients before any, or certainly before any extensive, surgery. Surgery is known to alter lymph drainage patterns markedly.

21.6 RADIONUCLIDE LYMPHOGRAPHY

In addition to the investigation of the lymphatics in the assessment of unrelated (usually malignant) disease lymphoscintigraphy has been used to answer questions about the adequacy of the lymphatic system itself (Rijke *et al.*, 1990). Using the same radiopharmaceuticals and sites of injection it is possible to obtain information about the anatomical integrity of the lymphatic system and to estimate flow in the lymphatic channels. This is important mainly in relation to oedematous limbs. Repeated imaging over 3 h with quantification of residual activity at the site of injection and accumulation in the drainage nodes provides an indication of the potential lymphatic contribution to the swelling of affected limbs. The technique is particularly applicable to the paediatric age group because of its simplicity (Sty and Starshak, 1982). It immediately differentiates between venous and lymphatic obstruction (Stewart *et al.*, 1985). Differing patterns of lymphatic inadequacy have been shown to be helpful in identifying patients who may benefit from lymphatic microsurgery (Vaqueiro *et al.*, 1986).

21.7 POTENTIAL NEW RADIOACTIVE AGENTS FOR LYMPHOSCINTIGRAPHY

Some preliminary publications have considered the extension of radiocolloid lymphoscintigraphy by the use of specific anti-tumour antibodies (Thompson *et al.*, 1984). Progress in this direction will depend on the introduction of suitable antibodies and particularly a move away from long-lived radioiodine as the labelling agent, which causes a high radiation dose at the site of injection. This has proved difficult owing to relatively long preparation and separation procedures necessary to provide a product of high specific activity which is not denatured. ^{123}I is a possible substitute for ^{131}I but is less freely available. With other radionuclides it has proved difficult to match the high levels of predictability and reliability routinely achieved with radioiodine, which has been used for protein labelling for 40 years. When these problems have been solved a new field of lymphoscintigraphy will be opened for development.

REFERENCES

Bennett, L. R. and Lago, G. (1983) Cutaneous lymphoscintigraphy in malignant melanoma. *Semin. Nucl. Med.*, **13**, 61–9.

Black, R. B., Merrick, M. V., Taylor, T. V. *et al.* (1980) Prediction of axillary metastases in breast cancer by lymphoscintigraphy. *Lancet*, **ii**, 15–17.

Breit, A., Czempiel, H. and Koernig-Kron, K. (1969) Die lymphszintigraphie in der tumortherapie (Erfah rung an über 800 tumorpatienten). *Strahlen-therapie*, **138**, 74–84.

Brown, R. C., Buchsbaum, H. J., Tewfik, H. H. *et al.* (1979) Accuracy of lymphangiography in the diag-

nosis of paraaortic lymph node metastases from cervical carcinoma. *Obstet. Gynecol.*, **54**, 571–5.
Collier, B. D., Palmer, D. W., Wilson, J. F. *et al.* (1983) Internal mammary lymphoscintigraphy in patients with breast cancer. *Radiology*, **147**, 845–8.
Cox, P. H. (1971) The preparation of mercuric sulphide suspension for lymphatic investigations and the influence of particle size on its physiological properties. *Radioisotopy*, **12**, 997–1010.
Cox, P. H. (1974) The use of radiocolloids for the evaluation of lymphnode function, Doctoral thesis, University of Utrecht, Holland.
Ege, G. N. (1977) Internal mammary lymphoscintigraphy in breast carcinoma: a study of 1072 patients. *Int. J. Radiat. Oncol. Biol. Phys.*, **2**, 755.
Ege, G. N. and Clark, R. M. (1985) Internal mammary lymphoscintigraphy in the conservative management of breast carcinoma: an update and recommendations for a new TMN staging. *Clin. Radiol.*, **36**, 469–72.
Ege, G. N. and Warbrick, A. (1979) Lymphoscintigraphy: A comparison of 99mTc antimony sulphide colloid and 99mTc stannous phytate. *Br. J. Radiol.*, **52**, 124–9.
Fairbanks, V. F., Tauxe, W. N., Kiely, J. M. *et al.* (1972) Scintigraphic visualization of abdominal lymph nodes with 99mTc pertechnetate labelled sulfur colloid. *J. Nucl. Med.*, **13**, 185–90.
Glassburn, J. R., Prasasvinichia, S., Nuss, R. C. *et al.* (1972) Correlation of 198 Au abdominal lymph scan with lymphangiograms and lymph node biopsies. *Radiology*, **105**, 93–6.
Handley, R. S. (1975) Carcinoma of the breast. *Ann. R. Coll. Surg. Engl.*, **57**, 59–66.
Juma, N., Audrey, T. and Ege, G. N. (1985) Comparison as a lymphoscintigraphic agent between 99mTc dextran and 99mTc antimony sulphide colloid. *Br. J. Radiol.*, **58**, 325–30.
Kaplan, W. D. (1983) Iliopelvic lymphoscintigraphy. *Semin. Nucl. Med.*, **13**, 42–53.
Kaplan, W. D., Bloomer, W. D., Jones, A. G. *et al.* (1981) Mediastinal lymphoscintigraphy in ovarian cancer using intra peritoneal autologous technetium-99m-labelled erythrocytes. *Br. J. Radiol.*, **54**, 126–31.
Kazem, I., Nedwick, A., Mortel, R. *et al.* (1971) Comparative histological changes in the normal lymph node following ethiodol lymphography and colloidal gold 198 lymph scanning. *Clin. Radiol.*, **22**, 382–8.
Kimmonth, J. B., Taylor, G. W. and Harper, R. A. K. (1955) Lymphangiography: a technique for its clinical use in the lower limb. *Br. Med. J.* **1**, 940–2.
MacLean, R. G. and Ege, G. M. (1986) Prognostic value of axillary lymphoscintigraphy in breast carcinoma patients. *J. Nucl. Med.*, **27**, 1116–24.
McIvor, J. (1980) Changes in lymph node size induced by lymphography. *Clin. Radiol.*, **31**, 541–4.
Rijke, A. M., Croft, B. Y., Johnson, R. A., Jongste, A. B. and Camps, J. A. (1990) *J. Nucl. Med.*, **31**, (6).
Sadek, S., Dayem, H. A., Owunwanne, A. *et al.* (1987) 99Tc m hydroxyethyl starch: a potential radiopharmaceutical for lymphoscintigraphy. *Nucl. Med. Commun.*, **8**, 395–405.
Stewart, G., Gaunt, J. I., Croft, D. N. *et al.* (1985) Isotope lymphography: a new method of investigating the role of lymphatics in chronic limb oedema. *Br. J. Surg.*, **72**, 906–9.
Sty, J. R. and Starshak, R. J. (1982) Atlas of paediatric radionuclide lymphography. *Clin. Nucl. Med.* **7**, 428–33.
Thompson, C. H., Lichtenstein, M., Stacker, S. A. *et al.* (1984) Immunoscintigraphy for detection of lymph node metastases from breast cancer. *Lancet*, **ii**, 1245–47.
Thornton, A. and Pickering, D. (1985) Abdominal lymphoscintigraphy: an effective substitute for lymphography? *Br. J. Radiol.*, **58**, 603–10.
Vaqueiro, M., Gloviczki, P., Fisher, J. *et al.* (1986) Lymphoscintigraphy in lymphoedema: an aid to microsurgery. *J. Nucl. Med.*, **27**, 1125–30.
Wanebo, H. J., Harpole, D. and Teates, C. D. (1985) Radionuclide lymphoscintigraphy with technetium 99m antimony sulfide colloid to identify lymphatic drainage of cutaneous melanoma at ambiguous sites in the head and neck and trunk. *Cancer*, **55**, 1403–13.

CHAPTER TWENTY-TWO

Clinical applications of positron emission tomography

H. N. Wagner Jr

22.1 INTRODUCTION

Advances in positron emission tomography (PET) make it possible to measure the rate of chemical reactions within the human body. This makes it possible to identify disease at the molecular as well as the cellular level in living human beings. PET imaging is revolutionizing medicine by making it possible for the first time to measure *in vivo* chemistry, expressing the results in absolute units of metres, kilograms and seconds (the MKS system), rather than in relative terms, such as the percentage of the administered dose of radioiodine accumulated by the thyroid, or the amount of thallium-201 in one part of the myocardium compared to another. PET is bringing about a new way of looking at disease, by making it possible to define disease in terms of regional chemistry, measuring regional chemistry in normal persons to provide standards. Then diseases are defined as deviations from the norm by statistical analysis. Although the use of radioactive tracers to measure regional chemistry was first introduced for the study of the thyroid gland with radioactive iodine almost 50 years ago, only recently has the concept been applied widely in the study of other organs, such as the brain and heart. In theory, when we can measure the rate of a chemical process in an organ or part of an organ, there is the possibility of at least two diseases: one in which the rate of the chemical process is abnormally slow, and another in which the process is abnormally fast.

PET imaging provides information about *in vivo* regional chemistry with a sensitivity and specificity comparable to that obtained by radioimmunoassay in studies of body fluids. Other imaging modalities, such as computed tomography (CT) scanning and magnetic resonance imaging (MRI), provide predominantly anatomical information. By measuring regional chemistry, PET can at times detect abnormalities before anatomical changes have occurred, for example, in epilepsy (Engel *et al.*, 1982), Huntington's disease (Kuhl *et al.*, 1982) or cerebrovascular disease (Frackowiak *et al.*, 1983). PET scanning can also help in the care of patients with cancer, by providing information useful in the planning and monitoring of treatment. PET can be used to measure the rate of utilization of important biochemical substrates that supply energy to tumours, such as sugars and amino acids, and in pharmacokinetic and pharmacodynamic studies of cancer chemotherapeutic agents. PET can be used to assess the effectiveness of surgery, radiation and chemotherapy. PET can document the extent of tumours, and progression or regression with different forms of treatment at a time when modifications can be made in the treatment plan. Up to now, treatment has been based primarily on histopathological examination of biopsies; biochemical characterization may be an even better way to classify tumours.

22.2 THE LANGUAGE OF CHEMISTRY

PET helps us to understand the 'chemical language' of the body. The studies fall into three categories: regional blood flow, substrate metabolism, and information transfer. In the latter category, PET makes it possible to identify 'recognition' sites involved in the energy supply to the cell or in regulatory processes, for example, via neurotransmitters and neuroreceptors (Plate 14). Since most drugs act by blocking or stimulating these recognition sites, PET imaging can be used to monitor the effects of drugs on receptors, and show promise in improving the treatment of depression, Parkinson's disease, epilepsy, tardive dyskinaesia, Alzheimer's disease and substance abuse. The use of simple probe detector systems makes it possible to monitor the response of a given patient to drug treatment. Such measurements can increase the effectiveness and decrease the incidence of untoward side effects.

22.3 BRAIN TUMOURS

One of the first uses of PET imaging was measurement of the rate of ^{18}F-fluorodeoxyglucose (FDG) uptake in lesions in the brain seen by CT or MRI after therapy for brain tumours in order to discriminate between recurrence of brain tumour and radiation necrosis (Patronas, 1982). Sebsequently, another substrate, ^{11}C-methionine, began to be used to delineate the boundaries of brain tumours, providing information of value in directing stereotactic biopsy, planning the approach and extent of brain surgery, and permitting differentiation of the metabolizing brain tumour from simple disruption of the blood–brain barrier (Wagner, 1986) (Plate 15).

In some tumours, such as pituitary adenomas, PET imaging can detect the presence of receptors in the tumour. Using the dopamine receptor binding agent ^{11}C-*N*-methylspiperone, it has been possible to classify pituitary adenomas according to whether they possess dopamine receptors (Muhr, 1986). If the tumours contain such receptors, they can be treated chemically rather than surgically, i.e. by administering the dopamine receptor agonist bromocryptine (Plate 16).

Another example of the use of PET to assess the presence of receptors in tumours is breast cancer. ^{18}F-labelled oestradiol accumulation as determined by PET makes it possible to tailor the treatment of a specific patient on the basis of the number of oestrogen and progesterone receptors. A tumour containing oestrogen receptors is more likely to be treated successfully with oestrogen-receptor blocking drugs, such as tamoxifen, than cancers which do not contain oestrogen receptors. The presence of progesterone receptors as well as oestrogen receptors is the best prognostic sign. Radioactive tracers that bind to oestrogen receptors make it possible to assess the status of the primary breast cancer and regional metastatic deposits (Mathias, 1985; Mintun, 1987). This is an example of the new biochemical approach to the characterization of disease, an approach directly related to prognosis and therapy. Histopathology alone need no longer be the only criterion for diagnosis, prognosis and therapy.

22.4 STROKE

Stroke is another disease in which PET/SPECT can aid in the care of the patient. In stroke, metabolic abnormalities seen on PET frequently are more extensive than the corresponding CT findings (Kushner *et al.*, 1987), and the pattern of metabolic abnormalities in PET correlate with the clinical syndrome and with the degree of eventual recovery.

PET imaging provides a powerful method for quantitative, non-invasive measurement of the physiological and biochemical consequences of cerebral ischaemia. In addition to being an important prognostic test, PET imaging can lead to more effective treatment of an individual patient, as well as providing a better understanding of the pathogenesis of the disease.

22.5 DEMENTIA

Dementias fall broadly into two categories: those treated successfully by specific medical means, and those in whom the only treatment consists of supportive care. Thirty per cent of demented elderly patients suffer from impairment of brain blood flow from blocked blood vessels. Another 20% of dementias are caused by diseases for which there are specific treatments, one of the most common being drug intoxication. Older people often take many medicines which singly or in combination can cause dementia. Depression is also common in the elderly and can be associated with increased forgetfulness and confusion. If diagnosed correctly, depression is often treated successfully. Hyper- or hypothyroidism and vitamin B12 deficiency are other causes of dementia which, if recognized, can be treated. Subdural haematomas can lead to dementia and may be the result of unrecognized or minor trauma.

The diagnosis of Alzheimer's disease is usually made by exclusion of the other causes. Because the disease is so progressive, it is important to make the diagnosis in the early stages, which can be made with a 90% accuracy on the basis of clinical and psychological testing in about 50% of the patients who first come to medical attention because of memory loss. Usually, the diagnosis is not made before thousands of dollars have been spent on diagnostic tests.

Alzheimer's disease accounts for about 50% of demented patients. The disease is characterized by abnormally accelerated neuronal death, especially pronounced in the hippocampus, parietal, temporal and, to a lesser degree, frontal lobes. As a result of the neuronal degeneration, there is a secondary loss of blood flow, oxygen and glucose metabolism to the involved regions (Plate 10).

22.6 EPILEPSY

Epilepsy is one of the most common diseases of the brain. Many patients have partial epilepsy, i.e. seizures that begin in a focus, often in the temporal lobe, and then spread over large areas of the cortex. For most patients with partial epilepsy, diagnosis and classification depend on the use of surface electroencephalography (EEG), which records the summation of electrical activity associated with neuronal activity. For the approximately 20% of patients whose seizures are uncontrolled by medication, surgical therapy becomes a possibility if the site of origin of the seizure can be determined. Anatomical imaging techniques such as CT or MRI reveal lesions in only a minority of patients, so that certainty of diagnosis may require intraoperative electrocorticography and chronic direct recordings from stereotaxically implanted depth electrodes. The results are often conflicting, and the procedure is invasive and accompanied by certain risks. PET imaging can provide independent confirmatory information about the site of the epileptogenic lesion.

During focal seizures, brain metabolism and blood flow are increased at the site of onset of the epileptic activity, which spreads as the seizure activity is propagated. Between the seizures (interictal state), both metabolism and blood flow are reduced at the site where the seizures begin. PET was first applied in epilepsy in 1980 (Kuhl, 1980). It was found that PET imaging could localize the focal changes in cerebral metabolism and perfusion and provide unique diagnostic information which would be useful in the management of patients with epilepsy. A variety of examinations have proved to be useful: glucose utilization (FDG), oxygen utilization ($^{15}O_2$), and cerebral perfusion ($^{13}NH_3$ and $^{15}H_2O$).

PET scans made during partial seizures have shown marked increases in local brain metabolism and perfusion at the site of seizure onset, but because of propagated neuronal activity the ictal scans are less useful in predicting epileptic origin than those made during the interictal state (Kuhl, 1980; Engel, 1982, 1983); PET scans made during non-focal seizures showed generalized increase in brain metabolism and perfusion (Kuhl, 1980; Engel, 1982, 1983, 1985; Theodore, 1985). In patients with petit mal seizures, there is a diffuse increase of metabolism at the time of the petit mal seizure.

PET scans made during the interictal state are better in delineating the offending focus from which the seizure originates, rather than measuring the increased regional blood flow or metabolic activity during the seizures themselves. The results of interictal PET scans in patients with partial epilepsy have been compared with the results of CT and EEG in multiple reports (Bernardi, 1983; Chugani, 1984; Depresseux, 1984; Engel, 1981, 1982, 1983, 1984, 1985; Gur, 1982; Kuhl, 1980, 1981, 1983, 1984; Mazziotta, 1984; Newmark, 1981; Ochs, 1984; Sperling, 1985; Szelies, 1983; Theodore, 1983, 1984, 1985, 1986). Similar results were found in the patient series reported from UCLA (Kuhl, 1980; Engel 1982d), from NIH (Theodore, 1983), and from the Montreal Neurological Institute (Ochs, 1984). Approximately 70% of the patients with partial complex epilepsy demonstrate zones of hypometabolism or decreased cerebral blood flow at the site of origin of the seizure. At times, focal abnormalities may be identified with PET even if EEG data do not reveal a clear-cut focus. In such cases, PET is particularly useful in localizing the site. In most cases, however, EEG will verify the site as being the source of the seizures. Furthermore, there has been an excellent correlation between the site of hypometabolism as determined by PET and the presence of a pathological abnormality in the surgical specimen, even in cases where lesions have not been detectable by MRI or CT.

22.7 HEART

While many PET studies of the heart, such as measurements of regional glucose metabolism, involve the use of cyclotron-produced radionuclides, measurements of regional myocardial blood flow can be measured with a tracer available from a generator. Rubidium-82 has a 76 s half-life and is obtained from the parent radionuclide strontium-82, which has a 25-day half-life (Yano *et al.*, 1979). For studies of myocardial blood flow, rubidium-82 is administered in ionic form as it is eluted from the generator (Yano *et al.*, 1981).

Coronary artery disease often is present in persons with no symptoms, although chest pain may be the presenting complaint. The first sign of heart disease in many persons is sudden death. Approximately 60% of patients who have coronary artery disease die suddenly from heart disease or have a myocardial infarction without prior symptoms (Midwall *et al.*, 1982; Reunanen *et al.*, 1983; Kannel and Abbott, 1984; Lown, 1979). The accuracy of exercise thallium-201 imaging for detecting coronary artery disease is approximately 80–90% in symptomatic patients, but is much lower in asymptomatic individuals. Rest–exercise ventricular function studies with technetium-99m tracers have a sensitivity similar to that of ^{201}Tl imaging (Jones *et al.*, 1981). Gould and colleagues have advocated the use of PET imaging with rubidium-82 as a means of screening high-risk patients to detect asymptomatic coronary artery disease. PET scanning has also been used to differentiate damaged from necrotic myocardium in patients with myocardial infarction. This presence of damaged myocardium is an important consideration in selecting patients for revascularization procedures.

Several studies have documented the accuracy of myocardial perfusion imaging with PET in the diagnosis of coronary artery disease (Schelbert *et al.*, 1982; Gould *et al.*, 1986; Tamaki *et al.*, 1985; Deanfield *et al.*, 1984a, 1984b; Deanfield *et al.*, 1986; Selwyn *et al.*, 1982; Camici *et al.*, 1986; Goldstein *et al.*, 1986; Grover-McKay *et al.*, 1986; Selwyn *et al.*, 1985). The patients are examined during supine bicycle exercise (Tamaki *et al.*, 1985) or after intravenous administration of dipyridamole (Gould *et al.*, 1978).

Gould *et al.* have found the sensitivity of PET for diagnosing coronary artery disease is greater than 95% and the specificity is similarly high, even in asymptomatic individuals. PET perfusion studies are more accurate than the non-invasive studies presently being used in the evaluation of patients with suspected coronary artery disease.

Myocardial viability is determined with ^{18}F-FDG (Schwaiger *et al.*, 1986; Marshal *et al.*, 1983; Tillisch *et al.*, Brunken *et al.*, 1986; Schelbert *et al.*, 1982; Schelbert *et al.*, 1983, 1986). One can identify areas that are ischaemic but contain viable myocardium. Although in the fasting state 95% of the energy requirements of the myocardium are normally supplied by fatty acids, ischaemic myocardium shifts from fatty acid to glucose metabolism. ^{18}F-FDG accumulation in ischaemic myocardium is greater than in normally perfused myocardium. In contrast, necrotic myocardium does not accumulate ^{18}F-FDG (Marshal *et al.*, 1983; Tillisch *et al.*, 1986; Brunken *et al.*, 1986). Prior to coronary artery bypass graft surgery, viable myocardium can be characterized as regions of decreased blood flow and increased FDG accumulation. Such regions often have decreased mobility. Myocardial scar is characterized by both decreased regional blood flow and FDG accumulation. In a UCLA study, regional wall motion improved after bypass grafting in 85% of the segments identified as viable by their metabolism of glucose. On the other hand, 96% of segments identified as scar did not improve regional wall motion. In another study of patients with previous infarction, PET studies identified viable myocardium in many segments with fixed defects on ^{201}Tl imaging. In patients with acute infarction, areas of matching decreases in flow and FDG did not recover contractile function. In approximately 50% of segments with FDG accumulation but decreased flow, regional function was improved six weeks later.

REFERENCES

Bernardi, S., Trimble, M. R., Frackowiak, R. S. *et al.* (1983) An interictal study of partial epilepsy using positron emission tomography and the oxygen-15 inhalation technique. *J. Neurol. Neurosurg. Psych.*, **46**, 473–7.

Brunken, R., Tilisch, J., Schwaiger, M. *et al.* (1986) Regional perfusion, glucose metabolism, and wall motion in patients with chronic electrocardiographic Q wave infarcations: evidence for persistence of viable tissue in some infarct regions by positron emission tomography. *Circulation*, **73**, 951–63.

Camici, P., Araujo, L. I., Spinks, T., *et al.* (1986) Increased uptake of 18 F-fluorodeoxyglucose in postischemic myocardium of patients with exercise-induced angina. *Circulation*, **74**, 81–8.

Chugani, H. T., Engel, J. Jr, Mazziotta, J. C. and Phelps, M. E. (1984) ^{18}F-2-fluorodeoxyglucose positron emission topography in medically refractory childhood epilepsy. *Neurol.*, **34**, (Supply 1) 107.

Deanfield, J. E., Kensett, M., Wilson, R. A. (1984) Silent myocardial ischaemia due to mental stress. *Lancet*, **i**, 1001–5.

Deanfield, J. E., Shea, M., Ribiero, P. *et al.* (1984b) Transient ST-segment depression as a marker of myocardial ischemia during daily life, *Am. J. Cardiol.*, **54**, 1195–200.

Deanfield, J. E., Shea, M. J., Wilson, R. A. (1986) Direct effects of smoking on the heart: silent ischemic disturbances of coronary flow. *Am. J. Cardiol.*, **57**, 1005–9.

Depresseux, J. C., Granck, G. and Sadzot, B. (1984) Regional cerebral blood flow and oxygen uptake rate in human focal epilepsy, in *Current Problems in Epilepsy* (eds M. Blady-Moulinier, D. H. Ingvar and B. S. Meldrum) pp. 76–81, John Libby, London.

Engel, J. Jr, Rausch, R., Lieb, J. P. *et al.* (1981) Correlation of criteria used for localizing epileptic foci in patients considered for surgical therapy of epilepsy. *Ann. Neurol.*, **9**, 215–24.

Engel, J. Jr, Kuhl, D. E., Phelps, M. E. and Mazziotta, J. C. (1982) Interictal cerebral glucose metabolism in partial epilepsy and its relation to EEG chantes. *Ann. Neurol.*, **12**, 510–17.

Engel, J. Jr, Kuhl, D. E., Phelps, M. E. and Crandall, P. H. (1982) Comparative localization of epileptic foci in partial epilepsy by PCT and EEG. *Ann. Neurol.*, **12**, 529–37.

Engel, J. Jr (1984) The use of PET scanning in epilepsy. *Ann. Neurol.*, **15**, (Suppl), 5180–5191.

Engel, J. Jr, Lubens, P., Kuhl, D. E. and Phelps, M. E. (1985) Local cerebral metabolic rate for glucose during petit mal absences. *Ann. Neurol.*, **17**, 121–28.

Frackowiak, R. S. F., Wise, R. J. (1983) Positron tomography in ischemic cardiovascular disease. *Neurol. Clin.*, **1**, 183–200.

Goldstein, R. A., Kirkeeide, R., Demer, L. *et al.* (1986) Assessment of coronary flow reserve with quantitative coronary arteriography. *J. Nucl. Med.*, **27**, 943.

Gould, K. L. (1978) Noninvasive assessment of coronary stenosis by myocardial perfusion imaging during pharmacological coronary vasodilation. I. *Am. J. Cardiol.*, **41**, 267–8.

Gould, K. L., Goldstein, R. A., Mullani, N. A. *et al.* (1986) Noninvasive assessment of coronary stenoses by myocardial perfusion imaging during pharmacologic coronary vasodilation. VIII. Clinical feasibility of positron cardiac imaging without a cyclotron using generator-produced rubidium-82. *J. Am. Coll. Cardiol.*, 775–89.

Grover-McKay, M., Schelbert, H. E., Schwaiger, M. *et al.* (1986) Identification of impaired metabolic reserve by atrial pacing in patients with significant coronary artery stenosis. *Circulation*, **74**, 281–92.

Gur, R. C., Sussman, N. M., Alavi, A. *et al.* (1982) Positron emission tomography in two cases of childhood epileptic encephalopathy (Lennox-Gastaut syndrome). *Neurology*, **32**, 1191–4.

Jones, R. H., McEwan, P., Newam, G. E. *et al.* (1981) Accuracy of diagnosis of coronary artery disease by measurement of left ventricular function during rest and exercise. *Circulation*, **64**, 586–601.

Kannel, W. B. and Abbott, R. D. (1984) Incidence and prognosis of unrecognized myocardial infarction. An update on the Framingham study. *N. Engl. J. Med.*, **311**, 1114–47.

Kuhl, D. E., Engel, J. Jr, Phelps, M. E. and Selin, C. (1980) Epileptic patterns of local cerebral metabolism and perfusion in humans determined by emission computed tomography of ^{18}FOG and $^{15}NH_3$. *Ann. Neurol.*, **8**, 348–60.

Kuhl, D. E., Engel, J. Jr and Phelps, M. E. (1983) Emission computed tomography in the study of human epilepsy. *Res. Publ. Assoc. Res. Nerv. Ment. Dis.*, **61**, 327–40.

Kuhl, D. E., Phelps, M. E., Markham, C. E. *et al.* (1983) Cerebral metabolism and atrophy in Huntington's disease determined by FDG and computed tomographic scan. *Ann. Neurol.*, **12**, 425–34.

Kuhl, D. E., Metter, E. J., Riege, W. H. *et al.* (1983) Local cerebral glucose utilization in elderly patients with depression, multiple infarct dementia and Alzheimer's disease. *J. Cereb. Bid. Flow. Met.*, **3**, (Suppl 1), 494–5.

Kuhl, D. E. (1984) Annual Oration 1982: Imaging local brain function with emission computed tomography. *Radiology*, **150**, 625–31.

Kushner, M., Reivich, M., Fieschi, C. *et al.* (1987) Metabolic and clinical correlates of acute ischemic infarction. *Neurology*, **37** (7), 1103–10.

Lown, B. (1979) Sudden cardiac death: The major challenge confronting contemporary cardiology. *Am. J. Cardiol.*, **43**, 313–28.

Marshall, R. C., Tillisch, J. H., Phelps, M. E. *et al.* (1987) Identification and differentiation of resting myocardial ischemia and infarction in man with position computed tomography; F-18 labelled fluorodexyglucose and N-13 ammonia. *Circulation*, **67**, 766–78.

Mathias, C. J., Broadack, J. W., Kilbourn, M. R. *et al.* Biodistribution and metabolism of 16-alpha-(18-F)-fluoro-17-beta-estradiol. *J. Nucl. Med.*, **26**, 127.

Mazziotta, J. C. and Engel, J. Jr (1984) The use and impact of PET scanning in epilepsy. *Epilepsia*, **25** (Suppl 2),s86–s104.

Midwall, J., Ambrose, J., Pichard, A. (1982) Angina pectoris before and after mycardial infarction. *Chest*, **81**, 681–6.

Mintun, M. A., Welch, M. J., Mathias, C. J. *et al.* (1987) Application of 16-alpha-(18-F) fluoro-17-beta estradiol for the assessment of estrogen receptors in human breast carcinoma. *Society of Nuclear Medicine Annual Meeting Abstracts*.

Muhr, C., Bergstrom, M., Lundberg, P. O. *et al.* (1986) Dopamine receptors in pituitary adenomas: PET visualization. *JCAT*, **10**, 175–80.

Newmark, M. E., Theodore, W., DeLaPaz, R. *et al.* (1981) Positron emission tomography in refractory complex partial seizures. *Ann. Neurol.*, **10**, 73–4.

Ochs, R. E., Yamamoto, Y. L., Gloor, R. *et al.* (1984) Correlation between the PET measurement of glucose metabolism and oxygen utilization with focal epilepsy. *Neurol.*, **34** (Suppl 1), 125.

Patronas, N. J., Di Chiro, G., Brooks, R. A. *et al.* (1982) Work in progress. 18-F-fluorodeoxyglucose and PET in the evaluation of radiation necrosis of the brain. *Radiology*, **144**, 885–9.

Reunanen, A., Aromaa, A, Pyorala, K. (1983) Social Insurance Institution's coronary heart disease study: Baseline data and 5-year mortality experience. *Acta Med. Scand.*, Suppl 673, 67–81.

Schelbert, H. R., Henze, E., Phelps, M. E. and Kuhl, D. E. (1982) Assessment of regional myocardial ischemia by positron-emission computed tomography. *Am. Heart J.*, **103**, 588–97.

Schelbert, H. R., Phelps, M. E. and Shina, K. I. (1983) Imaging metabolism and biochemistry – a look at the heart. *Am. Heart. J.*, **105** (3), 522–6.

Schelbert, H. R. (1986) Evaluation of 'metabolic fingerprints' of myocardial ischaemia *Can. J. Cardiol.*, Suppl. A. 121A–30A.

Schwaiger, M., Brunken, R., Grover-McKay, M. *et al.* (1986) Regional myocardial metabolism in patients with acute myocardial infarction assessed by positron emission tomography. *J. Am. Coll. Cardiol.* **8**, 800–8.

Selwyn, A. P., Allan, R. M., L'Abbate, A. L. *et al.* (1982) Relation between regional myocardial uptake of rubidium-82 and perfusion: absolute reduction of cation uptake in ischemia. *Am. J. Cardiol.*, **50**, 112–21.

Selwyn, A. P., Shea, M., Deanfield, J. *et al.* (1985) The character of transient myocardial ischemia: Clinical studies and progress using positron emission tomography. *Inter. J. Card. Imag.*, **1**, 61–72.

Sperling, M. R., Engel, J. Jr, Bradley, W. and Wilson, G. (1985) MRI, PET, and CT in complex partial epilepsy. *Epilepsia*, **26**, 534–5.

Szelies, B., Herholz, K., Heiss, W. D. *et al.* (1983) Hypometabolic cortical lesions in tuberous sclerosis with epilepsy: Demonstration by positron emission tomography. *J. Comput. Assist. Tomogr.*, **7**, 945–53.

Tamaki, N., Yonekura, Y., Senda, M. *et al.* (1985) Myocardial positron computed tomography with ^{13}N-ammonia at rest and during exercise. *Eur. J. Nucl. Med.* **1**, 246–51.

Theodore, W. H., Newmark, M. E., Sato, S. *et al.* (1983) Fluorodeoxyglucose positron emission computed tomography in refractory complex partial seizures. *Ann. Neurol.*, **13**, 419–28.

Theodore, W. H., Brooks, R., Sata, S. *et al.* (1984) The role of positron emission tomography in the evaluation of seizure disorders. *Ann. Neurol.*, **15** (Suppl), s176–9.

Theodore, W. H., Brooks, R., Margolin, R. *et al.* (1985) Positron emission tomography in generalized seizures. *Neurol.*, **35**, 684–90.

Theodore, W. H., Dorwart, R., Holmes, M. *et al* (1986) Neuroimaging in refractory partial seizures. Comparison of PET, CT, and MRI. *Neurol.*, **36**, 60–4.

Tillisch, J., Brunken, R., Marshall, R. *et al.* (1986) Reversibility of cardiac wall-motion abnormalities predicted by positron tomography. *N. Engl. J. Med.*, **314**, 884–8.

Wagner, H. N. (1986) Chemical neurotransmission in man. *Curr. Conc. Diagn. Nucl. Med.*, **3**, 14–18.

Yano, Y., Budinger, T. E., Chiang, G. *et al.* (1979) Evaluation and application of alumina-based Rb-82 generators charged with high levels of Sr-82/85. *J. Nucl. Med.*, **20**, 961–6.

Yano, Y., Cahoon, J. L. and Budinger, T. F. (1981) A precision flow-controlled Rb-82 generator for bolus or constant-infusion studies of the heart and brain. *J. Nucl. Med.*, **22**, 1006–10.

CHAPTER TWENTY-THREE

Radiopharmaceuticals

C. Lazarus

23.1 INTRODUCTION

A radiopharmaceutical can be defined as 'a radioactive material in a form suitable for administration to a human for the purposes of therapy or diagnostic investigation'. The majority of these materials are for diagnostic purposes, and this chapter is mainly concerned with those radiopharmaceuticals which are designed or formulated such that after administration they will localize in the body organ or system under investigation. The radiations from the radionuclide within the body can be detected externally using appropriate equipment and usually an image obtained of the normal or abnormal distribution.

23.2 IDEAL PROPERTIES OF RADIONUCLIDES FOR USE IN MEDICINE

Table 23.1 shows some radionuclides which are commonly used in nuclear medicine, together with their physical properties.

For external imaging of a radionuclide deposited within a body the energy of the γ-rays must be high enough to be detected, but not so high that the radiations cannot be effectively collimated. This means that the energy should be somewhere within the range of 20–400 keV. A radionuclide with a low γ-ray energy of about 30 keV is suitable for the external detection of emissions from a fairly superficial organ such as the thyroid. For organs lying deeper within the body more energetic emissions are required. The ideal radionuclide should emit γ-rays of about 150 keV.

The physical half-life ($t_{1/2}$) of a radionuclide should be such that there is sufficient time to produce the radionuclide and its radiopharmaceutical in a form suitable for human use, transport it to the site of use, administer it to the patient, and obtain the necessary images and data. Cyclotron-produced radionuclides such as ^{11}C ($t_{1/2}$ = 20 min), ^{15}O ($t_{1/2}$ = 2 min) and ^{13}N ($t_{1/2}$ = 10 min) are only available to those departments within a short distance from the cyclotron. Ideally the physical half-life should be only a few hours and not much longer than the time necessary to obtain the data. Radioactivity remaining within the body after the completion of imaging will deliver an undesired radiation dose to the body, without benefit of any useful data. The use of a radionuclide with a fairly short $t_{1/2}$ of minutes or hours enables studies to be repeated at reasonable intervals, when either an intervention can be performed and its effect studied, or the progress of, for example, a transplanted kidney can be observed.

An ideal radionuclide should be readily available, at a reasonable cost, and in a sufficiently high specific activity that the administration of the required dose of radioactivity does not produce a physiological, toxic or pharmacological response. The use of radionuclides with shorter physical $t_{1/2}$ has necessitated the production of the radionuclide at its site of use. Thus the radionuclides ^{99m}Tc ($t_{1/2}$ = 6 h), ^{113m}In ($t_{1/2}$ = 100 min), ^{81m}Kr ($t_{1/2}$ = 13 s), ^{191m}Ir ($t_{1/2}$ = 4.96 s) and ^{195m}Au ($t_{1/2}$ = 30.5 s) are now available from generators located within a nuclear medicine department. Regular elutions from the generator supply sufficient quantities of radionuclide to perform tests in several patients. Although the generators themselves may be costly, the cost per patient can be reduced by taking many patient doses from any one generator. Other radionuclides, such as ^{201}Tl ($t_{1/2}$ = 3.1 days), ^{67}Ga ($t_{1/2}$ = 78.1 h) and ^{111}In ($t_{1/2}$ = 67.4 h) are produced by a more expensive process using a cyclotron. These radionuclides are not always readily available within a department, may have to be obtained specially for a patient, and

Table 23.1 Some radionuclides used in nuclear medicine

Radionuclide	*Principal emissions and energies (keV)*	*Half-life ($t_{1/2}$)*	*Uses*
^{99m}Tc	γ 140	6 h	Widespread organ imaging
^{131}I	γ 364	8.04 d	Thyroid function tests
	β^- 600		Treatment of thyrotoxicosis and thyroid cancer
^{125}I	γ 35, 27	60 d	*In vitro* assays
^{123}I	γ 159	13.3 h	Thyroid tests. Labelling of fatty acids, monoclonal antibodies, proteins
^{67}Ga	γ 91, 185, 300	78.1 h	Localization of infection and some tumours
^{68}Ga	β^+ 1900	68 min	Positron tomography
^{51}Cr	γ 320	27.7 d	Labelled red blood cell studies, gastrointestinal blood and protein loss, glomerular filtration rate
^{75}Se	γ 265	120 d	Adrenal gland imaging
	280		Pancreas imaging
^{201}Tl	X 81	3.1 d	Myocardial visualization, bone tumour imaging
^{81m}Kr	γ 191	13 s	Lung ventilation
^{127}Xe	γ 172, 203, 375	36.4 d	Lung ventilation
^{133}Xe	γ 809	5.3 d	Lung ventilation
^{111}In	γ 171	67.4 h	Cisternography
	245		Platelet labelling
^{113m}In	γ 393	100 min	Brain, liver and blood pool imaging
^{11}C	β^+ 1000	20.4 min	Metabolic and pharmacological studies
^{13}N	β^+ 1200	10 min	Metabolic and pharmacological studies
^{15}O	β^+ 1700	2 min	Blood flow, blood volume and metabolic studies
^{18}F	β^+ 600	110 min	Labelled glucose analogues for regional cerebral blood flow and myocardial metabolism
^{32}P	β^- 1710 (E_{max})	14.3 d	Polycythaemia rubra vera, bone pain therapy
^{89}Sr	β^- 1460 (E_{max})	52.0 d	Bone pain therapy
^{90}Y	β^- 2270 (E_{max})	2.7 d	Intracavity therapy
^{198}Au	β^- 960	2.7 d	Intracavity therapy
^{186}Re	β^- 1070 (E_{max}); γ 137	3.7 d	Bone pain therapy
^{76}Br	β^+ 3700	16.2 h	Brain receptor imaging
^{75}Br	β^+ 1700	98 min	Brain receptor imaging
^{153}Sm	β^- 810, 710, 640; γ 103	46.8 h	Bone therapy
^{109}Pd	β^- E_{max} 1000	13.4 h	Antibody therapy

consequently their cost per patient dose is considerably greater than with the use of generator-produced shorter-lived radionuclides.

It should be possible to formulate the radionuclide into a range of radiopharmaceuticals so that the same radionuclide can be used to study many body organs, the localization occurring by virtue of the alteration in chemical structure or physical form. Thus ^{99m}Tc, ^{113m}In and ^{111}In can be formulated as dozens of different radiopharmaceuticals.

It is also desirable that the radionuclide does not produce any significant waste-disposal problems. With the shorter-lived radionuclides a short period of storage of radioactive waste will be sufficient to reduce the level of radioactivity so that liquids, vials, syringes, etc. can be readily disposed of. Short-lived materials where the $t_{1/2}$ is of the order of seconds or minutes usually present no problem, although radioactive gases such as ^{81m}Kr ($t_{1/2}$ = 13 s) may need to be ducted or blown away from air-cooling inlets of gamma cameras in expired air from patients. The longer-lived radionuclides such as ^{75}Se ($t_{1/2}$ = 120 days) may present some storage problems if they are used in any great quantities.

23.3 DEVELOPMENTS WITH GENERATORS

The radionuclide ^{99m}Tc continues to be the most widespread in use in nuclear medicine. It is produced from the decay of ^{99}Mo and the ^{99}Mo–^{99m}Tc provides a convenient, easily used, cheap and readily available source of ^{99m}Tc, an almost ideal radionuclide for imaging. Several generator systems have been developed which produce very short-lived radionuclides useful in cardiac studies. Gold-195m (^{195m}Au) is a radionuclide with a physical half-life of 30.5 s, allowing first-pass cardiac, lung perfusion and cerebral blood flow investigations, which can be repeated at short intervals of 3–5 min. This radionuclide is constantly formed by decay (electron capture) of mercury-195m (^{195m}Hg) loaded as mercuric nitrate onto a column. The $t_{1/2}$ of ^{195m}Hg is 40.5 h. ^{195m}Au is eluted from the generator with 2 ml of a sodium thiosulphate–sodium nitrate solution. Within 3 min over 98% of ^{195m}Au is regenerated and the generator is ready to be eluted again. The preparation of a ^{195m}Hg–^{195m}Au generator for medical use was described by Bett *et al.* (1981), and its use for sequential first-pass ventriculography was reported by Mena *et al.* (1983). The 262 keV γ-rays emitted by ^{195m}Au in 68% of its decays are suitable for imaging with gamma cameras.

Osmium-191 (^{191}Os) decays to iridium-191m (^{191m}Ir), a radionuclide with a physical half-life of 4.96 s. ^{191m}Ir decays by isomeric transition to stable ^{191}Ir emitting a 129 keV γ-ray. The $t_{1/2}$ of ^{191}Os (15.4 days) is sufficiently long to allow transportation of a generator. The ^{191}Os is loaded onto an anion-exchange column and ^{191m}Ir is eluted with 0.9% sodium chloride solution at pH 1. The very short $t_{1/2}$ of ^{191m}Ir is too short for adult cardiology, but is useful in paediatric cardiology. The generator system was described by Cheng *et al.* (1980).

Ehrhardt *et al.* (1983) reported on a new cadmium-115 (^{115}Cd) indium-115m (^{115m}In) generator. ^{115m}In decays with a physical half-life of 4.5 h emitting γ-rays of 336 keV (45.9%), conversion electrons (300 keV, 49.1%) and β^--particles (840 keV, 5.0%). Parent ^{115}Cd can be produced by neutron irradiation of enriched ^{114}Cd and, as the iodide, is loaded onto an anion-exchange resin column. ^{115m}In is eluted with 0.05 M hydrochloric acid as the chloride. The authors investigated the use of ^{115m}In to label canine platelets and image induced canine thrombus.

Many other generators for the production of short-lived radionuclide have been investigated, and their potential and limitations have been reviewed by Panek (1986). A generator-produced radionuclide which has enormous clinical potential is gallium-68 (^{68}Ga). This positron-emitting radionuclide ($t_{1/2}$ = 68 min) is produced from the decay of germanium-68 (^{68}Ge) and can be eluted from an organic anion-exchange resin column (Neirinckx and Davis, 1980). The $t_{1/2}$ of ^{68}Ge (290 days) gives the generator a long working life of about one year. The commercially available generators of ^{68}Ga are eluted with an ethylenediaminetetraacetic acid (EDTA) solution to give ^{68}Ga-labelled EDTA, which, although suitable for brain and kidney imaging, must be chemically altered for other imaging purposes. Loc'h *et al.* (1980) have described a system which produces ionic ^{68}Ga. By elution of the generator under reduced pressure with tin dioxide/1N hydrochloric acid, ionic ^{68}Ga can be obtained. In this form ^{68}Ga can be used to label a wide range of materials including phosphates, chelating agents, proteins, oxine and colloids.

Yttrium-90 (^{90}Y) has many favourable properties for radioimmunotherapy, and can be produced from its parent ^{90}Sr in a radionuclide generator (Chinol and Hnatowich, 1987). These authors have reported on the use of ^{90}Y labelled to diethylenetriaminepentaacetic acid (DTPA)-coupled antibodies for therapy. The physical half-life of ^{90}Y is 64 h, and is consistent with the rate of antibody accumulation in tumour. The generator consists of a Dowex 50 cation exchange resin onto which is loaded ^{90}Sr ($t_{1/2}$ 28 years). ^{90}Y is eluted with 0.003 M EDTA which is subsequently destroyed and the radioactivity dissolved in 0.05 M

Table 23.2 Some generator systems of clinical interest

Parent radionuclide		*Daughter radionuclide*		*Decay product*
^{99}Mo	$\xrightarrow[2.7\ d]{\beta^-,\gamma}$	^{99m}Tc	$\xrightarrow[6\ h]{IT}$	^{99}Tc
^{113}Sn	$\xrightarrow[118\ d]{EC}$	^{113m}In	$\xrightarrow[1.7\ h]{IT}$	^{113}In
^{81}Rb	$\xrightarrow[4.7\ h]{EC,\beta^+}$	^{81m}Kr	$\xrightarrow[13\ s]{IT}$	^{81}Kr
^{195m}Hg	$\xrightarrow[40.5\ h]{EC}$	^{195m}Au	$\xrightarrow[30\ s]{\gamma}$	^{195}Au
^{191}Os	$\xrightarrow[15.4\ d]{\beta^-}$	^{191m}Ir	$\xrightarrow[4.9\ s]{\gamma}$	^{191}Ir
^{68}Ge	$\xrightarrow[290\ d]{EC}$	^{68}Ga	$\xrightarrow[68\ min]{\beta^+,\gamma}$	^{68}Zn
^{115}Cd	$\xrightarrow[53.4\ h]{\beta^-}$	^{115m}In	$\xrightarrow[4.49\ h]{\beta^-,\gamma}$	^{115}In

IT = isomeric transition; EC = electron capture.

acetate, pH 6. In this form ^{90}Y can be used to label DTPA-coupled proteins at specific activities of 37–111 MBq mg^{-1}.

Some newly developed generator systems of current clinical interest are shown in Table 23.2.

23.4 DEVELOPMENTS WITH RADIOPHARMACEUTICALS

23.4.1 LUNG IMAGING

Radiopharmaceuticals for routine perfusion lung imaging consist of human serum albumin (HSA) particles labelled with ^{99m}Tc. The sizes of the particles should be in the range of 10–100 μm, and can be as microspheres or more commonly as macroaggregates. Preparations of macroaggregates of albumin (MAA) have a wider particle size distribution (10–100 μm) than microspheres (20–50 μm), but are cheaper to buy. Both preparations are commercially available in kit form, and the reconstituted products are stable for 6–8 h.

Developments in radiopharmaceuticals have mostly been for ventilation lung imaging. ^{81m}Kr and ^{133}Xe are still the most widely used radioactive gases, but the problems with availability of ^{81m}Kr generators, and the inconvenience in use of ^{133}Xe, requiring a method of trapping expired radioactive gas, has led to the development of radioactive aerosols. Recently ^{127}Xe has been introduced but, although it offers superior physical characteristics for lung imaging, it suffers from a longer physical half-life ($t_{1/2}$ = 36.4 days), and is far more expensive. Images obtained with radioactive gases are, however, considered superior to those produced with aerosols. This may be due to excessive mucous retention of aerosol droplets affecting their distribution in the lungs, which is not the case with gases.

Images with radioaerosols can be formed from the deposition of aerosol droplets in the lung airways by several mechanisms, including deposition, gravitational sedimentation, Brownian motion, interception and electrostatic precipitation. These mechanisms are reviewed by Pavia *et al.* (1986) and Pillay (1985). Various factors will influence the deposition of the aerosol droplets in the lungs. Perhaps the most important of these factors is the physical properties of the aerosol. Generally the larger the particle (greater than 0.5 μm) the greater the tendency for the particles to lodge in the proximal airways. Hygroscopic particles are deposited more centrally in the lungs than non-hygroscopic particles of the same dry size. Electrical charge on the particles can also influence the site of deposition. Other factors affecting droplet deposition in the lungs are the inhalation mode and airway characteristics. The volume of inhalation, inspiratory flow rate, breath holding and degree of lung inflation will affect the amount of inhaled aerosol deposited and its distribution in the lungs. The structure of the airways also influences the deposition of aerosol droplets, e.g. the dimensions of the airways.

To produce radioaerosols physical forces are required to overcome liquid surface tension and produce droplets. Compressed air jet nebulizers are the most popular devices for producing radioaerosols in nuclear medicine. The varieties of these nebulizers have been described by Francis *et al.* (1986) and Pillay (1985). A high-efficiency ultrasound nebulizer has been described by Pillay *et al.* (1987) to produce an aerosol of ^{99m}Tc-labelled HIDA. In routine practice ^{99m}Tc-labelled DTPA is the radiopharmaceutical most commonly used, although ^{99m}Tc-labelled rhenium sulphur has been used by Peltier and Chatal (1986), who showed it to be preferable in patients suspected of increased bronchoalveolar permeability, because of its slower lung clearance. Huchon *et al.* (1987) studied eight radiopharmaceuticals to determine the effect of molecular weight on respiratory clearance of radioaerosols in dogs. They found that respiratory clearance of large-molecular-weight compounds, such as ^{111}In-labelled transferrin, was negligible at 30 min, and that clearance of molecules between 347 (^{99m}Tc-labelled glucoheptonate) and 5099 daltons (^{99m}Tc-labelled dextran) differed greatly, suggesting that binding and/or intrapulmonary retention affects transfer. Liposolubility, however, probably did not have a major influence on the respiratory clearance compounds of the eight radiopharmaceuticals. Wollmer *et al.* (1987) showed ^{113m}In to be useful for ventilation scintigraphy in the diagnosis of pulmonary embolism, but ^{99m}Tc was the radionuclide of choice.

Schuster *et al.* (1987) have identified two factors to produce high-quality aerosols. They suggest the use of 10% ethanol added to the ^{99m}Tc-labelled DTPA in order to decrease the surface tension of the radioactive fluid in the nebulizer. This almost doubles the droplet density, without affecting the size of the droplets, resulting in high-quality ventilation images. Secondly, accurate air flow rates are important; rates lower than those recommended produce droplets with diameters too large, whereas those higher than those recommended do not greatly affect the droplet size.

In order to maximize the effectiveness of aerosol ventilation studies it is necessary to reduce the radiation dose to the patient and personnel administering the dose and the cost of procedure, by producing a uniform peripheral aerosol deposition in the lungs. This can be achieved by reducing as much as possible the duration of administration and the unusable portion of the radioactive aerosol i.e. the droplets depositing in the delivery tubing, oropharynx, central airways and that exhaled by the patient. Phipps *et al.* (1987) have developed a rapid method to evaluate the rate of delivery of usable droplets (up to 3.3 μm) and wasted delivery droplets (above 3.3 μm) generated in four commercially available aerosol delivery systems.

A further criterion for a diagnostically effective aerosol is that the bond between ^{99m}Tc and the ligand, e.g. DTPA, should be stable. The intact aerosol ^{99m}Tc-labelled DTPA is cleared from normal human lungs with a half-time of 60–80 min (Lippmann and Albert, 1969), whereas dissociated pertechnetate, $^{99m}TcO_4$, clears with a half-time of a few minutes. The implications of a faulty radiopharmaceutical resulting in an incorrect image interpretation are obvious. Waldman *et al.* (1987) studied the radiochemical purity of ^{99m}Tc-labelled DTPA aerosols produced by jet nebulizers and ultrasonic nebulizers. Paper and liquid

Table 23.3 Radiopharmaceuticals fo

Perfusion	
^{99m}Tc-labelled MAA	
^{99m}Tc-labelled microspheres	
Ventilation	
Gases	^{81m}Kr
	^{133}Xe
	^{127}Xe
Aerosols	^{99m}Tc: DTPA, HIDA, GH, albumin, TcO_4, rhenium sulphur, dextran, polystyrene
	^{113m}In: colloid
	^{111}In: DTPA, transferrin
	^{51}Cr: EDTA
	^{67}Ga: desferoxaminemesylate
Particles	^{99m}Tc-labelled carbon ('Technegas')

chromatography of the aerosols produced by these nebulizers showed greater than 90% of radioactivity bound to DTPA with the jet nebulizer, but less than 10% bound to DTPA with the ultrasonic nebulizer. They recommend that the radiochemical purity of aerosols should be checked before use in lung ventilation imaging and clearance studies.

Two serious practical limitations of aerosols, namely particle size and specific activity, have stimulated the search for a more acceptable ^{99m}Tc-labelled radiopharmaceutical for ventilation imaging. Burch *et al.* (1986a) reported on lung ventilation studies using ^{99m}Tc-labelled 'Pseudogas'. This radiopharmaceutical, now known as 'Technegas', is a structured ultra-fine dispersion of ^{99m}Tc-labelled carbon. The carbon particles of size 5 nm and less are produced by heating $^{99m}TcO_4$ in a graphite crucible at 2500 °C in an atmosphere of pure argon for 15 s. The resulting vapour and argon mixture is inhaled by the patient (Burch *et al.*, 1986b).

Some radiopharmaceuticals used in routine lung imaging, and others which have been investigated, are shown in Table 23.3.

23.4.2 BONE IMAGING

In 1971 Subramanian and McAfee introduced ^{99m}Tc-labelled polyphosphate, the predecessor to a range of radiolabelled phosphate compounds which are now the agents of choice for bone imaging.

Polyphosphates are condensed phosphates linked to form chains of –P–O–P– units. Improved scans with better bone to background ratios were obtained in animals and patients using

…erez *et al.*, 1972). …wed by another …st of which to …ed ethylene- …t present …(MDP) is …y used …her new …developed in …nity and improve … Studies with ^{99m}Tc- …ymethylenediphosphonate …rated a faster blood clearance …, 1980) and high skeletal uptake … *al.*, 1980; Francis *et al.*, 1980; Fogelman *et* …1981) than MDP. Similarly ^{99m}Tc-labelled …dicarboxypropane diphosphonate (DPD) has been shown by Schwartz and Kloss (1981) to have 15% higher bone uptake than MDP in rats. Hale *et al.* (1981) found improved skeletal visualization and higher bone to soft tissue ratio with DPD compared with MDP in a study of 60 patients. Although the later ^{99m}Tc-labelled diphosphonates are improvements on the earlier ^{18}F, ^{99m}Tc-labelled pyrophosphate and ^{99m}Tc-labelled polyphosphate for bone imaging, there is no evidence that they are superior to ^{99m}Tc-labelled EHDP with respect to lesion detection in malignancy (Fogelman, 1986).

More recently ^{99m}Tc-labelled dimethylamino-diphosphonate (DMAD) has been reported, which demonstrates very low uptake by normal bone with high uptake in lesions. Several lesions seen with ^{99m}Tc-labelled DMAD were not seen with ^{99m}Tc-labelled MDP in the same patient (Rosenthall *et al.*, 1982; Smith *et al.*, 1984). However, this material is not commercially available, and was provided by Prof. Subramanian. The

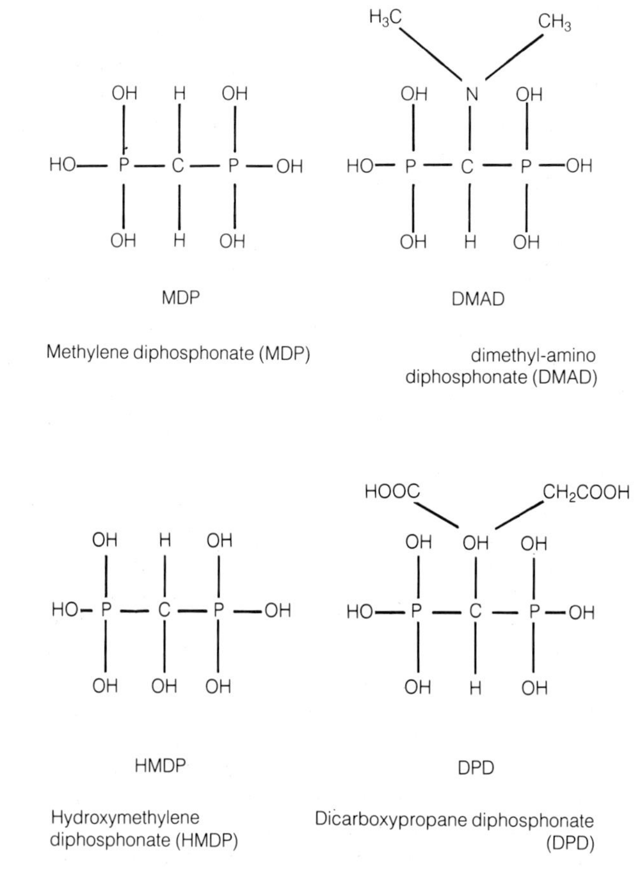

Figure 23.1 Chemical structures of methylenediphosphonate and some newer diphosphonate compounds for skeletal imaging.

chemical structures of some of the newer bone imaging agents are shown in Figure 20.1.

23.4.3 KIDNEY IMAGING

For many years ^{197}Hg-labelled chlormerodrin was the usual agent for renal scanning studies, but because of the poor imaging characteristics of ^{197}Hg, and the toxicity of mercury, a ^{99m}Tc-labelled agent was sought as a replacement. Now static kidney images are usually performed using ^{99m}Tc-labelled dimercaptosuccinic acid (DMSA). After injection approximately 60–70% of the radioactivity becomes indefinitely bound to the kidney parenchyma, the remainder being excreted. After injection ^{99m}Tc-labelled DMSA is almost completely bound to plasma proteins, mainly serum albumin and α-globulins. The blood radioactivity decreases from 20% to 30% after 10 min to about 2% 24 h after injection. ^{99m}Tc-labelled aprotinin, a polypeptide of low molecular weight which inhibits kallikrein and other proteases, has been studied (Bianchi *et al.*, 1981). The biodistribution of this radiopharmaceutical is highly sensitive to pH variations as well as the aprotinin dose. The high renal uptake, and extremely low urinary excretion in normal patients, shows this to be a promising radiopharmaceutical which is less sensitive to high serum creatinine levels than DMSA or chlormerodrin.

^{131}I Orthoiodohippurate (OIH) and ^{99m}Tc-labelled DTPA have been widely used and recently research into the development of a ^{99m}Tc complex which would combine the properties of ^{99m}Tc-labelled DTPA and ^{131}I OIH has resulted in the introduction of some new radiopharmaceuticals.

In 1981 Fritzberg *et al.* reported on chemical and biological studies of ^{99m}Tc-labelled *N,N′*-bis (mercaptoacetamido)-ethylenediamine (DADS). This compound is an example of a series of tetradentate, dimercaptoamide ligands which chelate to the technetium (V) TcO^{3+} core (Davison *et al.*, 1981). The biological studies of Fritzberg *et al.* (1981) in mice, rats and rabbits showed that ^{99m}Tc-labelled DADS was cleared by the kidneys significantly faster than ^{99m}Tc-labelled DTPA, but slightly slower than ^{131}I OIH, with no evidence of significant renal retention. All the species studied excreted 70–75% of the injected dose in 30 min through the kidneys, 7% in the bile in rats with normal renal function, and 18% in 90 min in the absence of renal function. Analysis has shown ^{99m}Tc-labelled DADS to be a robust complex, and is excreted unchanged in the urine and bile (Jones *et al.*, 1982). Fritzberg *et al.* (1982) have also evaluated ^{99m}Tc-labelled CO_2–DADS as a potential renal agent. This radiopharmaceutical is a mixture of two forms, or epimers, of ^{99m}Tc-labelled CO_2–DADS: one as effective as ^{131}I OIH in normal and diseased patients (Klingensmith *et al.*, 1983), whereas the other epimer has inferior biological properties. Because the two epimers are only separable by high-performance liquid chromatography (HPLC), ^{99m}Tc-labelled CO_2–DADS is not suitable for routine clinical use. Schneider *et al.* (1984) have synthesized 21 different compounds in this series in an effort to establish a relationship between their structure and renal imaging properties.

To overcome the problem of formation of stereoisomers produced with the core donor ligand of N_2S_2, as in the DADS series of compounds, further research led to the synthesis of the N_3S ligand ^{99m}Tc-labelled mercaptoacetyltriglycine (MAG3) (Eshima *et al.*, 1985). This radiopharmaceutical can be produced in a single stereochemical form, as a kit formulation. Fritzberg *et al.* (1986) synthesized MAG3 and evaluated its biodistribution in mice, comparing it with ^{131}I OIH and ^{125}I iothalamate, and its renal clearance in rats. The results in mice indicated excretion rates faster than OIH both in normal and in probenecid-treated animals. The clearance study results for MAG3 were 2.84 ml min^{-1} 100 g^{-1}, compared with 2.17 for OIH and 1.29 for iothalamate. Extraction efficiencies were 85% for MAG3, 60% for OIH and 39% for iothalamate. In a study involving ten normal volunteers blood clearance of ^{99m}Tc-labelled MAG3 was more rapid than ^{131}I OIH (mean clearance of 1.30 l min^{-1} for MAG3, and 0.88 l min^{-1} for OIH). Further, 73% of the injected dose of MAG3 was excreted by 30 min compared with 66.8% of OIH. In all subjects imaged, the quality of ^{99m}Tc-labelled MAG3 images were considered to be superior to those of ^{131}I OIH (Taylor *et al.*, 1986).

Eshima *et al.* (1987) synthesized a series of 12 new N_3S complexes, and screened them in mice and rats. This series of compounds differed from MAG3 in having different terminal amino acids, such as glycine, alanine, asparagine and glutamine. The purpose of the study was to evaluate the effect of the different amino acids on renal clearance of the complexes, and to assess their potential as ^{99m}Tc tubular function agents as possible replacements for ^{131}I-OIH. The renal excretion of all these complexes compared favourably with simultaneously administered ^{131}I OIH and ^{125}I-iothalamate.

The involved preparation methods of Fritzberg *et al.* (1986) might inhibit the use of MAG3 for routine clinical work (Coveney and Robbins, 1987). These latter workers compared a ^{99m}Tc-labelled MAG3 kit preparation with an HPLC pure ^{99m}Tc-labelled MAG3 preparation and simultaneously administered ^{131}I-OIH in rats. They found no significant difference in mean renal whole-blood clearance between the two ^{99m}Tc-labelled MAG3 preparations, and no significant difference in renal whole-blood clearance ratios for both ^{99m}Tc-labelled MAG3 preparations and co-administered ^{131}I-OIH. They concluded that a kit formulation, prepared by addition of eluate from a commercial ^{99m}Tc generator, produced ^{99m}Tc-labelled MAG3 with similar biological properties to those of ^{131}I-OIH in the rat. The preparation of ^{99m}Tc-labelled MAG3 from a commercial kit requires an inconvenient boiling step. Two alternative methods of preparation, a 'wet labelling' and a 'pre-reconstituted' method, have been described by Solanki *et al.* (1988). The latter method has the advantages that the kit could be reconstituted at the desired time, left at room temperature for the ^{99m}Tc-labelled MAG3 complex to accumulate (at the rate of 0.14% per minute) and used up to 1.5 h (95% labelling), and even 4 h (90% labelling). Millar *et al.* (1988) have studied the stability of a commercial ^{99m}Tc-labelled MAG3 kit by determining the radiochemical purity using HPLC. At 6 h after reconstitution 94.2% and 95.2% of radioactivity was found to be associated with the principal HPLC peak.

The chemical structures of some of the renal agents discussed in this section are shown in Figure 23.2.

23.4.4 CARDIOVASCULAR IMAGING

^{201}Tl has been the tracer of choice for myocardial blood flow studies. Research has been directed towards the development of ^{99m}Tc-labelled compounds for regional myocardial blood flow scintigraphy. New tracers of myocardial blood flow which have been developed include those for use with positron emission tomography (PET) and those for use with planar and single-photon emission computed tomography (SPECT).

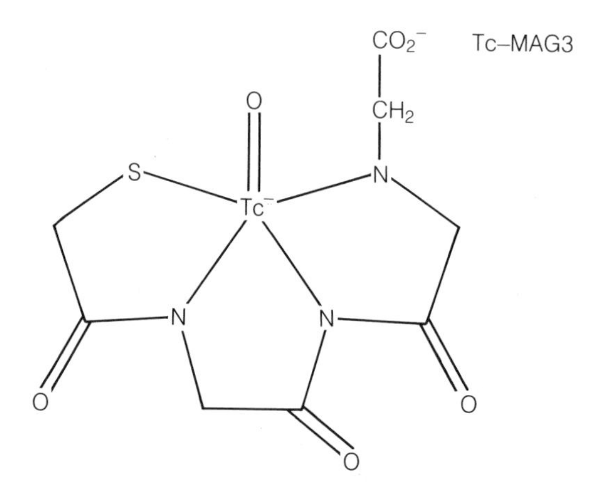

Figure 23.2 Chemical structures of some new ^{99m}Tc-labelled renal imaging agents.

Positron-emitting radiopharmaceuticals include ^{13}N-ammonia (Schelbert *et al.*, 1981) and ^{82}Rb, an analogue of potassium, exhibiting high myocardial and low blood concentrations (Budinger *et al.*, 1983). The availability of ^{82}Rb from a generator system, and the ease of use of the delivery system, make it clinically practical. ^{15}O-H_2O is metabolically inert, and its extraction by the myocardium is independent of metabolic changes or disruption of cationic exchange across membranes.

The properties of an ideal myocardial perfusion agent have been described by English *et al.* (1987) and include no pharmacological effects, distribution proportional to myocardial blood flow over the physiological range, rapid blood clearance, no myocardial clearance or redistribution, a suitable γ-ray energy, low absorbed dose, short effective physical half-life, and readily available at a reasonable cost. Previous ionic tracers of potassium, rubidium and thallium have not matched these ideal properties. Their extraction efficiencies are 70–90% with only 3–4% of radioactivity in the heart at imaging.

The search for ^{99m}Tc-labelled radiopharmaceuticals has centred on cationic complexes since many cationic species are known to be efficiently taken up by normal myocardial muscle (Deutsch *et al.*, 1982). Excellent myocardial images of the canine heart were obtained by Deutsch *et al.* (1981a, 1981b) using radiopharmaceuticals with the general formula $[^{99m}Tc(diars)_2X_2]^+$ where X = Cl or Br, and diars = O-phenylenbis (dimethylarsine). Of 19 cationic complexes tested by Deutsch *et al.* (1981a) in a resting beagle dog, $[^{99m}Tc(diars)_2Cl_2]^+$ showed the highest uptake in normal myocardium, about half as well as ^{201}Tl (0.022% compared with 0.038% dose per gram). The compounds are, however, almost insoluble in water, and a similar complex $[^{99m}Tc(DMPE)Cl_2]^+$, with the less lipophilic ligand DMPE (= 1,2-bis(dimethylphosphinoethane) was proposed (Deutsch *et al.*, 1981b). This compound (^{99m}Tc-labelled DMPE) showed faster overall kinetics than ^{201}Tl, with a higher heart:lung ratio, and high liver uptake. The mean heart uptake of ^{201}Tl was 4.3% and 2.9% with ^{99m}Tc-labelled DMPE at peak myocardial uptake, but with only 0.9% of ^{99m}Tc-labelled DMPE in the lung compared with 3.3% of ^{201}Tl. ^{99m}Tc-labelled DMPE gave better images in both normal and infarcted dog heart than ^{201}Tl. The hepatic uptake was, however, high (Nishiyama *et al.*, 1982). In man the intense hepatic uptake of ^{99m}Tc-labelled DMPE proved it to be unsatisfactory (Gerson *et al.*, 1983), and was greater than for any other species studied.

Another class of myocardial imaging agent was developed by Nunn *et al.* (1986). This compound was a neutral seven-coordinate technetium complex with the chemical formula chloro-(methylboron(1−)-tris[1,2-cyclohexanedionedioxime])technetium. It is one of a series of boronic acid adducts of technetium complexes (BATOs). ^{99m}Tc-BATO showed high myocardial uptake in the first minutes after injection in patient studies. The washout from the myocardium, however, was shown to be high, with a half-time of 3–4 min.

A number of ^{99m}Tc-labelled radiopharmaceuticals based on derivatives of isonitrile complexes have been developed and these appear to hold the greatest promise for imaging the human myocardium. In 1984, Holman *et al.* reported on the first of the isonitrile complexes, ^{99m}Tc-labelled hexakis-*t*-butylisonitrile) (TBI). Diagnostic images were, however, only obtained between 1 h and 4 h after injection of this radiopharmaceutical, due to early high lung uptake. Clearance of ^{99m}Tc-labelled TBI through the hepatobiliary system, and its high lung uptake, led to alterations in the basic isonitrile complex, in order to produce a superior myocardial imaging agent. Holman *et al.* (1987) described their initial experience in humans with ^{99m}Tc-labelled carbomethoxyisopropyl isonitrile (CPI), which has high accumulation in normal myocardium, and rapid clearance from the lung and liver. However, unlike ^{99m}Tc-labelled TBI, ^{99m}Tc-labelled CPI does not redistribute in the myocardium, and a second dose at 3–4 h later is necessary for a resting study. Early gall-bladder and bowel activity are seen, as with ^{99m}Tc-labelled TBI. Another in the series to be developed was ^{99m}Tc-labelled methoxyisobutyl isonitrile (MIBI). This radiopharmaceutical retains the myocardial uptake of ^{99m}Tc-labelled TBI and ^{99m}Tc-labelled CPI, but has greater blood, liver and lung clearance. Its greater heart : lung and heart : liver ratios, despite a slightly lower myocardial uptake, make it a superior imaging agent.

As mentioned earlier one of the problems with ^{99m}Tc-labelled DMPE was its intense uptake into the liver which interfered with imaging of the cardiac apex. One of the causes of this uptake occurs when Tc(III) in ^{99m}Tc-labelled DMPE undergoes *in vivo* reduction to Tc(II), a neutral and non-cationic form. This reduction leads to myocardial washout and increased liver uptake of the more lipophilic Tc(II) form. Deutsch *et al.* (1987), in order to avoid the effects of reduction, studied a series of 15 non-reducible $^{99m}Tc(III)$

cationic complexes with the general formula $[^{99m}TcL(Y)_2]^+$. These complexes are mixed ligand complexes containing a tetradentate Schiff base ligand (L) and monodentate phosphine, phosphite or isonitrile ligand (Y). Of the 15 complexes none showed detectable myocardial washout. However, a typical complex, $[^{99m}Tc(en)(P(CH_3)_3)_2]^+$, proved to be only a mediocre myocardial imaging agent in a study of seven normal human volunteers.

Long-chain fatty acids are an important source of energy for the heart. Extraction of fatty acids from blood by normal myocardium is high, with rapid conversion of the fatty acid to CO_2, or incorporation into several different tissue lipids. However, uptake into ischaemic regions is lower, enabling these areas to be delineated by imaging with radiolabelled long-chain fatty acids. Work with single-photon emitters, such as ^{131}I, has produced less successful radiopharmaceuticals as metabolic tracers than those produced with positron emitters such as ^{18}F and ^{11}C.

Radiolabelling tracers of myocardial metabolism has, broadly speaking, progressed on three fronts. First attempts involved the radiolabelling of the oleic acid across a double bond with radioiodine (Evans *et al.*, 1965). This resulted in a reduction in myocardial extraction. Poe *et al.* (1976) attempted to overcome this problem by substituting the terminal methyl groups with radioiodine to produce ^{123}I-labelled hexadecanoic acid. These radiopharmaceuticals do, however, tend to become deiodinated rather rapidly, producing high blood levels of radioactivity. Other radioiodinated fatty acids were therefore developed which had lower blood radioactivity levels, e.g. 15(*p*-^{123}I-iodophenyl) pentadecanoic acid, where the iodophenyl group is on the terminal carbon atom of the pentadecanoic acid molecule (Machulla *et al.*, 1980). Other examples, more recently developed, are 15(*p*-^{123}I-iodophenyl)-6-telluraheptadecanoic acid (Goodman *et al.*, 1982), 15(*p*-^{123}I-iodophenyl)-3, 3-dimethylpentadecanoic acid, and 15(*p*-^{123}I-iodophenyl)-3-methylpentadecanoic acid (Yamamoto *et al.*, 1986). These latter compounds do appear to offer advantages over the halogenated compounds in having lower blood activities.

Other attempts at radiolabelling fatty acids with radioactive tellurium and iodine have resulted largely in a loss of biological properties of the fatty acid (Knapp *et al.*, 1981). These authors proposed that by placing a large heteroatom in the fatty acid chain oxidation would be inhibited and the biological properties retained. Examples of the radiopharmaceuticals are radioiodinated 18-iodotellura-17-octadecanoic acid (Knapp *et al.*, 1984) and 9-^{123m}Te-telluraheptadecanoic acid (Okada *et al.*, 1982). These latter workers further studied the effects of the position of the tellurium atom on myocardial fatty acid kinetics in a series of ^{123m}Te-labelled heptadecanoic acid analogues in dogs. Their results suggested that as the ^{123m}Te atom was positioned further from the carboxyl portion of the molecule there was progressive increase in myocardial clearance. Further, selection of the position of ^{123m}Te depends on whether initial fatty acid distribution or subsequent clearance rates are being studied (Okada *et al.*, 1985).

Another approach to the development of new radiopharmaceuticals for myocardial imaging has involved the use of radiolabelled monoclonal antibodies. These have now been prepared and can be used to localize areas of myocardial infarction because the antibody binds exclusively to intracellular myosin, which is only exposed on the death of the cell. The localization of an antimyosin antibody in myocardial infarction was described as early as 1976 by Khaw *et al.* These studies were performed with radioiodinated antibodies and later with radioiodinated antibody fragments (Khaw *et al.*, 1978). The use of antibody fragments rather than whole antibody helped to reduce adverse reactions and speed the clearance of radiolabel from the blood, thus improving target to background ratios and allowing earlier imaging.

Later developments resulted in ^{99m}Tc-labelled antibody fragments which retained immunoreactivity, yet had the advantages for imaging of the ^{99m}Tc radiolabel (Khaw *et al.*, 1982). Antimyosin fragment was also radiolabelled with ^{111}In by use of the bifunctional chelating agent DTPA (Khaw *et al.*, 1980) to produce a product which is now commercially available.

The structures of some radiopharmaceuticals for heart imaging are shown in Figure 23.3.

23.4.5 BRAIN IMAGING

Radiopharmaceuticals which have been used for brain imaging, e.g. ^{99m}Tc-pertechnetate, ^{99m}Tc-labelled DTPA and ^{99m}Tc-labelled glucoheptonate (GHA), do not cross an intact blood–brain barrier (BBB), but detect changes in the barrier. Radio-

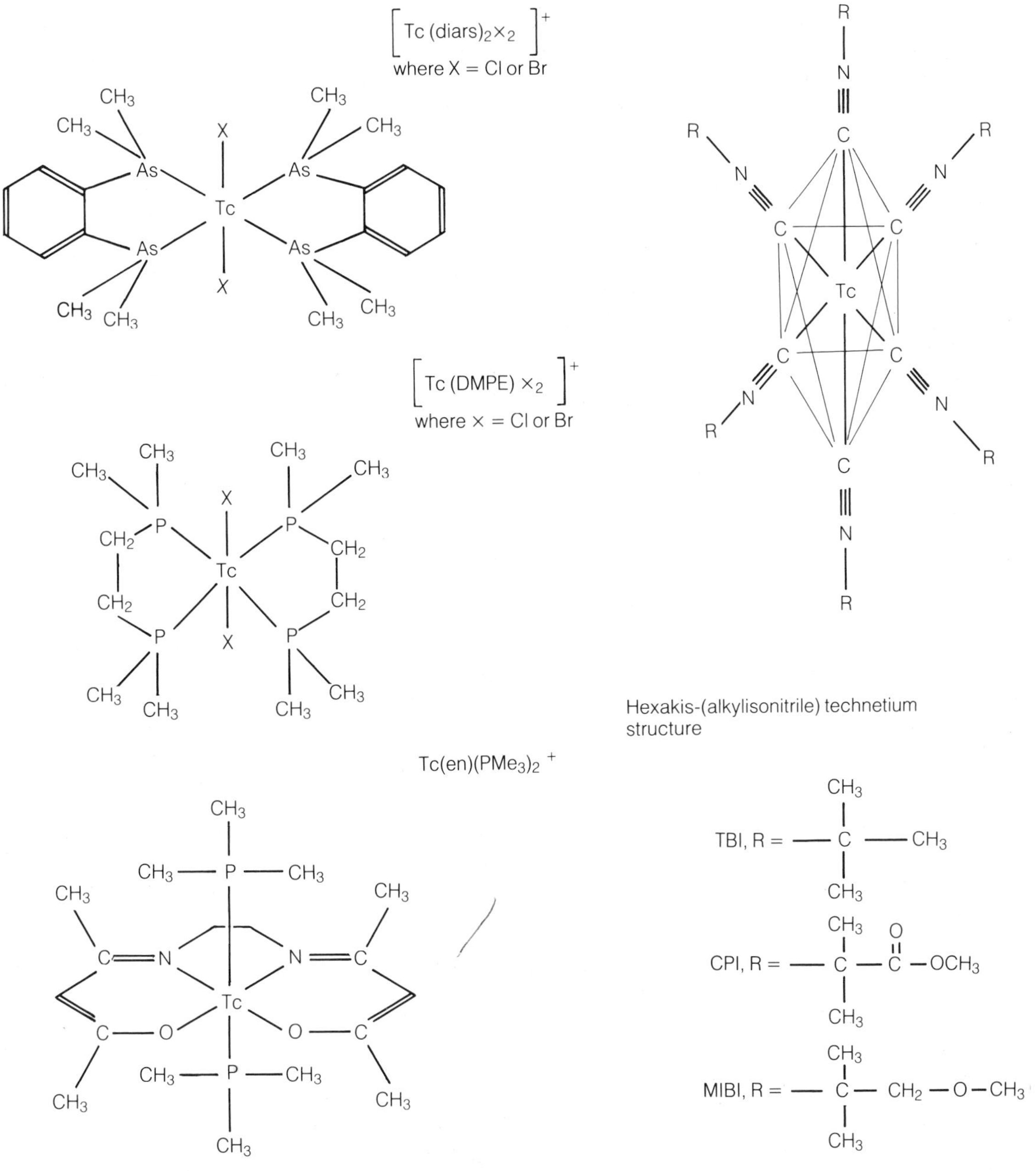

$[Tc(diars)_2X_2]^+$
where X = Cl or Br

$[Tc(DMPE)X_2]^+$
where X = Cl or Br

$Tc(en)(PMe_3)_2{}^+$

Hexakis-(alkylisonitrile) technetium structure

TBI, R = $-C(CH_3)_2-CH_3$

CPI, R = $-C(CH_3)_2-C(=O)-OCH_3$

MIBI, R = $-C(CH_3)_2-CH_2-O-CH_3$

Figure 23.3 Chemical structures of some new ^{99m}Tc-labelled cationic myocardial imaging agents.

pharmaceuticals have been developed which will cross the BBB, some being subsequently trapped in the brain parenchyma, whereas others will diffuse back across the barrier into the blood. These radiopharmaceuticals can provide functional data such as regional perfusion and metabolism, and information on receptor sites within the brain.

(a) Cerebral blood flow

Some compounds, e.g. glucose, will cross the BBB by specific mechanisms, whereas others are required to be neutral, lipid-soluble, and with a molecular weight less than 500 to achieve passage across the barrier. Some diffusible radiopharmaceuticals, e.g. ^{127}Xe, ^{133}Xe, are not trapped within the brain and diffuse out again. Amines are important chemical mediators of brain function, and radiolabelled amines are lipophilic, moving across the BBB with almost complete extraction during a single passage through the brain circulation. Once across the barrier these radiopharmaceuticals are trapped, either by binding to non-specific receptors or metabolized to non-diffusible non-lipophilic compounds. There is no redistribution of radioactivity within the brain for at least an hour after injection, thus allowing tomographic imaging of regional cerebral perfusion to be achieved.

One of the most widely studied radiopharmaceuticals for regional cerebral perfusion imaging is *N*-isopropyl-*p*-^{123}I-iodoamphetamine (^{123}I-IMP), which was one of several iodophenylalkylamines studied in rat brain by Winchell *et al.* (1980). Another radioiodinated compound to receive extensive study is *N,N,N'*-trimethyl-*N'*-(2-hydroxy-3-methyl-5-iodobenzyl)-1,3-propanedamine (^{123}I-HIPDM). This radiopharmaceutical, developed by Kung *et al.* (1983), is an example of a 'pH shift' agent. These materials readily cross the BBB from the neutral blood pH 7.4 to the more acid pH 7.0 environment of the brain. Here the molecule picks up an H^+ and the resulting charged form cannot recross the BBB. ^{123}I-IMP and ^{123}I-HIPDM have similar molecular structures and behave similarly in humans.

The high cost and limited availability of ^{123}I led to a search for ^{99m}Tc-labelled compounds which would have similar imaging characteristics to the radiolabelled agents in that they would be readily available, be retained in the brain parenchyma for at least 1 h, be suitable for imaging by SPECT, and be relatively inexpensive. Many compounds were developed for ^{99m}Tc labelling without a high degree of success in that uptake into the brain was low. More recently Kung *et al.* (1984) developed derivatives based on bis-aminoethanethiol (BAT), which were neutral, lipophilic and crossed the BBB. A six-coordinate, neutral, lipophilic complex, propyleneamineoxime (PnAO) was synthesized by Troutner *et al.* (1983). Both the BAT and PnAO ring systems require alteration to provide retention in the brain. Kung *et al.* (1985) have achieved this by synthesizing complexes of BAT with amine side-chains, and Chaplin *et al.* (1985) have prepared derivatives of PnAO.

Holmes *et al.* (1985) developed ^{99m}Tc-labelled hexamethylpropyleneamineoxime (HMPAO), which demonstrates good brain uptake, prolonged retention of activity in the brain and slow regional redistribution. The results, obtained in rats and one human volunteer, suggested this radiopharmaceutical to be ideal for SPECT imaging of cerebral blood flow. Two diastereoisomers, the 'meso' and '*d,l*' forms, were subsequently isolated from HMPAO (Nowotnik *et al.*, 1985). The latter form showed 4.1% uptake of the dose in the brain of nine normal volunteers, a level which remained constant over 8 h (Sharp *et al.*, 1986). The '*d,l*' form is a neutral lipophilic complex which converts slowly to a secondary complex, which may account for the prolonged brain retention (Neirinckx *et al.*, 1987). This conversion also happens *in vitro* and limits the time after preparation for which ^{99m}Tc-labelled HMPAO can be used to about 30 min. Efange *et al.* (1987) have developed two new BAT ligands containing amines in the side chain: ^{99m}Tc-labelled DEA and ^{99m}Tc-labelled TMPDA. Two isomers of each material were prepared, the *syn* and *anti*. Both isomers of ^{99m}Tc-labelled TMPDA showed little brain uptake, whereas the *anti* form of ^{99m}Tc-labelled DEA showed brain uptake of 0.99% and 0.26% at 2 min and 15 min, and the *syn* form 2.27% and 0.64% of dose per organ respectively.

An alternative radiopharmaceutical to the iodinated amine compounds was developed by Vyth *et al.* (1983). ^{201}Tl-labelled diethyldithiocarbamate (DDC) is a highly lipophilic complex with a distribution similar to the radiolabelled amines. Van Royen (1987) has reviewed the pharmacology and uses of this agent, and reported it to be a suitable radiopharmaceutical for SPECT studies of cerebral blood flow (van Royen *et al.*, 1987).

Moretti *et al.* (1987) have reviewed amines for brain tomoscintigraphy, their structure–biodistribution relationship and their value in ischaemic diseases.

(b) Indicators of metabolism

Fluorodeoxyglucose (FDG) is transported into the brain by a specific facilitated transported system, and then phosphorylated to a form which cannot recross the BBB. ^{18}F-FDG has been used to calculate local glucose metabolism (Reivich *et al.*, 1979), and ^{11}C-deoxyglucose has been used for the same purpose when the 20 minute half-life of ^{11}C allows repeated measurements (Reivich *et al.*, 1982).

Oxygen metabolism and oxygen extraction has been measured using ^{15}O-oxygen (Frakowiak *et al.*, 1980).

(c) Receptor imaging

Cerebral muscarinic acetylcholine receptors have been imaged using ^{123}I-3-quinuclidinyl-4-iodobenzilate (^{123}I-QNB) by Eckleman *et al.* (1984). Positron tomography with ^{11}C-3-*N*-methylspiperone has been used by Wagner *et al.* (1983) for imaging dopamine receptors. Shiue *et al.* (1987) developed no-carrier-added ^{18}F-*N*-(3-fluoropropyl)spiroperidol, and studied its biodistribution in mice, where 1.1% of administered dose was found in the brain. Their results suggested that this radiopharmaceutical may be suitable for PET studies of the dopamine receptors in humans.

The structures of some radiopharmaceuticals for brain imaging are shown in Figure 23.4.

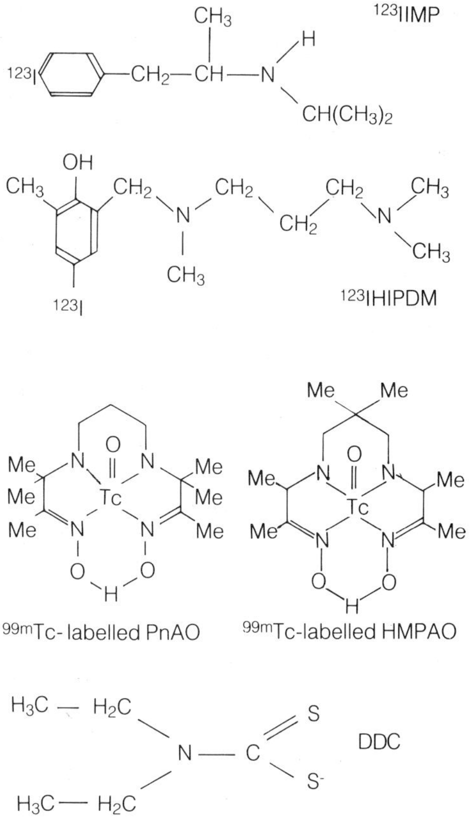

Figure 23.4 Chemical structures of some new brain imaging agents.

23.4.6 CELL LABELLING

Radiolabelled granulocytes, monocytes, platelets and red cells have wide clinical applications. The main disadvantages which inhibit wider application of these techniques are the cost of the radiolabel, usually ^{111}In, and the time of a skilled operator required for cell separation and radiolabelling. Many workers have attempted over the last few years to develop techniques to replace ^{111}In with ^{99m}Tc, which would considerably reduce the cost. Other groups have developed monoclonal antibodies for the specific labelling of cells *in vivo*, thus avoiding lengthy cell separation procedures.

A crucial consideration in cell labelling is that the radiolabelled cells behave in the same way as unlabelled cells, i.e. they are not modified or damaged during the labelling procedure, otherwise their required performance *in vivo* may be lost. The radiolabel must also remain associated with the cells *in vivo*, or else images will reflect the biodistribution of the radiolabel and not the cells. In 1976 McAfee and Thakur introduced ^{111}In-labelled oxine, a lipid-soluble neutral complex, which labels all blood cells. This radiopharmaceutical has been widely used to radiolabel a mixed leucocyte population of cells, after their separation from red cells and platelets. Concern that ^{111}In-labelled oxine preparations, which usually contain ethanol or a detergent, may damage cells led to the search for a water-soluble ligand which would chelate ^{111}In. Danpure and Osman (1981) introduced ^{111}In-labelled acetylacetone (acac) which satisfied this requirement. Later Danpure *et al.* (1982) developed ^{111}In-labelled tropolonate which, unlike ^{111}In-labelled oxine and ^{111}In-labelled acac, radiolabels leucocytes while still in a plasma environment. However, it was not until 1986 that Peters *et al.* introduced ^{99m}Tc-labelled HMPAO, which effectively labelled leucocytes. A clinical protocol for radiolabelling mixed leucocytes with ^{99m}Tc has been developed by Danpure *et al.* (1987), which results in a preparation with the radionuclide firmly attached to the cells for the length of the clinical investigation. A comparison of ^{99m}Tc and ^{111}In-labelled leukocytes is given by Mountford *et al.* (1990).

Attempts have been made to develop selective cell-labelling radiopharmaceuticals which will label specific cell populations in whole blood, thus avoiding the costly and time-consuming cell separation techniques. McAfee and Thakur (1976b) attempted to utilize the phagocytic properties of monocytes and granulocytes to introduce radiolabelled particles into these cells. The radiolabelled particles, however, also attached non-specifically to other cells. Schroth *et al.* (1981) used ^{99m}Tc-labelled tin colloid in a technique to label cells which were successfully used in patients. Others, however, could not achieve the same level of success in their patients owing to cell damage during the labelling procedure (McAfee *et al.*, 1984). Mock and English (1987) showed that ^{99m}Tc-labelled tin colloid would only label mixtures of leucocytes and not granulocytes in whole blood, which meant there was no advantage over existing techniques.

In a review on methods of separation and radiolabelling of human leucocytes, Danpure and Osman (1988) feel that the main hope for useful selective agents lies with monoclonal antibodies directed against surface antigens of particular blood cells. Such preparations have been developed (Danpure *et al.*, 1987; Locher *et al.*, 1986), but problems of achieving high enough specific activity and immune response to foreign proteins, particularly with repeated injections, are yet to be overcome. Seybold (1988) has reported on an anti-CEA monoclonal antibody which selectively reacts with surface glycoprotein of normal human granulocytes, without affecting their vital functions. However, this author does not consider the method suitable for general use, but restricts its use to immunoscintigraphy of infectious lesions, until a clinically relevant immunization can be excluded. Joseph *et al.* (1988) have successfully looked for inflammatory lesions in patients using a ^{99m}Tc-labelled murine antibody reacting with non-specific crossreacting antigen (NCA) and CEA. The antibody can be stored in a freeze-dried form and radiolabelled when required.

Peters (1988a) has reviewed methods of platelet labelling and kinetics. The platelets must first be separated from other blood cells by simple differential centrifugation, prior to radiolabelling. Activation of platelet function, which can occur during a concentration procedure, can be inhibited by adjustment of the pH to 6.5 with an acid–citrate–dextrose buffer, or by the use of prostaglandins. The separated cells can be labelled with ^{111}In-labelled oxine, ^{111}In-labelled acac or ^{111}In-labelled tropolonate. Platelets have also been labelled with ^{99m}Tc-labelled HMPAO and using radiolabelled monoclonal antibodies directed against platelet surface antigens (Oster *et al.*, 1985).

The radiolabelling of both granulocytes and platelets can activate the function of these cells, similar to the processes occurring at sites of inflammation. Assessment of the functional status before and after labelling of the cells should be performed by techniques reviewed by Peters (1988b).

23.4.7 TUMOUR IMAGING

(a) MONOCLONAL ANTIBODIES

The biggest advance in the detection of tumours has been the development and introduction of radiolabelled monoclonal antibodies into nuclear medicine.

The development of a radiolabelled antibody which is clinically useful involves several steps: the development and preparation of an antibody, relevant to the disease process under study, in a form suitable for human use; the radiolabelling of the antibody; the administration of the antibody to the patient and subsequent gamma camera imaging after a suitable period has elapsed for localization.

There are many factors which will affect the localization of a radiolabelled monoclonal antibody in a tumour (Goodwin, 1987). The first requirement is that the antibody should reach the tumour. Blood flow to some tumours, and particularly necrotic centres, is often very low, resulting in only 0.1–0.001% of the dose per gram of tumour tissue. The antibody must cross the blood capillary wall and diffuse through interstitial fluid to reach the tumour. The large size of the antibody molecule slows down these processes, resulting in imaging times of days after administration to the patient. Antibody fragments have now been used because of their more rapid diffusion due to their smaller size. Once the antibody reaches the tumour it must then bind to the tumour antigen, a process which requires a high specific activity of radiolabelled antibody due to the large number of competing non-specific binding sites. For satisfactory imaging it is necessary to achieve a high ratio of radioactivity in the tumour to that in the surrounding tissues. This ratio depends on several factors including the rate of excretion of the antibody, its metabolism, non-specific binding to non-tumour targets and specificity of the antibody for the antigen.

Monoclonal antibodies are well covered in various reviews (Sikora *et al.*, 1984; Keenan *et al.*, 1985; Strudler and Larson, 1985; Mather, 1985) and in Chapter 20. A review of radiolabelling methods and quality control of radiolabelled antibodies is described by Mather (1986). Both ^{123}I and ^{131}I have been widely used to label antibodies, where ^{123}I is often preferred because of its greater photon yield, more suitable γ-ray energy and better dosimetry resulting in images with superior definition and improved statistics. ^{111}In has become very popular more recently when its three day half-life permits imaging up to a week or more after administration, and the photon energies give good-quality images but ^{99m}Tc is now the label of choice (Mather and Ellison, 1990; Granowska *et al.*, 1990a, b).

(b) RADIOIODINATED MIBG

Sisson *et al.* (1981) reported on the use of ^{131}I-*m*-iodobenzylguanidine (^{131}I-MIBG), a guanethidine analogue, to detect and localize adrenal medullary and extra-adrenal phaeochromocytoma pre-operatively. However, the radiolabel ^{131}I is not ideal for detection using a gamma camera, and there is evidence that ^{123}I-MIBG may be clinically superior to ^{131}I-MIBG in visualizing normal adrenal glands and secondaries (Lynn *et al.*, 1984).

MIBG is concentrated in neurosecretory storage granules of chromaffin cells, and is therefore of potential use in tumours that derive from the neural crest and are capable of production or storage of catecholamines. Thus ^{131}I-MIBG has been used in the diagnosis and follow-up of children with neuroblastoma (Hoefnagel *et al.*, 1985), detection of carcinoid tumours (Feldman *et al.*, 1986), uptake in primary medullary thyroid carcinoma (Endo *et al.*, 1984; Connell *et al.*, 1984) and uptake in metastatic medullary thyroid carcinoma (Sone *et al.*, 1985).

In addition to the diagnosis of carcinoid tumours ^{131}I-MIBG has also been used in the treatment of this disease (Hoefnagel *et al.*, 1986) as well as phaeochromocytoma (Sisson *et al.*, 1984), medullary thyroid carcinoma (Hoefnagel *et al.*, 1988) and neuroblastoma in children (Kimmig *et al.*, 1984).

(c) ^{201}TI-Thallous chloride

Lebowitz *et al.* (1974) suggested that ^{201}Tl might be useful for tumour localization in addition to its use as a myocardial imaging agent. The uptake of ^{201}Tl into tumours as a possible complication in heart imaging was reported by Cox *et al.* in 1976. Since then ^{201}Tl has been used to image a variety of benign and malignant tumours, including brain, parathyroid, thyroid, lung and liver (Krasnow *et al.*, 1988). The uptake kinetics of ^{201}Tl into primary tumours of lung, breast and mediastinal lymphoma have been studied by Sehweil *et al.* (1988), who reported the maximum tumour uptake to be 8–20 min after injection for the three types of tumour. The authors conclude that the uptake mechanism of ^{201}Tl into tumours is similar to that in the myocardium. Hoefnagel *et al.* (1988) report the use of ^{201}Tl total body imaging, in combination with calcitonin and CEA assays, to be a reliable parameter in the follow-up of medullary thyroid carcinoma.

(d) Pentavalent DMSA

For tumour imaging dimercaptosuccinic acid (DMSA) is prepared in the pentavalent (V) form rather than the more familiar trivalent (III) form, which is widely used for renal imaging. ^{99m}Tc-labelled (V) DMSA is prepared using alkaline rather than the acid conditions necessary for the trivalent form. Yokoyama *et al.* (1985) investigated other parameters involved in the preparation and concluded that optimum labelling conditions occurred at pH 8.0 with an Sn:Tc molar ratio of 1.0. The resulting complex contains a $T_cO_4^{-3}$ core, which exhibits similar characteristics *in vivo* to the orthophosphate ion PO_4^{-3}, which has been shown to accumulate in tumours (Yokayama and Saji, 1980). Hesslewood *et al.* (1988) have shown that the stannous ion to DMSA ratio does not need to be altered from the ratio used in the preparation of the trivalent form. The use of ^{99m}Tc-labelled (V)DMSA for tumour imaging was first reported by Ohta *et al.* (1984), when they found significant uptake of the radiopharmaceutical in four patients with pathologically confirmed medullary thyroid carcinoma and elevated serum calcitonin levels.

Clarke *et al.* (1987a) showed ^{99m}Tc-labelled (V)DMSA to be superior to ^{131}I-MIBG as an imaging agent for medullary thyroid carcinoma in an initial series of four patients. Although the main role of ^{99m}Tc-labelled (V)DMSA appears to be in the investigation of primary and recurrent medullary thyroid carcinoma, its use in imaging other tumours, particularly those of the head and neck, has been reported (Ohta *et al.*, 1988; Watkinson and Maisey, 1988).

23.5 THERAPY WITH RADIONUCLIDES

Radionuclides such as ^{131}I, ^{32}P and ^{90}Y have been used to treat benign and malignant disease for many years. Recently, however, these radionuclides have been under evaluation as new radiopharmaceuticals for the treatment of bone metastases, adrenal tumours and other tumours with radiolabelled antibodies. In addition other radionuclides have been introduced for therapy purposes, including rhenium-186 (^{186}Re), palladium-109 (^{109}Pd) and samarium-153 (^{153}Sm) (see Table 23.1).

Many nuclear medicine centres have attempted radiotherapy with ^{131}I-labelled monoclonal antibodies either administered intravenously or intracavitary. However, the *in vivo* deiodination of the antibody with rapid appearance of radioactivity in the urine may help to explain the low levels of radioiodine found in patient tumours. Further, ^{131}I does emit several unwanted abundant γ-rays. Wessels and Rogus (1984) have described ^{90}Y as one of the best radionuclides for therapy with antibodies owing to its suitable $t_{1/2}$ of 64 h, absence of γ-rays, stable daughter, intermediate β-particle energy ($E_{max} = 2.3$ MeV), and chemical properties for forming conjugates with DTPA. Chinol and Hnatowich (1987) have described the use of ^{90}Y prepared by the decay of ^{90}Sr in a radionuclide generator, and the preparation of radiolabelled antibodies with this radionuclide (Hnatowich *et al.*, 1985). Snook *et al.* (1987) have also labelled antibodies with ^{90}Y for the effective intraperitoneal treatment of ovarian cancer with minimal toxic problems for the patient. ^{109}Pd is a predominantly β-emitting radionuclide ($E_{max} = 1$ MeV; $t_{1/2}$, = 13.4 h) which has been used by Fawwaz *et al.* (1984) to radiolabel monoclonal antibodies to a human melanoma-associated antigen of high molecular weight. Their studies with this radiolabelled antibody in nude mice bearing human melanoma resulted in 19% per gram of the dose being taken up into the tumour. The visualization of tumours with radiolabelled monoclonal antibodies presents difficulties such as low antigenic specificity of malignant cells, cross-reactivity of antibodies with other tissues as well as tumour, poor radiolabelling of antibody and immune response of patients to foreign protein. These difficulties are also true for therapy, but other problems, in addition to selection of the most suitable radionuclide, must be addressed. Antigens are unevenly expressed over the surface of the tumour mass which will, in turn, result in an uneven distribution of the radiolabelled antibody and subsequent irradiation of the tumour. Pauwels and Van Kroonenburgh (1988) have suggested the use of α-particle emitters, such as astatine-211 (^{211}As) and bismuth-212 (^{212}Bi), as radiolabels because of their high cytotoxic effect due to the short range of the particles. Therapy with radiolabelled monoclonal antibodies still has a long way to go before it can be described as an effective tool.

Medullary carcinoma of the thyroid (MCT) is an uncommon tumour accounting for 2–9% of all thyroid malignancies. Until recently nuclear medicine procedures were of limited use in the localization of MCT. More recently, however, ^{131}I-MIBG has been shown to be taken up in these tumours (Connell *et al.*, 1984) as well as phaeochromocytoma (Wieland *et al.*, 1980), neuroblastoma (Trennor *et al.*, 1984; Geatti *et al.*, 1985) and carcinoid tumours (Fischer *et al.*, 1984). Clarke *et al.* (1987b) have used ^{131}I MIBG to treat two patients with MCT with symptoms of diarrhoea and severe pain from known bone metastases. Both patients showed marked improvement in both pain and diarrhoea, but no significant biochemical response. The authors suggest there may be a palliative role for ^{131}I-MIBG in patients with MCT. Therapy, however, should be considered earlier in the disease and doses given at two-monthly intervals. Sisson *et al.* (1984) used this radiopharmaceutical to treat five patients with malignant phaeochromocytoma using two to four doses. Two patients exhibited benefits with tumours declining in size to 28% and 30% of their original volumes, and hormone secretion decreasing to 50% or less of baseline rates. The other three patients were mostly asymptomatic and showed little improvement after treatment. The tumours of those patients who did respond seemed to be more rapidly growing and more predominantly in soft tissue than in those patients obtaining little benefit. Hoefnagel *et al.* (1986) treated a patient with liver metastases from a carcinoid gastric tumour using ^{131}I MIBG in two doses administered over four weeks. Although the disease progressed the patient experienced temporary relief from pain, fever and nausea.

Bone pain is a frequent complication of bone metastases. Until recently ^{32}P in the form of orthophosphate and later diphosphonates was used to treat the pain, but with inconsistent results. Mathieu *et al.* (1979) investigated the use of ^{186}Re to label EHDP and studied its biodistribution in bone. Weininger *et al.* (1983) reported on the preparation of ^{186}Re-labelled EHDP with a high labelling efficiency. Although the radiopharmaceutical localized in bone in a variety of animal species, it was cleared very slowly from blood and soft tissue. In an attempt to overcome some of these disadvantages Eisenhut (1984) radiolabelled α-amino-(4-hydroxybenzylidene)-disphosphonate (BDP3) with ^{131}I and studied its biodistribution in rats. ^{131}I-labelled BDP3 exhibited high bone affinity with rapid blood clearance and renal excretion. The author suggested that because of the reasonable biokinetic results and simple labelling procedure ^{131}I-labelled BDP3 would be useful for palliative treatment of bone pain. Pecher (1942) was the first to report a possible therapeutic role for ^{89}Sr in the palliation of disseminated carcinoma of the prostate. It has been shown that about three-quarters of patients benefit from ^{89}Sr therapy (Robinson 1986; McEwan *et al.*, 1986), and some patients obtain complete relief. The use of ^{89}Sr, as strontium chloride, is now under study by several groups. A series of stable complexes of ^{153}Sm has been studied in rats by Goeckeler *et al.* (1987). Of these complexes ethylendiaminetetramethylenephosphonate (EDTMP) showed the best combination of high bone uptake, low non-osseous uptake and rapid blood clearance. In rabbits the blood clearance was found to be more rapid than ^{99m}Tc-labelled MDP. The authors suggest that ^{153}Sm-labelled EDTMP could be therapeutically useful in treating metastatic bone cancer.

23.6 COMPLICATIONS IN THE USE OF RADIOPHARMACEUTICALS

Most studies performed in the nuclear medicine department are free of unexpected problems. However, over the years information has been collated describing incidents that were unforeseen.

23.6.1 ADVERSE REACTIONS TO RADIOPHARMACEUTICALS

An adverse reaction to a radiopharmaceutical can be defined as an unexpected reaction or unusual and undesirable clinical manifestation to the vehicle, and not the radiation itself, of an administered radiopharmaceutical. The reaction does not result from an overdose, nor injury caused by poor injection technique (Cordova *et al.*, 1984). The majority of adverse reactions are mild, transient, and require little or no treatment. Occasionally, however, serious reactions such as cardiorespiratory arrest, tachycardia, dyspnoea and hypotension have been reported. Fatalities have on rare occasions also been reported.

Adverse reactions to radiopharmaceuticals fall into one of several groups with a variety of symptoms (Table 23.4). The usual types of reactions are anaphylaxis, allergic, pyrogen and vasovagal. Miscellaneous reactions such as phlebitis, metallic taste and chills have on occasions been reported. Four groups of radiopharmaceuticals account for most of the reported reactions, i.e. diphosphonates, colloids, albumin particulates and DTPA. The frequency of reports of reactions to these groups of radiopharmaceuticals is shown in Table 23.5. The remainder of the reported reactions were covered by a variety of radiopharmaceuticals including sodium ^{131}I-iodide, ^{67}Ga-gallium citrate, ^{111}In-labelled DTPA and ^{201}Tl-thallous chloride. Some examples of reported reactions to commonly used radiopharmaceuticals are shown in Table 23.6.

The US Society of Nuclear Medicine has main-

Table 23.4 Some examples of clinical manifestations observed in adverse reactions to radiopharmaceuticals

Manifestation	*Examples*
Anaphylaxis (anaphylactoid) (immediate reactions)	Nausea, vomiting Hypotension Incontinence Syncope Flushing tachycardia
Allergic (delayed reaction)	Rash, urticaria Pruritus Dyspnoea Chest pain Palpitation Tachycardia
Pyrogen	Fever, headaches
Vasovagal	Faintness Blanching Sweating
Miscellaneous	Phlebitis Metallic taste Chills Cyanosis

Cordova *et al.* (1984).

Table 23.5 Radiopharmaceuticals associated with most commonly reported reactions

Radiopharmaceutical	*Period*	*Frequency*	*Reference*
Diphosphonates	1984	8/28	Kristensen (1987a)
	1985	11/34	Kristensen (1987a)
	1986	5/24	Kristensen (1987b)
	1977–86	UK 34/102	Keeling and Sampson (1987)
	1984	US 7/21	Atkins (1986)
Colloids	1984	2/28	Kristensen (1987a)
	1985	2/34	Kristensen (1987a)
	1986	2/24	Kristensen (1987b)
	1977–86	22/102	Keeling and Sampson (1987)
	1984	3/21	Atkins (1986)
Albumin particulates	1984	3/28	Kristensen (1987a)
	1985	5/34	Kristensen (1987a)
	1986	0/24	Kristensen (1987b)
	1977–86	12/102	Keeling and Sampson (1987)
	1986	3/21	Atkins (1986)
DTPA	1984	7/28	Kristensen (1987a)
	1985	3/34	Kristensen (1987a)
	1986	7/24	Kristensen (1987b)
	1982–86	16/102	Keeling and Sampson (1987)

Frequency refers to the number of reactions caused by that radiopharmaceutical as a fraction of the total reactions in the year.

Table 23.6 Some reported reactions to commonly used radiopharmaceuticals

Radiopharmaceutical	*Reported reactions*
^{99m}Tc-labelled sulphur colloid	Nausea and vomiting, decreased blood pressure, rash and urticaria, pruritus, incontinence, dyspnoea, wheezing, cyanosis, dizziness, palpitations, pallor, flushing, pyrogen reactions
^{99m}Tc-labelled antimony sulphide colloid	Severe headaches, dyspnoea, tachycardia, cyanosis, cardiorespiratory arrest
^{99m}Tc-labelled human albumin preparations	Flushing, nausea, vomiting, pallor, dyspnoea, chest pain, hypotension, cardiocirculatory collapse, wheezing, pruritus, cyanosis, chills, sweating, tachycardia
^{99m}Tc-labelled MDP	Macropapular erythematous rashes (often late onset), pruritus, flushing, headache, dyspnoea, dizziness, nausea, hypotension, fever, chills
^{99m}Tc-labelled DTPA	Dizziness, hypotension, loss of consciousness, blurred vision, weakness, low back pain, respiratory distress, nausea, pallor
^{99m}Tc-labelled DMSA	Epigastric pain, flushing, nausea
^{99m}Tc-labelled GHA	Nausea, dizziness, flushing, tachycardia
Sodium ^{131}I-iodide	Pruritus, urticaria, rash, swelling, nausea, vomiting, headache, hot and cold flushes
^{131}I-Orthoiodohippurate	Urticaria, hypotension
^{67}Ga-Gallium citrate	Pruritus, rash, nausea, vomiting
^{111}In-labelled DTPA	Pyrogen reactions, aseptic, meningitis
^{201}Tl-Thallous chloride	Pruritus, rash, flushing

tained a registry of adverse reactions since 1970 and publishes an annual report. From the data collected they have been able to estimate the overall incidence of adverse reactions to radiopharmaceuticals as between 1 and 6 reactions per 10 000 administrations (Rhodes and Cordova, 1980; Cordova *et al.*, 1982). A similar reporting system is run in the UK by the British Institute of Radiology, who estimated an overall incidence of between 1 and 20 reactions per 100 000 administrations (Keeling and Sampson, 1984). The European Nuclear Medicine Society also operates a reporting system for adverse reactions, and publishes annual figures.

From their data Keeling and Sampson (1984) describe a changing pattern of reported reactions. This is partly due to decreased use of older radiopharmaceuticals of doubtful formulation, improved quality-control measures, and introduction of methylene diphosphonate which accounts for nearly one-half of their reports. The overall incidence of reporting adverse reactions is suspected to be low, and this may be due to the possibility that many reactions go unrecognized by nuclear medicine personnel, and reactions occurring outside the nuclear medicine department may not be reported.

23.6.2 ALTERATIONS IN RADIOPHARMACEUTICAL BIODISTRIBUTIONS

An intentional procedure in some nuclear medicine studies is the administration of a drug to alter the biodistribution of a radiopharmaceutical. Dipyridamole, for example, is sometimes used to stress the heart prior to imaging with ^{201}Tl. However, many patients are on medication when they present for a nuclear medicine study. The clinician should be aware that there are many instances reported in the literature where this medication has unexpectedly altered the way in which the radiopharmaceutical has been handled by the body. Failure to recognize alterations may lead to missed or incorrect diagnosis.

During the past decade over 400 reports have been published on drug–radiopharmaceutical incompatabilities. Sampson and Hesslewood (1989) have classified these effects as: unusual handling of the radiopharmaceutical as a result of the pharmacological effect of the drug; physicochemical interaction between the radiopharmaceutical and the drug; and drug-induced disease. In addition other causative agents have been reported to affect radiopharmaceutical biodistribution, e.g. therapeutic irradiation, surgery and haemodialysis (Lazarus and Maisey, 1987). Some examples of the above are shown in Table 23.7.

Radiolabelling of red blood cells with ^{99m}Tc is a common procedure in nuclear medicine. Many drugs have been reported to decrease the labelling efficiency (see Table 23.7). Various mechanisms have been postulated for these effects. Tatum and Burke (1983) described three patients who showed poor labelling of red cells after administration of iodinated contrast media in the previous 24 h. However, Finkel *et al.* (1988) studied red cell labelling with ^{99m}Tc in 25 patients, before and after administration of intravenous contrast agent, and could find no significant differences in the percentage labelling yields.

23.6.3 EXCRETION OF RADIOACTIVITY IN BREAST MILK

Occasionally in the nuclear medicine department it is considered necessary to perform a study on a nursing mother. The hazard to the suckling infant from ingestion of milk contaminated with radioactivity must be borne in mind. A decision must then be made either to instruct the mother to interrupt breast-feeding for a suitable length of time, or recommend that breast-feeding should cease altogether in certain circumstances. Difficulties are often met in making such a decision because the available data for guidance are often inadequate. There are several factors which complicate the situation and these include: the effective half-life of the radionuclide to be administered; the dose of the radionuclide; the chemical form in which the radionuclide is administered to the mother; the route of administration to the mother; the chemical form in which the radionuclide appears in the milk; and the frequency of breast-feeding and the volume of milk ingested at each feed.

There are many reports in the literature describing cases where radiopharmaceuticals have been administered to nursing mothers, and attempts have been made to assess the risk to the infant, and make a recommendation. Much of the data in these reports have been presented in different ways, making it difficult to assess risks and recommendations from one report to another. However, recently several publications have attempted to collate the literature reviews and assess the

Table 23.7 Some causes and examples of alterations in radiopharmaceutical biodistribution

Cause	*Effect*	*Reference*
Chemotherapeutic agents		
Adriamycin	Change in myocardial biodistribution of ^{99m}Tc-labelled pyrophosphate	Chacko *et al.* (1977)
	Increased uptake of ^{67}Ga in adriamycin-damaged myocardium	Hatfield *et al.* (1986)
Bleomycin	Uptake of ^{67}Ga into pulmonary lesions	Rickman *et al.* (1975)
Methotrexate	Increased uptake of ^{99m}Tc-pertechnetate in cerebral ventricles	Makler *et al.* (1978)
Cyclophosphamide and doxorubicin	Intense renal uptake of ^{99m}Tc-labelled pyrophosphate	Lutrin *et al.* (1978)
Doxorubicin	Decreased red cell labelling with ^{99m}Tc	Ballinger *et al.* (1988)
Therapeutic irradiations	Increased uptake of ^{67}Ga in irradiated soft tissue	Van der Schoot *et al.* (1972)
	Uptake of ^{99m}Tc-labelled phosphate analogues in soft tissue, particularly myocardium	Soin *et al.* (1977)
Surgery	Uptake of ^{67}Ga in scar	Jackson *et al.* (1976)
	Extra-osseous uptake of ^{99m}Tc-labelled pyrophosphate	Poulose *et al.* (1975)
Other drugs		
Anaesthetics	Reversed liver to spleen ratio with ^{99m}Tc-labelled sulphur colloid	Lentle *et al.* (1979)
Sodium bicarbonate	Decreased renal uptake of ^{99m}Tc-labelled DMSA	Yee *et al.* (1981)
Cortisone preparations	Suppression of ^{67}Ga uptake in brain tumours	Stebner (1975) Waxman *et al.* (1977)
	Reduced uptake of tracer into abscess	Hladik *et al.* (1987)
Oral contraceptives	Increased adrenal uptake of ^{131}I-iodomethylnorcholesterol	Gross *et al.* (1981)
Sex hormones	Uptake of ^{67}Ga in male breast	Kim *et al.* (1977)
Phenylbutazone	Delayed renal uptake of ^{67}Ga	Lin *et al.* (1983)
Erythromycin	False-positive ^{99m}Tc-labelled DISIDA study	Swayne and Kolc (1986)
Phenothiazines	Increased breast uptake of ^{67}Ga	Ajmani and Pircher (1978)
Aluminium hydroxide	Lung uptake of ^{99m}Tc-labelled sulphur colloid	Bobinet *et al.* (1974)
	Altered distribution of ^{99m}Tc-labelled EHDP	Chaudhuri (1976)
Miscellaneous		
Haemodialysis	Excess uptake of ^{67}Ga in bone	Lentle *et al.* (1979)
Iodinated antiseptics	Release of ^{99m}Tc from some radiopharmaceuticals	Fisher *et al.* (1977)
Methyldopa, hydralazine	Decreased ^{99m}Tc labelling of red blood cells *in vivo*	Zimmer *et al.* (1981)
Digoxin	Inhibits uptake of ^{86}Rb by red blood cells	Zanad *et al.* (1981)
Prazosin, digoxin	Decreased binding of red blood cells with ^{99m}Tc	Lee *et al.* (1983)
Nifedipine	Altered red blood cell labelling with ^{99m}Tc	Sampson (1988)

risks and make recommendations on a more scientific basis. Lazarus and Edwards (1988) have determined the concentrations of radioactivity in milk samples at the times at which maximum concentration is estimated to occur, and at a second time when the authors recommend that breast-feeding can recommence. Their calculations are based on the assumption of a 150 ml volume milk feed consumed, and the absorbed radiation doses for various infant body organs estimated. Unless otherwise specified in the literature report, they have in many cases assumed the chemical form of the radionuclide in the milk to be the same as that administered to the mother.

Table 23.8 Recommendations for interruption of breast-feeding after administration of some radiopharmaceuticals to nursing mothers

	Recommendations for interruption			
Radiopharmaceutical	A *(h)*	B *(h)*	C *(MBq ml^{-1})*	D *(h, MBq)*
^{99m}Tc-Pertechnetate	16	III, 36	30.34×10^{-4}	24, 740
^{99m}Tc-labelled macroaggregated albumin	14	II, 6	30.34×10^{-4}	24, 740
^{99m}Tc-labelled erythrocytes	20	III, 13	30.34×10^{-4}	24, 740
^{99m}Tc-labelled DTPA	4	I	30.34×10^{-4}	24, 740
^{99m}Tc-labelled DMSA	–	I	30.34×10^{-4}	24, 740
^{99m}Tc-labelled glucoheptonate	–	I	30.34×10^{-4}	24, 740
^{99m}Tc-labelled MDP	12	I	30.34×10^{-4}	24, 740
^{75}Se-Selenomethionine	168	IV, 467	–	–
^{67}Ga-Gallium citrate	264	IV, 427	7.77×10^{-5}	720, III
^{51}Cr-labelled EDTA	4	I	–	–
Chromic ^{32}P-phosphate	1000	–	–	–
Sodium ^{32}P-phosphate	1000	–	–	–
^{111}In-labelled leukocytes	24*	I	–	–
^{125}I-labelled fibrinogen	264	IV, 540	–	–
^{125}I-labelled human serum albumin	240	IV, 260	–	–
^{125}I-Orthoiodohippurate	16	III, 18	–	–
^{123}I-Orthoiodohippurate	–	III, 8	–	–
^{131}I-Orthoiodohippurate	15	III, 30	6.10×10^{-7}	108, 7.4
^{123}I-Iodide	–	III, 5	4.44×10^{-6}	48–72, 0.37–1.11
^{131}I Iodide	–	IV, 1727	15.17×10^{-9}	1344, 0.185

A. Lazarus and Edwards (1988). Time to reduce risk by a factor of 10 (*by 25%).
B. Mountford and Coakley (1989). I, interruption not essential; II, interruption for number of hours shown; III, interruption to reduce effective dose equivalent to below 1 mSv; IV, cessation.
C. Breast milk activity at which nursing considered safe (Romney *et al.*, 1986).
D. Maximum delay recommended after maternal dose shown (Romney *et al.* 1986).

With ^{99m}Tc-labelled radiopharmaceuticals they have assumed the radioactivity to be in the form of $^{99m}TcO_4$, and calculated the absorbed radiation dose to the whole body, stomach wall and thyroid of the infant. In their treatment of the problem, Romney *et al.* (1986) have reviewed the literature and proposed a mathematically derived approach taking into account the effective half-life of the tracer in breast milk, the daily volume of milk produced, a dose factor relating the relevant radionuclide to its critical organ in the infant, and some criterion for the maximum permissible dose to that organ. Mountford and Coakley (1989) have also taken the available data and attempted to calculate the fraction of the administered dose which appears in feeds, and the total fractional activity ingested for all the feeds the infant would ingest, assuming 850 ml milk are ingested each day.

In all the above reviews the authors have attempted to estimate the absorbed radiation dose to the critical organs and effective dose equivalent to the infant. Based on these estimations they have calculated the breast milk activity at which breast-feeding is considered safe to recommence where appropriate, and the delay required before nursing is resumed. In an attempt to provide a common basis for comparing the different radiopharmaceuticals, Lazarus and Edwards (1988) have calculated a risk factor based on the effective dose equivalent to the infant per megabecquerel administered to the mother, assuming the resumption of breast-feeding at some stated time after the radioactivity was administered to the mother. Where possible they have also given an estimate of the time delay to reduce the risk by a factor of ten. Romney *et al.* (1986) have theoretically derived maximum delays required before nursing resumes for several radionuclides. Mountford and Coakley (1989) have calculated the time after administration of various radiopharmaceuticals to the mother to reduce the effective dose equivalent to the infant to below 1 mSv. They have then assigned each radiopharmaceutical to one of four categories: interruption of feeding not essential; interruption for a fixed period of time; interruption until measurements indicate feeding can be resumed; and complete cessation of breast-feeding. Some examples where radioactivity has been measured in breast milk following the administration of radiopharmaceuticals to nursing mothers are shown in Table 23.8. In almost all of these cases no milk was ingested by the infant, and the recommendations are made based on calculations of the radiation dose the infant would have received if the milk had been consumed.

REFERENCES

Ajmani, S. K. and Pircher, F. J. (1978) Ga-67 citrate in gynecomastia. *J. Nucl. Med.*, **19**, 560–1.

Atkins, H. L. (1986) Reported adverse reactions to radiopharmaceuticals remain low in 1984. *J. Nucl. Med.*, **27**, 327.

Ballinger, J. R., Gerson, B., Gulenchyn, K. Y. *et al.* (1988) Technetium-99m red blood cell labelling in patients treated with doxorubicin. *Clin. Nucl. Med.*, **13**, 169–70.

Bett, R., Coleman, G. H., Cunninghame, J. G. *et al.* (1981) Preparation of a ^{195m}Hg–^{195m}Au isotope generator for medical use. *Nucl. Med. Commun.*, **2**, 75–9.

Bevan, J. A., Tofe, A. J., Benedict, J. J. *et al.* (1980) Tc-99m HMDP (hydroxymethylene disphosphonate): a radiopharmaceutical for skeletal and acute myocardial infarct imaging. 1. Synthesis and distribution in animals. *J. Nucl. Med.*, **21**, 961–6.

Bianchi, C. (1981) in: *Secondary Forms of Hypertension: Current Diagnosis and Management* (ed. M. D. Blaufox), Grune and Stratton, New York, pp. 289–308.

Bobinet, D. D., Sevrin, R., Zurbriggen, M. T. *et al.* (1974) Lung uptake of 99mTc-sulphur colloid in patient exhibiting presence of Al^{3+} in plasma. *J. Nucl. Med.*, **15**, 1220–2.

Budinger, T. F., Yano, Y., Moyer, B. *et al.* (1983) Myocardial extraction of Rb-82 vs flow determined by positron emission tomography. *Circulation*, **68**, (Suppl. 3), III-81 (abstr.).

Burch, W. M., Sullivan, P. J., Lomas, F. E. *et al.* (1986a) Lung ventilation studies with technetium-99m 'Pseudogas'. *J. Nucl. Med.*, **27**, 842–6.

Burch, W. M., Sullivan, P. J. and McLaren, C. J. (1986b) Technegas: a new ventilation agent for lung scanning. *Nucl. Med. Commun.*, **7**, 865–71.

Chacko, A. K., Gordon, D. H. and Bennett, J. M. (1977) Myocardial imaging with Tc-99m pyrophosphate in patients on adriamycin treatment of neoplasia. *J. Nucl. Med.*, **18**, 680–3.

Chaplin, S. B., Oberle, P. O., Hoffman, T. J. *et al.* (1985) Regional brain uptake and retention of Tc-99m-propylene amine oxine derivatives. *J. Nucl. Med.*, **26**, 18 (abstr.).

Chaudhuri, T. K. (1976) The effect of aluminium and pH on altered body distribution of 99mTc-EHDP. *Int. J. Nucl. Med.*, **3**, 37.

Cheng, C., Treves, S., Samuel, A. *et al.* (1980) A new osmium-191–iridium-191m generator. *J. Nucl. Med.*, **21**, 1169–76.

Chinol, M. and Hnatowich, D. J. (1987) Generator-produced yttrium-90 for radioimmunotherapy. *J. Nucl. Med.*, **28**, 1465–70.

Clarke, S. E. M., Fogelman, I., Lazarus, C. R. *et al.* (1987a) in *Nuklearmedizin – Nuclear Medicine in Research and Practice* (eds H. A. E. Schmidt and D. Emrich), Schattauer-Verlag, Stuttgart, pp. 475–6.

Clarke, S. E. M., Lazarus, C. R., Edwards, S. *et al.* (1987b) Scintigraphy and treatment of medullary carcinoma of the thyroid with iodine-131 meta-iodobenzylguanidine. *J. Nucl. Med.*, **28**, 1820–5.

Connell, J. M. C. Hilditch, T. G., Elliott, A. *et al.* (1984) ^{131}I MIBG and medullary carcinoma of the thyroid. *Lancet*, **ii**, 273–4.

Cordova, M. A., Rhodes, B. A., Atkins, H. L. *et al.* (1982) Adverse reactions to radiopharmaceuticals. *J. Nucl. Med.*, **23**, 550–1.

Cordova, M. A., Hladik, W. B. III and Rhodes, B. A. (1984) Validation and characterization of adverse reactions to radiopharmaceuticals. *Non-invasive Med. Imaging*, **1**, 17–24.

Coveney, J. R. and Robbins, M. S. (1987) Comparison of technetium-99m MAG_3 kit with HPLC-purified technetium-99m MAG_3 and OIH in rats. *J. Nucl. Med.*, **28**, 1881–7.

Cox, P. H. Belfer, A. J. and Van der Pompe, W. B. (1976) Thallium-201 chloride uptake in tumours, a possible complication in heart scintigraphy. *Br. J. Radiol.*, **49**, 767–8.

Danpure, H. J. and Osman, S. (1981) Cell labelling and cell damage with In-111-acetylacetone: an alternative to In-111 oxine. *Br. J. Radiol.*, **54**, 596–601.

Danpure, H. J., Osman, S. and Brady, F. (1982) The labelling of blood cells in plasma with In-111 tropolonate. *Br. J. Radiol.*, **55**, 247–9.

Danpure, H. J., Osman, S. and Carroll, M. J. (1987a) *In vitro* studies to develop a clinical protocol for radiolabelling mixed leucocytes with Tc-99m HM-PAO. *Nucl. Med. Commun.*, **8**, 280 (abstr.).

Danpure, H. J., Osman, S., Hogg, N. *et al.* (1987b) The clinical use of I-123 labelled leucocyte-specific monoclonal antibody to detect inflammatory lesions. *Nuklearmedizin* (Suppl. 23), 492–4.

Danpure, H. J. and Osman, S. (1988) A review of methods of separating and radiolabelling human leucocytes. *Nucl. Med. Commun.*, **9**, 681–5.

Davison, A., Jones, A. G., Orvig, C. *et al.* (1981) A new class of oxotechnetium (5+) chelate complexes containing a $TcON_2S_2$ core. *Inorg. Chem.*, **20**, 1629–32.

Deutsch, E., Glavan, K. A., Sodd, V. J. *et al.* (1981a) Cationic Tc-99m complexes as potential myocardial imaging agents. *J. Nucl. Med.*, **22**, 897–907.

Deutsch, E., Bushong, W., Glavan, K. A. *et al.* (1981b) Heart imaging with cationic complexes of technetium. *Science*, **214**, 85–6.

Deutsch, E. (1982) in *Applications of Nuclear and Radiochemistry* (eds R. M. Lambrecht and N. Morcos), Pergamon Press, New York, pp. 139–51.

Deutsch, E., Vanderheyden, J.-L., Gerundini, P. *et al.* (1987) Development of nonreducible technetium-99m (III) cations as myocardial perfusion imaging agents: initial experience in humans. *J. Nucl. Med.*, **28**, 1870–80.

Eckleman, W. C., Reba, R. C., Rzeszotarski, B. *et al.*

(1984) External imaging of cerebral muscarinic acetylcholine receptors. *Science*, **223**, 291–2.

Efange, S. M. N., Kung, H. F., Billings, J. *et al.* (1987) Technetium-99m bis (aminoethanethiol) complexes with amine sidechains: potential brain perfusion imaging agents for SPECT. *J. Nucl. Med.*, **28**, 1012–19.

Ehrhardt, G. J., Volkert, W., Goeckeler, W. F. *et al.* (1983) A new Cd-115 → In-115m radionuclide generator. *J. Nucl. Med.*, **24**, 349–52.

Eisenhut, M. (1984) Iodine-131-labelled diphosphonates for the palliative treatment of bone metastases: 1. Organ distribution and kinetics of I-131BDP3 in rats. *J. Nucl. Med.*, **25**, 1356–1361.

Endo, K., Shiomi, K., Kasagi, K. *et al.* (1984) Imaging of medullary thyroid carcinoma with ^{131}I-MIBG. *Lancet*, **ii**, 233.

English, R. J., Kozlowski, J., Tumeh, S. S. and Holman, B. L. (1987) Technetium myocardial perfusion agents: an introduction. *J. Nucl. Med. Technol.*, **15**, 138–43.

Eshima, D., Fritzberg, A. R., Kasina, S., Johnson, D. L. and Taylor, A. Jr (1985) Comparison of a new Tc-99m renal function agent, Tc-99m-mercaptoacetyltriglycine, with I-131 OIH. *J. Nucl. Med.*, **26**, P56–7 (abstr.).

Eshima, D., Taylor, A. Jr, Fritzberg, A. R. *et al.* (1987) Animal evaluation of technetium-99m triamide mercaptide complexes as potential renal imaging agents. *J. Nucl. Med.*, **28**, 1180–6.

Evans, J. R., Gunton, R. W., Baker, R. G. *et al.* (1965) Use of radioiodinated fatty acid for photoscans of the heart. *Circ. Res.*, **16**, 1–10.

Fawwaz, R. A., Wang, T. S. T., Srivastava, S. C. *et al.* (1984) Potential of palladium-109-labelled antimelanoma monoclonal antibody for tumour therapy. *J. Nucl. Med.*, **25**, 796–9.

Feldman, J. M., Blinder, R. A., Lucas, K. J. *et al.* (1986) Iodine-131 metaiodobenzylguanidine scintigraphy of carcinoid tumours. *J. Nucl. Med.*, **27**, 1691–6.

Finkel, J., Chervu, L. R., Bernstein, R. G. *et al.* (1988) Red blood cell labelling with technetium-99m: effect of radiopaque contrast agents. *Clin. Nucl. Med.*, **13**, 166–8.

Fischer, M., Kamanabroo, D., Sondorkamy, H. *et al.* (1984) Scintigraphic imaging of carcinoid tumours with ^{131}I-metaiodobenzylguanidine. *Lancet*, **ii**, 165.

Fisher, S. M., Brown, R. G. and Greyson, N. D. (1977) Unbinding of Tc-99m by iodinated antiseptics. *J. Nucl. Med.*, **18**, 1139–40.

Fogelman, I., Pearson, D. W., Bessent, R. G. *et al.* (1981) A comparison of skeletal uptake of three diphosphonates by whole-body retention: concise communication. *J. Nucl. Med.*, **22**, 880–3.

Fogelman, I. (ed.) (1986) in *Bone Scanning in Clinical Practice*, Springer-Verlag, London, p. 11.

Frakowiak, R. S. J., Lenzi, G.-L., Jones, T. *et al.* (1980) Quantitative measurement of regional cerebral blood flow and oxygen metabolism in man using O-15 and positron emission tomography: theory, procedure and normal values. *J. Comput. Assist. Tomogr.*, **4**, 727–36.

Francis, M. D., Ferguson, D. L., Tofe, A. J. *et al.* (1980) Comparative evaluation of three diphosphonates: *in vitro* adsorption (C-14 labelled) and *in vivo* osteogenic uptake (Tc-99m complexed). *J. Nucl. Med.*, **21**, 1185–1189.

Francis, R. A., Agnew, J. E. and Clarke, S. W. (1986) in *Progress in Radiopharmacy* (eds P. H. Cox, S. J. Mather, C. B. Sampson and C. R. Lazarus), Martinus Nijhoff, Dordrecht, p. 590.

Fritzberg, A. R., Klingensmith W. C. III, Whitney, W. P. and Kuni, C. C. (1981) Chemical and biological studies of Tc-99m *N, N'*-bis (Mercaptoacetamido)-ethylenediamine: a potential replacement for I-131 iodohippurate. *J. Nucl. Med.*, **22**, 258–63.

Fritzberg, A., Kuni, C. C., Klingensmith, W. C. *et al.* (1982) Synthesis and biological evaluation of Tc-99m *N,N'*-bis (mercaptoacetyl)-2,3-diaminopropanoate: a potential replacement for 131-I-o-iodohippurate. *J. Nucl. Med.*, **23**, 592–8.

Fritzberg, A. R., Kasina, S., Eshima, D. and Johnson, D. L. (1986) Synthesis and biological evaluation of technetium-99m MAG_3 as a hippuran replacement. *J. Nucl. Med.*, **27**, 111–16.

Geatti, O., Shapiro, B., Sisson, J. *et al.* (1985) Iodine-131 metaidobenzylguanidine scintigraphy for the location of neuroblastoma: preliminary experience in ten cases. *J. Nucl. Med.*, **26**, 736–42.

Gerson, M. C., Deutsch, E. A., Nishiyama, H. *et al.* (1983) Myocardial perfusion imaging with 99mTc-DMPE in man. *Eur. J. Nucl. Med.*, **8**, 371–4.

Goeckeler, W. F., Edwards, B., Volkert, W. A. *et al.* (1987) Skeletal localization of samarium-153 chelates: potential therapeutic bone agents. *J. Nucl. Med.*, **28**, 495–504.

Goodman, M. M., Knapp, F. F. Jr, Callahan, A. P. *et al.* (1982) A new well-retained myocardial imaging agent: radioiodinated 15-(*p*-iodophenyl)-6-tellurapentadecanoic acid. *J. Nucl. Med.*, **23**, 904–8.

Goodwin, D. A. (1987) Pharmacokinetics and antibodies. *J. Nucl. Med.*, **28**, 1358–62.

Granowska, M., Mather, S. J., Britton, K. E. *et al.* (1990a) ^{99m}Tc radioimmunoscintigraphy of colorectal cancer. *Br. J. Cancer*, **62**, Suppl. X, 30–3.

Granowska, M., Mather, S. J., Jobling, T. *et al.* (1990b) Radiolabelled mucin, SM3, monoclonial antibody for immunoscintigraphy of ovarian tumours. *Int. J. Biol. Mech.*, **5**, 89–96.

Gross, M. D., Valk, T. W., Swanson, D. P. *et al.* (1981) The role of pharmacologic manipulation in adrenal cortical scintigraphy. *Semin. Nucl. Med.*, **11**, 128–48.

Hale, T. I., Jucker, A., Vgenopoulos, K., Sauter, B., Wacheck, W. and Bors, L. (1981) Clinical experience with a new bone seeking 99mTc radiopharmaceutical. *Nucl. Compact*, **12**, 54–5.

Hatfield, M. K., Martin, W. B., Ryan, J. W. *et al.* (1986) Increased uptake of 67-gallium citrate activity in a patient with adriamycin-damaged myocardium. *Clin. Nucl. Med.*, **11**, 756–7.

Hesslewood, S. R., Dahir, N. D. and Jack, D. B. (1988) Pentavalent technetium DMSA: preparation and protein binding studies. *Nucl. Med. Commun.*, **9**, 191 (abstr.).

Hladik, W. B., Ponto, J. A., Lentle, B. C. *et al.* (1987) in *Essentials of Nuclear Medicine Science* (eds W. B. Hladick, and G. P. Saha), Williams and Wilkins, London.

Hnatowich, D. J., Virzi, F. and Doherty, P. W. (1985) DTPA-coupled antibodies labelled with yttrium-90. *J. Nucl. Med.*, **26**, 503–9.

Hoefnagel, C. A., Voûte, P. A., de Kraker, J. *et al.* (1985)

Total body scintigraphy with ^{131}I-*meta*-iodobenzylguanidine for detection of neuroblastoma. *Diagn. Imag. Clin. Med.*, **54**, 21–7.

Hoefnagel, C. A., den Hartog Jager, F. C. A., van Gennip, A. H. *et al.* (1986) Diagnosis and treatment of a carcinoid tumour using Iodine-131 *meta*-iodobenzylguanidine. *Clin. Nucl. Med.*, **11**, 150–2.

Hoefnagel, C. A., Delprat, C. C., Zanin, D. *et al.* (1988) New radionuclide tracers for the diagnosis and therapy of medullary thyroid carcinoma. *Clin. Nucl. Med.*, **13**, 159–65.

Holmes, R. A., Chaplin, S. B., Royston, K. G. *et al.* (1985) Cerebral uptake and retention of ^{99}Tc^{m}-hexamethylpropyleneamine oxime (^{99}Tc^{m}-HM-PAO). *Nucl. Med. Commun.*, **6**, 443–7.

Holman, B. L., Jones, A. G., Lister-James, J. *et al.* (1984) A new Tc-99m-labelled myocardial imaging agent hexakis (*t*-butyl-isonitrile)-technetium (I) [Tc-99m TBI]: initial experience in the human. *J. Nucl. Med.*, **25**, 1350–5.

Holman, B. L., Sporn, V., Jones, A. G. *et al.* (1987) Myocardial imaging with technetium-99m CPI: initial experience in the human. *J. Nucl. Med.*, **28**, 13–18.

Huchon, G. J., Montgomery, A. B., Lipavsky, A. *et al.* (1987) Respiratory clearance of aerosolized radioactive solutes of varying molecular weight. *J. Nucl. Med.*, **28**, 894–902.

Jackson, F. I., Dierich, H. C. and Lentle, B. C. (1976) Gallium-67 citrate scintiscanning in testicular neoplasia. *J. Canad. Assoc. Radiol.*, **27**, 84–8.

Jones, A. G., Davison, A., La Tegola, M. R. *et al.* (1982) Chemical and *in vivo* studies of the anion oxo-(*N,N'*-ethylenebis (2-mercaptoacetamido) technetate. *J. Nucl. Med.*, **23**, 801–9.

Joseph, K., Höffken, H., Bosslett, K. *et al.* (1988) Imaging of inflammation with granulocytes labelled *in vivo*. *Nucl. Med. Commun.*, **9**, 763–9.

Keeling, D. H. and Sampson, C. B. (1984) Adverse reactions to radiopharmaceuticals: United Kingdom, 1977–1983. *Br. J. Radiol.*, **57**, 1091–1096.

Keeling, D. H. and Sampson, C. B. (1987) Adverse reactions to radiopharmaceuticals: incidence, reporting, symptoms, treatment. *Nuklearmedizin Suppl.*, **23**, 478–82.

Keenan, A. M., Harbert, J. C. and Larson, S. M. (1985) Monoclonal antibodies in nuclear medicine. *J. Nucl. Med.*, **26**, 531–7.

Khaw, B. A., Beller, G. A., Haber, E. *et al.* (1976) Localisation of cardiac myosin-specific antibody in myocardial infarction. *J. Clin. Invest.*, **58**, 439–46.

Khaw, B. A., Beller, G. A. and Haber, E. (1978) Experimental myocardial infarct imaging following intravenous administration of iodine-131 labelled antibody $(Fab^1)_2$ fragments specific for cardiac myosin. *Circulation*, **57**, 743–50.

Khaw, B. A., Fallon, J. T., Strauss, H. W. *et al.* (1980) Myocardial infarct imaging with indium-III-diethylenetriaminepentaacetic acid anticanine cardiac myosin antibodies. *Science*, **209**, 295–7.

Khaw, B. A., Strauss, W., Carvalho, A. *et al.* (1982) Technetium-99m labelling of antibodies to cardiac myosin Fab and to human fibrinogen. *J. Nucl. Med.*, **23**, 1011–19.

Kim, Y. C., Brown, M. L. and Thrall, J. H. (1977) Scintigraphic patterns of gallium-67 uptake in the breast. *Radiology*, **124**, 169–175.

Kimmig, G., Brandeis, W. E., Eisenhut, M. *et al.* (1984) Scintigraphy of a neuroblastoma with I-131 *meta*-iodobenzylguanidine. *J. Nucl. Med.*, **25**, 773–5.

Klingensmith, W. C., Fritzberg, A. R., Spitzer, V. M. *et al.* (1983) Clinical evaluation of Tc-99m-*N,N'*-bis(mercaptoacetyl)-2,3-diaminopropanoate (component A) (Tc-99m-CO_2-DADS-A) as a replacement for I-131-hippuran. *J. Nucl. Med.*, **24**, 80 (abstr.).

Knapp, F. F. Jr, Ambrose, K. R., Callahan, A. P. *et al.* (1981) Effects of chain length and tellurium position on the myocardial uptake of Te-123m fatty acids. *J. Nucl. Med.*, **22**, 988–93.

Knapp, F. F. Jr, Srivastava, P. C., Callahan, A. P. *et al.* (1984) Effect of tellurium position on the myocardial uptake of radioiodinated 18-iodotellura-17-octadecanoic acid analogues. *J. Med. Chem.*, **27**, 57–63.

Krasnow, A. Z., Collier, B. D., Isitman, A. T. *et al.* (1988) The clinical significance of unusual sites of thallium-201 uptake. *Semin. Nucl. Med.*, **18**, 350–8.

Kristensen, K. (1987a) European system for reporting of adverse reactions and drug defects: third report 1984–1985. *Eur. J. Nucl. Med.*, **13**, 487–90.

Kristensen, K. (1987b) European system for reporting of adverse reactions and drug defects: fourth report 1986. *Eur. J. Nucl. Med.*, **13**, 491–2.

Kung, H. F., Tramposch, K. M. and Blau, M. (1983) A new brain perfusion imaging agent: (^{123}I)HIPDM: *N,N,N'*-trimethyl-*N*-[2-hydroxy-3-methyl-5-iodobenzyl]-1,3-propanediamine.) *J. Nucl. Med.*, **24**, 66–72.

Kung, H. F., Molnar, M., Billings, J. *et al.* (1984) Synthesis and biodistribution of neutral lipid-soluble Tc-99m complexes that cross the blood–brain barrier. *J. Nucl. Med.*, **25**, 326–32.

Kung, H. F., Efange, S., Yu, C. C. *et al.* (1985) Synthesis and biodistribution of Tc-99m bisaminoethanethiol (BAT) complexes with amine sidechains. *J. Nucl. Med.*, **26**, 18 (abstr.).

Lazarus, C. R. and Edwards, S. (1988) in *Drugs and Human Lactation* (ed. P. N. Bennett), Elsevier, Amsterdam, pp. 495–549.

Lazarus, C. R. and Maisey, M. N. (1987) in *Complications in Diagnostic Imaging*, 2nd ed. (eds G. Ansell and R. A. Wilkins), Blackwell, Oxford, pp. 373–90.

Lebowitz, E., Greene, M. W. and Fairchild, R. (1974) Thallium-201 for medical use. *J. Nucl. Med.*, **16**, 151–5.

Lee, H. B., Wexler, J. B., Scharf, S. C. *et al.* (1983) Pharmacologic alterations in Tc99m binding by red blood cells. *J. Nucl. Med* **24**, 397–401.

Lentle, B. C., Scott, J. R., Noujaim, A. A. *et al.* (1979) Iatrogenic alterations in radionuclide biodistributions. *Semin. Nucl. Med.*, **9**, 131–43.

Lin, D. S., Sanders, J. A. and Patel, B. R. (1983) Delayed renal localisation of Ga-67. *J. Nucl. Med.*, **24**, 894–7.

Lippmann, M. and Albert, R. E. (1969) The effect of particle size on the regional deposition of inhaled aerosols in the human respiratory tract. *Am. Ind. Hyg. Assoc. J.*, **30**, 257–75.

Loc'h, C., Mazière, B. and Comar, D. (1980) A new generator for ionic gallium-68. *J. Nucl. Med.*, **21**, 171–3.

Locher, J. T. H., Seybold, K., Andres, R. Y. *et al.* (1986)

Imaging inflammation and infectious lesions after injection of radioiodinated monoclonal antigranulocyte antibodies. *Nucl. Med. Commun.*, **7**, 659–70.
Lutrin, C. L., McDougall, I. R. and Goris, M. L. (1978) Intense concentration of technetium-99m pyrophosphate in the kidneys of children treated with chemotherapeutic drugs for malignant disease. *Radiology*, **128**, 165–7.
Lynn, M. D., Shapiro, B., Sisson, J. C. *et al.* (1984) Portrayal of pheochromocytoma and normal human adrenal medulla by *m*-[^{123}I]iodobenzylguanidine. *J. Nucl. Med.*, **25**, 436–40.
Machulla, H. J., Marsmann, M. and Dutschka, K. (1980) Biochemical synthesis of a radioiodinated phenyl fatty acid for *in vivo* metabolic studies of the myocardium. *Eur. J. Nucl. Med.*, **5**, 171–3.
Makler, P. T. Jr, Gutowicz, M. F. and Kuhl, D. E. (1978) Methotrexate-induced ventriculitis: appearance on routine radionuclide scan and emission computed tomography. *Clin. Nucl. Med.*, **3**, 22–3.
Mather, S. J. (1985) in *Radiopharmacy and Radiopharmaceuticals* (ed. A. E. Theobold), Taylor and Francis, London, pp. 29–50.
Mather, S. J. (1986) in *Progress in Radiopharmacy* (eds P. H. Cox, S. J. Mather, C. B. Sampson and C.R. Lazarus), Martinus Nijhoff, Dordrecht, pp. 512–29.
Mather, S. J., Ellison, D. (1990) Reduction mediated Techetium 99m-labelling of monoclonal antibodies. *J. Nucl. Med.*, **31**, 692–7.
Mathieu, L., Chevalier, P., Galy, G. *et al.* (1979) Preparation of rhenium-186 labelled EHDP and its possible use in the treatment of osseous neoplasms. *Int. J. Appl. Radiat. Isot.*, **30**, 725–7.
McAfee, J. G. and Thakur, M. L. (1976a) Survey of radioactive agents for in vitro labelling of phagocytic leucocytes. I. Soluble agents. *J. Nucl. Med.*, **17**, 480–7.
McAfee, J. G. and Thakur, M. L. (1976b) Survey of radioactive agents for *in vitro* labelling of phagocytic leucocytes II. Particles. *J. Nucl. Med.*, **17**, 488–92.
McAfee, J. G., Subramanian, G. and Gagne, G. (1984) Techniques of leucocyte harvesting and labelling: problems and perspectives. *Semin. Nucl. Med.*, **14**, 83–106.
McEwan, A. J., Zivanovic, M. A., Blake, G. M. *et al.* (1986) Sr-89 therapy: clinical response in metastatic bone disease. *Nucl. Med. Commun.*, **7**, 293 (abstr.).
Mena, I., Narahara, K. A., de Jong, R. *et al.* (1983) Gold-195m, an ultra-short-lived generator-produced radionuclide: clinical application in sequential first pass ventriculography. *J. Nucl. Med.*, **24**, 139–44.
Millar, A. M., Wilkinson, A. G. and Best, J. J. K. (1988) ^{99}Tc^{m}-MAG3: *in vitro* stability and *in vivo* behaviour at different times after preparation. *Nucl. Med. Commun.*, **9**, 190 (abstr.).
Mock, B. H. and English. D. (1987) Leucocyte labelling with technetium-99m tin colloids. *J. Nucl. Med.*, **28**, 1471–7.
Moretti, J. L., Cinotti, L., Cesaro, P. *et al.* (1987) Amines for brain tomoscintigraphy. *Nucl. Med. Commun.*, **8**, 581–95.
Mountford, P. J. and Coakley, A. J. (1989) A review of the secretion of radioactivity in human breast milk: data, quantitative analysis and recommendations. *Nucl. Med. Commun.*, **10**, 15–27.
Mountford, P. J., Kettle, A. G., O'Doherty, M. J. *et al.* (1990) Comparison of Techetium 99m leukocytes with Indium III oxime leukocytes of localising intra-abdominal sepsis. *J. Nucl. Med.*, **31**, 311–15.
Neirinckx, R. D. and Davis, M. A. (1980) Potential column chromatography for ionic Ga-68, 11. Organic ion exchangers as chromatographic supports. *J. Nucl. Med.*, **21**, 81–3.
Neirinckx, R. D., Canning, L. R., Piper, I. M. *et al.* (1987) Technetium-99m *d,l*-HM-PAO: a new radiopharmaceutical for SPECT imaging of regional cerebral blood perfusion. *J. Nucl. Med.*, **28**, 191–202.
Nishiyama, H., Deutsch, E., Adolph, R. J. *et al.* (1982) Basal kinetic studies of Tc-99m DMPE as a myocardial imaging agent in the dog. *J. Nucl. Med.*, **23**, 1093–101.
Nowotnik, D. P., Canning, L. R., Cumming, S. A. *et al.* (1985) Development of a Tc-99m-labelled radiopharmaceutical for cerebral blood flow imaging. *Nucl. Med. Commun.*, **6**, 499–506.
Nunn, A. D. Treher, E. N. and Feld, T. (1986) Boronic acid adducts of technetium oxine complexes (BATOs): a new class of neutral complex with myocardial imaging capabilities. *J. Nucl. Med.*, **27**, 893 (abstr.).
Ohta, H., Yamamoto, K., Endo, K. *et al.* (1984) A new imaging agent for medullary carcinoma of the thyroid. *J. Nucl. Med.*, **25**, 323–5.
Ohta, H., Endo, K., Fujita, T. *et al.* (1988) Clinical evaluation of tumour imaging using ^{99}Tc(V)^{m} dimercaptosuccinic acid, a new tumour-seeking agent. *Nucl. Med. Commun.*, **9**, 105–16.
Okada, R. D., Knapp, F. F. Jr, Elmaleh, D. R. *et al.* (1982) Tellurium-123m-labelled 9-telluraheptadecanoic acid: a possible cardiac imaging agent. *Circulation*, **65**, 305–10.
Okada, R. D., Knapp, F. F. Jr, Goodman, M. M. *et al.* (1985) Tellurium-labelled fatty-acid analogs: relationship of heteroatom position to myocardial kinetics. *Eur. J. Nucl. Med.*, **11**, 156–61.
Oster, Z. H., Srivastava, S. C., Som, P. *et al.* (1985) Thrombus radioimmunoscintigraphy: an approach using monoclonal antiplatelet antibody. *Proc. Natl Acad. Sci. USA*, **82**, 346–8.
Panek, K. J. (1986) in *Progress in Radiopharmacy* (eds P. H. Cox, S. J. Mather, C. B. Sampson and C. R. Lazarus), Martinus Nijhoff, Dordrecht, pp. 3–20.
Pauwels, E. K. J. and Van Kroonenburgh, M. J. P. G. (1988) Prospects of radioimmunoimaging and radioimmunotherapy in oncology. *Nucl. Med. Commun.*, **9**, 867–9.
Pavia, D., Agnew, J. E. and Clarke, S. W. (1986) in *Progress in Radiopharmacy* (eds P. H. Cox, S. J. Mather, C. B. Sampson and C. R. Lazarus), Martinus Nijhoff, Dordrecht, pp. 579–89.
Pecher, R. (1942) Biological investigations with radioactive calcium and strontium: preliminary report on the use of radioactive strontium in the treatment of bone cancer. *Univ. Calif. Publ. Pharmacol.*, **11**, 117–49.
Peltier, P. and Chatal, J.-F. (1986) ^{99m}Tc-DTPA and ^{99m}Tc-rhenium sulphur aerosol compared as adjuncts to perfusion scintigraphy in patients with suspected pulmonary embolism. *Eur. J. Nucl. Med.*, **12**, 254–7.
Perez, R., Cohen, Y., Henry, R. and Panneciere, C. (1972) A new radiopharmaceutical for 99mTc bone scanning. *J. Nucl. Med.*, **13**, 788–9 (abstr.).

Peters, A. M. (1988a) Review of platelet labelling and kinetics. *Nucl. Med. Commun.*, **9**, 803–8.

Peters, A. M. (1988b) Granulocyte kinetics and methods of evaluating cell performance. *Nucl. Med. Commun.*, **9**, 687–92.

Peters, A. M., Danpure, H. J., Osman, S. *et al.* (1986) Preliminary clinical experience with Tc-99m-HM-PAO for labelling leucocytes and imaging infection. *Lancet*, **ii**, 945–9.

Phipps, P., Borham, P., Gonda, I. *et al.* (1987) A rapid method for the evaluation of diagnostic radioaerosol delivery systems. *Eur. J. Nucl. Med.*, **13**, 183–6.

Pillay, M. (1985) in *Radiopharmacy and Radiopharmacology Yearbook* (ed. P. H. Cox), Gordon and Breach, New York, p. 123.

Pillay, M., Akkermans, J. A. and Cox, P. H. (1987) A high efficiency ultrasound nebuliser for radioaerosol studies of the lungs. *Eur. J. Nucl. Med.*, **13**, 331–4.

Poe, N. D., Robinson, G. D. Jr, Graham, L. S. *et al.* (1976) Experimental basis for myocardial imaging with I-123-labelled hexadecanoic acid. *J. Nucl. Med.*, **17**, 1077–82.

Poulose, K. P., Reba, R. C., Eckelman, E. C. *et al.* (1975) Extraosseous localisation of 99m Tc-pyrophosphate. *Br. J. Radiol.*, **48**, 724–6.

Reivich, M., Kuhl, D., Wolf, A. P. *et al.* (1979) The F-18-fluorodeoxyglucose method for the measurement of local cerebral glucose utilization in man. *Circ. Res.*, **44**, 127–37.

Reivich, M., Alavi, A., Wolf, A. P. *et al.* (1982) The use of 2-deoxy-D (1-C-11) glucose for the determination of local cerebral glucose metabolism in humans. *J. Cereb. Blood Flow Metab.*, **2**, 307–20.

Rhodes, B. A. and Cordova, M. A. (1980) Adverse reactions to radiopharmaceuticals: incidence in 1978 and associated symptoms. Report of the Adverse Reactions Subcommittee of the Society of Nuclear Medicine. *J. Nucl. Med.*, **21**, 1107–9.

Rickman, S. D., Levenson, S. M., Bunn, P. A. *et al.* (1975) ^{67}Ga accumulation in pulmonary lesions associated with bleomycin toxicity. *Cancer*, **36**, 1966–72.

Robinson, R. G. (1986) Radionuclides for the alleviation of bone pain in advanced malignancy. *Clin. Oncol.*, **5**, 39–49.

Romney, B. M., Nickoloff, E. L., Esser, P. D. *et al.* (1986) Radionuclide administration to nursing mothers: mathematically derived guidelines. *Radiology*, **160**, 549–54.

Rosenthall, L., Stern, J. and Arzoumanian, A. (1982) A clinical comparison of MDP and DMAD. *Clin. Nucl. Med.*, **7**, 403–6.

Sampson, C. B. (1988) Personal communication.

Sampson, C. B. and Hesslewood, S. R. (1989) in *Radiopharmaceuticals: Using Radioactive Compounds in Pharmaceutics and Medicine* (ed. A. E. Theobald), Ellis Horwood, Chichester, pp. 132–51.

Schelbert, H. R., Phelps, M. E., Huang, S. C. *et al.* (1981) *N*-13 ammonia as an indicator of myocardial blood flow. *Circulation*, **63**, 1259–72.

Schneider, R. F., Subramanian, G., Feld, T. A. *et al.* (1984) *N,N'*-bis (*S*-Benzoylmercaptoacetamido) ethylenediamine and propylenediamine ligands as renal function imaging agents. 1. Alternate synthetic methods. *J. Nucl. Med.*, **25**, 223–9.

Schroth, H. J., Oberhausen, E. and Berberich, R. (1981) Cell labelling with colloidal substances in whole blood. *Eur. J. Nucl. Med.*, **6**, 469–72.

Schuster, K., Peterson, J., Sirr, S. and Stuart, D. (1987) Quality control in the production of aerosols. *J. Nucl. Med. Technol.*, **15**, 97–8.

Schwartz, A. and Kloss, G. (1981) Technetium-99m DPD: a new skeletal imaging agent. *J. Nucl. Med.*, **22**, 77 (abstr.).

Sehweil, A., McKillop, J. H., Ziada, G. *et al.* (1988) The optimum time for tumour imaging with thallium-201. *Eur. J. Nucl. Med.*, **13**, 527–9.

Seybold, K. (1988) *In vivo* labelling of granulocytes using ^{123}I-tagged anti-granulocyte antibodies. *Nucl. Med. Commun.*, **9**, 745–52.

Sharp, P. F., Smith, F. W., Gemmell, H. G. *et al.* (1986) Technetium-99m HM-PAO stereoisomers as potential agents for imaging regional cerebral blood flow: human volunteer studies. *J. Nucl. Med.*, **27**, 171–7.

Shiue, C.-Y., Bai, L.-Q., Teng, R.-R. *et al.* (1987) No-carrier-added *N*-(3-[^{18}F] fluoropropyl) spiroperidol: biodistribution in mice and tomographic studies in a baboon. *J. Nucl. Med.*, **28**, 1164–70.

Sikora, K., Smedley, H. and Thorpe, P. (1984) Tumour imaging and drug targeting. *Br. Med. Bull.*, **40**, 233–9.

Sisson, J. C., Frager, M. S., Valk, T. W. *et al.* (1981) Scintigraphic localization of pheochromocytoma, *N. Engl. J. Med.*, **305**, 12–17.

Sisson, J. C., Shapiro, B., Beierwaltes, W. H. *et al.* (1984) Radiopharmaceutical treatment of malignant pheochromocytoma. *J. Nucl. Med.*, **25**, 197–206.

Smith, M. L., Martin, W., McKillop, J. H. and Fogelman, I. (1984) Improved lesion detection with dimethyl-amino-diphosphonate: a report of two cases. *Eur. J. Nucl. Med.*, **9**, 519–20.

Snook, D., Rowlinson, G. and Epenetos, A. A. (1987) Preparation and *in vivo* study of yttrium-90 labelled immunoconjugates. *Nucl. Med. Commun.*, **8**, 257 (abstr.).

Soin, J. S., Cox, J. D., Youker, J. E. *et al.* (1977) Cardiac localisation of Tc-99m-(Sn)-pyrophosphate following irradiation of the chest. *Radiology*, **124**, 165–8.

Solanki, K. K., Al-Nahhas, A. and Britton, K. E. (1988) Alternative methods for the preparation of ^{99}Tc^{m}-mercaptoacetyltriglycine (MAG3). *Nucl. Med. Commun.*, **9**, 190 (abstr.).

Sone, T., Fukunaga, M., Otsuka, N. *et al.* (1985) Metastatic medullary thyroid cancer: localization with iodine-131 metaiodobenzylguanidine. *J. Nucl. Med.*, **26**, 604–80.

Stebner, F. C. (1975) Steroid effect on the brain scan in a patient with cerebral metastases. *J. Nucl. Med.*, **16**, 320–1.

Strudler, P. K. and Larson, S. M. (1985) Radiolabelled monoclonal antibodies: a 'decisive' technology. *J. Nucl. Med. Technol.*, **13**, 46–52.

Subramanian, G. and McAfee, J. G. (1971) A new complex of ^{99m}Tc for skeletal imaging. *Radiology*, **99**, 192–6.

Subramanian, G., McAfee, J. G., Blair, R. J., Kallfeltz, F. A. and Thomas, F. D. (1975) Technetium-99m-methylene diphosphonate: a superior agent for skeletal imaging: comparison with other technetium complexes. *J. Nucl. Med.*, **16**, 744–55.

Swayne, L. C. and Kolc, J. (1986) Erythromycin hepatotoxicity: a rare case of a false positive technetium DISIDA study. *Clin. Nucl. Med.*, **11**, 10–12.

Tatum, J. and Burke, T. (1983) Pitfalls to modified *in vivo* method of Tc-99m red blood cell labelling: iodinated contrast media. *Clin. Nucl. Med.*, **8**, 585.

Taylor, A. Jr, Eshima, D., Fritzberg, A. R. *et al.* (1986) Comparison of iodine-131 OIH and technetium-99m MAG_3: renal imaging in volunteers. *J. Nucl. Med.*, **27**, 795–803.

Trennor, J., Feine, U. and Neighammer, D. (1984) Scintigraphic imaging of neuroblastoma with ^{131}I metaiodobenzylguanidine. *Lancet*, **i**, 333–4.

Troutner, D. E., Volkert, W. A., Hoffman, T. J. *et al.* (1983) A tetra-dentate amine oxine complex of Tc-99m. *J. Nucl. Med.*, **24**, 10 (abstr.).

Van der Schoot, J. B., Groen, A. S. and Dejong, J. (1972) Gallium-67 scintigraphy in lung diseases. *Thorax*, **27**, 543–6.

Van Royen, E. A. (1987) Thallium-201 DDC, an alternative radiopharmaceutical for rCBF. *Nucl. Med. Commun.*, **8**, 603–10.

Van Royen, E. A., de Bruine, J. F., Hill, Th. C. *et al.* (1987) Cerebral blood flow imaging with thallium-201 diethyldithiocarbamate SPECT. *J. Nucl. Med.*, **28**, 178–83.

Vyth, A., Fennema, P. J. and van der Schoot, J. B. (1983) 201-Tl diethyldithiocarbamate: a possible radiopharmaceutical for brain imaging. *Pharm. Weekbl. Sci. Ed.*, **5**, 213–26.

Wagner, H. N., Burns, H. D., Dannals, R. F. *et al.* (1983) Imaging dopamine receptors in the human brain by positron tomography. *Science*, **221**, 1264–6.

Waldman, D. L., Weber, D. A. Oberdorster, G. *et al.* (1987) Chemical breakdown of technetium-99m DTPA during nebulization. *J. Nucl. Med.*, **28**, 378–82.

Watkinson, J. C. and Maisey, M. N. (1988) Imaging head and neck cancer using radioisotopes: a review. *J. R. Soc. Med.*, **81**, 653–7.

Waxman, A. D., Beldon, J. R., Richli, W. R. *et al.* (1977) Steroid induced suppression of gallium uptake in tumours of the central nervous system. *J. Nucl. Med.*, **18**, 617.

Weininger, J., Ketring, A. R., Deutsch, E. *et al.* (1983) Re-186 HEDP: a potential therapeutic bone agent. *J. Nucl. Med.*, **24**, 125.

Wessels, B. W. and Rogus, R. D. (1984) Radionuclide selection and model, absorbed dose calculations for radiolabelled tumor associated antibodies. *Med. Phys.*, **11**, 638–45.

Wieland, D. M., Wu, J. L., Brown, L. E. *et al.* (1980) Radiolabelled adrenergic neuroblocking agents: adrenomedullary imaging with iodine-131-*meta*-iodobenzylguanidine. *J. Nucl. Med.*, **21**, 349–53.

Winchell, H. S., Baldwin, R. M. and Lin, T. H. (1980) Development of I-123 labelled amines for brain studies: localisation of I-123 iodophenylalkylamines in rat brain. *J. Nucl. Med.*, **21**, 940–6.

Wollmer, P., Andersson, L. and Eriksson, L. (1987) Tracers for aerosol ventilation scintigraphy: Tc-99m versus In-113m. *Eur. J. Nucl. Med.*, **13**, 155–8.

Yamamoto, K., Som, P., Brill, A. B. *et al.* (1986) Dual tracer autoradiographic study of β-methyl-(1-^{14}C) heptadecanoic acid and 15-*p*-(^{131}I)-iodophenyl-β-methylpentadecanoic acid in normotensive and hypertensive rats. *J. Nucl. Med.*, **27**, 1178–83.

Yee, C. A., Lee, H. B. and Blaufox, M. D. (1981) Tc-99m DMSA renal uptake: influence of biochemistry and physiologic factors. *J. Nucl. Med.*, **22**, 1054–8.

Yokoyama, A. and Saji, H. (1980) in *Metal Ions in Biological Systems*, Vol. 10 (ed. H. Sigel), Marcel Dekker, New York 313–40.

Yokoyama, A., Hata, N., Horiuchi, K. *et al.* (1985) The design of a pentavalent ^{99m}Tc-dimercaptosuccinate complex as a tumour imaging agent. *Int. J. Nucl. Med. Biol.*, **12**, 273–9.

Zanad, F., Royer, R. G. and Robert, J. (1981) Changes in 86–rubidium uptake in erythrocytes of digoxin-treated patients, in heart failure with sinus rhythm: relationship to clinical effects. *Eur. J. Cardiol.*, **12**, 275–84.

Zimmer, A. M., Spies, S. M. and Majewski, W. (1981) Effect of drugs on *in vivo* RBC labelling: a proposed mechanism of inhibition. *Proceedings of Second International Symposium on Radiopharmacy*, Chicago, USA.

FURTHER READING

Britton, K. E. (1990) The development of new radiopharmaceuticals. *Eur. J. Nucl. Med.*, **16**, 373–85.

Mather, S. J. and Britton, K. E. (1990) Recent developments in radiopharmaceuticals. *Pharm. J.*, **244** (Suppl.) HS8–HSH.

McAfee, J. G. (1989) Update on radiopharmaceuticals for medical imaging. *Radiology*, **171**, 593–601.

Sampson, C. B. (1990) *Textbook of Radiopharmacy, Theory and Practice*. Gordon and Breach, London.

CHAPTER TWENTY-FOUR

Practical instrumentation

A. T. Elliott

24.1 SCINTILLATION DETECTORS

The radiation detector used in almost all nuclear medicine equipment is the scintillation crystal coupled to one or more photomultiplier tubes (PMTs). When ionizing radiation interacts with a scintillator, light is emitted in a short flash or pulse, the magnitude of which is proportional to the amount of energy deposited in the scintillator by the radiation. By using a material of high atomic number, γ-rays can be detected by the light pulses due to electrons secondary to the photoelectric, Compton scattering and pair production processes; for the γ-energies encountered in nuclear medicine, the pair production process may be neglected.

Several scintillators are in use, but by far the most common is sodium iodide, activated by the addition of 0.1% of thallium and denoted NaI(Tl). The scintillator is contained in a light-tight can, usually of thin aluminium, the inside of which is coated with a powdered titanium dioxide reflector to direct all the light through a glass window in the rear of the can (Figure 24.1). The light output is viewed by the PMT, an evacuated glass tube containing a number of electrodes; the PMT is coupled to the window by an optical coupling grease or oil. The first electrode in the PMT is the photocathode, a semi-transparent coating of photoemissive material maintained at ground potential, which absorbs the light and emits photoelectrons. The latter are accelerated by a DC voltage to the first of a series of electrodes known as dynodes, where each incident electron causes the emission of two to three electrons, which are accelerated to the next dynode. The last dynode, the anode, provides the output pulse. A typical PMT has ten dynodes with a potential difference of 100 V between successive dynodes and gives a gain of 10^4–10^6. The gain is highly dependent on the applied voltage and varies also with the ambient temperature.

A theoretical frequency diagram (spectrum) of the output pulse amplitudes obtained from a crystal/PMT assembly exposed to the radiation emitted from a monoenergetic γ-emitter is shown in Figure 24.2(a). The single line to the right, the photopeak, is the result of photoelectric interactions in the crystal, in which all the energy of the γ-photon is absorbed. The remainder of the spectrum arises from the detection of Compton scattering events, in which only a portion of the γ-photon energy is absorbed; the right-hand cut-off of the Compton portion, the Compton edge,

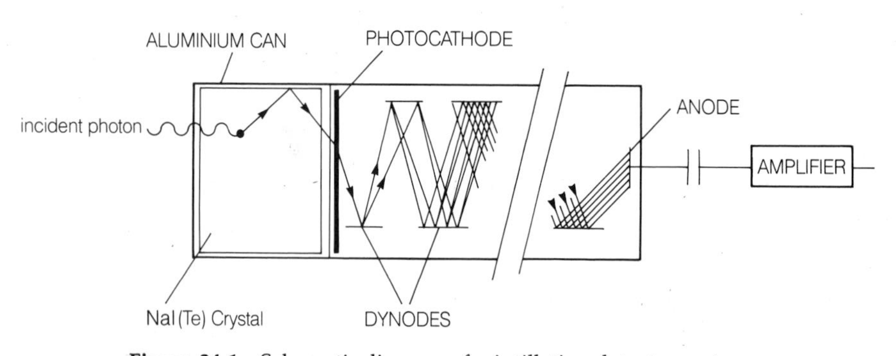

Figure 24.1 Schematic diagram of scintillation detector system.

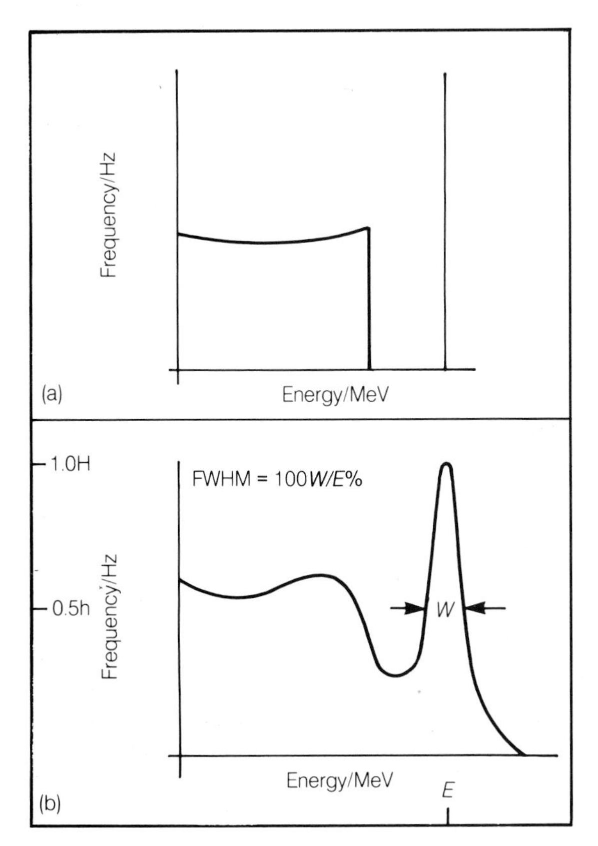

Figure 24.2 Theoretical (a) and practical (b) gamma ray pulse height spectrum in NaI(Tl).

corresponds to the detection of photons involved in 180° scattering events (maximum energy transfer). In practice, effects such as fluctuations in the crystal's light output and the statistical nature of the processes within the photomultiplier lead to a blurring of the system's response, to yield the spectrum shown in Figure 24.2(b). When the source radioactivity is distributed in the body of a patient, the spectrum obtained is degraded still further, since scattering takes place in the body as well as in the crystal, reducing the photopeak/ Compton ratio.

A measure of the performance of a radiation detector is its energy resolution. This is obtained by measuring the full width at half maximum (FWHM) of the photopeak (W in Figure 24.2b). W is then expressed as a percentage of the photopeak energy E. Since the percentage FWHM decreases as the photopeak energy increases, both parameters must be specified as, for example, a FWHM of 12% at 141 keV.

24.2 GAMMA CAMERAS

24.2.1 ANGER CAMERAS

The most common imaging device in current use is the scintillation camera. The conventional design (Anger, 1958) uses a single NaI(Tl) crystal, 6–9 mm thick and with a field of view (FoV) of between 250 mm and 550 mm diameter. The crystal is viewed by a number of PMTs arranged in concentric hexagonal rings around a central tube, a typical arrangement being shown in Figure 24.3. The patient field of view is defined by the collimator, of which there are four major types as shown in Figure 24.4. The parallel hole collimator, which is used in the great majority of studies, gives a 1:1 relationship between the object and the image. The diverging, commonly used only with 250 mm FOV cameras, allows an object larger than the FOV to be imaged, while the converging is used to give enlarged images of smaller organs. The

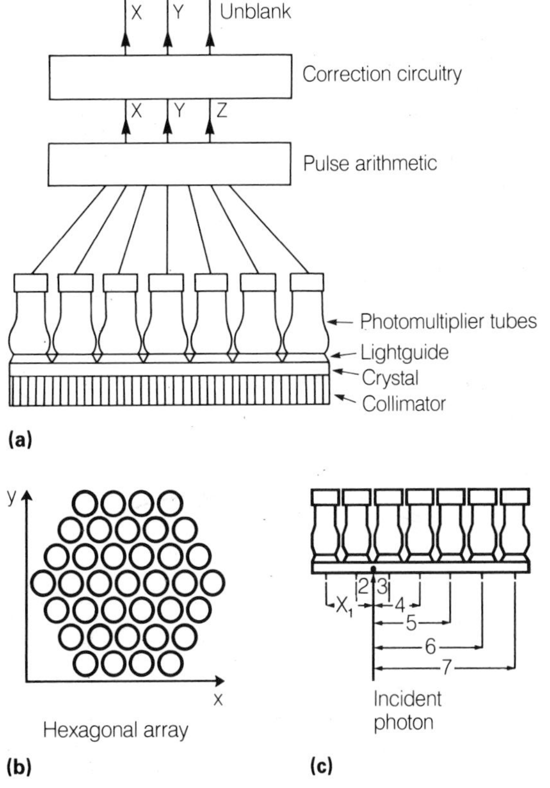

Figure 24.3 Schematic diagram of gamma camera detector; (a) cross-section and (b) plan view of PMT layout, (c) position sensing (one dimensional).

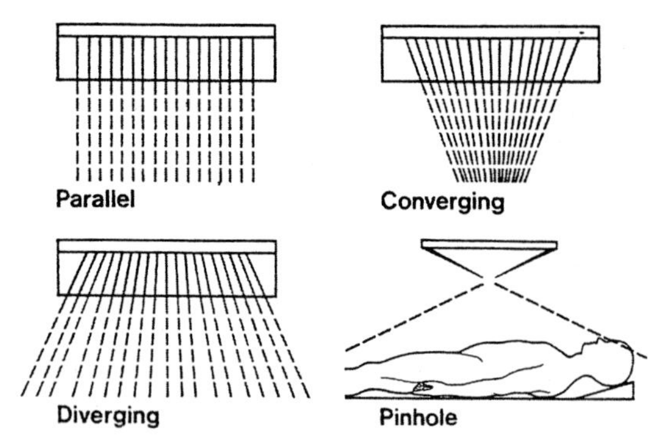

Figure 24.4 Schematic diagram of gamma camera collimator types.

pinhole can be used either to magnify a small organ (e.g. the thyroid) positioned close to the collimator or to minify a large area (e.g. the whole body) positioned farther away. Collimators are designed for specific energy ranges; current designs are rated for energies <160, <300 and <400 keV. Typically, a camera will be purchased with two low-energy (all-purpose and high-resolution) and one medium-energy collimators.

A γ-photon passing through the collimator may interact to produce a light flash in the crystal. If the effect of crystal depth is neglected, and this is the reason for the thin crystal, the intensity of the light received by a given PMT will be dependent on the distances x_1 shown in Figure 24.3(c). If x and y axes are chosen arbitrarily as shown, the electronic signals from the PMTs can be processed by ratio circuits to yield the positional coordinates of the event in the crystal. By summing the outputs of all the PMTs, an 'energy' signal is obtained which can be submitted to pulse-height analysis to determine the energy deposited in the interaction. An 'energy window' is set by the operator (usually ± 7.5%, centred on the photopeak energy) which is used by the pulse-height analyser to select photopeak pulses, those arising from photoelectric (full energy) absorption of unscattered incident photons. Ideally, all other pulses, arising from photons which have undergone scattering within the patient, in the collimator or within the crystal itself, are rejected: their inclusion would lead to a blurring of the image as depicted in Figure 24.5. In practice, because of the imperfect energy resolution of the detector, some scatter photons will fall within the energy pulse-height analyser window.

If a pulse is accepted by the energy analyser, the event is recorded as a dot on an oscilloscope screen at a location determined by the positional coordinates. The analogue image is obtained by making a time exposure photograph of the oscilloscope screen.

The overall system performance of a camera can be considered in two parts: that of the collimator and that of the detection/display equipment. A collimator is specified by two parameters – its sensitivity (which can be defined as the proportion of incident photons transmitted) and its spatial resolution – each of which can be improved only at the expense of the other. A parallel hole collimator for use with ^{99m}Tc is typically 25 mm thick and perforated by up to 35 000 holes. Collimators for use with higher-energy radionuclides have thicker septa (the lead wall between adjacent holes), larger diameter and fewer holes. A commonly accepted design criterion is that crosstalk from one collimator hole into an adjacent hole should be less than 5%.

The overall spatial resolution of the system, R_s is given, to a good approximation, by

$$R_s^2 = R_i^2 + R_c^2$$

Where R_c is the collimator resolution and R_i is the intrinsic resolution of the detector and electronics. R_s is measured by imaging a narrow (0.5 mm

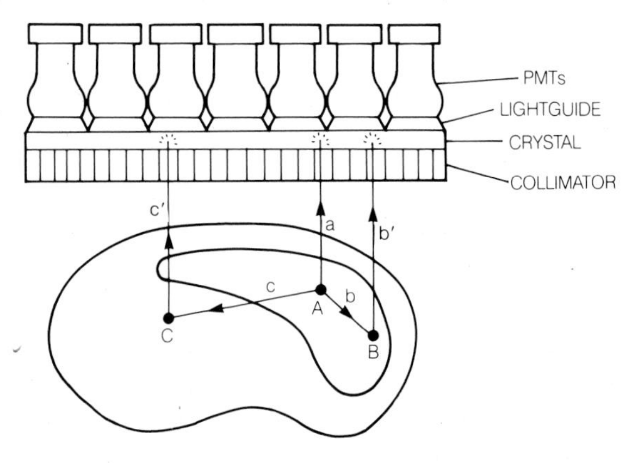

Figure 24.5 Consider a source at point A, emitting gamma-rays isotropically. Photon a is unscattered and is absorbed in the crystal, generating a z-signal which is accepted by the energy analyser. Photons b and c undergo scattering within the patient, giving rise to lower energy photons b′ and c′; by chance, these reach the crystal. If these events were not rejected by the energy analyser, they would be plotted as originating from points B and C, giving a false image of the radionuclide distribution.

Table 24.1 System resolution data (typical high resolution collimator)

Depth in scattering medium	*FWHM*	*FWTM*
(mm)	(mm)	(mm)
10	4.4	8.1
30	5.2	9.4
50	6.0	10.9
100	8.4	15.3
150	11.6	21.2

FWHM = Full width at half maximum, FWTM = Full width at tenth maximum

internal diameter) tube filled with a radioactive solution aligned parallel to, say, the x axis shown in Figure 24.3. A profile of the image parallel to the y axis is then obtained; the profile has a 'Gaussian' shape, the FWHM of this curve being quoted as a measure of resolution. The FWHM is dependent on the energy window used, increasing with increasing window width due to the acceptance of pulses arising from scattered photons. Resolution deteriorates also with increasing depth in tissue as shown in Table 24.1.

Gamma cameras are presently available with either 6 mm or 9 mm thick crystals. The thinner crystal offers a slightly superior intrinsic resolution (Royal *et al.*, 1979) but is some 10% less efficient for ^{99m}Tc. This loss of sensitivity may negate any resolution advantage since, as pointed out by Muehllehner (1979), the same overall result could be achieved by fitting a higher resolution collimator to a camera having the thicker crystal. Since the sensitivity difference becomes more important at higher energies, cameras with a 9 mm crystal are to be preferred.

The main disadvantage of the Anger design is its inherent non-uniformity across the field of view, which arises from non-uniformities in the NaI(Tl) crystal itself, defects in optical coupling between the crystal and the PMTs, variations in the performance of the PMTs and non-linearity in the processing circuitry. Various efforts have been made to overcome this problem, earlier methods being based on the technique of 'flood field' correction. An image of a uniform ('flood field') source was obtained and stored in matrix form, initially in an associated computer and later in a microprocessor integral with the position processing circuitry; the pixel count in subsequent images was subject to a correction factor based upon the ratio between the corresponding pixel count and mean pixel count in the flood image. This approach produced cosmetically improved images but was flawed in that the technique assumed non-uniformity to be due entirely to variations in detector sensitivity. Wicks and Blau (1979) have shown, however, that 60% of non-uniformity is due to errors in the positioning circuitry with only 40% due to sensitivity variations. Modern systems employ multiple microprocessors integral with the positioning circuitry which carry out on-line (real-time) corrections for spatial distortion (Muehllehner *et al.*, 1980) and variations in PMT performance (Todd-Pokropek *et al.*, 1977). The processes are depicted schematically in Figure 24.6.

If the energy spectrum is measured at a number of points over the FOV, the position of the photopeak is found to vary. An energy window positioned correctly for the photopeak at one point in the FOV may thus wrongly reject a photopeak event at another location. At manufacture an image of a test phantom comprising an array of orthogonal holes (either 64 × 64 or 128 × 128) is acquired. For each hole image, the energy spectrum is measured and the photopeak locations determined. For each point in the correction matrix (64 × 64 or 128 × 128 dependent on the phantom), a correction multiplier is obtained which adjusts the amplitude of the energy signal to give a constant photopeak amplitude over the entire FOV; thus all valid events will be accepted by the energy analyser wherever their origin within the FOV. Fortunately, the correction multipliers obtained for, say, technetium are valid over the radionuclide energy range encountered in clinical practice.

The second part of the correction process takes account of spatial distortion, systematic errors in calculating the event coordinates. Again at manufacture, calibration transmission images of either orthogonal slit patterns or of an orthogonal hole phantom are obtained. Since the correct position of the slit or hole images are known, computer

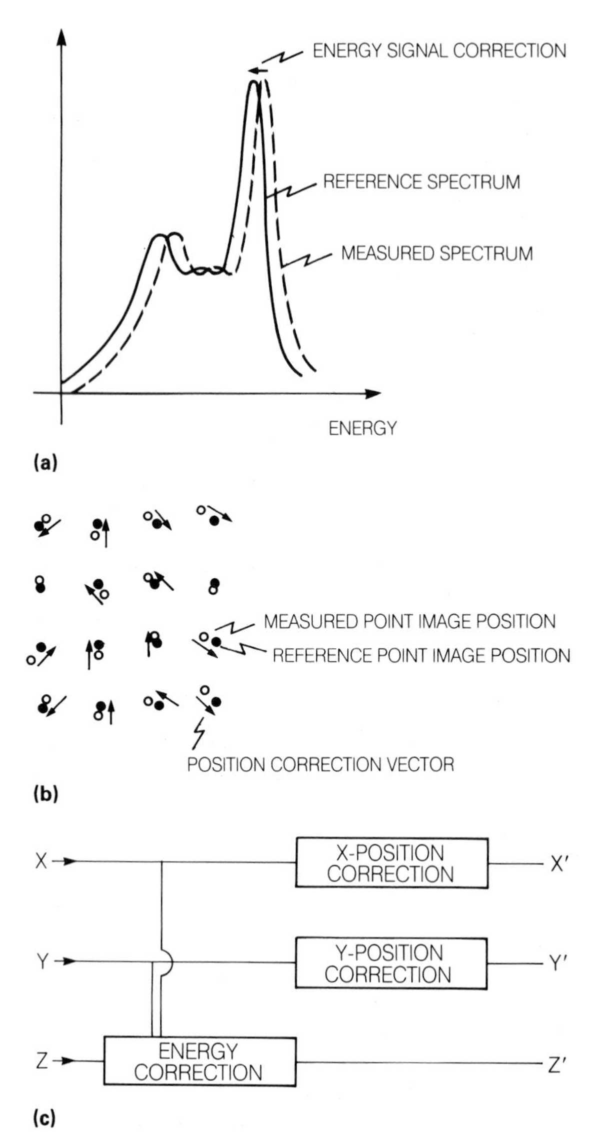

Figure 24.6 Schematic of real-time correction system: (a) energy spectrum is measured at each point and a correction value obtained; (b) the centroid of each point image is calculated and compared with the known reference position to obtain a correction vector, which is split into x and y components; (c) incoming signals are corrected on the basis of the above by reference to stored look-up tables.

measurement of their actual positions in the calibration image permits the computation of a set of correction vectors (again usually on a 64×64 or 128×128 matrix) over the FoV. The initial x and y coordinates are then used to access a look-up table which calculates the appropriate correction vector from the four nearest nodes. The corrected x and y coordinates are those fed to the display system.

Both the energy and spatial distortion corrections are applied in real-time. In some of the latest integrated camera/computer systems, the corrections are applied in the computer rather than in the detector head. The look-up tables can be accessed by software, which may have advantages in that recalibration is easy. In the latter connection, it should be remembered that PMTs 'burn in' over the first few hundred hours' operation, while pre-amplifiers may do the same over some six months.

Some cameras also feature continuous retuning of the PMT gains, since these are subject to random drift with time. One method of measuring drift is based on the responses of the PMTs to standard amplitude light pulses fed to the crystal. Light from a very stable LED (light-emitting diode) is fed down a bundle of optical fibres typically one fibre per 3 PMTs, and the responses measured. In one design, this is accomplished in a calibration mode prior to imaging while in another, the calibration is carried out several times per second even during imaging. An alternative method is to use a second, narrow energy window on the high-energy side of the photopeak, which is assumed not to contain any scattered photons; the count rate within this window is highly sensitive to gain changes. In both methods, any change in the response of a PMT is compensated by altering its gain through an adjustment of its high-voltage supply.

The above corrections are applied to compensate for defects in the detector performance and have a sound theoretical basis. One further correction which has been introduced lately attempts to compensate for the effects on the final image of scattered photons on an empirical basis. A further look-up table is provided, in which each value of the corrected energy signal is associated with a given numerical weighting factor, which may be negative for those energy signals corresponding to scattered photons. A storage matrix, interposed ahead of the hardcopy or computer output, is used for temporary accumulation; the pixel specified by the x and y coordinates is incremented by the fraction of a count specified by the weighting factor. Whenever a pixel value exceeds 1, a count with that x and y coordinate is passed to the hardcopy device and/or computer. The end product is a 'scatter free' image, the main application of which lies in SPECT.

24.2.2 SPECIALIZED DESIGNS

(a) Scanning cameras

Scanning gamma cameras have been developed to facilitate whole-body imaging. In most cases, the patient bed remains stationary and the detector is moved; in addition to the standard positional coordinates for each event, the display system is fed coordinates specifying the detector position in order to generate images as shown in Figure 24.7.

Initial models, utilizing 250 mm FOV detectors, built up the image from a series of two or three adjacent longitudinal scans. This required a high degree both of stability in the display system and of patient cooperation in remaining still for the duration of the scan. Single-pass scanning was achieved by fitting a 400 mm FOV detector with a special collimator which was parallel-holed in the longitudinal direction (that of motion) but divergent in the transverse direction. The degree of divergence was greater at the edge of the field than at the centre in an attempt to maintain good resolution for the trunk. This system did not achieve wide acceptance. The latest systems employ a 550 mm FOV detector fitted with a standard parallel hole collimator. The FOV is masked electronically to a rectangle and the scan may be obtained either in continuous motion or in 'step and shoot' mode; in the latter, an image is obtained with the detector static, the detector is moved by the length of the rectangle and another image obtained for the same time as the first. The process is repeated until the desired area has been covered. In general, the resolution of a continuous motion system deteriorates somewhat in the direction of motion.

(b) Mobile cameras

To extend the availability of nuclear medicine investigations, several manufacturers have developed mobile gamma cameras. These find use in coronary and intensive care units, in accident and emergency departments and in operating theatres (e.g. Elliott *et al.*, 1979). They have been fitted also into vehicles and used to provide a mobile nuclear medicine service.

Initial models were restricted to 250 mm FoV detectors, but 400 mm detectors are now available. In order to cut down the weight of the machine, the detector shielding is lighter than static systems and the range of collimators is limited; the maximum γ-ray energy is usually restricted to approximately 200 keV. The level of computing required will be determined by the level of service to be provided – static imaging only or static and dynamic studies, on-site reporting or off-line reporting in the base department.

In choosing a mobile camera, consideration should be given to its manoeuvrability and ease of detector positioning; the space beneath and between beds in, say, the coronary care unit should be checked carefully. It should be noted that many hospital lifts have a maximum load capacity of 800 kg or less, while the wheel diameter of the camera should be sufficient to give a point loading which will not damage the floor screed. The wheel diameter should be large enough also to cope with any gaps between lift and building floors. The collimator should be left in place during transport to provide a measure of protection against both thermal and mechanical shock; if taking the machine out of doors, the manufacturer's advice should be sought as to whether further thermal protection (e.g. an insulating cover) should be provided for the detector.

(c) Multicrystal camera

The alternative to the Anger design is the multicrystal camera, introduced by Bender and Blau (1963). The detector of this device uses 294 separate NaI(Tl) crystals each 8 mm square and 38 mm deep arranged in a 21 × 14 matrix with an 11 mm crystal spacing. Light from the crystals is fed to 35 PMTs, one for each row and each column of the matrix.

The light from each crystal is split and fed to the appropriate row and column PMTs, the location of an event in the detector being determined by coincidence analysis of the row and column signals. Counts are stored initially in a 294-element, 16-bit deep semiconductor buffer memory, data from which are transferred into the integral computer for subsequent disc or magnetic tape storage. Since each crystal is independent of all others, the flood-field uniformity correction is valid for this configuration: it is possible also to apply a dead-time correction, which extends the count-rate capability to some 500 000 events per second, in comparison to the 80 000–100 000 events per second of typical Anger cameras, making it extremely useful for high-speed dynamic studies, of which the most common is the first-pass nuclear angiocardiogram.

Because of the relatively low number of sample points over the 230 × 150 mm FoV, together with its poor energy resolution (60% FWHM at 141 keV

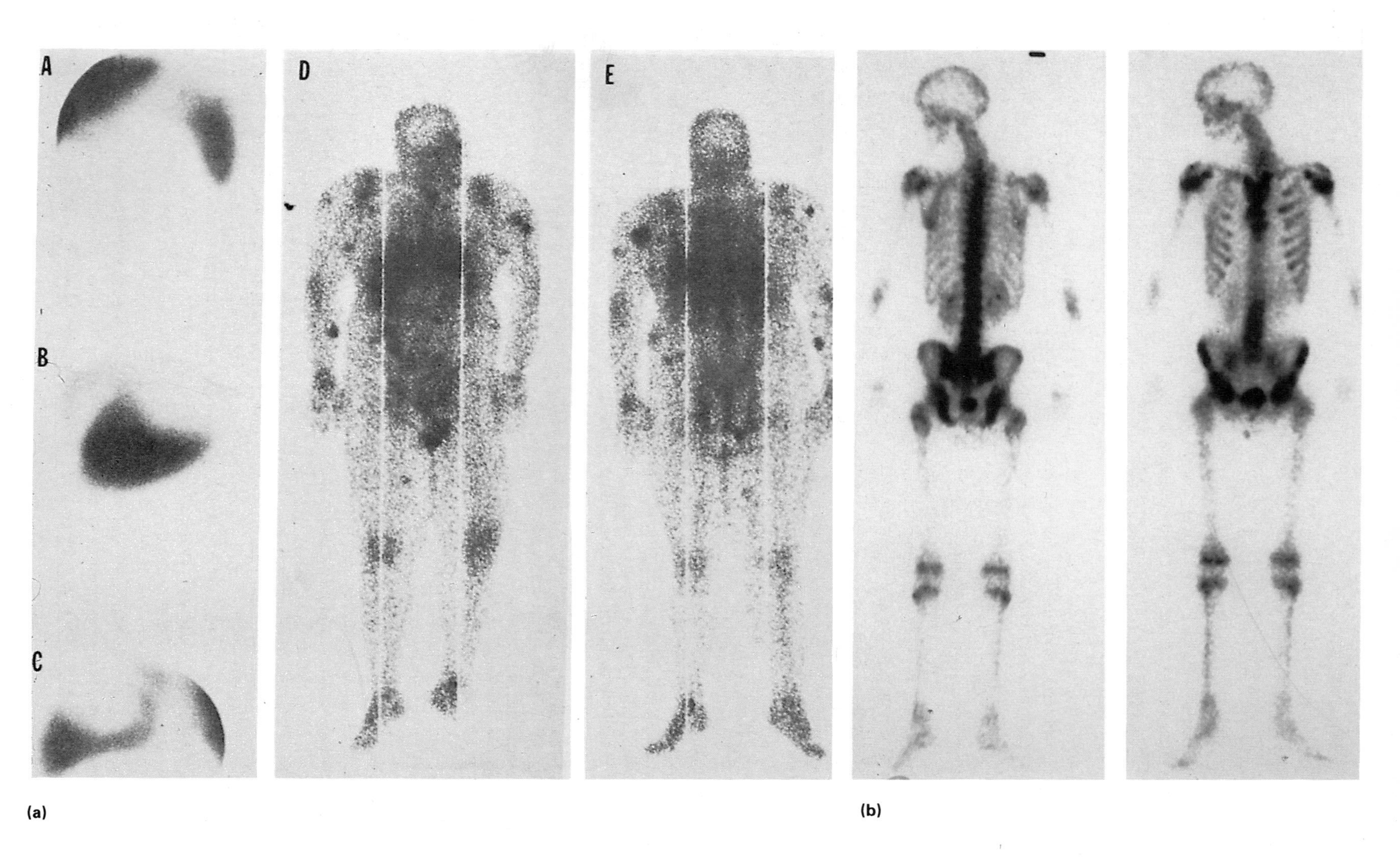

Figure 24.7 Whole body scans; (a) early three-pass system, showing gaps between strips of image and (b) single-pass system.

compared to 10–13% for Anger cameras), the spatial resolution of the machine is poor. This renders it less than optimal for static imaging. The sensitivity of the multicrystal camera is, however, superior to that of the Anger design: the thicker crystals of the former make the difference even more marked for medium- and high-energy radionuclides.

(d) Other designs

Newer designs of gamma camera have replaced the NaI(Tl) detector with a germanium crystal (Ewins *et al.*, 1977) or a multiwire proportional counter (Bateman and Connolly, 1978; Lacy *et al.*, 1984). The former suffers the disadvantages of high cost, small FoV and low sensitivity. The latter has a poor sensitivity for ^{99m}Tc but may be used effectively with low-energy radionuclides such as ^{201}Tl and ^{133}Xe. Both designs offer an intrinsic resolution markedly superior to the Anger design, but neither seems set to succeed the Anger camera.

24.3 EMISSION TOMOGRAPHY

In conventional radionuclide imaging, two-dimensional projections are obtained of the three-dimensional distribution of the radiopharmaceutical within the patient. Three-dimensional visualization of the distribution must be accomplished by the observer, usually on the basis of a set of orthogonal images. Early attempts to produce an image of a sectional plane within the body used radiographic focal plane tomography, the first radionuclide methods using rectilinear scanners fitted with highly focusing collimators: both techniques produced longitudinal sections.

The image reconstruction techniques used in transaxial tomography were introduced by Bracewell (1956) in radioastronomy and although their most widely known medical application today lies in the radiographic transmission scanner (CAT scanner), Oldendorf (1961) used a ^{131}I source in his apparatus for transmission imaging, while Kuhl and Edwards developed the first radionuclide emission tomograph in 1963. There are two approaches to emission tomography; single-photon emission computed tomography (SPECT) and positron emission tomography (PET).

As the name implies, the PET technique relies on the coincidence counting, in opposing detectors, of the 511 keV γ-photons arising from positron annihilation. To achieve a high counting efficiency, signals are not submitted to full pulse-height analysis, but a low-level discriminator is used to eliminate detector noise. Since it can be shown that the net attenuation for a pair of γ-rays is constant, independent of where the emission point is located along the ray path between the opposing detectors, attenuation corrections can be applied easily by making transmission measurements for each ray path prior to the emission scan. The resolution and quantification capabilities of PET are thus markedly superior to those of SPECT systems. Detector configurations include the dual head scintillation camera (Muehllehner *et al.*, 1976) and the hexagonal scanner (Ter-Pogossian *et al.*, 1975). Recently, time-of-flight PET systems have been designed (Mullani *et al.*, 1984).

The major disadvantage of PET systems, other than the cost of the tomographs themselves, is the need for positron-emitting radiopharmaceuticals; since the most useful (^{11}C, ^{13}N, ^{15}O and ^{18}F) have very short half-lives, an on-site cyclotron is required. In order to minimize this problem, so-called 'baby' or 'benchtop' cyclotrons have been developed, often with automated radiochemistry 'cells' to synthesize radiopharmaceuticals. These are purpose-built to produce the above radionuclides only and require both fewer operating staff and less complex installations than conventional machines, substantially lowering operating costs. Together with positron generator systems such as ^{82}Rb (Yano *et al.*, 1981) and ^{68}Ga (Loc'h *et al.*, 1980), the baby cyclotron has been instrumental in bringing the cost of a PET installation within the realms of possibility for larger hospitals. Despite the claims of manufacturers, however, operation of these systems is not easy (Harby, 1988).

The most common systems encountered clinically are SPECT systems based upon a conventional gamma camera detector mounted on an arm capable of 360° rotation around the patient (Figure 24.8). These have the advantage of being dual purpose – capable of both conventional planar imaging and emission tomography – and of cost; the addition of SPECT capability adds only some 15–20% to the cost of a basic gamma camera/computer system. In comparison, a dedicated SPECT machine with ring geometry (Jarritt *et al.* 1979) costs more than twice the price of a basic camera/computer system. While the single-slice machines offer theoretically superior resolution, the difference clinically is not significant; they do

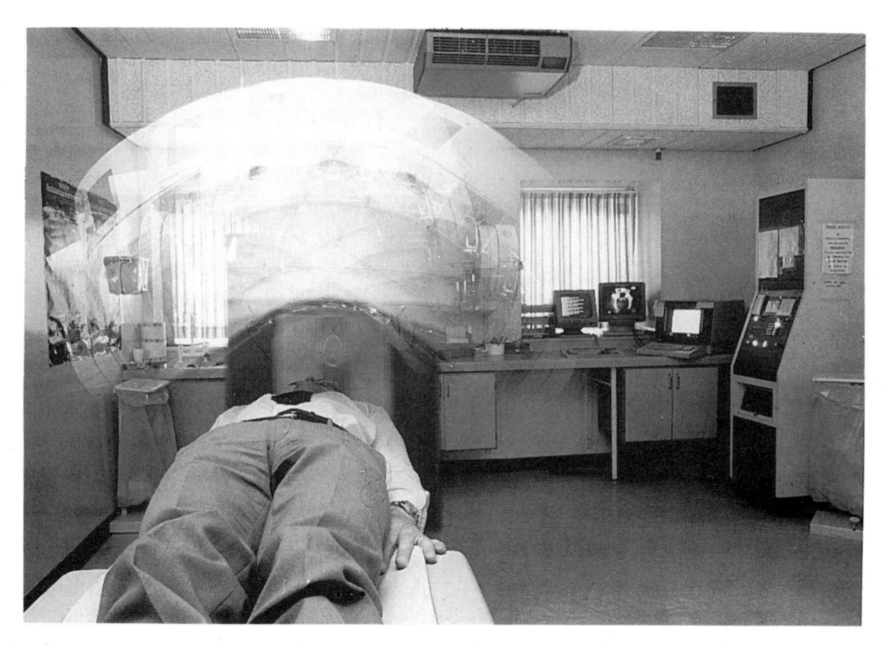

Figure 24.8 Rotating gamma camera SPECT system.

have the capability, due to their higher sensitivity within the slice, of being able to acquire the raw data in 2–3 min whereas a rotating camera takes typically 20–30 min to complete a rotation. This may be of importance if dynamic studies of a rapidly varying radiopharmaceutical distribution are to be carried out. The rotating camera, however, acquires the data to reconstruct a set of parallel, contiguous axial slices in a single rotation; these represent the three-dimensional distribution of the radiopharmaceutical within a patient volume and these data may be reconfigured to yield coronal, sagittal or oblique planar slices.

The reconstruction algorithms used in most nuclear medicine computer systems are variants of a technique known as filtered back projection (Budinger and Gullberg, 1974) in which the data are subject to a mathematical filter prior to the reconstruction process. Most systems permit the operator to define the filter or select one from a range of pre-programmed functions, among the most common of which are:

1. The ramp filter, which preserves the high-frequency (i.e. fine-resolution) detail of the input data but leaves any statistical noise present to be amplified by the reconstruction process. It is best used, therefore, only with data having a high count density, typically phantom data.
2. The Shepp–Logan with Hanning window, which damps the higher spatial frequencies in the raw data, leading to a loss of resolution in the final image. It has the benefit of reducing markedly the noise level in the final image and so may be employed when the raw data has a low count density.
3. The Shepp–Logan filter, which is a compromise between the first two and is the one of choice for most clinical studies.

The other problem in SPECT reconstruction is that of applying an attenuation correction. Most systems use post-reconstruction techniques such as the first-order Chang correction (Chang, 1978), which is based upon the way in which a point source would be attenuated by the body contour. It is adequate for most clinical images but is not accurate enough to permit quantification of radiopharmaceutical concentration.

Quantitative accuracy is dependent on scatter, attenuation, the reconstruction filter, the slice shape and partial volume effects. The latter is an apparent reduction in the pixel count corresponding to a given radioactive concentration in a small volume relative to the pixel count from the same concentration in a larger volume. It may occur when the object is thinner than the slice thickness or only partly lies within the slice. The absolute quantification of radioactive concentration is difficult for objects whose linear dimensions are less than twice the corresponding FWHM. For measurements of volume, the limits appear to be similar in the clinical situation, although Todd-Pokropek and Jarritt (1982) have shown that, in a high signal-to-noise situation, 'hot' objects could be sized down to one FWHM while 'cold' objects could be sized down to one half FWHM. Corrections for the partial volume effect may be made to either of the volume or concentration if the other can be estimated independently (e.g. by CT scanning). Volumes of larger organs have been estimated successfully (Tauxe *et al.*, 1982; Underwood *et al.*, 1985). While not an absolute method, the so-called 'bullseye' method of quantification of thallium tomograms (Garcia *et al.*, 1985) has been widely used.

In performing SPECT, it is vital to choose a detector with good energy resolution and planar uniformity and low spatial distortion; the FWHM of a point source in air in a reconstructed image will be some 10% worse than the planar resolution and so, where the count rate is adequate, a high-resolution collimator should be fitted; since resolution deteriorates with depth, the smallest practicable radius of rotation should be selected. The setting of the energy window is of crucial importance and a value of ±7.5% of the photopeak energy should be employed and checked carefully prior to data acquisition. Further operational details are given in Section 24.10.

24.4 WHOLE-BODY COUNTERS

For certain tests, such as the investigation of vitamin B12 metabolism, it is necessary to measure the absolute amount of radioactivity retained within the patient's body as a function of time. The machine used to obtain this information is the whole-body counter, which was actually the first nuclear medicine machine to be developed. Modern systems can assay activities of 185 Bq with a standard error of 5%.

A whole-body counter can be specified in terms of two parameters:

1. Detection sensitivity, which is the minimum quantity of radioactivity which can be assayed with a given statistical accuracy and is dependent on the counter's efficiency and the background counting rate;
2. Uniformity of spatial response, which is a measure of the independence of the distribution of the radiopharmaceutical within the body and is dependent on the geometry of the monitor and, to a limited extent, on the method of operation.

In clinical use, one must specify the minimum acceptable detection sensitivity and the maximum tolerable variation in spatial response. The former parameter is determined by considerations of radiation dose to the patient, the effective half-life of the radiopharmaceutical being used and the time-scale of the physiological process being investigated. The spatial response must be considered in the light of the possibly abnormal, unpredictable and extremely non-uniform distribution of tracers encountered in clinical use. The distribution will probably vary also as a function of time after administration and so even successive measurements on the same patient may produce misleading data unless the spatial response is uniform to within certain limits. These limits will be determined by the magnitude of the change in body content of the tracer which is of clinical significance. Corrections for non-uniformity of spatial response can be obtained from phantom studies or by using the patient as his/her own reference. In phantom studies, the count obtained from the patient is compared to that from a radionuclide distribution assumed to be similar to that in the patient with regard to geometry, attenuation and scatter. Alternatively, a second radionuclide, having biodistribution and radiation emission properties similar to the primary radionuclide, is administered, an example being the use of ^{42}K to allow accurate quantification of ^{40}K.

Whole-body monitors fall into two classes: shielded-room and shadow-shield types. In the shielded room configuration (e.g. Cohn *et al.*, 1969), the counter is constructed within a room whose walls, floor and ceiling are lined with radiation shielding material, the detectors themselves being unshielded (Figure 24.9a). Typically, 120 cm of chalk, 15 cm of steel or 10 cm of lead is the required thickness of shielding. In all cases, the material must be of low radioactive content itself: shields using concrete and cement may require an inner lining of 2 cm of lead. Steel is usually pre-Hiroshima and uncontaminated by nuclear fallout (obtained from ships sunk prior to 1945).

Shadow shields (e.g. Boddy *et al.*, 1975) are constructed usually of lead and, in this case, only the detectors themselves are enclosed in shielding

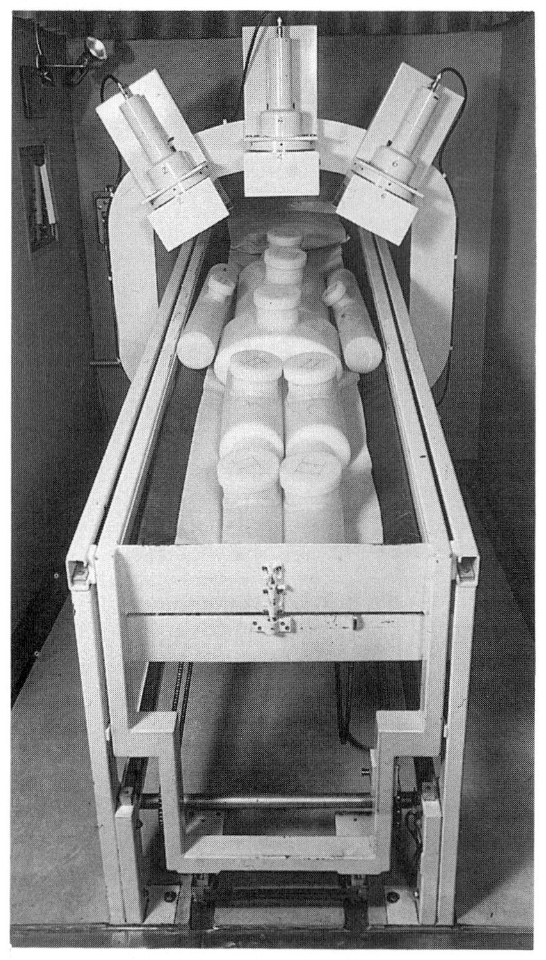

(a)

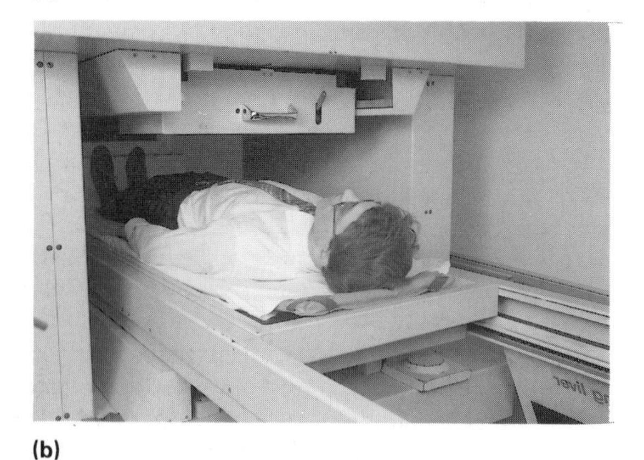

(b)

Figure 24.9 Whole body counters; (a) shielded room type and (b) shadow shield type.

(Figure 24.9b). Since the shielding is concentrated in a small volume, the resulting floor loading may be substantial and require the load to be spread by building the central portion on a steel base plate. Since 'line of sight' background radiation can still reach the detectors in this design, they must be orientated carefully with respect to external radiation sources such as passing patients to whom radiopharmaceuticals have been administered, X-ray sources, etc.

The performance of a 10 cm lead shadow-shield monitor is approximately the same as that of a steel shielded-room type, lying between that of chalk and lead shielded-room monitors. Shadow-shield types are satisfactory for most routine clinical applications although, if extensive studies of natural ^{40}K are to be undertaken, a shielded-room type would be preferred.

24.5 PROBE SYSTEMS

24.5.1 NUCLEAR STETHOSCOPE

This is a modern version of the single probe, now coupled to a microprocessor (Wagner *et al.*, 1976). This instrument generates a real-time left-ventricular time–activity curve, from which the ejection fraction can be assessed on a beat-to-beat basis. Correct probe positioning is crucial but, with practice, results correlate well with those from imaging studies (Berger *et al.*, 1981; Strashun *et al.*, 1981) and the probe system appears useful in the continuous assessment of ventricular function in response to drugs.

24.5.2 MINIATURE DETECTORS

In order to carry out ambulatory studies, small cadmium telluride (Cd-Te) detectors have been developed, the output of which is fed into a solid-state data logger. The total weight is some 600 g, permitting its use in ambulatory measurement.

The sensitivity of the Cd–Te detector decreases rapidly with depth in tissue and so a thallium-activated caesium iodide detector has been developed for nuclear cardiology studies. This probe utilizes a solid-state photodiode rather than a PMT to measure the light output of the crystal and so does not require a high voltage supply. Like the nuclear stethoscope, it is microcomputer-based, but its software is not as well developed.

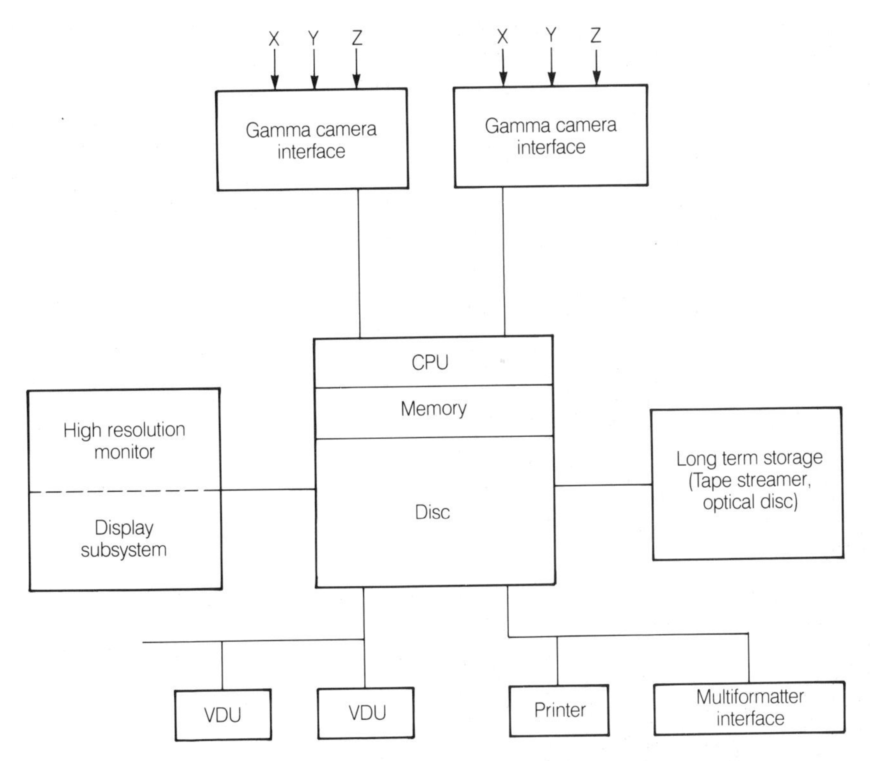

Figure 24.10 Block diagram of nuclear medicine computer system.

24.6 COMPUTER SYSTEMS

Most gamma cameras are interfaced to computer systems. Nuclear medicine computer systems are usually built around microprocessors and a block diagram of a typical system is shown in Figure 24.10. The system can be used for the acquisition, display and processing of both static and dynamic images (see below), but its greatest advantage lies in the potential for evaluating physiological parameters from dynamic studies such as nuclear angiocardiography, renography and cerebral blood flow determinations. In SPECT systems, it also performs the reconstruction process.

In order to input the data from the gamma camera, the x and y analogue coordinate signals are converted into numeric form by analogue-to-digital converters (ADCs). The stability and linearity of the ADCs is of crucial importance if no distortions are to be introduced into the image; this is a fundamental requirement for SPECT. Data storage is accomplished in one of two modes: frame or list. In frame mode, which is used for the great majority of both static and dynamic studies, the image matrix is formed during data acquisition. Many computers carry out frame mode acquisition in a microprocessor-controlled subsystem comprising the ADCs and 64–256K words of memory, permitting acquisition to be independent of the central processor. This facilitates the connection of more than one camera to a single system and improves the access speed of the whole system. List mode is used for very high-speed data acquisition (e.g. first-pass nuclear angiocardiography) or where some pre-processing is to be carried out on the data prior to matrix formation. In this case, each event word (a concatenation of the x and y coordinates) is merely stored sequentially – usually on magnetic disc – along with timing markers and the image matrices are formed off-line.

In choosing the size of a matrix for data storage, a compromise between spatial resolution and pixel statistics must be reached. An image recorded into, say, a 32 × 32 matrix would have low spatial resolution but the pixel count would be high, giving a good statistical accuracy. The same image, recorded into a 512 × 512 matrix, would have good spatial resolution but poor statistical validity due to the low number of counts in each pixel. Within limits, spatial resolution is less important than high pixel counts for dynamic studies, since the quality of subsequent mathematical processing is dependent on the statistical goodness of the raw data; in practice, most dynamic studies are acquired into 64 × 64 matrices. In static imaging, the required matrix size can be derived from consideration of sampling theory, which suggests that a pixel size of one-third of the spatial resolution FWHM is required. For a 400 mm FOV detector, a typical FWHM is approximately 7–10 mm at clinically important depths, suggesting that between 120 and 170 pixels would be required across the FoV. Static images are thus acquired typically into 128 × 128 or 256 × 256 matrices (the latter if the count rate is sufficiently high to obtain adequate pixel counts). For SPECT studies, pixel statistics in the two-dimensional projection images are extremely important since the reconstruction process acts as a noise amplifier; raw data are usually acquired into 64 × 64 matrices.

From dynamic study data, time–activity curves can be generated by delineating a region-of-interest around an area of an image in the series and instructing the computer to sum the pixel counts within the selected area in all images of the series. Such curves can then be subjected to further analysis (e.g. two kidney curves and a blood curve form the input to deconvolution in renography). The computer can be used also to synchronize data collection with a repetitive physiological process, such as the cardiac cycle (as monitored by the patient's ECG) in gated cardiac imaging or the respiratory cycle in lung imaging. Clearly, SPECT cannot be carried out without an adequate computer system.

Most current systems use a display subsystem with 128–512 kbytes of memory and a high-resolution, studio-quality television monitor. This will be capable of displaying a true 256 × 256 image interpolated to 512 × 512, with a minimum of 64 intensity levels. For hard-copy output of curves or processed images, it is desirable to include an interface to the gamma camera's multiformatter. If colour output is required, Polaroid film is probably the fastest and most convenient method.

As the relative cost of hardware decreases, it is not uncommon to find systems comprising 2–4 Mbytes of main memory, capable of operating at rates of 2 Mips (million instructions per second), with magnetic discs having a capacity of 80–400 Mbytes. Given the volume of data held on a single disc, and the volume of data which may be associated with a single SPECT study, the preferred medium for data archival is becoming the tape streamer, which can read/write data at rates of up to 20 Mbytes per minute. As yet, optical discs have not been widely used, but this will change as erasable models, permitting over-writing in the same manner as current magnetic discs, become available.

The computations required by SPECT reconstruction have led to the inclusion of array processors (devices which can perform complex operations, such as Fourier transformation, on complete images while the main processor executes other tasks) in some systems. Modern 32-bit processors, however, can carry out the calculations in approximately 0.6 s per slice, rendering array processors unnecessary for typical SPECT matrix sizes.

24.7 DATA DISPLAY AND PROCESSING

24.7.1 STATIC IMAGES

The theoretical performance capabilities of an imaging device cannot be realized in practice since the image is produced in the form of electronic signals that cannot be viewed directly but must be used as the input to a display system, which introduces its own distortions into the images.

Considering first the conventional analogue film output, the detection of a lesion is dependent on the change in grey-scale level caused by the different count density over the lesion. Three factors are important: the absolute magnitude of the difference, its statistical significance with respect to background fluctuations and the minimum change detectable by the human visual system, the physiology of which has been discussed by Campbell (1976). It can be shown that the perceived difference ΔD expressed as an optical density change between a lesion and its surrounding background is given by

$$\Delta D = \gamma \log(1 + S/B)$$

where γ is the slope of the film characteristic (plot of optical density against log(exposure)), B is the average background count density and S the incremental increase (or decrease) in count density over the lesion. Whitehead (1978) found that for spherical lesions in a uniform background the minimum detectable value of D is 0.07 units and showed that a signal-to-noise ratio of 4.25 : 1 yields an error rate of 2% in detection of 20–40 mm lesions for images obtained from a 400 mm FoV camera. Since these results are dependent on the film γ, the use of high-contrast (high γ) film is advantageous: several manufacturers have developed high γ single-emulsion films for use in multiformat devices.

The properties of the cathode-ray tube being photographed are of prime importance. It should have a small dot size and provide uniform dot intensity over the field, the emission wavelength of the phosphor being suitable for the film in use. It is vital that the film be properly exposed, the resulting optical densities in the developed film lying on the linear portion of the film characteristic curve; this implies a high stability also in the cathode-ray tube dot intensity. Viewing conditions are important and it is advantageous to black out uncovered sections of the viewing screen when using transparency film.

Analogue imaging has the major disadvantage that if the film has not been properly exposed, or has not been properly developed, the study must be repeated. Further, no processing of the image is possible. Some centres have adopted the practice of storing all images directly into the computer without any analogue output. The image which best transmits the diagnostic information is then selected from the digital display and, if deemed necessary, output onto film; note that since the optimum display settings may vary from one portion of the image to another it may be necessary to output more than one image to transmit all the data contained therein.

As detailed above, the most common display format is in matrix form, using a discrete number of grey-scale or colour levels to represent the pixel count. Less common formats include contour mapping and isometric display.

Todd-Pokropek and Pizer (1977) have suggested, from considerations of visual acuity, that the display pixel size should be less than the data pixel size and recommend the use of at least a 256 × 256 pixel matrix to display static images from current gamma cameras. A linear interpolation can be used to generate the intermediate values for the larger matrix, but it should be noted that extra precision in the pixel counts is required.

In considering the number of grey-scale or colour levels necessary, the purpose of the display must be taken into account. If it is desired to transmit the maximum amount of 'pattern' information, a sufficient number of levels must be used so that boundaries between levels are not readily distinguishable, since a clear boundary 'contour' may suggest a structure where none is present. If, on the other hand, it is intended to make quantitative measurements, comparing the pixel count in one part of an image with that in another, a much smaller number of clearly recognizable levels is required. For the former purpose, a minimum of 64 levels appears to be necessary while, for the latter, Brown *et al* (1975) showed that eight levels are sufficient. For the 'pattern' information display, the heated object spectrum (Milan and Taylor, 1976) appears particularly suitable; increasing pixel values are represented by hues of black, red, orange, yellow and white. It is naturally interpretable and can be used by the colour-blind.

The simplest form of data processing is smoothing to reduce the effects of statistical fluctuations, the most commonly used being the 9-point weighted smooth with weights of 4, 2 and 1. Several, more complex smoothing techniques have been developed, such as the non-stationary filter of Gustafsson and Pizer (1975). Among image enhancement techniques in use are those of maximum convexity (Neill and Hutchinson, 1971), zero summation filters (Houston, 1976) and the Canterbury filter (Corfield, 1976). The last of these is an optical unsharp masking technique adapted for use in nuclear medicine, which highlights regions of changing count density (e.g. edges of lesions).

These techniques have been used extensively, with the aim of increasing the detection rate of lesions without an increase in the false-positive detection rate. In general, however, efforts have proved unrewarding when compared with results from raw data images recorded directly onto transparency film. The only images which are generally accepted to benefit from computer processing are those of poor statistical quality, such as thallium cardiac images or those from monoclonal antibody imaging.

Efforts have been made to make the process of lesion detection more objective by dividing the task into two parts: the identification of an apparently abnormal region and the quantitative comparison of the count density in this region, either with other areas of the same image (e.g. contralateral areas) or with expected values obtained from the study of 'normal' images.

The relative usefulness of computer data processing can be evaluated by the method of receiver operating characteristic (ROC) analysis (Goodenough *et al.*, 1974), which takes account only of whether a lesion is identified as present or not in an image, and localization receiver operating characteristic (LROC) analysis (Starr *et al.*, 1975). In the latter, the position of any lesion must be identified also. LROC analysis has been used by Houston and Macleod (1977) in an extensive intercomparison of processing and display methods. Metz and Kronman (1980) and Metz *et al.* (1984) have developed statistical tests to evaluate the resulting curves.

24.7.2 DYNAMIC IMAGES

The greatest utility of computers in the clinical environment is in the acquisition, display and analysis of dynamic studies, in which a time series of images is obtained. In most cases, the sequence starts simultaneously with the administration of the radiopharmaceutical (e.g. cerebral blood flow or renal studies) and continues for a period determined by the time span of the physiological process being studied. In other cases, a repetitive phenomenon (e.g. the heart cycle) is being studied and acquisition is gated by a marker (the ECG) to produce a number of images depicting the organ at various stages in the cycle; data acquisition can be continued until a sufficient number of counts has been obtained.

In all cases, a suitable image (or summation of images) of the organ under study is displayed from the series. The operator delineates a region-of-interest (ROI) within the image, most usually using a trackerball or joystick control, and the computer is instructed to generate a graph of the summation of pixel counts within the ROI as a function of time – the activity–time curve. This curve, or several curves derived from different ROIs from the same study, may be subject to further processing to yield parameters measuring, or related to, the physiological process.

The most common technique is that of deconvolution analysis, as applied to renography (e.g. Diffey *et al.*, 1976). Many different algorithms have been proposed for deconvolution, including direct Fourier transformation, but the most widely used is to derive the transfer function by successive weighted stripping of the input function from the output function. This technique is prone to oscillation if the input function suffers statistical fluctuations and so a good bolus administration of the radiopharmaceutical is desirable.

An alternative is the method of principal components/factorial analysis (e.g. Houston *et al.*, 1979; Schmidlin, 1979). In this technique, curves are generated for each region and the mean curve is computed; the mean curve is then subtracted from the original curves and the principal discriminating features extracted from the resulting set of data.

Other methods which have been employed to analyse dynamic studies include cluster analysis (Griffin *et al.*, 1979) and the random walk function (Hart *et al.*, 1987).

A technique widely applied to gated cardiac studies is that of functional imaging. It is possible to derive activity–time curves on an individual pixel basis; these curves may be referred to as 'dixels' or 'trixels'. A parameter associated with these curves, such as maximum amplitude, time to maximum or initial slope, may be derived and the value plotted in the corresponding pixel of a 'functional' image. In cardiac studies, the assumption is made that each trixel may be approximated by a curve of the form

$$A = a + r.\sin(\theta + \phi)$$

where r is the amplitude and θ the phase (e.g. Pavel *et al.*, 1980).

24.8 CHOICE OF EQUIPMENT

24.8.1 IMAGING DEVICES

Traditionally, nuclear medicine imaging equipment has been purchased to fill a general-purpose role. As detailed above, special-purpose systems are now available for those departments which have a sufficient workload to justify an instrument dedicated to a particular investigation or group of investigations. For the department dependent upon a single gamma camera, a 400 mm FoV Anger camera will still be the instrument of choice, although it would now be standard practice to purchase one capable of SPECT. Such a general-purpose machine may be 'customized' for particular investigations by a suitable collimator selection; 'cutaway' collimators are available to facilitate neurological studies, while 'bilateral' collimators (capable of viewing the heart simultaneously from two directions) are available for cardiac work.

When choosing a collimator, several factors

must be considered. In general, static studies should be undertaken with a high-resolution collimator to provide the best possible spatial resolution. Sensitivity is a less important factor since imaging can be continued for a longer time if necessary to accumulate sufficient counts. Exceptions to this rule are studies involving radiopharmaceuticals which give rise to very low count rates. Examples are ^{201}Tl, where the low energy of the photons leads to a high scattered/unscattered ratio for detected photons and considerations of toxicity and radiation dose preclude the use of increased amounts of radiopharmaceutical, ^{75}Se for adrenal imaging, where the uptake fraction is extremely small, and radiolabelled monoclonal antibodies for tumour imaging, where the uptake may be low and imaging may have to be carried out more than a half-life after administration. In such cases, emphasis should be placed on the sensitivity of the collimator.

Sensitivity is usually the more important factor in choosing a collimator for dynamic studies, particularly those involving short frame durations, to ensure that each frame contains a sufficient number of counts.

It must be remembered that, in imaging a radionuclide which emits γ-photons of more than one energy, the collimator chosen must be that appropriate to the highest energy emission, irrespective of whether this energy is to be used for imaging. As an example, ^{67}Ga emits γ-photons at energies of 93, 185, 300 and 394 keV; the collimator used must be suitable for use at 394 keV.

Many manufacturers offer two or three versions of a given type of collimator, for example high-resolution, general-purpose and high-sensitivity low-energy parallel-hole collimators. Data for a typical set of collimators are given in Table 24.2.

The problem of radionuclides with emissions at more than one energy has led to the evolution of cameras fitted with dual- or triple-channel pulse-height analysis capability. Rather than use a single wide window to encompass, say, two photopeaks, it is preferable to use two energy windows, one centred on each photopeak, thus eliminating scattered photons having energies between the photopeak values. For ^{67}Ga, the optimum arrangement is to use triple windows, selecting the 93, 185 and 300 keV photopeaks; if only a single window is available, it should be set on the 93 keV photopeak, since this has the highest abundance of the three. Systems fitted with multiple energy windows can be used also for studies involving the simultaneous administration of more than one radionuclide, an example being the measurement of the gastric emptying of a test meal, the liquid component being labelled with one radionuclide and the solid component with another.

The image produced by a gamma camera has been recorded traditionally on film by a time exposure of an oscilloscope display. A multiformat device should be installed as standard, since this gives considerable flexibility for recording both static and dynamic images onto transparency film; as detailed earlier, it should be capable also of accepting images from the computer system. Polaroid film has little to offer for the recording of analogue images.

24.8.2 COMPUTER SYSTEMS

Almost all departments, irrespective of size, will require a computer system. The characteristics of available systems, together with the detailed requirements of the user, must be considered

Table 24.2 Collimator data

Collimator	*Hole dia (mm)*	*Number of holes*	*Sensitivity (relative)*	*Maximum energy (keV)*
Low energy				
high sensitivity	3.5	9 000	1.49	160
general purpose	2.5	18 000	1.00	160
high resolution	1.9	29 000	0.45	160
converging	2.6	13 000	1.40	160
Medium energy				
general purpose	4.0	4 000	1.00	300
pinhole	4.0	1	0.35	300
^{131}I	4.0	2 600	0.69	400

carefully prior to purchase. Most camera manufacturers offer their own computer systems and some have been made an integral and essential part of the camera. Now in a numerical minority, there are independent computer suppliers, whose systems can be interfaced to any camera.

Some systems are capable of being interfaced to, and acquiring data simultaneously from, two or more cameras and are thus suitable for larger departments. These systems can become very complex and the whole department then becomes vulnerable to a major failure. A measure of redundancy must be designed into such a system for this reason.

Another approach favours the installation of a number of smaller computer systems, each capable of acquiring data from only one camera. To keep costs down, the systems need not be of the same level of sophistication or performance, some being capable only of data-logging with subsequent transfer of data to the analysis system by floppy disc or magnetic tape. In this case, the department will still be able to operate following a failure.

If the computer is an integral part of the camera, then the choice of system must include consideration of whether both components meet the user's requirements.

It is good practice to have the results of each investigation, both images and quantitative analysis, available before the patient leaves the department. This requires multiple ground operation, even when the maximum data acquisition demands are being made on the system – remote acquisition subsystems facilitate this. If a department has an extensive research and development programme, a smaller separate computer system, linked to the main system, is highly desirable; this is particularly so if a large amount of programming is to be undertaken.

As hospital 'patient administration systems' are now being implemented, it is advantageous for the computer system to be capable of running a departmental patient database; it should be provided also with communication interfaces (such as X25 or Ethernet) to exchange information with other systems.

24.9 ENVIRONMENT

For most imaging devices, the performance is less stable if the room temperature varies markedly and, in extreme cases, the crystal of an Anger camera may suffer thermal fracture (Figure 24.11a). This happens most often if a window in the room is left open during the winter when there is a rapid drop in temperature overnight. It should be noted that it is the rate of temperature change, and not the absolute temperature, which is important. A gamma camera has a heat load of some 2.5 kW (including the console), which must be taken into account also. It is necessary, therefore, to utilize air-conditioning systems to maintain the temperature at, say, 22–25 °C with a maximum change of 3 °C per hour. For a single room installation, window-mounted units are satisfactory; for larger departments, a full air-conditioning system may be more economic. If it is intended to discharge radioactive gases (e.g. ^{133}Xe), the extract ducts should be led to the roof level of the building containing the department.

Ideally, the air-conditioning system should maintain a non-condensating humidity of 45 ±5%. Magnetic tape will stretch when variations in temperature and humidity occur and condensation on magnetic hard disc surfaces can cause the disc to 'crash', damaging the read/write head and permanently destroying the data on the disc.

Although gamma cameras tend to be quiet devices, computers are frequently noisy due to cooling fans and motors sucking air through filters in magnetic disc drives and magnetic tape units. Cheaper printers can be noisy also. This noise can be unpleasant for staff and patients and is another reason for placing the computer in a separate room if possible. It is easier to keep the computer free from dust if it is not positioned in the camera room, which contains sheets and blankets that inevitably create fibres and dust.

The dimensions and weight of equipment will be supplied by the manufacturer. A typical 400 mm FoV camera weighs some 1200 kg and the hospital architect/engineer should be consulted to ensure that the floor will take the load. If a scanning type camera is to be installed, it should be noted that the point floor loading may be substantially higher than in the static case and consideration may have to be given to plating the system. For a scanning camera, the maximum tolerable floor slope is 2° over the length of the scanning track. A room area of some 30 m^2 will be required and, if an emission tomography system is being installed, care should be taken to ensure that sufficient space is available for ease of patient access and transfer in both planar and tomographic modes of operation.

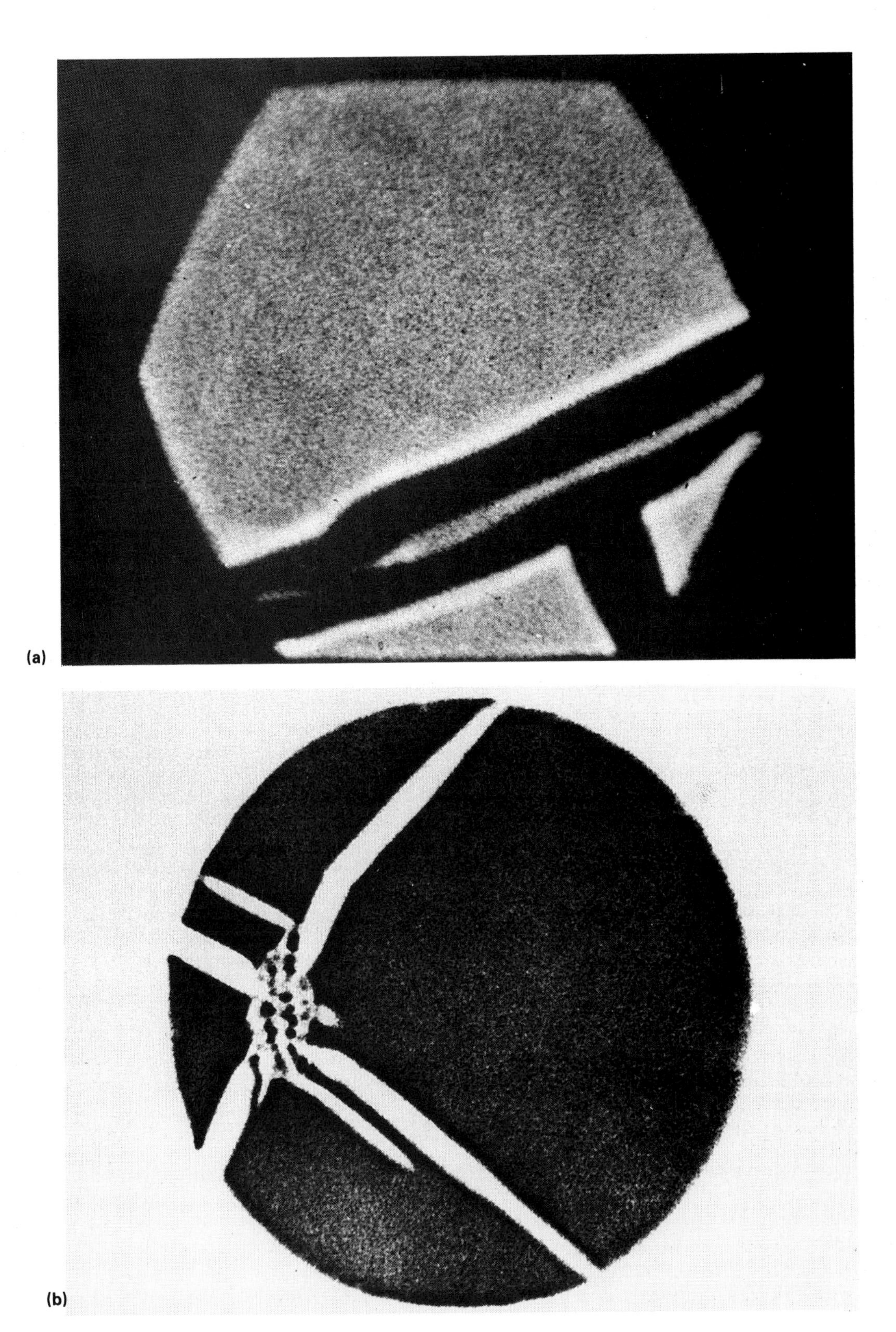

Figure 24.11 Flood field images following (a) thermal fracture and (b) impact fracture of the crystal.

If a mobile camera is being purchased, the loading of floors and lifts, height clearances, door widths and corridor gradients should be checked.

In addition to a measure of thermal protection (see above) for the crystal, a collimator provides mechanical protection (Figure 24.11b) and should not be left off longer than necessary. It should be remembered that, in current generation cameras, the crystal, PMTs and electronics form a matched set and the entire detector assembly may have to be replaced if the crystal is damaged – the cost is not insubstantial.

If, as is common, the nuclear medicine facility is installed as part of, or adjacent to, the radiology department, care must be taken to ensure that no interference will be caused to the cameras, counters etc. by X-ray sources.

24.10 QUALITY CONTROL

This is a topic more written about than carried out. Nevertheless, it is of vital importance if the best possible patient service is to be provided. It should begin at the time of placing an order for equipment, when a performance specification should be drawn up and form part of the order; for cameras, data to assist in this may be obtained from a series of reports published by DHSS/SHHD (1980, 1982, 1985, 1986) or from the manufacturer's NEMA data, although the latter are less applicable to the clinical situation. Following installation, the user should undertake comprehensive testing to ensure that the performance complies with the specification. A close physical inspection of the mechanical and electrical aspects of the equipment should be made; it is worthwhile arranging to X-ray the collimators on delivery to check for defects.

With the instrument in regular clinical use, simple but regular checks should be made to ensure that the device continues to perform within specification. Some of these checks should be made daily, while others need be made only on a quarterly or annual basis. All quantitative data should be archived carefully and, where appropriate, subjected to trend analysis. Among publications offering guidance are those of the US Department of Health, Education and Welfare (1976), the Hospital Physicists' Association (1978, 1983) and the World Health Organization (1982).

The following practices can help to maintain stable and optimal operating conditions:

1. The high-voltage supply to the PMTs should always be maintained. Some users advocate leaving all power supplies permanently on but, if this practice is adopted, the display and persistence oscilloscopes should be switched off overnight or for long periods when the camera is not in use; this will prolong their useful life.
2. As detailed above, a collimator should be attached to the detector at all times to provide thermal and mechanical protection.
3. Check for damage to the detector head, collimator mountings and collimator cart each time collimators are changed. Ensure that the correct fixing bolts are used and that the collimator is secured properly before moving the detector head. Be careful that no foreign objects are trapped between the collimator and the detector when collimators are fitted.
4. Ensure that photographic cameras are fastened securely to their mountings and are in the correct focus position. If using a multiformat device take care that the intensity is adjusted properly whenever the format is changed.
5. Avoid radioactive contamination of the collimators and detector head. It is good practice to seal phantoms containing radioactivity in a plastic bag before placing them on a collimator surface.

24.10.1 DAILY CHECKS

(a) Display system

If accessible, the display and persistence oscilloscopes should be checked to ensure that the dot size and shape are satisfactory. If a multiformat device is in use, the intensity setting should be checked with the photometer if fitted. If a Polaroid camera or multiformat camera back is attached to the display oscilloscope, the lens system should be checked for foreign matter and cleaned if necessary.

(b) Energy settings

The single most important factor in the operation of a gamma camera is the correct setting of the energy analyser peak and window and this must be impressed upon users. The exact way in which this is achieved varies among the types of camera available.

Some cameras have aids to help achieve this such as displaying the output from the energy amplifier on the display oscilloscope while simultaneously modulating or blanking off the beam intensity with the output from the pulse-height analyser (Figure 24.12a) or adding a simple multichannel analyser (MCA) to the camera's electronics with the selected energy window indicated by intensification of the display as shown in Figure 24.12(b). Under minimum scatter conditions, i.e. with the collimator off and a point source of activity at least five times the FOV away on the camera axis, the MCA display on a peaked camera will appear as in Figure 24.12(b), where the lowest left and right intensified channels are at the same height and equal numbers of intensified channels are on either side of the peak's maximum. Under clinical conditions, a collimator is fitted to the camera and the activity is distributed throughout the patient's body. Considerable Compton scattering will therefore occur, distorting the low-energy side of the peak so that the MCA display will appear as shown in Figure 24.12(c). There are again equal numbers of intensified channels either side of the maximum but the lowest channels on each side are no longer at the same height. Any adjustment to the peaking to position the lowest left and right channels at the same height will produce a small shift of the energy window to lower energies, with a consequent asymmetry of the energy window about the photopeak. Fortunately, this shift is so small (approximately 2–3 keV for the 141 keV photopeak of ^{99m}Tc) that no serious problems arise.

(c) Uniformity check: flood field image

All users should be familiar with the best flood field image that is possible with their camera so that any deterioration is recognized. The flood field should be larger than the camera's FOV in order to avoid edge effects and should be well mixed; since the performance of modern cameras can vary between 122 and 141 keV, it is preferable to use a ^{99m}Tc flood source. The quantity of radioactivity added to the source and the time of preparation should be noted.

The same collimator (preferably the highest resolution ^{99m}Tc collimator available) should be used each day and the source placed on its surface. Both analogue and digital images containing a fixed number of counts (at least 1 000 000) should be obtained and the acquisition time noted. An index of sensitivity can be obtained by calculating the counting rate per megabecquerel of activity in the source. The most likely cause for discrepancy

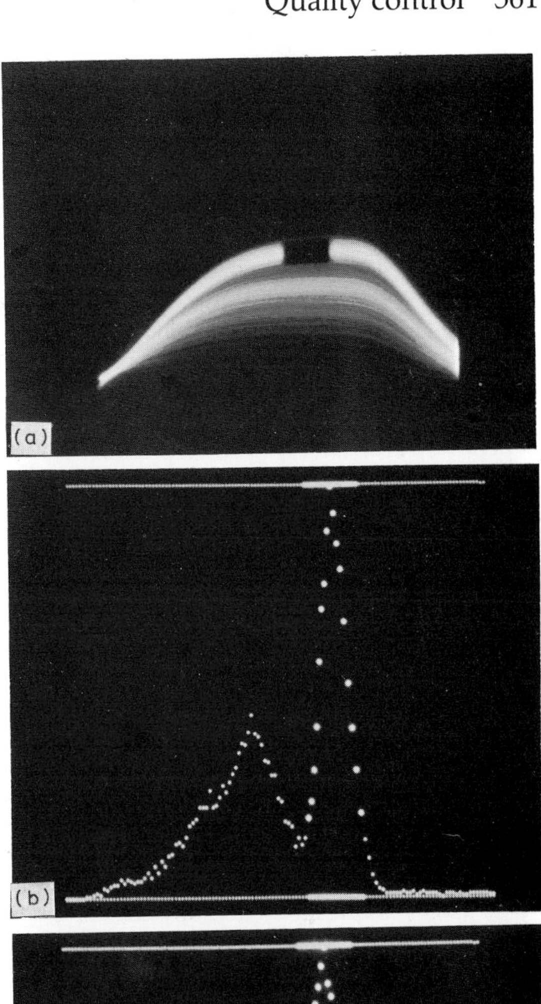

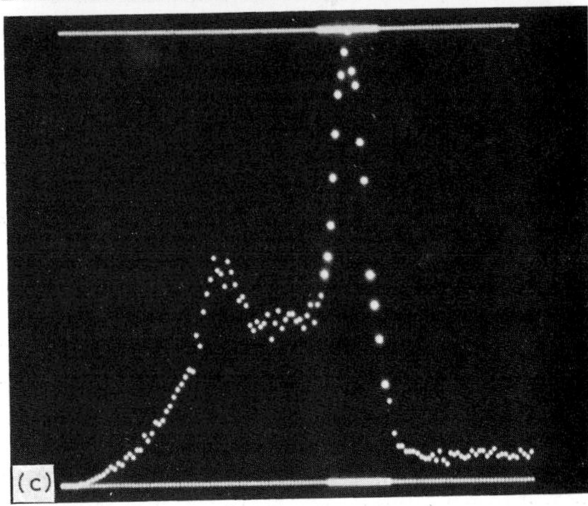

Figure 24.12 Detector pulse height energy spectra; (a) analogue display, the blanked-off portion indicating the position of the energy analyser window. Multichannel analyser display with the camera peaked using a ^{99m}Tc source in air (b) and subsequently viewing a ^{99m}Tc distribute source in the presence of scattering medium (c).

in this figure is inaccuracy in setting the energy window.

The analogue image should be examined for intensity and the dot size and shape should be inspected in addition to a visual assessment of the uniformity of the image. Any adjustments to camera or display settings should be logged. The digital image should be examined for any gross abnormality.

Some causes of poor flood fields are easily remedied. Figure 24.13(a) shows the effect of mis-peaking the camera; cameras from different manufacturers differ in their response to this type of error. Figure 24.13(b) shows a poor flood field caused by the non-uniform build-up of dirt on the face plate of the oscilloscope. This should not occur if the cleaning schedule above is adopted. Other than these simple causes, there are no adjustments which the user can make to a modern camera and a service engineer should be called.

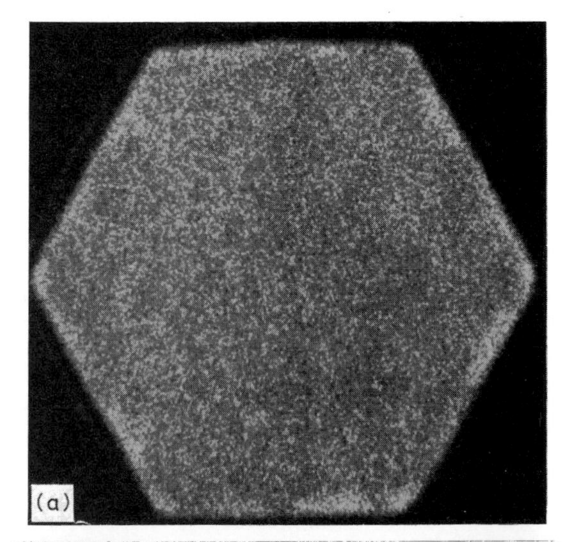

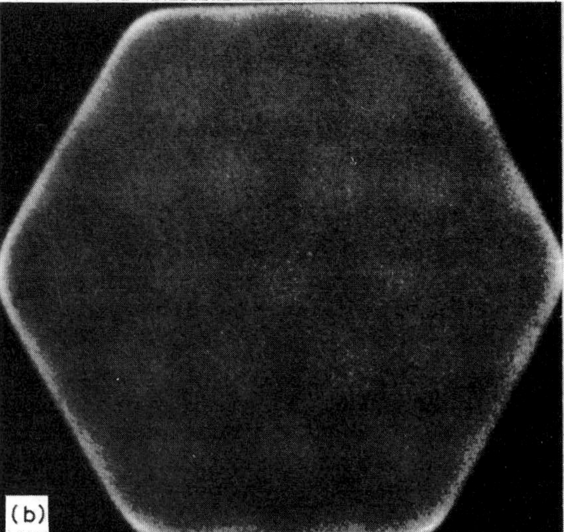

Figure 24.13 Examples of flood field images; (a) result of incorrect setting of the energy analyser window and (b) artefact due to accumulation of dust behind CRT implosion shield.

24.10.2 WEEKLY CHECKS

(a) Uniformity check: flood field image

While the daily test specified above is adequate for its purpose of determining whether the camera is usable clinically, it is necessary to make closer investigation of the machine's performance to yield quantitative data from which any more insidious problems can be identified; it also provides benchmark data against which the effect of any adjustment can be checked.

In addition to the daily test, a flood field image containing at least 20 000 000 counts should be acquired into the computer system once per week; it is convenient to carry out this acquisition overnight or, if scheduling permits, over a lunch break – at a count rate of 10 000 counts per second, the acquisition will take approximately 45 min. The data should be collected into a 64 × 64 matrix to give high statistical accuracy and analysed to yield integral and differential uniformity as specified in the IEC Standard 789. For modern cameras, it is useful to compile a histogram of pixel counts at intervals of 1% from the mean as shown in Figure 24.14. This distribution is more sensitive to changes in performance than the global uniformity figures. It is advisable to archive these flood field images and the resulting data for trend analysis.

(b) Resolution check

On a modern system, resolution is unlikely to deteriorate rapidly and so a qualitative test is sufficient. An image of a modified Anger phantom, an 'Anger + 3', obtained with the collimator removed as detailed in, for example, DHSS Report STB/86/9 (1986) should be scrutinized visually for evidence of worsening resolution and spatial distortion.

NO OF PIXELS = 2559.0 MEAN COUNTS = 8396.2
RANGE = + 8.2 PERCENT TO - 7.5 PERCENT
SD = 152.8 COUNTS COV = 1.8 PERCENT
MAX COUNT = 9087.0 MIN COUNT = 7768.0
DIFF UNIF = 10.53 PERCENT AT 5,28 AND 4,29

% OF MEAN	NO OF PIXELS	% OF PIXELS
80	0.0	0.0
81	0.0	0.0
82	0.0	0.0
83	0.0	0.0
84	0.0	0.0
85	0.0	0.0
86	0.0	0.0
87	0.0	0.0
88	0.0	0.0
89	0.0	0.0
90	0.0	0.0
91	0.0	0.0
92	1.0	0.0
93	2.0	.1
94	9.0	.4
95	47.0	1.8
96	117.0	4.6
97	250.0	9.8
98	408.0	15.9
99	458.0	17.9
100	488.0	19.1
101	345.0	13.5
102	248.0	9.7
103	112.0	4.4
104	43.0	1.7
105	23.0	.9
106	4.0	.2
107	3.0	.1
108	1.0	.0
109	0.0	0.0
110	0.0	0.0
111	0.0	0.0
112	0.0	0.0
113	0.0	0.0
114	0.0	0.0
115	0.0	0.0
116	0.0	0.0
117	0.0	0.0
118	0.0	0.0
119	0.0	0.0
120	0.0	0.0

% PIXELS WITHIN 1% OF MEAN = 37.0
% PIXELS WITHIN 2% OF MEAN = 66.4
% PIXELS WITHIN 3% OF MEAN = 85.9
% PIXELS WITHIN 4% OF MEAN = 94.8
% PIXELS WITHIN 5% OF MEAN = 98.3
% PIXELS WITHIN 6% OF MEAN = 99.6
% PIXELS WITHIN 7% OF MEAN = 99.8
% PIXELS WITHIN 8% OF MEAN = 100.0
% PIXELS WITHIN 9% OF MEAN = 100.0
% PIXELS WITHIN 10% OF MEAN = 100.0

Figure 24.14 Results of uniformity analysis of flood field image.

(c) SPECT systems

The most critical parameter, apart from the performance of the detector head itself, for a rotating camera SPECT system is the centre of rotation (CoR) offset. This should be measured by placing a point source, in air, within 20 mm of the axis of rotation and within 20 mm of the centre of the FOV. A 32-angle tomographic acquisition should be performed into a 128 × 128 matrix, collecting a minimum of 10 000 counts at each angle. The data should be analysed by the standard method (e.g. Todd-Pokropek *et al.*, 1987). The mean value of the CoR offset after correction should be less than 1 mm. If the CoR offset is not independent of the position of the point source within the FOV, it may be an indication that the y axis is not aligned with the axis of rotation.

For systems used routinely for tomography, it is recommended that a total performance phantom (e.g. Jaszczak) is imaged also. Tomographic uniformity and resolution may be assessed from the resulting tomograms.

24.10.3 ANNUAL CHECKS

The following parameters should be assessed annually, or following major servicing.

(a) Uniformity

This should be carried out as specified above for the weekly check.

(b) Intrinsic resolution

This should be measured by the method specified in the IEC (1984) and NEMA (1986) standards, using a phantom comprising 0.5 mm wide parallel slits, spaced 30 mm apart. Data analysis should yield the mean and range of values found over the FOV.

(c) Spatial distortion

This can be obtained from the same raw data as the intrinsic resolution measurement. Data may be analysed either by the NEMA method or that contained in the DHSS Reports.

(d) Energy resolution

The energy resolution for ^{99m}Tc should be measured as specified in the IEC standard.

(e) System resolution

A single measurement of overall system resolution should be made as specified in the IEC standard, using a given collimator at a depth of 100 mm in scatter and compared to the value obtained at installation.

(f) Computer

Tests of the computer system should be undertaken as recommended by Todd-Pokropek (1983).

24.11 EQUIPMENT SERVICING

When choosing equipment, reliability should be an important criterion. Nevertheless, it must be realized that breakdowns will occur and so the servicing arrangements offered by the manufacturer should be examined; the service record of a company may be the deciding factor in the choice of equipment.

Service contracts are based usually on a percentage of the installed capital cost of the equipment, although some are based on a percentage of the current replacement cost. The latter should be examined carefully, since they could be linked to a 'list' price higher than would actually be paid for new equipment. In general, computers attract a higher percentage than cameras.

It is important to ensure that the contract specifies the response time to a fault call, the range of faults and parts replacement covered by the agreement (e.g. whether PMT replacement is covered for a camera) and the preventative maintenance schedule. The cost of a service contract should be balanced against the likelihood of a breakdown and the charges made by the manufacturer for non-contract service. Note that, in most cases, contract customers take precedence over non-contract customers and so the response time to a fault call may be quite long for the latter. The availability of service advice over the telephone should be ascertained also.

A third alternative, viable only in a large department or on a group basis (where hospitals have agreed to standardize equipment), is to employ an in-house service engineer. In this case, training will be necessary and the manufacturer should be consulted to ensure that this is available and to ascertain the cost. The issue of spare parts availability is a vital one to resolve and both this and training should form part of the purchase contract if in-house maintenance is contemplated. One potential drawback of this approach is that, if the engineer is of high quality, he/she is very likely to be offered a more lucrative job by the manufacturer.

For complex computer systems, the average department is best advised to take out a maintenance contract since, because of the modular architecture of modern machines, fault correction is frequently accomplished by module replacement and it is uneconomic for a department to carry the spare boards required to cover all eventualities. It is still worthwhile, however, to negotiate with the supplier for a discount on the basis of local staff carrying out first-line maintenance. This is advantageous not only in cost, but also in minimizing downtime. It should be borne in mind that, as the system ages, the point may be reached (typically at ten years old) where the company may refuse to provide contract maintenance or to guarantee the availability of spare parts.

For small 'data-logger' type systems, where downtime is less crucial, and for word-processor systems, a service contract is not good value.

In the case of gamma cameras, the question is more difficult to resolve, particularly as so-called 'digital cameras' have begun to appear. It must be remembered that, as described above, a modern camera has its correction circuitry calibrated at manufacture; small corrections can be made thereafter to compensate for deteriorating performance but some systems require replacement of the correction circuitry when physical adjustments are made to the detector. This is difficult for the user to accomplish. An ideal solution (assuming the camera to be covered by guarantee in the first year) would be to pay for service on an as-required basis in the second and third years, when the system is unlikely to suffer a major fault, taking out a service contract thereafter. Understandably, manufacturers are not keen on such an arrangement.

A service contract is probably best for a film processor, but other equipment such as air-conditioning, fume cupboards and laminar flow cabinets can usually be maintained by the hospital engineering department.

Problems can arise where a system (including third-party software for a computer) has been assembled from equipment supplied from more than one manufacturer. The user must ensure that areas of responsibility are clearly defined and, if at all possible, endeavour to deal with a single service organization willing to service the entire system. Otherwise the situation may arise in which each of two manufacturers tries to blame the other, with the user becoming 'pig in the middle'.

24.12 RADIATION PROTECTION

The UK requirements are set out in The Ionising Radiations Regulations (HMSO, 1985), the associated Approved Code of Practice (HMSO, 1985) and Guidance Notes (HMSO, 1988) and the Ionising Radiation (Protection of Persons Undergoing Medical Examination or Treatment) Regulations (HMSO, 1988). These implement EC Council Directive 84/466 Euratom.

Good radiation protection practice may be considered under four headings:

1. the adoption of careful and tidy working procedures;
2. careful, systematic and regular contamination monitoring;
3. the establishment of a comprehensive training programme;
4. the provision of a clear set of local rules.

The local rules for the handling of radioactive materials should be prepared in consultation with the local radiation protection adviser, health and safety inspector and pollution inspector. It should include detailed method sheets for each procedure involving radionuclides undertaken in the department and should contain also clear instructions for the action to be taken in the case of an emergency.

Entry to any area of the department identified as a controlled area by virtue of dose rate or potential contamination levels, and where staff are not classified personnel, will be permissible only under a written system of work. These systems of work must cover the department's own staff and also other groups (e.g. escort nurses, porters, engineering and maintenance staff) who may occasionally enter the department. Consideration should be given to issuing all staff working in a department with a film badge dosimeter, including secretarial, portering and domestic staff. Since the minimum reported dose is usually 0.2 mSv per badge, the frequency of changing badges should not be too great for staff exposed to low doses, otherwise an artificially high radiation dose will appear in the records of such staff. It will be found that a film badge change each month is adequate for most staff, with a fortnightly change for staff exposed to higher radiation levels (e.g. those dispensing radiopharmaceuticals). Personnel working in the radiopharmacy should be provided with two additional types of dosimeter: a pocket dose-rate meter, preferably of the 'bleeper' type, and TLD finger badge dosimeters, which should be worn on the index finger of each hand beneath disposable gloves. The gloves themselves should be assessed for their permeability to radioactive materials – latex types are to be preferred.

Appropriate radiation contamination monitors should be provided in each laboratory in which radionuclides are handled; these will generally include the radiopharmacy, the radioiodination laboratory, the patient injection room and the radionuclide store. Staff should be instructed to monitor their hands, clothing and work surfaces on completion of every session during which radionuclides have been handled. A convenient method of attempting to ensure that this is done is to provide a log book at each site to record the results of monitoring. The departmental radiation protection supervisor should carry out an independent survey of all staff and laboratories at least once each week. For staff handling radioiodine, particularly the high specific activity ^{125}I used for protein iodination, particular attention should be paid to regular thyroid monitoring.

Particular care should be taken when introducing a new procedure or when a new member of staff takes up post. Since reduction of exposure time can be an easier way of reducing radiation dose than introducing extra shielding to cut down dose rate, the procedure(s) should be practised with 'cold' materials to gain familiarity with the handling techniques and to identify potential problems. Extra film badge dosimeters and surface monitoring may be used to measure the radiation dose associated with the particular procedure and the working method accepted or modified on the basis of the results.

Adequate shielding must be used, particularly around a radionuclide generator; the elution vial shields should be checked for efficacy also. Provision must be made for the convenient transport of patient doses of radiopharmaceuticals, particularly therapy doses, between the radiopharmacy and the patient injection room, either by a shielded trolley or in individual containers. To reduce the radiation dose to staff injecting radiopharmaceuticals, syringe shields should be used wherever possible; tungsten shields are easier to use than lead. If necessary, a butterfly should be inserted into a difficult vein rather than handling an active syringe for protracted periods.

Note that, under the Patient Protection Regulations, medical practitioners are required to have undergone training in a 'core of knowledge' prior to administering radiopharmaceuticals, to keep patient radiation exposures as low as reasonably practicable and to maintain adequate records of equipment. Although not strictly a radiation protection requirement, it is worthwhile reiterating the need for appropriate certification by the Administration of Radioactive Substances Advisory Committee (ARSAC).

REFERENCES

Anger, H. O. (1958) Scintillation camera. *Rev. Sci. Instr.*, **29**, 27–33.

Bateman, J. E. and Connolly, J. F. (1978) A multiwire proportional gamma camera for imaging Tc-99m radionuclide distributions. *Phys. Med. Biol.*, **23**, 445.

Bender, M. A. and Blau, M. (1963) The autofluoroscope. *Nucleonics*, **21**, 52–59.

Berger, H. J., Davies, R. A., Batsford, W. P. *et al.* (1981) Beat-to-beat left ventricular performance assessed from the equilibrium cardiac blood pool using a computerised nuclear probe. *Circulation*, **63**, 133–42.

Boddy, K., Elliott, A. T., Robertson, I. *et al.* (1975) A high sensitivity dual-detector shadow-shield whole-body counter with an invariant response for total body *in vivo* neutron activation analysis. *Phys. Med. Biol.*, **20**, 296–304.

Bracewell, R. N. (1956) Strip integration in radio astronomy. *Aust. J. Phys.*, **9**, 198–217.

Brown, N. J. G., Budd, T. and Britton, K. E. (1976) in *Proceedings of the 13th Internationale Jahrestagung der Gesellschaft fur Nuclearmedizin EV*, Copenhagen.

Budinger, T. F. and Gullberg, G. T. (1974) Three dimensional reconstruction in nuclear medicine by iterative least-squares and Fourier transform techniques. *IEEE Trans. Nucl. Sci.*, **NS-21**, 2–20.

Campbell, F. W. (1976) in *Medical Images: Formation, Perception and Measurement* (ed. G. A. Hay), John Wright, Bristol.

Chang, L. T. (1978) A method for attenuation correction in radionuclide computed tomography. *IEE Trans. Nucl. Sci.*, **NS-25**, 638–43.

Cohn, S. H., Dombrowski, S., Pate, H. R. and Robertson, J. S. (1969) A whole-body counter with invariant response to radionuclide distribution and body size. *Phys. Med. Biol.*, **14**, 645.

Corfield, J. R. (1976) in *Proceedings of the 13th International Jahrestagung der Gesellschaft fur Nuclearmedizin EV*, Copenhagen.

DHSS (1980) *Performance Assessment of Gamma Cameras – Part I, Report STB/11/80*, Department of Health and Social Security, London.

DHSS (1982) *Performance Assessment of Gamma Cameras – Part II, Report STB/13/82*, Department of Health and Social Security, London.

DHSS (1985) *Performance Assessment of Gamma Cameras – Part III, Report STB6D/85/6*, Department of Health and Social Security, London.

DHSS (1986) *Performance Assessment of Gamma Cameras – Part IV, Report STB/86/9*, Department of Health and Social Security, London.

Diffey, B. L., Hall, F. M. and Corfield, J. R. (1976) The Tc-DTPA dynamic renal scan with deconvolution analysis. *J. Nucl. Med.*, **17**, 352–5.

Elliott, A. T., Langford, R. M., Corbishley, T. P. *et al.* (1979) Peroperative nuclear medicine: the portable gamma camera on-line to a computer as a diagnostic service to the surgeon. *Nuklearmedizin*, **17**, 78–80.

Ewins, J. H., Armantrout, G. A., Camp, D. C. *et al.* (1977) in *Medical Radionuclide Imaging*, Vol. 1, IAEA, Vienna, pp. 149–6.

Garcia, E. V., Van Train, K., Maddahi, J. *et al.* (1985) Quantification of rotational thallium-201 myocardial tomography. *J. Nucl. Med.*, **26**, 17–26.

Goodenough, D. J., Rossmann, K. and Lusted, L. E. (1974) Radiographic applications of receiver operating characteristic (ROC) curves. *Radiology*, **110**, 89–95.

Griffin, D. W., Donovan, I. A., Harding, L. K. and White, C. M. (1979) Liquid gastric emptying in four minutes, 7th Annual Meeting, British Nuclear Medicine Society, London.

Gustafsson, T. R. and Pizer, S. M. (1975) in *Information Processing in Scintigraphy*, CEA, Orsay, pp. 56–64.

Harby, K. (1988) Clinical PET: is it time to take the plunge? *J. Nucl. Med.*, **29**, 1751–7.

Hart, G. C., Bunday, B. and Kiri, V. (1987) The random walk function in the analysis of time–activity curves from dynamic radionuclide studies. *Nucl. Med. Commun.*, **8**, 189–97.

HMSO (1985) *The Ionising Radiations Regulations 1985*, Statutory Instrument 1333, HMSO, London.

HMSO (1985) *Approved Code of Practice; The Protection of Persons Against Ionising Radiation Arising from Any Work Activity*, HMSO, London.

HMSO (1988) *Guidance Notes for the Protection of Persons Against Ionising Radiations Arising from Medical and Dental Use*, HMSO, London.

HMSO (1988) *The Ionising Radiation (Protection of Persons Undergoing Medical Examination or Treatment) Regulations*, Statutory Instrument 778, HMSO, London.

Hospital Physicists' Association (1978) *The Theory, Specification and Testing of Anger Type Gamma Cameras*, HPA, London.

Hospital Physicists' Association (1983) *Quality Control of Nuclear Medicine Instrumentation*, HPA, London.

Houston, A. S. (1976) An attempt to optimise two zero summation filters for use in radioisotope scintigraphy. *Int. J. Nucl. Med. Biol.*, **3**, 111–14.

Houston, A. S. and MacLeod, M. A. (1977) An intercomparison of computer assisted data processing and display methods in radioisotope scintigraphy using mathematical tumours. *Phys. Med. Biol.*, **22**, 1097–114.

Houston, A. S., MacLeod, M. A. and Sampson, W. (1979) Principal components analysis as an aid to classification of renal dynamic studies. *Eur. J. Nucl. Med.*, **4**, 295–9.

International Electrotechnical Commission (1984) *Char-*

acteristics and test conditions of radionuclide imaging devices – IEC789. IEC, Geneva.

Jarritt, P. H., Ell, P. J., Myers, M. J., Brown, N. J. G. and Deacon, J. M. (1979) A new transverse-section brain imager for single-photon gamma emitters. *J. Nucl. Med.*, **20**, 319–27.

Kuhl, D. E. and Edwards, R. Q. (1963) Image separation radioisotope scanning. *Radiology*, **80**, 653–62.

Lacy, J. L., LeBlanc, A. D., Babich, J. W. *et al.* (1984) A gamma camera for medical applications, using a mutiwire proportional counter. *J. Nucl. Med.*, **25**, 1003–12.

Loc'h, C., Maziere, B. and Comar, D. (1980) A new generator for ionic gallium-68. *J. Nucl. Med.*, **21**, 171–3.

Metz, C. E. and Kronman, H. B. (1980) in *Information Processing in Medical Imaging*, Les Colloques de l'INSERM, 88, pp. 647–658.

Metz, C. E., Wang, P. and Kronman, H. B. (1984) in *Information Processing in Medical Imaging* (ed. F. Deconinck), Martinus Nijhoff, The Hague.

Milan, J. and Taylor, K. J. W. (1976) The application of the temperature scale to ultrasonic imaging. *J. Clin. Ultrasound*, **3**, 171–3.

Muehllehner, G. (1979) Effect of crystal thickness on scintillation camera performance. *J. Nucl. Med.*, **20**, 992–3.

Muehllehner, G., Buchin, M. P. and Dudek, J. H. (1976) Performance parameters of a positron imaging camera. *IEEE Trans. Nucl. Sci.*, **23**, 528–37.

Muehllehner, G., Colsher, J. G. and Stoub, E. W. (1980) Correction for field nonuniformity in scintillation cameras through removal of spatial distortion. *J. Nucl. Med.*, **21**, 771–76.

Mullani, N. A., Gaeta, J. and Yerian, K. (1984) Dynamic imaging with high-resolution time-of-flight PET camera – TOFPET I. *IEEE Trans. Nucl. Sci.*, **S-31**, 609–13.

National Electrical Manufacturers' Association (1986) *Performance measurements of scintillation cameras*, Publication NU1-1986, NEMA, Washington.

Neill, G. D. S. and Hutchinson, F. (1971) Computer detection and display of focal lesions on scintiscans. *Br. J. Radiol.*, **44**, 962–9.

Oldendorf, W. H. (1961) Isolated flying spot detection of radiodensity discontinuities: displaying the internal structural pattern of a complex object. *IRE Trans. Bio-Med. Elect.*, **8**, 68–72.

Pavel, D., Byron, E., Swiryn, S. *et al.* (1980) in *Medical Radionuclide Imaging*, IAEA, Vienna, pp. 253–9.

Royal, H. D., Brown, P. H. and Claunch, B. C. (1979) Effects of a reduction in crystal thickness on Anger-camera performance. *J. Nucl. Med.*, **20**, 977–80.

Schmidlin, P. (1979) Quantitative evaluation and imaging of functions using pattern recognition methods. *Phys. Med. Biol.*, **24**, 385–95.

Starr, S. J., Metz, C. E., Lusted, L. B. and Goodenough, D. J. (1975) Visual detection and localisation of radiographic images. *Radiology*, **116**, 533–8.

Strashun, A., Horowitz, S. F., Goldsmith, S. J. *et al.* (1981) Noninvasive detection of left ventricular dysfunction with a portable electrocardiographic gated scintillation probe device. *Am. J. Cardiol.*, **47**, 61–17.

Tauxe, W. N., Soussaline, F., Todd-Pokropek, A. E. *et al.* (1982) Determination of organ volume by single-photon emission tomography. *J. Nucl. Med.*, **23**, 984–7.

Ter-Pogossian, M. M., Phelps, M. E., Hoffman, E. J. and Mullani, N. A. (1975) A positron emission transaxial tomograph for nuclear medicine imaging (PETT). *Radiology*, **114**, 89–98.

Todd-Pokropek, A. E. (1983) in *Quality Control of Nuclear Medicine Instrumentation*, HPA, London, pp. 54–73.

Todd-Pokropek, A. E. and Jarritt, P. H. (1982) in *Computed Emission Tomography* (eds P. J. Ell and B. L. Holman), Oxford University Press, London, pp. 361–89.

Todd-Pokropek, A. E. and Pizer, S. M. (1977) in *Medical Radionuclide Imaging*, Vol. 1, IAEA, Vienna, pp. 505–38.

Todd-Pokropek, A. E., Erbsmann, F. and Soussaline, F. (1977) in *Medical Radionuclide Imaging*, Vol. 1, IAEA, Vienna, pp. 67–82.

Underwood, S. R., Walton, S., Laming, P. J. *et al.* (1985) Left ventricular volume and ejection fraction determined by gated blood pool emission tomography. *Br. Heart J.*, **53**, 216–22.

US Department of Health, Education and Welfare (1976) *Workshop Manual for Quality Control of Scintillation Cameras in Nuclear Medicine*, USDHEW, Washington.

Wagner, H. N., Wake, R., Nickoloff, E. and Natarajan, T. K. (1976). The nuclear stethoscope: A simple device for generation of left ventricular volume curves. *Am. J. Cardiol.*, **38**, 747–50.

Wicks, R. and Blau, M. (1979) Effect of spatial distortion on Anger camera field-uniformity correction. *J. Nucl. Med.*, **20**, 252–4.

Whitehead, F. R. (1978) Minimum detectable gray-scale differences in nuclear medicine images. *J. Nucl. Med.*, **19**, 87–93.

World Health Organization (1982) *Quality Assurance in Nuclear Medicine*, WHO, Geneva.

Yano, Y., Cahoon, J. L. and Budinger, T. F. (1981) A precision flow-controlled Rb-82 generator for bolus or constant infusion studies of the heart and brain. *J. Nucl. Med.*, **22**, 1006–10.

BIBLIOGRAPHY

Computed Emission Tomography (1982) (eds P. J. Ell and B. L. Holman), Oxford University Press, Oxford.

Tracer techniques and nuclear medicine (1986), in *Mathematical Methods in Medicine, Part 1* (editors D. Ingram and R. Bloch), John Wiley, Chichester.

Imaging (1986), in *Mathematical Methods in Medicine, Part 2* (eds D. Ingram and R. Bloch), John Wiley, Chichester.

The Physics of Medical Imaging (1988) (ed. S. Webb), Adam Hilger, Bristol.

CHAPTER TWENTY-FIVE

The evaluation of diagnostic methods

M. N. Maisey and J. Hutton

Radiological investigations over the years have generally been introduced with very little evaluation of either the diagnostic performance or the influence they have on patient management. This deficiency has become particularly important over the last two decades as major new diagnostic technologies, including magnetic resonance, computed tomography, ultrasound and nuclear medicine have been introduced into clinical medicine. The Council on Science and Society report in 1983 noted the haphazard manner in which expensive technologies were introduced and also that assessment is considered with very little concern for patient reactions or to the social and psychological consequences. Although the overriding reason for an evaluation is to confirm a positive benefit in patient care there are other practical reasons for increasing effort in this area. Increasingly there are constraints on the resources available within health services together with a general demand to achieve better value for money. Clinicians have the right, and indeed should demand to know, whether the diagnostic services that are offered make a real contribution to patient care and the assessments should be based on well-documented facts.

This chapter will set out some of the methodologies involved in diagnostic technology performance evaluation, to draw attention to common inadequacies in published studies and to provide a bibliography of the subject.

25.1 INTRODUCTION

The general methodology for evaluation is common to most diagnostic applications, although the emphasis will alter depending on the specific purpose for which the diagnostic method is used. Diagnostic imaging techniques can broadly be divided into four categories.

1. *Screening of asymptomatic patients for disease*: in this application, (e.g. breast screening by mammography), the prevalence of disease in the referred population is usually low; the goal is to detect all patients who have early disease and usually to accept the need to investigate a proportion of patients without the disease as the cost of not missing any individuals with disease.
2. *The detection and diagnosis of disease in symptomatic patients*: this is the conventional area of diagnostic imaging techniques in hospital. The patients are symptomatic, the prevelance of disease in the investigated population is intermediate and the goal is to detect and characterize disease.
3. *Staging of disease*: in this instance the presence of disease has usually been established by alternative methods (e.g. staging investigations for lymphoma or cancer); the usual goal is to identify further sites of disease and to establish the nature of the disease. A further example is in the search for a primary tumour when a metastatic adenocarcinoma of unkown origin has presented clinically and has been confirmed by biopsy.
4. *Assessment of change*: imaging techniques are frequently used to assess the progress of disease for prognostic purposes or the response to treatment (e.g. radionuclide liver scans to measure the effectiveness of chemotherapy in the treatment of cancer).
5. Targeting disease: the use of imaging to target lesions by ultrasonic guided biopsy or PET/SPECT brain studies for stereotactic surgery in partial epilepsy.

25.1.1 THE GOALS OF DIAGNOSTIC TESTS

The preceding section classified the applications of diagnostic tests; in order for them to be effective there must be a gain to the individual and to society when they are used, if the diagnostic technology is not to do more harm than good. The demonstration of pathology in a patient as a goal in itself is not sufficient: it must provide new information which will ultimately benefit the patient in one of the following ways.

1. Save lives.
2. Restore health, i.e. it will result in a useful treatment or change of treatment.
3. Alleviate suffering (physical and/or psychological), for example by detecting a metastatic bone lesion, permitting radiotherapy to relieve pain. A negative investigation may also relieve psychological suffering in this context by diminishing anxiety associated with the possibility of metastatic disease.
4. Prevent symptomatic disease occurring, for example breast screening which results in early treatment or by diagnosing an unsuspected metastatic bone disease which by prompt palliative measures could prevent a debilitating pathological fracture.
5. Predict the course of disease, which will contribute towards the prognosis and thereby aid the social and general management.

It can therefore be seen that, particularly in the case of screening, the investigation of symptomatic patients and for staging investigations, the test is being used to detect or exclude disease and the test must be able to do this more effectively than simpler methods.

25.1.2 THE COSTS AND BENEFITS OF EVALUATION

Although it appears self-evident that soundly based evaluation of the role of diagnostic methods in clinical medicine would be beneficial, an argument has to be made for the increasing use of these methods, as they have costs of their own.

The potential benefits of careful evaluation include: the better use of limited resource in patient care within the health service; the withdrawal of tests which cannot be shown to be of value and could even do more harm than good; and the prevention of early diffusion of unproven tests into widespread clinical practice. On the other hand there are costs including the direct costs of evaluation itself which may be high because the methods are difficult and studies are time-consuming to undertake. Further costs may include the delay in the introduction of a truly effective test. Similar evaluation costs apply to drug trials and these have undoubtedly been broadly beneficial.

The timing of evaluations is often critical; early evaluation studies are like 'trying to hit a moving target' because technology changes so rapidly that the results are regarded as irrelevant. On the other hand, early evaluation may prevent the widespread application of a test or purchase of equipment and dissemination of a method that is ultimately shown to be useless or at best non-contributory. Early evaluation by a well-designed study may detect an unsuspected morbidity associated with the diagnostic technique, which would have taken much longer to uncover if proper evaluation had not been undertaken. On the other hand, too early evaluation could lead to the premature rejection of a potentially valuable technique. Evaluation which is too late may be unable to prevent the use of a technology which cannot be shown to be useful but is 'believed in' by clinicians and therefore difficult to dislodge. The advantage of late evaluation is usually that the technology is stable and therefore the results of evaluation more credible.

25.1.3 HOW SHOULD NEW TECHNOLOGY BE INTRODUCED?

There are broadly three ways that new technology can be introduced.

1. *Random diffusion*: at the present time new technology is largely introduced on a random basis depending on a variety of factors such as: source of finance; clinical pressure on the assumption that the medical professionals 'know best' even when data are not available to support an opinion. Other factors include institutional prestige to have the newest equipment, commercial interests and outside pressures (Young, 1988).
2. *Evaluation of every technique:* with the rapid change of technology and the number of established diagnostic methods this is clearly impractical, would not be a cost-effective exercise and is probably not realistically achievable.
3. *Selective evaluation:* this is probably the ideal for deciding on the introduction and application of

diagnostic methods. Both new and old tests can be selectively examined especially if they are expensive, widely used and applied to disease with a high prevalence. Subsequent resource decisions can then be made on well-established quantifiable data. The choice of what should be evaluated should also be influenced by therapeutic implications and downstream costs.

25.3 METHODOLOGY AND TECHNIQUES FOR THE EVALUATION OF DIAGNOSTIC PERFORMANCE

The performance of diagnostic tests can be measured at several well-defined hierarchical levels, which have been categorized by Feinberg *et al.* (1977, 1979), and form the basis of a useful classification which assists in the understanding of the evaluation procedures. The six levels are:

1. Technical capacity;
2. Diagnostic accuracy;
3. Diagnostic impact;
4. Therapeutic impact;
5. Patient outcome;
6. Optimal usage.

For the most part diagnostic tests, when they have been evaluated, have been evaluated at the first and second levels, very rarely at the third level, and almost never at the fourth, fifth or sixth levels.

25.3.1 TECHNICAL CAPACITY

Evaluation of test performance at this level is essentially a pilot study or, in drug evaluation terms, a phase one trial. It is concerned with questions of safety; are there major hazards? Is there any morbidity associated with the test? What is the patient acceptability? Does the test perform reliably, i.e. is it repeatable, is it consistent and does it measure what it claims to measure, for example a myocardial perfusion radiopharmaceutical may be used to measure regional myocardial blood flow, but does it only depend on this, or are there other factors involved, such as cell metabolism? What is the reproducibility of the test and the precision of the test? These studies should include an assessment of the engineering reliability of the equipment and the frequency of non-diagnostic tests, test failures or patient failures.

25.3.2 DIAGNOSTIC ACCURACY

At this level of evaluation the purpose is to assess how good the test is at discriminating between patients with the disease from those without the disease. The test used will usually detect an indicator of the presence of disease, such as an area of increased density on a chest x-ray which will be present in both normal and diseased populations. It is very rare for a test of any sort in medicine to distinguish totally between a diseased population and a non-diseased population; this overlap means that a criterion has to be developed for the optimal separation of the two populations. One of the consequences of this overlap means that there will always be false-negative (FN) and false-positive (FP) diagnoses arising from the use of the test. Figure 25.1 illustrates this general principle graphically.

Figure 25.2 is, however, more realistic because it would be unusual for 50% of the population studied to be diseased and 50% normal. In this case there are fewer diseased than normal people, i.e. the prevalence of disease in the population is less than 50%.

The diagnostic criterion that is used to separate diseased from non-diseased populations may be quantitative in nuclear medicine (e.g. thyroid uptake or ejection fraction), but more often qualitative and reported as positive or negative with varying degrees of confidence or probability, e.g. thallium scans. Figure 25.3 shows how changing the criterion or threshold for diagnosing disease alters the numbers of false negatives and false positives.

For any one value of the diagnostic criterion used to separate diseased from non-diseased populations, we can consider the outcome as a 2 × 2 matrix;

		DISEASE Present	Absent	Total
DIAGNOSTIC TEST	Positive	TP	FP	TP + FP
	Negative	FN	TN	FN + TN
	Total	TP + FN	FP + FN	TP + FN + FP + TN

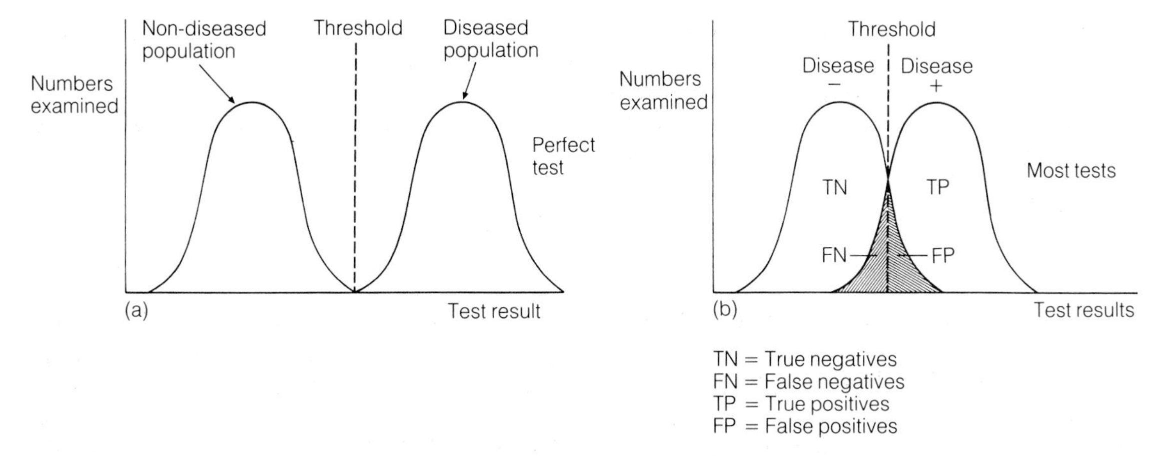

Figure 25.1 The two graphs show how a threshold may be used to separate normal from diseased populations; however (a) is almost unknown in medicine; the overlap in (b) is the more usual finding.

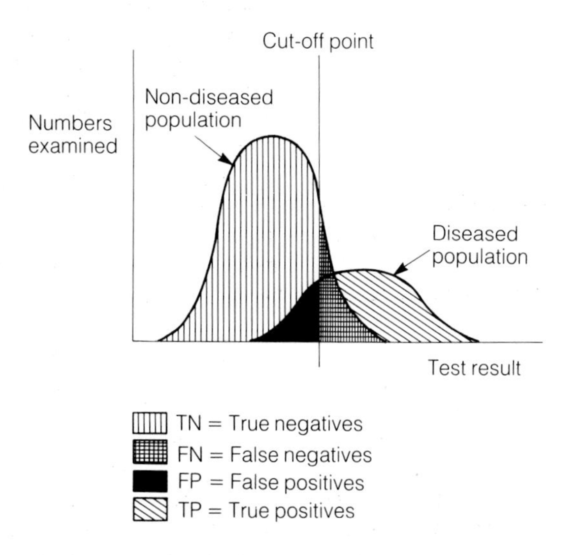

Figure 25.2 This shows the overlap with false-positive and false-negative results when the prevalence in the population studied is less than 50%.

Different ways of measuring accuracy of a diagnostic test have been developed which have advantages and disadvantages and will now be considered.

(a) Accuracy

The accuracy of a test is defined as the ratio of true-positive results (TP) plus true-negative results (TN) to the total number of patients studied.

$$\text{Accuracy} = \frac{\text{TP} + \text{TN}}{\text{TP} + \text{FP} + \text{TN} + \text{FP}} \times 100\%$$

This is a global measure of accuracy and does not distinguish between positives and negatives, is therefore often misleading as a measure of test performance and is rarely of any value. This problem can be seen graphically from Figure 25.3, in which the accuracy of the test is the unshaded areas relative to the total area under both curves.

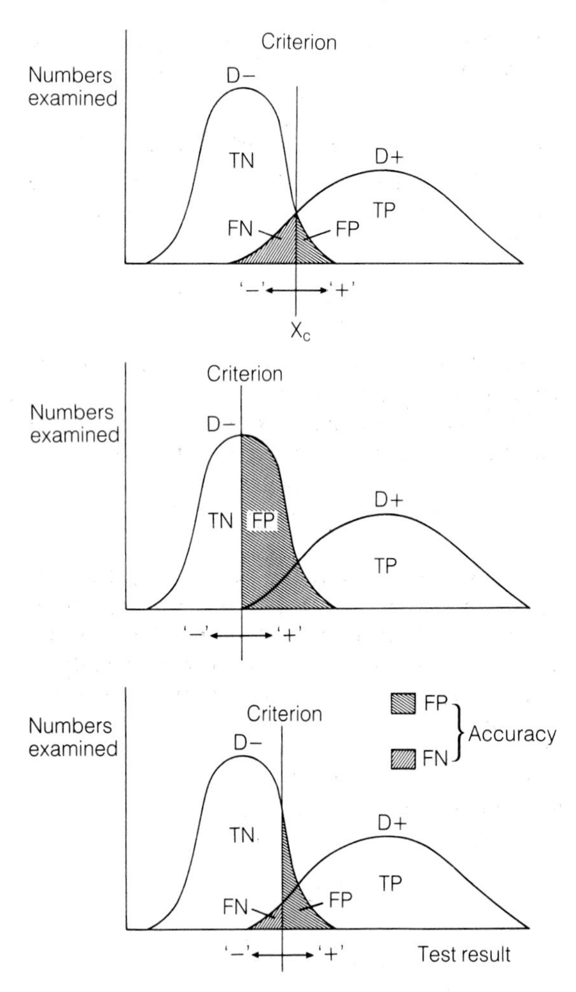

Figure 25.3 These three graphs show how when the population prevalence and the test remain constant the sensitivities and specificities can alter by adjusting the diagnostic criterion.

The prevalence of the disease in the population studied will also affect the accuracy of the test:

Example 1 Prevalence 50%

		Disease +	Disease −
Test	+	450	200
	−	50	300

$$\text{Accuracy} = \frac{450 + 300}{1000} = 75\%$$

Example 2 Prevalence 2%

		Disease +	Disease −
Test	+	18	392
	−	2	588

$$\text{Accuracy} = \frac{18 + 588}{1000} \times 100\% = 60.6\%$$

This effect is illustrated graphically in Figure 25.4, where the disease prevalence is lower but the threshold remains unchanged.

(b) Sensitivity and specificity

The information from the matrix can be translated into measurements referred to as the sensitivity and the specificity of the test. These are defined as: *sensitivity*; the ratio of true positive to true positive plus false negative, or

$$\text{Sensitivity} = \frac{\text{TP}}{\text{TP} + \text{FN}} \times 100\%$$

This can be expressed as 'the proportion of people with the disease that will be detected by the test' (diagnosed by the test set at a particular threshold or criterion).

Specificity; the ratio of true negative, to true negative plus false positive, or

$$\text{Specificity} = \frac{\text{TN}}{\text{TN} + \text{FP}} \times 100\%$$

This can be expressed as 'the proportion of people without the disease that will be confirmed to be free of the disease'. The closer to 100% each of these measurements approaches the better the test is performing.

It can be seen from Figure 25.3 that as the criterion or threshold is changed, the number of true-positive and false-positive cases, and therefore the sensitivity and specificity of the test, varies. When the sensitivity and specificity of the test have been measured using a broad enough spectrum of patients with the disease and without the disease, and with a wide range of disease presentations and severity, the prevalence of disease in the test population *does not* influence the sensitivity and specificity of the test. This can be shown by recalculating the figures in the previous section for sensitivity and specificity.

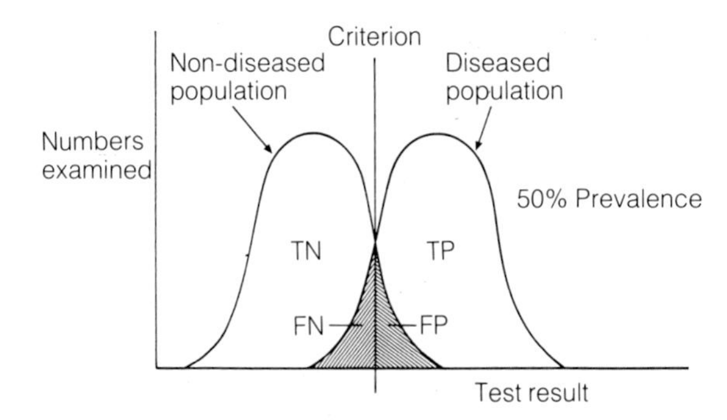

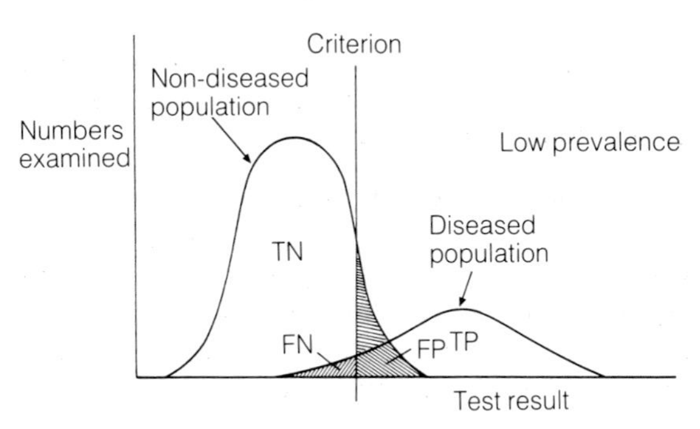

Figure 25.4 These two graphs show the effect on the test performance changing the disease prevalence in the population when the diagnostic criterion remains constant.

Example 1 Prevalence 50%

$$\text{Sensitivity} = \frac{450}{450 + 50} = 90\%$$

$$\text{Specificity} = \frac{300}{300 + 200} = 60\%$$

Example 2 Prevalence 2%

$$\text{Sensitivity} = \frac{18}{18 + 2} = 90\%$$

$$\text{Specificity} = \frac{588}{588 + 392} = 60\%$$

This effect can be seen graphically in Figure 25.4 where these ratios remain constant in spite of much lower disease in the population. Although sensitivity and specificity are good objective measures of the performance of a test they do not provide any information as to the likelihood of an individual patient whose test is positive or negative being normal or having the disease, and this is the information needed by a clinician for decision making. The measures which provide this information are called the positive and negative predictive accuracies (PPA and NPA) or positive and negative predictive values (PPV and NPV).

(c) Positive and negative predictive accuracies

The positive predictive accuracy is the ratio of true positive, to true positive plus false positive results;

$$\text{PPA} = \frac{\text{TP}}{\text{TP} + \text{FP}} \times 100\%$$

or the likelihood of a patient with a positive test actually having the disease.

The negative predictive accuracy is the ratio of true negative, to true negative plus false negative:

$$\text{NPA} = \frac{\text{TN}}{\text{TN} + \text{FN}} \times 100\%$$

or the likelihood of a patient with a negative test being free of the disease. These post-test probabilities are dependent on the prevalence of the disease in the population (pre-test probability of disease), which can be seen by working the same example.

Example 1 *Prevalence 50%*
Predictive value of positive test =
(PPA)

$$\frac{450}{450 + 200} \times 100\% = 69\%$$

Predictive value of negative test =
(NPA)

$$\frac{300}{300 + 50} \times 100\% = 86\%$$

Example 2 *Prevalence 2%*
Predictive value of positive test =
(PPA)

$$\frac{18}{18 + 392} \times 100\% = 4.4\%$$

Predictive value of negative test =
(NPA)

$$\frac{588}{588 + 2} \times 100\% = 99.7\%$$

The measures so far discussed are sometimes expressed as probabilities:

Sensitivity (true positive ratio) = $P(T+|D+)$ where P = the probability of an event occurring

T+ = the positive result to a test
| = given
D+ = disease present
i.e. the probability of disease being present given a positive test result.

Similarly:
Specificity (true negative ratio) = $P(T-|D-)$
where P = the probability of an event occurring
T− = the negative result to a test
| = given
D− = disease absent

and
False positive ratio = $P(T+|D-)$
False negative ratio = $P(T-|D+)$
Predictive value of a positive test = $P(D+|T+)$
Predictive value of a negative test = $P(D-|T-)$
Prevalence = $P(D+)$

(d) Bayes' theorem

Bayes' theorem (McNeil *et al.*, 1975) provides a general basis for decision theory from which a mathematical formula can be derived of how sensitivity and specificity combine with probability of disease to give a predictive value of a positive or negative test, i.e. how positive predictive value or negative predictive value can be calculated from sensitivity, specificity and prevalence.

For example:

$$P(D+|T+) = \frac{P(T+|D+) \times P(D+)}{P(T+)}$$

or

$$= \frac{P(T+|D+) \times P(D+)}{P(T+|D+) \times P(D+) + P(T+|D-) \times P(D-)}$$

where

P = probability
D+ = disease present
D− = disease absent
T+ = positive test result
| = given

The measures of accuracy which have been discussed only apply to disease being present or absent. When the possibility of various different diseases is introduced (i.e. an ordered differential diagnosis) the problem becomes more complex. For example a chest X-ray may be abnormal because of tuberculosis, cancer or infection. Further discussion of this situation is beyond the scope of this report, more details can be found in Friedman (1987).

When two tests (X and Y) are used then the two sensitivities can be combined as shown below.

Test	Sensitivity (%)	Specificity (%)
Ultrasound (X)	80	60
CT Scan (Y)	90	90
X or Y positive*	98	54
X and Y positive^	72	96

*Positive X+ and/or Y+
Negative X− and Y−
Sensitivity = sens X + ((100 − sens X) × sens Y) / 100
Specificity = spec X × spec Y / 100

^ Positive X+ and Y+
Negative X− and/or Y−
Sensitivity = sens X × sens Y / 100
Specificity = spec X + ((100 − spec X) × spec Y) / 100

(e) Test selection

The choice of which test to use as well as the threshold for calling a test positive will depend on the use to which the test is being put.

High SENSITIVITY picks up most of the abnormals (few false negatives).
Good for
- excluding disease;
- screening especially if there is high morbidity associated with missing the disease.

High SPECIFICITY picks up most of the normals (few false positives).
Good for
- confirming the presence of disease;
- cases when there is high risk associated with treating unnecessarily.

Or

$$PPV = \frac{\text{Sensitivity} \times \text{Prevalence}}{\text{Sensitivity} \times \text{Prevalence} + (1 - \text{Specificity}) \times (1 - \text{Prevalence})}$$

and

$$NVP = \frac{\text{Specificity} \times (1 - \text{Prevalence})}{1 - \text{Sensitivity}) \times \text{Prevalence} + \text{Specificity} \times (1 - \text{Prevalence})}$$

If two or more tests are very sensitive and the primary purpose is to exclude disease, the gain in sensitivity obtained by using two or more tests may be offset by the decrease in specificity.

RECEIVER-OPERATING CHARACTERISTIC (ROC) CURVE

A useful measure of the performance of a diagnostic test is the receiver-operating characteristic curve (ROC curve) because it measures the sensitivities and specificities over a wide range of altered thresholds. These curves will demonstrate graphically how the sensitivities and the specificities change when the diagnostic criterion used is altered, i.e. the threshold for reporting a test as positive is raised or lowered. If the test has a quantitative measure, the diagnostic criterion for abnormality may be set at different levels, e.g. in the case of lymph nodes on CT we can say they are pathological if they are larger than *x* mm or only if they are larger than *y* mm or *z* mm etc. Although most imaging techniques are reported qualitatively, it is still possible to express the likelihood of their being abnormal semi-quantitatively with different levels of confidence. For example, a chest X-ray may be absolutely normal or there may be something suspicious or something almost certainly abnormal or a gross abnormality. Conventionally these different levels of likelihood of disease being present are divided into five categories:

0 – definitely normal
1 – probably normal
2 – possibly abnormal
3 – probably abnormal
4 – definitely abnormal

The evaluation of a test will use these different levels of likelihood and are included in the reporting of the films. From these data the ROC curves can be constructed and each test, X-ray or imaging method will have its own characteristically shaped curve which will express the performance of the test quantitatively.

To produce such a curve for an imaging test a series of scans (using a minimum of 100) are obtained from a representative population with an intermediate prevalence of disease and a wide range of severity of disease. The scans will be read by one individual or a group of radiologists and put into one of the categories above (i.e. graded 0–4). The positivity of the test is then created five times, i.e. the test is called positive:

1. Only when the definitely abnormals are called positive i.e. very strict threshold;
2. Only when definitely abnormal and probably abnormal are called positive;
3. When definitely abnormal, probably abnormal and possibly abnormal are called positive, i.e. lax threshold;
4. Even when cases categorized as probably normal are included and called positive;
5. Even when cases categorized as definitely normal are included, i.e. all cases are called abnormal, in which case no diseased patient will go undetected (100% sensitivity), but all the patients free of disease will be called diseased (0% specificity).

These results are then plotted in the ROC space, the vertical axis being true positive ratio (the sensitivity correct detection of disease or 'hits') and the horizontal axis being the false-positive ratio (1 − Specificity or the 'false alarms'). This is shown in Figure 25.5.

(e) Typical characteristic curves

These curves can be used to compare the overall performance of tests (Figure 25.6). Curve A would result from randomly assigning results to one of the categories referred to above and using the outcome to report whether the test was normal or

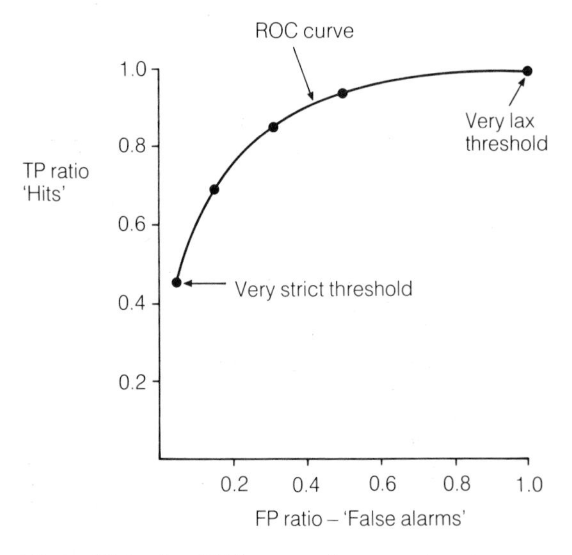

Figure 25.5 An ROC curve from an imaging procedure with five levels of diagnostic probability.

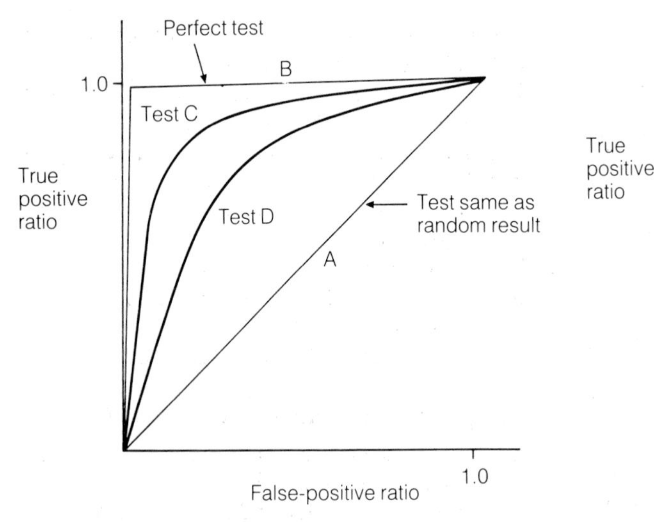

Figure 25.6 Four theoretical ROC curves showing test performance from perfect (B) to random (A); C and D are typical for many imaging procedures.

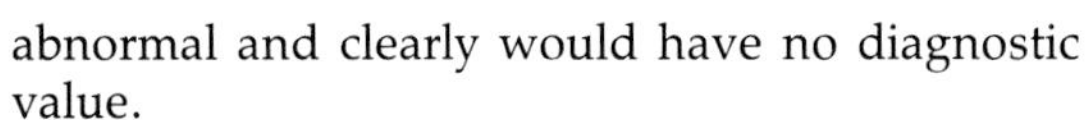

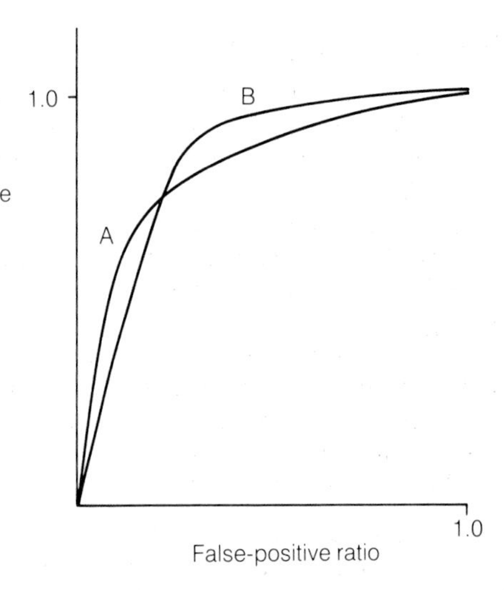

Figure 25.7 An example of an ROC curve when the total accuracy may be similar but performance differs in different areas of the curve.

abnormal and clearly would have no diagnostic value.

Curve B describes the shape of a perfect curve when there are no false-positive and no false-negative results and, as we have already seen, for practical purposes never occurs in radiological practice. Most tests will have shapes approximating to C and D, where C is a better test for detecting a particular condition than D, because at every threshold or criterion there are more true positives and less false positives than for curve D. It can be seen from this that if the result of the scan has to be unequivocally abnormal before it is reported to the clinician as abnormal, then the sensitivity of detection of disease will be low, but the specificity will be high. On the other hand, if we report as positive anything which is possibly abnormal, probably abnormal or definitely abnormal, then the sensitivity for detection of the disease will be much higher but with decreased specificity, i.e. there will be more false positives, increasing the number of patients who are actually free of disease, but whom we are diagnosing as having the disease.

The performance of the tests can be assessed by simply inspecting the curves' shapes; however, quantitative values can also be derived from them. The most commonly used method for this is to integrate the entire area below the curve and express this as a proportion – the nearer to 1.0, the better the test.

The shape of the ROC curves may be more complex than indicated previously and may cross over as indicated in Figure 25.7. This illustrates how two tests may be similar in accuracy because the areas under the curves are identical but the characteristics are different. In this instance neither of the tests is necessarily better overall, but performance will depend on the use to which it is put. If false positive results are to be avoided, e.g. when the consequences of a positive diagnosis would be dangerous treatment, test A would be a better test, provided a strict threshold is used. Whereas test B may be better (provided a lax threshold were used) for screening tests because the sensitivity is better in this area of the curve.

Showing that a test has a good sensitivity and specificity and performs well using ROC curve measurement does not prove that it is clinically useful. It is only by measuring diagnostic impact, therapeutic impact and outcome that this can be assessed.

25.3.3 DIAGNOSTIC IMPACT

The diagnostic impact of an imaging procedure is a further measure of performance and is used to measure the extent by which a test is able to influence the pattern of subsequent diagnostic testing. Does it replace other diagnostic tests? Does it significantly alter the need for or choice of other tests afterwards?

The following may occur:

1. The new test may be more accurate and thereby render previously used tests redundant: e.g. bone scanning rendering skeletal surveys redundant.
2. The test may be equivalent to two or more other tests, in which case other factors such as morbidity and cost would determine any change.
3. The new test may be equal to the old test in accuracy and information content, but have other characteristics such as significantly decreased morbidity or cost: e.g. CT scanning of the brain replacing pneumoencephalography.

The general tendency is for more tests to be performed on patients for any particular disease rather than replacing redundant tests because of the lack of good evaluation procedures and a clear understanding of the diagnostic process. New investigations, unless they have a significantly decreased morbidity, are too often used as 'add-on tests'. It is usually not possible to consider a technology in its entirety because it may have one characteristic in one clinical situation and another for another clinical situation; e.g. MRI can replace CT for posterior fossa disease but has less advantage in supratentorial disease. It is also possible for the introduction of a new test to increase the use of other diagnostic tests. For example, non-specific findings on MR examinations in patients with multiple sclerosis who would not previously have had the diagnostic imaging technique may increase the necessity for subsequent CT examinations.

In this category of evaluation the concepts of costs and morbidities which did not figure in the measurement of accuracy are a necessary part of the evaluation. There are two types of costs and benefits that have to be considered: the costs and benefits in health terms, sometimes known as health costs (risks) and benefits; and those measured in purely financial terms.

(a) Diagnostic test health costs (risks)

1. The pain and discomfort of the test to the patient;
2. The anxiety generated both about having the test performed and the potential result;
3. The radiation dose from the test;
4. Complications of the test, both morbidity and mortality;
5. Social costs (the time in hospital, the disruption of family life, loss of work, etc.);
6. The downstream costs: these include the risks of treatment which may result from a false-positive diagnosis, missed therapeutic opportunities from a false-negative diagnosis, complications associated with delay in making the diagnosis;
7. The opportunity costs: these are the costs due to a loss of the available resource (e.g. scanning time available to other patients who would benefit more from the use of that time).

(b) Diagnostic test benefits (health benefits)

1. The avoidance of other tests which have their own risks associated with them;
2. The potential for early and effective treatment;
3. Increased confidence both of the patient in the doctor and the doctor in the diagnosis. It should be emphasized here that negative results may have equally strong benefits as positive results.

(c) Financial costs

1. The direct costs of the tests (capital, staffing, consumables, etc.);
2. The indirect costs to the hospital (e.g. the need for overnight stay);
3. Patient costs (travel cost, lost earnings, etc.);
4. Downstream costs: these are the costs of the therapy if a false-positive diagnosis is made and treatment instituted inappropriately.

(d) Financial benefits

1. The avoidance of other tests and their associated costs can sometimes be achieved, but only if current clinical routines are altered with the advent of the new test.
2. Early diagnosis can avoid the extra costs associated with later and more intensive treatment, or extended diagnostic processes for conditions for which there is no effective treatment. This is not always the case, however, as for some cancers early detection leads to aggressive and expensive curative treatment, as opposed to palliative therapy for cancers detected in late stages. Earlier detection of currently incurable diseases such as multiple sclerosis may reduce the need for other diagnostic tests, but often leads to earlier counselling, nursing and rehabilitative services (Conomy, 1987).

(e) What information do we need to know about a test which is needed to assess costs and benefits?

1. Pain and discomfort: these can be measured by various psychological and other scales.
2. Anxiety: there are methods for measuring anxiety and studies have been performed in association with MRI (Brennan *et al.*, 1988).
3. Complications: it is necessary to know the incidence of complications causing morbidity and mortality.
4. The radiation doses received from the diagnostic test and a measure of their associated risk need to be known.
5. The accuracy of the test as discussed in Section 25.3.2 must be known and should have been derived from appropriate populations.
6. Measures of the health risks as well as the benefits of subsequent treatment resulting from the test need to be appreciated and quantified.

It can be seen from the above that not only can diagnostic tests fail to be beneficial, but they can be quite harmful when the entire balance of costs and benefits is considered. When the patient's views are also incorporated into the equation the results may change markedly (McNeil and Parker, 1979).

25.3.4 THE THERAPEUTIC IMPACT

The performance of diagnostic tests can be measured by assessing the effect they have on therapy and management of the patient, i.e. decisions that are altered about patient management on the basis of the test result. Does the test result influence the selection and the delivery of treatment? The resource costs and patient risks associated with these downstream costs have been indicated in the previous section.

25.3.5 THE PATIENT OUTCOME

This is quite clearly the most important or 'bottom line' of any evaluation of the impact of diagnostic methods in clinical care. The question being asked is: 'Does the peformance of the test contribute to the improved health of the patient?' If the tests do not in some way materially affect the patient in such a way as to lessen mortality, alleviate suffering, restore health, prevent symptomatic disease or predict prognosis, then in the final analysis the test, however accurate, becomes worthless and may be harmful. Equally this is the most difficult and least often attempted measurement of the performance of diagnostic tests. Indicators or measures which can be used to measure this patient outcome include:

1. The total lives saved;
2. Life years saved;
3. Quality-adjusted life years saved;
4. Disability days avoided;
5. Age-adjusted disability days saved.

25.3.6 METHODS FOR MEASURING THE CLINICAL BENEFIT FROM THE PERFORMANCE OF A DIAGNOSTIC TEST

It has usually been regarded as sufficient to measure the accuracy of the diagnostic test and from this infer a consequential benefit as a result of an accurate test. Clearly this is not necessarily the case and methods are available and should be increasingly used in an attempt to measure the diagnostic impact, the therapeutic impact and patient outcome. The methods currently available are shown in Table 25.1.

The first three methods – diagnostic trials, prospective measurement of impact and consensus evaluation – are the most important and relevant to diagnostic radiology.

(a) Diagnostic clinical trial

An editorial in the *British Medical Journal* in 1983 said: 'Slowly and painfully over the last twenty years most doctors have learned that proper clinical trials are the only way of assessing new drugs . . . The same critical process needs to be applied to new operations, new treatments and *new diagnostic tests*' (Editorial, 1983). Six years later, very few clinical diagnostic trials have been undertaken successfully and many poor attempts at assessing the clinical value of a technology have

Table 25.1 Methods for testing clinical value

1. The clinical trials
2. Prospective measurement of clinical impact
3. Consensus evaluation

Other methods available but generally less accurate:

4. Databases
5. Mathematical modelling
6. Meta-analysis
7. Case studies (individual series or samples)
8. Epidemiology

Table 25.2 Classification of trials

	Drug	Imaging
Phase I	Toxicity Feasibility	Feasibility Promise
Phase II	Screen of effectiveness against the disease	Diagnostic accuracy
Phase III	Randomized clinical controlled trial	Studies of clinical value (diagnostic, treatment or outcome)
Phase IV	Monitoring routine usefulness	Before and after introduction studies

been made. In the review by Cooper *et al.* (1988) in the *Journal of the American Medical Association*, not one of the 54 studies of magnetic resonance had used a prospective randomized clinical trial. Of the studies of MRI incorporating economics alongside clinical evaluation which was funded by the MRC in the UK only two have adopted a randomized controlled design (MRC Report, 1987). The classification of diagnostic trials can be best compared with the more widely used drug trials and are shown in Table 25.2.

In exactly the same way as drug trials have had to approach the ethical problems, these must also be considered in diagnostic evaluation trials. The trial can only be conducted if the investigator is genuinely unsure as to the clinical value of the test, for example it would now be unethical to compare pneumoencephalography with CT scanning of the brain. The same ethical criteria of patient consent used in all other clinical experiments must be adhered to, together with ethical committee approval. There are, however, methods for overcoming some of the ethical problems. For example, in the trial of MRI versus CT, it may be unethical to deny patients a CT scan which was felt by the clinician to be of accepted benefit, and therefore provision can be made for double scanning of the patients on request after the initial randomization. Ideally they will be randomized, prospective and compare either one test with another with measures of outcome or one test with no test, again with the appropriate measure of outcome. Details of the statistical analysis and numbers required for the trials are similar to those of drug trials and will not be discussed further, but reference can be made to standard works (Armitage, 1971).

To calculate the outcome measures usually requires assessment of patient health states and quality of life. These can be used as outcome measures themselves in some circumstances, e.g. to indicate improvement versus non-improvement in health. They can be combined with survival data to produce 'quality-adjusted' life-years saved.

There are many methods for measuring health status including general health status indicators (Hurst, 1984) such as:

1. Nottingham health profile;
2. Rosser and Kind health classification;
3. Sickness impact profile.
4. Methods specific to patient groups, e.g. Karnovsky Index, Guttman Scale for the elderly and the New York Heart Association (NYHA) Activity Scale. As well as distinguishing the outcomes by the above methods, the trial is also capable of measuring the diagnostic and therapeutic impact in one of the following ways:

1. Measuring the utilization of all tests in the two randomized groups, both imaging studies and other tests;
2. Measuring the use of subsequent therapy, for example the amount of corticosteroid suppression therapy in the treatment of renal transplant patients when radionuclide or ultrasound scans are used;
3. Hospital days used;
4. Days off work or disability days;
5. Frequency of visits to hospital or Practitioner.

(b) Prospective measurement of clinical impact on management

The principle of this technique is that a questionnaire is completed by the referring clinician before the test is performed which records the pre-test diagnostic likelihoods and the current management plan and any other tests which are planned. This is then repeated after the test result is available and the two are compared. This method measures the impact of the test on subsequent management but does not measure the final outcome. A good example is the CT study performed by Wittenberg *et al.* (1980). The flow of this technique is shown in Figure 25.8 and in Table 25.3. This technique can provide very sound information, but is less rigorous than the randomized trial as it relies on subjective data from the first form as the main comparison. However, if the forms are

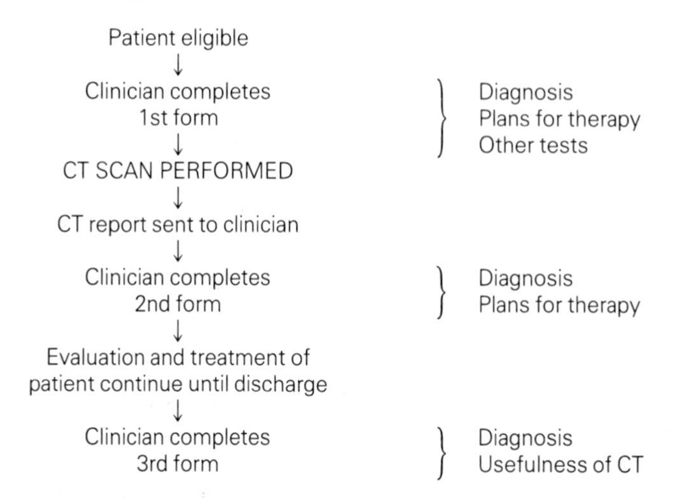

Figure 25.8 Flow diagram of the design of a study of clinical value, adapted from Wittenberg *et al.* (1980) and Friedman (1988). This technique can provide very sound information, but is less rigorous than the randomized trial as it relies on subjective data from the first form as the main comparison. However, if the forms are completed conscientiously at the appropriate time, the potential bias of subjective assessment can be minimized.

Table 25.3 Scale for usefulness of CT

Diagnostic understanding
1. CT confused my understanding of this patient's disease and led to investigations I would not otherwise have done
2. CT confused my understanding of this patient's disease but did not lead to any additional investigations
3. CT had little or no effect on my understanding of this patient's disease
4. CT provided information which substantially improved my understanding of this patient's disease
5. My understanding of this patient's disease depended upon diagnostic information provided only by CT (unavailable from any other non-surgical procedure)

Choice of therapy
1. CT led me to choose therapy which in retrospect was not in the best interests of the patient
2. CT was of no influence in my choice of therapy
3. CT did not alter my choice of therapy but did increase my confidence in the choice
4. CT contributed to a change in my chosen therapy but other factors (other imaging tests, other diagnostic tests, changes in patient status) were equally or more important
5. CT was very important compared with other factors in leading to a beneficial change in therapy

Adapted from Wittenberg *et al.* (1980), which is adapted from a modification by Friedman.

completed conscientiously at the appropriate time, the potential bias of subjective assessment can be minimized.

(c) Consensus evaluation

The introduction of consensus conference evaluation may be applied to diagnostic and therapeutic regimes.

MRI has been evaluated by this method (Consensus Development Conference, 1987). The main advantage of this method is that it is quick and relatively cheap. The main disadvantage is that it is subjective, dependent on received wisdom and critically dependent on the choice of participants as though the subjectivity can be minimized if the focus is on scientific evaluation and not wholly on subjective judgements. It does not provide new factual information because it is dependent on existing information only. They are, however, being very widely used in the USA and Europe.

(d) Databases

This is a source of retrospective case comparison and has been well reviewed in *Assessing Medical Technologies*. They also require meticulous attention to detailed data collection and therefore can be expensive. One advantage is that they may be used to measure effectiveness.

(e) Mathematical modelling

Can be very powerful and inexpensive, allowing the investigation of predicted usefulness under a variety of 'what if' situations.

(f) Meta-analysis

Analysing the data from several published or unpublished series with similar designs will increase the statistical power of a conclusion about the evaluation. There are, however, numerous sources of error and it has not been applied systematically to diagnostic methods.

(g) Case studies

These are of limited value but are the commonest method of reporting the 'clinical performance' of tests.

(h) Epidemiology

These are studies of the impact of a diagnostic technology before and after the introduction of the technology into an institution or a district. Alternatively, comparisons can be made between a hospital or region with another hospital where the technology is available. These studies are fraught with difficulties, including local variations (a) between institutions, (b) in the population of patients and (c) of clinical practice irrespective of the diagnostic technology. These variables may also change during the timespan of the study.

It is important to appreciate that studies of accuracy, impact and outcome undertaken under controlled and ideal circumstances, which may be referred to as efficacy studies, may produce results which may not always apply when the technique is more widely dispersed to a less specialized hospital. Studies which measure the performance in more general applications may be referred to as effectiveness studies. An example might be the performance of ultrasound examinations in a specialized unit with an enthusiast who has become highly skilled. Publication of impressive performance under these circumstances may lead others using the same technology but with less experience, training and enthusiasm to assume that the results will apply in their own practice, which in turn may lead to a significant deterioration in patient care.

25.3.7 OPTIMAL UTILIZATION

The previous sections have addressed the problems of measuring the clinical benefits derived from the use of tests and the resource costs involved in changing diagnostic methods and introducing new ones. A further important question is to decide whether the benefits are worth the extra costs and these involve economic comparisons. That is to say, which patients should have the tests, where the facility should be sited and how many facilities there should be; finally, how to implement the changes which may be necessary as a result of measuring the performance of the tests.

(a) Economic analyses

Although the comparison of benefits and costs is usually the last stage of an evaluation, to be useful the economic element must be built into the study design from the beginning. Many of the items on which data are collected for the assessment of diagnostic and therapeutic impact involve resource use, so that the rigour of the research design also influences the confidence which can be placed in the economic element of any comparison.

(b) Costing

The direct cost of a technology under evaluation is often easy to identify, particularly for a new technique being provided under special funding arrangements. However, just as care must be taken in projecting effectiveness from studies of efficacy conducted in 'laboratory' conditions, the use of cost data derived from studies of technologies used in a 'research mode' may not reflect the actual cost of provision in the 'service mode'. The size and direction of this cost difference may be unpredictable. For example, investigations carried out under a research protocol may take longer because more information is required than is strictly necessary for immediate diagnosis, and patient processing may take longer. On the other hand, use of technology in a research unit may use hidden resources, such as special technical and maintenance expertise, the cost of which cannot readily be separated from other overhead costs.

In using any costing information the appropriate form of presentation varies with the question being addressed. If it is proposed that a new technology should be introduced to replace completely an existing service, then comparison can be made on the basis of total costs. It is more often the case that a new method is a partial replacement for several existing techniques, none of which will completely disappear. Here a careful assessment of the marginal (or incremental) cost is necessary. The full cost of the new service is still relevant, but the estimates of resource savings from avoidance of other tests will be much reduced, reflecting only the direct operating costs which can be avoided, while maintaining capital equipment and trained staff.

(c) Evaluation methods

Two forms of economic evaluation have been used in this area.

(i) Cost–benefit analysis (CBA) This approach is intended to demonstrate 'social efficiency' in the sense of whether something is worth doing *per se*. It is based on the idea that through the market system the value placed by individuals on goods and services is reflected in their willingness to pay for them. Where no market transactions take place, as in the NHS, it is necessary to estimate values indirectly for the various benefits accruing to patients. Given the nature of these benefits as outlined above, this approach applied to health care is riddled with methodological pitfalls and ethical difficulties. A common approach has been to value life years gained in terms of the potential gain in earnings in those years. This allows a comparison of costs and benefits on a purely monetary basis, a surplus of the latter over the former indicating social benefit from the activity. As will be seen from the previous section, this includes only a limited part of the potential benefits, and the appropriateness of the earnings measure to many patients has been called into question.

(ii) Cost-effectiveness analysis (CEA) Given the problems of using CBA in the health care field, most evaluations use the more limited techniques of cost-effectiveness analysis. Although the cost element is the same as for CBA, no attempt is made to place financial measures on the benefits. Effectiveness is measured quantitatively using a single indicator of outcome, e.g. quality-adjusted life years saved. This means that CEA can only be used to compare options whose effectiveness is best measured in the same way, based on the pre-judgement that benefits of the type are socially valuable. CEA is therefore most suited to identifying the best solution to tightly defined problems such as 'which is the best technique for the diagnosis of demyelinative disease?' rather than broader question such as 'how much should be spent on health care services as opposed to other forms of public expenditure?'

'Cost-effective' has become a grossly misused term, as pointed out recently (Doubilet *et al.*, 1986). They recommend, and we agree, that a test should be defined as cost-effective if it has 'an additional benefit worth the additional cost'. It should be noted that this implies that the 'most effective' tests may not be 'cost-effective' if its additional costs are very high, nor will the 'cheapest' test be 'cost-effective' if its relative effectiveness is very low.

(d) The time factor

A crucial element in any economic analysis is the time at which costs are incurred and benefits accrue. For many diagnostic tests the recource use and the immediate benefits from any therapeutic intervention may occur very quickly, but, if there are any effects on long-term survival, the benefits of these extra life years will not be experienced for a considerable time. This problem is most evident in the case of screening applications. The immediate cost of screening whole populations can be very high. The alternative strategy of waiting for disease to present may lead to much more expensive therapeutic intervention. However, these latter costs may not occur until well into the future. Generally, people prefer benefits sooner and costs later, and economic analysis takes this into account by discounting future costs and benefits, i.e. by applying a declining weight to effect the further into the future they occur (see DHSS, 1988, for detailed explanation).

(e) Presentation of results

If the costs of different technologies are equal then cost-effectiveness can be judged solely on the effectiveness data. Similarly, the choice between two equally effective methods can be made on cost. When both differ it is usual to express the results in ratio form, e.g. cost per quality-adjusted life year saved (QUALY). It should be remembered that this ratio will depend on the level of activity envisaged in the analysis, e.g. cost per QALY saved from mammographic screening of women over 50 would depend on the take up rate as well as cost per scan and expected benefit. Cost per QALY would also be expected to change if the screened population group were to be altered. Marginal cost and effectiveness analysis can be used to identify the most appropriate target group.

Presenting the results in their proper decision context is very important, particularly for diagnostic technologies which may be used very early in a long management process. There has been a tendency to restrict evaluation to the diagnostic impact by using cost per correct diagnosis as the decision criterion. Unless a clear link can be established between use of a technology and patient outcome the case for its use is not proven.

25.3.8 IMPLEMENTATION OF CHANGES

When the measures of accuracy, impact, outcome and cost-effectiveness have been completed, the final problem is one of implementation. Several methods have been adopted for implementation and attempts to measure their effectiveness have been undertaken which include education, feedback, financial, decision aids and control (Fowkes, 1985).

(a) Education

By making the results of investigations widely known, and by introducing this information into undergraduate and postgraduate education, it should be possible to influence the use of diagnostic tests. For example, in the study of the guidelines for pre-operative chest X-rays and skull X-rays (Royal College of Radiologists, 1976–86; Fowkes *et al.*, 1984), it was possible to show a reduction after the guidelines were introduced. It is clearly necessary to consider the expansion of education about methods of diagnosis and the assessment of management impact into the undergraduate and postgraduate curricula.

(b) Feedback

By regular discussion between doctors, particularly between senior and junior doctors, a form of audit can result in the more appropriate use of the diagnostic resources. In a recent study (Martin *et al.*, 1980) it was shown that the numbers of tests used on patients could be reduced in an institution by regular audit and feedback discussions.

(c) Financial

In the same study (Martin *et al.*, 1980), a group of junior doctors as a control group to the feedback group were given a personal financial incentive. Interestingly this failed to achieve results as good as educational review and feedback. With the introduction of clinical budgeting and resource management within the health service, financial restraint on the clinical use of diagnostic resources should become more sensitive to the effective use of these resources. Clinicians should be demanding accurate data about the performance of diagnostic tests and their impact and respond more rapidly to this information. No studies as yet have been undertaken to measure the effects of these new financial and organisational changes.

(d) Decision aids

Decision aids can take the form of charts, microcomputers or calculators used to introduce a quantitative measure of the usefulness of tests under particular clinical circumstances. These are usually Baysian probability studies, and an example is the work on diagnosis of abdominal pain by the use of a decision aid in the diagnosis of the acute abdomen (de Dombal, 1989).

(e) Control

Finally, the value of control by radiologists to restrict the use of tests to those which are of proven value has been assessed. Methods may include the establishment of agreed protocols and checking back to the referring clinician whenever these are not followed, the choice by a department to follow an agreed protocol whatever the test requested, and limiting the number of tests to a fixed number per patient or per clinician.

Even a change of layout of request forms (Wong *et al.*, 1983; Lundberg, 1983) can reduce unnecessary investigations.

25.4 ERRORS ASSOCIATED WITH MEASURING DIAGNOSTIC PERFORMANCES

These sources of error and bias are well-known methodological problems but despite this there are consistent errors in reported evaluation procedures.

25.4.1 INTER- AND INTRA-OBSERVER VARIATIONS

As a part of every test performance evaluation, information about the variations in reporting the images or making the measurements between different radiologists (inter-observer variation) and for the same observer on different occasions (intra-observer variation) must be incorporated as these errors can lead to inconsistent test performances.

25.4.2 INADEQUATE RANGE OF PATIENTS

When a new test is evaluated it is frequently applied to patients with well-advanced, well-documented disease. When this is the case and then the use is subsequently extended to patients with milder disease and a broader range of disease severity, the results of the initial evaluation will no longer apply.

25.4.3 NON-MATCHED CONTROLS

Controls must always be used in a good scientific evaluation. Frequently, however, inappropriate controls are chosen. For example, a test may be performed for elderly patients with heart disease and the controls are young fit individuals. In most instances they should at least be age and sex matched.

25.4.4 EXCLUSION OF UNINTERPRETABLE RESULTS OR UNCOOPERATIVE PATIENTS

Frequently, these are excluded before the calculations are made. This is wrong and will give quite inaccurate and often optimistic measures of the performance of the test. Such patients should always be included and it is only possible to exclude them if the exclusion is done before the test is undertaken (Simel *et al.*, 1987).

25.4.5 READING THE IMAGES BLIND OR OPEN

For the best non-subjective results the reading should be blind, i.e. the reporting radiologist should not be aware of the clinical history of the patient. Ideally they should be read blind and then on a subsequent occasion open, with the other clinical information available. Many studies do not comment on this point and do not specify which was used.

25.4.6 PREVALENCE OF THE DISEASE IN THE POPULATION

As mentioned previously, in a well-conducted study with a broad range of patients and disease stages, sensitivities and specificities will not change with prevalence. However, if positive predictive accuracies are calculated, these are acutely dependent on the prevalence in the population, which must be stated.

25.4.7 THE GOLD OR REFERENCE STANDARD IS INADEQUATE

It is often impossible to obtain a final diagnosis on the basis of well-established gold standards such as histology, and the diagnosis may be assessed with another non-invasive test. When this is so, it is essential to know the test performance parameters of the gold standard.

25.4.8 INADEQUATE SAMPLE SIZE

Too frequently, sensitivities, specificities and even ROC curves are calculated from inadequate small numbers. There are well-defined rules based on the prevalence of the disease and the likely accuracy of the test which enable investigators to estimate the sample sizes needed for accurate sensitivity and specificity measurements. In addition, the confidence range of these sensitivities must be calculated. The size of samples needed was discussed recently: the size should be such that the SE is less than ½ of (100% − estimated sensitivity %) (Friedman, 1987) but will also depend on the measured parameter of performance of competing tests.

25.4.9 CONCORDANCE WITH HISTOLOGY

Histology is often regarded as the gold standard. However, if the only patients are those that have final histology available are used for assessing the test performance, this may have introduced a major source of bias because of referral patterns.

25.4.10 CLINICAL FOLLOW-UP (FINAL OUTCOME)

Clinical follow-up is often used as the gold standard, which may be entirely appropriate where histology is not available. The follow-up must be long enough to detect disease that may have been present and missed by the diagnostic test, but more importantly, the results of the test must not have been incorporated into this final diagnosis. This is a frequent source of error.

25.4.11 STATISTICAL CALCULATIONS

These are often inappropriate, the commonest error being the use of parametric statistics when the numbers are too small and the information inadequate to know that the data are normally distributed. In these instances, non-parametric statistics are usually more appropriate.

25.4.12 LOGISTIC PROBLEMS

The logistic problems of performing evaluation tests are not to be underestimated.

25.4.13 ETHICAL FACTORS

Ethical approval is necessary for most studies, particularly randomized control trials. The patients must give their consent, preferably in writing. This fact should be incorporated in reports of the study design.

25.4.14 RANDOM ORDER

When two tests are compared, the order in which this is done should be randomized.

25.4.15 PUBLICATION BIAS

There is a natural bias towards enhancing the value of a test because of the tendency to report positive findings and not write up negative ones.

25.5 GLOSSARY OF TERMS

Cost–benefit analysis Places a monetary value on the benefits and non-monetary costs and compares them with the monetary costs, to produce a net present value. Also net social benefit.

Cost-effective Additional benefits worth the additional costs.

Cost–effectiveness analysis Outcome measure is chosen and expressed as a ratio to the cost.

Diagnostic efficiency Capacity of a test to meet its immediate objectives, i.e. correct diagnosis.

Downstream costs Costs consequent on the result of the test, e.g. treatment costs.

Effectiveness The usefulness when widely applied.

Efficacy The usefulness of a procedure under ideal or pilot conditions.

Incremental cost The additional cost of changing the level of activity or the type of activity. Often referred to as marginal cost, to distinguish it from the total cost of the whole activity.

Opportunity costs The value of a resource in its best alternative use.

Predictive tests Risk/assessment, e.g. tests to assess risk of myocardial infarction.

ROC curve Receiver-operating characteristic curve.

Specificity Measures the ability of a test to correctly exclude disease in non-diseased patients.

Sensitivity Measures the ability of a test to detect disease when it is present.

REFERENCES

Armitage, P. (1971) *Statistical Methods in Medical Research.* Blackwell Scientific Publications, Oxford.

Brennan, S. C., Redd, W. H., Jacobsen, P. B. *et al.* (1988) Anxiety and panic during magnetic resonance scans. *Lancet*, **ii**.

Consensus Development Conference (1987) Magnetic Resonance Imaging. CDC Statement, Vol. 6, No. 14.

Committee for Evaluating Medical Technologies in Clinical Use (1985) *Assessing Medical Technologies*, National Academy Press, Washington DC.

Conomy, J. P. (1987) *Designation of Patient Services in a Comprehensive Multiple Sclerosis Centre*, Paper presented to International Society for Technology Assessment in Health Care, 3rd Annual Meeting, Rotterdam.

Cooper, L. S., Chalmers, T. C., McCally, M. *et al.* (1988) The poor quality of early evaluations of magnetic resonance imaging. *JAMA*, **259**, 3277–80.

Council for Science and Society (1983) Expensive medical techniques: Report of a working party, London.

de Dombal, F. T. (1989) Computer aided decision support in clinical medicine. *Int. J. Biomed. Comput.*, **24**, 9–16.

DHSS (1988) *Option Appraisal: Medical and Scientific Equipment, A Guide for the NHS.*

Doubilet, P., Weinstein, M. C. and McNeil, B. J. (1986) Use and misuse of the term 'cost effective' in medicine. *N. Engl. J. Med.*, **314**, 253–5.

Editorial (1983) Expensive innovations. *Br. Med. J.*, **286**, 417–18.

Feinberg, H. V., Bauman, R. and Sosmon, M. (1977) Computerised cranial tomography: effect on diagnostic and therapeutic plans. *JAMA*, **238**, 224–7.

Feinberg, H. V. (1979) The case for evaluating high technology. *N. Engl. J. Med.*, **301**, 1086–91.

Fowkes, F. G. R. (1985) Containing the use of diagnostic tests. *Br. Med. J.*, **290**, 488–9.

Fowkes, F. G. R., Evans, R. C., Williams, L. A. *et al.* (1984) Implementation of guidelines for the use of skull radiographs in patients with head injuries. *Lancet*, **ii**,

Hillman, B. J. (1988b) The value of imaging technology to patients' health. *AJR*, **150**, 1191–2.

Hurst, J. W. (1984) Health status review. Measuring the benefits and costs of medical care: the contribution of health status measurements. *Health Trends*, **16**, 16–19.

Lundberg, G. D. (1983) Laboratory request forms (menus) that guide and teach. *JAMA*, **249**, 3075.

Martin, A. R., Walfe, M. A., Thibodeau, L. A. *et al.* (1980) A trial of two strategies to modify the test ordering behavior of medical residents. *N. Engl. J. Med.*, **303**, 1330–6.

McNeil, B. J., Keeler, E., Adelstein, S. J. (1975) Primer on certain elements of medical decision making. *N. Engl. J. Med.*, **293**, 211–5.

McNeil, B. J. and Parker, S. G. (1979) The patient's role in assessing the value of diagnostic tests. *Radiology*, **132**, 605–10. Also: Patient's attitudes in assessing medical technologies, p. 535.

MRC Report (1987) Review of the clinical evaluation of MRI.

Royal College of Radiologists (1976–86) Towards the more effective use of diagnostic radiology: A review of the work of the Royal College of Radiologists working party on the more effective use of diagnostic radiology.

Simel, D. L., Feussner, J. R., Delong, E. R. and Matchar, D. B. (1987) Intermediate, indeterminate, and uninterpretable diagnostic test results. *Med. Decis. Making*, **7**, 107–14.

Wittenberg, J., Fienberg, H. V., Ferrucc, J. T. *et al.* (1980) Clinical efficacy of computed body tomography. *AJR*, **134**, 1111–20.

Wong, E. T., McCarron, M. M. and Shaw, S. T. (1983) Ordering of laboratory tests in a teaching hospital: can it be improved? *JAMA*, **249**, 3076–80.

Young, I. (1988) Time to bring on the scanners. *Health Service Journal*, 20 October.

GENERAL REVIEWS AND FURTHER READING

Begg, C. B. and McNeil, B. J. (1988) Assessment of radiologic tests: control of bias and other design considerations. *Radiology*, **167**, 565–9.

Cochrane, A. J. (1972) *Effectiveness and Efficiency*, Nuffield Provincial Hospital Trust, London.

Culyer, A. J. and Hariskerger, B. (eds) (1983) *Economic and Medical Evaluation of Health Care Technologies*. Springer-Verlag, Berlin.

Doubliet, P., Weinstein, M. C. and McNeil, B. J. (1986) Use and misuse of the term 'cost effective' in medicine. *N. Engl. J. Med.*, **314**, 253–5.

Drummond, M. F. (ed.) (1987) *Economic Appraisal of Health Technology in the European Community*, Oxford Medical Publications, Oxford.

Freedman, L. S. (1987) Evaluating and comparing imaging techniques: a review and classification of study designs. *BJR*, **60**, 1071–81.

Jennett, B. (1986) *High Technology Medicine: Benefits and Burdens*, 2nd edn, Oxford University Press, Oxford and New York.

Kelsey-Fry, I. (1984) Who needs high technology? *Br. J. Radiol.*, **57**, 765–72.

National Academy Press (1986) Assessing medical technologies: Institute of medical committee for evaluating medical technologies in clinical use.

Roberts, C. J. (1988) Towards the more effective use of diagnostic radiology: a review of the work of the Royal College of Radiologists working party on the more effective use of diagnostic radiology, 1976–1986. *Clin. Radiol.*, **39**, 3–6.

Russell, J. G. B. and Webb, G. A. M. (1987) Valuing the man-sievert in X-ray diagnosis. *BJR*, **60**, 681–4.

Steinberg, E. P., Sisk, J. E. and Locke, K. E. (1985) X-ray CT and magnetic resonance imagers. *N. Engl. J. Med.*, **313**, 859–64.

Swets, J. A. (1988) Measuring the accuracy of diagnostic systems. *Science*, **240**, 1285–93.

Wagner, J. L. (1983) The feasibility of economic evaluation of diagnostic procedures. *Soc. Sci. Med.*, **17**, 861–9.

CASE STUDIES

Bristow, M. R., Marcia, B. L., Mason J. W. *et al.* (1982) Efficacy and cost of cardiac monitoring in patients receiving doxorubicin. *Cancer*, **50**, 32–41.

Case study No. 13 (1982) *Cardiac Radionuclide: Imaging and cost effectiveness*. US Government Printing Office, Washington DC.

de Lacey, G., Johnson, S. and Mee, D. (1988) Prostatism: how useful is routine imaging of the urinary tract?

Dixon, A. K., Fry, I. K., Kingham, J. G. C. *et al.* (1981) Computed tomography in patients with an abdominal mass: effective and efficient. *Lancet*, **i**, 1199–201.

Forrest Report (1987) *Breast Cancer Screening Report to the Health Ministers of England, Wales, Scotland and Northern Ireland*. HMSO, London.

Hamilton, C. S. and Langlands, A. O. (1983) ACUPS (adenocarcinoma of unknown primary site): a clinical and cost benefit analysis. *Int. J. Radiat. Oncol. Biol. Phys.*, **13**, 1497–503.

Houston, G. A., Sanders, J. A., Little, D. D. *et al.* (1985) Staging of lung cancer: a cost-effective analysis. *Am. J. Clin. Oncol.*, **8**, 224–30.

Hubbell, F. A., Greenfield, S., Tyler, J. L. *et al.* (1985) The impact of routine admission chest x-ray films on patient care. *N. Engl. J. Med.*, **312**, 209–13.

Jacobs, I., Stabile, I., Bridges, J. *et al.* (1988) Multimodal approach to screening for ovarian cancer. *Lancet*, **i**, 268–71.

Lacey, G. D., Gajjar, B., Twomey, B. *et al.* (1984) Should choloecystography or ultrasound be the primary investigation for gallbladder disease? *Lancet*, **i**, 205–7.

Masters, S. J., McClean, P. M., Arcarese, J. S. *et al.* (1987) Skull X-ray examinations after head trauma: recommendations by a multidisciplinary panel and validation study. *N. Engl. J. Med.*, **316**, 84–91.

McNeil B. J., Varady, P. D., Burrows, B. A. and Adelstein, S. J. (1975) Measures of clinical efficacy. *N. Engl. J. Med.*, **293**, 216–21.

Specker, B. L., Saenger, E. L., Buncher, C. R. and

McDevitt, R. A. (1987) Pulmonary embolism and lung scanning: cost-effectiveness and benefit: risk. *J. Nucl. Med.*, **28**, 1521–30.
Todd, N. V., McDonagh, T. and Miller, J. D. (1987) What follows diagnosis by computed tomography of solitary brain tumour. *Lancet*, 611 and 605.
Wassertheil-Smoller, S., Steingart, R. M., Wexler, J. P. *et al.* (1987) Nuclear scans: a clinical decision making tool that reduces the need for cardiac catheterization. *J. Chron. Dis.*, **40**, 385–97.
Wickerham, L., Fisher, B., Cronin, W. *et al.* (1984) The efficacy of bone scanning in the follow-up of patients with operable breast cancer. *Breast Cancer Res. Treatment*, **4**, 303–7.

APPENDIX ONE

Protocols for clinical practice

R. Mistry

This is not intended to be a textbook of nuclear medicine science or technology. We have, however, included an outline of the major procedures for reference. Needless to say, a more complete description should be studied before starting a new method. There is more than one way of doing any one investigation but we have included methods that we use and are generally found to be workable in routine clinical use. More details of some techniques will be found where appropriate in individual chapters.

Patient preparation	*Radiopharmaceutical/s and dose*	*Patient position*	*Route of administration and delay*	*Equipment*	*Technique*	*Quantitative analysis*	*Comment*
Thallium myocardial scan							
None for resting study Maximum exercise (bicycle ergometer or treadmill) for stress study	^{201}Tl chloride 1.5-2mCi (50–75 MBq)	Supine	I.V. injection (at peak of stress); continue exercise for 1 minute, image after a delay of 5 minutes for stress and 20 minutes for a rest study	Standard field of view gamma camera, GAP collimator. Computer	10 min images screening the extra-cardiac structures with lead sheet. Views are A, LAO (45 and 55°), LL. Delayed views at 4 hours as indicated	Varies from background subtraction to various filters and count density measurements	Pharmacological stress with dipyridamole may be substituted for exercise. SPECT may be substituted
^{99m}Tc MIBI myocardial scan							
Exercise as per thallium scan	300-500 MBq	Supine	I.V. injection at peak of exercise; continue exercise for 1 min. Image at 1–2 hours following	Standard field of view gamma camera with GAP or high resolution collimator and computer and gating unit	10 min images (gated) view – ANT, LAO45 LAO70 or elliptical tomography 180° using high resolution collimator		Rest and stress may be performed on the same day
For rest MIBI							
Wait for 48 hrs following Exercise study	300–500 MBq	Supine	Patients rested for 1 hour prior to injection	Standard field of view Gamma camera with GAP or high resolution collimator and computer and gating unit	+ elliptical 180° tomography using high resolution collimator		
Multiple gated blood pool scan							
None	20 mCi (750 MBq) ^{99m}Tc-Autologous red blood cells labelled *in vivo* or *in vitro*	Supine. Prone for LPO	Careful i.v. injection or bolus first pass study performed simultaneously. No delay	Standard field of view gamma camera, high resolution, GAP or slant hole collimator and computer with R wave trigger	Image to attain a count density of greater than 250 counts/pixel over the left ventricle in each frame. Views are RAO, A, LAO, possibly LPO. Repeat LAO.	Measure ejection fraction routinely. There are many other parameters which may be used	

Myocardial infarct imaging							
None	10 m Ci (350 MBq) ^{99m}Tc-pyrophosphate or equivalent	Supine	I.V. injection (Avoid use of indwelling catheters). 3 hour delay	Standard field of view gamma camera with high resolution collimator. Possibly computer	5 min images in A, LAO 45° and 70°	Not routine	Single photon emission tomography is helpful
First pass isotope angiogram							
None (Children sedated)	20 mCi (750 MBq) ^{99m}-Tc-pertechnetate or autologous red blood cells (Reduce childrens' dose on the basis of body surface area)	Supine	Rapid i.v. bolus with saline flush. No delay	Standard field of view gamma camera with high resolution collimator. (High sensitivity or GAP collimator for small children.) Computer. Possibly R wave trigger	Rapid sequence imaging during first pass with data acquisition in list, frame, or histogram mode. View depends on clinical problem; RAO or A. If using autologous red blood cells proceed to routine gated blood pool study	Measure ejection fraction and L – R shunting	
Perfusion lung scan							
None	1–3 mCi (30–100 MBq) approximately 200 000 particles of ^{99m}Tc-labelled microspheres or macroaggregates	Lying or sitting	Slow i.v. injection during quiet breathing while lying supine. Do not draw back blood into syringe. No delay	LFOV gamma camera with GAP or High resolution collimator	500 000 count images of A, P, RL, LL, RPO, LPO	Useful in determining relative pulmonary arterial perfusion in patients with compromised lung function.	This is usually done with ventilation scan.

(cont'd over)

(cont'd)

Patient preparation	*Radiopharmaceutical/s and dose*	*Patient position*	*Route of administration and delay*	*Equipment*	*Technique*	*Quantitative analysis*	*Comment*
Ventilation scan							
None	^{81m}Kr from ^{81}Rb generator or 10–20 mCi (350–700 MBq) ^{133}Xe via dispenser, ^{99m}Tc DTPA aerosol or ^{99m}Tc Technegas	Lying or sitting	Inhalation either before perfusion scan (^{133}Xe) or simultaneously (^{81}Kr). No delay	LFOV Gamma camera with GAP collimator (^{133}Xe) or medium collimator (^{81m}Kr)	^{81m}Kr-views obtained immediately after each perfusion scan view with camera peaked to ^{81m}Kr. ^{133}Xe – view depending on clinical problem. (^{99m}Tc DTPA aerosol or Technegas – views immediately followed by ^{99m}Tc MAA perfusion at 1–2 hours later.)	Not routinely, but use is increasing	This examination is usually done with a perfusion lung scan. The combination of these tests increases the sensitivity and specificity of the findings
Radionuclide venogram							
None	2 doses of 4mCi ^{99m}Tc (150 MBq) labelled microspheres or macroaggregates	Supine, camera over abdomen for inferior vena cava flow, or over calves for leg venogram	Simultaneously i.v. bilateral in dorsum of feet, leave tourniquets on around ankles	Large field of a view gamma camera with GAP collimator	With tourniquets on, move patient to obtain sequential 6000–10 000 count images of calves, knees, thighs and abdomen. Repeat with tourniquets off, and again after lung scan or after leg raising	Nil	Performed in conjunction with lung scan

Mediastinal venogram							
None	Any ^{99m}Tc labelled radiopharmaceutical. May be done in conjunction with liver, bone, or lung scan, etc., 2–5 mCi (100–200 MBq)	Supine, camera positioned over mediastinum	Right antecubital vein for SVC assessment. Left antecubital vein for innominate and SVC assessment	Large field of view camera with GAP collimator	Sequential 2 second images until bolus has passed the heart	N/A	
^{125}I-labelled fibrinogen thrombus localization							
Block thyroid with Lugols Iodine. Mark legs at 5 cm intervals from ankle to thigh	100 μCi (4MBq) ^{125}I or ^{131}I fibrinogen i.v.	Supine	I.V. 5 – 10 minutes delay	Collimated scintillation detector and recorder	Spot counts at each 5 cm point after equilibration and daily	There should not be > 20% difference between adjacent points on a limb or between symmetrical points between the two limbs	Relatively insensitive above mid-thigh
Peripheral perfusion							
None or may be during an arteriogram	^{99m}Tc labelled microspheres (500 000 spheres, approx. 1.4 mCi) (50–150 MBq)	Supine	Intra-arterial injection via syringe and needle or catheter	LFOV gamma camera with GAP collimator	300 000 count images to cover the lower limbs immediately after injection of microspheres	None	May be combined with peripheral AV shunt calculation
Glomerular filtration							
None	^{51}Cr EDTA. Adult 3 MBq, Child 2 MBq, Infant 1 MBq	Resting	Careful complete i.v. injection. First sample after 2 hours from opposite arm	Sample counting (well scintillation counter)	Timed 10 ml venous blood samples at 2, 3 and 4 hours (extra samples at 6 and 8 hours if renal function severely impaired)	Centrifuge and measure radioactivity of plasma samples and standard of ^{51}Cr EDTA. Plot counts/time on semi log calculate T 1/2 and estimate intercept at Time = 0 Calculate GFR	Great care must be taken to inject exact measured volume and to time the blood samples accurately. If urine collections are included GFR may be calculated from UV/P formula

(cont'd over)

(cont'd)

Patient preparation	*Radiopharmaceutical/s and dose*	*Patient position*	*Route of administration and delay*	*Equipment*	*Technique*	*Quantitative analysis*	*Comment*
Static renal image							
None	5 mCi (200 MBq) ^{99m}Tc-DMSA	Supine with knees bent to reduce lumbar lordosis	I.V. 3 hour delay	LFOV gamma camera with high resolution collimator	5 min images. Anterior and posterior view oblique and lateral views as indicated using zoom on camera/computer	Analysis of differential uptake with background subtracted and geometric mean of A and P views	Using large doses, an early flow image may be obtained
Dynamic renal scan							
200 ml fluid 30 min prior to study	(a) ^{99m}Tc DTPA (10 mCi, 175 MBq) (b) ^{123}I Hippuran (2 mCi, 75 MBq) (c) ^{99m}TcMAG3 3 mCi, 100 MBq	Sitting supine, or reclining	I.V. bolus injection. Immediate imaging	LFOV gamma camera, GAP collimator. Computer	Posterior views (anterior for transplant) 0–30s, 400 000 counts at 1 min fixed time, 5, 10, 20 minutes. Bladder views at end	Analysis of relative blood flow, divided GFR, parenchymal transit time	Fluids ++ and empty bladder frequently after study to reduce bladder dose
Dynamic renal scan with Frusemide washout							
First 20 minutes as per dynamic renal scan with ^{99m}Tc DTPA. Inject Frusemide i.v. (0.5 mg kg^{-1} body weight for adults. For children 20 mg if > 10 kg 2 mg/kg if < 10 kg	As per dynamic renal scan with ^{99m}Tc DTPA	As per dynamic renal with ^{99m}Tc DTPA	As per dynamic renal scan with ^{99m}Tc DTPA	As per dynamic renal with ^{99m}Tc DTPA	Image kidneys at 0 time 2 min, 5 min, 10 min, for fixed time	Measure percentage and rate of washout from renal pelvis. Output efficiency %	Warn patient of diuretic effect Frusemide

Vesico-ureteric reflux							
First 20 minutes as per dynamic renal scan with ^{99m}Tc DTPA	As per dynamic renal scan with ^{99m}Tc DTPA	Sitting on commode with gamma camera behind over bladder and renal areas	As per dynamic renal scan with ^{99m}Tc DTPA	LFOV gamma camera with GAP collimator and computer	Record data on to computer before, during and for 2 minutes post micturition	Measure change in activity in kidneys and ureters before, during and after micturition	Female technicians for females and vice versa males. Try to operate equipment by remote control with maximum privacy. Only suitable for 3 years and older children.
Residual urine volume							
This may be performed after standard dynamic ^{99m}Tc renal scan	^{99m}Tc DTPA 1 mCi (35 MBq)	N/A	I.V. 30–60 minute delay	LFOV gamma camera with computer	Anterior bladder view recorded for 1 minute (A) Bladder emptied into disposable urinal and volume recorded. Anterior bladder review recorded for 1 minute (B)	Residual volume (ml) $= \frac{\text{(bladder counts (A) − Bladder counts (B))}}{\text{(ml of urine passed)}} \times B$	
Bone scan							
Hydration of patient at the time of injection	^{99m}Tc-Methylene Diphosphonate (MDP) 15 mCi (500 MBq)	Lying or sitting	I.V. injection. 3 hours or more delay	LFOV gamma camera, high resolution collimator or converging collimator pinhole for hips or whole body imaging device	750,000 count image of posterior chest. Fixed time for remainder of images to cover the body anteriorly and posteriorly or equivalent count density for whole body imaging device	Routinely none. Sacro-iliac activity quantitation if indicated	Advise patient to drink and empty bladder frequently for the remainder of the day to reduce bladder dose.

(cont'd over)

(cont'd)

Patient preparation	*Radiopharmaceutical/s and dose*	*Patient position*	*Route of administration and delay*	*Equipment*	*Technique*	*Quantitative analysis*	*Comment*
3 phase bone scan for specific site							
None	15 mCi ^{99m}Tc-MDP (500 MBq)	Specific site positioned under/over camera	I.V. bolus injection (foot injection for imaging hands) Begin immediately 20–40 sec image for 'flow' study. Static images commenced within 1 minute for 'blood pool' phase, then 3 hour delay for static bone scan images	LFOV or standard field camera, depending on size of area to be examined. High resolution or converging collimator	500 000 count delayed images of involved side. Comparison contralateral side for same time. (15 min if single view only)	Routinely none	May be done in association with whole body images for additional assessment of particular symptomatic site
Cisternogram							
None	500 μCi (20 MBq) ^{111}In-DTPA	Lying	Intrathecal or cisterna magna injection: 2 hour delay	Standard field of view gamma camera with high energy collimator	5 minute images of cisterns (A, P, RL, LL, Vertex) views at 2 hours, 6 hours, 24 hours, 48 hours	Not routinely	Nasal or ear packs may be used to detect and measure CSF leakage

Brain scan							
None	20 mCi (750 MBq) ^{99m}TcGHA or equivalent	Lying	I.V. rapid bolus injection. No delay for dynamic study. 90 minute delay for static scan	Standard field of view gamma camera with GAP collimator and computer	1 second images for 1 min in the anterior or vertex view during the first pass. Equilibrium blood pool image immediately after dynamic scan for 300 000 counts. At 90 minutes 300 000 count images in A, P, LL, RL and vertex positions	Time activity curves plotted from ROI over the two hemispheres	Delayed views may be helpful in equivocal cases, patients suspected of having subdural haematoma should be scanned at 3 hours post injection. SPECT imaging may contribute.
SPECT Brain							
	10 mCi (350 MBq) ^{99m}TcHMPAO ^{99m}TcECD	Supine in a dimly lit room, with I.V. cannula for 5–10 mins prior to injection	I.V. wait 20 min before starting scan	LFOV gamma camera and computer for tomography with a high resolution collimator	64, 20 second images using circular tomography around 360° (using 64 × 64 matrix) reconstruct 2 pixel thick slices.		
Thyroid scan							
None	5 mCi (180 MBq) ^{99m}Tc Pertechnetate or 500μ Ci (20 MBq) ^{123}I sodium iodide	Supine with neck extended	I.V. injection with 20 minute delay (^{99m}Tc pertechnetate) or oral administration with 3 hour delay (^{123}I)	Standard gamma camera with pinhole or 'snout' collimator computer if measuring uptake simultaneously. Use parallel hole GAP collimator for retrosternal extensions	Wash oesophagus with glass of water; anterior view with maximum magnification 100 000 counts for 15 minutes. LAO and RAO if indicated. Repeat with ^{57}Co marker on nodule or suprasternal notch if indicated	Measure uptake using ROI around thyroid and also a background ROI and express as percentage of a standard or the syringe measured in a thyroid phantom at a set distance from the gamma camera	Scan must be combined with manual examination of the gland ± ultrasound

(cont'd over)

(cont'd)

Patient preparation	*Radiopharmaceutical/s and dose*	*Patient position*	*Route of administration and delay*	*Equipment*	*Technique*	*Quantitative analysis*	*Comment*
Perchlorate discharge							
As per thyroid scan using ^{123}I	As per thyroid scan using ^{123}I	As per thyroid scan using ^{123}I	As per thyroid scan using ^{123}I	As per thyroid scan using ^{123}I	Give KC104 1 g orally; image the thyroid at constant distance at 15 minute intervals for one hour	Measure uptake at each point and plot on graph paper. 10% discharge of ^{123}I or more is abnormal indicating failure of organification	
Whole body scan for thyroid cancer							
4 weeks off T4 or 2 weeks off T3 replacement therapy with a low iodine diet; serum TSH level above 40 mU ml^{-1}	5–15 mCi (180–550 MBq) ^{131}I-sodium iodide	Lying	Oral administration; 72 hours delay	LFOV gamma camera with high energy collimator or whole body imaging device	5 minute images to cover whole body	Not usual	Simultaneous serum thyroglobulin levels will improve accuracy
Adrenal scan							
Renal outline and depth may be marked by prior imaging with ^{99m}Tc-DMSA or ^{99m}Tc-DTPA	250 μCi (10 MBq) ^{75}Se methyl cholesterol 1–2 mCi (35–75 MBq) of ^{131}I-iodocholesterol is alternative	Prone	I.V. 7 day delay, repeat at 14 days	LFOV gamma camera medium energy high sensitivity collimator and computer	At 7 days a 15 min image is obtained centred over the upper poles	The percentage uptake in each gland may be made measuring the syringe containing ^{75}Se-cholesterol and depth correction	Iodocholesterol scan may be made after 5 days of suppression with dexamethasone for detection of aldosterone secreting tumour

Salivary gland scan							
None	5 mCi (180 MBq) ^{99m}Tc pertechnetate	Supine with neck extended	I.V. injection. No delay	Standard field of view gamma camera with GAP or high resolution collimator and computer	1 minute images of anterior neck to include all 4 glands for 15 minutes. Continuous data collection. Stimulant (acid drop or lemon) is given at 10 min after start. If mass lesion suspected magnified images of the gland	Using ROI over glands, measure rate of accumulated activity and rate of discharge with stimulant	
Oesphaegeal transit studies							
Nil by mouth 4 hours	500 μCi (20 MBq) ^{99m}Tc sulphur colloid in 15 ml water	Supine. Repeat erect if bolus does not reach stomach	Oral	LFOV gamma camera with computer	Swallowed as bolus with camera positioned anteriorly to show oesophagus and upper stomach. 15 second images for 10 minutes	Analyse time activity curves for upper, middle and lower thirds of oesophagus and stomach. Measure total transit to stomach	
Gastro-oesophageal reflux							
Clear fluids orally for 6 hours	500 μCi (20 MBq) ^{99m}Tc sulphur colloid in 300 ml acidified orange squash	Supine with abdominal binder	Oral administration. No delay	LFOV gamma camera and computer	Single image erect to exclude retention of activity in the oesophagus, then anterior abdomen/chest view 30 second images at 20 mm, 40 mm, 60 mm, 80 mm, 100 mm Hg pressure in inflatable abdominal binder	Optimize image for oesophagus and record changing activity in oesophagus with ROI	Record presence of symptoms during test

(cont'd over)

(cont'd)

Patient preparation	*Radiopharmaceutical/s and dose*	*Patient position*	*Route of administration and delay*	*Equipment*	*Technique*	*Quantitative analysis*	*Comment*
Gastric emptying							
Nil by mouth for 6 hours	1 mCi (35 MBq) ^{111}In DTPA in 100 ml milk (liquid meal); 1 mCi (35 MBq) ^{99m}Tc labelled bran or chicken liver labelled *in vivo* (solid)	Standing, sitting or lying (depending on standardization)	Oral administration. No delay	LFOV with similar gamma camera with dual isotope recording facility and high energy collimator. Computer	Continuous recording of stomach activity anteriorly for 60 minutes. Simultaneous acquisition in dual isotope mode	ROI over stomach contents, plot time activity curve and calculate log time and $T_{1/2}$ emptying	This is a very variable technique. It must be standardized locally
Duodeno-gastric bile reflux							
Nil by mouth for 6 hours	6 mμCi (200 MBq) ^{99m}Tc HIDA. 500 Ci (20 MBq) ^{111}In DTPA in fatty meal	Supine	I.V. injection ^{99m}Tc HIDA. No delay. Oral ^{111}In-DTPA at 30 minutes after HIDA (20 minutes if post cholecystectomy)	LFOV gamma camera with dual isotope recording facility and high energy collimator. Computer	Following HIDA injection 60 second anterior abdominal images at 2, 5, 10, 15, 20 and 30 minutes. Give ^{111}In-DTPA fatty meal, record 60 second images every 5 minutes for 60 minutes	Display images corrected for cross-over activity. Using ROI measure the amount of ^{99m}Tc-HIDA in gastric area outlined by ^{111}In-DTPA	
Localization of G.I. bleeding							
None	10 mCi (400 MBq) ^{99m}Tc labelled autologous red blood cells	Supine	I.V. injection. No delay	LFOV gamma camera with GAP or high resolution collimator	Anterior abdomen images every 5 minutes for 30 minutes. Then as indicated up to 24 hours lateral views as necessary		

Meckel's diverticulum							
6 hours nil by mouth	5 mCi (200 MBq) ^{99m}Tc pertechnetate	Supine	I.V. injection. No delay	LFOV gamma camera	Anterior abdominal images every 5 minutes up to 30 minutes. Lateral and posterior images as indicated	N/A	Pentagastrin with or without nasogastric suction may also be used to enhance ectopic uptake while removing intragastric activity
Gastrointestinal blood loss measurement							
None	200 μCi (7 MBq) ^{51}Cr labelled autologous red blood cells. Prepare standard solution	N/A	I.V.	Well scintillation counter, large specimen scintillation counter	Blood samples at 15 minutes, 7 and 14 days. Faecal collection collected and radioactivity measured over 2 week period	ml of blood sample $= \frac{\text{\% administered dose in faeces} \times 1000}{\text{\% litre administered dose in blood}}$	Large specimen scintillation counter makes the technique acceptable
Liver/spleen scan							
None	4 mCi (150 MBq) ^{99m}Tc HSA colloid	Standing or lying	I.V. injection, 15 minutes delay	LFOV gamma camera with GAP or high resolution collimator	Standard 4 views (A, P, RL, LL). 500 000 counts each with extra anterior view with costal margin marker	Usually none	May be combined with 'first pass' blood flow study

(**cont'd over**)

(cont'd)

Patient preparation	*Radiopharmaceutical/s and dose*	*Patient position*	*Route of administration and delay*	*Equipment*	*Technique*	*Quantitative analysis*	*Comment*
Hepatobiliary scan							
6 hours nil by mouth	5 mCi (200 MBq) ^{99m}Tc HIDA or equivalent	Supine	I.V. injection. No delay	LFOV gamma camera with high resolution collimator	400 000 count image of liver anteriorly at 2 minutes. Repeat for the same time every 5 minutes to 30 minutes. Rt lateral view after 30 mins. If gallbladder and duodenum are not visualized continue intermittently up to 4 hours	Usually not done	Gallbladder response to cholecystokinin or fatty meal may be measured after gallbladder filling
Spleen scan							
None	1 mCi (40 MBq) ^{99m}Tc Autologous denatured red blood cells	Standing or lying	I.V. injection, 45 minutes delay	Standard or LFOV gamma camera with GAP collimator. Standard well counter	250 000 count images A, P, LAO, LL, LPO views. Blood samples taken at 3, 10, 20 and 30 minutes. These are haemolysed and 2 ml samples measured	Results plotted on paper taking 3 min as 100%. Record time to 50% activity (normal 9–18 minutes)	
Bone marrow							
None	^{99m}Tc HSA colloid 10 mCi (370 MBq) per 1.73 m^2 body surface	Lying	I.V. injection. 15–30 minutes delay	LFOV gamma camera with GAP collimator or whole body imaging device	5 minute images of posterior thoracic and lumbar spine, posterior pelvis, both shoulders, both upper femora (distal limbs if indicated) lateral skull.	Routinely none	Do routine liver/ spleen scan

Plasma volume						
None	10 μCi (0.3 MBq) ^{125}I human serum albumin. Preparation of standard solution	N/A	I.V.	Well scintillation counter	10 ml heparinized blood sample before injection. Administration of ^{125}I HSA. 10 ml heparinized blood samples at 10, 20, 30 minutes. Count 1 ml plasma samples and standard from opposite to injection	Plasma volume $= \frac{\text{vol injected (10)} \times \text{CPM standard} \times \text{dilution of standard}}{\text{extrapolated CPM/1 ml plasma at time 0}}$ Normal range 30–40 ml kg^{-1} body weight.
Red cell mass						
None	10 μCi (0.3 MBq) ^{51}Cr sodium chromate tagged to 20 ml of patient's whole blood	N/A	16 ml of labelled blood injected i.v. with no extravasation. Remainder used for standard preparation	Well scintillation counter	Preinjection 10 ml heparinized blood sample then samples 10, 20 minutes. Whole blood and plasma samples are counted	Red cell volume = vol. injected $\times \frac{\text{WB std CPM/1 ml} \times \text{dilution} - \text{plasma std CPM/1 ml} \times \text{std plasmacrit WB CPM/1 ml} - \text{plasma CPM/1 ml} \times \text{plasmacrit}}{\text{haematocrit}}$ Normal red cell volume: males 25–35 ml kg^{-1}; females 20–30 ml kg^{-1}; Total blood volume: males 55–80 ml kg^{-1}, females 50–75 ml kg^{-1}

(cont'd over)

(cont'd)

Patient preparation	*Radiopharma-ceutical/s and dose*	*Patient position*	*Route of administration and delay*	*Equipment*	*Technique*	*Quantitative analysis*	*Comment*
Red cell survival and sequestration							
None	1.5 μCi (0.05 MBq) kg^{-1} body weight of ^{51}Cr sodium chromate tagged to 20 ml blood	Supine	16 ml injection intravenously	Well scintillation counter. Collimated scintillation detector	Blood sample taken at 24 hours and then 3 times each week for 3 weeks. Counts are recorded over the precordium, spleen and liver at the same times as blood samples	Plot blood sample count rates on semi log paper and estimate $T_{1/2}$. Sequestration results expressed as ratio of precordial to spleen and spleen to liver ratio	Normal value 25–35 days
B_{12} absorption (Schilling Test)							
Fasting from midnight and 2 hours after oral vitamin B_{12} administration	0.5 μCi (0.02 MBq)	N/A	Oral	Well scintillation counter	Administer ^{57}Co B_{12}, Inject 1 mg stable B_{12} 1–2 hours later. Collect urine for 24 hours twice. Prepare a ^{57}Co B_{12} standard	Measure radioactivity of a 5 ml aliquot of urine and standard.	Normal value 9% in 1st 24 hours, < 1% in 2nd 24 hours. If less than 6% excreted repeat with intrinsic factor. The two tests can be combined with two different radioactive cobalt labels

$$\% \text{ in 24 hours} = \frac{\text{CPM in 5 ml of urine} \times \text{urine vol/5}}{\text{CPM in 5 ml of std} \times \text{dilution factor} \times 100}$$

Ferrokinetics							
None	5 μCi (0.2 MBq) ^{59}Fe citrate incubated with plasma (use donor compatible blood) if the iron binding capacity is $< 10\ g\ dl^{-1}$. Prepare standard solution	N/A	Intravenous injection of 5 ml of labelled plasma	Well scintillation counter	Draw 6 ml sample heparinized blood at 10, 30, 60, 90 minutes after injection from another vein and then at 24 hours and alternate days for 3 weeks	Plot on semi log paper determine $T_{1/2}$.	Normal $T_{1/2} = 6$–120 minutes. Red cell incorporation = 60–80% of dose in 7–10 days Red cell mass and survival and sequestration can be measured simultaneously
						% RBC incorporation of ^{59}Fe per day $= \frac{\text{CPM 5 cc blood} \times \text{red cell mass}/5 \times 100\%}{\text{CPM} \times 20 \times \text{decimal haematocrit}}$	
Lymph node imaging							
None	1 mCi (50 MBq) ^{99m}Tc HSA micro colloid	Supine	Subcutaneous injection at site depending on nodes to be examined. 2 hour delay	LFOV gamma camera with GAP or high sensitivity collimator	Image regional lymph nodes, cover the injection site with lead if in field of view	Usually none	
^{67}Gallium whole body scan							
Mild purgation during course of study	50 μCi (1.85 MBq) kg^{-1} body weight of ^{67}Ga citrate	Lying	I.V. injection: 48 hour delay (occasionally 6 hours)	LFOV gamma camera with 1, 2 or 3 pulse height analysers and high energy collimator or whole body imaging device	200 000 count images. Views to cover whole body or local areas as clinically appropriate. Repeat at 72 hours	Possibly use subtraction technique for liver lesions	Usually combine with liver/spleen scan
White cell localization study							
None	500 μCi (20 MBq) ^{111}In-autologous oxine labelled leucocytes	Supine	Intravenous, 3 hours and 24 hours	LFOV gamma camera preferably with dual PHA, with high energy collimator	Anterior and posterior views of chest and abdomen. Record images 5 min each at 1 and 3 hr. Other views as clinically indicated. Repeat at 24 hours for 7 min per view.	N/A	

APPENDIX TWO

Risk factors and dosimetry

A. B. Brill

A2.1 INTRODUCTION

The practice of medicine, like many other disciplines, is inextricably involved with benefit–risk decision making. This relates to actions taken or deferred in all areas of patient management, i.e. both diagnosis and therapy. Heightened radiation concerns now affect and could increasingly impact on the practice of radiation-related specialties. Public concern derives in part from increasing awareness of the fact that we live in an increasingly complex world in which obvious and subtle risks are a natural part of life, and also that many of these risks are increasing in both developed and developing nations.

Exposures to some of these risks have significant potential impact on human health. Medical radiations have a strong positive impact on health. On the other hand, chemical toxins found in increasing amounts in food and human tissues are likely to confer significant negative effects. Whereas it is very easy to measure minuscule amounts of radiation, it is very difficult to measure organ contents of chemicals even when tissues are available for assay. The fear of things 'nuclear' arises in part from the mysterious non-touchable aspects of the atom and its forces, plus deep-seated anxieties regarding nuclear weapons and the possibility of their use in war or terrorist acts. Unfortunately, nuclear medicine, radioactive waste disposal, nuclear power, and reactors in general, are all lumped together in many people's minds. In nuclear medicine, doses administered to patients usually exceed natural background by several fold, and many patients ask questions concerning risks from our studies. Nuclear medicine staff members need to be well informed concerning these issues to answer these questions correctly, and in such a way as to inspire patient confidence.

The choice and manner of conduct of procedures requires a balance between benefit and risk. We strive to conduct only needed procedures, i.e. those that could make a difference regarding choices of patient management. We need to strive to have the best equipment and the appropriate isotopes available to use in such circumstances, and to choose the best combinations and doses to provide needed information (NCRP 70, 1982). A patient who realizes that careful attention is being paid to these issues is likely to feel reassured. When called upon to answer a patient's specific risk-related question, one has a unique opportunity to provide information to a person whose full attention you have. At such a time, one has the greatest chance of getting beyond superficial barriers and emotional biases and maybe even allay some misplaced fears regarding radiation risk. In these discussions, it is sometimes useful to relate procedural exposures to doses and risks from common generally accepted life circumstances. As practitioners we need to be knowledgable concerning the risk for the average patient and for patients at unusual risk, whether this be from their disease, from the particular radiation exposure they will receive, or from the anxiety that they may have. A knowledge of the base upon which current knowledge rests is of importance for one's confidence in the reliability of current dogma, and also so that explanations can be given in appropriate depth to persons of differing backgrounds when such discussions arise.

The press is quick to pick up on and report issues relating to radiation health. Recent concern has focused on radon, and we need to learn enough about that issue to compare it to other potential exposures, including ^{133}Xe, for example, used in nuclear medicine. If possible, we should be able to discuss such issues in sufficient depth to win listener confidence of our expertise. The problem that arises is that when such matters are first reported there is often too little information generally available. At that point we may not have the needed level of understanding of the issues involved, and if this is the case we should say so. National and international radiation protection bodies, and nuclear medicine, and health physics societies all have groups which focus on these matters, and which can be called upon to answer specific questions as they arise. Even when one cannot answer a patient's question immediately, a quick follow-up after obtaining the needed information may be very useful, and certainly more so than a hastily given imprecise answer to a thoughtful question.

The level and variations in natural background radiation in different places is often given as a reference point relative to potential risks of specific procedures. Recent information and publicity regarding the significant contribution ^{222}Rn makes to individual radiation exposure has attracted great attention. Variations in local geology, water supply and home construction practices result in significant differences in radiation exposure depending on specific factors which are home and region specific, and hence the use of natural background as the reference for acceptable dose levels is a less stable number than previously realized. Recent revisions of accepted sea level mid-latitude assessments of natural background, for example in the USA, places this at 300 mrem (NCRP 93, 1987), **effective** dose equivalent (EDE). Note: the EDE weights the rem dose by a set of organ dose weighting factors to estimate the whole-body risk equivalent of partial body exposures. Natural background was previously given at 80 mrem dose equivalent (DE) for many regions in the USA (NCRP 45, 1975). This four- to fivefold increase in our estimate of the level of natural background exposure does not suggest that natural background is increasing, but that we now have new ways of computing dose, i.e. the effective dose equivalent, which makes it possible to add the radon lung dose to whole-body and partial-body dose from other contributions to natural background dose, as discussed below. A discussion of the notions underlying additivity of dose contributions is presented in Lam (1988).

Among the rationale for the development of the EDE notion was the need in occupational safety programmes to calculate the integrated dose to workers exposed to various internal and external doses during a working career. Further, the risk to workers comes from radiation and chemical exposures, and in principle the EDE permits the integration of risks from multiple sources. If one accepts the whole-body radiation risk figures from the Japanese A-bomb survivors, those numbers (cancers per million per rem whole-body dose) can be multiplied by the whole-body dose equivalent (EDE), to estimate the fractional lifetime increase in cancer risk to the individual. As one develops data on internal exposures to chemicals, and the risk associated therewith, the risks from chemical exposures could be calculated and summed with the propagated radiation risk data.

The increasing gap between natural background and nuclear medicine doses could be used to suggest that nuclear medicine procedural risks are less than previously believed, relative to natural background. However, at the same time as assessments of natural background point to an increase, evidence of an increasing cancer risk emerges from continued follow-up of the Japanese A-bomb survivors. Recent studies from Japan are consistent with a two- to threefold increase in low linear energy transfer (LET) risk coefficients (Sinclair, 1987). Thus, it appears that our previous assessment of the 'relative risk' of nuclear medicine procedures, i.e. relative to natural background radiation, is essentially unchanged, based on changes in our understanding of both dose and risk coefficients.

A2.2 DOSE ASSESSMENT

A2.2.1 GENERAL

Dose estimation involves the measurement of absorbed dose received by tissues, and is expressed in various units based upon energy deposited by the various primary and secondary radiations. Macroscopic dosimetry provides estimates of average dose received in the different organs. The question often arises as to how a particular patient's condition will influence the dose, i.e. will the dose be more or less than average values for normal subjects? A second level of uncertainty that complicates the dosimetry of internal emitters arises from nonuniform spatial distribution, and the techniques and data needed to calculate dose distribution at the cellular level (microdosimetry) are not well established. Doses from radiopharmaceuticals that accumulate intracellularly, and particularly those that accumulate inside the cell nucleus, are significantly higher than predicted by 'macro'-dosimetry, i.e. average dose calculations. We need to know more about the mechanisms of carcinogenesis, and the nature of initiation and promotion processes and radiosensitive sites, to know how to compute and use microdosimetry data for risk prediction analyses. An excellent discussion of theoretical and practical aspects of dosimetry, including microdosimetric considerations is presented in a two-volume series edited by Kase *et al.* (1987).

Great interest focuses on the use of increasingly used new classes of intracellular tracers, including short-lived cyclotron-produced ^{11}C, ^{13}N and ^{15}O, and such tracers as ^{111}In-labelled white cells. This has led to an increased need for dosimetry data, and particularly for microdosimetry data from diagnostic studies. The recognition of the fact that short-range Auger electrons emitted during radioactive decay can convey high radiation doses to the radiosensitive cell nucleus, when incorporated into DNA, suggests care in the use of high diagnostic doses, but supports consideration of their potential utility in higher administered doses for radiotherapy. Because the margin between safe and effective doses is narrow in radiotherapy, careful attention needs to be given to the measurement and assessment of radiation dose in these circumstances. For diagnostic studies, electron emissions result in unwanted radiation dose, whereas they provide the rationale for therapeutic protocols. Choices affecting the design of such procedural combinations will be illustrated for monoclonal antibody diagnosis and therapy.

A2.2.2 MEASUREMENT OF MACROSCOPIC DOSE FROM INTERNAL EMITTERS

The calculation of radiation doses from internal emitters requires data on the radioactivity distribution following administration in the different organs in which the material is distributed. The area under the activity–time curve (given in MBq h (μCi h)) and referred to as the A tilda in the notation used by the Medical Internal Radiation Dose (MIRD) Committee of the SNM provides the first of the two pieces of information needed. The second is radionuclide-specific data (S factors in MIRD notation) which is given in (cGy MBq^{-1} h {rads μCi^{-1} h}) for the different source organs measured in terms of dose contribution to the various target organs in the body. For γ-rays, the source–target contributions to distant regions needs to be calculated, whereas for short-range radiations absorbed dose comes only from the activity that concentrates in the organ plus dose from blood flowing through the organ.

The biological testing of a new radiopharmaceutical starts with animal studies. Small animals, frequently mice, are given small doses, and the animal sacrificed at various times to obtain biodistribution data. The calculations of dose for human studies take the mouse data, and scale the activity measured in terms of fraction of the injected dose per organ to humans by adjusting for weight differences. These preliminary dose estimates guide initial human trials in which direct information on dosimetry and potential utility is obtained from human studies. The hardest part of dosimetry studies is the collection of good data from human studies. The best studies employ opposed detectors which are used to collect emission and transmission data from the various organs of interest, along with reference standards for dose calibration. Multiple measurements are required over times that span at least two effective half-lives of the tracer. In addition to organ counts, whole-body counter, blood and urine data are needed. In the past, specialized equipment was needed, and relatively few institutions were in a position to collect and analyse such data. The situation is now different, and computer-based gamma cameras are capable of being used for such studies, and computer programs are now widely available for use in the analyses.

Tabulated dosimetry data almost always indicate the average dose to various organs based on studies done in normal volunteers. Little data are available for persons with abnormalities that may influence dose significantly (NCRP 70, 1982). The greatest changes between dose received by normal and diseased subjects come when normal excretory channels are blocked. Thus, patients with anuria receive higher doses (per unit administered dose) from renal studies than do normal subjects. A similar situation applies to patients with biliary atresia, infiltrated administered doses, etc. There is a need to broaden the number of institutions doing careful dosimetry studies if such data are to become available. For this reason, we will be more explicit on the methods that we have found most useful, and will illustrate this using recently collected data on ^{111}In-labelled antibodies.

Accurate standards, needed to calibrate *in vivo* and in *in vitro* sample counts, are easily made by weighing radioisotope-containing syringes before and after delivery of measured (i.e. counted) amounts of radioactivity into tubes (for standard preparation) and into the patient. One needs to avoid flushing syringes in these studies. Alternatively, one can count syringes before and after delivery, but this requires carefully calibrated systems to cover the wide range in activities accurately. The techniques for blood and urine measurements are well established in all nuclear medicine laboratories. The complete collection of urine and the measurement of urine losses is difficult to achieve. In many cases, where stool losses are negligible, or the time of measurements is short with respect to faecal excretion, whole-body counts can be very useful. Since imaging studies require the administration of many microcuries, traditional whole-body counters are of little value, as they are too sensitive. Instead of a traditional whole-body counter, we use an uncollimated gamma camera, with the patient >5 m in front of the detector, and count the patient, a standard, and room background for less than 1 min, to obtain retention data. Alternatively, any reasonably good scintillation detector (high data rate capability) can be used for such studies. Initial measures at 15–30 min (counts in patient/standard) are used as the 100% reference against which subsequent whole-body counts are compared.

For organ activity determinations, a collimated gamma camera can be used which has been calibrated for the particular low-energy γ-emitting radionuclide under investigation. Calibration studies are accomplished by transmission and emission imaging of a known activity source embedded in different amounts of scattering material. Correction factors derived from such studies are obtained and used with the measured emission and transmission data sets from patients. Analyses are based on geometric means of the emission data from selected regions of interest including organs, background sites and standards (Doherty *et al.*, 1986). Other groups in many countries have used specialized counters to collect data for dosimetry of higher-energy nuclides than can be measured effectively with gamma cameras because of scanty side shielding and thin, low-efficiency crystals.

A2.2.3 DOSE ESTIMATES

Organ doses for different radiopharmaceuticals are given in package inserts for all radiopharmaceuticals approved for use in humans. A number of tabulations have been published which bring together these useful data. Doses are given in absorbed dose per administered amount (Gy Bq^{-1} or rads mCi^{-1} administered). Since the quality factor for γ- and high-energy β-emitters is 1.0, these doses are also equal to dose quivalent (cSv or rem dose).

The relative risk of X-ray and nuclear medicine studies has been presented in various ways. The problem is complicated by different distributions of dose and dose rate. A logical basis for summing the risks of partial body exposures and comparing these to the risks of whole-body exposures was needed, and several approaches, have been suggested. The International Council for Radiation Protection (ICRP, 1977) established a series of weighting factors to accomplish that task. These weighting factors are based on the relative contribution of cancers of different organs to the total somatic risk based on whole-body exposures. Thus, for example, if 15% of the cancer risk in women following whole-body exposures involves the breast, then the weighting factor on breast

Table A2.1 Comparison of doses from lung studies/exposures

Procedure or nuclide	*Amount administered*	*Lung dose (mrem)*	*Effective dose equiv. (mrem)*
^{127}Xe p.o.	10 mCi	47[a]	17[b]
^{133}Xe p.o.	10 mCi	110[a]	25[b]
^{222}Rn p.o.	Nat. background	2500[d]	200[c]
Chest X-ray	–	20[e]	6[e]

[a] NCRP 70 (1982).
[b] Johansson *et al.* (1984).
[c] NCRP 93 (1987). The lung dose comes from α-particles from radon daughters to the tracheal bronchial epithelium.
[d] BEIR (1988). The dose of 2500 mrem is to the tracheobronchial epithelium.
[e] Kereiakes and Rosenstein (1980).

dose would be 0.15. If a woman receives a 1 rem breast exposure, this is assigned a whole-body dose equivalent of 0.150 cSv (mrem), which is denoted as the effective dose equivalent (EDE). In radionuclide studies which deliver dose to a series of organs, the weighting factors are applied to these doses and summed to estimate the whole-body dose equivalent. Exposures to the gonads are also included and weighted in with somatic risk, based on theoretical risk projections based on animal studies (ICRP, 1977; NCRP 91, 1987). An example of the use of EDE in comparing doses from environmental exposures and diagnostic lung studies is presented in Table A2.1. The EDE from environmental ^{222}Rn is approximately ten times higher than from the other tabulated exposures, whereas, when considering lung doses alone, it is two to ten times higher than the referenced procedures tablulated. For detailed examples that illustrate the EDE computation, see ICRP (1977).

A2.3 EFFECTS OF RADIATION: HIGH DOSES (WANTED EFFECTS)

A2.3.1 GENERAL

The effects of radiation therapy are wanted effects. In that situation our objective is to kill cells, with the goal of killing abnormal cells, and preserving normal cells as much as possible. Effects of high doses of ionizing radiation have been well known and well documented for many years. This comes from occupational data (miners exposed to pitchblende, radium dial painters, and accidents in the workplace), untoward effects in patients receiving high-dose radiation therapy, and more recently from the effects of A-bomb exposure in Japan. Early effects depend on the part of the body exposed, the kind and amount of radiation, and the rate at which it is administered. Following doses in the range of 50–100 rads or higher whole-body dose, changes can be observed in several body systems. Rapidly proliferating tissues show the greatest effects, since rapidly turning-over cell populations have a larger probability of being in radiosensitive mitotic stages than do resting cells. This accounts for the high radiosensitivity of haematopoeitic cells and gastrointestinal lining cells. Some tumour cells fall into this same category, and for this reason there has been a long history of efforts to target radionuclides to tumour tissue. The whole-body dose that killed 50% of the people exposed to A-bomb radiations in 30 days (the $LD\text{-}50_{30}$) is variously reported as being in the range 155–350 rads (Adelstein, 1987). The numerical value of the LD-50 that relates to medical practice, however, is quite different and many patients have survived deliberate doses of 1000 rads, whole-body, in managed therapy situations, but at very significantly lower dose rates than from an A-bomb. There is a significant difference between the outcome of accidental exposures and planned medical exposures for various reasons. The proper choice of therapy depends critically on the absorbed dose, and timing of treatment is of cardinal importance. Dose is well established and planned in radiotherapy and is almost never as well established early in the management of accidents. Much has been written on this subject (Hubner and Fry, 1980) which we will not repeat here but will direct our attention to issues relating to radiotherapy with radionuclides.

A2.3.2 RADIOTHERAPY CONSIDERATIONS (EXAMPLE FROM RADIOIMMUNOTHERAPY)

Early investigators used ^{32}P to treat polycythaemia vera (PV), and ^{131}I to treat thyroid disorders (thyroid cancer and hyperthyroidism). The fact that high doses can be useful in treating disease is now well established. It is also true that high doses can cause deleterious effects, such as leukaemia in both PV and thyroid cancer patients treated with high doses, but the benefit–risk ratio still favours the use of these therapies. A number of targeting strategies have been attempted to achieve higher therapeutic concentrations in tumour tissues. Compounds that are strongly localized in tumour tissue are under intensive search. ^{131}I-*meta*-iodobenzylguanidine (MIBG) is an example of one such compound being used for adrenal medullary tumour therapy (McEwan *et al.*, 1985). With the development of hybridoma technology, great impetus has been given to the use of monoclonal antibodies for diagnosis and more impetus toward therapy. High tumour to normal tissue ratios are required for successful therapy, and at the same time dose to the bone marrow and other critical organs needs to be kept at acceptable levels.

For many years there has been a recognition of the need for better means of treating ovarian cancer, a radiosensitive common cancer, and we will use this as an example in our discussions. Isotope therapy with ^{32}P-CrPO, and ^{198}Au-labelled colloid has been given intraperitoneally with varying success in many clinical trials. Complications which arise in the course of these treatments includes bowel necrosis, presumably due to high local doses from poorly distributed radionuclides, i.e. loculated injections, and marginal success has been generally reported. Recently, there has been increasing enthusiasm for the use of radiolabelled monoclonal antibodies in treatment of this disease. Several antibodies are being used. In Britain, ^{90}Y-labelled HMFG1, a monoclonal antibody targeted to ovarian cancer, is being used in clinical trials (Epenetos *et al.*, personal communication). In the USA, a feasibility study is now beginning, using a different ovarian cancer targeted antibody, intraperitoneally injected ^{90}Y-labelled OC-125(Hnatowich *et al.*). The considerations that dictate the choice of radionuclide and antibody include the effective half-life and emissions from the radionuclide, and antibody-related factors that influence the pharmacokinetics, both of which factors determine the radiation dose distribution. It is generally believed that a therapeutic nuclide should have a radioactive half-life of the order of two to seven days. Ideally blood levels should be high, to provide a driving force pushing tracer into the tumour, and non-target tissues should have low uptake and retention. Excretion of the isotope should be slow, and should occur through the kidney, in the case of intraperitoneal therapy of ovarian cancer, to minimize added dose to the gastrointestinal tract. Radionuclidic considerations depend on the type of tumour distribution and the size of the masses to be treated. The emissions should be particulate, so as to deliver high dose over a short range, ideally confined to the tumour volume. The maximum range of the 2.2 MeV β-emissions from ^{90}Y is 1.0 cm in tissue (average = 0.36 cm). The utility of ^{90}Y for treatment depends on kinetics of the tracer, target to background ratios, and geometry of the target with respect to radiosensitive normal tissues.

The primary treatment of ovarian cancer is surgery, along with traditional radiotherapy directed at the tumour area, including known local pathways of dissemination. Chemotherapy and radioimmunotherapy are directed at metastases which have evaded the surgeon and the radiotherapist. The anticipated role of immunotherapy is to find and kill cells that have left the treatment field. Ideally these would be isolated cells, seeding the peritoneal cavity. If this is the case, then cell surface directed antibodies need to be tagged with an emitter whose radiations penetrate on the order of one cell diameter, i.e. approximately 10 μm (0.001 cm). Thus, using ^{90}Y, the largest fraction of its β-energy will deposit in the normal tissue to which the malignant cell is juxtaposed. This can be to omentum or bowel, typically, in the peritoneal space, or in bone, to which ^{90}Y that breaks free from its antibody binding site may attach, and which could pose a hazard to bone marrow. If the tumour masses are larger, then the deep penetration by energetic β-radiations would be needed to treat cells that are distant from the site of attachment of the antibody. Since one of the objectives in therapy is to kill all tumour cells, and since it is unlikely that any antibody will target all cells, then a particle whose range is greater than one cell diameter is needed.

A further problem that faces intraperitoneal therapy is that this route of administration delivers material primarily to the surface of the tumour cells. When they are isolated cells, that can be effective. When tumour masses are larger, then it is important to get to the deep portions of the tumour as well, and two different approaches can be considered. The first was referred to above, and that involves the use of energetic β-emitters. The other possibility that needs to be explored involves the use of two different routes of administration, i.e. intraperitoneal for surface targeting, and intravenous for delivery of dose to deeper sites in the tumour. One could use the same nuclide, or a different one, whose properties are a better match to the kinetics and biodistribution of the particular antibody to which it is attached. Clearly, dosimetry considerations will play an important role in selection of appropriate combinations, and experience gained in animal and human research studies will determine the potential role of such combined approaches.

A2.4 LATE EFFECTS OF RADIATION (UNWANTED EFFECTS)

A2.4.1 GENERAL

The effects of radiation encountered in radiation therapy are wanted effects. In that situation our objective is to kill cells, with the goal of killing abnormal cells, and preserving normal cells as much as possible. In the discussion we are now embarking upon, we focus on the late effects of low doses of radiation, where these effects are not what we are seeking to achieve but are unwanted side effects. Since the objective of nuclear medical diagnostic procedures is to obtain clinically needed information with minimum risk to the patient, any late effect of the radiation we deliver has to be looked upon as unwanted. The information we have on radiation effects of low doses of radiation is based on extrapolations down into the low-dose region from data obtained at high doses. Because of the uncertainty in making these extrapolations, we always state that our knowledge in the low-dose region is imprecise. This creates the impression in the general public that we do not know what is happening at those doses, and that there may be significant unexpected risk from procedures which deliver low doses. That is misleading because, in fact, given present radiobiology knowledge the larger concern in the low-dose region is whether the risk is as high as extrapolated from high doses, or less.

It is generally conceded that there is more known about radiation risks than about any other potentially deleterious agent. Extensive radiobiology information comes from a long series of careful animal and plant radiobiology studies conducted over many years. The ability to separate the importance of the different factors, i.e. dose, radiation quality, dose rate and other co-factors, can be assessed only in animal systems, and this has been done. Observations at high doses provide data that are useful for interspecies comparisons at high doses. Knowledge of mechanisms of radiation action is needed to provide insight into the expected rates at lower levels than can be experimentally resolved. The results of animal studies establish the principles upon which human radiation data are assessed. The need for human data arises in order to facilitate scaling the results of animal studies to humans, and also to be sure that similar mechanisms operate. An example of the latter is in the area of radiation repair mechanisms. In cell culture systems, radiation repair mechanisms have now been clearly demonstrated. In these processes, abnormal segments of DNA are excised and replaced with normal segments. For many years theory has associated such processes with the shoulder region of experimental dose–response curves. Now we know from studies on radiation repair mechanisms that there are animals and persons with heightened radiation sensitivity, a phenomenon associated with deficient radiation repair mechanisms (Patterson *et al.*, 1984). These observations provide direct confirmation of the existence of repair mechanisms in man. Fortunately, diseases involving defective radiation repair mechanisms (such as ataxia telangiectasia and xeroderma pigmentosa) are sufficiently rare that it is not deemed necessary to make adjustments in population exposure guidelines (BEIR, 1980). However, when such persons come for radiation therapy, it is very important that they be identified as individuals, as they can be expected to sustain serious injury or death from doses which are well tolerated by 'normal' individuals.

Information on the relation between dose and subsequent expression of radiation-induced disease in humans relies heavily on findings from the follow-up of the Japanese A-bomb survivors. Unlike most other human data, exposure to different doses of radiation in the survivors was not confounded with prior health status, age or sex, and long-term follow-up has been achieved with unprecedented success. Additional support for the findings from these studies comes from very similar results derived from follow-up in the UK of the effects of partial-body, fractionated, high-dose-rate radiation therapy of ankylosing spondylitis, a disease affecting young males predominantly (Darby *et al.*, 1984).

Epidemiology studies are difficult and expensive to conduct, and require many years before conclusions can be reached. The strength of these conclusions is often diminished by inherent limitations in human research. A healthy worker effect has been noted in some occupational exposure studies where employment selection factors can lead to underestimated risk of radiation with respect to the general population. Even in the Japanese studies, where there should be minimum bias, the question has been raised concerning the possibility that the 'weakest' persons exposed had the highest probability of dying from early effects, and hence the surviving population represents a healthier cohort than average. Despite the various problems associated with the Japanese A-bomb survivors study, it provides the best human radiation effects data, and represents the major source of information used by national and international bodies responsible for radiation policy making.

A2.4.2 DOSE–RESPONSE CURVES

Statistically valid data on the effects of radiation in irradiated human subjects are available primarily following high-dose, high-dose-rate exposures. Analysis of effects at whole-body doses lower than 50 rads requires the extrapolation of data gained at higher doses into the low-dose region. Various models have been used for this purpose. These can be classified in a number of ways. These include linear, greater than linear, and less than linear models, and there is greatest radiobiological support for the less than linear models for low-dose predictions. No good human data have been presented which justify the use of greater than linear models. Based on extensive animal and plant data, the US NAS BEIR Committee (BEIR, 1980) based its best estimates of low-dose low-LET human radiation effects on a linear quadratic model. In that model, a linear dose component adds to a quadratic component, with the latter becoming dominant in the high-dose region. Risk predictions from this model were intermediate between lower estimates from a quadratic model, and higher estimates from a linear dose response model, and all these estimates were tabulated. The data were also presented based on absolute risk and relative risk models. The former assume that radiation risks add to the baseline expectancy of disease, while relative risk models assume that radiation increases risk in a multiplicative fashion. Thus, relative risk projections assume that children, for example, who have a given increment of cancer above expectancy for their age cohort will continue to express that relative increase throughout life. Thus, when they achieve older ages in which spontaneous rates of cancer are high, they will express rates which are a multiple thereof. Thus, relative risk models result in significantly higher risk projections than do absolute risk models.

In 1990, the US NAS BEIR Comm. issued a new report (BEIR, 1990) in which they projected approx. 4 fold higher risk from low level ionizing radiation exposures than previously considered. These were based on continued follow up of Japanese A-bomb survivors, and reflected changes in dosimetry, which are still being debated, and additional cancer mortality in the years since the 1980 report. Two decisions by that committee account for the major change in their estimate of the risk, and these are the use of the relative risk model, instead of the absolute risk model, and second, they based their calculations on the linear risk model, and failed to include a correction for the lower radiobiological hazard from low dose rate radiations. These have been documented extensively in animal and plant research and the effects of low dose rate radiations as from occupational, medical and environmental radiations are believed to lie between 2 and 10 times less than from high dose rate radiations. As they could not decide on a particular value for that correction factor, they ignored dose rate considerations, and estimated the risk of whole body radiation from low dose rate sources at 3–4 times higher than previously accepted. This has had a large impact on public perception of risk, as the issues are complex, and the public is ill-prepared to cope with details regarding such emotionally charged matters. Regulatory agencies in many countries are in process of reevaluating exposure guidelines, and in view of the continuing debates concerning these values, we have not included tabulations from that report in late editing of this chapter just prior to publication. The interested reader is referred to the BEIR (1990) report for further information concerning this controversial matter.

At low doses, it is generally accepted that the limiting slope of somatic and genetic effect curves is linear in the low-dose region. However, for some end-points, skin cancer, and effects that require damage to multiple cells, a threshold is known to exist. Some data suggest that there may be beneficial effects of radiation delivered at low doses, the so-called hormesis effect, and this is presumed to be due to stimulation of immunological or other reparative processes. Such effects are manifest by a dose–response curve which dips below the baseline spontaneous risk values at low doses (Hickey *et al.*, 1983).

At approximately 100 rads, linear and quadratic components are believed to be of approximately equal magnitude. This cross-over point is demonstrated in many radiobiology experiments (Brown, 1977), but there are little data in humans in which this value can be established. The one circumstance for which this can be justified is in the Japanese leukaemia data, as reviewed in BEIR (1980). The strength of such analyses rests on the extensive experimental radiobiology data cited above, rather than on the statistical robustness of the human data. At higher doses, all models, including the linear quadratic, need to include a saturation term, i.e. where additional doses are associated with decreasing effect rates, due to the phenomenon of 'wasted radiation', i.e. a fraction of the extra radiation kills or transforms already damaged cells.

A.2.4.3 RADIATION RISK COEFFICIENTS

(a) Data

There are extensive data on somatic risks of radiation in human subjects. Much of it comes from the studies on the Japanese A-bomb survivors, but an appreciable amount of data are available from the review of data on persons who received radiation therapy. There are no good human data relating radiation exposure to genetic risks. The extensive data collected on the A-bomb survivors have not demonstrated a significant increase in genetic effects following high-dose-rate whole-body doses which in the heavily exposed averaged greater than 25 rads. Thus, projections of human genetic risk are based entirely upon experimental cell and animal radiobiology data. However, based on analysis of the Japanese data, and statistical and radiobiology plausibility considerations, the low-LET low-dose-rate doubling dose for genetic effects is estimated at approximately 480 rads (Schull *et al.*, 1987).

Risk coefficients for somatic effects based on data available in 1980 from Japan were in close agreement with the ankylosing spondylitis data, and data from other human experience. Data presented in BEIR (1980) were recalculated by John Boice for an NCRP Committee Report for different tumours for different age groups, and these appear in Table A2.2 (presented in Sinclair, 1987).

(b) Use of risk coefficients to estimate probability of causation

The above-referenced data describe the prospective risk of radiation-induced effects, i.e. the probability that an effect will be observed following whole-body radiation exposures. An alternative means of encoding this information attempting to relate observed illness to antecedent radiation exposures was developed in the USA in response to the need for data that could be used in courts of law to adjudicate radiation injury cases. This was motivated largely in response to attempts by persons living in southern Utah near the Nevada weapons test site to recover damages they attributed to radiation injury. The NIH was instructed to develop tables that would relate the increased probability of malignant disease that had supervened with respect to estimated exposure dose, for different types of cancer, and different ages, sex and time intervals since irradiation. The attributable risk or probability of causation (PC) they defined was based on the notion that radiation adds linearly to the natural risk (NR), and that percentage increment is tabulated as the PC (NAS, 1984; NIH 85).

$$\text{Probability of causation (PC)} = [\text{Radiation risk (RR)} \div (\text{RR} + \text{NR})] \times 100$$

Given a 30-year-old male exposed to 10 rads whole-body low-LET radiation, who at age 40 develops leukaemia, the tabulated PC is 26%. Examples for other malignancies, given the same age/latency and dose, include the following:

TUMOUR	*PC (%)*
Bone	81
Oesophagus	0.83

Table A2.2 Risk of fatal cancer

Age (years)	*Leukaemia*	*Lung*	*Breast*	*Thyroid*	*Total cancers*	*Risk (×10/Sv)*
Male						
25	1.72	6.15	–	0.32	19.9	2.0
35	1.88	4.30	–	0.22	12.0	1.2
45	2.00	3.13	–	0.14	9.2	0.9
55	1.83	2.18	–	0.08	7.5	0.8
Female						
25	1.07	4.80	8.14	0.57	29.3	2.9
35	1.24	4.19	3.32	0.44	17.0	1.7
45	1.46	3.73	0.81	0.31	11.9	1.2
55	1.45	2.92	0.35	0.20	9.9	1.0

Note: Fatal cases per 1000 persons after 0.1 Gy per year for ten years (1 Gy). From Sinclair (1987).

Stomach	2.8	
Colon	0.83	
Liver	8.4	
Pancreas	1.9	
Lung	3.8	Non-smokers
	0.35	Smokers
Breast	2.6	(female)
Kidney	0.69	
Thyroid	11	

The above numbers are very high with respect to the numbers of cases of a disease predicted a priori, i.e. at the time of radiation exposure. For example, the lifetime increment in risk of leukaemia following a 10 rad whole-body exposure is approximately $2–4 \times 10^{-4}$ (Sinclair, 1987). This is far less than the 26% number cited as the PC. The reason for the discrepancy is that the PC starts from the fact that the person has leukaemia, or some other specific radiation-relatable disease, and looks backward in time to estimate the relative contribution of radiation versus all other causes lumped together (the spontaneous risk). This assumes that the individual is comparable to the 'general population', although in one tabulated case special attention is given to cigarette smoking as a potent identifiable predictor.

It is clear that caution has to be used in interpreting the above numbers. The fact that the PC is less in smokers than in non-smokers is not because radiation is less hazardous to smokers, but because their spontaneous risk is much higher, leaving less of a contribution for radiation. The hope had been that courts would be guided by these tables in adjudicating accidental and occupational exposures. It was expected that the 'more likely than not' notion would have been used by courts, and PCs greater than 50% attributed to radiation, and those at lesser levels would have been discounted. However, to date, the tabulated data have been used quixotically in the US. In one notable case in California, damage was awarded to a patient with lymphoma following a low-dose occupational exposure with a PC less than 1%. The court based its decision on the belief that the exposure, small as it was, had increased the probability of cancer, and since no other cause could be identified it was assumed to be radiation related, and damages were awarded (Shaffer, 1985).

Whether PCs are useful for their intended purpose remains to be demonstrated. Nonetheless, the tabulations do provide an excellent source of data on the relative sensitivity of different tumours as indicators of prior radiation exposure at different ages from low-LET exposures. This type of detailed information is not available in the usual tabulations of specific types of cancer observed following radiation exposure. Epidemiological studies which allege radiation as the cause of injury should be cast in doubt if based on enhanced occurrence of low-probability cancers in the presence of a diminished frequency of higher-probability cancers in the appropriate age, sex, dose and latent periods.

(c) Changing values of risk coefficients

Risk coefficients for various solid tumours are in the process of being adjusted upward, probably by factors of two to three. This is based on continuing follow-up of the A-bomb survivors which is now showing an increasing incidence of tumours in survivors who were in the younger age groups at time of exposure. Increased risk apparently awaited these individuals growing into the age groups at which those tumours are most frequently seen (Preston and Pierce, 1987).

The second reason for the increase is that there have been adjustments in the estimated radiation dose yields from the bombs, and the propagation of radiation as a function of distance. Further, it was previously believed that neutrons accounted for more of the Hiroshima exposures than is now believed, and hence the weighting factors on the γ-radiations has increased to account for the observed cancer incidence/mortality (Preston and Pierce, 1987; *Science*, 1987).

The third factor that has received attention in the discussions regarding revisions of risk factors is the increasing availability of incidence data from the A-bomb survivor studies. Since at least 50% of cancers are cured by modern medical therapy, it is clear that incidence rates are two times higher than mortality. Only in recent years have cancer registries been incorporated effectively into the A-bomb survivors follow-up studies. Thus, an increase in cancer risk coefficients which are based on incidence is a computational restatement of risk, and not a true increase in disease rates. Radiation-induced thyroid cancer is one of the more commonly induced cancers, usually papillary, a type that is rarely fatal. Thus, thyroid cancer appears in incidence statistics, but not in mortality data, and therefore the switch from mortality to incidence inherently would lead to an increase of greater than two in risk coefficients based on incidence data.

Lastly, lifetime risk projections require a completed follow-up for all individuals from birth to death. Since only 45 years have elapsed since the August 1945 A-bomb explosions in Hiroshima and Nagasaki, the youngest exposed persons have a number of years left to live, before their pattern of mortality will be known with certainty. In the case of leukaemia, the expression of increased risk was no longer evident after 1970, 25 years following exposure. For other conditions, beside bone cancer, the period of increased risk has not yet been completed and for some solid tumours the risk appears to increase in proportion to the natural risk observed at a given age (relative risk model). As the population ages, one then projects a continuing increase in radiation effect with time and this risk projection model leads to the highest estimated risk for this population (i.e. a 15-fold increase for some cancers according to Preston and Pierce, 1987).

Nonetheless, given the pattern of changes noted above, the National Radiation Protection Board (NRPB) in the UK now advocates revising occupational dose standards downward by a factor of three, i.e. from 5 rem to 1.5 rem per year (*Science*, 1987). It is a matter of history that radiation protection standards have been lowered sequentially over the years, not because of increased knowledge of radiation risk but because it was possible to do the same work with lower dose to workers, without unduly restricting the availability or quality of needed procedures (or societal benefits). The interpretation of the meaning of maximum permissible dose has also undergone recent revision. In the past, this was assumed to be an acceptable dose limit, whereas now it is taken as the upper limit of acceptable dose, and one is encouraged to strive to keep doses as low as reasonably achievable (ALARA).

A2.5 RISK AND PERCEPTION OF RISK

The risk of exposure to ionizing radiation has been assessed in a systematic way by scientists and physicians in intensive and extensive fundamental and applied research. More is known about radiation and its risks than any other agent known to impact on human health. Nonetheless, given the opportunity to rank the hazards of radiation and other life circumstances, the average person greatly overestimates the risk of ionizing radiations.

Many factors are likely to be responsible for risk perception. Among these are whether it is a risk to you as an individual, whether you anticipate a direct benefit, and whether it is risk which you accept voluntarily. Another is whether you understand and believe the magnitude of the risk as told to you. Third, you may accept the benefit of the particular exposure or circumstance leading to it, but be fearful of related processes, such as an association of things 'nuclear' with the threat of nuclear war or terrorist actions. It is not surprising that there is a widespread distrust of radiation, despite the many good things it affords.

Numerous sources document numerical comparisons between the risks of ionizing radiation and other life circumstances. A medical perspective is presented in Brill (1985), and the nuclear scientist perspective is documented in a book focusing on risk perception with respect to nuclear power (Cohen, 1983). Table A2.3 presents a listing of different life circumstances which carry a one in a million risk. Present data suggest that these risks are equal to the increase in cancer mortality risk during a lifetime following a single 10 mrem whole-body exposure.

Shortening of lifespan is an easily understood

Table. A2.3 One-in-a-million risks

	Risk	*Nature*
Existence		
Male, age 60	20 min	CVD[a] cancer
in New York	2 days	Air pollution
in Denver	2 months	Cosmic radiation
in stone building	2 months	Natural radioactivity
Miami water	1 year	Carcinogens
Near PVC plant	10 years	Carcinogens
Travel		
Canoe	6 min	Accident
Bicycle	10 miles	Accident
Car	300 miles	Accident
Airline	1000 miles	Accident
Airline	6000 miles	Cosmic radiation
Work		
Coal mine	1 h	Black lung
Coal mine	3 h	Accident
Typical factory	10 days	Accident
Miscellaneous		
Cigarettes	1.4	CVD[a] cancer
Wine	500 ml	Cirrhosis
Diet soda	30 cans	Carcinogens

[a] Cardiovascular disease.
From Brill (1985).

Table A2.4 Lifespan shortening associated with varying conditions

Condition	*Days*
Unmarried (male)	3500
Cigarette smoking (male)	2250
Heart disease	2100
30% overweight	1300
Cancer	980
Stroke	700
Motor vehicle accidents	207
Alcohol (US average)	130
Accidents in home	95
Average job (accidents)	74
Drowning	41
Job with radiation exposure	40
Illicit drugs (US average)	18
Natural radiation (Beir, 1972)	8
Medical X-rays	6
Diet drinks	2
Reactor accidents (UCS, 1977)	2[a]
Reactor accidents (Wash-1400, 1975)	0.02[a]
Smoke alarm in home	−10
Air bags in car	−50

[a] These items assume that all US power is nuclear. UCS is Union of Concerned Scientists, the most prominent group of nuclear critics.
From Brill (1985).

concept, and Table A2.4 presents a ranked listing of various conditions associated with lifespan shortening. There is a wide divergence (4000-fold difference) between the risks of cigarette smoking, and average annual medical radiation exposures (53 mrem per year). Accidents (motor vehicles, accidents in the home and in the workplace) are far more hazardous than medical diagnostic radiation procedures, and the normal operations of nuclear power plants (including nuclear waste disposal). Accidents do occur, and the accidents at TMI and Chernobyl have severely impacted on public attitudes toward nuclear power. The accident at Bhopal once again reminds us of the risks of accidents in non-nuclear areas, in this case involving chemicals. Such exposure can come from production plants, uses in agriculture and food processing, and waste disposal. The magnitude and severity of the health effects of the Bhopal accident have been compared to the effects of the Hiroshima A-bomb (Kurzman, 1987). The hazard of carcinogens from living for ten years near a PVC plant was cited in Table A2.3 as a one in a million risk. It is not clear that this number is greatly different from the Bhopal type of disaster, which makes one uneasy about the magnitude of such probability assignments. Large effects and low-event probabilities are hard to rank against better-known phenomena, and this no doubt influences public fears.

Statistical analyses, including factor analysis, have been applied to the risk perception problem and two factors were identified by Slovic (1987). He graphed and labelled the first factor, dread risk, defined at its high end (right side) by such expressions as lack of controllability, the dreadfulness of the event, the extent of its impact, and the inequitable distribution of risks and benefits (Figure A2.1). Nuclear weapons and nuclear power score highest on the characteristics that make up this factor. Factor 2 is plotted on the y axis, labelled as unknown risk, and at the high end lie hazards judged as unknown, unobservable, new, and delayed manifestations of harm. Smoking as a cause of disease lies at the centre of the diagram, as do the well-known hazards of Pb, Hg, DDT and coal exhausts. The largest concerns focus on the issues at the right end of the factor 1 scale, and appear to be independent of factor 2. This includes various nuclear-associated activities, along with nerve gas accidents, coal and uranium mining. The size of the dot encodes the attitudes toward regulation of each of the hazards. The larger the dot, the greater the desire for strict regulation to reduce risk. Again, radiation-associated phenomena receive the greatest concern. It is instructive to rank the cost of increased regulation per projected life saved in each circumstance. At present, the US Nuclear Regulatory Committee requires the expenditure of approximately 5 million dollars per life saved from low-level radioactive waste disposal, site design and management, whereas it is difficult to find societal approval for more than 10 000–100 000 dollars for medical therapies (renal dialysis or renovascular hypertension screening) or safety appliances (auto seat bags).

A2.6 SUMMARY

Radiation doses from diagnostic nuclear medicine procedures have decreased in recent years because of the increasing use of short-lived low-energy γ-emitting tracers. At the same time, increased use of tracers which enter into the intracellular space raises questions concerning the microscopic distribution of dose, particularly when tracers with significant Auger emissions, like ^{111}In, ^{125}I or ^{201}Tl are used. Additional information on mechanisms of carcinogenesis will

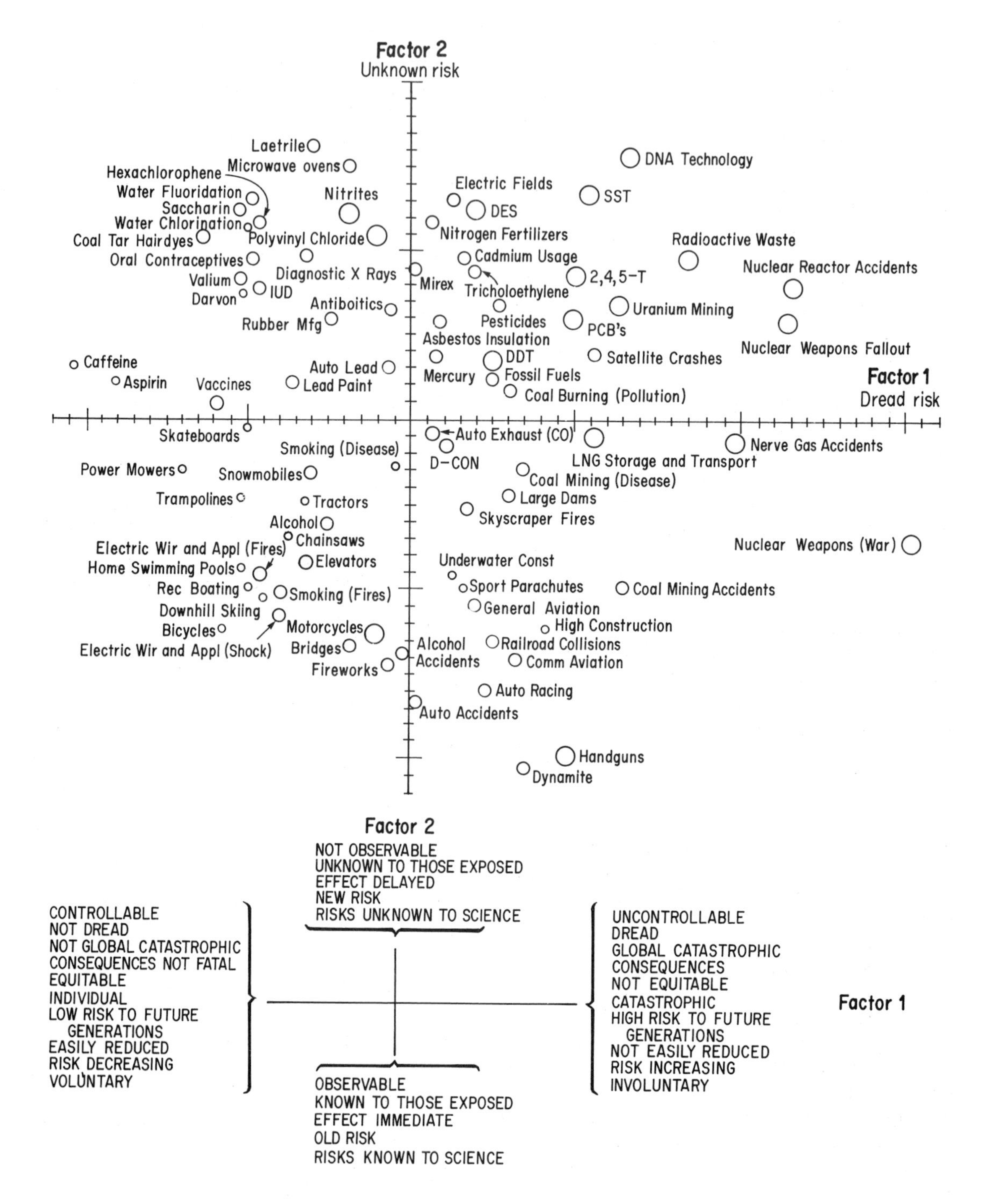

Figure A2.1 Location of 81 hazards on factors 1 and 2, based on the relationships among 18 risk characteristics. Each factor is made up of a combination of characteristics, as indicated in the lower diagram. The larger the circle, the greater the desire for strict regulation to reduce risk. (Modified from Slovic, 1987.)

be needed before risks of these procedures are likely to be understood. It is well recognized that the benefits derived from the administration of tracers in clinical nuclear medicine are far greater than the theoretical risks associated with the low doses used in diagnostic studies. Nonetheless, increasing estimates of radiation hazard are certain to be followed by heightened concern on the part of patients and regulatory agencies. It is important to realize that the increase in risk projections, based on linear extrapolations from A-bomb exposure data, fail to account for the big difference in dose rates, and that data are entirely lacking following low doses, such as received from diagnostic medical radiation procedures. Further, the major factor responsible for the increase in risk coefficients is not the new dosimetry, but is the high future risk projected for the youngest A-bomb survivors. If these projections turn out to be valid, then our long-established policies in medicine of minimizing radiation exposures to children will prove to have been prudent, and exposures delivered to the general population which involve significant exposures to children will have to be reconsidered.

In any case, continuing effort needs to be devoted toward the development of better targeting strategies to increase the target-to-background ratios to increase the quality of diagnostic judgements and to improve therapeutic results as well. This will include the development of new chemical compounds that enter into tissue-specific metabolic processes, improved tumour-specific monoclonal antibodies for improved diagnosis, and even more so for successful therapy, along with improvements in instrumentation, image analysis techniques, and diagnostic decision strategies that utilize available information optimally.

More information concerning the mechanism of radiation effects and repair is needed. This is primarily motivated by the hope that if one understands how radiation acts as a carcinogen we will then know how other carcinogens work, and be able to block the process at early stages by appropriate therapy. Along the way we will need to obtain better information on dosimetry of agents we use, at the macroscopic and microscopic levels.

Public perception of risk now focuses on nuclear power and other nuclear-related activities. The deletion of the term 'nuclear' from nuclear magnetic resonance imaging systems was motivated by the desire to avoid public misunderstanding about the word 'nuclear' if it were associated with the process. In retrospect, the inclusion of 'nuclear' in MRI designations would have afforded an opportunity to educate the public to better understand the nature of such phenomena. Such an opportunity could have been used to convey the minuscule or negligible risk associated with nuclear magnetic resonance, where the risk is from the magnetic and/or radiofrequency fields rather than from ionizing nuclear emissions, which are not part of the magnetic resonance process.

REFERENCES

Adelstein, S. J. (1987) Uncertainty and relative risks of radiation exposure. *JAMA*, **258**, 655–7.

BEIR (1980) *The Effects on Populations of Exposure of Low Levels of Ionizing Radiation*, National Academy Press, Washington DC.

BEIR (1988) *Health Risks of Radon and Other Internally Deposited Alpha-Emitters*, National Academy Press, Washington DC.

BEIR (1990) *Health Effects or Exposure to Low Levels of Ionizing Radiation*. BEIR V, National Academy Press, Washington DC.

Brill, A. B. (ed.) (1985) *Low-Level Radiation Effects: A Fact Book*, SNM Press, New York.

Brown, J. M. (1977) The shape of the dose–response curve for radiation carcinogenesis: extrapolation to low doses. *Radiat. Res.*, **71**, 34–50.

Cohen, B. L. (1983) *Before It's Too Late: A Scientists's Case for Nuclear Energy*. Plenum Press, New York.

Darby, S. C. Nakashima, E. and Kato, H. (1984) A parallel analysis of cancer mortality among atomic bomb survivors and patients with ankylosing spondylitis given X-ray therapy. *RERF Technical Report*, TR 4-84.

Doherty, P., Schwinger, R., King, M. and Gionet, M. (1986) Distribution and dosimetry of In-111 Labeled $F(ab')_2$ fragments in humans In *Fourth International Radiopharmaceutical Dosimetry Symposium: Dosimetry for Ultrashort-lived Radionuclides, Radiolabeled Blood Cells, Monoclonal Antibodies, Positron Emitters, Microdosimetry, Children, Fetus*, Oak Ridge, Nov. 5–8, 1985, CONF-851113, ORAU, pp. 464–76.

Epenetos, A. A. *et al.* (personal communication) Hammersmith Hospital, London.

Hickey, R. J., Bowers, E. E. and Clelland, R. C. (1983) Radiation hormesis, public health and public policy. *Health Phys.*, **44**, 207–19.

Hnatowich, D. *et al.* University of Massachusetts Medical Center, Worcester, MA.

Hubner, K. F. and Fry, S. A. (1980) *The Medical Basis for Radiation Accident Preparedness*, Elsevier/North-Holland, Amsterdam.

ICRP (1977) *Recommendations of the International Commission on Radiation Protection*, Publication 26.

Johansson, L., Mattson, S. and Nosslin, B. (personal

communication) Effective dose equivalent from radiopharmaceuticals.

Kase, K. R., Bjarngard, B. E. and Attix, F. H. (eds) (1987) *The Dosimetry of Ionizing Radiations*, Academic Press, London.

Kereiakes, J. G. and Rosenstein, M. (1980) *Handbook of Radiation Doses in Nuclear Medicine and Diagnostic X-ray*. CRC Press,

Kurzman, D. (1987) *A Killing Wind: Inside Union Carbide and the Bhopal Catastrophy*, McGraw Hill, New York.

Lam, G. K. Y. (1988) On the general validity of linear summation of dose equivalents for mixed radiation. *Health Phys.*, **54**, 57–61.

McEwan, A. J., Shapiro, B., Sisson, J. C. *et al.* (1985) Radio-iodobenzylguanidine for the scintigraphic location and therapy of adrenergic tumors. *Sem. Nucl. Med.*, **15**, 132–53.

MIRD. Medical Internal Radiation Dose Committee, Society of Nuclear Medicine. (Publishes data on decay scheme for tracers used in nuclear medicine, tables of computational factors needed for dose analyses, guidance on accepted analytic methodology, and periodic reports of dosimetry analyses for particular radiopharmaceuticals.)

NAS (1984) *Assigned Share for Radiation as a Cause of Cancer. Review of Radioepidemiologic Tables Assigning Probabilities of Causation. Oversight on Radioepidemiologic Tables*, National Academy of Sciences Press.

NCRP 45 (1975) *Natural Background in the United States.*

NCRP 70 (1982) *Nuclear Medicine: Factors Influencing the Choice and Use of Radionuclides in Diagnosis and Therapy.*

NCRP 91 (1987) *Recommendations on Limits For Exposure to Ionizing Radiation.*

NCRP 93 (1987) *Ionizing Radiation Exposure of the Population of the United States.*

NIH 85. *Report of the National Institutes of Health. Ad Hoc Working Group to Develop Radioepidemiological Tables.* NIH Publication No. 85–2748.

Patterson, M. C. Bech-Hansen, N. T., Smith, P. J. and Mulvihill, J. J. (1984) in *Radiation Carcinogenesis: Epidemiology and Biological Significance* (eds J. D. Boice Jr and J. F. Fraumeni, Jr) Raven Press. New York.

Preston, D. L. and Pierce, D. A. (1976) *The Effect of Changes in Dosimetry on Cancer Mortality Risk Estimates in the Atomic Bomb Survivors*, RERF Technical Report, TR 9-87.

Regan, J. D. and Setlow, R. B. (1976) in *Biology of Radiation Carcinogenesis* (eds J. M. Yuhas and J. D. Regan), Raven Press, New York.

RERF (1987) *US–Japan Joint Reassessment of Atomic Bomb Radiation Dosimetry in Hiroshima and Nagasaki, Final Report, 1987*, available from RERF Office, NRC, Washington DC.

Schull, W. J., Otake, M. and Neel, J. V. (1987) *A Reappraisal of the Genetic Effects of the Atomic Bombs. Summary of a 34 year Study*, RERF Technical Report, TR 7-81.

Science (1987) **236**, 1649–51.

Science Radiation Limits, News and Comment (1987) **236**, 1349.

Shaffer, W. G. (1985) Law review: letter to editor. *Health Phys.*

Sinclair, W. (1987) Risk, research, and radiation protection: Failla memorial lecture. *Radiat. Res.*, **112**, 191–216.

Slovic, P. (1987) Perception of risk. *Science*, **236**, 280–5.

Absorbed radiation in patients: a memorandum for the ethical committee

K. E. Britton

A2.7 INTRODUCTION

Radiation is a natural phenomenon. The current method of measuring absorbed radiation is the effective dose equivalent in units called millisieverts (mSv). This allows different types of radiation from different sources, X-rays, γ-rays, cosmic rays etc., to be compared. Normal exposure in London is about 0.15 mSv per month, including that from our bodies. The computed risk of death from 0.1 mSv is one in a million which is the same risk as smoking one and a half cigarettes in a lifetime or drinking half a litre of wine in a life time, or indeed that risk of death for a man aged 42 living for a day or a man aged 60 living for 20 min (Brill, 1985).

A2.8 PERCEPTION OF RISK

The popular perception of radiation risk is much greater than in fact it is. Studies in the USA of league of women voters and college students put the risk of nuclear power first and business and professional club members put the risk at eighth of a list of 30 agents, whereas in fact it was 20th (the risk was 1500 times less than average cigarette smoking, 1000 times less than average alcohol consumption, 500 times less than motor vehicle driving, 30 times less than swimming and 10 times less than bicycling (Brill, 1985). The lifespan shortening on a population basis associated with medical X-rays is 6 days, of which the nuclear medicine contribution is 4 h, as compared with: natural background radiation 8 days; accidents in the home 95 days; accidents at work 74 days; heart disease 2100 days as examples (Brill, 1990).

A2.9 ICRP

The International Commission on Radiation Protection (ICRP) has defined annual limits for the absorbed radiation to be received by various populations (ICRP, 1977/8). The level of exposure for pregnant women should be less than 0.5 mSv, for members of the public less than 5 mSv (and preferably no more than 1 mSv) and for occupationally exposed workers less than 50 mSv (natural background is 1.87 mSv per year). Typical diagnostic studies and their effective dose equivalents are given in Table A2.5 (Shrimpton and Wall, 1986; DHSS, 1988; Sheilds *et al.*, 1987).

It is normal nuclear medicine practice to relate the absorbed radiation dose from the nuclear medicine procedure to that of the same organ undergoing an X-ray procedure, partly because many patients are familiar with X-ray studies of the organ about which they are concerned and partly because it serves as a familiar frame of reference to the referring clinician. It is usually not appropriate to relate absorbed radiation dose to that of a chest X-ray since for a chest X-ray, depending upon the machinery used, it varies from 0.01 to 0.1 mSv.

The risks from the injection of contrast media and radiopharmaceuticals are shown in Table A2.6. It can be seen that the risks from the radiation involved for diagnostic X-ray and nuclear medicine studies are much less than those from the pharmaceutical preparation itself. Given this information, the question is how to get over the very low risk associated with diagnostic X-ray and nuclear medicine procedures to the public with an exaggerated perception of risk from radiation.

Lord Rothschild gave in his Reith lectures a statement that only if a risk was greater than 1 in 2000 was it a risk worth worrying about and radiation risks are much below this level (Table A2.5).

A2.10 PREGNANCY AND RADIATION

The radiation sensitivity of the fertilized ovum is of the same order as that of the unfertilized ovum, so that the so-called ten-day rule (that studies of the lower abdomen involving the use of X-rays should be limited to the first ten days after the start of the last menstrual period) was never radiobiologically sound (Mole, 1987) and not directly applicable to nuclear medicine procedures (Longmead *et al.*, 1983).

Women of child-bearing age who are pregnant are most sensitive to radiation during the period of fetal organogenesis between seven and 17 weeks of pregnancy, at which time most women know that they are pregnant. No pregnant patients should be considered for a research study and any patient who was uncertain as to whether or not she was pregnant should not normally be considered for a research study involving the diagnostic use of radiation. However, the effective dose equivalent of 0.5 mSv absorbed radiation in any women of reproductive age who turned out subsequently to be pregnant would give a 1:100 000 risk of damage to the fetus and 5 mSv a 1:10 000 risk as compared to the current risk of congenital abnormality in a delivered baby of about 1:40. The legal requirements set out in the Ionising Radiations Regulations 1987 is that the dose limit for the abdomen of a women of reproductive capacity 'shall be 13 mSv in any consecutive three-month interval', and for the abdomen of a pregnant women 'shall be 10 mSv during the declared term of pregnancy' (Ionising Radiation Regulations, 1987).

A2.11 CONSENT FORMS

It is proposed that for investigations involving an absorbed radiation dose of less than 5 mSv the phrase in consent form is:

> The study involves administration of (X-rays) (a tiny amount of radioactivity) at a level considered to be of negligible risk for members of the public by the International Commission on Radiation Protection.

Table A2.5 Effective dose equivalents

Test	*Activity (MBq)*	*Absorbed dose (mSv)*	*Risk*
Chest X-ray	–	0.01–0.1	Less than 1 per million
Renography (^{123}I)	12	0.4	
Lung ventilation (Tc)	80	0.6	
Thoracic spine	–	0.8	
Thyroid imaging (Tc)	80	1.0	Less than 1 per 100 000
Plain X-ray, abdomen	–	1.0	
Lung perfusion (Tc)	100	1.0	
Liver scan (Tc)	80	1.0	
Annual natural background		1.87	
Lumbar spine X-ray	–	2.0	
Renal radionuclide study (Tc)	400	2.0–3.8	
Bone scan (Tc)	400	4.0	
Barium meal	–	4.2	
Kidney X-ray	–	4.5	
Dynamic cardiac imaging (Tc)	800	5.6	
Thallium cardiac scan	75	7.0	
Barium enema	–	7.7	
X-ray computed tomography		2–10	Less than 1 per 10 000
Coronary angiography		10–20	Less than 1 per 5000

Table A2.6 Risks of contrast material and radiopharmaceuticals

Material	*Risk*	*Reference*
Death from routinely used water-soluble intravenous X-ray contrast material	1 in 40 000	Ansell *et al.* (1984)
Reaction to routinely used water-soluble intravenous contrast material	1 in 15 1 in 6	Ansell *et al.* (1984) Panto *et al.* (1986)
Reaction to radiopharmaceutical injections	1 in 2500	Keeling and Sampson (1975a)
Reaction to penicillin	1 in 10	Keeling and Sampson (1975b)

and for 5–15 mSv:

> The study involves administration of (X-rays) (a small amount of radioactivity) at a level considered to be of negligible risk for workers in the field of radiation by the International Commission on Radiation Protection.

In the text of a submission to the Ethical Committee, it is proposed that the effective dose equivalent in millisieverts should be stated for each study which involves the diagnostic use of X-rays or of a nuclear medicine procedure.

A2.12 RADIATION HORMONES

Current absorbed radiation dose assessment is based on the assumption that all radiation, however low, represents a risk and that no radiation represents no risk. Such an argument would not apply to any other physical environment affecting human beings. Indeed there is experimental evidence of the beneficial effects of low-level radiation in animals and plants on longevity and fecundity, even ignoring the supposed benefits of radon-containing hot-spring spa water. This beneficial effect is called radiation hormesis and the prestigious radiation protection journal *Health Physics* has devoted a special issue to this subject (Radiation hormesis, 1987).

A2.13 CONCLUSION

Radiation is a natural phenomenon with disadvantages and benefits to man. The principle is to keep diagnostic medical radiation exposures as low as reasonably practicable consistent with achieving a diagnostic result of good quality. This is best defined as the absorbed dose in millisieverts where 1 mSv exposure carries a risk of 17 in one million. The risks of radiation used diagnostically are generally negligible as compared to the risks from the administration of standard medicines and from invasive or operative procedures.

REFERENCES

Ansell, G. *et al.* (1984) *Br. J. Radiol.*, **57**, 548 (abstr.).

Brill, A. R. (1985) *Low Level Radiation Effects: A Fact Book*, Society of Nuclear Medicine, New York.

DHSS (1988) Notes for guidance on the administration of radioactive substances to persons for purposes of diagnosis, treatment or research, Administration of Radioactive Substances Advisory Committee, Department of Health and Social Security, Alexander Fleming House, London, pp. 1–32.

ICRP (1977/8) Recommendations of the International Commission on Radiological Protection, ICRP Publication 26, *Ann. ICRP* 1977, **1**, No. 3; *Ann. ICRP*, 1978, **2**, No. 3.

Ionising Radiation Regulations (1987) Health and Safety 1985, No. 1333, HMSO, London, p. 36.

Keeling, D. H. and Sampson, C. B. (1975a) *Br. J. Radiol.*, **57**, 1091–6.

Keeling, D. H. and Sampson, C. B. (1975b) *Drug Ther. Bull.*, **13**, 9.

Longmead, W. A., Crown, V. P. D., Jewkes, R. J. *et al.* (1983) *Radiation Protection of the Patient in Nuclear Medicine: A Manual of Good Practice*, Oxford Medical Publications, Oxford, pp. 79–83.

Mole, R. H. (1987) The so called 10-day rule. *Lancet*, **ii**, 1138–40.

Panto, P. N. and Davies, P. (1986) *Br. J. Radiol.*, **59**, 41–4.

Radiation hormesis. *Health Phys.*, **52**, 517–680.

Sheilds, R. A. and Lawson, R. S. (1987) Effective dose equivalent. *Nucl. Med. Commun.*, **8**, 851–85.

Shrimpton, P. C. and Wall, B. F. (1986) Doses to patients from medical radiological examinations in Great Britain. *Rad. Prot. Bull.*, **7**, 10–14.

APPENDIX THREE

Quantitative analysis in clinical nuclear medicine

H. D. Royal and B. J. McNeil

A3.1 INTRODUCTION

Clinicians who are either enthralled by numbers or who are somewhat in awe of them frequently fail to be sufficiently critical of tests with numerical outputs. They assume that such tests have a value or accuracy higher than do tests which have only subjective or qualitative outputs. While this situation is sometimes the case, it is clearly not always the case. In this chapter on quantitative nuclear medicine, we shall focus first on objective measurements of regional physiology and secondly on measurements of the efficacy of diagnotic tests. In both sections we shall try to emphasize basic principles, the likely effects of errors in analysis and the extent to which mathematical approximations provide accurate answers to clinical problems. Since this chapter provides only an introduction to these quantitative techniques, the interested reader is encouraged to consult other more detailed sources which are listed in the references.

A3.2 QUANTITATIVE TRACER STUDIES

Although nuclear medicine has its origins in utilizing basic radiotracer principles to study non-invasively a variety of physiology processes, the clinical specialty has consisted primarily of subjectively evaluated static images in which changes in structure are often as important as changes in function. Two forces are now at work to mould clinical nuclear medicine into a more quantitative, more physiological, more dynamic specialty. Firstly, for the first time in nuclear medicine's short history, sophisticated digital data acquisition and analysis capabilities are becoming widely available in clinical units. The impetus for rapid dissemination of digital capabilities has come from nuclear cardiology and from high-technology developments which have made sophisticad data analysis systems available at a reasonable cost. Secondly, improvements in spatial resolution of other non-invasive modalities (computed tomography and ultrasound) are re-directing nuclear medicine to exploit its unique capability for studying regional pathophysiology. In this climate, quantitative physiological studies will surely flourish; therefore the need for radiologists and nuclear medicine physicians to become aware of the fundamentals of quantitative tracer studies is more acute than ever.

The examples of quantitative clinical studies which will be presented in subsequent sections have been chosen for a variety of reasons. The cerebrospinal fluid shunt flow study has limited application; however, its simplicity as a quantitative model is attractive for didactic purposes. An understanding of physical, biological and effective half-lives is essential in any quantitative study; therefore these have been discussed. Measurement of glomerular filtration rate provides an example of a quantitative *non-imaging* physiological test. Regional blood flow has many potential clinical applications although it has until now been primarily a research tool. Cardiac output and transit time determination undoubtedly will be routinely obtained as nuclear cardiology becomes more refined. Finally, more sophisticated methods of data analysis such as deconvolution are likely to be widely applied in the future.

Although the details of each section of this half of the chapter differ, the reader should recognize the similarity of approach in each section. When faced with the task of determining a quantitative solution to a problem, the following approach should be taken. First, define the assumptions upon which the solution to the problem is based. Secondly, assess how accurately each assumption is met in reality. Thirdly, test the technique in a broad spectrum of patients to determine what limitations might exist.

A3.2.1 CEREBROSPINAL FLUID (CSF) SHUNT FLOW

Measurement of CSF flow through ventriculoperitoneal or ventriculovenous shunts in patients with non-communicating hydrocephalus is useful in differentiating disease progression from shunt failure (Rudd *et al.*, 1973; Harbert, Haddad and McCullough, 1974). To perform this study, 500 μCi of pertechnetate in a small volume (<0.1 ml) are rapidly injected into the reservoir of the one-way valve of the shunt appliance. Sequential digital images are then acquired at a rate of 12 frames min^{-1} for 5 min using a pinhole or parallel-hole collimator and a gamma camera interfaced to a minicomputer. An activity-time curve is generated using an operator-defined region of interest over the reservoir (see Fig. A3.1).

Shunt flow (ml min^{-1}) can be measured with this system if the effective volume of the reservoir is known and if two assumptions are made (see Fig. A3.2). First, there is instantaneous, uniform mixing of the tracer within the reservoir. Secondly, the volume of the reservoir is constant, and, therefore, flow into and out of the reservoir are equal. Under these conditions, the change in the tracer activity of the reservoir during any small time interval is equal to the flow times the tracer activity of the reservoir divided by the effective volume of the reservoir, all times the time interval. That is:

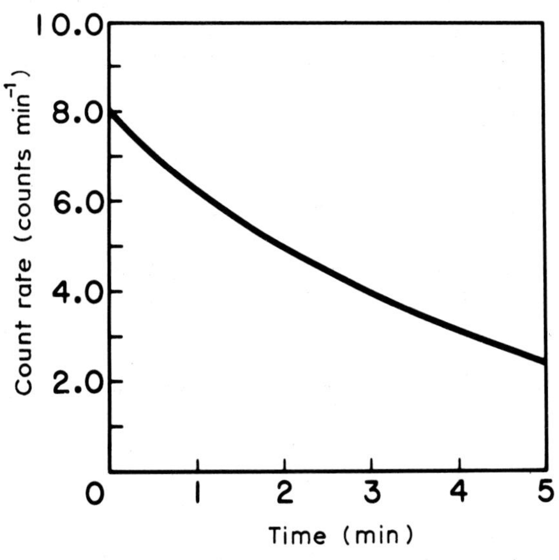

Figure A3.1 Measurement of CSF shunt flow. An activity–time curve obtained from a region of interest over a shunt reservoir is shown. The ordinate is the count rate recorded by the scintillation camera and the abscissa is time. Both scales are linear, and a mono-exponential curve is seen. This curve becomes a straight line when plotted on a semi-logarithmic graph (see Figure A3.3).

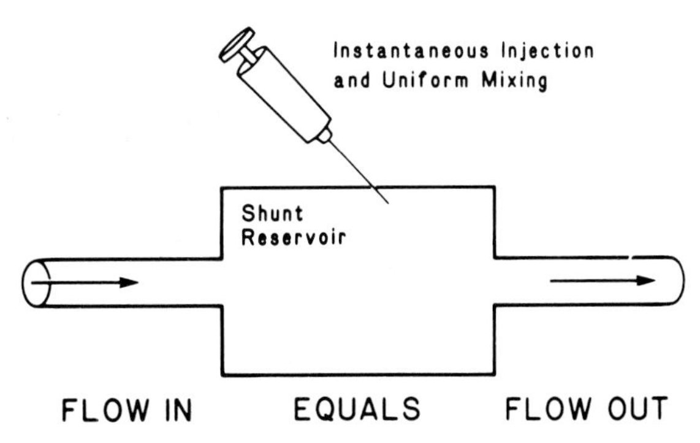

Figure A3.2 Assumptions underlying CSF flow calculation. This diagram shows schematically a shunt reservoir with an entrance (Flow in) from the ventricles and an exit (Flow out), first into the shunt tubing and ultimately into the peritoneum. The injection site for the radiotracer is also illustrated. Calculation of CSF shunt flow assumes that there is instantaneous injection and uniform mixing of the tracer and also that flow into and out of the reservoir are equal. The latter implies that the volume of the reservoir is constant.

$$\Delta Q(t) = -F\frac{Q(t)}{V}\Delta t \qquad \text{(A3.1)}$$

where

$Q(t)$ = tracer activity of the reservoir (mCi)
$\Delta Q(t)$ = the change in the tracer activity in the reservoir at time t (mCi)
F = CSF shunt flow (ml min^{-1})
V = effective volume of the reservoir (ml)
Δt = a small time interval (min).

The minus sign indicates that tracer is lost from the reservoir system.

Since the change in activity of tracer in the reservoir is equal to the change in concentration times the volume, equation (A3.1) can be rewritten in terms of concentration

$$\Delta Q(t) = -\Delta C(t)V = -FC(t)\Delta t \qquad \text{(A3.2)}$$

where

$C(t)$ = tracer concentration of the reservoir (mCi ml^{-1})

$\Delta C(t)$ = the change in tracer concentration of the reservoir at time t (mCi ml^{-1})

If Δt approaches 0, equation (A3.2) can be rearranged and written in differential form as

$$\frac{dC(t)}{C(t)} = -\frac{F}{V}dt \quad (A3.3)$$

Integration results in

$$\int_0^t \frac{dC(t)}{C(t)} = -\int_0^t \frac{F}{V}dt \quad (A3.4)$$

The solution to equation (20.4) can be found in standard tables of solutions to integrals and is

$$\ln C(t) \Big|_0^t = -\frac{F}{V}t \Big|_0 \quad (A3.5)$$

Substituting the limits of the integral into equation (A3.5) and simplifying, yields

$$\ln C(t) = -\frac{F}{V}t + \ln C(0) \quad (A3.6)$$

Since equation (20.6) has the form of a linear equation, a graph of the logarithm of the concentration against time produces a straight line with a slope of F/V and an intercept of $C(0)$ (see Fig. A3.3). The slope of the straight line can be calculated using a least squares fit; therefore, since the effective reservoir volume, V, can be determined experimentally, CSF shunt flow, F, can be calculated from

$$F = -\text{slope} \times V \quad (A3.7)$$

Equation (A3.6) is sometimes expressed in exponential form

$$C(t) = C(0)e^{(-F/V)t} \quad (A3.8)$$

Even in this simple example of quantitative analysis, the critical reader will appreciate that the assumptions upon which the analysis was based are not strictly met. For example, flow through the reservoir is more likely to be pulsatile than constant; there may not be instantaneous uniform mixing; and the injection of even a small volume of tracer will cause a transient increase in flow. Moreover, in the more elaborate shunt appliances, eddy currents and turbulence may make the *effective* reservoir volume differ from the *physical* reservoir volume. Despite these differences between the model and the actual situation, this technique has been found to be clinically useful (Rudd *et al.*, 1973; Harbert, Haddard and McCullough, 1974).

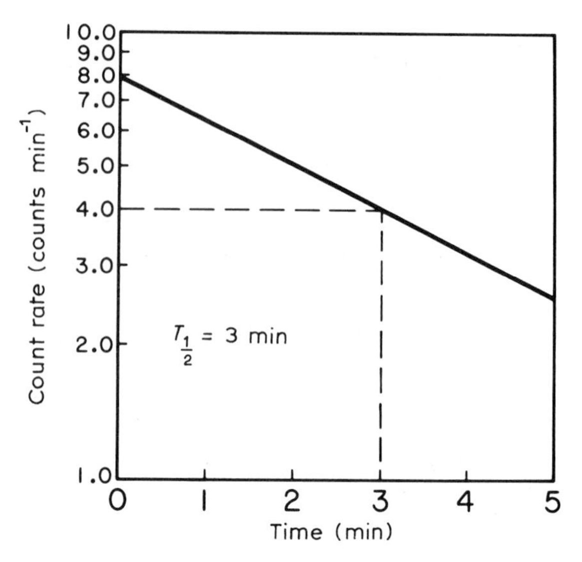

Figure A3.3 Calculation of CSF flow from data presented in Fig. A3.1. The ordinate is the activity recorded on a logarithmic scale and the abscissa is time (min). If the volume of the reservoir is known, the slope of the resulting straight line can be used to calculate CSF flow. CSF shunt flow (F) equals the slope times the effective volume (V) of the reservoir. For a Holter valve with an effective volume of 0.18 ml, the flow is 0.042 ml min^{-1}; this is within the range of normal.

CSF shunt flow determination

F = (Slope) (V)

$$\text{Slope} = \frac{0.693}{T_{\frac{1}{2}}} = \frac{0.693}{3\ \text{min}} = 0.231\ \text{min}^{-1}$$

V = 0.18ml

F = (0.231 min^{-1}) (0.18 ml) = 0.042 ml min^{-1}

A3.2.2 HALF-LIVES

Quantitative analysis of CSF shunt flow described in the previous section is an example of *first-order kinetics* where the rate of change of a substance is directly proportional to the quantity of substance present. That is

$$\frac{dQ(t)}{dt} = kQ(t) \quad (A3.9)$$

where

$Q(t)$ = the quantity of substance present at time t (mCi)

$\frac{dQ(t)}{dt}$ = instantaneous rate of change of $Q(t)$ ($mCi\ s^{-1}$)

k = proportionality constant (s^{-1})

Many physical processes demonstrate the first-order kinetics described by equation (20.9). For example, the rate of radionuclide decay is directly proportional to the number of atoms present, that is

$$\frac{dN(t)}{dt} = -kN(t) \quad \text{(A3.10)}$$

where

$N(t)$ = number of atoms present at time t (atoms)

$\frac{dN(t)}{dt}$ = the decay rate (atoms s^{-1})

k = decay constant (s^{-1})

Integration and simplification, analogues to equations (A3.3–6) and (A3.8) results in

$$N(t) = N(0)e^{-kt} \quad \text{(A3.11)}$$

where $N(0)$ = initial number of atoms. Since the physical half-life of a radionuclide is well known, equation (20.11) is more useful when k is expressed in terms of physical half-life ($T_{\frac{1}{2}p}$). By definition

$$\frac{N(0)}{N(T_{\frac{1}{2}p})} = \frac{1}{0.5} = 2 = \frac{N(0)}{N(0)e^{-k(T_{\frac{1}{2}})}} = \frac{1}{e^{-k(T_{\frac{1}{2}})}} \quad \text{(A3.12)}$$

Thus, k is defined in terms of $T_{\frac{1}{2}p}$ by taking the natural logarithm of equation (A2.12) and rearranging

$$k = \frac{-\ln 2}{T_{\frac{1}{2}p}} = \frac{-0.693}{T_{\frac{1}{2}p}} \quad \text{(A3.13)}$$

In biological systems, the disappearance of a tracer is often the result of both its physical decay and its biological clearance (see Fig. A3.4). If the biological clearance follows first-order kinetics, the effective or observed clearance of the tracer will be equal to the sum of the amount cleared biologically and that lost by physical decay

$$\frac{dQ(t)}{dt} = \frac{-\ln 2}{T_{\frac{1}{2}p}} Q(t) + \frac{-\ln 2}{T_{\frac{1}{2}b}} Q(t) \quad \text{(A3.14)}$$

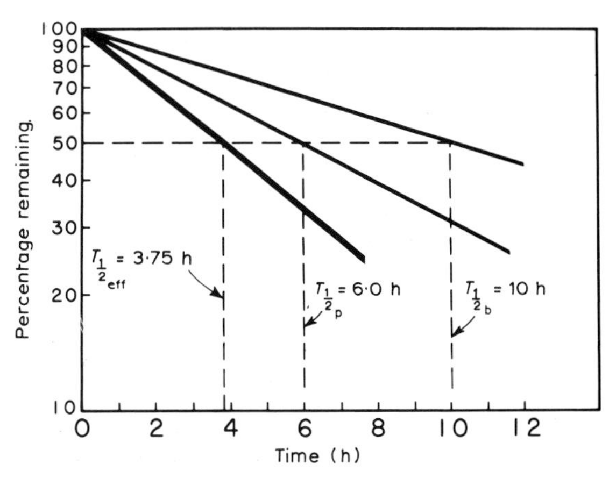

Figure A3.4 Effective ($T_{\frac{1}{2}eff}$), physical ($T_{\frac{1}{2}p}$) and biological half-lives ($T_{\frac{1}{2}b}$). In this graph, the percentages of radionuclide remaining if only physical decay or biological clearance was considered are plotted as the light lines. The heavy black line indicates the actual percentage remaining assuming that both physical decay and biological clearance occur. Typically the physical half-life is known and the effective half-life is measured. Biological half-life is then calculated. As shown in the sample calculations, any of the half-lives can be calculated if the other two are known.

Half-life determination

$$T_{\frac{1}{2}eff} = \frac{T_{\frac{1}{2}p} \times T_{\frac{1}{2}b}}{T_{\frac{1}{2}p} + T_{\frac{1}{2}b}} = \frac{(10h)96h)}{10\,h + 6\,h} = 3.75\,h$$

$$T_{\frac{1}{2}b} = \frac{T_{\frac{1}{2}p} \times T_{\frac{1}{2}eff}}{T_{\frac{1}{2}p} - T_{\frac{1}{2}eff}} = \frac{(6.0\,h)\,(3.75\,h)}{6.0\,h - 3.75\,h} = 10\,h$$

$$T_{\frac{1}{2}p} = \frac{T_{\frac{1}{2}b} \times T_{\frac{1}{2}eff}}{T_{\frac{1}{2}b} - T_{\frac{1}{2}eff}} = \frac{(10\,h)\,(3.75\,h)}{10\,h - 3.75\,h} = 6\,h$$

where

$Q(t)$ = quantity at time t (mCi)

$\frac{dQ(t)}{dt}$ = *total* rate of loss of activity ($mCis^{-1}$)

$T_{\frac{1}{2}p}$ = physical half-life (s)

$T_{\frac{1}{2}b}$ = biological half-life (s)

Collected terms yields

$$\frac{dQ(t)}{dt} = -\left(\frac{\ln 2}{T_{\frac{1}{2}p}} + \frac{\ln 2}{T_{\frac{1}{2}b}}\right)Q(t) \quad \text{(A3.15)}$$

By definition, the effective clearance rate is equal to the sum of the biological and physical clearance rates

$$\frac{\ln 2}{T_{\frac{1}{2}eff}} = \frac{\ln 2}{T_{\frac{1}{2}b}} + \frac{\ln 2}{T_{\frac{1}{2}p}} \quad \text{(A3.16)}$$

where

$T_{\frac{1}{2}\text{eff}}$ = effective half-life (s).

Simplifying equation (A3.16) yields

$$T_{\frac{1}{2}\text{eff}} = \frac{T_{\frac{1}{2}\text{b}} \times T_{\frac{1}{2}\text{p}}}{T_{\frac{1}{2}\text{b}} + T_{\frac{1}{2}\text{p}}} \qquad \text{(A3.17)}$$

Since the physical half-life is usually known and the effective half-life is usually measured, equation (A3.17) can be written in terms of the unknown biological half-life

$$T_{\frac{1}{2}\text{b}} = \frac{T_{\frac{1}{2}\text{p}} \times t_{\frac{1}{2}\text{eff}}}{T_{\frac{1}{2}\text{p}} + T_{\frac{1}{2}\text{eff}}} \qquad \text{(A3.18)}$$

A3.2.3 GLOMERULAR FILTRATION RATE

Although the clinical usefulness of measuring glomerula filtration rate (GFR) is widely accepted, the existence of multiple methodologies to measure GFR (for example, 24-h endogenous creatinine clearance, inulin clearance, radiotracer clearance) indicates that each one has limitations. One commonly used radiotracer method is based on Sapirstein's mode (Sapirstein, Vidt, Mandel and Hanusek, 1955) to measure GFR after a single intravenous injection of non-radioactive creatinine. The simplified method discussed here requires three hourly venous blood samples beginning 2 h after a single intravenous injection of a suitable radiopharmaceutical. Although controversy exists regarding the radiopharmaceutical of choice for this study, the ideal radiotracer would have the following four characteristics: (a) no loss of the tracer due to in-vivo metabolism; (b) no protein binding of the tracer preventing free filtration by the glomerulus; (c) small molecular size; (d) no secretion or absorption of the radiotracer by the renal tubular cell.

Sapirstein's model of GFR measurement is based on five assumptions. First, the tracer mixed instantly and uniformly in the intravascular space. Secondly, the tracer mixed uniformly in the extravascular space. Thirdly, the volumes of the intra- and extravascular spaces are constant. Fourthly, the rate of loss from the intravascular compartment due to GFR is equal to the glomerular filtration rate times the concentration in the intravascular space. Finally, the tracer diffusion rate between the intravascular and extravascular space varies directly with the difference in tracer concentration in these areas. These assumptions are schematically illustrated in Fig. A3.5.

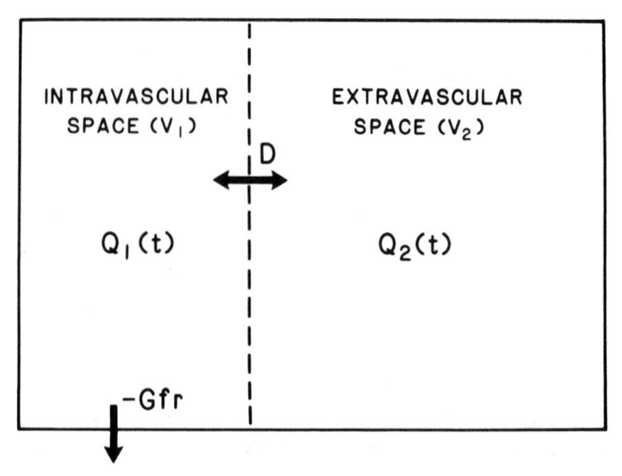

Figure A3.5 Sapirstein's model for measurement of glomerular filtration rate. This model assumes instantaneous intravascular injection with uniform mixing within the intravascular (V_1) and extravascular (V_2) space. The rate of transfer of the tracer between spaces equals the difference between the concentrations in two spaces times the diffusion constant (D) (equation (A3.20)). The rate of tracer loss due to glomerular filtration equals the intravascular concentration of tracer times the glomerular filtration rate (GFR) (equation (A3.19)).

The assumption that the rate of tracer loss due to GFR is equal to the intravascular tracer concentration times the GFR can be stated mathematically

$$\left(\frac{dQ_1(t)}{dt}\right)_{\text{GFR}} = \text{GFR}C_1(t) \qquad \text{(A3.19)}$$

where

$\left(\frac{dQ_1(t)}{dt}\right)_{\text{GFR}}$ = the rate of tracer loss from the intravascular space due to GFR at time t (mCi min^{-1})

GFR = glomerular filtration rate (ml min^{-1})

$C_1(t)$ = intravascular tracer concentration at time t (mCi min^{-1})

Likewise, the assumption that the rate of tracer loss due to diffusion is equal to the diffusion constant time the intravascular and extravascular tracer concentration differences can be stated mathematically

$$\left(\frac{dQ_1(t)}{dt}\right)_{\text{Diff}} = -D(C_1(t) - C_2(t)) \qquad \text{(A3.20)}$$

where $\left(\frac{dQ_1(t)}{dt}\right)_{Diff}$ = rate of loss of tracer from the intravascular compartment due to diffusion at time t (mCi min^{-1})

D = Diffusion constant (ml min^{-1})

$C_2(t)$ = extravascular tracer concentration at time t (mCi ml^{-1})

Furthermore, the left sides of equations (A3.19) and (A3.20) can be expressed in terms of changes in concentration since the change in quantity of a substance is equal to the change in concentration times the volume of distribution

$$\left(\frac{dQ_1(t)}{dt}\right)_{GFR} = V_1\left(\frac{dC_1(t)}{dt}\right)_{GFR} \quad (A3.21)$$

where V_1 = the intravascular volume (ml)

$\frac{dC_1(t)}{dt}_{GFR}$ = rate of change in concentration due to GFR (mCi $ml^{-1}s^{-1}$)

An analogous relationship exists for changes due to diffusion,

$$\left(\frac{dQ_1(t)}{dt}\right)_{Diff}$$

Therefore, equations (A3.19) and (A3.20) can now be rewritten solely in terms of concentration

$$\left(\frac{dC_1(t)}{dt}\right)_{GFR} = \frac{-GFR}{V_1}C_1(t) \quad (A3.22)$$

and

$$\left(\frac{dC_1(t)}{dt}\right)_{Diff} = \frac{-D}{V_1}(C_1(t) - C_2(t)) \quad (A3.23)$$

Since the total rate of change in concentration of tracer equals the sum of the rate of change due to GFR and to diffusion, the following equation emerges

$$\left(\frac{dC_1(t)}{dt}\right)_{Total} = \left(\frac{dC_1(t)}{dt}\right)_{GFR} + \left(\frac{dC_1(t)}{dt}\right)_{Diff} = \frac{-GFR}{V_1}C_1(t) - \frac{D}{V}(C_1(t) - C_2(t)) \quad (A3.24)$$

The equation is not practical to work with since it contains the term $C_2(t)$ which represents the concentration of the tracer in the extravascular space. Since this value cannot be measured clinically, some mathematical manipulations of equation (A3.24) are needed to eliminate this term. The interested reader is referred to Sapirstein *et al.* (1955), Bianchi (1972) and Morgan, Birks and Singer (1977) for a full derivation which bridges the gap between equation (A3.24) and the following equation which states that the concentration in the intravascular compartment is equal to the sum of two monoexponentials

$$C_1(t) = A_1e^{\alpha_1 t} + A_2e^{\alpha_2 t} \quad (A3.25)$$

where

A_1 = effective initial concentration for diffusion (mCi ml^{-1})

α_1 = effective transfer rate for diffusion (min^{-1})

A_2 = effective initial concentration for GFR (mCi ml^{-1})

α_2 = effective transfer rate for GFR (min^{-1})

The logarithm of equation (A3.25) shown below, is used to calculate GFR since it is the simplest form of the equation

$$\ln C_1(t) = \ln A_1 + \alpha_1 t + \ln A_2 = \alpha_2 t \quad (A3.26)$$

As shown in Fig. A3.6 equation (A3.26) is in the form of the sum of two linear equations. The initial rapid decrease in the intravascular tracer concentration is due to the rapid diffusion of the tracer from the intravascular space to the extravascular space. Once the extravascular tracer concentration approximately equals the intravascular concentration (point P), loss of tracer from the intravascular compartment is due solely to glomerular filtration. Analogous to the calculation of F/V in the GSF shunt flow study

$$\alpha_2 = \frac{GFR}{V_{eff}} \quad (A3.27)$$

where

α_2 = slope of the slow component shown in Figure (A3.5) (min^{-1})

V_{eff} = effective volume of distribution (ml)

α_2 can be calculated using a least squares fit through the data points after point P. The effective volume of distribution can be calculated from the extrapolated y-intercept, A_2, the effective initial concentration, since the effective volume of dis-

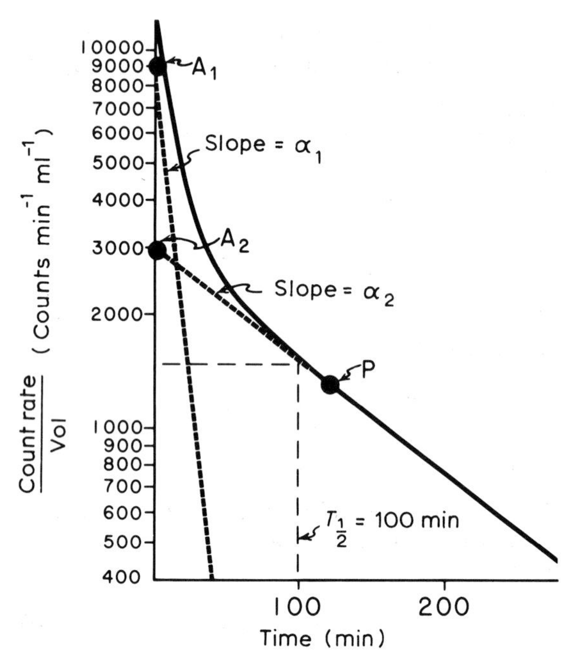

Figure A3.6 Calculation of GFR. GFR is calculated by determining the slope (α_2) and Y intercept (A_2) of the slow component of the blood clearance curve following a single injection of an appropriate radiopharmaceutical. After point P (usually 2 h after injection) the effects of the fast component on the blood clearance curve are negligible; therefore the slope of the slow component can be determined using a semi-logarithmic plot of the concentration–time curve. Extrapolation of this curve identifies A_2 as the Y intercept. The amount of activity injected (I) is determined by measuring the counts g^{-1} of a diluted standard multiplied by the actual number of grams of the injectate and the dilution factor.

GFR determination

$$\text{GFR} = \left(\frac{I}{A_2}\right)\left(\alpha_2\right)$$

$$\alpha_2 = \frac{0.693}{T_{\frac{1}{2}}} = \frac{0.693}{100\ \text{min}} = 0.00693\ \text{min}^{-1}$$

$$\text{I} = 45\,000\,000\ \text{counts min}^{-1}$$

$$A_2 = 3000\ \text{counts min}^{-1}\ \text{ml}^{-1}$$

$$\text{GFR} = \frac{45\,000\,000\ \text{counts min}^{-1}}{3000\ \text{cts min}^{-1}\text{ml}^{-1}}(0.00693\ \text{min}^{-1})$$

$$= 104\ \text{ml min}^{-1}$$

tribution equals the injected dose divided by the effective initial concentration, that is

$$V_{\text{eff}} = \frac{I}{A_2} \qquad \text{(A3.28)}$$

where

V_{eff} = effective volume of distribution (ml)
I = dose injected (mCi)
A_2 = effective initial concentration (mCiml^{-1})

Substituting equation (A3.28) into equation (A3.27) and rearranging yields

$$\text{GFR} = \frac{I}{A_2}\alpha_2 \qquad \text{(A3.29)}$$

Routine clinical use of this technique is promising; however, two obstacles must be overcome. Firstly, the accuracy of this method in patients with moderate to severe renal failure who had expanded extravascular spaces needs further validation. Secondly, an easily prepared chemically stable radiopharmaceutical which meets the previously described criteria for an optimal GFR agent for all pathological states is needed.

A3.2.4 REGIONAL BLOOD FLOW

The measurement of regional blood flow is based on principles similar to the ones used for calculation of CSF shunt flow. The main difference between the two techniques is the type of tracer used – diffusible in the case of blood flow measurement and non-diffusible in the case of shunt flow measurements (Fig. A3.7). Regional blood flow is measured after the intra-arterial injection of a poorly soluble gas such as ^{133}Xe, which does not recirculate because of rapid elimination by the lungs (Kety, 1951). The injection is frequently given as part of a contrast angiogram; to avoid the effects of contrast on blood flow, a delay of 30–40 min between the injection of contrast agent and Xe is common.

Measurement of regional blood flow using this technique is based on four assumptions. Firstly, instantaneous injection of the tracer into the organ; secondly, instantaneous equilibrium between blood and tissue; thirdly, no recirculation of tracer; and fourthly, an accurate measurement of organ concentration by external monitoring.

Under these conditions, the regional rate of tracer loss at time t, is equal to the regional blood

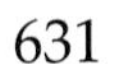

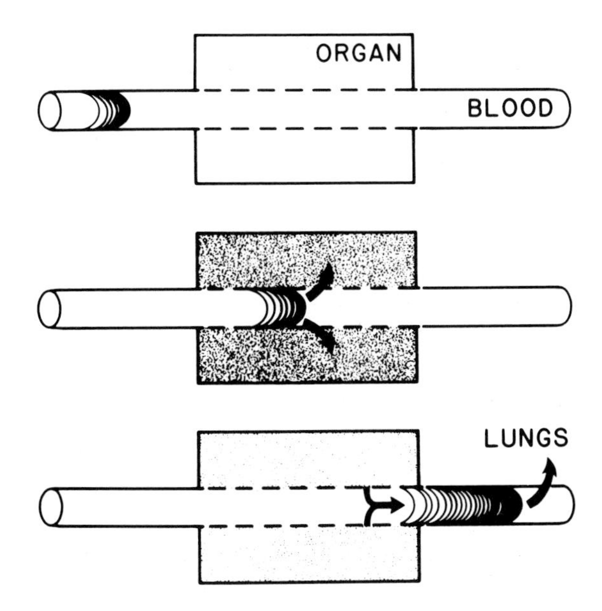

Figure A3.7 Assumptions underlying regional blood flow measurement. (a) Instantaneous injection of the diffusible radioactive tracer into the arterial blood supply of the organ of interest. (b) Rapid diffusion of the tracer into the organ during the first passage of the bolus of radioactivity. (c) Washout of the tracer from the organ into the veins. Note that recirculation of the tracer is prevented by elimination through the lungs.

flow times the regional concentration of the tracer in the venous blood, that is

$$\frac{dQ(t)}{dt} = -FC_v(t) \qquad \text{(A3.30)}$$

where

$Q(t)$ = regional amount of tracer (mCi)

$\frac{dQ(t)}{dt}$ = the regional rate of loss of the tracer ($mCi\ s^{-1}$)

F = regional blood flow ($ml\ s^{-1}$)

$C_v(t)$ = concentration of tracer within the venous blood ($mCi\ ml^{-1}$)

Since external monitoring measures organ concentration (assumption 4), not venous concentration, equation (A3.30) must be expressed in terms of organ concentrations. Venous blood-organ concentrations are related in the following manner

$$\lambda = \frac{C_o(t)}{C_v(t)} \qquad \text{(A3.31)}$$

where λ = blood/organ partition coefficient
$C_o(t)$ = organ tracer concentration ($mCi\ mg^{-1}$)

In addition, the organ tracer concentration equals the quantity of tracer, $Q(t)$, in the organ divided by the organ weight, W; thereore equation (A3.30) can be rewritten

$$\frac{dQ(t)}{dt} = -F\frac{Q(t)}{W\lambda} \qquad \text{(A3.32)}$$

This can be re-expressed in a form analogous to equation (A3.6)

$$\ln Q(t) = \frac{-F}{W\lambda}t + \ln Q(0) \qquad \text{(A3.33)}$$

where $Q(0)$ = initial organ activity (mCi)

A plot of the logarithm of activity against time yields a single straight line with a slope of $-F/W\lambda$. Thus

$$\frac{F}{W} = -\lambda \times \text{slope} \qquad \text{(A3.34)}$$

Equation (A3.34) applies to regional organ flow for organs with homogeneous blood flow. Generally, however, organs are more complex and consist of several types of tissues, each with their own characteristic blood flow. In the brain (Hoedt-Rasmussen, Aveisdotter and Lasser, 1966), for example, a plot of activity against time does *not* yield a single straight line. Rather, a biexponential curve results (Fig. A3.8). This occurs because of differences in blood flow between grey and white matter. Grey matter has a high blood flow (78.0–80.5 ml min^{-1} per 100 g tissue) which causes a rapid washout of the tracer. White matter has a lower blood flow (18.7–21.1 ml min^{-1} per 100 g) and hence a slower washout. These two components can be separated mathematically either by simple curve stripping or by a more complicated procedure using a non-linear least squares fit (Dell, Sciacca, Lieberman, Case and Cannon, 1973).

An alternative mathematical approach to the measurement of regional systemic blood flow using washout has been proposed by Zierler (1965). It is based on the principle that over all time, the change in the amount of tracer, dQ(t), must equal the efferent flow times the efferent concentration, that is

$$\int_0^\infty dQ(t) = -\int_0^\infty FC_v(t)dt \qquad \text{(A3.35)}$$

Equation (A3.35) is identical to equation (A3.30), except that integration has been per-

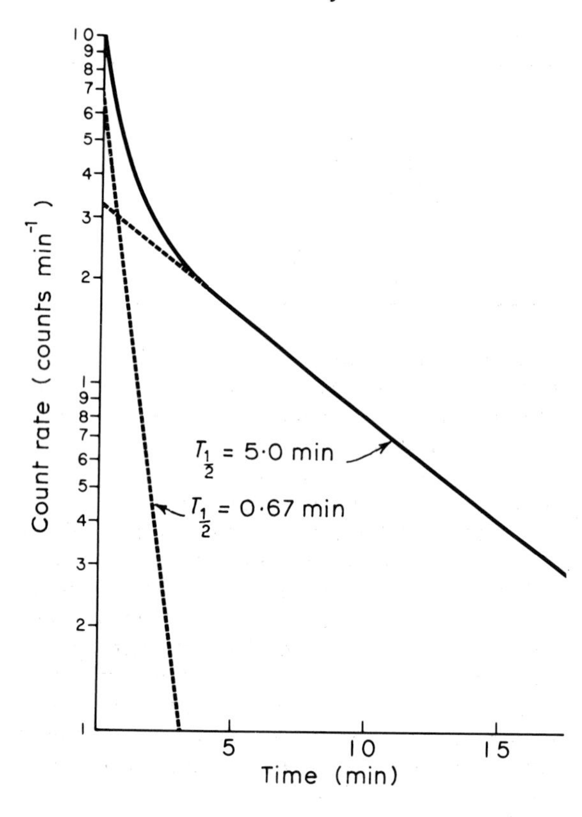

Figure A3.8 Typical brain washout curve after an internal carotid injection of ^{133}Xe. The count rate–time curve representing washout of activity from the brain following an intra-arterial injection of radioactive xenon is plotted on a semi-logarithmic graph. Two components representing blood flow to the white and grey matter are apparent. The relative blood flow can be determined from the slopes of the two components of the washout curve if the blood/tissue partition coefficients are known. These blood/tissue partition coefficients can be determined experimentally and tables containing their values are available. Blood flow is customarily determined per 100 g of tissue.

Regional blood flow determining (slope method)
$F/W = (-\lambda)$ (Slope)
Grey matter

$$\lambda = 0.77 \frac{\text{ml}}{\text{g grey matter}}$$

$$\text{Slope} = \frac{-0.693}{T_{\frac{1}{2}}} = \frac{0.693}{0.67 \text{ min}} = 1.03 \text{ min}^{-1}$$

$$F/W = 0.77 \frac{\text{ml}}{\text{g grey matter}} (1.03 \text{ min}^{-1})$$

$$(100 \text{ g grey matter})$$

$$= 79.3 \text{ ml min}^{-1}$$

White matter

$$\lambda = 1.44 \frac{\text{ml}}{\text{g white matter}}$$

$$\text{Slope} = \frac{-0.693}{T_{\frac{1}{2}}} = \frac{0.693}{5.0 \text{ min}} = 0.139 \text{ min}^{-1}$$

$$F/W = 1.44 \frac{\text{ml}}{\text{g white matter}} (0.139 \text{ min}^{-1})$$

$$= (100 \text{ g grey matter})$$

$$= 20.0 \text{ ml min}^{-1}$$

formed. Substituting $(1/(\lambda Q)/Q(t)$ for $C_v(t)$ (see equation (A3.31)) and rearranging terms, yields

$$\int_0^{\infty} \mathrm{d}Q = \frac{-F}{\lambda W} \int_0^{\infty} Q(t)\mathrm{d}t \qquad \text{(A3.36)}$$

Solving the integration of the left-hand side of equation (A3.36) yields

$$Q(0) = \frac{F}{\lambda W} \int_0^{\infty} Q(t)\mathrm{d}t \qquad \text{(A3.37)}$$

Rearrangement yields equation (20.38) which expresses relative flow (F/W) in terms of the measured variables, $Q(0)$ and $\int_0^{\infty} Q(t)\mathrm{d}t$

$$\frac{F}{W} = \frac{Q(0)}{\int_0^{\infty} Q(t)\mathrm{d}t} = \frac{\lambda H}{A} \qquad \text{(A3.38)}$$

where

H = height ($Q(0)$) of the washout curve

A = area ($\int Q(t)\mathrm{d}t$) under the washout curve from t equals 0 to ∞.

The tissue blood coefficient (λ) can be determined experimentally.

The height of the washout curve is proportional to $Q(0)$ and the area under the washout curve is proportional to $\int_0^{\infty} Q(t)\mathrm{d}t$. Since the same detector geometry is used to measure both, relative flow (F/W) is equal to the blood tissue coefficient (λ) times the height of the washout curve divided by its area. In Fig. A3.9 shows component of the washout curve from Fig. A3.8 ($T_{\frac{1}{2}}$ = 5.0 min) has been replotted on a linear graph. The height over area method yields the same relative flow as was obtained using the slope method.

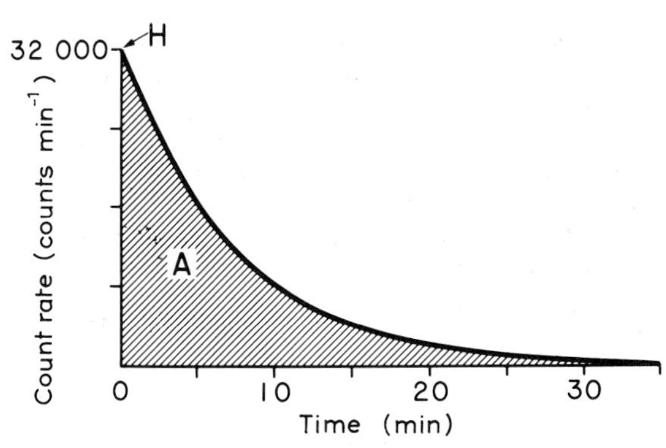

Figure A3.9 Regional blood flow determination (height/area method). The slow component from the biexponential curve obtained in Fig. 14.8 is plotted here on linear paper. Note that the same relative flow which was obtained using the slope method in Fig. A3.8 is obtained using the height over area method. Regional blood flow determination (height/area method)

$$F/W = (\lambda)\ \frac{H}{A}$$

$$\lambda = 1.44\ \frac{\text{ml}}{\text{g white matter}}$$

$$H = 32\,000 \text{ counts min}^{-1}$$

$$A = 229\,200 \text{ counts}$$

$$F/W = \left(1.44\ \frac{\text{ml}}{\text{g white matter}}\right)\left(\frac{32\,000 \text{ counts min}^{-1}}{229\,000 \text{ counts}}\right)(100 \text{ g white matter})$$

$$= 20.0 \text{ ml min}^{-1}$$

A3.2.5 CARDIAC OUTPUT

During the past several years, cardiovascular nuclear medicine has grown dramatically. See also chapter 1. An important index of cardiac function, cardiac output, can be obtained non-invasively in conjunction with a first-pass radionuclide angiocardiogram performed alone or performed prior to grated equilibrium cardiovascular studies. In fact, if cardiac output, ejection fraction, mean transit time (see the next section) and total blood volume are known, all of the cardiac indices listed in Table A3.1 can be determined non-invasively.

Two problems need to be solved, however, before the simultaneous radionuclide measurement of cardiac output and ejection fraction is widespread. Firstly, a ^{99m}Tc-labelled radiopharmaceutical which can be used for both of these measurements is needed. In-vitro labelled red cells prepared with the Brookhaven kit currently come closest to meeting this need. Secondly, externally monitored activity-time curves must accurately reflect intravascular concentration-time curves. Problems related to detector geometry and deadtime at high count rates with an Anger camera need to be resolved.

Table A3.1

Measured
Cardiac Output
Ejection Fraction
Mean Pulmonary Transit Time
Total Blood Volume
Derived
End Diastolic Volume
End Systolic Volume
Pulmonary Blood Volume

Cardiac output determinations are based on the principle of conservation of mass (Donato *et al.*, 1962a, b; Lewis, Guintini, Donato, Harvey and Cournand, 1962; Kaikka, Timisjarvi and Tuominen, 1979). If a non-diffusible, non-metabolizable tracer is used, the amount of tracer entering the heart must equal the amount of tracer leaving the heart. The amount of tracer entering the heart is equal to the total amount of the tracer injected. The amount of tracer leaving the heart region of interest in any small time interval is equal to the concentration of the tracer at that time times the cardiac output times the time interval. The *total* amount leaving the heart is equal to the sum of all the amounts that left during all of the small time intervals. Mathematically

$$Q = \Sigma FkC(t)\Delta T \qquad \text{(A3.39)}$$

where

Q = the total amount of tracer injected (mCi)
F = cardiac output (ml min^{-1})
k = proportionality constant to convert counts min^{-1} to mCi ml^{-1}

$$\left(\frac{\text{mCi}}{\text{ml}} \Big/ \frac{\text{counts}}{\text{min}}\right)$$

$C(t)$ = externally monitored count rate of the tracer leaving heart region of interest at time t (counts min^{-1})
Δt = small time interval (min)

As Δt approaches 0, equation (A3.39) can be integrated

$$Q = Fk\int_0^\infty C(t)\mathrm{d}t \qquad \text{(A3.40)}$$

Estimation of cardiac output requires knowledge of the proportionality constant k. This is difficult to measure since it changes with each patient and with each detector. However, if equilibrium measurements are made using the same detector geometry used to measure concentration changes, then the following relationship exists

$$Q = kC_{eq}V \qquad (A3.41)$$

where

C_{eq} = count rate at equilibrium in the heart region of interest (counts min^{-1})
V = total blood volume (ml).

Substituting equation (A3.41) into (A3.40), simplifying and rearranging leads to the elimination of k in the final expression. Thus

$$F = \frac{C_{eq}V}{\int_0^\infty C(t)dt} \qquad (A3.42)$$

The total blood volume can be determined by simple dilution principles if the red cells have been labelled *in vitro* with high efficiency.

The use of equation (A3.42) in measured cardiac output is described in Fig. A3.10. In this example 15 mCi of Tc-labelled red cells were injected (Q). A blood sample obtained at equilibrium contained 3 $\mu Ci\ ml^{-1}$; therefore, the total blood volume (V) was 5000 cm^3. To calculate cardiac output the equilibrium concentration, C_{eq}, and the area under the activity–time curve are needed. The curve has two peaks representing the passage of the bolus through the right and left side of the heart (see Fig. A3.10). When corrections for background and recirculation were made by extrapolating to zero, the area was found to be 130 000 counts-s. The count rate at equilibrium, C_{eq}, was determined several minutes after the injection of the tracer using the same region of interest and without moving the patient. In performing this technique, it is important to note that the gamma camera must have a linear response over a severalfold range in count rates (that is, 2000–18 000 counts s^{-1}) if accurate results are to be obtained. Excessive deadtime will result in underestimation of the denominator of equation (A3.42) and therefore will overestimate cardiac output.

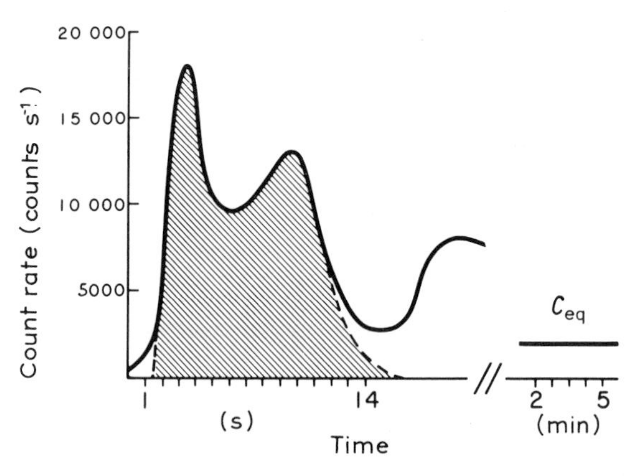

Figure A3.10 Cardiac output determination. The count rate–time curve from a region of interest of the heart is plotted. The crosshatched area under the curve is a graphic representation of the area under the curve when the upslope and downslope have been extraplated to zero. The total blood volume (V) is calculated from simple dilution principles. Since the injected dose (Q) contains several thousand times the amount of activity as the equilibrium sample (E), an aliquot of the injected dose is usually carefully diluted one thousandfold to assure a linear response of the well counter. Once total blood volume is known, cardiac output can be determined by measuring the count rate at equilibrium (C_{eq}) and the area under the count rate–time curve. In order to eliminate the effects of background and recirculation the count rate–time curve must be extrapolated to zero.

Cardiac output determination

$$F = \frac{(C_{eq})(V)}{\int_0^\infty C(t)dt}$$

$$V = \frac{Q}{E} = \frac{15\ mCi}{3\mu Ci\ ml^{-1}} = 5000\ ml$$

$$C_{eq} = (2000\ counts\ s^{-1})(60\ s\ min^{-1})$$
$$= 120\,000\ counts\ min^{-1}$$

$$\int_0^\infty C(t)dt = 130\,000\ counts$$

$$F = \frac{(120\,000\ counts\ min^{-1})(5000\ ml)}{(130\,000\ counts)}$$
$$= 4615\ ml\ min^{-1}$$

A3.2.6 TRANSIT TIMES

The current popularity of first-pass radionuclide angiocardiography has stimulated interest in transit times because they can be used to estimate pulmonary blood volume. The calculation of transit times can be understood if the flow of a nondiffusible radioactive marker travelling with a velocity, v, through a pipe of length, L, and an area, A, is considered (Fig. A3.11) (McNeil, Holman and Adelstein, 1976). If the quantity of

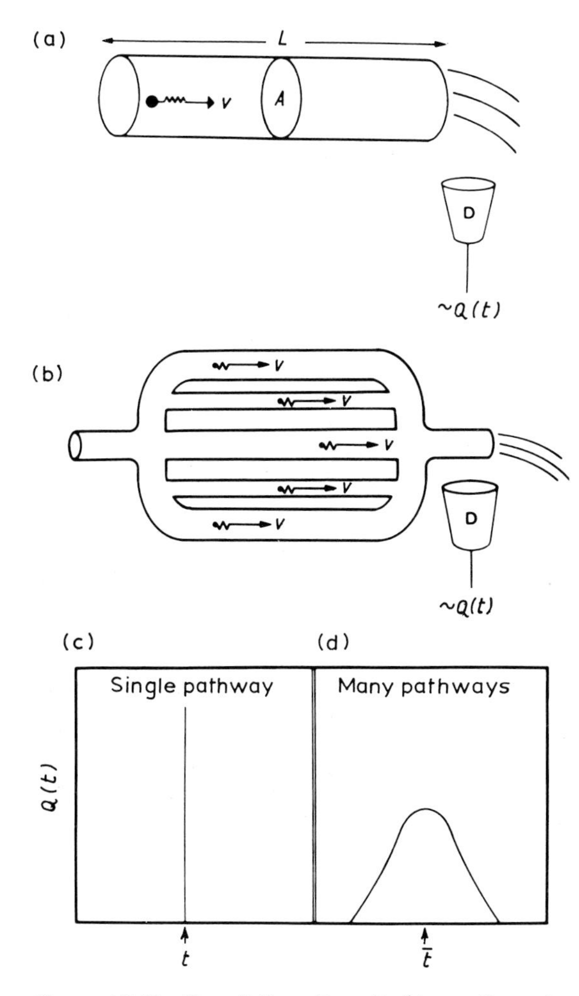

Figure A3.11 Transit time. Transit of tracer through a single pathway (a) yields a single transit time, t (c). Transit of tracer through many pathways (b) yields a mean transit time, t (d). (Reprinted with permission from *Diagnostic Nuclear Medicine* edited by Alexander Gottschalk and E. J. Potchen, MD, Williams and Wilkins Company, Baltimore.)

nuclide appearing at the exit is monitored as a function of time, no activity is registered at the exit while the marker is in the pipe; once the tracer leaves the pipe, counts are registered. The time to transverse the system from entrance to exit is the transit time (Fig. A3.11c).

Because flow, F, can be related to velocity by

$$F = vA \tag{A3.43}$$

where

F = flow of the tracer (mls^{-1})
v = velocity of flow (cm s^{-1})
A = cross-sectional area of the pipe (cm^2)

and because $v = L/t$ (A3.44)
where L = length of the pipe (cm)
t = transit time (s)

$$F = \frac{LA}{t} = \frac{V}{t} \tag{A3.45}$$

where V = volume (ml)

and, on rearranging,

$$t = \frac{V}{F} \tag{A3.46}$$

The transit time, t, then equals the volume of the pipe divided by its flow. This generality applies to all intravascular (non-diffusible) indicators.

For real systems the situation is more complex because several paths through the conduit are possible (Fig. A3.11b). In such cases, a distribution of counts against time is expected at the exit (Fig. A3.11d); those tracer molecules appearing at earlier times will have traversed a shorter total path length than those appearing at later times. Thus, there is no single transit time but rather many transit times with a mean transit time, $\bar{t}$. located at the centre of gravity of the activity–time plot. Mean transit time is equal to the integral of the activity at time t times the time divided by the integral of the acitivity–time curve

$$\bar{t} = \frac{\int_0^\infty Q(t)t\mathrm{d}t}{\int_0^\infty Q(t)\mathrm{d}t} \tag{A3.47}$$

where

$\bar{t}$ = mean transit time
$Q(t)$ = activity at time t (mCi)
t = time from the initial input of activity (s)

Equation (A3.47) is called the first moment of the activity–time curve.

An example of the calculation of mean pulmonary transit time is shown in Fig. A3.12. A time activity plot from a region of interest over the lungs is obtained. The upslope and downslope of the pulmonary curve must be extrapolated to zero activity to eliminate the effects of background and recirculation and, thus, obtain a finite value from the integral of the curve, Typically, the extrapolation of the upstroke is linear, whereas the extrapolation of the downslope is monoexponential. Once this extrapolation has been

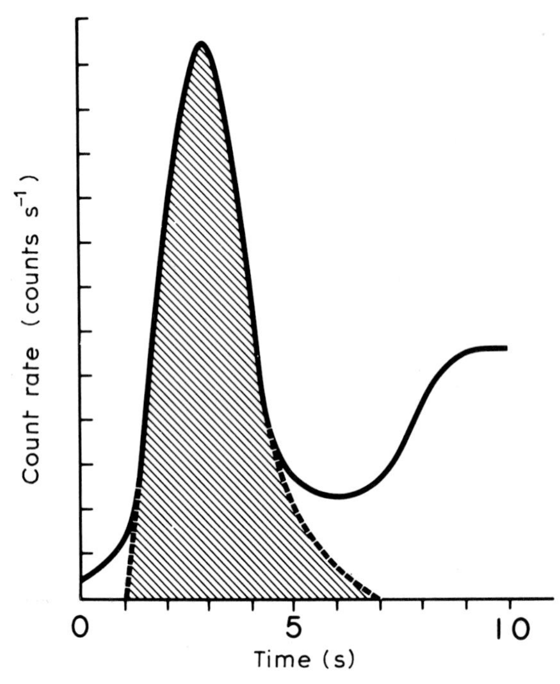

Figure A3.12 Calculation of mean pulmonary transit time. A count rate–time curve is obtained over the lungs after a bolus injection of radiotracer. The activity–time curve is extrapolated to zero to eliminate the effects of background and recirculation (dashed curve). The crosshatched area graphically represents the integral of the extrapolated count rate–time curve. The integrals in equation (A3.47) are calculated from this extrapolated curve and are used to determine mean pulmonary transit time.

Mean pulmonary transit time determination

$$\text{MPTT} = \frac{\int_0^\infty Q(t)t\,dt}{\int_0^\infty Q(t)\,dt}$$

$$\int_0^\infty Q(t)t\,dt = 180\,000 \text{ counts s}^{-1}$$

$$\int_0^\infty Q(t)\,dt = 30\,000 \text{ counts}$$

$$t = \frac{180\,000 \text{ counts s}^{-1}}{30\,000 \text{ counts}} = 6 \text{ s}$$

performed, mean transit time can be calculated using equation A3.47.

Furthermore, as implied in equation (A3.46), pulmonary blood volume can be calculated if pulmonary flood flow and mean transit time are known. Mathematically, pulmonary blood volume equals pulmonary blood flow times mean pulmonary transit time. In patients without shunts, pulmonary blood flow equals cardiac output; therefore

$$V_p = F\bar{t}_p \qquad \text{(A3.48)}$$

where V_p = pulmonary blood volume (ml)
F = cardiac output (mls^{-1})
$\bar{t}_p$ = mean pulmonary transit time (min)

Since cardiac output and mean pulmonary transit time can be calculated using first-pass radionuclide angiocardiography, an estimate of pulmonary blood volume, which may be useful in evaluation of left ventricular failure, can also be obtained.

An alternative approach to the measurement of mean transit time has been proposed, analogous to that described in the measurement of regional blood flow (Zierler, 1965). It states that

$$\bar{t} = \frac{A}{\lambda\sigma H} \qquad \text{(A3.49)}$$

where

A = area under the washout curve
H = initial height of washout curve
λ = the blood/tissue partition coefficient
σ = tissue density, which for most tissues is approximately 1. Therefore, equation (A3.49) can be simplified to

$$\bar{t} = \frac{A}{\lambda H} \qquad \text{(A3.50)}$$

The concept of transit time has been confused because two other indices which can easily be calculated have been popularized. In addition to mean transit time, peak-to-peak transit time and mean pool transit time are routinely calculated by one major manufacturer's software for first-pass radionuclide angiocardiograms. Although these two indices are *proportional* to mean pulmonary transit time, the proportionality constant is unknown; therefore, the desired measurement of pulmonary blood volume cannot be made.

Measurement of peak-to-peak transit time is illustrated in Fig. A3.13. For this purpose, activity–time curves from right and left ventricular regions of interest are superimposed. The peak-to-peak transit time is equal to the difference in the times that peak activity is in the right and left ventricles.

Calculation of the mean pool transit time is slightly more complex than calculation of peak-to-peak transit time. This index measures the difference between the time when the maximum activity enters and the time when it leaves the

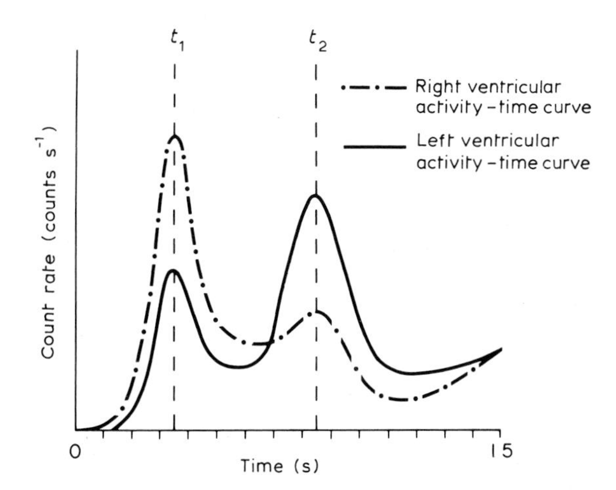

Figure A3.13 Peak-to-peak transit time (T). The dashed curve represents activity–time curve from a region of interest over the right heart. The solid curve represents an activity–time curve from a region of interest over the left heart. The peak to peak transit time is calculated by subtracting the time that peak activity occurs in the right ventricle (t_1) from the time that peak activity occurs in the left ventricle (t_2). These times are determined from right (_._.) and left (—) ventricular activity-time curves following a bolus injection of a radiotracer.

Peak to peak transit time determination

$$T = t_2 - t_1 = 8.5\,\text{s} - 3.5\,\text{s} = 5.0\,\text{s}$$

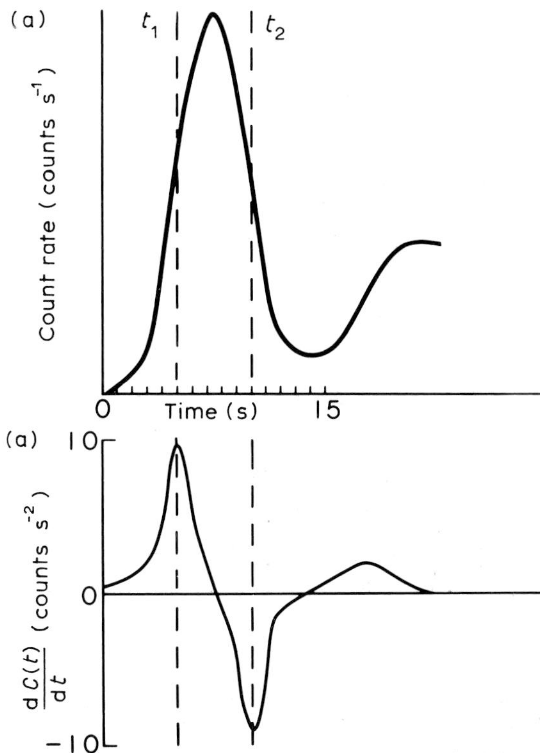

Figure A3.14 Mean pulmonary pool transit time. Curve A represents an activity–time curve from a region of interest over the lungs. Curve b represents the first derivative of curve a. Mean pulmonary transit time equals the difference between the time when the maximum activity enters (t_1) and leaves the lung. Since the first derivative (curve b) corresponds to the instantaneous slope of the pulmonary activity–time curve (curve a), the times of maximum upslope and downslope can be easily calculated from the peaks and valleys of the first derivative.

Mean pulmonary pool transit time determination

$$T = t_2 - t_1$$
$$T = 10\,\text{s} - 5\,\text{s} = 5\,\text{s}$$

region. The upper curve in Fig. A3.14 is the pulmonary activity–time curve; the lower curve is the first derivative of the upper curve. The pool transit time is equal to the difference between the time of maximum upslope and maximum downslope. Since the first derivative (the lower curve) corresponds to the instantaneous slope of the upper curve, the times of maximum upslope and maximum downslope of the upper curve can easily be calculated from the peaks and valleys of the lower curve.

A3.2.7 CONVOLUTION AND DECONVOLUTION

Although convolution and deconvolution analysis has been widely applied in many quantitative fields, these techniques have only recently been utilized in the analysis of cardiac (Alderson *et al.*, 1979) and renal radiotracer studies (Kenny, Ackery, Fleming, Goddard and Grant, 1975; Diffey, Hall and Corfield, 1976). In all dynamic studies, observed organ activity–time curves depend not only on the organ function (the organ response) but also on the manner in which the tracer arrives in the organ (the input function). Deconvolution analysis eliminates the effects of the input function and, therefore, allows more accurate investigation of organ response.

To understand this analysis, let us first look at the interaction of a hypothetical input function and organ response function (see Fig. A3.15). Assume that the input to the organ is instantaneous and that the area under the input function is equal to 1.0. This theoretical input function is

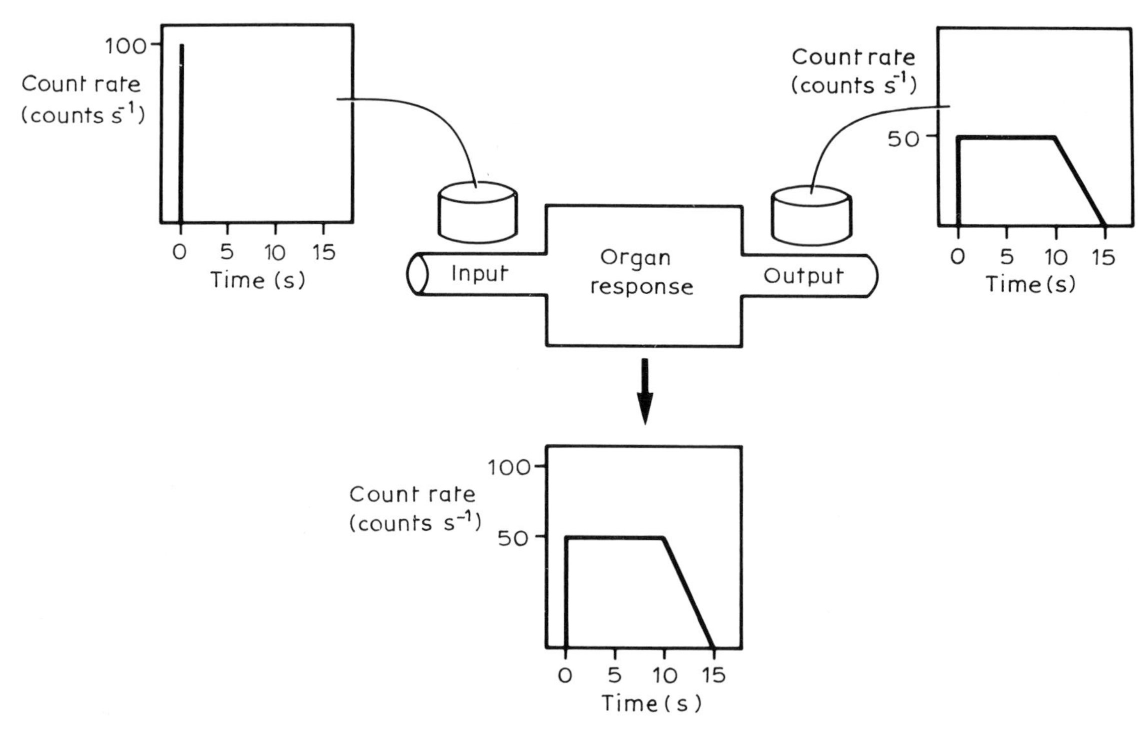

Figure A3.15 The relationship of the input function, organ response and output function. If the input function (the bolus injection) illustrated in the upper left and the output fraction (the activity–time curve for the organ of interest), illustrated in the upper right, are externally monitored, the organ response (below) can be calculated. In the example shown here, the output function is identical to the organ response since the input function is instantaneous (spike or delta function).

called a delta or spike function. Let us further assume that the organ of interest instantaneously extracts 50 per cent of the injected tracer, that the minimum time it takes for the tracer to pass through the organ is 10s, and that the elimination of the tracer from the organ is linear. With an instantaneous input, the output function is equal to the organ response. Generally, instantaneous input functions do not exist; therefore, in practice, the output function never equals the organ response.

A continuous input function can be approximated by multiple instantaneous input functions. In Fig. A3.16a, five instantaneous input functions, 10s apart, have been used to approximate a continuous input function (dashed curve). The organ response from each of these five instantaneous inputs is shown in Fig. A3.16b. Under these conditions the output function equals the *sum* of the organ responses to multiple instantaneous inputs. The sum of the organ responses in Fig. A3.16b at six different times is indicated in Fig. A3.16c. This process of summing the organ response and input product is called *convolution*. A dashed line connecting the points in Fig. A3.16c reveals that the shape of the output function can be affected much more by the input function than by the organ response.

Mathematically, a continuous input function can be treated as an infinite number of instantaneous inputs; therefore any input function can be convoluted with any organ response to yield an output function. Likewise any output function can be deconvoluted so that the organ response is identified if the input function is known. The actual mathematics of the convolution and deconvolution processes are beyond the scope of this text. The formal mathematical statement of the convolution process is as follows

$$C(t) = \int_0^\infty I(T)H(t-T)\mathrm{d}T \qquad \text{(A3.15)}$$

where $C(t)$ = output function
$I(T)$ = input function
$H(T)$ = system (organ) response

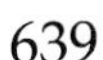

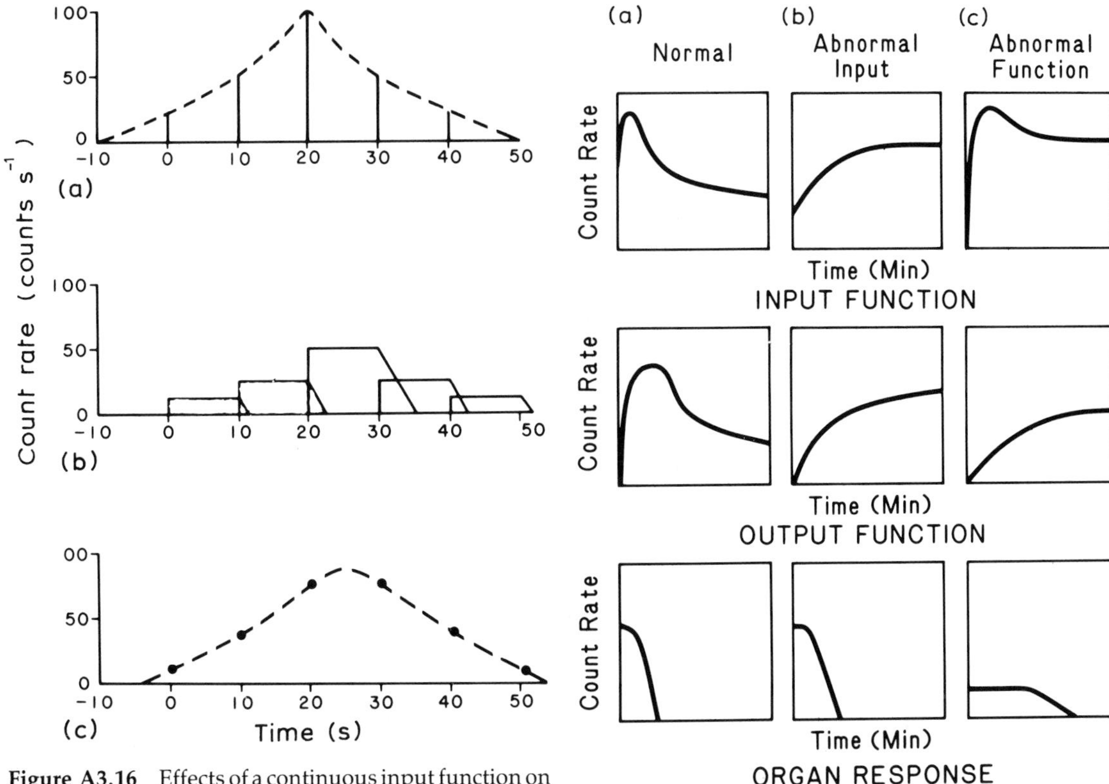

Figure A3.16 Effects of a continuous input function on the output function. (a) The count rate–time curve of a continuous input function is illustrated. A continuous input function can be treated mathematically as an infinite series of instantaneous input functions. For simplicity only five of the instantaneous input functions used to approximate the continuous input function are shown. (b) The instantaneous organ response to the five instantaneous input is illustrated. (c) The externally monitored output function equals the sum of the organ responses illustrated in (b). The shape of output function can be more profoundly affected by the input function than by the organ response.

Figure A3.17 Usefulness of deconvolution analysis of renograms. The count rate–time curves for the input function, the output function and the organ response are illustrated for a normal renogram, an abnormal renogram due to an abnormal input function, and an abnormal renogram on all graphs. Column (a), normal input function, normal output function (renogram), normal organ response. Column (b), abnormal input function due to the subcutaneous injection of the radiopharmaceutical. Abnormal output function (renogram) due to the abnormal input function. Normal organ response after deconvolution. Column (c), abnormal input function revealing delayed blood clearance due to poor renal function. Abnormal output function (renogram) due to abnormal organ response and the resulting abnormal input function. Organ response is clearly abnormal after deconvolution indicating the abnormal output function was not due soley to an abnormal input function.

These calculations are performed relatively easily on computers by using fast Fourier transforms which change the complex process of convolution/deconvolution to multiplication and division, respectively.

An obvious but sometimes overlooked limitation of deconvolution analysis is that this technique is valid only if the input and output functions are accurately known. If the externally monitored activity–time curves from regions of interest are inaccurate due to poor statistics or due to contamination by activity from surrounding structures, then the deconvolution will be meaningless. Since bolus injections are generally used, determination of the input function can be particularly difficult. Monitoring activity from a region of interest over the heart would give the best counting statistics but would not accurately reflect the input function of an organ which is some distance from the heart. By the time the bolus reached the organ it would have spread out. The time delay from the heart to the organ would also be unknown. Because of these problems, the input function is measured as close to the organ of interest as possible. For renal studies, a region of interest over the abdominal aorta is used to determine the input function. This approach introduces uncertainties because the counting statistics are poor, background activity is high and small changes in position will cause great changes in the detected activity. Since the deconvolution analysis is very sensitive to aberrations in the input function, some processing of the raw data to remove some of these aberrations is often needed before the deconvolution can be performed (Fleming and Kenny, 1977).

Examples of the clinical usefulness of deconvolution analysis of renograms is shown in Fig. A3.17. A normal input function, renogram and deconvoluted renogram are shown in (a), an abnormal input function (due to a subcutaneous injection), the resulting abnormal renogram and the deconvoluted renogram are shown in (b), and an abnormal input function (due to poor renal function), and abnormal renogram and the deconvoluted renogram are shown in (c). Since the height of the deconvoluted renogram is proportional to renal function, and since the transit time increases with decreased renal function, the deconvoluted renogram can be used to differentiate between normal and abnormal renal function independent of the input function. Note that not only does an abnormal input function cause an abnormal renogram (b) but also that abnormal renal function causes an abnormal input function (c) because of slower blood clearance.

REFERENCES

Alderson, P. O., Douglass, K. H., Mendenhall, K. G., Guadini, V. A., Watson, D. C., Links, J. M. and Wagner, H. N. (1979), Deconvolution analysis in radionuclide quantitation of left and right cardiac shunts. *J. nucl. Med.*, **20**, 502.

Bianchi, C. (1972), *Radionuclides in Renal Evaluation*, Vol. 2, Basel and University Park Press, Baltimore, pp. 21–53.

Dell, R. B., Sciacca, R., Lieberman, K., Case, D. and Cannon, P. J. (1973), A weighted least-squares technique for the analysis of kinetic data and its application in the study of renal 133 Xenon washout in dogs and man. *Circ. Res.*, **32**, 71–84.

Diffey, B. L., Hall, F. M. and Corfield, J. R. (1976), The ^{99m}Tc-DTPA dynamic renal scan with deconvolution analysis. *J. nucl. Med.*, **17**, 352–5.

Donato, L., Guintini, C., Lewis, M. L., Durand, J., Rochester, D. F., Harvey, R. M. and Cournand, A. (1962a), Quantitative radiocardiography – I theoretical considerations. *Circulation*, **26**, 174–82.

Donato, L., Rochester, D. F., Lewis, M. D., Durand, J., Parker, J. O. and Harvey, R. M. (1962b), Quantitative Radiocardiography – II technical analysis of curves. *Circulation*, **26**, 183–8.

Fleming, J. S. and Kenny, R. W. (1977), A comparison of techniques for filtering noise in the renogram. *Phys. Med. Biol.*, **22**, 359–64.

Harbert, J., Haddad, D. and McCullough, D. (1974), Quantitation of cerebrospinal fluid shunt flow. *Radiology*, **112**, 379–87.

Hoedt-Rasmussen, K. Aveisdotter, E. and Lasser, N. (1966), Regional cerebral blood flow in man determined by intra-arterial injection of inert gas. *Circ. Res.*, **18**, 237–47.

Kaikka, J., Timisjarvi, J. and Tuominen, M. (1979), Quantitative radiocardiographic evaluation of cardiac dynamics in man at rest and during exercise. *Scand. J. clin. Lab. Invest.*, **39**, 423–34.

Kenny, R. W., Ackery, D. M., Fleming, J. S., Goddard, B. A. and Grant, R. W. (1975), Deconvolution analysis of the scintillation camera renogram. *Br. J. Radiol.*, **48**, 481–6.

Kety, S. S. (1951), The theory and applications of the exchange of inert gas at the lungs and tissues. *Pharmac. Rev.*, **3**, 1–47.

Lewis, M. L., Guintini, G., Donato, L., Harvey, R. M. and Cournand, A. (1962), Quantitative radiocardiography – III results and validation of theory and method. *Circulation*, **26**, 189–99.

McNeil, B. J., Holman, B. L. and Adelstein, S. J. (1976). In *Theoretical Basis for Blood Flow Measurement in Diagnostic Nuclear Medicine* (eds A. Gottschalk and J. Potchen), Williams and Wilkins, Baltimore, ch. 13.

Morgan, W. D., Birks, J. L. and Singer, A. (1977), An efficient technique for the simultaneous estimation of GFR and ERPF, involving a single injection and two blood samples. *Int. J. nucl. Med. Biol.*, **4**, 79–83.

Rudd, T. G., Shurtleff, D. B., Loeser, J. D. and Nelp, W. B. (1973), Radionuclide assessment of cerebrospinal fluid shunt flow in children. *J. nucl. Med.*, **14**, 683–6.

Sapirstein, L. A., Vidt, D. G., Mandel, M. J. and Hanusek, G. (1955), Volumes of distribution and clearances of intravenously injected creatinine in the dog. *Am. J. Physiol.*, **181**, 330–6.

Zierler, K. L. (1965), Equations for measuring blood flow by external monitoring of radioisotopes. *Circ. Res.*, **16**, 309–21.

Index

Page numbers in *italics* refer to figures and tables